Tuberculosis
and the Tubercle Bacillus

Tuberculosis
and the Tubercle Bacillus

Editors

Stewart T. Cole
Unité de Génétique Moléculaire Bactérienne
Institut Pasteur
Paris, France

Kathleen Davis Eisenach
Mycobacteriology Research Laboratory
University of Arkansas for Medical Sciences
Central Arkansas Veterans Healthcare System
Little Rock, Arkansas

David N. McMurray
Department of Medical Microbiology and Immunology
Texas A&M University System Health Science Center
College Station, Texas

and

William R. Jacobs, Jr.
Department of Microbiology and Immunology
Howard Hughes Medical Institute
Albert Einstein College of Medicine
New York, New York

ASM
PRESS

Washington, DC

Address editorial correspondence to ASM Press, 1752 N St. NW, Washington, DC 20036-2904, USA

Send orders to ASM Press, P.O. Box 605, Herndon, VA 20172, USA
Phone: (800) 546-2416 or (703) 661-1593
Fax: (703) 661-1501
E-mail: books@asmusa.org
Online: www.asmpress.org

Library of Congress Cataloging-in-Publication Data

Tuberculosis and the tubercle bacillus / editors, Stewart T. Cole   ... [et al.].
     p. ; cm.
   Includes bibliographical references and index.
   ISBN 1-55581-295-3
   1. Tuberculosis.   I. Cole, Stewart T.
   [DNLM: 1. Tuberculosis--microbiology. 2. Mycobacterium
tuberculosis. 3. Tuberculosis--immunology.   WF 200 T8854
2005]
   QR201.T6T83 2005
   616.9'95--dc22

                                                    2004017059

10 9 8 7 6 5 4 3 2 1

Cover: The cover design is a montage of images, each symbolizing some aspect of past or present tuberculosis research and history. Starting from the top center and proceeding clockwise: the crystal structure of *Mycobacterium tuberculosis* antigen 85b, a researcher working in a biosafety level 3 facility, the chemical structure of mycobactin (courtesy David Young), circular map of the *M. tuberculosis* genome, a false color scanning electron micrograph of *M. tuberculosis*, the structure of mycolic acid, three panels showing successive views of a tuberculous lung (back: chest X-ray of TB patient with right lobe disease; center: a granuloma from a tuberculous lung [hematoxylin and eosin]; front: acid fast bacilli in a lung biopsy), portrait of Robert Koch, green fluorescent protein expressing H37Rv *M. tuberculosis*-infected human dendritic cell stained with monoclonal antibody to CD1a (red) and nucleus (blue) (fluorescence microscopy courtesy of Carme Roura-Mir), the chemical structure of isoniazid, crystal structure of human CD1a, microarray data, mother and child (the young girl was treated successfully for tuberculosis). The circular arrow is meant to symbolize the continuum between basic research, clinical medicine, and public health that is required to meet the challenges of tuberculosis. Cover art and concept: Chris Bickel. Design studio: Naylor Design Inc.

CONTENTS

CONTRIBUTORS

Jose A. Ainsa
Departamento de Microbiologia, Facultad de
Medicina, Universidad de Zaragoza, 50009
Zaragoza, Spain

Peter Andersen
Department of Immunology, Statens Serum
Institute, Copenhagen, Denmark

Yossef Av-Gay
Division of Infectious Diseases, University of British
Columbia, Vancouver, British Columbia, Canada
V5Z 3J5

Peter F. Barnes
Center for Pulmonary and Infectious Disease
Control, Department of Medicine, and Department
of Microbiology and Immunology, The University of
Texas Health Center, Tyler, TX 75708-3154

Joyoti Basu
Department of Chemistry, Bose Institute, Kolkata
700 009, India

Marcel A. Behr
McGill University Health Centre, Division of
Infectious Diseases and Medical Microbiology,
Montreal General Hospital, Montreal, Quebec,
Canada H3G 1A4

John T. Belisle
Mycobacteria Research Laboratories, Department
of Microbiology, Immunology, and Pathology,
Colorado State University, Fort Collins, CO 80523-
1682

Gurdyal S. Besra
School of Biosciences, The University of
Birmingham, Edgbaston, Birmingham B15 2TT,
United Kingdom

William R. Bishai
Center for Tuberculosis Research, Johns Hopkins
University School of Medicine, Baltimore, MD
21231-1001

John S. Blanchard
Department of Biochemistry, Albert Einstein College
of Medicine, Bronx, NY 10461

Martine Braibant
BioAgresseurs, Santé et Environnement (BASE),
INRA de Tours, F-37380 Nouzilly, France

Miriam Braunstein
Department of Microbiology, University of North
Carolina, Chapel Hill, NC 27599

Michael J. Brennan
Center for Biologics Evaluation and Research, Food
and Drug Administration, Bethesda, MD 20892

Patrick J. Brennan
Department of Microbiology, Immunology, and
Pathology, Colorado State University, Fort Collins,
CO 80523-1682

Michael B. Brenner
Division of Rheumatology, Immunology and
Allergy, Brigham and Women's Hospital and
Harvard Medical School, Boston, MA 02115

Priscille Brodin
Unité de Génétique Moléculaire Bactérienne, Institut
Pasteur, 75724 Paris Cedex 15 France

Roland Brosch
Unité de Génétique Moléculaire Bactérienne, Institut
Pasteur, 75724 Paris Cedex 15, France

Bryce M. Buddle
AgResearch, Wallaceville Animal Research Centre,
Upper Hutt, New Zealand

Michael Buckstein
Division of Infectious Diseases, Department of Medicine, University of Pennsylvania Medical Center, Philadelphia, PA 19104-6073

Arturo Casadevall
Division of Infectious Diseases, Department of Medicine and Microbiology and Immunology, Albert Einstein College of Medicine, Bronx, NY 10461

M. Donald Cave
Department of Neurobiology and Developmental Sciences, University of Arkansas for Medical Sciences, Little Rock, AR 72205

John Chan
Department of Microbiology and Immunology, Albert Einstein College of Medicine, Bronx, NY 10461

Stewart T. Cole
Unité de Génétique Moléculaire Bactérienne, Institut Pasteur, 75724 Paris Cedex 15 France

Nancy D. Connell
Department of Microbiology and Molecular Genetics, New Jersey Medical School, Newark, NJ 07103-3535

Jean Content
Institut Pasteur de Bruxelles, Brussels B-1180, Belgium

Andrea M. Cooper
Trudeau Institute, Inc. Saranac Lake, NY 12983

Liz Corbett
Biomedical Research and Training Institute, University of Zimbabwe, Mount Pleasant, Harare, Zimbabwe

Dean C. Crick
Department of Microbiology, Immunology, and Pathology, Colorado State University, Fort Collins, CO 80523-1682

Mamadou Daffé
Department of Molecular Mechanisms of Mycobacterial Infections, Institute of Pharmacology and Structural Biology, CNRS-University Paul Sabatier Mixed Research Unit, 31077 Toulouse Cedex 04, France

Christopher C. Dascher
Division of Rheumatology, Immunology, and Allergy, Brigham and Women's Hospital, and Harvard Medical School, Boston, MA 02115

Caroline Demangel
Unité de Génétique Moléculaire Bactérienne, Institut Pasteur, 75724 Paris Cedex 15 France

Vojo Peter Deretic
Department of Molecular Genetics and Microbiology, University of New Mexico Health Sciences Center, Albuquerque, NM 87131

Edward Desmond
Microbial Diseases Laboratory, Division of Communicable Disease Control, California Department of Health Services, Berkeley, CA 94704

Philip Draper
Philip@borehamh.demon.co.uk (Retired)

Kathleen D. Eisenach
Mycobacteriology Research Laboratory, University of Arkansas for Medical Sciences, Central Arkansas Veterans Healthcare System, Little Rock, AR 72205

David Eisenberg
UCLA-DOE Institute of Genomics and Proteomics, Los Angeles, CA 90095-1570

Marcos Espinal
Stop TB Partnership, World Health Organization, 1211 Geneva 27, Switzerland

Clara Espitia
Departamento de Inmunología, Instituto de Investigaciones Biomédicas, Universidad Nacional Autónoma de México, Mexico D.F., Mexico

Matthew J. Fenton
Departments of Medicine, Microbiology, and Immunology, University of Maryland School of Medicine, Baltimore, MD 21201

JoAnne L. Flynn
Department of Molecular Genetics and Biochemistry, University of Pittsburgh School of Medicine, Pittsburgh, PA 15261

Betty A. Forbes
Department of Pathology, Medical College of Virginia, VCU Health System, Richmond, VA 23298-0210

Aharona Glatman-Freedman
Division of Infectious Diseases, Department of Pediatrics, Children's Hospital at Montefiore, Albert Einstein College of Medicine, Bronx, NY 10461

Stephen V. Gordon
TB Research, Veterinary Laboratories Agency (Weybridge), New Haw Addlestone, Surrey KT15 3NB, United Kingdom

Celia W. Goulding
UCLA-DOE Institute of Genomics and Proteomics, Los Angeles, CA 90095-1570

Willem Hanekom
Departments of Pediatrics, Microbiology, and Immunology, University of Miami School of Medicine, Miami, FL 33101

Graham F. Hatfull
Pittsburgh Bacteriophage Institute and Department of Biological Sciences, University of Pittsburgh, Pittsburgh, PA 15260

Leonid Heifets
Mycobacteriology Laboratory, National Jewish Medical and Research Medicine, Denver, CO 80206

R. Glyn Hewinson
TB Research Group, Department of Bacterial Diseases, VLA Weybridge, Addlestone, Surrey KT15 3NB, United Kingdom

Philip C. Hopewell
Dean's Office, University of California, San Francisco, San Francisco General Hospital, San Francisco, CA 94110

Angelo A. Izzo
Department of Microbiology, Immunology, and Pathology, Colorado State University, Ft. Collins, CO 80523

William R. Jacobs, Jr.
Howard Hughes Medical Institute, Department of Microbiology and Immunology, Albert Einstein College of Medicine, New York, NY 10043

Robert M. Jasmer
Division of Pulmonary and Critical Care Medicine, San Francisco General Hospital, San Francisco, CA 94110

Beate Kampmann
Department of Pediatrics, Imperial College, London, United Kingdom

Gilla Kaplan
Laboratory of Mycobacterial Immunity and Pathogenesis, Public Health Research Institute, International Center for Public Health, Newark, NJ 07103-3535

Stefan H.E. Kaufmann
Department of Immunology, Max-Planck-Institute for Infection Biology, D-10117 Berlin, Germany

Laurent Kremer
Laboratoire des Mécanismes Moléculaires de la Pathogénie Microbienne, INSERM U447, Institut Pasteur de Lille/IBL, 59 000 Lille, France

Suman Laal
Department of Pathology, New York University School of Medicine, VA Medical Center, New York, NY 10010

Sebabrata Mahapatra
Department of Microbiology, Immunology, and Pathology, Colorado State University, Fort Collins, CO 80523-1682

Marc Mendelson
Laboratory of Mycobacterial Immunity and Pathogenesis, Public Health Research Institute, International Center for Public Health, Newark, NJ 07103-3535

Valerie Mizrahi
Molecular Mycobacteriology Research Unit, School of Pathology, National Health Laboratory Service and University of Witwatersrand, Johannesburg 2000, South Africa

Megan Murray
Departments of Epidemiology and Pulmonary Medicine, Harvard School of Public Health, Harvard Medical School, Boston, MA 02115

Valakunja Nagaraja
Department of Microbiology and Cell Biology, Indian Institute of Science, Bangalore, India 560012

Edward Nardell
Departments of Epidemiology and Pulmonary Medicine, Harvard School of Public Health, Harvard Medical School, Boston, MA 02115

Ian M. Orme
Department of Microbiology, Immunology, and Pathology, Colorado State University, Ft. Collins, CO 80523

Debnath Pal
UCLA-DOE Institute of Genomics and Proteomics, Los Angeles, CA 90095-1570

Gaby Pfyffer
Department of Medical Microbiology, Kantonsspital, Luzern 16 6000, Switzerland

John M. Pollock
Veterinary Sciences Division, Department of Agriculture and Rural Development for Northern Ireland, Belfast, United Kingdom

Christopher L. Pritchett
Biology Department, Northeastern State University, Tahlequah, OK 74464

Luis E. N. Quadri
Department of Microbiology and Immunology, Weill Medical College of Cornell University, New York, NY 10021

Colin Ratledge
Department of Biological Sciences, University of Hull, Hull HU6 7RX, United Kingdom

Mario Raviglione
Stop TB Department, World Health Organization, CH 1211 Geneva 27, Switzerland

Renate Reimschuessel
Center for Veterinary Medicine, Food and Drug Administration, Laurel, MD 20857

Jean-Marc Reyrat
Faculté de Médecine Necker-Enfants Malades, INSERM U570, 75730 Paris Cedex 15, France

Lee W. Riley
Division of Infectious Diseases, School of Public Health, University of California, Berkeley, CA 94720

Ida Rosenkrands
Department of Immunology, Statens Serum Institute, Copenhagen, Denmark

Harvey Rubin
Division of Infectious Diseases, Department of Medicine, University of Pennsylvania Medical Center, Philadelphia, PA 19104-6073

David G. Russell
Department of Microbiology and Immunology, College of Veterinary Medicine, Cornell University, Ithaca, NY 14853

Max Salfinger
Department of Biomedical Sciences, School of Public Health, University at Albany, New York State Department of Health, Wadsworth Center, Albany, NY 12201-0509

Peter Sander
Institut für Medizinische Mikrobiologie, Universität Zürich, CH-8028 Zurich, Switzerland

Larry S. Schlesinger
Departments of Medicine and Molecular Virology, Immunology, and Medical Genetics, The Ohio State University, Columbus, OH 43210

Richard F. Silver
Department of Medicine, Case Western Reserve University, Cleveland, OH 44106

Yasir A. W. Skeiky
Aeras Global TB Vaccine Foundation, Bethesda, MD 20814

Issar Smith
TB Center, The Public Health Research Institute, The International Center for Public Health, Newark, NJ 07103-3535

Neil G. Stoker
Department of Pathology and Infectious Diseases, Royal Veterinary College, London NW1 0TU, United Kingdom

Philip Supply
Laboratoire des Mécanismes Moléculaires de la Pathogenèse Bactérienne, INSERM U447, Institut Pasteur de Lille, F-59019 Lille Cedex, France

Michele Trucksis
Division of Infectious Diseases and Immunology, University of Massachusetts Medical School, Worcester, MA 01605

Ramakrishna Vankayalapati
Center for Pulmonary and Infectious Disease Control and Department of Microbiology and Immunology, The University of Texas Health Center, Tyler, TX 75708-3154

Nico C. Gey van Pittius
US/MRC Centre for Molecular and Cellular Biology, Department of Medicinal Biochemistry, Faculty of Health Sciences, Stellenbosch University, Tygerberg 7505, South Africa

Catherine Vilchèze
Howard Hughes Medical Institute, Department of Microbiology and Immunology, Albert Einstein College of Medicine, New York, NY 10043

Robert S. Wallis
Department of Medicine, UMDNJ-New Jersey Medical School, Newark, NJ 07103

Paul R. Wheeler
Tuberculosis Research Unit, Veterinary Laboratories Agency (Weybridge), New Haw Addlestone, Surrey KT15 3NB, United Kingdom

Ying Zhang
Department of Molecular Microbiology and Immunology, Bloomberg School of Public Health, Johns Hopkins University, Baltimore, MD 21205

PREFACE

Even at that early date, Dr. Janeway's great skill in physical diagnosis was recognized, and he had a class at Bellevue for physical diagnosis to which I belonged. He received me cordially and began the examination at once. When this was concluded he said nothing. So I ventured, "Well, Dr. Janeway, you can find nothing the matter?" He looked grave and said, "Yes, the upper two-thirds of the left lung is involved in an active tuberculosis process." . . . I think I know something of the feelings of the man at the bar who is told he is to be hanged on a given date, for in those days pulmonary consumption was considered as absolutely fatal. I pulled myself together, put as good a face on the matter as I could, and escaped from the office after thanking the doctor for his examination. When I got outside, as I stood on Dr. Janeway's stoop, I felt stunned. It seemed to me that the world had suddenly grown dark. The sun was shining, it is true, and the street was filled with the rush and noise of traffic, but to me the world had lost every vestige of brightness. I had consumption—that most fatal of diseases.

He had such a very full translation of Dr. Koch's famous paper made in English for me and presented it to me at Christmas. Surely, I have never had a Christmas present that meant more to me than that big handwritten copybook. I read every word of it over and over again. Koch's paper on 'The Aetiology of Tuberculosis' is certainly, one of the greatest, if not the greatest, medical papers ever written and a model of logic of the new experimental method to the study of disease.

Edward Livingston Trudeau, *An Autobiography*, 1916

In 1994, the World Health Organization declared tuberculosis (TB) to be a global health emergency. Despite this alarm, the problem has intensified worldwide, even though a TB vaccine exists and an effective regimen of short-course chemotherapy is available for treating *Mycobacterium tuberculosis* infections. The increasing global health burden of TB has resulted primarily from widespread poverty and social inequality and has been compounded by the growing AIDS epidemic and by the emergence of multi-drug-resistant tuberculosis. Despite this gloomy outlook, there is reason for hope that these trends can

be reversed. The hope comes from a growing body of new knowledge about the disease tuberculosis. This book seeks to extend the classic work edited by Dr. Barry Bloom in 1994 entitled *Tuberculosis: Pathogenesis, Protection, and Control*. We, the editors, have sought to build upon Dr. Bloom's opus by bringing together the latest developments in many areas of TB research to provide the reader with the state of the art in 2004.

This volume is divided into three sections and begins with a realistic look at the problems posed by TB today, including clinical as well as epidemiological features of the *M. tuberculosis* strains causing disease. Detecting *M. tuberculosis* infections requires excellent diagnostics, and three chapters are devoted to the latest methodologies. TB control requires effective chemotherapies as well as an understanding of the mechanisms by which therapies fail, and these are described in two chapters.

The second section focuses on the *M. tuberculosis* bacillus and explores genetics, genomics, cell structure, and metabolism. Tremendous progress has been made in our understanding of *M. tuberculosis* as a result of interpretation of the genome sequence. This interpretation involves functional genomic approaches as well as knowledge of genome evolution, the proteome, and the basic principles of gene transfer and gene expression. A large portion of this section describes the current understanding of the cell wall of *M. tuberculosis* as well as many important aspects of mycobacterial metabolism.

The last section of the book details the interaction of *M. tuberculosis* with its host, beginning with the entry and survival of *M. tuberculosis* in its primary residence—a macrophage. The next few chapters focus on the way the host defends itself from the growing bacillus. The last chapters of this section describe existing animal models and their application to the elucidation of the pathogenic mechanisms of TB and to the development and preclinical evaluation of new TB vaccines.

Edward Livingston Trudeau was devastated the day he was diagnosed with TB. Since he was doomed to die, he traveled to Saranac Lake to hunt and fish to enjoy his remaining days on earth. In the process, he discovered that fresh air and sunlight helped control the TB infection and he therefore established "cure cottages" for treating TB. His life changed forever, though, the day he read Dr. Koch's work describing the method of acquiring knowledge of the enemy. He was filled with optimism, as he knew that knowledge could overcome despair. Knowledge of TB is expanding with the development of better genetic tools, the application of genomics, and deeper insight into host-pathogen interactions. We share the optimism of Koch and Trudeau that the TB problem can be overcome and believe that this will be best achieved by enlarging the knowledge base. Thus, we trust that clinicians, basic scientists, and all those working for the demise of tuberculosis will benefit from this book.

Stewart T. Cole
Kathleen Davis Eisenach
David N. McMurray
William R. Jacobs, Jr.
July 2004

INTRODUCTION

I. HISTORICAL PERSPECTIVES

Chapter 1

Global Burden of Tuberculosis: Past, Present, and Future

LIZ CORBETT AND MARIO RAVIGLIONE

Tuberculosis (TB) was catapulted back onto the center stage of international health at the beginning of the 1990s, when New York City and Miami were affected by multiple institutional outbreaks of multidrug-resistant TB (MDR-TB), mainly affecting hospitalized human immunodeficiency virus (HIV)-positive persons and associated with extremely high case fatality rates (7). There had also been a more general breakdown of TB control in New York City, with a doubling in TB incidence rates during the previous decade (25), alarmingly high treatment default rates (5), and an increase in drug resistance to high levels, including a 7% prevalence of MDR-TB among patients never previously treated for TB (25).

Once international attention had refocused on TB, it became apparent that renewed efforts were required worldwide. The New York City epidemic was successfully controlled, but at an estimated cost of $110 million (26). Even in the poorest countries, however, excellent results had been achieved during the 1980s by a number of TB control programs operating at very low cost. These used an approach that has since been packaged by the World Health Organization (WHO) as the directly observed treatment, short course (DOTS) (Table 1), which by 2001 had been adopted by 155 countries and covered 62% of the world's population (69). DOTS is particularly effective in improving treatment outcomes and preventing deaths (21). In some countries, implementation of DOTS has led to reductions in the prevalence of TB disease (40). TB incidence rates then start to decline as transmission rates are affected by the lower burden of infectious TB in the community, as has been most clearly demonstrated in Peru (Fig. 1) (58).

Unmet challenges remain. TB is the second most common infectious cause of adult mortality and is ranked 10th of all causes of loss of healthy life world-wide. Over 98% of deaths from TB occur in developing countries (19), with case fatality rates of HIV-related TB being particularly high (70). Estimated per capita TB incidence rates for 2000 varied from below 6 per 100,000 per year in the United States to over 600 per 100,000 per year in six African countries (13). Not one country in Africa has managed to reduce TB incidence rates to pre-HIV levels (69), strategies for managing drug-resistant TB in resource-poor settings are still in development (59), and weak health care systems, resulting in lack of adequate primary services and human resources, have inhibited progress in many of the countries with the highest TB burden (44).

This chapter aims to summarize our current understanding of the global epidemiology of TB, including regional estimates and trends in the burden of morbidity and mortality, and to detail the main recent events and persisting obstacles towards improving control in the coming decade.

THE EARLY 1990s: TUBERCULOSIS CONTROL IN CRISIS

The problems affecting New York City were not isolated. In the United States as a whole, TB case notification rates had been increasing since 1984 after many decades of steady decline (53), and other industrialized countries in Europe were also reporting increases or a leveling-off in the rate of decline of TB case notification rates (49). Disease among foreign-born residents was identified as a major factor behind these trends in both the United States and Western Europe (38, 49), drawing attention to the minimal rate of progress being made in many resource-poor settings and the need to consider TB control as a global rather than a national challenge.

Liz Corbett • Department of Infectious and Tropical Diseases, London School of Hygiene and Tropical Medicine, London WC1E 7HT, United Kingdom, and Biomedical Research and Training Institute, University of Zimbabwe, Mount Pleasant, PO Box CY 1753, Causeway, Harare, Zimbabwe. Mario Raviglione • StopTB Department, World Health Organization, 20 Avenue Appia, CH 1211 Geneva 27, Switzerland.

Table 1. WHO TB control strategies

Strategy	Description
DOTS	A five-point strategy consisting of a. Government commitment to sustainable TB control b. Diagnosis through sputum smear microscopy, mainly among symptomatic patients self-referring to health services c. Standardized short-course chemotherapy provided under proper case management conditions, including DOT d. A functioning drug supply system e. A recording and reporting system allowing assessment of treatment results
DOTS-Plus	A strategy, under development, to manage MDR TB by using second-line drugs in low- and middle-income countries within the DOTS strategy. Guidelines for diagnosis and management are available, and access to low-cost drugs can be obtained through the Green Light Committee.
ProTEST	Promotion of VCT as the entry point for intensified TB case detection and IPT.

In two global regions, TB control was deteriorating rapidly. The socioeconomic collapse that accompanied the end of the Communist era was accompanied by a rapid resurgence of TB, with high rates of drug resistance, in the previously low-incidence states of the Baltic region and former USSR (50). In sub-Saharan Africa, the severity and consequences of the HIV epidemic were becoming increasingly apparent (15). TB was identified as the major cause of death among HIV-positive Africans (36),

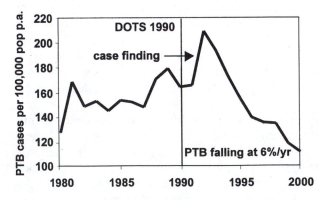

Figure 1. DOTS and trends in pulmonary TB case notifications in Peru. DOTS was implemented in Peru in 1990 and is now performed countrywide. After an initial peak of case notifications attributable to increased case detection, there has been a progressive decrease in case notifications that is likely to reflect decreasing TB transmission rates secondary to reduction in the prevalence of infectious TB (58). From reference 21 with permission.

and there was growing recognition that HIV was leading to a fundamental change in the epidemiology of TB throughout the continent (15).

The more attention that was paid to global TB control, the more it became apparent that merely making treatment available had proved inadequate, particularly in resource-poor settings (29). It was against this stark background that the World Health Assembly adopted in 1991 the global targets of reaching a 70% case detection rate and an 85% cure rate for smear-positive TB by the year 2000, using the WHO strategy (52). These goals were not met, but they have been reaffirmed with a new target date of 2005.

GLOBAL TUBERCULOSIS EPIDEMIOLOGY

Estimating the Global Burden of Tuberculosis

Estimates of the burden of TB in developing countries were published in 1981 (57) and 1990 (42). Although based mainly on indirect data derived from regional estimates of annual risk of TB infection, they drew attention to the massive burden of morbidity and mortality still being exacted by the disease. Among the main conclusions from the 1990 estimates were that the global case detection rate (proportion of all new TB patients who are ever diagnosed) was only 55% and that high default and failure rates compromised therapy and increased case fatality rates further (29).

A more detailed country-by-country assessment for 1997 placed global case detection rates even lower, at 35% (19). The number of incident TB cases was estimated to be 8.0 million, with 16.2 million prevalent cases of TB disease and 1.86 million deaths, giving an overall case fatality rate of 23%. The global prevalence of *Mycobacterium tuberculosis* infection was estimated to be 32%, with 0.18% of the world's population dually infected with *M. tuberculosis* and HIV. Twenty-two high-burden countries were identified as having more than 80% of the new cases of TB worldwide (Fig. 2). Reducing the burden of disease in these countries is clearly a prerequisite for improved global control.

Regional Trends and Associations with HIV Infection in 2000

Updated estimates for 2000 (13, 69) indicate that incident cases have risen to nearly 8.5 million, with over 1.8 million deaths. Global incidence rates increased by 0.4% per year between 1997 and 2000 (Table 2; Color Plate 1A). Two regions, sub-Saharan Africa and the former USSR, were mainly responsible for the upward trend in incidence rates, with incidence falling in the Americas, Eastern Mediterranean

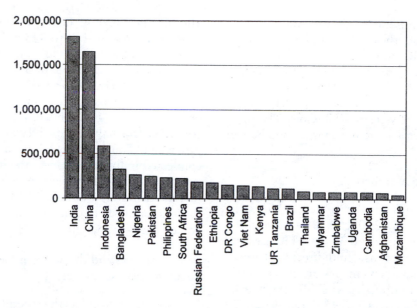

Figure 2. Number of new TB cases in each of the 22 high-burden countries at the start of 2000. Numbers are estimated from case notifications and estimated case detection rates in each country (67).

Table 2. Regional trends, burdens of morbidity and mortality, and associations with HIV infection at the start of 2000

Characteristic	Result in WHO region						
	Africa[a]	Americas	Eastern Mediterranean	Europe	Southeast Asia	Western Pacific	Global
Population (millions)	640	832	485	874	1,536	1,688	6,053
Trends in TB incidence 1997–2000 (% per yr)	3.9	−4.1	−1.4	2.8	−1.3	0.0	0.4
New cases of TB, all forms							
No. of cases (thousands)	1,857	382	587	468	2,986	2,031	8,311
Incidence rate (per 100,000)	290	46	121	54	194	120	137
HIV prevalence in new adult cases (%)	38	5.9	1.8	2.8	3.2	1.3	11
Attributable to HIV (thousands)	421	12	5.2	8.2	53	13	511
Attributable to HIV (% of adult cases)	31	5.1	1.5	2.6	2.7	1.1	9
New smear-positive cases of TB[b]							
No. of cases (thousands)	785	169	264	210	1,338	913	3,679
Prevalence of smear-positive TB (per 100,000)	185	27	103	35	209	117	122
% of smear-positive cases that are HIV+ (%)	7.5	1.0	0.2	0.5	0.3	0.1	1.4
Infection prevalence among adults							
Prevalence of *M. tuberculosis* infection (%)	31	15	27	14	46	32	30
Prevalence of *M. tuberculosis*/HIV coinfection (%)	2.7	0.1	0.1	0.0	0.3	0.0	0.4
Deaths from TB							
Deaths from TB (thousands)	482	55	135	72	727	368	1,839
Deaths from TB (per 100,000)	75	6.6	28	8.3	47	22	30
Deaths from TB in HIV+ adults (thousands)	203	3.9	3.0	1.6	29	5.7	246
% of adult AIDS deaths due to TB[c]	12	4.1	11	10	8.1	17	11
TB deaths attributable to HIV (%)	39	6.5	2.0	2.1	3.7	1.4	12

[a]WHO African Region comprises sub-Saharan Africa and Algeria. The remaining North African countries are in the Eastern Mediterranean region.
[b]"Smear-positive" is sputum smear positive.
[c]Adults are defined as persons aged 15 to 69 years.

Region (which contains most of North Africa and the Middle East), and Southeast Asia and stagnating in the Western Pacific Region.

Morbidity and mortality rates by WHO region are shown in Table 2. Although Africa has the highest per capita incidence rates (Color Plate 1A) and the highest incidence of HIV-related TB (Color Plate 1B), Asia and the Western Pacific have larger numbers of cases (Table 2; Fig. 2).

Africa: documenting a deepening crisis

TB control in Africa is dominated by the worsening HIV epidemic. By 2000, 38% of African TB patients were HIV positive and 31% of TB cases and 39% of TB deaths were considered directly attributable to HIV (13). These percentages are much higher in southern African countries severely affected by HIV; for example, in Botswana 77% of African TB patients were HIV positive and 64% of TB cases were directly attributable to HIV. The HIV epidemic was the cause of 421,000 new TB cases and 203,000 deaths from TB during 2000. Only 37% of Africans with TB were diagnosed and treated. TB was the cause of at least 12% of all deaths among HIV-positive Africans (13). This may well be an underestimate because of the difficulties in quantifying deaths from undiagnosed TB, which is still a major hazard for HIV-positive persons in this region (2, 48).

TB incidence for the region was 290 per 100,000 per year, with an upward trend of 3.9% per year between 1997 and 2000 and a huge range from 85 per

100,000 per year in Benin, a low-HIV-prevalence country in West Africa, to 823 per 100,000 per year in Swaziland, a country in southern Africa with an adult HIV prevalence rate of 33% and a high prevalence of latent TB infection (57%).

M. tuberculosis-HIV coinfection rates were 5% or more in the general adult population of eight countries and have reached 14% in Swaziland and Botswana. South Africa alone has over 2 million coinfected individuals. Given the high risk of breakdown to active TB disease in coinfected persons, a lifetime risk of approximately 30 to 40% if no treatment is received (13), the magnitude of the crisis becomes starkly apparent.

Southeast Asia and the Western Pacific: health systems challenges

Southeast Asia has the second highest per capita incidence rate, at 194 per 100,000 per year, and contains a number of large and densely populated countries, including India, Indonesia and Bangladesh. The Western Pacific region includes China, the country with the second highest burden after India. Southeast Asia has the highest estimated point prevalence rate of smear-positive TB globally (13, 60), and prevalence is also known to be high in China (40) and the Philippines (61), reflecting lengthy delays in diagnosis and low case detection rates. This is attributable mainly to weaknesses in the public health system and the difficulties of standardizing care in the private sector (43, 62).

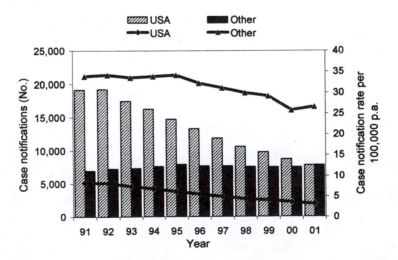

Figure 3. Time trends in TB case notification numbers and rates in the United States from 1991 to 2001 according to place of birth. Bars show the number of case notifications among U.S. born (cross-hatched bars) and foreign-born (grey bars) residents. Lines show the corresponding case notification rates per 100,000 population. The number of case notifications and case notification rates among U.S.-born residents has declined progressively during the last decade, whereas disease among foreign-born residents has changed relatively little (CDC, 2002: http://www.cdc.gov/nchstp/tb/surv/surv2001/default.htm). For 2001, case notification rates were 3.1 and 26.6 per 100,000 population for U.S.-born and foreign-born residents, respectively.

India had 1.8 million incident TB cases and over 450,000 TB deaths in 2000, the highest burden of any single country worldwide. DOTS was adopted in 1993 and now covers 65% of the population, with marked improvements in case detection rates and treatment outcomes and prevention of an estimated 200,000 deaths (35). HIV prevalence is increasing, and although it is low by African standards at 0.7% of adults (32), there were 4 million HIV-positive persons and an HIV prevalence of 5% in TB patients by 2000 (13). Surveillance in two limited geographical areas showed prevalence rates of MDR-TB of between 1 and 3.4% in new TB patients (23).

China started a DOTS project in 1991 that now covers over half of the population (20) and has achieved a 37% reduction in disease prevalence since 1990, with improvement limited to DOTS areas (40). However, the prevalence of smear-positive disease in DOTS areas was 128 per 100,000 population in 2000, which is 5.8 times the annual case notification rate for the same districts. The country also has MDR-TB "hot spots." In the worst affected province, Henan, 11% of TB patients never previously treated had MDR-TB during a 1996 survey, and other surveyed provinces not implementing DOTS also had worryingly high rates of primary MDR-TB (23).

By 2000, over 1% of the adult population were HIV infected in Cambodia (4.0%), Thailand (2.1%), and Myanmar (2.0%), all of which are also countries with a high burden of TB (Fig. 2). Otherwise, these two regions have relatively low burdens of HIV-related TB.

Eastern Europe and the former Soviet States: declining TB control and a rapidly growing HIV epidemic in IVDUs

Following the collapse of Communism, most of the newly independent states of Eastern Europe suffered rapid impoverishment and health system fragmentation. Between 1997 and 2000, the incidence of TB in the former USSR increased by 5 to 7% per year (13), and incidence rates now range between 70 and 150 per 100,000 per year. The subregion also has the fastest-growing HIV epidemic and the most severe MDR-TB problem worldwide (23).

The explosive epidemic of HIV among intravenous drug users (IVDUs) (18) deserves special attention because there are epidemiological links between drug use and TB. First, being an IVDU seems to be a strong risk factor for becoming infected with TB, regardless of HIV status (47, 55). Second, the rate of imprisonment among IVDUs is high, and this carries its own risks of institutionally transmitted TB (9). For these reasons, IVDUs may act as a bridging group, linking the growing HIV and TB epidemics in

Eastern Europe more closely than would otherwise occur.

Established market economies: the increasing importance of high-risk groups

TB case notification rates are slowly falling in most of the established market economies following the intensification of TB control efforts in the 1990s (67). TB transmission rates are now extremely low, and most disease occurs in persons with identifiable risk factors for having been infected with *M. tuberculosis*: most commonly older age or foreign birthplace (4, 38, 54). Serial TB caseloads and case notification rates from the United States are illustrated in Fig. 3: the caseload of TB from U.S.-born residents fell progressively during the 1990s, while the caseload among foreign-born residents has remained static and now accounts for half of all cases of notified TB disease in the United States (CDC, 2002: http://www.cdc.gov/nchstp/tb/surv/surv2001/default.htm). When expressed as case notification rates, the difference between the two groups is even more striking.

HIV infection, alcohol or drug dependency, homelessness, and previous imprisonment are also associated with an increased risk of TB. Social interaction between individuals with multiple risk factors can result in very high rates of disease, for example 270 per 100,000 person-years in the homeless of San Francisco (41).

Recommendations for improving control include intensified case detection and infection control measures in institutional settings, risk group management, and maintenance of awareness of TB to enable effective detection of symptomatic persons in the community (4).

PROGRESS AND PROSPECTS IN TUBERCULOSIS CONTROL

International Policy and Strategies

At the start of the 1990s, only a handful of countries were running TB control programs using the strategy recommended by WHO. By 2001, however, 155 countries had adopted the strategy that was by then known as DOTS (52). DOTS is possibly the best known and perhaps also the most misunderstood health intervention acronym: the five key elements are listed in Table 1. DOTS, even before its branding in 1995, was endorsed by the World Health Assembly in 1991, when global targets were adopted, and again in 1993 by the World Bank (65). In the mid-1990s, a global monitoring system was put in place by WHO (51) and a multicountry surveillance project of drug resistance was initiated (46). These have resulted in a much clearer picture of global epidemiology than exists for other major infectious diseases.

The Stop TB Partnership, a broad coalition of government, nongovernment organizations, and individuals, was formed in 1998 as part of the attempts to accelerate the pace at which DOTS was being implemented across the globe. This was in response to the identification of a lack of political will and commitment, inadequate financing, weak health care systems, and irregular drug supplies as major barriers to the rate at which TB control can be improved (52). A Global Drugs Facility has since been established to assist the poorest countries in procuring high-quality first-line TB drugs (44), and the Green Light Committee has since been introduced to provide access to and rational use of drugs for treatment for MDR-TB in countries with limited resources (30).

Initiatives to tackle weakness in health care systems are also ongoing. These include the Practical Approach to Lung Health and the Integrated Management of Adult Illnesses, which are WHO-coordinated primary health care projects along the same lines as the Integrated Management of Childhood Illnesses. In some regions, notably Asia, private practitioners diagnose and treat most TB patients but commonly provide suboptimal and nonstandard management (43, 62). In Hyderabad, India, case notifications were increased fourfold and 90% cure rates were achieved by direct interaction with private practitioners, showing that this sector can and must be more fully engaged to maximize control efforts (43).

Recommendations for reducing TB transmission in institutional settings such as prisons and hospitals have also been developed (9, 31). TB transmission and incidence rates in prisons can be extremely high (9, 24, 45). Prisons can be an important source of TB infection and disease in the community, as in the former USSR, where a high proportion of circulating *M. tuberculosis* strains are drug resistant, and prison-acquired TB may account for a surprisingly high percentage of new TB cases (56).

Progress under DOTS

By 2001, DOTS covered 62% of the global population, and by the end of 2002 the cumulative number of patients treated under DOTS exceeded 10 million (21). DOTS is particularly effective in improving treatment outcomes and reducing mortality (20, 35). The example of Peru, where DOTS led to an increased number of incident TB cases attributable to increased case detection and then to decreased incidence rates attributable to falling TB transmission rates, represents the ultimate successful application of DOTS (58) (Fig. 1). However, progress in improv-

ing the detection of smear-positive TB has been slow in other parts of the world (Fig. 4). Global case detection rates in 2001 were estimated to be 43% for smear-positive cases, of which three-quarters were from DOTS program (69). Thus, only 32% of all estimated infection cases in the world were detected by DOTS program in 2001, leaving the remaining 68% undetected, managed under non-DOTS standards, or unnotified. Rapidly increasing the rate at which infectious TB cases are detected, notified, and treated under DOTS, so that the global 70% target is reached by 2005, is the main challenge for TB control today. It is increasingly clear that besides the engagement of private for-profit practitioners in standard DOTS practices, interventions to standardize practice in all parts of the public health sector are necessary to achieve this target. For instance, in large high-burden countries such as China and Indonesia, linkages between parallel governmental care services, such as those delivered in hospitals and prisons, are weak and need to be strengthened to ensure that DOTS is implemented everywhere and not just in the officially designated national program sites. In contrast, cure or treatment completion was achieved in 82% of those treated under DOTS in 2001, so that significant progress has been made toward the 85% target for 2005. WHO has an ambitious Global DOTS Expansion Plan that aims to accelerate the rate at which

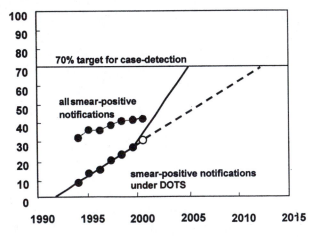

Figure 4. Rate of progress toward the 70% global case detection target for smear-positive TB. Black points mark the number of smear-positive cases notified under DOTS from 1994 to 2000, expressed as a percentage of all estimated smear-positive cases for each year. Projected lines show the rate at which case detection under DOTS would have to increase from 2000 to meet the 2005 targets of 70% global case detection (solid line). There has been a steady increase in the rate of case detection under DOTS, but at the current rate of progress targets will not be met until the year 2013 (dashed line). The estimate for 2001 (white point) is more compatible with the 2013 than the 2005 projection, however, and the overall rate of case detection under any strategy (grey points) appears to be leveling off at about 40%. From reference 68a with permission.

DOTS is implemented and increase case detection rates so that the 2005 global targets can be met.

DOT and care in the community

Direct observation of therapy (DOT), one of the core elements of DOTS, is intended to reduce the default rate and minimize the risk of acquired drug resistance due to selective noncompliance with one or more of the different drugs. DOT is recommended for all patients in the intensive phase, for patients with new TB being treated with the rifampin-based continuation phase, and throughout the regimen in retreatment cases. In practice, many DOTS programs do not meet the minimum recommendations for DOT, because it is labor-intensive for both the patient and the health care providers. The feasibility of recruiting treatment supporters other than TB clinic nurses has been investigated in a number of countries (37, 64) and has been found to be a highly cost-effective way of achieving good outcomes in resource-poor settings with a high burden of TB (44). Guidelines for management of TB patients, including recruitment and training of community treatment supporters, are included in the guidelines for Integrated Management of Adult Illnesses being developed for use in primary health care settings.

DOTS, DOTS-Plus, and drug-resistant TB

There is good evidence that standardized regimens given under direct observation result in minimal generation of drug resistance and that drug susceptibility patterns are then maintained or improved, even in settings with very high HIV prevalence and TB incidence rates (8, 34). Moreover, the majority of patients with drug-resistant TB that is not resistant to both isoniazid and rifampin (MDR-TB) are adequately managed by the standard DOTS regimens (22), although high relapse rates are seen in patients with MDR-TB (39).

As detailed more fully in chapter 7, sentinel surveys were carried out under the WHO/IUATLD Global Drug Resistance Surveillance Project during the early 1990s (23, 46). Some sites were chosen to be representative of their region, whereas others were included because there was already evidence of a local problem with drug-resistant TB. A few settings, named hot spots, were identified as having a major drug resistance problem, with an MDR-TB prevalence of 3% or more. These included the Baltic republics of Estonia and Latvia, parts of Russia and China, Iran, and the Dominican Republic (23).

Subsequently, a DOTS-Plus strategy has been piloted, starting in Peru, Latvia, Estonia, the Philippines, and three oblasts in Russia, to test the feasibility, out-come, and cost-effectiveness of different approaches to managing MDR-TB. Results from a countrywide project in Peru are promising and suggest that MDR-TB can be effectively managed with second-line drugs under routine program conditions, with reasonable compliance and cure rates (59).

Tuberculosis Control in Areas with High HIV Prevalence

TB control programs can and should have a special place in HIV care provision, because of the strong epidemiological link between the two diseases and the high prevalence of HIV infection among TB patients. Until recently, however, policy was directed predominantly toward coping with the massive increases in caseloads and diagnostic demands that have been generated by the HIV epidemic (66), at the expense of integration between TB and HIV services. Even today, many African TB patients will not have any discussion about HIV with their health care providers, on the grounds that providing sufficient counseling is impractical. This denies any possibility of accessing interventions aimed at preventing subsequent opportunistic infections and misses an opportunity for HIV prevention (17).

TB control programs in Africa have been greatly strengthened during the 1990s, and increased collaboration between HIV and TB control programs is now recommended (68). Interventions with relevance to both HIV and TB control include the ProTEST initiative, a multicountry study linking voluntary counseling and testing (VCT) services to active TB case finding and provision of isoniazid preventive therapy (IPT) and co-trimoxazole prophylaxis (28). Access to antiretroviral therapy, which may reduce the risk of TB to a greater extent than IPT (3, 6, 27, 33), will have to be added to this package of care. The impact on TB incidence from interventions targeted to HIV-positive persons is, however, limited by the need to diagnose HIV before TB has developed, and so these interventions are currently viewed as being of individual rather than public health benefit (28). For antiretroviral therapy (ART) there is also the risk of TB occurring in the interval between diagnosis of HIV and starting therapy, since median CD4 counts in ambulant African TB patients are much higher than in the United States or Europe (1, 11, 63) and are in the same range as the currently recommended threshold for starting ART (200×10^6 per ml). Reducing mortality in HIV-infected TB patients is another priority area, and in this respect ART is likely to be highly effective (10, 14). Co-trimoxazole prophylaxis also improves the survival of HIV-infected TB patients (63, 70).

Improving TB control in the wider community may be the most effective way of protecting HIV-infected persons. In this respect, the experience with DOTS in areas with high HIV prevalence has been disappointing, with steeply rising TB incidence and mortality rates even in countries with model programs (16). This may not be a fair test, however, because observation has so far been limited to a period when HIV prevalence rates were rising. DOTS clearly cannot prevent HIV-infected individuals who are already infected with *M. tuberculosis* from becoming more susceptible to TB disease, even if ongoing TB transmission rates are being successfully reduced. It can be argued that the burden of mortality and morbidity in the community is already so high that a more vigorous intervention than DOTS is needed (16). Research to identify strategies capable of substantially reducing morbidity and mortality from TB in countries with high HIV prevalence is under way. Possible approaches include greatly intensified case detection of symptomatic TB patients, active case detection (mass screening of asymptomatic as well as symptomatic individuals), and mass delivery of preventive therapy either coupled to intensive promotion of VCT or given to all members of the community regardless of HIV status (12).

CONCLUSIONS

Considerable progress has been made during the last decade toward the improvement of global TB control; the establishment of a global surveillance mechanism means that it is now possible to monitor trends and progress. DOTS, a clear strategy that is cost-effective, prevents drug resistance, and reduces TB mortality and incidence in countries with low HIV prevalence, has been developed and widely implemented. Strategies for managing MDR-TB and reducing the prevalence of drug resistance are in the late stage of development and have produced promising results in pilot projects. Despite these gains, there were still 8.5 million TB cases and 1.8 million deaths from TB in 2001. The epidemic of HIV-associated TB continues to grow and drive global incidence rates upward. Universal access to DOTS has not yet been achieved. Coverage is still incomplete in some countries with high HIV prevalence and in a number of countries with the highest burden, including India and China, which together were home to 39% of the new TB patients in 2001. Operational challenges for the coming decade are to achieve rapid expansion of access to DOTS and to accelerate the pace at which case detection is improving through more timely and complete diagnosis of smear-positive TB patients

while maintaining high cure rates. The principal research challenge, however, will be to identify new strategies that are capable of regaining control and reducing mortality from TB in areas with high HIV prevalence.

Acknowledgment. We thank Chris Dye for providing Fig. 1, 2, and 4.

REFERENCES

1. Ackah, A. N., D. Coulibaly, H. Digbeu, K. Diallo, K. M. Vetter, I. M. Coulibaly, A. E. Greenberg, and K. M. De Cock. 1995. Response to treatment, mortality, and CD4 lymphocyte counts in HIV-infected persons with tuberculosis in Abidjan, Cote d'Ivoire. *Lancet* 345:607–610.
2. Ansari, N. A., A. H. Kombe, T. A. Kenyon, N. M. Hone, J. W. Tappero, S. T. Nyirenda, N. J. Binkin, and S. B. Lucas. 2002. Pathology and causes of death in a group of 128 predominantly HIV-positive patients in Botswana, 1997–1998. *Int. J. Tuberc. Lung Dis.* 6:55–63.
3. Badri, M., D. Wilson, and R. Wood. 2002. Effect of highly active antiretroviral therapy on incidence of tuberculosis in South Africa: a cohort study. *Lancet* 359:2059–2064.
4. Broekmans, J. F., G. B. Migliori, H. L. Rieder, J. Lees, P. Ruutu, R. Loddenkemper, and M. C. Raviglione. 2002. European framework for tuberculosis control and elimination in countries with a low incidence. Recommendations of the World Health Organization (WHO), International Union Against Tuberculosis and Lung Disease (IUATLD) and Royal Netherlands Tuberculosis Association (KNCV) Working Group. *Eur. Respir. J.* 19:765–775.
5. Brudney, K., and J. Dobkin. 1991. Resurgent tuberculosis in New York City. Human immunodeficiency virus, homelessness, and the decline of tuberculosis control programs. *Am. Rev. Respir. Dis.* 144:745–749.
6. Bucher, H. C., L. E. Griffith, G. H. Guyatt, P. Sudre, M. Naef, P. Sendi, and M. Battegay. 1999. Isoniazid prophylaxis for tuberculosis in HIV infection: a meta-analysis of randomized controlled trials. *AIDS* 13:501–507.
7. Centers for Disease Control and Prevention. 1991. Nosocomial transmission of multidrug-resistant tuberculosis among HIV-infected persons—Florida and New York, 1988–1991. *Morb. Mortal. Wkly. Rep.* 40:585–591.
8. Churchyard, G. J., E. L. Corbett, I. Kleinschmidt, D. Mulder, and K. M. De Cock. 2000. Drug-resistant tuberculosis in South African gold miners: incidence and associated factors. *Int. J. Tuberc. Lung. Dis.* 4:433–440.
9. Coninx, R., D. Maher, H. Reyes, and M. Grzemska. 2000. Tuberculosis in prisons in countries with high prevalence. *Br. Med. J.* 320:440–442.
10. Conti, S., M. Masocco, P. Pezzotti, V. Toccaceli, M. Vichi, S. Boros, R. Urciuoli, C. Valdarchi, and G. Rezza. 2000. Differential impact of combined antiretroviral therapy on the survival of Italian patients with specific AIDS-defining illnesses. *J. Acquir. Immune Defic. Syndr.* 25:451–458.
11. Corbett, E. L., G. J. Churchyard, S. Charalambous, B. Samb, V. Moloi, T. C. Clayton, A. D. Grant, J. Murray, R. J. Hayes, and K. M. De Cock. 2002. Morbidity and mortality in South African gold miners: impact of untreated HIV infection. *Clin. Infect. Dis.* 34:1251–1258.
12. Corbett, E. L., R. W. Steketee, F. O. ter Kuile, A. S. Latif, A. Kamali, and R. J. Hayes. 2002. HIV-1/AIDS and the control of other infectious diseases in Africa. *Lancet* 359:2177–2187.

13. Corbett, E. L., C. J. Watt, N. Walker, D. Maher, S. Lazzari, B. G. Williams, M. C. Raviglione, and C. Dye. 2003. The growing burden of tuberculosis: global trends and interactions with the HIV epidemic. *Arch. Intern. Med.* **163:**1009–1021.

14. Dean, G. L., S. G. Edwards, N. J. Ives, G. Matthews, E. F. Fox, L. Navaratne, M. Fisher, G. P. Taylor, R. Miller, C. B. Taylor, A. de Ruiter, and A. L. Pozniak. 2002. Treatment of tuberculosis in HIV-infected persons in the era of highly active antiretroviral therapy. *AIDS* **16:**75–83.

15. De Cock, K. M., B. Soro, I. M. Coulibaly, and S. B. Lucas. 1992. Tuberculosis and HIV infection in sub-Saharan Africa. *JAMA* **268:**1581–1587.

16. De Cock, K. M., and R. E. Chaisson. 1999. Will DOTS do it? A reappraisal of tuberculosis control in countries with high rates of HIV infection. *Int. J. Tuberc. Lung Dis.* **3:**457–465.

17. De Cock, K. M., D. Mbori-Ngacha, and E. Marum. 2002. Shadow on the continent: public health and HIV/AIDS in Africa in the 21st century. *Lancet* **360:**67–72.

18. Dehne, K. L., V. Pokrovskiy, Y. Kobyshcha, and B. Schwartlander. 2000. Update on the epidemics of HIV and other sexually transmitted infections in the newly independent states of the former Soviet Union. *AIDS* **14**(Suppl. 3):S75–S84.

19. Dye, C., S. Scheele, P. Dolin, V. Pathania, and M. C. Raviglione. 1999. Global burden of tuberculosis: estimated incidence, prevalence, and mortality by country. *JAMA* **282:**677–686.

20. Dye, C., F. Zhao, S. Scheele, and B. G. Williams. 2000. Evaluating the impact of tuberculosis control: number of deaths prevented by short-course chemotherapy in China. *Int. J. Epidemiol.* **29:**564.

21. Dye, C., C. J. Watt, and D. Bleed. 2002. Low access to a highly effective therapy: a challenge for international tuberculosis control. *Bull W. H. O.* **80:**437–444.

22. Espinal, M. A., S. J. Kim, P. G. Suarez, K. M. Kam, A. G. Khomenko, G. B. Migliori, J. Baez, A. Kochi, C. Dye, and M. C. Raviglione. 2000. Standard short-course chemotherapy for drug-resistant tuberculosis: treatment outcomes in 6 countries. *JAMA* **283:**2537–2545.

23. Espinal, M. A., A. Laszlo, L. Simonsen, F. Boulahbal, S. J. Kim, A. Reniero, S. Hoffner, H. L. Rieder, N. Binkin, C. Dye, R. Williams, and M. C. Raviglione. 2001. Global trends in resistance to antituberculosis drugs. World Health Organization—International Union against Tuberculosis and Lung Disease Working Group on Antituberculosis Drug Resistance Surveillance. *N. Engl. J. Med.* **344:**1294–1303.

24. Ferreira, M.M., L. Ferrazoli, M. Palaci, P. S. Salles, L. A. Medeiros, P. Novoa, C. R. Kiefer, M. Schechtmann, A. L. Kritski, W. D. Johnson, L. W. Riley, and J. O. Ferreira. 1996. Tuberculosis and HIV infection among female inmates in Sao Paulo, Brazil: a prospective cohort study. *J. Acquir. Immune Defic. Syndr. Hum. Retrovirol.* **13:**177–183.

25. Frieden, T. R., T. Sterling, A. Pablos-Mendez, J. O. Kilburn, G. M. Cauthen, and S. W. Dooley. 1993. The emergence of drug-resistant tuberculosis in New York City. *N. Engl. J. Med.* **328:**521–526.

26. Frieden, T. R., P. I. Fujiwara, R. M. Washko, and M. A. Hamburg. 1995. Tuberculosis in New York City—turning the tide. *N. Engl. J. Med.* **333:**229–233.

27. Girardi, E., G. Antonucci, P. Vanacore, M. Libanore, I. Errante, A. Mattelli, G. Ippolito, and Gruppo Italiano di Studio Tuberculosi e AIDS (GISTA). 2000. Impact of combination antiretroviral therapy on the risk of tuberculosis among persons with HIV infection. *AIDS* **14:**1985–1991.

28. Godfrey-Faussett, P., D. Maher, Y. D. Mukadi, P. Nunn, J. Perriens, and M. Raviglione. 2002. How human immunodeficiency virus voluntary testing can contribute to tuberculosis control. *Bull. W. H. O.* **80:**939–945.

29. Grzybowski, S., and D. A. Enarson. 1978. The fate of pulmonary tuberculosis under various treatment programmes. *Bull. Int. Union Tuberc.* **53:**70–75.

30. Gupta, R., J. P. Cegielski, M. A. Espinal, M. Henkens, J. Y. Kim, C. S. Lambregts-Van Weezenbeek, J. W. Lee, M. C. Raviglione, P. G. Suarez, and F. Varaine. 2002. Increasing transparency in partnerships for health—introducing the Green Light Committee. *Trop. Med. Int. Health* **7:**970–976.

31. Harries A. D., D. Maher, and P. Nunn. 1997. Practical and affordable measures for the protection of health care workers from tuberculosis in low-income countries. *Bull. W. H. O.* **75:**477–489.

32. Joint United Nations Programme on HIV/AIDS. 2000. *Report on the Global HIV/AIDS Epidemic.* UNAIDS/00.13E. United Nations, New York, N.Y.

33. Jones, J. L., D. L. Hanson, M. S. Dworkin, K. M. De Cock, and The Adult/Adolescent Spectrum of HIV Disease Group. 2000. HIV associated TB in the era of HAART. *Int. J. Tuberc. Lung Dis.* **4:**1026–1031.

34. Kenyon, T. A., M. J. Mwasekaga, R. Huebner, D. Rumisha, N. Binkin, and E. Maganu. 1999. Low levels of drug resistance amidst rapidly increasing tuberculosis and human immunodeficiency virus co-epidemics in Botswana. *Int. J. Tuberc. Lung Dis.* **3:**4–11.

35. Khatri, G. R., and T. R. Frieden. 2002. Controlling tuberculosis in India. *N. Engl. J. Med.* **347:**1420–1425.

36. Lucas, S. B., A. Hounnou, C. Peacock, A. Beaumel, G. Djomand, J. M. N'Gbichi, K. Yeboue, M. Honde, M. Diomande, C. Giordano, R. Doorly, K. Brattegaard, L. Kestens, R. W. Smithwick, A. Kadio, N. Ezani, A. Yapi, and K. M. De Cock. 1993. The mortality and pathology of HIV infection in a west African city. *AIDS* **7:**1569–1579.

37. Maher, D., J. L. van Gorkom, P. C. Gondrie, and M. Raviglione. 1999. Community contribution to tuberculosis care in countries with high tuberculosis prevalence: past, present and future. *Int. J. Tuberc. Lung Dis.* **3:**762–768.

38. McKenna, M. T., E. McCray, and I. Onorato. 1995. The epidemiology of tuberculosis among foreign-born persons in the United States, 1986–1993. *N. Engl. J. Med.* **332:**1071–1076.

39. Migliori, G. B., M. Espinal, I. D. Danilova, V. V. Punga, M. Grzemska, and M. C. Raviglione. 2002. Frequency of recurrence among MDR-tB cases "successfully" treated with standardised short-course chemotherapy. *Int. J. Tuberc. Lung Dis.* **6:**858–864.

40. Ministry of Health of the People's Republic of China. 2002. *Report on Nationwide Random Survey for the Epidemiology of Tuberculosis in 2000.* Ministry of Health of the People's Republic of China, Beijing, China.

41. Moss, A. R., J. A. Hahn, J. P. Tulsky, C. L. Daley, P. M. Small, and P. C. Hopewell. 2000. Tuberculosis in the homeless. A prospective study. *Am. J. Respir. Crit. Care Med.* **162:**460–464.

42. Murray, C. J., K. Styblo, and A. Rouillon. 1990. Tuberculosis in developing countries: burden, intervention and cost. *Bull. Int. Union Tuberc. Lung Dis.* **65:**6–24.

43. Murthy, K. J., T. R. Frieden, A. Yazdani, and P. Hreshikesh. 2001. Public-private partnership in tuberculosis control: experience in Hyderabad, India. *Int. J. Tuberc. Lung Dis.* **5:**354–359.

44. Nunn, P., A. Harries, P. Godfrey-Faussett, R. Gupta, D. Maher, and M. Raviglione. 2002. The research agenda for improving health policy, systems performance, and service delivery for tuberculosis control: a WHO perspective. *Bull. W. H. O.* **80:**471–476.

45. Nyangulu, D. S., A. D. Harries, C. Kang'ombe, A. E. Yadidi, K. Chokani, T. Cullinan, D. Maher, P. Nunn, and F. M. Sala-

niponi. 1997. Tuberculosis in a prison population in Malawi. *Lancet* **350:**1284–1287.

46. Pablos-Mendez, A., M. C. Raviglione, A. Laszlo, N. Binkin, H. L. Rieder, F. Bustreo, D. L. Cohn, W. C. Lambregts-van Weezenbeck, S. J. Kim, P. Chaulet, and P. Nunn. 1998. Global surveillance for antituberculosis-drug resistance, 1994–1997. World Health Organization—International Union against Tuberculosis and Lung Disease Working Group on Anti-Tuberculosis Drug Resistance Surveillance. *N. Engl. J. Med.* **338:**1641–1649.

47. Portu, J. J., M. Aldamiz-Etxebarria, J. M. Agud, J. M. Arevalo, M. J. Almaraz, and C. Ayensa. 2002. Tuberculin skin testing in intravenous drug users: differences between HIV-seropositive and HIV-seronegative subjects. *Addict. Biol.* **7:**235–241.

48. Rana, F. S., M. P. Hawken, C. Mwachari, S. M. Bhatt, F. Abdullah, L. W. Ng'ang'a, C. Power, W. A. Githui, J. D. Porter, and S. B. Lucas. 2000. Autopsy study of HIV-1-positive and HIV-1-negative adult medical patients in Nairobi, Kenya. *J. Acquir. Immune Defic. Syndr.* **24:**23–29.

49. Raviglione, M. C., P. Sudre, H. L. Rieder, S. Spinaci, and A. Kochi. 1993. Secular trends of tuberculosis in western Europe. *Bull. W. H. O.* **71:**297–306.

50. Raviglione, M. C., H. L. Rieder, K. Styblo, A. G. Khomenko, K. Esteves, and A. Kochi. 1994. Tuberculosis trends in eastern Europe and the former USSR. *Tubercle Lung Dis.* **75:**400–416.

51. Raviglione, M. C., C. Dye, S. Schmidt, and A. Kochi. 1997. Assessment of worldwide tuberculosis control. WHO Global Surveillance and Monitoring Project. *Lancet* **350:**624–629.

52. Raviglione, M. C., and A. Pio. 2002. Evolution of WHO policies for tuberculosis control, 1948–2001. *Lancet* **359:**775–780.

53. Rieder, H. L., G. M. Cauthen, G. W. Comstock, D. E. Snider, Jr. 1989. Epidemiology of tuberculosis in the United States. *Epidemiol. Rev.* **11:**79–98.

54. Rose, A. M., J. M. Watson, C. Graham, A. J. Nunn, F. Drobniewski, L. P. Ormerod, J. H. Darbyshire, and J. Leese. 2001. Tuberculosis at the end of the 20th century in England and Wales: results of a national survey in 1998. *Thorax* **56:**173–179.

55. Selwyn, P. A., D. Hartel, V. A. Lewis, E. E. Schoenbaum, S. H. Vermund, R. S. Klein, A. T. Walker, and G. H. Friedland. 1989. A prospective study of the risk of tuberculosis among intravenous drug users with human immunodeficiency virus infection. *N. Engl. J. Med.* **320:**545–550.

56. Shilova, M. V., and C. Dye. 2001. The resurgence of tuberculosis in Russia. *Philos. Trans. R. Soc. London B Ser.* **356:**1069–1075.

57. Styblo, K., and A. Rouillon. 1981. Estimated global incidence of smear-positive pulmonary tuberculosis. Unreliability of officially reported figures on tuberculosis. *Bull. Int. Union Tuberc.* **56:**118–126.

58. Suarez, P., C. J. Watt, E. Alarcon, J. Portocarrero, D. Zavala, R. Canales, F. Luelmo, M. A. Espinal, and C. Dye. 2001. The dynamics of tuberculosis in response to 10 years of intensive control effort in Peru. *J. Infect. Dis.* **184:**473–478.

59. Suarez, P. G., K. Floyd, J. Portocarrero, E. Alarcon, E. Rapiti, G. Ramos, C. Bonilla, I. Sabogal, I. Aranda, C. Dye, M. Raviglione, and M. A. Espinal. 2002. Feasibility and cost-effectiveness of standardised second-line drug treatment for chronic tuberculosis patients: a national cohort study in Peru. *Lancet* **359:**1980–1989.

60. Tuberculosis Research Centre CCI. 2001. Trends in the prevalence and incidence of tuberculosis in South India. *Int. J. Tuberc. Lung Dis.* **5:**142–157.

61. Tupasi, T. E., S. Radhakrishna, A. B. Rivera, M. L. Pascual, M. I. Quelapio, V. M. Co, M. L. A. Villa, G. Beltran, J. D. Legaspi, N. V. Mangubat, J. N. Sarol, A. C. Reyes, A. Sarmiento, M. Solon, F. S. Solon, and M. J. Mantala. 1999. The 1997 nationwide tuberculosis prevalence survey in the Philippines. *Int. J. Tuberc. Lung Dis.* **3:**471–477.

62. Uplekar, M., S. Juvekar, S. Morankar, S. Rangan, and P. Nunn. 1998. Tuberculosis patients and practitioners in private clinics in India. *Int. J. Tuberc. Lung Dis.* **2:**324–329.

63. Wiktor, S. Z., M. M. Sassan, A. D. Grant, L. Abouya, J. M. Karon, C. Maurice, G. Djomand, A. Ackah, K. Domoua, A. Kadio, A. Yapi, P. Combe, O. Tossou, T. H. Roels, E. M. Lackritz, D. Coulibaly, K. M. De Cock, I. M. Coulibaly, and A. E. Greenberg. 1999. Efficacy of trimethoprim-sulphamethoxazole prophylaxis to decrease morbidity and mortality in HIV-1-infected patients with tuberculosis in Abidjan, Cote d'Ivoire: a randomised controlled trial. *Lancet* **353:**1469–1475.

64. Wilkinson, D. 1994. High-compliance tuberculosis treatment programme in a rural community. *Lancet* **343:**647–648.

65. World Bank. 1993. *World Development Report 1993. Investing in Health.* World Bank, Washington, D.C.

66. World Health Organization, UNAIDS. 1999. Preventive therapy against tuberculosis in people living with HIV. *Wkly. Epidemiol. Rec.* **74:**385–398.

67. World Health Organization. 2002. *Global Tuberculosis Control: Surveillance, Planning, Financing.* WHO/TB/2002.287. World Health Organization, Geneva, Switzerland.

68. World Health Organization. 2002. *Strategic Framework to Decrease the Burden of TB/HIV.* WHO/CDS/TB/2002.296, WHO/HIV-AIDS/2002.2. World Health Organization, Geneva, Switzerland.

68a. World Health Organization. 2002. *Global Tuberculosis Control: Surveillance, Planning, Financing.* WHO Report 2002. WHO/TB/2002.295. World Health Organization, Geneva, Switzerland.

69. World Health Organization. 2003. *Global Tuberculosis Control: Surveillance, Planning, Financing.* WHO/TB/2003.316. World Health Organization, Geneva, Switzerland.

70. Ya Diul, M., D. Maher, and A. Harries. 2001. Tuberculosis case fatality rates in high HIV prevalence populations in sub-Saharan Africa. *AIDS* **15:**143–152.

II. CLINICAL AND EPIDEMIOLOGICAL PERSPECTIVES

Tuberculosis and the Tubercle Bacillus
Edited by Stewart T. Cole et al.
© 2005 ASM Press, Washington, D.C.

Chapter 2

Overview of Clinical Tuberculosis

PHILIP C. HOPEWELL AND ROBERT M. JASMER

FACTORS INFLUENCING THE CLINICAL EXPRESSION OF INFECTION WITH *MYCOBACTERIUM TUBERCULOSIS*

The clinical expression of infection with *Mycobacterium tuberculosis* is quite varied and depends on a number of identified factors. Table 1 lists both host- and microbe-related characteristics as well as the consequences of their interactions that influence the manifestations of tuberculous infection. Among generally healthy persons, infection with *M. tuberculosis* is highly likely to be asymptomatic. Data from a variety of sources suggest that the lifetime risk of developing clinically evident tuberculosis after being infected is approximately 10%, with a 90% likelihood of the infection remaining latent (20). Only a positive tuberculin skin test or a positive result from another validated test, such as whole-blood gamma interferon release, indicates the presence of the organism in persons with latent infections (55, 56).

Host factors play a major and obvious role in determining the risk of developing tuberculosis. In specific subpopulations, for example, persons with immunodeficiency states or infants, the proportions who develop evident tuberculosis once infected with *M. tuberculosis* are much higher than those in the general population (1, 20, 53, 70). For example, among persons infected with human immunodeficiency virus (HIV), rates of tuberculosis vary from 2 to 8% per year (15). Another host-related factor, immunization with bacillus Calmette-Guérin (BCG) (an attenuated strain of *Mycobacterium bovis*) in persons with intact cell-mediated immunity, minimizes the risk of early disseminated tuberculosis, especially in children.

In addition to host factors, there probably are factors related to the organism itself, such as its virulence or predilection for specific tissues, that influence the outcome and features of the infection; however, these features of the organism have not been characterized. For example, an outbreak of tuberculosis was reported in a rural community in which the growth characteristics of the strain involved greatly exceeded those of other clinical isolates (81). However, the magnitude of variations in the risk of disease by this strain of *M. tuberculosis* is not known.

The most obvious and important factor influencing the clinical features of tuberculosis is the site of involvement. Before the beginning of the epidemic of HIV infection, approximately 85% of reported tuberculosis cases were limited to the lungs, with the remaining 15% involving only nonpulmonary sites or both pulmonary and nonpulmonary sites (28) (Fig. 1). This proportional distribution is substantially different among persons with HIV infection. Although there are no national data that describe the sites of involvement in HIV-infected persons with tuberculosis, in one large retrospective study of tuberculosis in patients with advanced HIV infection, it was reported that 38% had only pulmonary involvement, 30% had infection at extrapulmonary sites, and 32% had both pulmonary and nonpulmonary involvement (36, 76). The multiplicity of sites in HIV-infected persons is typical of what is seen in individuals with an immune system whose ability to contain infection with *M. tuberculosis* is limited, and therefore such persons often have widely disseminated disease. Included in this category are infants, the elderly, and persons with primary or secondary immunodeficiency states resulting from coexisting diseases or malnutrition.

SYSTEMIC AND REMOTE EFFECTS OF TUBERCULOSIS

Tuberculosis occurring at any site may cause symptoms and findings that are not related specifically

Philip C. Hopewell • Dean's Office, University of California San Francisco, San Francisco General Hospital, Bldg. NH, SFGH Rm. 2A2, Box 0809, San Francisco, CA 94110. **Robert M. Jasmer** • San Francisco General Hospital, Division of Pulmonary and Critical Care Medicine, 1001 Potrero Ave., Rm. 5K-1, San Francisco, CA 94110.

Table 1. Factors influencing the clinical features of tuberculosis

Host factors	Microbial factors	Host-microbe interaction
Age Immune status Specific immunodeficiency states Malnutrition Genetic factors (?) Coexisting diseases Immunization with *M. bovis* (BCG)	Virulence of organism (?) Predilection (tropism) for specific tissues (?)	Sites of involvement Severity of disease

to the organ or tissue involved but, rather, are systemic in nature or are remote from the site of disease. Systemic manifestations of the disease, including fever, malaise, and weight loss, are probably mediated by cytokines, especially tumor necrosis factor alpha (TNF-α). Experimental data suggest that TNF-α is an important mediator of the systemic effects of the disease (26, 62, 79, 80). Of the systemic effects, fever is the most easily quantified. The frequency with which fever has been observed in patients with tuberculosis varies from approximately 37 to 80% (3, 44). In a study by Kiblawi et al. (44), in which the fever response was specifically examined, 21% of patients had no fever at any point in the course of hospitalization for tuberculosis. Of the febrile patients, 34% were afebrile within 1 week of hospitalization and 64% were afebrile within 2 weeks. The median duration of fever after beginning treatment was 10 days, with a range of 1 to 109 days. Weight loss, weakness, and malaise appear to be less common but are more difficult to quantify.

In addition to these generalized effects of tuberculosis, there are remote manifestations that are not a result of the anatomic site of involvement. These include hematologic abnormalities, hyponatremia, and psychological disorders. The most common hematologic manifestations of tuberculosis are increases in the peripheral blood leukocyte count and anemia, each of which occurs in approximately 10% of patients with apparently localized tuberculosis (14). The increase in leukocyte counts is usually slight, but leukemoid reactions may occur. Leukopenia has also been reported, often with disseminated tuberculosis. An increase in the peripheral blood monocyte and eosinophil counts also may occur in patients with tuberculosis. Anemia is common when the infection is disseminated. In some instances, anemia or pancytopenia may result from direct involvement of the bone marrow and may thus be a local rather than a remote effect.

Other than weight loss, the most frequent metabolic effect of tuberculosis is hyponatremia, which in one series was found to occur in 11% of patients (19). Hyponatremia is caused by the production of an antidiuretic hormone-like substance found within affected lung tissue (82) and can also be seen in patients with bacterial pneumonia, lung cancer, or central nervous system disorders. Because of this latter association, hyponatremia may be a feature of central nervous system tuberculosis. The poor prognosis associated with hyponatremia in the prechemotherapy era was probably related simply to the amount of lung involved and perhaps to adrenal involvement.

The psychological effects of tuberculosis are very poorly defined but were commonly recognized prior to the advent of effective therapy. These effects include depression and, on occasion, hypomania. The best descriptions of the psychological alterations in patients with tuberculosis are found in literary works, such as Thomas Mann's *The Magic Mountain*, rather than in the medical literature.

In many patients, tuberculosis is associated with other serious disorders, including HIV infection, alcoholism, chronic renal failure, diabetes mellitus, neoplastic diseases, and drug abuse, to name but a few. The signs and symptoms of these diseases and their

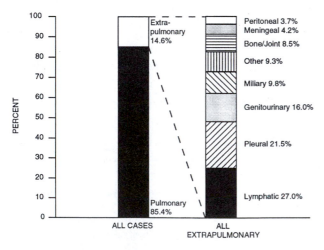

Figure 1. Distribution of sites of involvement in newly reported cases of tuberculosis in 1978 prior to the epidemic of infection with HIV.

complications can easily obscure or modify those of tuberculosis and can result in considerable delays in diagnosis or in misdiagnoses for extended periods, especially in patients with HIV infection (47). For this reason, it is important that clinicians have an understanding of the diseases with which tuberculosis may coexist and have a high index of suspicion for a combination of the two disorders.

DIAGNOSIS OF TUBERCULOSIS INFECTION

As noted above, a positive tuberculin skin test is usually the only evidence of latent tuberculous infection (40). Among persons with symptoms or clinical findings of tuberculosis, the tuberculin skin test may provide useful diagnostic information. However, in an individual patient, a positive test (usually defined as an induration of ≥10 mm in immunocompetent persons and ≥5 mm in persons with HIV infection) does not establish a diagnosis and a negative test does not exclude tuberculosis. False-positive tuberculin tests can occur due to infection with nontuberculous mycobacteria or immunization with BCG, and as many as 25% of apparently immunocompetent persons have negative tuberculin skin tests at the time of diagnosis of tuberculosis (37, 61). Among patients with tuberculosis and HIV infection, the frequency of positive tuberculin reactions varies considerably depending on the degree of immunocompromise (65).

The recent introduction of blood-based tests that assess levels of gamma interferon released from specific T cells infected with *M. tuberculosis* offers the promise of improved testing for tuberculosis infection (27, 55). However, blood tests that measure interferon levels are not currently recommended for use in those suspected of having active tuberculosis (56).

Pulmonary Tuberculosis

Symptoms and physical findings

Cough is the most common symptom of pulmonary tuberculosis. Early in the course of the illness, the cough may be nonproductive, but subsequently, as inflammation and tissue necrosis ensue, sputum is usually produced. Inflammation of the lung parenchyma adjacent to a pleural surface may cause pleuritic pain. Spontaneous pneumothorax may also occur, often causing chest pain and perhaps dyspnea. Dyspnea as a result of parenchymal lung involvement is unusual unless there is extensive disease. Tuberculosis may, however, cause severe respiratory failure (39, 60) (Fig. 2). Hemoptysis may also be a presenting symptom but does not necessarily indicate

active tuberculosis; it may result from posttuberculous bronchiectasis, rupture of a dilated blood vessel in the wall of an old cavity (Rasmussen's aneurysm), bacterial or fungal infection (especially *Aspergillus* infection in the form of a fungus ball or mycetoma) in a residual cavity, or erosion of calcified lesions into the lumen of an airway (broncholithiasis).

Physical findings in pulmonary tuberculosis are generally not particularly helpful in defining the disease. Rales may be heard in the area of involvement, and bronchial breath sounds may also be heard if there is lung consolidation. Amphoric breath sounds may be indicative of a cavity.

Radiographic features

In developed countries, radiographic examination of the chest is usually the first diagnostic study undertaken after history and physical examination. Pulmonary tuberculosis nearly always causes abnormalities on the chest radiograph, although an endobronchial lesion may not be associated with a radiographic finding. In primary tuberculosis occurring as a result of recent infection, the process is generally seen as a middle or lower lung zone infiltrate, often associated with ipsilateral hilar adenopathy (Fig. 3). Atelectasis may result from compression of airways by enlarged lymph nodes. If the primary process persists beyond the time when specific cell-mediated immunity develops, cavitation may occur (so-called progressive primary tuberculosis).

Tuberculosis that develops as a result of endogenous reactivation of latent infection usually causes abnormalities in the upper lobes of one or both lungs. Cavitation, resulting from destruction of lung tissue, is common in this form of tuberculosis. The most frequent sites of involvement are the apical and posterior segments of the right upper lobe and the apical-posterior segment of the left upper lobe (Fig. 4). Healing of the tuberculous lesions usually results in development of a scar with loss of lung parenchymal volume and, often, with calcification. In immunocompetent adults with tuberculosis, intrathoracic adenopathy is uncommon but may occur, especially in those with primary infection. As tuberculosis progresses, infected material may be spread via the airways into the lower portions of the lung or to the other lung. Erosion of a parenchymal focus of tuberculosis into a blood or lymph vessel may result in dissemination of the organism and a miliary pattern (consisting of evenly distributed small nodules 2 to 5 mm in diameter) on the chest radiograph (Fig. 5).

In patients with HIV infection, the nature of the radiographic findings depends to a certain extent on the degree of immunocompromise produced by the

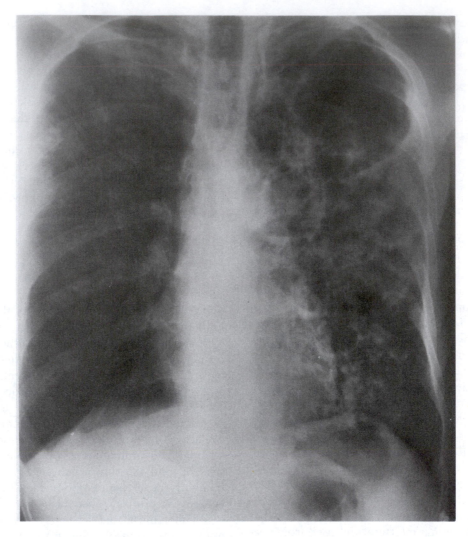

Figure 2. Frontal view chest radiograph showing extensive tuberculosis causing respiratory failure.

infection. Tuberculosis that occurs relatively early in the course of HIV infection tends to have the typical radiographic findings described above (17, 22, 63). In patients with more advanced HIV infection, the radiographic findings become more "atypical": cavitation is uncommon, and lower-lung-zone or diffuse infiltrates and intrathoracic adenopathy are frequent (Fig. 6).

Bacteriologic evaluation

At present, a definitive diagnosis of tuberculosis can be established either by the isolation of tubercle bacilli in culture or by tests that identify specific *M. tuberculosis* DNA. These latter tests, called nucleic acid amplification tests, are now approved for use with sputum specimens (16). When the lungs are involved, sputum is the initial diagnostic specimen of choice. Sputum specimens should be collected at the time of the initial evaluation. Single early-morning specimens have a higher yield of bacteria and a lower rate of contamination than pooled specimens. The sensitivity of sputum examination increases with the number of specimens, but there is no clinically significant increase in the cumulative recovery of organisms with more than three specimens (48). Therefore, most clinicians obtain three specimens collected on separate mornings to evaluate patients for active tuberculosis.

There are several ways of obtaining specimens from patients who are not producing sputum. The first and most useful is inducing sputum production by having the patient inhale a mist of hypertonic (3 to 5%) saline generated by an ultrasonic nebulizer. This is a benign and well-tolerated procedure, although bronchospasm is occasionally precipitated in asthmatics. Samples of gastric contents obtained via a nasogastric tube have lower yields than induced spu-

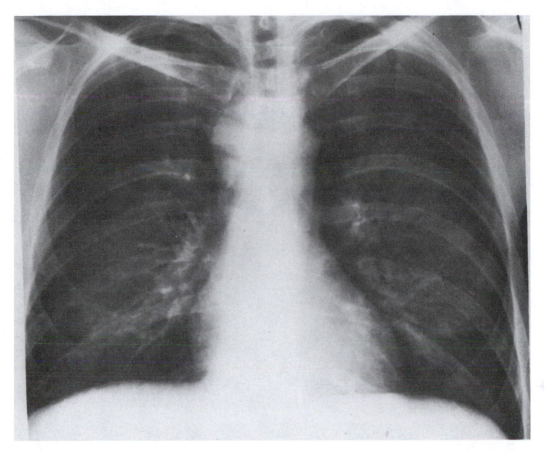

Figure 3. Frontal view chest radiograph showing right paratracheal adenopathy as a manifestation of recently acquired tuberculous infection.

tum, and the procedure is more complicated and uncomfortable for the patient. However, in children and some adults, gastric contents may be the only specimen that can be obtained.

Usually, fiberoptic bronchoscopy is the next diagnostic step if the sputum sample is negative or if sputum cannot be obtained by induction. In general, the bronchoscopic procedure should include bronchoalveolar lavage and transbronchial lung biopsy. The yield of bronchoscopy has been high both for miliary tuberculosis and for localized disease (12, 24, 77). For larger nodular lesions, needle aspiration biopsy may also provide specimens from which *M. tuberculosis* can be isolated. This technique is more suited to the evaluation of lesions when there is a suspicion of malignancy.

In situations in which the suspicion for active tuberculosis is high, a therapeutic trial of antituberculosis chemotherapy may be indicated before more invasive studies are undertaken (31). In the absence of another diagnosis, improvement in the chest radiograph concomitant with antituberculosis treatment would be sufficient for making a diagnosis of tuberculosis and continuing with a full course of therapy.

If a response is going to occur, it should be seen within 3 months of starting treatment. In the United States, the criteria for defining a case of tuberculosis allow for negative cultures if the patient in question has a positive tuberculin skin test and responds to multidrug chemotherapy in the absence of another diagnosis.

Extrapulmonary Tuberculosis

As noted above, prior to the epidemic of HIV infection, approximately 15% of newly reported cases of tuberculosis involved only extrapulmonary sites (28). For reasons that are not understood, as rates of pulmonary tuberculosis decreased, rates of extrapulmonary disease remained constant, resulting in an increasing proportion of cases being extrapulmonary. With the onset of the HIV epidemic, however, both absolute and relative rates of extrapulmonary involvement have increased.

Extrapulmonary tuberculosis presents more of a diagnostic and therapeutic challenge than pulmonary tuberculosis. In part, this problem relates to its being less common and therefore less familiar to

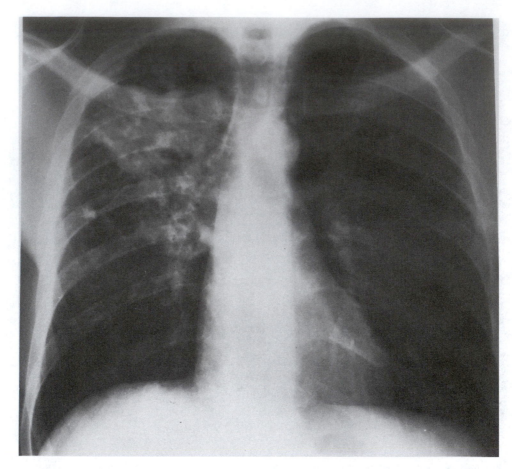

Figure 4. Frontal view chest radiograph showing the typical findings of endogenous reactivation tuberculosis in an immuno-competent patient. Note the upper lobe location and cavitation.

most clinicians (2, 83). In addition, extrapulmonary tuberculosis involves relatively inaccessible sites, and because of the nature of the sites involved, fewer bacilli can cause much greater damage. The combination of small numbers of bacilli and inaccessible sites makes bacteriologic confirmation of a diagnosis more difficult, and invasive procedures are frequently required to establish a diagnosis.

The relative frequencies of tuberculosis at various sites in persons without immunocompromise are shown in Fig. 1, and distribution by age is shown in Fig. 7 (28). As can be seen in the figures, in general the incidence for each extrapulmonary site increases with increasing age, except for lymphatic and meningeal tuberculosis, which are relatively more common in young children.

Extrapulmonary tuberculosis in HIV-infected patients

Presumably, the basis for the frequency of extrapulmonary tuberculosis among patients with HIV infection is the failure of the immune response to contain *M. tuberculosis*, thereby enabling hematogenous dissemination and subsequent involvement of single or multiple nonpulmonary sites. As evidence of this sequence, tuberculosis bacillemia has been documented in HIV-infected patients on a number of occasions (34, 47, 71). Because of the frequency of extrapulmonary tuberculosis among HIV-infected patients, diagnostic specimens from any suspected site of disease should be examined for mycobacteria. Moreover, cultures of blood and bone marrow may reveal *M. tuberculosis* in patients who do not have an obvious localized site of disease but who are being evaluated because of fever. Table 2 lists the sites from which *M. tuberculosis* was recovered in a group of patients with advanced HIV infection (76).

Disseminated tuberculosis

The epidemic of HIV infection has considerably altered the frequency and descriptive epidemiology of disseminated tuberculosis. Disseminated (or miliary) tuberculosis occurs because of the inadequacy of host defenses in containing tuberculous infection. This

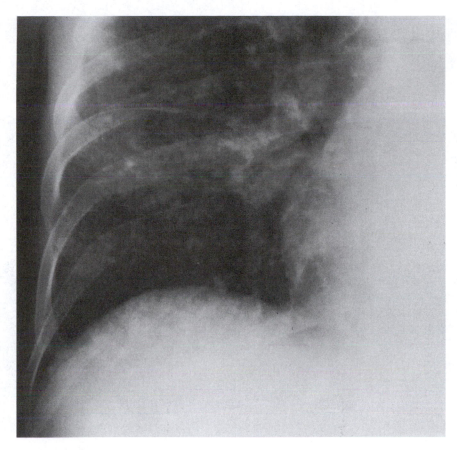

Figure 5. Portion of chest radiograph showing nodular lesions in a patient with disseminated tuberculosis.

failure of containment may occur in either latent or recently acquired tuberculous infection. Because of HIV or other causes of immunosuppression, the organism proliferates and disseminates throughout the body. Multiorgan involvement is probably much more common than is recognized because, generally, once *M. tuberculosis* is identified in any specimen, other sites are not evaluated. The term "miliary" is derived from the visual similarity of the lesions to millet seeds. Grossly, these lesions are 2- to 5-mm-diameter yellowish nodules that, histologically, are granulomas. Persons with HIV infection may not be able to form granulomas; hence, the individual lesions may not be present. Instead, a diffuse uniform pattern of lymphocytic infiltration and edema is seen.

Although disseminated tuberculosis nearly always involves the lungs, it is considered among the extrapulmonary forms of the disease because of the multiplicity of organs affected. In the past, miliary tuberculosis occurred mainly in young children; currently, however, except among HIV-infected persons, it is more common among older persons (28). The shift in age-specific incidence presumably has been caused by the paucity of new infections relative to the number of endogenous reactivations that take place in the United States. The sex incidence is nearly equal except in the HIV-infected population, wherein men predominate.

Because of the multisystem involvement in disseminated tuberculosis, the clinical manifestations are protean. The presenting symptoms and signs are generally nonspecific and are dominated by the systemic effects, particularly fever, weight loss, anorexia, and weakness (32, 45, 51, 59, 64, 67, 75). Other symptoms depend on the relative severity of disease in the organs involved. Cough and shortness of breath are common; headache and changes in mental status are less frequent and are usually associated with meningeal involvement (59). Physical findings are likewise variable. Fever, wasting, hepatomegaly, pulmonary findings, lymphadenopathy, and splenomegaly occur in descending order of frequency. The only physical finding that is specific for disseminated tuberculosis is the choroidal tubercle, a granuloma located in the choroid of the retina (54).

Initial screening laboratory studies are not particularly helpful for the diagnosis of miliary tuberculosis. Both leukopenia and leukocytosis may be seen,

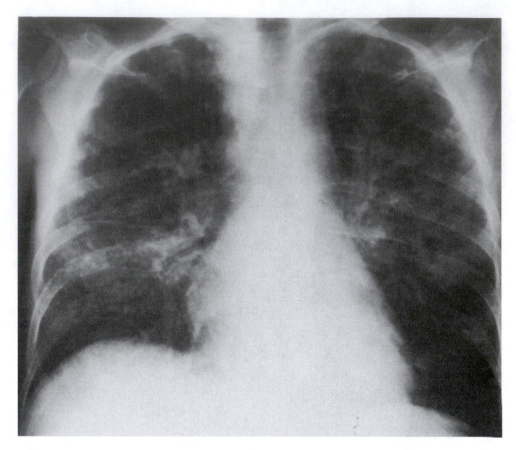

Figure 6. Frontal view chest radiograph showing diffuse infiltration caused by *M. tuberculosis* in a patient with HIV infection.

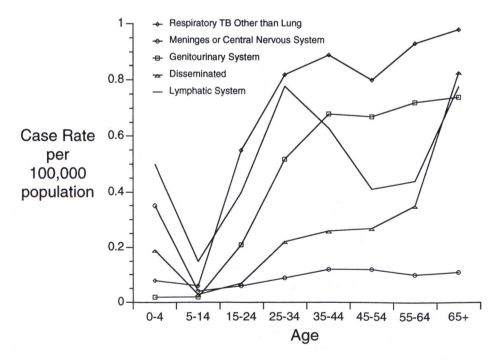

Figure 7. Age-specific case rates for the most frequent forms of extrapulmonary tuberculosis.

Table 2. Recovery of *M. tuberculosis* from various sites in patients with tuberculosis and HIV infection[a]

Specimen	No. positive/no. tested (%)	
	Smear	Culture
Sputum	43/69 (62)	64/69 (93)
Bronchoalveolar lavage fluid	9/44 (20)	39/44 (89)
Transbronchial biopsy specimen	1/10 (10)	7/10 (7)
Lymph node	21/44 (48)	39/44 (91)
Blood		15/46 (33)
Bone marrow	4/22 (18)	13/22 (62)
Cerebrospinal fluid		4/21 (19)
Urine		12/17 (71)
Other[b]	5/31 (16)	24/31 (76)

[a]Data from reference 76.
[b]Pleural fluid or tissue, pericardial fluid or tissue, liver peritoneal fluid, abscess drainage, or bone.

but the majority of patients have normal leukocyte counts. Anemia is common and may be normocytic, normochronic, or microcytic and hypochromic. Coagulation disorders are unusual, but disseminated intravascular coagulation has been found in association with miliary tuberculosis in severely ill patients (39, 60). Hyponatremia also occurs, as discussed above. The most frequent abnormality of liver function is an increased alkaline phosphatase concentration. Bilirubin and alanine aminotransferase levels may also be increased.

The chest radiograph is abnormal in most but not all patients with disseminated tuberculosis. In the series reported by Grieco and Chmel (32), only 14 (50%) of 28 patients had a miliary pattern on the chest radiograph, whereas 90% of 69 patients studied by Munt (59) had a miliary pattern. Overall, it appears that at the time of diagnosis, approximately 85% of patients have the characteristic radiographic findings of miliary tuberculosis. Other radiographic abnormalities may be present as well. These include upper-lobe infiltrates with or without cavitation, pleural effusion, and pericardial effusion. In patients with HIV infection, the radiographic pattern is one of diffuse infiltration rather than discrete nodules.

The tuberculin skin test is positive less frequently in patients with disseminated tuberculosis than in those with other forms of the disease. The rate of positivity at the time of diagnosis in apparently immunocompetent persons ranges from approximately 50 to 75% (32, 59, 67, 75). As the disease is treated, tuberculin reactivity tends to return unless there is systemic immunocompromise.

Autopsy series have shown the liver, lungs, bone marrow, kidneys, adrenals, and spleen to be the organs most frequently involved in miliary tuberculosis, but any organ can be the site of disease (48). Because of the multiplicity of sites involved, many potential sources of material can be used to provide a diagnosis. Acid-fast smears of sputum are positive in 20 to 25% of patients, and *M. tuberculosis* is isolated from sputum in 30 to 65% of patients (32, 59, 67, 75). Gastric washings or induced sputum samples may be positive when the patient is not expectorating spontaneously. In a patient with an abnormal chest radiograph and negative sputum examinations, bronchoscopy should be the next step. Combinations of bronchoalveolar lavage and transbronchial biopsy would be expected to have a high yield. Other potential sites for biopsy include the liver and bone marrow, each of which has a high likelihood (70 to 80%) of showing granulomas but only a 25 to 40% chance of providing bacteriologic confirmation (67). Urine is easy to obtain and may be positive in up to 25% of patients (67). Selection of other potential sources of diagnostic material should be guided by specific findings.

Lymph node tuberculosis

Prior to the HIV epidemic, lymph node tuberculosis made up approximately 20% of the cases of extrapulmonary tuberculosis in the United States (28). Although the basic descriptive epidemiology of tuberculosis applies to lymphatic tuberculosis, there are two main differences: lymphatic tuberculosis is relatively more common among children, and it occurs more frequently in women. It also appears to be more common among Asians and Pacific Islanders than among blacks and whites. Among HIV-infected persons, the demographic features of tuberculous lymphadenitis parallel those of HIV infection.

Tuberculous lymphadenitis usually presents as painless swelling of one or more lymph nodes. The nodes most commonly involved are those of the posterior or anterior cervical chain and those in the supraclavicular fossa. Frequently, the process is bilateral, and other noncontiguous groups of nodes can be involved (43). At least initially, the nodes are discrete and the overlying skin is normal. With continuing disease, the nodes may become matted and the overlying skin may become inflamed. Rupture of the node can result in formation of a sinus tract, which may be difficult to heal. Intrathoracic adenopathy may compress bronchi, causing atelectasis and leading to lung infection and perhaps bronchiectasis.

In HIV-non-infected persons with tuberculous lymphadenitis, systemic symptoms are not common unless there is concomitant tuberculosis elsewhere. The frequency of pulmonary involvement in reported series of patients with tuberculous lymphadenitis is quite variable, ranging from approximately 5 to 70%. In HIV-infected persons, lymphadenitis is commonly associated with multiple-organ involvement, although localized lymphadenitis, as described above, may occur as well. The diagnosis is established by lymph node biopsy or aspiration with histologic examination, including stains for acid-fast organisms, and culture of the material. Smears show acid-fast organisms in approximately 25 to 50% of biopsy specimens, and *M. tuberculosis* is isolated in roughly 70% of instances in which the diagnosis is tuberculosis (38). Caseating granulomas are seen in nearly all biopsy samples from immunocompetent patients. In immunodeficiency states, granulomas may be poorly formed or absent (52).

Pleural tuberculosis

The epidemiology of pleural tuberculosis parallels that of the overall pattern for tuberculosis, with the disease being more common among males and increasing in incidence with increasing age between the ages of 5 and 45 years (28). As noted above, this epidemiologic pattern is modified by the occurrence of HIV infection, although pleural involvement seems relatively less frequent among HIV-infected persons.

There are two mechanisms by which the pleural space becomes involved in tuberculosis, and the difference in pathogenesis results in different clinical presentations, approaches to diagnosis, treatment, and sequelae. Early in the course of a tuberculous infection, a few organisms may gain access to the pleural space, and in the presence of cell-mediated immunity they can cause a hypersensitivity response (6, 25). Commonly, this form of tuberculous pleuritis goes unnoticed and the process resolves spontaneously. In some patients, however, tuberculous involvement of the pleura is manifested as an acute illness with fever and pleuritic pain. This represents the first form of pleural tuberculosis. If the effusion is large enough, dyspnea may occur, although the effusions generally are small and rarely are bilateral. In approximately 30% of patients, there is no radiographic evidence of involvement of the lung parenchyma; however, parenchymal disease is nearly always present, as evidenced by the findings of lung dissections (78).

The diagnosis of pleural tuberculosis is generally established by analysis of pleural fluid and/or by pleural biopsy. A thoracentesis (aspiration of fluid from the chest) should be performed, and sufficient fluid for cell count, cytologic examination, biochemical analysis, and microbiologic evaluation should be obtained, leaving enough to allow a needle biopsy to be performed if the fluid is exudative and no diagnosis is evident. The fluid is nearly always straw col-

ored, although it may be slightly bloody. Cell counts are usually in the range of 100 to 5,000/μl (41). Early in the course of the process, polymorphonuclear leukocytes may predominate, but mononuclear cells soon become the majority. The fluid is exudative, with a protein concentration greater than 50% of the serum protein concentration, and the glucose level may be normal to low.

Because few organisms are present in the pleural space, smears of pleural fluid are rarely positive, and *M. tuberculosis* is isolated by culture in only 20 to 40% of patients with proved tuberculous pleuritis (50, 68). A single-blind-needle biopsy of the pleura confirms the diagnosis in approximately 65 to 75% of patients in whom tuberculous pleuritis is ultimately diagnosed (50, 68). The sensitivity of blind percutaneous needle biopsy of the pleura for diagnosis of tuberculous pleurisy is highest when more than six specimens are obtained (46). In a patient who has a pleural effusion that remains undiagnosed after a full evaluation, including pleural biopsy, and who has a positive tuberculin skin test reaction, antituberculosis treatment should be initiated. Because of the small number of organisms involved in tuberculous pleuritis, chest tube drainage is not required and antituberculosis medications alone will cure patients.

The second variety of tuberculous involvement of the pleura is a true empyema (pus in the pleural space). This condition is much less common than tuberculous pleurisy with effusion and results from a large number of organisms spilling into the pleural space, usually from rupture of a cavity or an adjacent parenchymal focus via a bronchopleural fistula (42). A tuberculous empyema is usually associated with evident pulmonary parenchymal disease on chest radiographs, and air may be seen in the pleural space. In this situation, the fluid is generally thick and cloudy and may contain cholesterol, causing the fluid to look like chyle (pseudochylous effusion). The fluid is exudative and usually has a relatively high leukocyte count, with nearly all of the leukocytes being lymphocytes. Acid-fast smears and mycobacterial cultures are usually positive, making pleural biopsy unnecessary. This type of pleural involvement has a tendency to burrow through soft tissues and may drain spontaneously through the chest wall. An example of this type of tuberculosis is shown in Fig. 8. In addition to antituberculosis medications, tuberculous empyema requires chest tube drainage, often with a large-bore chest tube, for adequate treatment of the pleural sepsis.

Genitourinary tuberculosis

As with pleural tuberculosis, the epidemiologic pattern of genitourinary tuberculosis parallels that of

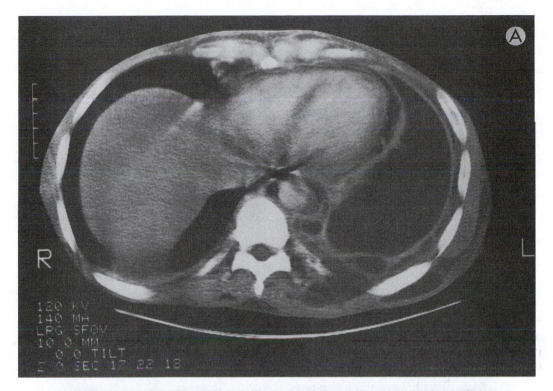

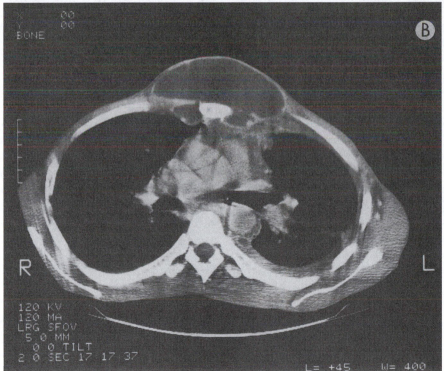

Figure 8. Computed tomographic scan of the chest showing a tuberculosis empyema with adjacent chest wall involvement (A) and a large chest wall abscess overlying the sternum with mediastinal involvement (B).

tuberculosis in general, except that the incidence is nearly equal in men and women. The pathogenesis appears to be one of seeding of the kidneys at the time of the initial infection and bacillemia.

In patients with genitourinary tuberculosis, local symptoms predominate and systemic symptoms are less common (18, 73). Dysuria, hematuria, and frequent urination are common, and flank pain may also be noted. However, the symptoms may be very subtle, and advanced destruction of the kidneys has often occurred by the time a diagnosis is established (49). Genital involvement without renal tuberculosis is more common in women than in men and may cause pelvic pain, menstrual irregularities, and infertility as presenting complaints (73). In men, a painless or only slightly painful scrotal mass is probably the most common presenting symptom of genital involvement, but symptoms of prostatitis, orchitis, or epididymitis may also occur (18). A substantial number of patients with any form of genitourinary tuberculosis are asymptomatic and are detected on the basis of evaluation for an abnormal routine urinalysis. In more than 90% of patients with renal or genital tuberculosis, urinalyses are abnormal, with the main finding being pyuria and/or hematuria. The finding of pyuria (pus in the urine) in an acidic urine with no organisms isolated from a routine urine culture should prompt an evaluation for tuberculosis. The suspicion of genitourinary tuberculosis should be heightened by the presence of abnormalities on the chest radiograph. In most series, approximately 40 to 75% of patients have chest radiographic abnormalities, although in many patients these abnormalities may be the result of previous, not current, tuberculosis (18, 73).

When genitourinary tuberculosis is suspected, at least three first-voided early-morning urine specimens should be collected for acid-fast stains and cultures. *M. tuberculosis* is isolated from the urine in 80 to 95% of cases of genitourinary tuberculosis (18, 73). Diagnosis of isolated genital lesions usually requires biopsy, because the differential diagnosis often includes neoplasia as well as other infectious processes.

Significant effects of tuberculosis on renal function are unusual, but renal failure may occur, especially in patients with preexisting renal disease. Nephrolithiasis and recurrent bacterial infections in seriously damaged kidneys also occur. Hypertension that responds to nephrectomy has also been described but is rare.

Skeletal tuberculosis

The incidence of tuberculosis involving the joints and bones increases with increasing age and is equally frequent in men and women, making up approximately 9% of cases of extrapulmonary tuberculosis overall (28). Compared to blacks and whites, other racial groups are less likely to have skeletal involvement. Skeletal tuberculosis does not appear to be frequent among persons with HIV infection.

It is presumed that most osteoarticular tuberculosis results from endogenous reactivation of foci of infection seeded during the initial bacillemia, although spread from paravertebral lymph nodes has been postulated to account for the common localization of spinal tuberculosis to the lower thoracic and upper lumbar vertebrae (13). It is also postulated that the predilection for tuberculosis to localize in the metaphyses of long bones is due to the relatively rich blood supply and the scarcity of phagocytic cells in this portion of the bone (7). After beginning in the subchondral region on the bone, the infection spreads to involve the cartilage, synovium, and joint space. This produces the typical findings of metaphyseal erosion and cysts and the loss of cartilage, with narrowing of the joint space. Typically, in the spine these changes involve two adjacent vertebrae and the intervertebral disk. Paravertebral or other para-articular abscesses may develop, with occasional formation of sinus tracts. Although weight-bearing joints are the most common sites of skeletal tuberculosis, any bone or joint may be involved (7). In most series, tuberculosis of the spine (Pott's disease) makes up 50 to 70% of the cases reported. In adults, the lower thoracic and upper lumbar vertebrae are most commonly involved, whereas in children, the upper thoracic spine is the most frequent site of vertebral tuberculosis. The hip or knee is involved in 15 to 20% of cases, and shoulders, elbows, ankles, wrists, and other bones or joints are also involved in 15 to 20% of cases. Usually only one bone or joint is involved, but occasionally the process is multifocal (21, 57). Evidence of either previous or current pulmonary tuberculosis is found in approximately one-half of the reported patients, and other extrapulmonary sites may also be involved.

The usual presenting symptom of skeletal tuberculosis is pain (7). Swelling of the involved joint may be noted, as may limitation of motion and, occasionally, sinus tracts. Systemic symptoms of infection are not common. Because of the subtle nature of the symptoms, diagnostic evaluations often are not undertaken until the process is advanced. Delay in diagnosis can be especially catastrophic in vertebral tuberculosis, in which compression of the spinal cord may cause severe and irreversible neurologic sequelae, including paraplegia.

The first diagnostic test undertaken is usually a radiograph of the involved area. The typical findings described above represent the more severe end of the spectrum. Early in the process, the only abnormality noted may be soft tissue swelling. Subsequently, subchondral osteoporosis, cystic changes, and sclerosis may be noted before the joint space is actually narrowed. The early changes of spinal tuberculosis may be particularly difficult to detect from standard radiographs of the spine. Computed tomography and magnetic resonance imaging of the spine are considerably more sensitive than routine radiography and should be performed when there is a high index of suspicion of an infectious process.

The diagnosis is confirmed by aspiration of joint fluid or periarticular abscesses or by biopsy of bone or synovium with histologic and microbiologic evaluation of the material obtained. Acid-fast stains of joint fluid are positive in 20 to 25% of samples examined, and M. tuberculosis is isolated in approximately 60 to 80% (7). Biopsy specimens of synovium or bone have a higher yield and allow histologic examination as well. Evidence of granulomatous inflammation even in the absence of bacteriologic proof of the diagnosis is sufficient evidence of tuberculosis to begin therapy unless another etiology is found.

Central nervous system tuberculosis

Meningitis is the most frequent form of central nervous system tuberculosis; solitary or multiple tuberculomas occur less commonly. The epidemiologic pattern of central nervous system tuberculosis is quite different from that of either pulmonary or other forms of extrapulmonary tuberculosis in that the peak incidence is in children younger than 4 years but an appreciable number of cases occur in adults (9, 28). Central nervous system disease accounts for only approximately 5% of all cases of extrapulmonary tuberculosis, and the cases are equally divided between males and females.

Central nervous system involvement, especially tuberculomas, seems to occur with greater frequency among HIV-infected persons. Tuberculomas have been found even in patients who are receiving what should be adequate chemotherapy (9). The findings produced by tuberculomas may be indistinguishable on computed tomography from those of toxoplasmosis. For this reason, a specific diagnosis should be sought when such lesions are noted.

Meningitis presumably can result from direct meningeal seeding and proliferation during a tuberculous bacillemia either at the time of initial infection or at the time of breakdown of an old pulmonary focus, or it can result from breakdown of an old parameningeal focus with rupture into the subarachnoid space. The consequences of contamination of the subarachnoid space include diffuse meningitis, a localized arteritis, encephalitis, or myelitis. With meningitis, the process takes place primarily at the base of the brain (4). Symptoms therefore include those related to cranial nerve involvement in addition to headache, decreased level of consciousness, and neck stiffness. The duration of illness prior to diagnosis is quite variable and relates in part to the presence or absence of

other sites of involvement. In most series, over 50% of patients with meningitis have abnormalities on chest radiographs that are consistent with an old or current tuberculous process, often miliary tuberculosis. At autopsy, disseminated disease is found in a very high percentage of patients with meningitis (4). Sputum cultures have been positive in 40 to 50% of patients with tuberculous meningitis; therefore, a substantial number of patients have pulmonary and systemic symptoms in addition to those referable to the central nervous system. Arteritis may be the predominant manifestation of meningitis and can result in a variety of focal ischemic syndromes in addition to the symptoms already described.

Physical findings and screening laboratory studies are not particularly helpful in establishing a diagnosis. In the presence of meningeal signs on physical examination, lumbar puncture is usually the next step in the diagnostic sequence. If there are focal findings on examination or if there are suggestions of increased intracranial pressure, a computed tomographic scan of the head, if it can be obtained expeditiously, should be performed before the lumbar puncture. In patients with meningitis the scan may be normal, but it can also show diffuse edema or obstructive hydrocephalus. Tuberculomas are generally seen as ring-enhancing mass lesions.

In tuberculous meningitis, the lumbar puncture usually shows increased opening pressure and the cerebrospinal fluid usually contains between 100 and 1,000 cells per μl. Lymphocytes predominate in approximately 65 to 75% of patients, whereas polymorphonuclear leukocytes predominate in the remainder of patients, generally early in the course of the illness. The protein concentration is elevated in nearly all patients. Very high (>300 mg/dl) protein concentrations have been associated with a poor prognosis (84). The glucose concentration in cerebrospinal fluid is usually low but not as low as concentrations that occur during pyogenic bacterial meningitis. Acid-fast organisms are seen on smears of cerebrospinal fluid from only 10 to 20% of patients, and the rate of culture positivity varies from 55 to 80% (5). Newer DNA-based tests directly on cerebrospinal fluid, using PCR, may improve the ability to make a rapid diagnosis of tuberculous meningitis (72). In a substantial number of patients, M. tuberculosis is isolated from other sources; in the presence of compatible cerebrospinal fluid findings, such isolation is sufficient to diagnose tuberculous meningitis. Given the severity of tuberculous meningitis, a presumptive diagnosis justifies empiric treatment if no other diagnosis can be established promptly.

The other major central nervous system form of tuberculosis, the tuberculoma, presents a more subtle clinical picture than tuberculous meningitis (23). The usual presentation is that of a slowly growing focal lesion, although a few patients have increased intracranial pressure and no focal findings. The cerebrospinal fluid is usually normal, and the diagnosis is established by computed tomography or magnetic resonance scanning and subsequent resection, biopsy, or aspiration of any ring-enhancing lesion.

Abdominal tuberculosis

Tuberculosis can involve any intra-abdominal organ as well as the peritoneum. The age distribution of abdominal tuberculosis shows a relatively higher incidence in young adults and a second peak in older persons. Males and females have a similar incidence. Intra-abdominal tuberculosis has not been common in HIV-infected persons.

Abdominal tuberculosis presumably results from seeding at the time of initial infection and then either direct or late progression to clinical disease. Peritonitis can also be caused by rupture of tuberculous lymph nodes within the abdomen. Intestinal tuberculosis may also result from ingested tubercle bacilli, with direct implantation in the gut. Before chemotherapy, tuberculous enteritis was quite common in patients with advanced pulmonary tuberculosis, presumably being caused by pulmonary bacilli that were swallowed. In a prospective study conducted between 1924 and 1949, intestinal abnormalities compatible with tuberculous enteritis were found by contrast radiography in 1, 4.5, and 24.7% of patients with minimal, moderately advanced, and far advanced pulmonary tuberculosis, respectively (58).

The clinical manifestations of abdominal tuberculosis depend on the areas of involvement. In the gut itself, tuberculosis may occur in any location from the mouth to the anus, although lesions proximal to the terminal ileum are unusual. The most common sites of involvement are the terminal ileum and the cecum, with other portions of the colon and the rectum being involved less frequently (8). In the terminal ileum or cecum, the most common manifestations are pain, which may be misdiagnosed as appendicitis, and intestinal obstruction. A palpable mass may be noted and, together with the appearance of the abnormality on barium enema or small-bowel radiographs, may easily be mistaken as a carcinoma. Rectal lesions usually present as anal fissures or fistulae or as perirectal abscesses. Because of the concern about carcinoma, the diagnosis often is made at surgery.

For tuberculous peritonitis, pain, often accompanied by abdominal swelling, is commonly the presenting manifestation (8, 10, 11, 74). Fever, weight loss, and anorexia are also common. Active pulmonary tuberculosis is uncommon in patients with tuberculous peritonitis. Because the process frequently coexists with other disorders, especially hepatic cirrhosis with ascites, the symptoms of tuberculosis may be obscured. The combination of fever and abdominal tenderness in a person with ascites should always prompt an evaluation for intra-abdominal infection, and a paracentesis should be performed. Ascitic fluid in patients with tuberculous peritonitis is exudative (the fluid protein content is higher than 50% of the serum protein concentration) and contains between 50 and 10,000 leukocytes per μl, the majority of them being lymphocytes, although polymorphonuclear leukocytes occasionally predominate (10, 74). Acid-fast organisms are rarely seen on smears of the fluid, and cultures are positive in only approximately 50% of patients. Because of the generally low yield from culture of the fluid, laparoscopic biopsy is often necessary to confirm the diagnosis.

Microscopic evidence of liver involvement is common in patients with all forms of tuberculosis, but actual hepatic tuberculosis of functional consequence is rare. A variety of histologic abnormalities may be seen, but none is specific for tuberculosis unless M. tuberculosis is isolated from hepatic tissue (29). For this reason, all liver biopsy specimens should be cultured for mycobacteria.

Pericardial tuberculosis

The descriptive epidemiology of pericardial tuberculosis is not well defined, but in general the disease tends to occur among older persons, with approximately 50% of patients being older than 55 years (28). Nonwhites and men have a relatively higher frequency of tuberculous pericarditis. Before the use of antituberculosis chemotherapy, tuberculous pericarditis was found in 0.4 to 1.0% of all autopsied patients and in 3 to 8% of autopsied patients in whom there was other evidence of tuberculosis (69). A clinical diagnosis of tuberculous pericarditis was made in 0.35% of approximately 10,000 patients with any form of tuberculosis admitted to Kings County Hospital Center, Brooklyn, N.Y., between 1 January 1960 and 31 December 1966 (66).

The pericardium may become involved during the initial bacillemia, with early progression to clinically evident disease or recrudescence following a quiescent period. Hematogenous seeding may also occur during the course of endogenous reactivation. Alternatively, there may be direct extension of an adjacent focus of disease into the pericardium. This focus may be in lung parenchyma, pleura, or tracheobronchial lymph nodes. In fact, all of these mechanisms probably occur and may account for some of the variability in the characteristics of the pericardial fluid, the severity of the process, and the prognosis (69). It is likely that tuberculin hypersensitivity plays a role in producing the inflammatory response in the pericardium, as presumably occurs in the pleura. On the other hand, rupture of a gaseous lymph node into the pericardium may cause contamination with a much larger number of organisms; a greater inflammatory response with thicker, more purulent fluid; and a greater likelihood of either early or late hemodynamic effects.

The most common form or stage of tuberculous pericarditis is characterized by pericardial effusion with little pericardial thickening or epicardial involvement. The fluid itself is usually serosanguineous or occasionally grossly bloody, is exudative, and has a leukocyte count of 500 to as high as 50,000/mm^3, with an average of 5,000 to 7,000/mm^3 (35). The cells are predominantly mononuclear, although polymorphonuclear leukocytes occasionally predominate. Tubercle bacilli have been identified in pericardial fluid in approximately 25 to 30% of cases (smear and culture combined) (66). Biopsy of the pericardium, with both histologic and bacteriologic evaluation, is much more likely to provide a diagnosis, although a nonspecific histologic pattern and failure to recover the organisms do not exclude a tuberculous etiology.

With persistence of the inflammation, there is thickening of the pericardium and progressive epicardial involvement. Granulomas, various amounts of free or loculated fluid, and fibrosis may be present during this stage, and evidence of cardiac constriction may begin to appear. The necrosis associated with the granulomatous inflammation may involve the myocardium, with consequent functional and electrocardiographic manifestations.

Although it is not well documented, it appears that if the patient survives the subacute phase without treatment, chronic fibrotic pericarditis nearly always follows. Prior to the advent of antituberculosis therapy, 88% of one series of patients who had tuberculous pericarditis developed evidence of chronic constriction (35). Constriction has also been observed to develop during the course of antituberculosis chemotherapy, although this development appears to be uncommon in patients who have had symptoms for less than 3 months. In the series reported by Hageman et al. (33), 11 of 13 patients who had symptoms for more than 6 months required pericardiectomy.

The fibrotic reaction described above progresses to complete fusion of visceral and parietal pericardium and encasement of the heart in a rigid scar. There are various amounts of calcium within the fibrotic mass. Impairment of coronary circulation is common. At this point, the histologic pattern is usu-

ally nonspecific; therefore, confirmation of a tuberculous etiology is infrequent.

The symptoms, physical findings, and laboratory abnormalities associated with tuberculous pericarditis may be the result of either the infectious process per se or the pericardial inflammation causing pain, effusion, and eventually hemodynamic effects. The systemic symptoms produced by the infection are quite nonspecific. Fever, weight loss, and night sweats are common in reported series (35, 66, 69). Symptoms of cardiopulmonary origin tend to occur later and include cough, dyspnea, orthopnea, ankle swelling, and chest pain. The chest pain occasionally mimics angina but usually is described as being dull, aching, and often affected by position and by inspiration.

Apart from fever, the most common physical findings are those caused by the pericardial fluid or fibrosis-cardiac tamponade or constriction. Various proportions of patients in reported series have signs of full-blown cardiac constriction when first evaluated. It is assumed that in these patients, the acute phase of the process was unnoticed.

The definitive diagnosis of tuberculous pericarditis requires identification of tubercle bacilli in pericardial fluid or tissue. Although not conclusive, demonstration of caseating granulomata in the pericardium and consistent clinical circumstances is convincing evidence of a tuberculous etiology. Less conclusive but still persuasive evidence is the finding of another form of tuberculosis in a patient with pericarditis of undetermined etiology. Approximately 25 to 50% of patients with tuberculous pericarditis have evidence of other organ involvement, particularly pleuritis, at the time when pericarditis is diagnosed (30, 69). Still less direct and more circumstantial evidence of a tuberculous etiology is the combination of a positive intermediate-strength tuberculin skin test reaction and pericarditis of unproven etiology.

REFERENCES

1. Allen, S., J. Batungwanayo, K. Kerlikowske, A. R. Lifson, W. Wolf, R. Granich, H. Taelman, P. Van De Perre, A. Serufilira, J. Bogaerts, G. Slutkin, and P. C. Hopewell. 1992. Prevalence of tuberculosis in HIV-infected urban Rwandan women. *Am. Rev. Respir. Dis.* **146:**1439–1444.
2. Alvarez, S., and W. R. McCabe. 1984. Extrapulmonary tuberculosis revisited: a review of experience at Boston City and other hospitals. *Medicine* **63:**25–55.
3. Arango, L., A. W. Brewin, and J. F. Murray. 1978. The spectrum of tuberculosis as currently seen in a metropolitan hospital. *Am. Rev. Respir. Dis.* **108:**805–812.
4. Auerbach, O. 1951. Tuberculous meningitis: correlation of therapeutic results with the pathogenesis and pathologic changes. II. Pathologic changes in untreated and treated cases. *Am. Rev. Tuberc.* **64:**419–429.
5. Barrett-Connor, E. 1967. Tuberculous meningitis in adults. *South. Med. J.* **60:**1061–1067.

6. Bergen, H. W., and E. Mejia. 1973. Tuberculous pleurisy. *Chest* **63**:88–92.

7. Berney, S., M. Goldstein, and F. Bishko. 1972. Clinical and diagnostic features of tuberculous arthritis. *Am. J. Med.* **53**: 36–42.

8. Bhansali, S. K. 1977. Abdominal tuberculosis: experiences with 300 cases. *Am. J. Gastroenterol.* **67**:324–337.

9. Bishberg, E., G. Sunderam, L. B. Reichman, and R. Kapila. 1986. Central nervous system tuberculosis with the acquired immunodeficiency syndrome and its related complex. *Ann. Intern. Med.* **105**:210–213.

10. Borhanmanesh, F., K. Hekmat, K. Vaezzadeh, and H. R. Rezai. 1972. Tuberculous peritonitis: prospective study of 32 cases in Iran. *Ann. Intern. Med.* **76**:567–572.

11. Burack, W. R., and R. M. Hollister. 1960. Tuberculous peritonitis: a study of forty-seven proved cases encountered by a general medical unit in twenty-five years. *Am. J. Med.* **28**:510–523.

12. Burk, J. R., J. Viroslav, and L. J. Bynum. 1978. Miliary tuberculosis diagnosed by fiberoptic bronchoscopy and transbronchial biopsy. *Tubercle* **59**:107–108.

13. Burke, H. E. 1950. The pathogenesis of certain forms of extrapulmonary tuberculosis. *Am. Rev. Tuberc.* **62**:48–67.

14. Cameron, S. J. 1974. Tuberculosis and the blood. *Tubercle* **55**:55–72.

15. Centers for Disease Control and Prevention. 1998. Prevention and treatment of tuberculosis among patients infected with human immunodeficiency virus: principles of therapy and revised recommendations. *Morb. Mortal. Wkly. Rep.* **47**(RR-20): 1–58.

16. Centers for Disease Control and Prevention. 2000. Update. Nucleic acid amplification tests for tuberculosis. *Morb. Mortal. Wkly. Rep.* **49**:593–594.

17. Chaisson, R. E., G. F. Schecter, C. P. Theuer, G. W. Rutherford, D. F. Echenberg, and P. C. Hopewell. 1987. Tuberculosis in patients with the acquired immunodeficiency syndrome: clinical features, response to therapy and survival. *Am. Rev. Respir. Dis.* **136**:570–574.

18. Christensen, W. I. 1974. Genitourinary tuberculosis: review of 102 cases. *Medicine* **53**:377–390.

19. Chung, D.-K., and W. W. Hubbard. 1969. Hyponatremia in untreated active pulmonary tuberculosis. *Am. Rev. Respir. Dis.* **99**:595–597.

20. Comstock, G. W. 1982. Epidemiology of tuberculosis. *Am. Rev. Respir. Dis.* **125**(Suppl.):8–16.

21. Cremin, B. J., R. M. Fisher, and M. W. Levinsohn. 1970. Multiple bone tuberculosis in the young. *Br. J. Radiol.* **43**:638–645.

22. Daley, C. L., P. M. Small, and G. F. Schecter. 1992. An outbreak of tuberculosis with accelerated progression among persons infected with the human immunodeficiency virus. An analysis using restriction fragment length polymorphisms. *N. Engl. J. Med.* **326**:2331–2335.

23. Damergis, J. A., E. Lefterich, and J. A. Cumin. 1979. Tuberculoma of the brain. *JAMA* **239**:413–415.

24. Danek, S. J., and J. S. Bower. 1979. Diagnosis of pulmonary tuberculosis by flexible fiberoptic bronchoscopy. *Am. Rev. Respir. Dis.* **119**:677–679.

25. Ellner, J. J. 1978. Pleural fluid and peripheral blood lymphocyte function in tuberculosis. *Ann. Intern. Med.* **89**:932–933.

26. Ernst, J. D. 1998. Macrophage receptors for *Mycobacterium tuberculosis. Infect. Immun.* **66**:1277–1281.

27. Ewer, K., J. Deeks, L. Alvarez, G. Bryant, S. Waller, P. Andersen, P. Monk, and A. Lalvani. 2003. Comparison of T-cell based assay with tuberculin skin test for diagnosis of *Mycobacterium tuberculosis* infection in a school tuberculosis outbreak. *Lancet* **361**:1168–1173.

28. Farer, L. S., L. M. Lowell, and M. P. Meador. 1979. Extrapulmonary tuberculosis in the United States. *Am. J. Epidemiol.* **109**:205–217.

29. Frank, B. R., and E. C. Raffensperger. 1965. Hepatic granulomata: report of a case with jaundice improving on antituberculous chemotherapy and review of the literature. *Arch. Intern. Med.* **115**:223–233.

30. Gooi, H. C., and J. M. Smith. 1978. Tuberculous pericarditis in Birmingham. *Thorax* **33**:94–96.

31. Gordin, F. M., G. Stutkin, G. F. Schecter, P. C. Goodman, and P. C. Hopewell. 1989. Presumptive diagnosis and treatment of pulmonary tuberculosis based on radiographic findings. *Am. Rev. Respir. Dis.* **139**:1090–1093.

32. Grieco, M. H., and H. Chmel. 1974. Acute disseminated tuberculosis as a diagnostic problem: a clinical study based on twenty-eight cases. *Am. Rev. Respir. Dis.* **109**:554–560.

33. Hageman, J. H., N. D. D'Esopo, and W. W. L. Glenn. 1964. Tuberculosis of the pericardium: a long-term analysis of forty-four proved cases. *N. Engl. J. Med.* **270**:327–332.

34. Handwerger, S., D. Mildvan, R. Sennie, and F. W. McKinley. 1987. Tuberculosis and the acquired immunodeficiency syndrome at a New York City hospital: 1978–1985. *Chest* **91**: 176–180.

35. Harvey, A. M., and M. R. Whitehill. 1937. Tuberculous pericarditis. *Medicine* **16**:45–94.

36. Havlir, D.V., and P. F. Barnes. 1999. Tuberculosis in patients with human immunodeficiency virus infection. *N. Engl. J. Med.* **340**:367–373.

37. Holden, M., M. R. Dubin, and P. H. Diamond. 1971. Frequency of negative intermediate-strength tuberculin sensitivity in patients with active tuberculosis. *N. Engl. J. Med.* **285**: 1506–1509.

38. Huhti, E., E. Brander, and S. Plohumo. 1975. Tuberculosis of the cervical lymph nodes: a clinical, pathological and bacteriological study. *Tubercle* **56**:27–36.

39. Huseby, J. S., and L. D. Hudson. 1976. Miliary tuberculosis and the adult respiratory distress syndrome. *Ann. Intern. Med.* **85**:609–611.

40. Jasmer, R. M., P. Nahid, and P. C. Hopewell. 2002. Latent tuberculosis infection. *N. Engl. J. Med.* **347**:1860–1866.

41. Jay, S. J. 1985. Diagnostic procedures for pleural disease. *Clin. Chest. Med.* **6**:33–48.

42. Johnson, T. M., W. McCann, and W. H. Davey. 1973. Tuberculous bronchopleural fistula. *Am. Rev. Respir. Dis.* **107**: 30–41.

43. Kent, D. C. 1967. Tuberculous lymphadenitis: not a localized disease process. *Am. J. Med. Sci.* **254**:866–874.

44. Kiblawi, S. S. O., S. J. Jay, R. B. Stonehill, and J. Norton. 1981. Fever response of patients on therapy for pulmonary tuberculosis. *Am. Rev. Respir. Dis.* **123**:20–24.

45. Kim, J. H., A. A. Langston, and H. A. Gallis. 1990. Miliary tuberculosis: epidemiology, clinical manifestations, diagnosis, and outcome. *Rev. Infect. Dis.* **12**:583–590.

46. Kirsch, C M., M. Kroe, R. Azzi, W. A. Jensen, F. T. Kagawa, and J. H. Wehner. 1997. The optimal number of pleural biopsy specimens for a diagnosis of tuberculous pleurisy. *Chest* **112**:702–706.

47. Kramer, F., T. Modelewsky, A. R. Walinay, J. M. Leedom, and P. F. Barnes. 1990. Delayed diagnosis of tuberculosis in patients with human immunodeficiency virus infection. *Am. J. Med.* **89**:451–456.

48. Kubica, G. P., W. M. Gross, J. E. Hawkins, H. M. Sommers, A. L. Vestal, and L. G. Wayne. 1975. Laboratory services for mycobacterial diseases. *Am. Rev. Respir. Dis.* **112**:773–787.

49. Lattimer, J. K. 1965. Renal tuberculosis. *N. Engl. J. Med.* **273**:208–211.

50. Levine, H., W. Metzger, and D. Lacera. 1970. Diagnosis of tuberculous pleurisy by culture of pleural biopsy specimen. *Arch. Intern. Med.* **126:**268–271.

51. Maartens, G., P. A. Wilcox, and S. R. Benatar. 1990. Miliary tuberculosis: rapid diagnosis, hematologic abnormalities, and outcome in 109 treated adults. *Am. J. Med.* **89:**291–296.

52. Marchevsky, A., M. J. Rosen, G. Chrystal, and J. Kleinerman. 1985. Pulmonary complications of the acquired immunodeficiency syndrome: a clinicopathologic study of 70 cases. *Hum. Pathol.* **16:**659–670.

53. Markowitz, N., N. I. Hansen, P. C. Hopewell, J. Glassroth, P. A. Kvale, B. T. Mangura, T. C. Wilcosky, J. M. Wallace, M. J. Rosen, L. B. Reichman, and The Pulmonary Complications of HIV Infection Study Group. 1997. Incidence of tuberculosis in the United States among HIV-infected persons. *Ann. Intern. Med.* **126:**123–132.

54. Massaro, D., S. Katz, and M. Sachs. 1964. Choroidal tubercles: a clue to hematogenous tuberculosis. *Ann. Intern. Med.* **60:**231–241

55. Mazurek, G. H., P. A. LoBue, C. L. Daley, J. Bernardo, A. A. Lardizabal, W. R. Bishai, M. F. Iademarco, and J. S. Rothel. 2001. Comparison of a whole-blood interferon-gamma assay with tuberculin skin testing for detecting latent *Mycobacterium tuberculosis* infection. *JAMA* **286:**1740–1747.

56. Mazurek, G. H., and M. E. Villarino. 2003. Guidelines for using the QuantiFERON®-TB test for diagnosing latent tuberculosis infection. *Morb. Mortal. Wkly. Rep.* **51**(RR02):15–18.

57. McTammany, J. R., K. M. Moser, and V. N. Houk. 1963. Disseminated bone tuberculosis: review of the literature and presentation of an unusual case. *Am. Rev. Respir. Dis.* **87:**889–895.

58. Mitchell, R. S., and L. J. Bristol. 1954. Intestinal tuberculosis: an analysis of 346 cases diagnosed by routine intestinal radiography on 5529 admissions for pulmonary tuberculosis, 1924–1949. *Am. J. Med. Sci.* **227:**241–249.

59. Munt, P. W. 1971. Miliary tuberculosis in the chemotherapy era with a clinical review in 69 American adults. *Medicine* **51:**139–155.

60. Murray, H. W., C. U. Tuazon, N. Kirmani, and J. H. Sheagren. 1978. The adult respiratory distress syndrome associated with miliary tuberculosis. *Chest* **73:**373.

61. Nash, D.-R., and J. E. Douglas. 1980. Anergy in active pulmonary tuberculosis: a comparison between positive and negative reactors and an evaluation of 5 TU and 250 TU skin test doses. *Chest* **77:**32.

62. Orme, I. M., and A. M. Cooper. 1999. Cytokine/chemokine cascades in immunity to tuberculosis. *Immunol. Today* **20:**307–312.

63. Pitchenik, A. E., and H. A. Rubinson. 1985. The radiographic appearance of tuberculosis in patients with the acquired immune deficiency syndrome (AIDS) and pre-AIDS. *Am. Rev. Respir. Dis.* **131:**393–396.

64. Prout, S., and S. R. Benatar. 1980. Disseminated tuberculosis: a study of 62 cases. *S. Afr. Med. J.* **58:**835–842.

65. Reider, H. L., G. M. Cauthen, A. B. Bloch, C. H. Cole, D. Holtzman, D. E. Snider, Jr., W. J. Bigler, and J. J Witte. 1989. Tuberculosis and the acquired immunodeficiency syndrome—Florida. *Arch. Intern. Med.* **149:**1268–1273.

66. Rooney, J. J., J. A. Crocco, and H. A. Lyons. 1970. Tuberculous pericarditis. *Ann. Intern. Med.* **72:**73–81.

67. Sahn, S. A., and T. A. Neff. 1974. Miliary tuberculosis. *Am. J. Med.* **56:**495–505.

68. Scharer, L., and J. H. McClement. 1968. Isolation of tubercle bacilli from needle biopsy specimens of parietal pleura. *Am. Rev. Respir. Dis.* **97:**466–468.

69. Schepers, G. W. H. 1962. Tuberculous pericarditis. *Am. J. Cardiol.* **9:**248–276.

70. Selwyn, P. A., B. M. Sckell, P. Alcabes, G. H. Friedland, R. S. Klein, and E. E. Schoenbaum. 1992. High risk of active tuberculosis in HIV-infected drug users with cutaneous anergy. *JAMA* **268:**504–509.

71. Shafer, R. W., R. Goldberg, M. Sierra, and A. E. Glatt. 1989. Frequency of *Mycobacterium tuberculosis* bacteremia in patients with tuberculosis in an area endemic for AIDS. *Am. Rev. Respir. Dis.* **140:**1611–1613.

72. Shankar P., N. Manjunath, K. K. Mohan, K. Prasad, M. Behari, Shriniwas, and G. K. Ahuja. 1991. Rapid diagnosis of tuberculous meningitis by polymerase chain reaction. *Lancet* **337:**5–7.

73. Simon, H. B., A. J. Weinstein, M. S. Pasternak, M. N. Swartz, and L. J. Lunz. 1977. Genitourinary tuberculosis: clinical features in a general hospital. *Am. J. Med.* **63:**410–420.

74. Singh, M. M., A. M. Bhargova, and K. P. Jain. 1968. Tuberculous peritonitis: an evaluation of pathogenetic mechanisms, diagnostic procedures and therapeutic measures. *N. Engl. J. Med.* **281:**1091–1094.

75. Slavin, R. E., T. J. Walsh, and A. D. Pollack. 1980. Late generalized tuberculosis: a clinical pathologic analysis of 100 cases in the preantibiotic and antibiotic eras. *Medicine* **59:**352–366.

76. Small, P. M., G. F. Schecter, P. C. Goodman, M. A. Sande, R. E. Chaisson, and P. C. Hopewell. 1991. Treatment of tuberculosis in patients with advanced human immunodeficiency virus infection. *N. Engl. J. Med.* **324:**289–294.

77. So, S. Y., W. K. Lam, and D. Y. C. Yu. 1982. Rapid diagnosis of suspected pulmonary tuberculosis by fiberoptic bronchoscopy. *Tubercle* **63:**195–200.

78. Stead, W. W., A. Eichenholtz, and H. K. Strauss. 1955. Operative and pathologic findings in 24 patients with the syndrome of idiopathic pleurisy with effusion presumably tuberculous. *Am. Rev. Respir. Dis.* **71:**473–502.

79. Takashima, T., C. Ueta, I. Tsuyuguchi, and S. Kishimoto. 1990. Production of tumor necrosis factor alpha by monocytes from patients with pulmonary tuberculosis. *Infect. Immun.* **58:**3286–3292.

80. Valone, S. E., E. Rich, R. S. Wallis, and J. J. Ellner. 1988. Expression of tumor necrosis factor in vitro by human mononuclear phagocytes stimulated with whole *Mycobacterium tuberculosis*, BCG, and mycobacterial antigens. *Infect. Immun.* **56:**3313–3315.

81. Valway, S. E., M. P. C. Sanchez, T. F. Shinnick, I. Orme, T. Agerton, D. Hoy, J. S. Jones, H. Westmoreland, and I. M. Onorato. 1998. An outbreak involving extensive transmission of a virulent strain of *Mycobacterium tuberculosis*. *N. Engl. J. Med.* **338:**633–639.

82. Vorken, H., S. G. Massy, R. Fallat, L. Kaplan, and C. R. Kleeman. 1970. Antidiuretic principle in tuberculous lung tissue of a patient with pulmonary tuberculosis and hyponatremia. *Ann. Intern. Med.* **72:**383–387.

83. Weir, M. R., and G. F. Thornton. 1985. Extrapulmonary tuberculosis: experience of a community hospital and review of the literature. *Am. J. Med.* **79:**467–478.

84. Weiss, W., and H. F. Flippin. 1961. The prognosis of tuberculous meningitis in the isoniazid era. *Am. J. Med.* **242:**423–430.

Tuberculosis and the Tubercle Bacillus
Edited by Stewart T. Cole et al.
© 2005 ASM Press, Washington, D.C.

Chapter 3

Molecular Epidemiology of *Mycobacterium tuberculosis*

M. Donald Cave, Megan Murray, and Edward Nardell

STRAIN IDENTIFICATION PROCEDURES FOR *MYCOBACTERIUM TUBERCULOSIS*

Unlike many of the methods for isolating and culturing *Mycobacterium tuberculosis*, most currently utilized methods of strain identification have developed since 1990. Prior to this, phenotypic markers such as mycobacterial phage susceptibility and drug resistance patterns were used to distinguish between strains (63). Epidemiologic investigations were limited because there are relatively few phage types, the most common of which are shared by many isolates, and antibiograms are useful only for drug-resistant strains. The modern genotyping methods and the relevance of these methods to the control and understanding of the pathogenesis of tuberculosis (TB) have recently been reviewed (4).

IS*6110*-Based Methods

The first extensively used strain identification methods were based on the insertion element IS*6110*. IS*6110* is a 1,365-bp insertion sequence (IS), the ends of which are defined by a 28-bp imperfect inverted repeat (73). The IS contains an open reading frame (ORF) that codes for a transposase related to the IS*3* family of enterobacterial IS elements. The IS is limited to the *M. tuberculosis* complex and is not present in other mycobacteria (15). The number of copies of IS*6110* varies from 1 to more than 20 per genome. A small number of strains (less than 0.1% of those analyzed) have no copies of IS*6110* (48). Individual strains vary in the number of copies of IS*6110* and in the sites into which IS*6110* is inserted. A standardized procedure that utilizes the restriction enzyme PvuII has been developed and is utilized worldwide (76). Southern blots of *M. tuberculosis* DNA electrophoresed on agarose gels and probed with a fragment

of IS*6110* that lies upstream of the single PvuII site provide restriction fragment length polymorphism (RFLP) patterns. The principles of the technique are demonstrated in Fig. 1. The RFLP patterns are entered into a computerized database and analyzed with an image analysis system.

A rapid technique, mixed-linker PCR, is based on PCR with one primer specific for IS*6110* and a second primer complementary to a linker ligated to restricted genomic DNA (39). The technique was automated by using a fluorescence-labeled IS*6110* primer and internal lane size standards with a DNA sequencer and Genescan software (13). As expected, the grouping of mixed-linker PCR fingerprints was consistent with the results of the standard IS*6110* RFLP procedure.

Many of the sites of IS*6110* insertion are highly conserved in strains having fewer than six copies of IS*6110* (29), leading to a lack of IS*6110*-based polymorphism in such low-copy-number strains. Moreover, most strains of *Mycobacterium bovis* including *M. bovis* BCG contain a single copy of IS*6110*. A number of secondary typing procedures for subtyping these low-copy-number strains have been developed. These techniques are based on other genetic elements such as the direct-repeat (DR) locus, variable-number tandem repeat (VNTR) sequences, and polymorphic GC-rich sequences. Another weakness of IS*6110* typing results from replicative transposition of the insertion sequence leading to the addition of insertion sites. Indeed, multiple isolates from a patient may demonstrate the gain or loss of a hybridizing fragment, and epidemiologic links among patients whose isolates differ by one or two copies of IS*6110* have been frequently noted (16, 52). Furthermore, IS*6110* analysis is inappropriate for evolutionary studies because there are several preferred sites of IS*6110* insertion or hot spots (27), strains may differ in the frequency of

M. Donald Cave • Department of Neurobiology and Developmental Sciences, University of Arkansas for Medical Sciences and Central Arkansas Veterans Healthcare System, Little Rock, AR 72205. **Megan Murray and Edward Nardell** • Departments of Epidemiology and Pulmonary Medicine, Harvard School of Public Health, Harvard Medical School, Cambridge, MA 02115.

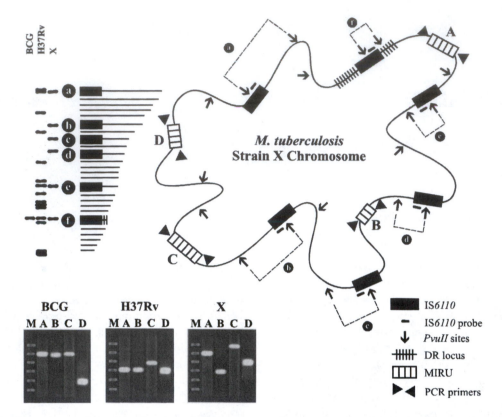

Figure 1. Chromosome of *M. tuberculosis* hypothetical strain X and genotyping of *M. bovis* BCG, the *M. tuberculosis* laboratory strain H37Rv, and strain X on the basis of IS*6110* insertion sites and MIRUs. The top right-hand panel shows the chromosome of hypothetical strain X. *Pvu*II sites are indicated by the arrows. The top left-hand panel shows the results of IS*6110*-based genotyping. Mycobacterial DNA is digested with the restriction enzyme *Pvu*II. The IS*6110* probe hybridizes to IS*6110* DNA to the right of the *Pvu*II site in IS*6110*. The size of each hybridizing fragment depends on the distance from this site to the next *Pvu*II site in the adjacent DNA (fragments a through f), as reflected by gel electrophoresis of the DNA fragments of BCG, H37Rv, and X. The horizontal lines to the right of the electrophoretic strip indicate the extent of the distribution of fragments in the gel, including *Pvu*II fragments that contain no IS*6110*. The three bottom panels show the results of MIRU-based genotyping. MIRUs contain repeat units, and MIRU analysis involves the use of PCR amplification and gel electrophoresis to categorize the number and size of the repeats at 12 independent loci, each of which has a unique repeated sequence. The sizes of molecular weight markers (lanes M) and PCR products for loci A, B, C, and D (lanes A to D, respectively), in BCG, H37Rv, and X are shown. The specific sizes of the various MIRUs in each strain result in a distinctive fingerprint for the strain. (Modified from reference 4 with permission. Copyright © 2003 Massachusetts Medical Society. All rights reserved.)

IS*6110* transposition, and IS*6110* is frequently inserted into ORFs and may therefore affect phenotype and or survival/fitness (5, 65).

Direct-Repeat Locus-Based Methods

The DR locus is a single region of the *M. tuberculosis* chromosome that contains multiple copies of a 36-bp direct repeat that is reiterated between 10 and 50 times (Figs. 1 and 2). Each repeat is separated from the next by a sequence of nonrepeated variable-spacer DNA, with each spacer containing 37 to 41 bp (40). Although the overall arrangement of the spacers in the DR is conserved among strains, polymorphisms result from deletion/insertion of segments of the DR locus. In all *M. bovis* BCG, strains, *M. bovis* strains, and most *M. tuberculosis* strains, a copy of

IS*6110* is inserted into a specific site in one of the 36-bp repeats (75). Even strains of *M. tuberculosis* that lack IS*6110* contain the DR locus. In its simplest format, the 36-bp repeat is used to probe genomic blots of DNA restricted with endonucleases for which there are no sites in the 36-bp repeat (PvuII, AluI and SmaI have been used) (79). Polymorphisms are generated by sequence differences in the spacer regions.

Spacer oligonucleotide typing, or spoligotyping, involves PCR of the DR locus with labeled primers (43). The two primers are directed outward from the 36-bp repeat, amplifying the variable spacers and repeats present in a particular strain. The labeled PCR products are then used to probe a membrane that contains covalently bound oligonucleotides corresponding to each of the 43 variable-spacer sequences present in *M. tuberculosis* strain H37Rv and *M. bovis*

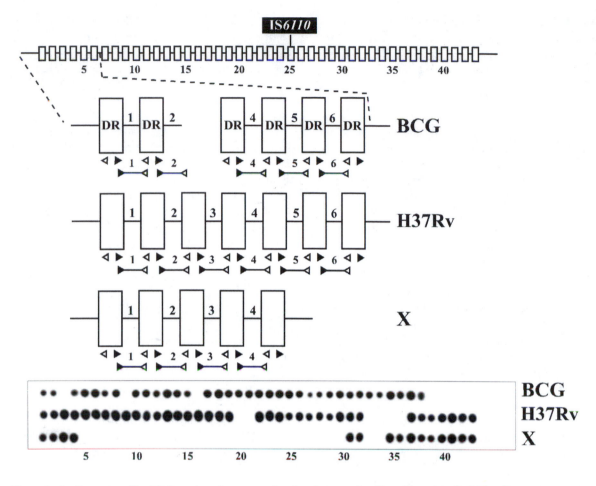

Figure 2. Spoligotyping. The DR locus is a chromosomal region that contains 10 to 50 copies of a 36-bp direct repeat, separated by spacer DNA with various sequences, each of which is 37 to 41 bp. A copy of IS*6110* is inserted within a 36-bp DR in the middle of the DR locus in most strains. *M. tuberculosis* strains have the same overall arrangement of spacers but differ in terms of the presence or absence of specific spacers. Spoligotyping involves PCR amplification of the DR locus, followed by hybridization of the labeled PCR products to a membrane that contains covalently bound oligonucleotides corresponding to each of 43 spacers. Individual strains have positive or negative signals for each spacer. The top section shows the 43 DR (rectangles) and spacers (horizontal lines) used in spoligotyping. The middle section shows the products of PCR amplification of spacers 1 through 6 in *M. bovis* BCG, *M. tuberculosis* strain H37Rv, and *M. tuberculosis* hypothetical strain X, with the use of primers (white and black arrows) at each end of the DR loci. The bottom section shows the spoligotypes of the three strains. (Reprinted from reference 4 with permission. Copyright © 2003 Massachusetts Medical Society. All rights reserved.)

BCG. These are arranged left to right on the blot in the same order that they are arranged in the DR loci of *M. tuberculosis* strain H37Rv and *M. bovis* BCG. Individual strains share various combinations of the variable spacers and are distinguished on the basis of their positive and negative signals for each spacer.

Spoligotyping can be applied directly to cultured cells and to clinical samples (43). The absence of five spacers (numbers 38 to 43) enables the *M. bovis* species to be determined. The results, expressed as positive or negative for each of the 43 spacers, can be readily digitalized (21). Polymorphisms in the DR locus do not discriminate *M. tuberculosis* strains as well as IS*6110* does (i.e., strains with different IS*6110* RFLP patterns may have the same spoligotype) or

low-IS*6110*-copy-number strains as well as polymorphic GC-rich sequences (85). Polymorphisms in the DR locus tend to group strains into larger groups than does IS*6110* analysis and have been used to link strains to specific geographic areas (80). A major criticism of spoligotyping is that it measures a small number of polymorphisms at a single genetic locus.

Tandem-Repeat Sequence-Based Methods

Polymorphisms in tandemly repeated minisatellite loci caused by unequal crossing over are the basis for human forensic DNA typing. Genotypes are based on the number of repeats in each of many tandem repeated loci, each of which is independent. Genome analysis of *M. tuberculosis* strain H37Rv has revealed 41 such independent loci, referred to as mycobacterial interspersed repeat units (MIRUs) (71). Loci consisting of multiple copies of these tandem repeats are distributed around the *M. tuberculosis* chromosome. The principles of MIRU are illustrated in Fig. 1.

The DR locus can be regarded as a tandem repeat in which each repeat unit (RU) consists of a conserved DR and a variable unique region that we referred to previously as spacer. Each RU measures 73 to 77 bp. In this case, the RU is not an exact repeat because each RU differs in the sequence of its spacer.

Exact tandem repeat (ETR) loci are composed of RUs that are identical copies of one another. In VNTR analysis, six different ETR loci that were distributed around the genome were selected from a search of the H37Rv genome (33). The ETR loci are amplified by PCR using primers complementary to sequences flanking each of the ETR loci. In its original format, the PCR primers are each run in separate reactions and the sizes of the products are analyzed by gel electrophoresis. Deducting the length of the primers or flanking DNA and then dividing the remainder by the size of the RU estimates the number of RUs at each locus. The sizes of the individual RUs in the six different ETRs ranged from 53 to 79 bp. The strains were polymorphic for the number of RUs at each locus. The number of RUs varied from one to seven per locus. At one locus, the number of RUs varied from one to six. Sequence analysis confirmed that the length polymorphisms corresponded to the insertion or deletion of complete tandem repeats. The data are digital in that each of the six ETR loci can be expressed in terms of the number of RUs in each locus, thereby generating a description of the six loci in a strain.

MIRU analysis employs the same principles to analyze 12 tandem repeat loci that are distributed around the chromosome. Sequence analysis of different strains of *M. tuberculosis* shows that these loci have some variation in tandem-repeat copy number and in sequence (71). From two to eight alleles were observed at each of the 12 loci, yielding approximately 1.6×10^6 possible combinations of alleles at the 12 loci (51). The correlation between the results of IS*6110* RFLP and MIRU typing carried out on the same isolates is highly significant. Automated high-throughput MIRU analysis has been developed using multiplex PCR, fluorescence-tagged PCR primers, and an automated DNA sequencer (70). The development of the automated MIRU analysis has enabled the establishment of a MIRU genotyping website that provides a means for laboratories to compare their data and generate a database that will facilitate global epidemiologic surveillance of TB.

The advantages of MIRU-VNTR analyses are that the results are intrinsically digital and analysis can be applied directly to cultures without the need for DNA purification. It has been postulated that the combined molecular clock of the 12 MIRU loci is slower than that of IS*6110* RFLP. Actually, each locus has a different molecular clock (70). This has proven useful in establishing relationships between isolates with similar but not identical IS*6110* patterns. MIRU-VNTR analysis appears to distinguish strains as well as IS*6110* analysis does, especially strains with fewer than six copies of IS*6110* (51). One of the shortcomings of VNTR-MIRU is that the tandem repeats can be lost or gained, making it difficult to establish convergence or divergence of strains.

GENOME-BASED ANALYSIS

Sequencing of the *M. tuberculosis* genome has provided additional means for comparing strains. Comparison of the sequence of the H37Rv laboratory strain (18) and of clinical strain CDC 1551 has revealed single-nucleotide polymorphisms (SNPs) as well as deletion, duplication, and insertion differences between the two strains (30). Such differences are exploited by SNP (68) and genomic deletion (44) analysis.

Deletion Mapping

Comparison of the genomes of H37Rv and CDC 1551 revealed sequences that were present in one strain but absent in the other. Using a high-density oligonucleotide array based on 1,500 ORFs present in the genome of *M. tuberculosis* strain H37Rv, 19 clinical strains of *M. tuberculosis* were analyzed by microarray analysis (44). The total number of deletions detected among the strains was 29. It was noted that the deleted genes represent ancestral genes no longer needed for strain survival. The likelihood that the tubercle bacillus would cause pulmonary cavitation decreased as the amount of the genome deleted increased. The obvious advantage of the microarray analysis technique is that it can relate the strain changes to gene function.

Although genomic microarray analysis can be used for genotyping based on genomic deletions, it is not, at present, practical for analyzing large numbers of isolates. To overcome this difficulty, a PCR-based reverse line probe assay similar to spoligotyping, termed delegotyping, has been developed (Y. O. Goguet de la Salmoniere, C. Kim, A. Tsolaki, S. Siegrist, and Small, *Abstr. Keystone Symp. Tuberc.*

Integrating Host Pathog. Biol. abstr. 418, p. 103, 2003). In this assay, 43 sequences that demonstrated deletion polymorphisms originally detected on genomic microarrays are amplified by multiplex PCR and a membrane containing oligomers complementary to those genes is used to detect the presence of those sequences in the PCR products of the amplified genes.

Single-Nucleotide Polymorphism Analysis

Recently, several groups have used synonymous SNPs as a tool to type *M. tuberculosis* strains. Point mutations are categorized as either nonsynonymous or synonymous, depending on whether the substitution leads to a change in amino acid sequence and thus in the protein for which the sequence codes. Synonymous mutations (sSNPs) are those that do not alter the amino acid sequence, and they are therefore usually considered neutral markers of ancestry that are not subject to selection pressure. In contrast, nonsynonymous SNPs (nsSNPs) may code for a trait that confers some survival advantage on an organism; in this case, one would expect that identical nsSNPs may have arisen independently through "homoplasy" and that they would not necessarily indicate shared ancestry.

Although some studies suggest that there is relatively little allelic variation among different strains of *M. tuberculosis*, the recent sequencing of four distinct *M. tuberculosis* complex genomes has led to the identification of more than 400 sSNPs (28). Subsets of these have been used to genotype isolates and generate phylogenetic trees demonstrating the genetic relationships among these strains (1). In addition, small groups of "highly informative" sSNPs have been used to differentiate strains with low copy numbers or unique IS*6110* profiles. When epidemiologically linked isolates were analyzed using sSNP genotyping, they were consistently shown to belong to the same cluster, while paired isolates from a single patient had identical sSNP genotypes. To date, sSNPs have not been routinely employed in the analysis of epidemiologic or population-based studies, but with the ease and availability of high through-put technology, this technique may provide a useful and relatively less laborious way to type *M. tuberculosis* isolates for molecular epidemiologic studies.

USES OF *M. TUBERCULOSIS* GENOTYPING

Identifying Laboratory Cross-Contamination

False-positive culture results were reported in 13 of 14 molecular epidemiologic studies that evaluated more than 100 patients. The median false-positive rate (the number of patients having a false-positive culture divided by the total number of patients with a positive culture) reported in these studies was 3.1% (12). False-positive cultures can result from clerical error, contamination of clinical devices (e.g., bronchoscopes) (which can also be a source of TB transmission), misidentification of the organism, or laboratory cross-contamination. Laboratory cross-contamination occurs when a viable tubercle bacillus is introduced into a specimen that does not contain *M. tuberculosis*. Among the factors that facilitate laboratory cross-contamination are the ability of the tubercle bacillus to survive harsh environmental conditions, the complexity of processing procedures requiring batch processing, and the use of automated growth detection systems that enable cross-contamination to occur (12).

Laboratory cross-contamination has been attributed to several causes. Aerosolization during sample processing can create droplets, and organisms contained in such aerosols can settle into other specimens. A contaminated tube cap or pipette used during batch processing can contaminate other specimens. Contaminated reagents can result in large numbers of false-positive cultures (64). Another opportunity for laboratory cross-contamination occurs when broth culture vials are examined by microscopy prior to demonstrating detectable growth or when broth cultures with fungal or bacterial contamination are removed from the tube and reprocessed. Specimens cross-contaminated by this means are difficult to identify because their initial processing occurred on different days.

The most common characteristic of false-positive cultures is the fact that the culture in question is the only positive culture from that patient (single positive culture). In one study, 44% of the patients with single positive cultures had false-positive cultures (31). However, there are documented cases of TB that show no evidence of cross-contamination and that have only single positive cultures. Since the inoculum of material that contaminates another specimen is small, containing few bacilli, growth in broth medium is slow and growth on solid medium shows only few colonies. Moreover, a false-positive culture is more likely to result from the sputum of a smear-negative patient unless the original sputum sample contained species of acid-fast bacilli other than those in the *M. tuberculosis* complex. However, specimens from patients with active TB can show the same characteristics.

Several factors can be used to screen for laboratory cross-contamination. Among these are single positive culture, growth in liquid media (which is more sensitive) but not on solid media, growth of only a few colonies on solid medium, and negative sputum smear. Moreover, clinicians should evaluate laboratory results in light of the patient's history and clinical presentation and consider the possibility of laboratory cross-contamination when the patient's diagnosis is not consistent with laboratory results. When cross-contamination is suspected, it is necessary to identify the occasions where it might have occurred. Good laboratory records are fundamental in determining when specimens were processed, positive cultures subcultured, and BACTEC vials read.

After the sites where laboratory cross-contamination might have occurred have been evaluated, genotyping can be used to confirm that the suspected false-positive culture is the same strain as the source of the cross-contamination. Moreover, genotyping can be useful in confirming causes of false-positive cultures other than those caused by laboratory cross-contamination (e.g., contamination of clinical devices [bronchoscopes] or clerical errors [mislabeling of specimens]).

False-positive cultures lead to patients being unnecessarily treated with antituberculous agents and may lead to further unnecessary diagnostic tests and hospitalizations. They may incorrectly indicate treatment failure or relapse, leading to subsequent treatment. Contact investigations and unnecessary treatment of LTBI can result from false-positive results. A specimen that contains drug-susceptible *M. tuberculosis* may be cross-contaminated with a drug-resistant strain, altering the susceptibility results and resulting in the patient being treated with second-line drugs.

Genotyping of suspected false-positive cultures plays an important role in confirming false-positive cases and possible sources of cross-contamination. In studies in which all of the isolates from a laboratory are genotyped, the finding of multiple isolates with an identical genotype can be the first indication that laboratory cross-contamination has occurred.

Differentiating Recurrent Tuberculosis Caused by Treatment Failure or Relapse from Exogenous Reinfection

Recurrence of TB can result from relapse of disease with the strain that caused the original episode or from infection by another strain, hence "exogenous reinfection." When isolates are available from both episodes of disease, this question can be resolved by genotyping. Since the genotypes of circulating strains are many, the genotypes of the strains causing original and recurrent episode of disease will probably be different in the case of exogenous reinfection. When the second episode results from relapse, the genotypes of the isolates causing the two episodes of disease are identical.

Although it has been long argued that exogenous reinfection made an important contribution to the burden of active TB in many high-prevalence communities, the relative frequency of exogenous reinfection has been the topic of contentious speculation over much of the past century. Styblo (69) cited the experience of Greenland in the 1950s as evidence of the role of exogenous reinfection. He noted that a vigorous intervention program in that country led to a decline in clinical TB, not only among the young people, in whom a first infection was averted, but also among the elderly, who had almost certainly been previously infected. Had most disease in the elderly been due to reactivation of remote TB, he argued, the incidence in that population would not have been affected by a reduction in transmission. A few years later, Nardell et al. (59) provided further circumstantial evidence for exogenous reinfection. In a TB outbreak in a Boston homeless shelter, 25 cases were linked by both identical drug resistance pattern and phage type. Seven of these patients had documented previous infection or disease, providing evidence for reinfection by the outbreak strain.

With the availability of molecular fingerprinting, the debate about the existence of exogenous reinfection has been put to rest. Early studies of human immunodeficiency virus (HIV)-infected patients demonstrated extensive TB transmission, accelerated progression to disease, and recurrent TB caused by exogenous reinfection (22, 67). Several recent studies in countries with high to moderate TB case rates showed that approximately half of the recurrent TB cases in HIV-noninfected patients result from reinfection with another strain (14, 77).

The frequency with which exogenous reinfection occurs and the context in which it may contribute substantially to TB dynamics can be readily identified by molecular epidemiologic techniques. For example, in a high-incidence South African community, 698 consecutive TB patients were enrolled over a 6-year period; 16 of these patients experienced recurrent disease after completing curative therapy, and 12 were infected with a strain different from that isolated during their first episode of disease (77). Similar studies have been conducted in areas with a lower prevalence of infection; these have shown that in low-risk areas, reinfection accounts for fewer of the second episodes of disease (3, 14).

While these studies suggest that exogenous reinfection occurs more commonly than was previously thought, most cases of exogenous reinfection are expected to occur in people who have been infected in the past but in whom clinical TB did not result from that initial infection. These people will not have *M. tuberculosis* isolates from two distinct episodes of disease and therefore cannot be counted by simply typing incident cases. One way to assess the burden of reinfection would be to estimate the frequency of clustered cases in a cohort of people who were known to be infected on the basis of a previous tuberculin skin testing. However, this study design would require long-term follow-up of an infected cohort.

These findings indicate that infection provides limited protection from exogenous reinfection. Indeed, such limited protection is indicated in patients who are simultaneously infected with more than one strain of *M. tuberculosis*. Several descriptions of such patients have been documented by genotyping (11, 41). Genotype analysis is a discriminating tool for such analysis; however, a mix of strains demonstrates that of the predominant strain or a composite genotype. To identify the presence of more than one strain in a single sample, multiple individual colonies from the isolate are analyzed individually. Coinfections with multiple strains of *M. tuberculosis* may be responsible for conflicting drug susceptibility results.

Population-Based Studies

Soon after genotyping techniques were first developed, they were used to document the transmission of *M. tuberculosis* between contacts. In 1992, 12 cases of TB were discovered in a housing facility for HIV-infected people (22). Isolates from all 12 patients shared a single IS*6110* fingerprint, confirming the expectation that these cases were due to the recent transmission of *M. tuberculosis* in this institutional setting. While this initial study suggested that TB can both rapidly spread and progress to active disease in people infected with HIV, many subsequent molecular studies documented the transmission and progression of TB among immunocompetent people as well (37, 46). More recently, investigators have integrated molecular epidemiologic studies with social network analyses to develop new approaches to TB outbreak investigations and explore the social context in which tuberculosis is spread. Several such studies, conducted in very different contexts, have found that TB transmission often occurs in the setting of alcohol consumption in bars, suggesting that interventions that focus on these sites may be useful methods of TB control.

While these studies made it clear that contact tracing often failed to identify transmission networks, they also showed that many cases of TB previously classified as reactivation disease shared a DNA fingerprint with other contemporaneous cases. Generally, researchers interpret genotype clusters to indicate epidemiologically linked cases of recently transmitted disease and isolates with unique genotypes to indicate cases of reactivation disease resulting from "remote" TB infection. This is based on the assumption that reactivation tuberculosis would be more likely to produce varied genotypes, since those patients would have been infected with a variety of strains having different genotypes over a wide span of time and it would be unlikely that those infected at the same time with the same strain would reactivate concurrently. Clustering is likely to represent recent transmission, since it is expected that at a given time and place there are a limited number of strains available and those infected with the same strain have the same genotype. In its simplest form, one of the cases in a cluster develops from reactivation of a remotely infected case and the others result from transmission of that strain. Alternative explanations for a given cluster representing recent transmission are that the cases did indeed reactivate concurrently, the genotype represents an endemic strain, or the genotype observed is not adequately discriminatory. Alternative explanations for a unique genotype representing a remote case are that the case was infected at another place or that not all of the isolates in a population were genotyped.

The finding that a large proportion of cases were clustered challenged the "conventional wisdom" that the vast majority of TB cases in low-incidence countries was due to the reactivation of *M. tuberculosis* infection acquired in the remote past. In 1994, researchers in New York City (1) and San Francisco (67) addressed this issue by systematically enrolling patients with consecutive cases in a "population-based" approach. Using genotyping to identify clusters, they independently estimated that 40% of incident TB cases fell into clusters and were thus classified as recently acquired disease. Since the proportions of clustered cases were much higher than expected, these findings demonstrated the problem of TB transmission in urban centers in the United States and helped invigorate previously neglected TB control efforts. Studies in Europe have found that the proportion of clustered cases ranges from 16 to 46%, again suggesting that transmission of *M. tuberculosis* can be an important factor even in the areas of very low incidence (10, 61).

Although large population-based studies in low-incidence countries have estimated similar proportions of clustered and unique cases, the data from higher-incidence areas have been less consistent. The proportion of clustered cases reported from Africa (82, 83) has ranged from approximately 30 to 70%, while in China and Vietnam (2, 80), a single genotype defined by spoligotyping, the Beijing strain, accounts for 50 to 80% of the cases sampled. Smaller studies in other high-incidence areas (25, 62) have inferred a surprising lack of recent transmission, with only about 20% of cases belonging to clusters. These findings raise questions about the correct interpretation of cluster studies and have sparked a growing interest in methodological research on inference in molecular epidemiology.

Several investigators have approached this problem by simulating the process of sampling isolates from a hypothetical distribution of clusters of *M. tuberculosis* isolates and then measuring the impact of this sampling on estimates of the proportion of clustered cases. Computer simulations showed that recent transmission was increasingly underestimated as the fraction of all cases included in the sample was decreased (36). An analytic method was developed for estimating the bias incurred by sampling when the underlying cluster distribution is known (57). Although neither of these methods allows one to adjust estimates of recent transmission without knowledge of the sampling fraction and the distribution of cluster sizes prior to sampling, they do suggest that small studies in high-incidence areas will severely underestimate recent transmission.

Another strategy used to assess these molecular methods has been to develop epidemic models as tools for epidemiologic inference. Transmission of *M. tuberculosis* strains in The Netherlands over the past century was modeled, allowing DNA fingerprint patterns to change over time due to random mutation (81). Using age-specific rates of primary and reactivation disease, it was shown that clustering of cases based on identical fingerprints underestimated recent transmission among younger patients but tended to overestimate recent transmission in the elderly. A stochastic model of TB transmission was used to identify social and demographic determinants of cluster distribution and to observe the effect of transmission dynamics on the empiric data from molecular epidemiologic studies (57). This study showed that the proportion of clustered cases of TB varies with a variety of host and population characteristics and may not be a direct reflection of the incidence of recent transmission in a specific setting. These findings suggest that the results of molecular epidemiologic studies that attempt to estimate the burden of recently transmitted TB need to be interpreted with great caution.

Since molecular-biology techniques enabled researchers to classify cases as clustered or unique, they also made it possible to identify risk factors for clustering and, by extension, for the recent transmission and rapid progression of clinical tuberculosis. In the analysis of the data from New York City, the prevalence of sociodemographic and clinical risk factors in the clustered and unique cases was compared (1). Young age, U.S. birth, Hispanic ethnicity, and HIV infection were identified as risk factors for recently transmitted disease. While studies in different geographic settings have confirmed some of these risk factors, they have also found some discrepant results; HIV was not a risk factor for clustering among South African gold miners (37), nor did it predict clustering in hospitalized patients in Rio de Janeiro, Brazil (26). Similarly, attributes such as homelessness, alcoholism, and intravenous drug use have been identified as risk factors for recent transmission in some areas but are not associated with this outcome in others (50, 85).

Since social and demographic risk factors identify people at risk for exposure to TB, it is hardly surprising that they vary in different communities with differing disease dynamics; this emphasizes the need for genotyping to be implemented in individual sites or communities to identify the local transmission dynamics. Nonetheless, some of the differences may have resulted from the wide variation in the fraction of cases sampled in the various studies. Just as sampling can bias an estimate of the proportion of clustered cases in a community by underestimating that proportion, it can also bias estimates of the effect of risk factors for clustering by underestimating their effect. In a recent reassessment of the impact of HIV on clustering in New York City, in which adjustments were made for potential sample bias, the revised estimate of the odds ratio increased from 2.7 to 23.6 (58). Since sampling strategies have varied widely across studies, it follows that those odds ratios for risk factors for clustering will also vary and be more or less accurate depending on the total number of cases sampled.

Identifying Settings for Tuberculosis Transmission

Traditional settings for TB transmission include households, family members, and friends. In a recent investigation in the United States, DNA fingerprinting was used to evaluate epidemiologically linked pairs found during contact investigations. Of 538 case pairs in which a source case and secondary case(s) could be identified, 29% did not have matching DNA fingerprints. Among 260 case pairs that shared the same household, 30% did not have a DNA fingerprint matching that for other patients in the same household (6). These data indicate that transmission of infection and subsequent disease occurred at a site other than the home. Similar results have been reported from household studies in South Africa and Uganda, in which approximately 50% of the households with more than one case of TB demonstrated more than one RFLP pattern (17; C. Whalen, D. Guwatuddc, M. D. Cave, K. D. Eisenach, et al., Abstract, *Am. J. Epidemiol.* **153**:S217, 2001). There are several documented cases in which TB has been spread by casual contact (20, 38) or has occurred in nontraditional settings. Genotyping to identify patients in clusters and subsequent investigation of these clusters has played a key role in identifying TB in settings outside of the home, including homeless shelters, jails and prisons, hospitals, workplaces, social clubs, bars, stores, schools, and mortuaries (20).

Application of *M. tuberculosis* Genotyping to Public Health

If *M. tuberculosis* genotyping had absolutely no measurable public health benefits, its contribution to our understanding of the organism and its transmission would still justify its use as a research tool. However, a substantial list of public health benefits of genotyping has been suggested (53). Still, we suspect that it would be difficult to show that a well-functioning state or municipal TB control program with the benefit of routine molecular fingerprinting reliably achieves a greater reduction in case rates, higher treatment completion rates, less transmission, or more effective case finding and treatment of infected contacts than a similarly good program without the routine availability of fingerprinting, although such a study has not, to our knowledge, been reported. Rather than being an indictment of genotyping, this provocative statement simply reflects the multifactorial nature of each of the TB control outcome measures listed and the difficulty of demonstrating the effects of changing any one factor. Case rates, for example, are increasingly influenced by such factors as immigration rates from high-prevalence countries and indirectly by control measures in those countries. Treatment completion rates are influenced primarily by programs such as direct observation of treatment and by the resources available to properly implement them, such as having sufficient dedicated and well-trained nursing staff and community outreach workers. Transmission rates are influenced most importantly by effective treatment but also by the prevalence of vulnerable populations (e.g., HIV-infected persons) and congregate settings conducive to transmission (e.g., jails, prisons, and homeless shelters). Contact investigations and the treatment of infected contacts require both commitment and sufficient community-based staff. Because these factors and others are constantly changing in public health programs with and without access to routine fingerprinting and because the impact of changes is not immediate, it is likely to be difficult to discern the subtle impact of molecular fingerprinting. What, then, is the evidence for the public health benefits of routinely genotyping tuberculosis isolates?

In a special issue of *Emerging Infectious Diseases*, the Centers for Disease Control and Prevention documented in one place the results of having funded seven health departments as sentinel surveillance sites for a period of 5 years in the National Tuberculosis Genotyping and Surveillance Network (19). Two of the sites, Arkansas and Massachusetts, are represented by authors of this chapter (D.C. and E.N.). As examples of the public health utilization of fingerprinting data, we review some of the findings primarily from these two sites.

The impact of genotyping on public health practice in Massachusetts can be divided into three categories: (i) supporting or refuting the results of classic epidemiologic case finding, (ii) identifying unsuspected transmission, and (iii) identifying laboratory cross-contamination (55). Each of these has clear public health implications.

From 1 July 1996 to 31 December 2000, 984 isolates, representing 95% of all available culture-positive cases in Massachusetts, were genotyped. A total of 372 (38%) were clustered. Conventional contact investigations during this period had identified 92 epidemiologic relationships among these cases, but in only 72% of these was the genotype exact or similar (±1 hybridization band). Twenty-five epidemiologic relationships were not supported by genotyping. These included 11 contacts identified in homeless shelters, 5 in household contacts, 2 in nonhousehold family members, 3 in friends and social contacts, and 4 in coworkers. The five household contacts all involved persons from high-prevalence countries.

Of 15 homeless men with TB and identical or similar RFLP types (±1 hybridization band), 11 were available for a contact investigation interview. Only one definite epidemiologic link was established by the interviews, but examination of the shelter bed logs established epidemiologic linkages for 13 of the 15 cases linked by genotype. One of the unlinked cases was suspected as being a false-positive culture.

During the period of the Massachusetts surveillance study, genotyping confirmed laboratory cross-contamination in two related instances occurring 3 weeks apart. Genotyping of all isolates 2 weeks before and 2 weeks after the episodes and review of their clinical record failed to uncover any other instances of cross-contamination. Interventions to correct the problem were instituted. It was estimated that three instances of cross-contamination, confirmed by genotyping, resulted in unnecessary treatment and contact investigations at an average cost of $10,873 each (range, $1,033 to $21,306), in addition to the unnecessary anxiety, inconvenience, and risk of complications of drug therapy (60).

The public health lessons here are that classic epidemiologic case finding can both miss relationships and overestimate transmission, especially in high-risk settings such as homeless shelters and among persons from high-risk countries. In retrospect only, genotyping demonstrated both of these errors, hopefully leading to improvements in future case finding investigations. This application of molecular fingerprinting assumes that identical or nearly identical fingerprints means recent transmission, which is not always the case, as noted below and elsewhere in this chapter. Disproving epidemiologic connections by finding different DNA fingerprint patterns is a more powerful tool than is postulating connections based on isolates with similar fingerprints. Genotyping can, but only in retrospect, reliably confirm laboratory cross-contamination or mislabeling, the first step in correcting this ubiquitous problem (42). However, because the most specific current genotyping methods require weeks or months to complete, the public health benefits are usually delayed. Patients are usually well into a course of treatment before fingerprint evidence of a false-positive culture is available.

In mostly rural Alabama, however, routine genotyping of isolates and analysis of clusters appeared to have had substantial public health benefit. Between 1994 and 1998, a cluster of 25 cases was reported, with 12 patients living in one county and the rest distributed over nine other counties across the state (24). In response to this information, a second epidemiologic contact investigation was performed by health departments and revealed the source to be a corrections facility and two homeless shelters, where surveillance and control measures were intensified.

Similarly, in Arkansas, genotyping and classic epidemiology demonstrated that despite "determined" public health measures, TB remained endemic in a rural community for more than 54 years (23). Based on these findings, the health department began investigating novel approaches to TB control in this high-risk community. Clonal relationships were discovered among organisms in a shelter-associated outbreak of TB among Boston's homeless that spanned at least 14 years (56). In both of these studies, the notion that the finding of matched fingerprints implies recent transmission is called into question.

In Denver, Colo., genotyping was used to demonstrate the effectiveness of a new program of mandatory symptom and tuberculin screening in homeless shelters (47). The estimated TB incidence in the population decreased from 510 to 121 cases per 100,000, presumably due to reducing transmission through earlier detection and treatment. Clustering of cases within a 2-year period decreased from 49 to 14% in the homeless population.

As TB case rates fall in the resource-rich countries and as health departments shrink, it will be critical to identify which strategies are effective and which are not working. The routine use of genotyping, although not ideal for rapid intervention in its current form, appears to provide clues to unsuspected sites of transmission and critical feedback on time-honored surveillance and control strategies, including laboratory performance.

Identifying Strains of *M. tuberculosis* Responsible for Large Numbers of Cases to Identify Possible Microbial Factors that Affect Transmission and/or Disease

The advent of molecular typing also has allowed researchers to describe strain-specific variation in clinical phenotypes of *M. tuberculosis* such as virulence, growth characteristics, immunogenicity, and transmissibility. Although phenotypic differences among clinical isolates have long been recognized, it was not previously possible to determine whether such differences were stably associated with specific lineages of *M. tuberculosis* circulating in the population. Among strains identified in outbreaks, several have been associated with large clusters that are widely dispersed both geographically and temporally, raising the possibility that they are either more transmissible or more likely to cause disease once transmitted than are other strains. One such lineage is strain W, which has been responsible for over 500 reported cases in the New York/New Jersey area since 1991 (7). DNA fingerprints from this strain closely resemble those from a large family of related lineages which represent a significant proportion of the isolates that have been genotyped throughout Asia, Russia, and Eastern Europe, designated the Beijing family (80), and a strain that is widely distributed throughout the United States, designated strain 210 (85). The identification of this highly successful strain has led to laboratory-based efforts to identify bacterial factors that may distinguish this lineage from other, less widely disseminated clones. Strain 210 has an enhanced capacity to replicate in human macrophages, and this function may be associated with its success (87).

Despite these findings, recent attempts to fully characterize specific clinical strains suggest that the assessment of "notorious" *M. tuberculosis* isolates can be problematic. Host factors clearly affect the behavior of strains and can be difficult to disentangle from bacterial traits. Laboratory studies measuring the growth rates of such strains must compare these to the growth rates of uniform reference strains, which vary substantially in different environments. Finally, it can be challenging to use epidemiologic patterns to differentiate microbial virulence from other bacterial factors such as immunogenicity and/or transmissibility. These problems have been exemplified by strain CDC 1551, an *M. tuberculosis* isolate that was identified as the culprit in a microepidemic reported in a rural area in the United States. In this largely susceptible community, 80% of the contacts of the index case were found to be tuberculin skin test (TST) positive, which led investigators to propose that the organism was more virulent than other strains (74). This hypothesis was supported by the early observation that CDC 1551 grew to very large numbers of bacilli in the lungs of infected animal models. Subsequent studies, however, found that other reference laboratory strains could also be induced to attain these bacterial numbers and, indeed, that CDC 1551 grew more slowly than these strains later in the course of an infection (45). Nonetheless, in other experiments, CDC 1551 was found to differ from standard laboratory strains in that it induced a more vigorous cytokine-mediated immune response in human monocytes (49) and produced smaller tubercles in the lungs of infected rabbits (9). These results raise the possibility that the high conversion rate among contacts might reflect the heightened immunogenicity of this strain, which would increase the sensitivity of the TST. This experience has made it clear that it will be important to distinguish between virulence, transmissibility, and immunogenicity in future studies of strain-specific phenotypes.

Relative Transmissibility of Drug-Sensitive and -Resistant *M. tuberculosis*

The fact that strain W was originally associated with an outbreak of multidrug-resistant TB (MDR-TB) confounds the issue of transmissibility/virulence and drug resistance. Earlier studies had suggested that strains characterized by isoniazid (INH) resistance mutations grew less vigorously in guinea pigs than did drug-sensitive (DS) strains (54). Subsequent work, however, has shown that resistance to INH is encoded by a number of different point mutations, raising the possibility that the behavior of different drug-resistant (DR) strains may be quite heterogeneous (88).

Epidemiologic studies designed to address this question have compared the number of TST positives and/or cases of clinical TB in household contacts exposed to DS and DR source cases. Using this method, an earlier study found no difference in the infectiousness of DS and DS sources (66). A similar 2001 study also reported a comparable prevalence of TB infection and progression to active disease in both groups (72).

Other molecular biology studies have taken a different approach to estimating the relative transmissibility of strains. These compare the sizes of clusters of isolates that are DR and DS, respectively. One

such study, conducted in The Netherlands (34), showed that INH resistance was negatively associated with clustering, while a second (78) found that being infected with MDR-TB was a factor associated with a decreased likelihood of being in a cluster. Conflicting results were reported in New York City, where drug resistance was a strong predictor of clustering, with some clusters belonging to the W strain (1). Many descriptive studies have documented the widespread transmission of DR organisms and have also noted that these disseminated DR strains belong disproportionately to the W family (8, 32, 35). These results may again raise the question whether molecular "cluster" studies can be used to infer the risk of infection or disease, in this case among those exposed to DS and DR strains, respectively. There are many possible reasons why clusters of cases of single-DR or MDR-TB may be smaller than clusters of DS cases. People infected with DR *M. tuberculosis* strains may have poorer access to health care and be less likely to be sampled than people infected with DS strains of the organism. They may also have fewer susceptible contacts than do people infected with DS strains, either because they have fewer social interactions in general or because the people they do contact are more likely to have been infected with TB in the past. Finally, since specific DR and DS strains probably differ at a variety of other genetic loci, observed differences in transmissibility and virulence may be related to strain differences that are independent of drug resistance phenotypes. These potentially confounding factors make such studies difficult to interpret and reemphasize the need for careful thought and innovative approaches to the design of epidemiologic studies that use molecular methods.

REFERENCES

1. Alland, D., T. S. Whittam, M. B. Murray, M. D. Cave, M. H. Hazbon, K. Dix, M. Kokoris, A. Duesterhoeft, J. A Eisen, C. M. Fraser, and R. D. Fleischmann. 2003. Modeling bacterial evolution with comparative-genome-based marker systems: application to *Mycobacterium tuberculosis* evolution and pathogenesis. *J. Bacteriol.* 185:3392–3399.
2. Anh, D. D., M. W. Borgdorff, L. N. Van, N. T. Lan, T. van Gorkom, and K. Kremer. 2000. *Mycobacterium tuberculosis* Beijing genotype emerging in Vietnam. *Emerg. Infect. Dis.* 6:302–305.
3. Bandera, A., A. Gori, L. Catozzi, A. Degli Esposti, G. Marchetti, C. Molteni, G. Ferrario, L. Codecasa, V. Penati, A. Matteelli, and F. Franzetti. 2000. Molecular epidemiology study of exogenous reinfection in an area with a low incidence of tuberculosis. *J. Clin. Microbiol.* 39:2213–2218.
4. Barnes, P. F., and M. D. Cave. 2003. Molecular epidemiology of tuberculosis. *N. Engl. J. Med.* 349:1149–1156.
5. Beggs, M. L., K. D. Eisenach, and M. D. Cave. 2000. Mapping of IS6110 insertion sites in two epidemic strains of *Mycobacterium tuberculosis*. *J. Clin Microbiol.* 38:2923–2928.

6. Bennett, D. E., I. M. Onorato, B. A. Ellis, J. T. Crawford, B. Schable, R. Byers, J. S. Kammerer, and C. R Braden. 2002. DNA fingerprinting of *Mycobacterium tuberculosis* isolates from epidemiologically linked case pairs. *Emerg. Infect. Dis.* 8:1224–1229.

7. Bifani, P. J., B. Mathema, N. E. Kurepina, B. N. Kreiswirth. 2002. Global dissemination of the *Mycobacterium tuberculosis* W-Beijing family strains. *Trends Microbiol.* 10:45–52.

8. Bifani, P. J., B. Mathema, Z. Liu, S. L. Moghazeh, B. Shopsin, B. Tempalski, R. Driscol Frothingham, J. M. Musser, P. Alcabes, and B. N. Kreiswirth. 1999. Identification of a W variant outbreak of *Mycobacterium tuberculosis* via population-based molecular epidemiology. *JAMA* 282:2321–2327.

9. Bishai, W. R., A. M. Dannenberg, Jr., N. Parrish, R. Ruiz, P. Chen, B. C. Zook, W. Johnson, J. W Boles, and M. L Pitt. 1999. Virulence of *Mycobacterium tuberculosis* CDC1551 and H37Rv in rabbits evaluated by Lurie's pulmonary tubercle count method. *Infect. Immun.* 67:4931–4934.

10. Borgdorff, M. W., N. Nagelkerke, D. van Soolingen, P. E. de Haas, J. Veen, and J. D. van Embden. 1998. Analysis of tuberculosis transmission between nationalities in the Netherlands in the period 1993–1995 using DNA fingerprinting. *Am. J. Epidemiol.* 147:187–195.

11. Braden, C. R., G. P. Morlock, C. L. Woodley, K. M. Johnson, A. C. Colombel, M. D. Cave, Z. Yang, S. E Valway, I. M. Onorato, and J. T Crawford. 2001. Simultaneous infection with multiple strains of *M. tuberculosis. Clin. Infect. Dis.* 33:e42–e47.

12. Burman, W. J., and R. Reves. 2000. Review of false-positive cultures for *Mycobacterium tuberculosis* and recommendations for avoiding unnecessary treatment. *Clin. Infect Dis.* 31:1390–1395.

13. Butler, W. R., W. H. Hass, and J. T. Crawford. 1996. Automated DNA fingerprinting analysis of *Mycobacterium tuberculosis* using fluorescent detection of PCR products. *J. Clin. Microbiol.* 34:1801–1803.

14. Caminero, J. A., M. J. Pena, M. I. Campos-Herrero, J. C. Rodriguez, O. Afonso, C. Martin, J. M. Pavon, M. J. Torres, M. Burgos, P. Cabrera, P. M. Small, and D. A Enarson. 2001. Exogenous reinfection with tuberculosis on a European island with moderate incidence of disease. *Am. J. Respir. Crit. Care. Med.* 163:717–720.

15. Cave, M. D., K. D. Eisenach, P. F. McDermott, J. J. Bates, and J. T. Crawford. 1991. IS*6110*: conservation of sequence in the *Mycobacterium tuberculosis* complex and its utilization in DNA fingerprinting. *Mol. Cell. Probes* 5:73–80.

16. Cave, M. D., K. D. Eisenach, G. Templeton, M. Salfinger, G. Mazurek, J. Bates, and J. T. Crawford. 1994. Stability of DNA fingerprint pattern produced with IS*6110* strains of *Mycobacterium tuberculosis. J. Clin. Microbiol.* 32:262–266.

17. Classen, C.N., R. Warren, M. Richardson, J. H. Hauman, R. P. Gie, J. H. Ellis, P. D. van Helden, and N. Beyers. 1999. Impact of social interactions in the community on the transmission of tuberculosis in a high incidence area. *Thorax* 54:136–140.

18. Cole, S. T., R. Brosch, J. Parkhill, T. Garnier, C. Churcher, D. Harris, S. V. Gordon, L. Eiglmeier, S. Gas, C. E. Barry, III, F. Tekaia, K. Badcock, D. Basham, D. Brown, T. Chillingworth, R. Connor, R. Davies, K. Devlin, T. Feltwell, S. Gentles, N. Hamlin, S. Holroyd, T. Hornsby, K. Jagels, J. Krogh, J. Mclean, S. Moule, L. Murphy, K. Oliver, J. Osborne, M. A. Quail, M. A. Rajandream, J. Rogers, S. Rutter, K. Seeger, J. Skelton, R. Squares, S. Squares, J. E. Sulston, K. Taylor, S. Whitehead, and B. G. Barrell. 1998. Deciphering the biology of *Mycobacterium tuberculosis* from the complete genome sequence. *Nature* 393:537–544.

19. Crawford, J. T., C. R. Braden, B. A. Schable, and I. M. Onorato. 2002. National Tuberculosis Genotyping and Surveillance Network: design and methods. *Emerg. Infect. Dis.* 8:1192–1196.

20. Cronin, W. A., J. E. Golub, M. J. Lathan, L. N. Mukasa, N. Hooper, J. H. Razaq, N. G. Baruch, D. Mulcahy, W. H. Benjamin, L. S. Magder, G. T. Strickland, and W. R. Bishai. 2002. Molecular epidemiology of tuberculosis in a low-to moderate-incidence state: are contact investigations enough? *Emerg. Infect. Dis.* 8:1271–1279.

21. Dale, J. W., D. Brittain, A. A. Cataldi, D. Cousins, J. T. Crawford, J. Driscoll, H. Heersma, T. Lilleback, T. Quitugua, N. Rastogi, R. A Skuce, C. Sola, D. van Soolingen, and V. Vincent. 2001. Spacer oligonucleotide typing of bacteria of the *Mycobacterium tuberculosis* complex: recommendations for standardized nomenclature. *Int. J. Tuberc. Lung Dis.* 5:216–219.

22. Daley, C. L., P. M. Small, G. F. Schecter, G. K. Schoolnik, R. A. McAdam, and W. R. Jacobs, Jr. 1992. An outbreak of tuberculosis with accelerated progression among persons infected with the human immunodeficiency virus. An analysis using restriction-fragment-length polymorphisms. *N. Engl. J. Med.* 326:231–235.

23. Dillaha, J. A., Z. Yang, K. Ijaz, K. D. Eisenach, M. D. Cave, F. J. Wilson, W. W. Stead, and J. H. Bates. 2002. Transmission of *Mycobacterium tuberculosis* in a rural community, Arkansas, 1945–2000. *Emerg. Infect. Dis.* 8:1246–1248.

24. Dobbs, K. G., K. H. Lok, F. Bruce, D. Mulcahy, W. H. Benjamin, and N. E. Dunlap. 2001. Value of *Mycobacterium tuberculosis* fingerprinting as a tool in a rural state surveillance program. *Chest* 120:1877–1882.

25. Doroudchi, M., K. Kremer, E. A. Basiri, M. R. Kadivar, D. van Soolingen, and A. A. Ghaderi. 2000. IS*6110*-RFLP and spoligotyping of *Mycobacterium tuberculosis* isolates in Iran. *Scand. J. Infect. Dis.* 32:663–668.

26. Fandinho, F. C., A. L. Kritski, C. Hofer, H. Conde, Jr., R. M. Ferreira, M. H. Saad, M. G. Silva, L. W. Riley, and L. S. Fonseca. 2000. RFLP patterns and risk factors for recent tuberculosis transmission among hospitalized tuberculosis patients in Rio de Janeiro, Brazil. *Trans. R. Soc. Trop. Med. Hyg.* 94:271–275.

27. Fang, Z., and K. J. Forbes. 1997. A *Mycobacterium tuberculosis* IS*6110* preferential locus (*ipl*) for insertion into the genome. *J. Clin. Microbiol.* 35:479–481.

28. Fleischmann, R. D., D. Alland, J. A. Eisen, L. Carpenter, O. White, J. Peterson, R. DeBoy, R. Dodson, M. Gwinn, D. Haft, E. Hickey, J. F. Kolonay, W. C. Nelson, L. A. Umayam, M. Ermolaeva, S. L. Salzberg, A. Delcher, T. Utterback, J. Weidman, H. Khouri, J. Gill, A. Mikula, W. Bishai, W. R. Jacobs, Jr., J. C. Venter, and C. M. Fraser. 2002. Whole-genome comparison of *Mycobacterium tuberculosis* clinical and laboratory strains. *J. Bacteriol.* 184:5479–5490.

29. Fomukong, N., M. Beggs, H. el Hajj, G. Templeton, K. Eisenach, and M. D. Cave. 1998. Differences in the prevalence of IS*6110* insertion sites in *Mycobacterium tuberculosis* strains: low and high copy number of IS*6110*. *Tubercle. Lung Dis.* 78:109–116.

30. Fraser, C. M., J. Eisen, R. D. Fleischmann, K. A. Ketchum, and S. Peterson. 2000. Comparative genomics and understanding of microbial biology. *Emerg. Infect. Dis.* 6:505–512.

31. Frieden, T. R., C. L. Woodley, J. T. Crawford, D. Lew, and S. M. Dooley. 1996. The molecular epidemiology of tuberculosis in New York City: the importance of nosocomial transmission and laboratory error. *Tubercle. Lung Dis.* 77:407–413.

32. Friedman, C. R., M. Y. Stoeckle, B. N. Kreiswirth, W. D. Johnson, Jr., S. M. Manoach, J. Berger, K. Sathianathan

A. Hafner, and L. W. Riley. 1995. Transmission of multidrug-resistant tuberculosis in a large urban setting. *Am. J. Respir. Crit. Care Med.* **152:**3

33. Frothingham, R., and W. A. Meeker-O'Connell. 1998. Genetic diversity in the *Mycobacterium tuberculosis* complex based on variable numbers of tandem DNA repeats. *Microbiology* **144:**1189–1196.

34. Garcia-Garcia, M. L., A. Ponce de Leon, M. E. Jimenez-Corona, A. Jimenez-Corona, M. Palacios-Martinez, S. Balandrano-Campos, L. Ferreyra-Reyes, L. Juarez-Sandino, J. Sifuentes-Osornio, H. Olivera-Diaz, J. L. Valdespino-Gomez, and P. M. Small. 2000. Clinical consequences and transmissibility of drug-resistant tuberculosis in southern Mexico. *Arch. Intern. Med.* **13:**630–636.

35. Githui, W. A., M. P. Hawken, E. S. Juma, P. Godfrey-Faussett, O. B. Swai, D. K. Kibuga, J. D. Porter, S. M. Wilson, and F. A. Drobniewski. 2000. Surveillance of drug-resistant tuberculosis and molecular evaluation of transmission of resistant strains in refugee and non-refugee populations in North-Eastern Kenya. *Int. J. Tuberc. Lung Dis.* **4:**947–955.

36. Glynn, J. R., E. Vynnycky, and P. E. Fine. 1999. Influence of sampling on estimates of clustering and recent transmission of *Mycobacterium tuberculosis* derived from DNA fingerprinting techniques. *Am. J. Epidemiol.* **149:**366–371.

37. Godfrey-Faussett, P., P. R. Mortimer, P. A. Jenkins, and N. G. Stoker. 1992. Evidence of transmission of tuberculosis by DNA fingerprinting. *Br. Med. J.* **305:**221–223.

38. Golub, J. E., W. A. Cronin, O. O. Obasanjo, W. Coggin, K. Moore, D. S. Pope, D. Thompson, T. R. Sterling, S. Harrington, W. R. Bishai, and R. E. Chaisson. 2001. Transmission of *Mycobacterium tuberculosis* through casual contact with an infectious case. *Arch. Intern. Med.* **161:**2254–2258.

39. Haas, W. H., W. R. Butler, C. L. Woodley, and J. T. Crawford. 1993. Mixed-linker polymerase chain reaction: a new method for rapid fingerprinting of isolates of the *Mycobacterium tuberculosis* complex. *J. Clin. Microbiol.* **31:**1293–1298.

40. Hermans, P. W. M., D. van Soolingen, E. M. Bik, P. E. W. de Haas, J. W. Dale, and J. D. A. van Embden. 1991. The insertion element IS*987* for *Mycobacterium bovis* BCG is located in a hot spot integration region for insertion elements in *M. tuberculosis* strains. *Infect. Immun.* **59:**2695–2705.

41. Horn, D. L., D. Hewlett, Jr., W. H. Haas, W. R. Butler, C. Alfalla, E. Tan, A. Levine, A. Nayak, and S. M. Opal. 1994. Superinfection with rifampin-isoniazid-streptomycin-ethambutol (RISE)-resistant tuberculosis in three patients with AIDS: confirmation by polymerase chain reaction fingerprinting. *Ann. Intern. Med.* **121:**115–116.

42. Jasmer, R. M., M. Roemer, J. Hamilton, J. Bunter, C. R. Braden, T. M. Shinnick, and E. P. Desmond. 2002. A prospective, multicenter study of laboratory cross-contamination of *Mycobacterium tuberculosis* cultures. *Emerg. Infect. Dis.* **8:**1260–1263.

43. Kamerbeek, J., L. Schouls, A. Kolk, M. van Agtervveld, D. van Soolingen, S. Kuijper, A. Bunschoten, H. Molhuizen, R. Shaw, M. Goyal, and J. D. A. van Embden. 1997. Simultaneous detection and strain differentiation of *Mycobacterium tuberculosis* for diagnosis and epidemiology. *J. Clin. Microbiol.* **35:**907–914.

44. Kato-Maeda, M., J. T. Rhee, T. R. Gingeras, H. Salamon, J. Drenkow, N. Smittipat, and P. M. Small. 2001. Comparing genomes within the species *Mycobacterium tuberculosis*. *Genome Res.* **11:**547–554.

45. Kelley, C. L., and F. M. Collins. 1999. Growth of a highly virulent strain of *Mycobacterium tuberculosis* in mice of differing susceptibility to tuberculous challenge. *Tubercle Lung Dis.* **79:**367–70.

46. Kline, S. E., L. L. Hedemark, and S. F. Davies. 1995. Outbreak of tuberculosis among regular patrons of a neighborhood bar. *N. Engl. J. Med.* **333:**222–227.

47. Kong, P. M., J. Tapy, P. Calixto, W. J. Burman, R. R. Reves, Z. Yang, and M. D. Cave. 2002. Skin-test screening and tuberculosis transmission among the homeless. *Emerg. Infect. Dis.* **8:**1280–1284.

48. Lok, K., W. Benjamin, M. E. Kimerling, V. Pruitt, M. Lathan, J. Raquez, N. Hooper, W. Cronin, and N. Dunlap. 2002. Molecular differentiation of *Mycobacterium tuberculosis* strains without IS*6110* insertions. *Emerg. Infect. Dis.* **8:**1310–1313.

49. Manca, C., L. Tsenova, C. E. Barry, III, A. Bergtold, S. Freeman, P. A. Haslett, J. M. Musser, V. H. Freedman, and G. Kaplan. 1999. *Mycobacterium tuberculosis* CDC1551 induces a more vigorous host response in vivo and in vitro, but is not more virulent than other clinical isolates. *J. Immun.* **162:**6740–6746.

50. March, F., P. Coll, R. A. Guerrero, E. Busquets, J. A. Cayla, and G. Prats. 2000. Predictors of tuberculosis transmission in prisons: an analysis using conventional and molecular methods. *AIDS* **14:**525–535.

51. Mazars, E., S. Lesjean, A.-L. Banuls, M. Gilbert, V. Vincent, B. Gicquel, M. Tibayrenc, C. Locht, and P. Supply. 2001. High-resolution minisatellite-based typing as a portable approach to global analysis of *Mycobacterium tuberculosis* molecular epidemiology. *Proc. Natl. Acad. Sci. USA* **98:**1901–1906.

52. Mazurek, C. H., M. D. Cave, K. D. Eisenach, R. J. Wallace, J. H. Bates, and J. T. Crawford. 1991. Chromosomal DNA fingerprint patterns produced with IS*6110* as a strain specific marker for the epidemiologic study of tuberculosis. *J. Clin. Microbiol.* **29:**2030–2033.

53. McNabb, S. J., C. R. Braden, and T. R. Navin. 2002. DNA fingerprinting of *Mycobacterium tuberculosis*: lessons learned and implications for the future. *Emerg. Infect. Dis.* 1314–1319.

54. Middlebrook, G., and M. L. Cohn. 1953. Some observations on the pathogenicity of isoniazid-resistant variants of the tubercle bacilli. *Science* **118:**297–299.

55. Miller, A.C., W. R. Butler, and B. McInnis. 2002. Clonal relationships in a shelter-associated outbreak of drug-resistant tuberculosis: 1983–1997. *Int. J. Tuberc. Lung Dis.* **6:**872–878.

56. Miller, A. C., S. Sharnprapai, R. Suruki, E. Corkren, E. A. Nardell, J. R. Driscoll, M. McGarry, H. Taber, and S. Etkind. 2002. Impact of genotyping of *Mycobacterium tuberculosis* on public health practice in Massachusetts. *Emerg. Infect. Dis.* **8:**1285–1292.

57. Murray, M. 2002. Sampling bias in the molecular epidemiology of tuberculosis. *Emerg. Infect. Dis.* **8:**363–369.

58. Murray, M. B., and D. A. Alland. 2002. Methodological problems in the molecular epidemiology of tuberculosis. *Am. J. Epidemiol.* **155:**565–571.

59. Nardell, E., B. McInnis, B. Thomas, and S. Weidhaas. 1986. Exogenous reinfection with tuberculosis in a shelter for the homeless. *N. Engl. J. Med.* **315:**1570–1574.

60. Northrup, J. M., A. C. Miller, E. Nardell, S. Sharnprapai, S. Etkind, J. Driscoll, M. McGarry, H. W. Taber, P. Elvin, N. L. Qualls, and C. R. Braden. 2002. Estimated costs of false laboratory diagnoses of tuberculosis in three patients. *Emerg. Infect. Dis.* **8:**1264–1270.

61. Pfyffer, G. E., A. Strassle, N. Rose, R. Wirth, O. Brandli, and H. Shang. 1998. Transmission of tuberculosis in the metropolitan area of Zurich: a 3 year survey based on DNA fingerprinting. *Eur. Respir. J.* **11:**804–808.

62. Pineda-Garcia, L., A. Ferrera, and S. E. Hoffner. 1997. DNA fingerprinting of *Mycobacterium tuberculosis* strains from patients with pulmonary tuberculosis in Honduras. *J. Clin. Microbiol.* 35:2393–2397.

63. Rado, T. A., J. H. Bates, H. W. Engel, E. Mankiewicz, T. Murohashi, Y. Mizuguchi, and L. Sula. 1975. World Health Organization studies on bacteriophage typing of mycobacteria. Subdivision of the species *Mycobacterium tuberculosis. Am. Rev. Respir. Dis.* 111:459–468.

64. Ramos, M. C., H. Soini, G. C. Roscanni, M. Jaques, M. C. Villares, and J. M. Musser. 1999. Extensive cross contamination of specimens with *Mycobacterium tuberculosis* in a reference laboratory. *J. Clin. Microbiol.* 97:916–919.

65. Sampson S., R. Warren, M. Richardson, G. van der Spuy, and P. van Helden. 2001. IS*6110* insertions in *Mycobacterium tuberculosis*: predominantly into coding regions. *J. Clin. Microbiol.* 39:3423–3424.

66. Snider, D. E., Jr., G. D. Kelly, G. M. Cauthen, N. J. Thompson, and J. O. Kilburn. 1985. Infection and disease among contacts of tuberculosis cases with drug-resistant and drug-susceptible bacilli. *Am. Rev. Respir. Dis.* 13:125–132.

67. Small, P. M., R. W. Shafer, P. C. Hopewell, S. P. Singh, M. J. Murphy, and E. Desmond. 1993. Exogenous reinfection with multidrug-resistant *Mycobacterium tuberculosis* in patients with advanced HIV infection. *N. Engl. J. Med.* 328: 1137–1144.

68. Sreevatsan, S., X. Pan, K. E. Stockbauer, N. D. Connell, B. N. Kreiswirth, T. S. Whittam, and J. M Musser. 1997. Restricted structural gene polymorphism in the *Mycobacterium tuberculosis* complex indicates evolutionary recent global dissemination. *Proc. Natl. Acad. Sci. USA* 94:9869–9874.

69. Styblo, K. 1984. *Epidemiology of Tuberculosis.* VER Gustav Fischer Verlag, Jena, Germany.

70. Supply, P., S. Lesjean, E. Savine, K. Kremer, D. van Soolingen, and C. Locht. 2001. Automated high-throughput genotyping for study of global epidemiology of *Mycobacterium tuberculosis* based on mycobacterial interspersed repetitive units. *J. Clin. Microbiol.* 39:3563–3571.

71. Supply, P., E. Mazars, S. Lesjean, V. Vincent, B. Gicquel, and C. Locht. 2000. Variable human minisatellite-like regions in the *Mycobacterium tuberculosis* genome. *Mol. Microbiol.* 36:762–771.

72. Teixeira, L., M. D. Perkins, J. L. Johnson, R. Keller, M. Palaci, and V. do Valle Dettoni. 2001. Infection and disease among household contacts of patients with multidrug-resistant tuberculosis. *Int. J. Tuberc. Lung Dis.* 5:321–328.

73. Thierry, D., M. D. Cave, K. D. Eisenach, J. C. Crawford, J. H. Bates, B. Gicquel, and J. L. Guesdon. 1990. IS*6110*, an IS-like element of the *Mycobacterium tuberculosis* complex. *Nucleic Acids Res.* 18:188.

74. Valway, S. E., M. P. Sanchez, T. F. Shinnick, I. Orme, T. Agerton, D. Hoy, J. S. Jones, H. Westmoreland, and I. M. Onorato. 1998. An outbreak involving extensive transmission of a virulent strain of *Mycobacterium tuberculosis. N. Engl. J. Med.* 338:633–639.

75. van Embden, J. D., T. van Gorkom, K. Kremer, R. Jansen, B. A. van Der Zeijst, and L. M. Schouls. 2000. Genetic variation and evolutionary origin of the direct repeat locus of *Mycobacterium tuberculosis* complex bacteria. *J. Bacteriol.* 182:2393–2401.

76. van Embden, J. D. A., M. D. Cave, J. T. Crawford, J. W. Dale, K. D. Eisenach, B. Gicquel, P. Hermans, C. Martin, R. McAdam, T. M. Shinnick, and P. M. Small. 1993. Strain identification of *Mycobacterium tuberculosis* by DNA fingerprinting: recommendation for a standardized methodology. *J. Clin. Microbiol.* 31:406–409.

77. van Rie, A, R. Warren, M. Richardson, T. C. Victor, R. P. Gie, D. A. Enarson, N. Beyers, and P. D. van Helden. 1999. Exogenous reinfection as a cause of recurrent tuberculosis after curative treatment. *N. Engl. J. Med.* 341:1174–1179.

78. van Soolingen, D., M. W. Borgdorff, P. E. de Haas, M. M. Sebek, J. Veen, M. Dessens K. Kremer, and J. D. van Embden. 1999. Molecular epidemiology of tuberculosis in the Netherlands: a nationwide study from 1993 through 1997. *J. Infect. Dis.* 18:726–736.

79. van Soolingen, D., E. W. Petra, P. de Haas, P. Hermans, P. Groenen, and J. D. van Embden. 1993. Comparison of various repetitive DNA elements as generic markers for strain differentiation and epidemiology of *Mycobacterium tuberculosis. J. Clin. Microbiol.* 31:1987–1995.

80. van Soolingen, D., L. Qian, P. E. de Haas, J. T. Douglas, H. Traore, F. Portaels, H. Z. Qing, D. Enkhsaikan, P. Nymadawa, and J. D. van Embden. 1995. Predominance of a single genotype of *Mycobacterium tuberculosis* in countries of East Asia. *J. Clin. Microbiol.* 33:3234–3243.

81. Vynnycky, E., N. Nagelkerke, M. W. Borgdorff, D. van Soolingen, and J. D. van Embden. 2001. The effect of age and study duration on the relationship between "clustering" of DNA fingerprint patterns and the proportion of tuberculosis disease attributable to recent transmission. *Epidemiol. Infect.* 126:43–62.

82. Warren, R., M. Richardson, G. van der Spuy, T. Victor, S. Sampson, N. Beyers, and P. van Helden. 1999. DNA fingerprinting and molecular epidemiology of tuberculosis: use and interpretation in an epidemic setting. *Electrophoresis* 20:1807–1812.

83. Wilkinson, D., M. Pillay, J. Crump, C. Lombard, G. R. Davies, and A. W. Sturm. 1997. Molecular epidemiology and transmission dynamics of *Mycobacterium tuberculosis* in rural Africa. *Trop. Med. Int. Health* 2:747–753.

84. Yang, Z., P. F. Barnes, F. Chaves, K. D. Eisenach, S. Weis, J. H. Bates, and M. D. Cave. 1998. Diversity of DNA fingerprints of *Mycobacterium tuberculosis* isolates in the United States. *J. Clin. Microbiol.* 36:1003–1007.

85. Yang, Z. H., K. Ijaz, J. H. Bates, K. D. Eisenach, and M. D. Cave. 2000. Spoligotyping and PGRS fingerprinting of *Mycobacterium tuberculosis* strains having few copies of IS*6110. J. Clin Microbiol.* 38:3572–3576.

86. Yang, Z. H., A. Rendon, A. Flores, R. Medina, K. Ijaz, J. Llaca, K. D. Eisenach, J. H. Bates, A. Villareal, and M. D. Cave. 2000. A clinic-based molecular epidemiologic study of tuberculosis in Monterrey, Mexico. *Int. J. Tuberc. Lung Dis.* 5:313–320.

87. Zhang, M., J. Gong, Z. Yang, B. Samten, M. D. Cave, and P. F. Barnes. 1999. Enhanced capacity of a widespread strain of *Mycobacterium tuberculosis* to grow in macrophages. *J. Infect. Dis.* 179:1213–1217.

88. Zhang, Y., B. Heym, B. Allen, D. Young, and S. Cole. 1992. The catalase-peroxidase gene and isoniazid resistance of *Mycobacterium tuberculosis. Nature* 358:591–593.

III. DIAGNOSTICS

Chapter 4

Clinical Mycobacteriology (Tuberculosis) Laboratory: Services and Methods

Leonid Heifets and Edward Desmond

The goal of this chapter is to present a broad picture of activities in a diagnostic mycobacteriology laboratory with a focus on *Mycobacterium tuberculosis* detection, identification, and drug susceptibility testing. Special issues pertinent to nontuberculous mycobacteria (NTM) are not included in this chapter. We address the methodology currently available in most laboratories as well as the techniques that require further standardization and therefore have been implemented in only a few laboratories, mostly in conjunction with research and development.

ORGANIZATION OF TUBERCULOSIS LABORATORY SERVICES

The role of the laboratory in the management of tuberculosis has been greatly underestimated in the past and is still not fully appreciated in the medical community. This underappreciation may have been a part of the greater problem, since it is now recognized that tuberculosis is the most neglected health crisis in the world. Since the tragic outbreaks of tuberculosis in the United States in the 1980s, and especially after the official definition of tuberculosis and other mycobacterial infections as AIDS related, these problems have attracted more attention. Development of rapid methods for mycobacterial species identification and drug susceptibility testing became especially important because of the extremely rapid progression of tuberculosis in human immunodeficiency virus (HIV)-positive individuals and because of the growing rates of drug resistance.

The laboratory can play an essential role in controlling the TB epidemic by achieving the following goals: (i) nearly complete case detection, with a realistic possibility of bacteriological confirmation of diagnosis in about 85% of adult patients with pulmonary tuberculosis; (ii) turnaround time of 24 h for a provisional diagnosis of tuberculosis by smear microscopy in about 60 to 70% of culture-positive patients; (iii) bacteriological diagnosis of tuberculosis, using various media for culture isolation and affordable rapid identification methods, within 2 weeks for 70 to 80% of patients; and (iv) turnaround time for laboratory reports of drug susceptibility test results within 3 weeks for 70% of patients and within 4 weeks for 80% of patients. These minimal goals can be easily achieved by modern clinical laboratories in most of the industrialized countries within reasonable financial restraints. The turnaround time for the laboratory reports can be further shortened by implementation of some molecular biology-based methods, if the cost-effectiveness of broad implementation of such methods can be justified. Therefore, the specific laboratory protocols and organization of tuberculosis laboratory services have to be individualized for each country or area within a country.

Laboratory Services in the United States

The concept of three-level laboratory services was introduced by the U.S. Centers for Disease Control and Prevention (CDC) in 1967 and was subsequently clarified and endorsed by the American Thoracic Society (4, 61, 94). According to this classification, the assignment of the laboratories was specified as follows. Laboratories at level I collect specimens, may examine smears for acid-fast bacilli (AFB), and forward the specimens to a higher-level laboratory. Laboratories at level II may perform the AFB smear examination, process specimens for cultures on standard egg-based and agar media, identify *M. tuberculosis,* and perform drug susceptibility tests with first-line drugs only. Level III laboratories may

Leonid Heifets • Mycobacteriology Laboratory, National Jewish Medical and Research Medicine, 1400 Jackson St., Denver, CO 80206.   **Edward Desmond** • Microbial Diseases Laboratory, Division of Communicable Disease Control, California Department of Health Services, 850 Marina Bay Parkway, Berkeley, CA 94704.

perform the same functions as level II laboratories but may also identify mycobacterial species other than *M. tuberculosis* and should perform susceptibility tests, including those with first- and second-line drugs.

The three-level structure of mycobacteriology services has been instrumental for proper management of tuberculosis in the past. The advantage of this system included the opportunity to have smear results closer to the physician and patient setting. This system survived for 25 years because the small number of level III laboratories could not possibly handle the huge number of specimens that would have been submitted directly to these laboratories instead of being handled first by level II laboratories for primary isolation. Among the disadvantages of the three-level system is extension of the turnaround time by transfer of specimens or cultures through the laboratory levels. Another problem is the relatively low predictive value of the AFB smear examination when performed in level I laboratories that are able to examine only direct smears (from nonconcentrated specimens) without the use of fluorescence microscopy. In addition, a large proportion of level II laboratories were (and still are) not properly equipped for rapid isolation, identification, and susceptibility testing and usually did (do) not perform direct susceptibility tests.

The disadvantages of the system and necessity for change became apparent only after the tragic outbreaks of multidrug-resistant (MDR) tuberculosis in the 1980s. Among the causes of extremely high mortality rates during these outbreaks were that (i) the drug susceptibility test results did not arrive early enough for clinicians to make changes in the treatment regimens and (ii) some of these delays were related to the time taken to transfer the specimens or cultures between laboratories. The extra time needed for the transfer between laboratories includes not only shipping time but also time for the reference laboratory to evaluate the purity, identification, and metabolic status of the specimen or culture. The direct susceptibility test on agar plates, the most reliable tool at that time for detecting drug resistance in new patients, with a turnaround time of only 2 to 4 weeks, was abandoned because the isolation was performed in one laboratory and the grown cultures were sent to another for susceptibility testing. In addition, many level II laboratories used only Löwenstein-Jensen medium for primary isolation, thus delaying the availability of the cultures for the indirect susceptibility test by 2 or 4 weeks compared with isolation by the BACTEC system (Becton Dickinson, Sparks, Md.) and also probably resulting in reduced sensitivity compared with BACTEC. This situation led to the misconception that the laboratories were not able to detect drug

resistance before 6 to 8 weeks. Changes in laboratory services systems were debated in April 1995 at the Second National Conference on Laboratory Aspects of Tuberculosis sponsored by the Association of State and Territorial Public Health Laboratory Directors and CDC (106). The conference recommended having only two levels of laboratory services. Level I laboratories, according to this recommendation, would perform AFB smear examinations of concentrated specimens only, with the mandatory use of the fluorescence microscopy, and would report within 24 h. In addition to these requirements, level II laboratories must use both solid and liquid media for primary isolation to achieve mycobacterial culture isolation within 14 days in most patients and identification of *M. tuberculosis* within 21 days. It was also recommended that such laboratories report the results of drug susceptibility testing for most patients within 28 days. Thus, the level II laboratory would be equivalent to level III in the earlier three-level system, with more responsibility and specific requirements. Direct centralized laboratory services, when the raw specimens are mailed directly to large mycobacteriology laboratories with the most skilled personnel in this field and with modern technology, have a number of significant advantages over the three-level structure, in which hundreds of laboratories are involved in testing mycobacterial specimens and cultures. Among these are better quality, better timing, and lower cost. The availability of a direct centralized service is especially important for new patients when both a bacteriological diagnosis of tuberculosis and drug susceptibility test results are essential for proper management of therapy.

Three- and two-level service systems will probably continue to coexist. At the same time, it is desirable that all sputum specimens from newly diagnosed patients or those suspected of having tuberculosis be submitted directly to a limited number of full-service laboratories. Such laboratories can be efficient if their work is focused on the first specimens (and cultures) from new patients and if the areas of their services are arranged according to the epidemiologic data for the anticipated incidence of tuberculosis.

Laboratory Services in Developing Countries

In many African and Asian countries, the availability of direct smear examinations of nonconcentrated sputum specimens has been (and remains) the level of service considered the "gold standard" necessary for the diagnosis of tuberculosis in most infectious patients. Even this goal has not yet been fully achieved, leaving substantial proportions of patients in these countries without access to this simple diagnostic tool because of a larger problem: the access to medical care in general. The necessity for isolation of *M. tuberculosis* and drug susceptibility testing in developing countries was recognized even in 1969 (16). At that time, the Committee on Bacteriology of the International Union Against Tuberculosis and Lung Disease (IUATLD) proposed the development of a reliable drug susceptibility test that was feasible for laboratories in developing countries (57). Although the AFB smear examination remained a reliable tool for diagnosis and for monitoring patient responses to therapy (7), it does not address the problem of drug resistance. According to the National Tuberculosis Control Program models recommended by the IUATLD (25), tuberculosis laboratory services are considered important elements of tuberculosis control in developing countries. A recommended laboratory network, as reviewed by Laszlo (63), should consist of three levels of service, similar to that implemented in the United States in 1967. In countries where no laboratory system exists, introduction of these three-level services represents a significant progress compared with the microscopy units alone. This system introduces, among other elements, cultivation of mycobacteria and limited drug susceptibility testing.

The resources available in most countries with high TB prevalence are very limited, and so detection of the most infectious cases by the direct smear examination as the main diagnostic tool constitutes one of the five elements of DOTS (directly observed therapy short course) strategy recommended by the World Health Organization (WHO). After effective implementation of the DOTS strategy (with only direct microscopy as a diagnostic tool), some countries will eventually face the need for culture isolation for better case detection and for drug susceptibility testing, particularly in areas with a high prevalence of drug resistance. Along with this, the issue of choosing the most effective and cost-effective ways to implement these procedures will inevitably emerge.

In the modern worldwide systems of information networks and effective transportation systems, laboratory service does not have to be in close proximity to the patient or physician. This, along with the implementation of new technologies and the need for personnel specialized in this field, requires centralization and direct services in large mycobacteriology laboratories to ensure cost-efficient, high-quality service with the shortest possible turnaround time.

Quality Assurance

Quality assurance (QA) is a system targeting continuous improvement of quality of laboratory services (88). A detailed description of QA issues pertinent to the mycobacteriology laboratory can be found in a special review (112). It is based on such components as quality control (QC), quality improvement (QI), and proficiency testing (PT).

Minimal QC testing and its frequency is mandated in the United States by the agencies authorized to issue accreditation of laboratories, either under the Clinical Laboratory Improvement Act or according to the programs of the College of American Pathologists (CAP). In addition, it should, as far as possible, address suggestions from the recommendations published in the professional and scientific literature and by the various product manufacturers (6, 48, 52, 68). Currently, QC procedures require the inclusion of positive and negative controls for such procedures as AFB smears (weekly) and each time DNA probe tests and biochemical identification procedures are performed. At least one QC susceptible strain should be included in each of the drug susceptibility test runs, along with checks for sterility and efficacy of culture media and comparison of each new batch of reagents and solutions with the previous one. The actual list of required QC procedures is changing over time, along with technical progress in the field.

A QI program needs to be developed for each laboratory and should address such issues as measures for improving the results of smear examination, prevention of cross-contamination, enforcement of biosafety measures, introduction of new methods and new technology, cross-training of technologists, improvement of turnaround time of laboratory reports, etc. The production of quarterly reports on the analysis of achieving the QI program goals is necessary for any conclusions about the efficacy of the laboratory operations, with a special emphasis on the turnaround time for the laboratory reports.

External PT was initially developed in the United States as a voluntary program, and since 1969 the primary provider of services in this area has been CAP. Analysis of the results of these activities by CAP can be found in a review by Woods and Witebsky (114). PT in the United States is being performed two or three times per year and usually includes smear examination, culture isolation, identification of major mycobacterial species, and drug susceptibility testing.

QA programs similar to that in the United States have been developed in many European countries. Worldwide, a major current concern about tuberculosis control programs is the need to implement QA programs guiding laboratory diagnosis and laboratory services in countries with high tuberculosis prevalence and limited resources. To this end, some laboratories have established informal arrangements with their city, state, or national reference laboratories for exchanging AFB-stained slides and *M. tuberculosis* strains for assessing proficiency in microscopy and drug susceptibility testing.

BIOSAFETY IN THE MYCOBACTERIOLOGY LABORATORY

The threat of contracting an infection in the laboratory is as old as the history of microbiology. A report from CDC reviewing a number of publications on this subject (78) suggested that infection in the laboratory was most commonly acquired through aerosols, mouth pipetting, and the use of syringes (74, 75, 92). Although tuberculosis was rarely found among the most frequent laboratory-related infections, some reports (3, 35, 77) suggest that tuberculosis occurs more frequently in laboratory personnel than in the general population. On the other hand, publicity about the higher virulence or contagiousness of the so-called "killer strains" from some recent outbreaks has led to the creation of some laboratory facilities that far exceed any reasonable necessity for containment. In fact, this "overkill" may have a negative effect on real biosafety, since the environment created by some of the implemented measures can be highly uncomfortable and tiring, increasing the probability of an accident or breach of technique. Sometimes such a facility becomes just a "showroom," while the actual work is done outside of the containment area. It is clear that along with the necessary specific protection measures, an appropriate work environment that is comfortable for personnel should be considered to be among the most important principles of biosafety. Detailed guidelines specific for mycobacteriology clinical laboratories were reviewed by Richmond et al. in 1996 (79). Biosafety level 2 (BL-2) practices, containment equipment, and facilities were required for preparation of smears and culturing of clinical specimens such as sputum, and BL-3 practices were applied to some other procedures. It seems rational today to apply BL-3 requirements to all procedures in the tuberculosis laboratory, including specimen processing, but we agree that it is the responsibility of the laboratory director to establish standards, which can realistically address the biosafety issues.

Biosafety Level 2

Basic requirements for BL-2 include standard microbiological practices, training in biosafety, protective laboratory clothing, protective gloves, annual tuberculin skin test, limited access, decontamination of all infectious waste, and class I or class II biosafety cabinets for any manipulative procedure. Either of these cabinets is equipped with a high-efficiency particulate air (HEPA) filter, and the airflow draws the aerosolized materials away from the worker into the exhaust system. Personal protection is therefore satisfactory in either class I or class II cabinets. In addition, class II type A cabinets filter the supply air through the second HEPA filter, thus providing near-sterile air to the work surface. This feature completely excludes any need to use open flames under the hood. More details can be found in a special review on this subject (79).

Biosafety Level 3

BL-3 practices require containment facilities (26, 52, 61, 79). Other requirements, in addition to those for level II, are special laboratory clothing, controlled access, and biosafety cabinets for all manipulations of infectious materials. Personnel and the laboratory environment (primary containment) are protected by observation of standard laboratory practices and techniques, selection and proper use of appropriate safety equipment, and design of a safe and practical laboratory layout, including proper air handling (directional airflow). The laboratory director may designate the actual safeguards, but the safety of personnel must be placed ahead of other factors.

Safety Equipment

Proper design by itself is not enough to provide a safe environment in the mycobacteriology laboratory. Safety equipment must be appropriate for the mycobacteriology laboratory and must be used properly. It serves mainly to prevent the dissemination of bacterial aerosols. Biological safety cabinets equipped with HEPA filters are important pieces of equipment in the mycobacteriology laboratory. All centrifuges must be equipped with aerosol containment by having safety caps for each bucket. They should be placed in a dedicated (BL-3) room so that, in the event of a centrifuge accident or leak, the produced aerosol will be contained. Another piece of safety equipment is a heating plate, which replaces flaming for fixation of smears. Use of disposable (instead of metallic) loops is another example of equipment to prevent aerosol formation and cross-contamination. Practices for the use of syringes, pipettes, and dispensers must be designed to minimize the production of aerosols.

Safety Practices

The most important principle of biosafety in the mycobacteriology laboratory is observance of standard and special practices. Standard microbiological practices include restricted access to the laboratory, especially to the areas where work is in progress; decontamination of the work surfaces every day; prohibition of mouth pipetting; prohibition of eating, drinking, smoking, and applying cosmetics; and washing hands before leaving the laboratory.

In addition, special practices in the mycobacteriology laboratory include the following: doors of the rooms where the work is in progress must be closed; all manipulations with cultures or specimens should be done with gloved hands; and personnel should wear special clothing while handling infectious materials. Protective clothing (including gloves) should not be worn outside of the laboratory. A respirator program must be in place, with appropriate training of the employees. Wearing a respirator in BL-3 facility serves as an additional protective barrier, but "this option is offered as a thoughtful consideration and not a recommendation" (79).

Personnel working in the mycobacteriology laboratory should be skin tested and given chest X rays on a regular schedule. Tuberculin-positive persons should be trained to identify the disease symptoms. Systematic training of personnel in biosafety issues and policy updates, all of which should be documented in the laboratory safety manual, is a necessary task in a safe laboratory. The laboratory director is responsible for specific application of the general principles of biosafety and for selecting any additional measures needed in each individual situation.

Specimen and Culture Shipment

For the best possible turnaround time, specimens for the recovery of *M. tuberculosis* and other mycobacteria, especially from newly diagnosed patients, should be mailed to a specialized mycobacteriology laboratory. Specimens of sputum, blood, or stool can be shipped without ice or cooling systems. *M. tuberculosis* and other organisms capable of causing disease in humans are called infectious substances or etiologic agents and are recognized, along with diagnostic specimens that may contain these organisms, as hazardous materials. Transportation of these materials is subject to special regulations by U.S. government agencies for the U.S. Postal Service and by the International Air Transport Association (IATA) for shipments via overnight delivery private couriers (e.g., Federal Express, Airborne Express, DHL).

Shipments by the U.S. Postal Service must be First Class, Priority, or Express Mail. According to the CDC instructions (52), a culture or diagnostic specimen mailed through the U.S. Postal Service must be packaged to withstand leakage, shock, and pressure changes. The primary receptacle must be watertight to prevent leakage (for example, a screw-cap tube with a culture on solid medium, a 50-ml Falcon

tube with a specimen, a flame-sealed glass ampoule, or a BACTEC 12B vial). Note that for primary containers, which have a screw cap, the cap must be held in place by adhesive tape. Several primary receptacles, each individually wrapped to prevent contact between them, along with a sufficient amount of absorbent material, must be placed in a watertight secondary packaging container constructed of metal, corrugated fiberboard, or other material of equivalent strength. Each secondary container, along with the itemized list of contents, must be placed in an outer package that has appropriate labeling. The label "Etiologic Agent/Biomedical Material" or its equivalent "Infectious Substance" must be affixed to the outside packages containing cultures of any mycobacterial species.

For shipments by private couriers, IATA requires that material classified as an "Infectious Substance" be packaged in a United Nations (UN) container with specific labeling. This applies both to international shipment and to those handled within the United States. This UN-approved container should carry an "Infectious Substance Affecting Humans, UN 2814 Mycobacterial Species" label and should be accompanied by a Shipper's Declaration for Dangerous Goods form. Packages with diagnostic specimens that do not qualify as an "Infectious Substance" (under UN 3733), packaged to withstand pressure and shock without leaking, can be placed for overnight delivery into special envelopes provided by the private couriers, such as a "Lab Pack" from Airborne Express or "Diagnostic Specimen Envelope" and "Clinical Pak" from FedEx.

For more details about biosafety regulations for mycobacteriology laboratories, see the review by Richmond et al. from CDC (79).

SPECIMEN COLLECTION AS THE FIRST STEP OF THE DIAGNOSTIC PROCEDURES

Specimens should be collected in sterile disposable containers, with maximum precautions to avoid contamination with environmental mycobacteria or non-AFB. This is especially true for specimens originating from sterile sites.

Sputum

Early-morning expectorates of 5 to 10 ml each are preferable to a daily collection. The volume should not exceed 10 ml because a larger specimen would be difficult to process in the laboratory. Small volumes, especially less than 2 ml, may lower the probability of detection of mycobacteria. Specimen quality is especially important. The patient should be instructed on the difference between saliva and sputum. The sputum should be brought up by deep productive cough or, if necessary, after inhalation of a warm, sterile, aerosolized 10% sodium chloride solution. The laboratory should be informed of the type of sputum submitted, because, in some laboratories such watery specimens may be mistaken for saliva and rejected. The laboratory report to the physician should contain information about the volume and quality of the specimen submitted. When the specimen does not look like true sputum or the volume is small, the laboratory should request an additional or replacement specimen. More than three specimens may be necessary when the smear examination detects only a small number of AFB or if the AFB are not found in all three initial specimens. If the patient cannot produce real sputum, a collection of an alternative type of specimen should be considered (laryngeal swabs, bronchial brushings, or gastric lavage). If the collection takes place in a medical facility (hospital or clinic), the patient should be placed in a well-ventilated or isolated outdoor area. The cap of the specimen container should be tightened, and the surface of the container should be wiped with a tuberculocidal disinfectant.

Laryngeal Swabs, Bronchial Brushings, and Gastric Lavage Fluid

Laryngeal swabs, bronchial brushings, and gastric lavage fluid are useful when sputum is difficult to collect or when the patient swallows it. Bronchoscopy may stimulate sputum production for several consecutive days, during which specimens should be collected. Laryngeal swabs can be placed in a sterile tube to be delivered to the laboratory immediately. If the swab is to be mailed, it should be washed by being dipped into about 2 ml of sterile 7H9 broth or sterile saline in a screw cap tube, followed by intense swirling. The swab then can be removed and the cap can be tightened. To collect gastric washings, 20 to 50 ml of sterile distilled water should be passed into the stomach through a plastic tube and the specimen can be collected through the tube with a 50-ml syringe. If there is any delay in processing the specimen, it should be neutralized by adding a 40% solution of disodium phosphate, about 1 to 1.5 ml per 20 to 50 ml of lavage fluid. In cases where the use of phosphate buffer must be avoided, 100 mg of sodium carbonate per specimen may be substituted.

Stool

Stool specimens should not be larger than 10 ml and should be placed in sterile, disposable, 50-ml plastic centrifuge tubes. Before being mailed, the specimens should be handled in the same way as sputum specimens. Special attention should be given to immediate mailing; the specimen should be refrigerated if there is any delay in shipment. If the volume exceeds 10 ml or if the laboratory technician suspects that there has been accumulated pressure, the tube should be disposed of without opening.

Urine

A midstream urine specimen should be collected after the external genitalia have been washed. The urine specimen should be processed in a local laboratory.

Tissue

Small pieces of tissue obtained from biopsy or during autopsy should be transferred aseptically into sterile screw cap tubes containing liquid (7H9 broth or saline). After packaging, the specimen should be stored in a refrigerator until shipment. It should be mailed to the laboratory in a box with ice by special overnight mail.

Body Fluids (Except Blood)

Spinal, pleural, joint, and other normally sterile body fluids should be collected aseptically in 50-ml plastic tubes containing 7H9 broth, with 1 ml of specimen per 4 to 5 ml of the medium. An alternative is to inject up to 1 ml of a specimen into a 12B BACTEC vial or MGIT tube containing selective liquid medium. To increase the probability of recovery of mycobacteria, these tubes or vials should be incubated on arrival in the laboratory without prior processing. If AFB are found during the systematic examination of samples taken from these cultures, a subculture to other media will be made. This sometimes requires prior decontamination.

Blood and Bone Marrow

Blood is the primary specimen for the bacteriologic diagnosis of disseminated mycobacterial infections, primarily in HIV-positive patients, including those with AIDS. In areas with high prevalence of TB, tuberculosis can be the first manifestation of HIV infection. Other mycobacterial infections, especially with *M. avium*, may cause disseminated infection in patients with advanced AIDS. Isolation of mycobacteria from blood is considered sufficient for diagnosis, but determination of the intensity of bacteremia may be of value to monitor the patient's response to therapy in cases of *M. avium* infection. There are different options for collection of the blood specimens

(i) for detection of mycobacteria and (ii) for quantification of mycobacteria. For isolation only, 5 ml of blood is taken with a syringe at the bedside or at the physician's office and injected into a 13A BACTEC vial. The vial should be labeled properly, wrapped in paper towel, and placed in a durable leak-proof secondary container with enough absorbent material to absorb the liquid if the vial breaks.

Other options can be more suitable for quantitative blood cultures. Blood can be collected in special Isolator tubes or Vacutainers containing sodium polyanethol sulfate (SPS) from Becton-Dickinson (Sparks, Md.). Either of these tubes, after being labeled, can be placed in a 50-ml plastic centrifuge tube, a combination that comprises a safe type of primary container (primary receptacle). At the National Jewish Center in Denver, we prefer SPS-containing Vacutainers over the Isolator tubes, for several reasons (87). First, there is less blood cell debris after processing a specimen from a Vacutainer, which allows better colony counts on agar plates. Second, inhibition of growth was observed in 12B BACTEC medium inoculated with a specimen from an Isolator tube (B. Wasilauskas and R. Morrel, Abstr. *93rd Gen. Meet Am. Soc. Microbiol.* 1993, abstr. U-78, 1993), whereas no such inhibition occurred with a specimen from the SPS-containing Vacutainer (87). Finally, the Vacutainer tubes are much less expensive.

See other reviews for more details on specimen collection and their primary processing in the laboratory (34, 52, 102).

SMEAR EXAMINATION AND CULTURE ISOLATION

Specimen Processing

On arrival in the laboratory, most specimens are homogenized with a mucolytic agent, but tissues and similar specimens may be ground in disposable homogenizers. Specimens from nonsterile sites (e.g., sputum) must be treated to kill contaminating organisms that may be present. Mycobacteria resist the bactericidal action of selected chemicals that kill contaminating bacteria; however, because even the mildest agents reduce the number of viable tubercle bacilli, all procedures must be carried out as quickly and as gently as possible to preserve viable bacilli (52). Many agents or combinations such as zephiran-trisodium phosphate, Petroff's sodium hydroxide, oxalic acid, sulfuric acid, and cetylpyridinium chloride-sodium chloride have been used for digestion and decontamination of specimens; however, the N-acetyl-L-cysteine–sodium hydroxide method is preferred in most laboratories in the United States (60,

62). Current descriptions of the method (52, 85) are basically unchanged from the original.

It is still traditional in many laboratories to perform specimen processing under BL-2 conditions. There are a number of reasons, some which have recently emerged, to switch to BL-3 practices. Among them are (i) increasing probability of dealing with specimens containing MDR strains, (ii) increasing probability that the specimens may contain HIV, (iii) necessity of processing tissue specimens by the grinding procedure that has the potential of creating aerosols (in this case, using proper masks should be mandatory), and (iv) the possibility of cross-contamination. Special mention is necessary regarding the prevention of cross-contamination occurrences in clinical laboratories, leading sometimes to a false diagnosis of tuberculosis (38). Implementation of BL-3 practices alone is not enough to prevent such events. It is necessary that each laboratory design its own specific protocol addressing this issue. One of the most important elements of such a protocol should be the use of aliquots of all reagent solutions mentioned above corresponding to the number of specimens to be processed. The laboratory manual should also include a description of circumstances when cross-contamination should be suspected and of the measures to be taken for confirmation or exclusion of such an occurrence.

Staining and Smear Examination

Procedures for smear preparation and staining, as well as the theoretical background of the stain reactions, are described elsewhere (52). Smears may be made directly from untreated specimens or from concentrated specimens. If a smear is made directly from sputum, areas that are most likely to contain mycobacteria, i.e., cheesy necrotic particles, or areas that are tinged with blood, should be selected. Smears of concentrates prepared as directed above are most often used when the specimen is to be cultured. If it is not cultured, an alternative to the direct smear is to add an equal volume of a 5% hypochlorite solution such as a common household bleach for a few minutes to kill bacilli before making the smear (93). However, when the hypochlorite method is used, two steps become critical to obtain good results—centrifugation at a speed sufficient to achieve $3,000 \times g$ and timing to prevent degradation of the AFB. Because quality control of these critical steps is required, the hypochlorite method may not be optimal for many laboratories. Generally, the smear can be considered noninfectious only after staining. The acid-fast staining procedure depends on the ability of mycobacteria and some other microorganisms to retain dye even when treated with mineral acid or an acid-alcohol solution. The procedure may involve application of heat or inclusion of a surfactant to allow penetration of the dye into the cell. Two procedures, those using the Ziehl-Neelsen stain and the auramine O fluorescence acid-fast stain, are the most widely used (Color Plates 2 and 3).

To avoid false-positive smear results, it is important that the slides placed on a rack for staining should have enough space between them to prevent overflow of the staining solutions and reagents. Carbol fuchsin-stained smears cannot be considered negative until the microscopy technician has examined a minimum of 100 oil immersion fields (some authorities recommend 300 fields). The smear must be examined in a standard manner, which is best accomplished by making three sweeps along its longest dimension. Alternatively, nine sweeps may be made along the narrowest dimension. Because auramine-stained slides can be screened at a lower magnification ($\times 250$ or $\times 400$), fewer fields may be read before the smear is considered negative. Reports of the results of smear examination should include a measure of quantity, such as actual number of bacilli seen per field or a 1+ to 4+ rating, which roughly estimates the same numbers (99). A graded smear is useful to the clinician for monitoring the results of therapy and for estimating the condition of the patient. Between 5×10^3 and 1×10^4 AFB per ml of sputum must be present to be detected by microscopy. Specimens that contain only three or fewer AFB in 100 oil immersion fields are considered doubtful and should be retested.

A sputum smear positive for AFB may represent either *M. tuberculosis* or some NTM. In conjunction with clinical and radiological data indicating that the patient has tuberculosis, the report of a positive smear result should trigger a number of prevention and control steps. Therefore, it is suggested that the results of the acid-fast stain be reported to the physician or clinic within 24 h of specimen collection (99).

Smear examination as a primary tool for case detection and tuberculosis diagnosis is one of five elements of the DOTS strategy introduced by the WHO and incorporated into national TB control programs in many countries. The purpose of this approach is to ensure detection of most infectious cases with minimal cost, which is essential for low-income developing countries that do not have any tuberculosis laboratory facilities and cannot afford them in the foreseeable future. On the other hand, acceptance of direct smear examination as the only diagnostic tool (rather than diagnosis of tuberculosis by culture), supposedly a prerequisite of DOTS implementation, is often a reflection of a misunderstanding of the DOTS strategy. The well-known fact that smears are positive in fewer than 50% of culture-positive sputum specimens in new tuberculosis patients should be taken into account. This rate is even lower (down to 30%) in patients who are coinfected with HIV and/or if only direct microscopy (without concentration) combined with light microscopy is being used. It is clear, on the other hand, that culture isolation cannot be recommended for laboratories that do not have proper biosafety protocols and equipment (for example, aerosol-contained centrifuges). Therefore, in middle-income countries that already have trained personnel and tuberculosis laboratories, emphasis should not be on abandoning culture isolation but, rather, should be on upgrading (and probably reorganizing) of the tuberculosis laboratories to make them more efficient and safe. It is especially important in areas with high prevalence of drug-resistance.

Primary Isolation of *M. tuberculosis*

Historically, the egg-based media, such as Löwenstein-Jensen, Ogawa, and American Trudeau Society media, were the best-known media for isolation of *M. tuberculosis*. The agar-based media (21, 65, 66) allow a more rapid recovery of growth (within 2 to 4 weeks) and offer a better opportunity to study colony morphology than the egg-based media do. Selective 7H10 or 7H11 agar, containing four antibiotics, inhibits the growth of nonmycobacterial contaminants, some of which may survive digestion-decontamination (64).

Liquid medium can be used for primary isolation of *M. tuberculosis* from sputum if it is a selective medium. The first medium of this type introduced for wide practical application was Middlebrook 7H12 broth (67) manufactured as BACTEC 12B vials by Becton Dickinson for radiometric detection of growth in the BACTEC 460 system. Five antimicrobial agents, under the acronym PANTA, are added to this medium to prevent the growth of nonmycobacterial contaminants. Growth of *M. tuberculosis* on this medium can usually be detected within 1 to 2 weeks, depending on the number of bacteria in the specimen. Isolation of mycobacteria in liquid media, used along with solid media, is dictated by the necessity for shortening the turnaround time for culture growth detection and other subsequent laboratory reports. Until recently, only one automated system—the BACTEC-460 system—was available for isolation of mycobacteria in a liquid medium. Its introduction changed laboratory protocols dramatically and allowed a relatively rapid diagnosis of tuberculosis and drug susceptibility testing. The main shortcoming of this system is the problem of disposal of its radioactive waste, the 12B vials containing [^{14}C]palmitic acid in 7H12 broth.

A number of suggestions were made to resolve this problem. One of them is the use of the Septi-Chek MB biphasic system (BBL, Becton Dickinson), in which each unit contains both liquid and solid media (46, 49, 101). The major problem is that it is not an automated system and hence requires substantial labor costs; its application therefore may be most suitable for lower-volume laboratories. A number of other suggestions were made to expedite isolation and drug susceptibility testing, for example, the microcolony method on thinly poured 7H10 agar plates (109), Redox tubes with liquid medium, and the MGIT (Mycobacterial Growth Indicator Tube) manual system, etc. These and other similar methods are nearly as effective as the BACTEC-460 system as regards turnaround time, but being nonautomated, they are suitable only for laboratories dealing with a small number of mycobacterial cultures (43).

One of the first nonradioactive automated systems was the MB/BacT (now BacT/Alert) microbial detection system from Organon-Teknika Corp. (now BioMérieux Inc., Durham, N.C.), employing broth with growth supplements and antibiotic agents. Bottles contain a colorimetric sensor reacting to the carbon dioxide production by the growing bacteria, which changes the color of the sensor from dark green to bright yellow in the growing culture. Growth is monitored by an integrated computer.

The ESP culture system from Trek Diagnostic Systems (Cleveland, Ohio) also employs a modified 7H9 broth with supplements and drugs. Detection of growth in this system is based on the consumption of oxygen by the growing bacteria. The negative pressure created in the bottle is recorded by the computer and printed.

The BACTEC 9000 TB system from Becton Dickinson employs BACTEC MycoF sputum culture vials containing modified 7H9 broth with antimicrobial agents. Each vial has a fluorescence sensor that reacts to the depletion of oxygen dissolved in the broth by the growing mycobacteria. The instrument is computerized, and the growth is detected and documented.

The same manufacturer has developed a new automated system, BACTEC 960, which employs 7-ml volumes of broth in an MGIT system. The bottom of each tube contains an oxygen-sensitive fluorescent indicator embedded in silicone. Consumption of oxygen by the growing bacteria results in fluorescence of the indicator, which is detected by exposure to UV lights in the instrument and recorded by the computer. This compact high-capacity system is currently gaining popularity in many countries, replacing the BACTEC-460.

According to our experience, a combination of four units of medium is optimal for primary isolation of mycobacteria from a processed sputum specimen. One of them is the liquid selective medium. National Jewish Medical and Research Center uses the BACTEC 12B vial, which is inoculated with 0.5 ml of concentrated specimen. The California Microbial Diseases Laboratory uses MGIT broth medium. Along with the liquid medium, both laboratories use a biplate containing plain and selective 7H11 agar, which is inoculated with 0.2 ml of the specimen on each side. The latter serves as a backup when digestion-decontamination of the specimen does not prevent the nonmycobacterial contaminants from growing in 12B vials or on plain 7H11 agar. Middlebrook agar plates offer the possibility of microscopic examination of colony morphologies, allowing early detection of mixed cultures and sometimes giving tentative information about which mycobacterial species might be present. The Löwenstein-Jensen slant, inoculated with 0.1 ml, serves as a backup for rare *M. tuberculosis* strains that may not grow on the other three media and is useful for storage or mailing of cultures. Inoculated tubes with solid media are incubated in a slanted position with the tube's screw cap loosened for at least the first week at 35 to 37°C in an atmosphere of 10% CO_2 and 90% air. The plates containing agar media are placed in CO_2-permeable polyethylene bags for incubation in CO_2 incubators. If no growth is detected in the liquid medium and on agar plates during the 6 weeks of incubation, the final report that the specimen is culture negative can be issued only after 8 weeks of incubation of the Löwenstein-Jensen slants.

METHODS FOR IDENTIFICATION OF *M. TUBERCULOSIS*

Differentiating Members of the *M. tuberculosis* Complex

Detection of AFB in a sputum smear in conjunction with certain clinical symptoms and X-ray findings leads to the suspicion of tuberculosis, the initiation of public health measures, and the start of therapy as early as 24 h after the sputum specimen was obtained from the patient. The AFB smear was an important tool in the past, but the current epidemiological situation, at least in industrialized countries, has greatly diminished its diagnostic value. It is now recognized that an AFB-positive smear is not sufficient evidence for the bacteriological diagnosis of tuberculosis. The probability that the AFB seen in a sputum smear represents *M. tuberculosis* depends on the frequency with which the laboratory isolates various

NTM. With the increasing rates of tuberculosis among HIV-infected persons, who frequently develop extrapulmonary tuberculosis, sputum may not be available, and specimens from other sources are frequently submitted for mycobacterial isolation. Additionally, HIV-infected persons may be coinfected with *M. avium* complex or other NTM.

Differentiation of *M. tuberculosis* from other mycobacteria represents an important health issue, since only tuberculosis is transmissible from person to person. To expedite the answer to the question ("TB or not TB"), the laboratory must rely on such methods as one of the amplification techniques, nucleic hybridization tests, DNA sequencing of the 16S ribosomal gene, or mycolic acid analysis using high-pressure liquid chromatography (HPLC) with a positive broth culture. Any of these tests, with a high level of sensitivity and specificity, tells whether the organism belongs to the *M. tuberculosis* complex, which includes five species— *M. tuberculosis*, *M. bovis* (and BCG), *M. canetti*, *M. africanum*, and *M. microti*. Therefore, differentiation of *M. tuberculosis* from other species of the complex requires further procedures.

Rarely, some of the NTM cause a false-positive signal for *M. tuberculosis*, even with the highly specific nucleic acid probes or HPLC analysis, requiring confirmation of *M. tuberculosis* by the conventional methods. Preliminary identification of *M. tuberculosis* complex in most laboratories can be reported for most isolates within 2 to 3 weeks of receipt of the specimen when DNA probes or HPLC are used with a broth culture. Final identification of *M. tuberculosis* by a few biochemical tests requires 2 weeks or more (Table 1). In the United States, other members of the complex are rarely found in human specimens. BCG is usually isolated as the result of BCG vaccine treatment of malignant tumors. Therefore, a patient's history can be helpful in alerting the laboratory that the isolate may not be *M. tuberculosis*. *M. bovis* usually grows poorly on agar media and produces dysgonic colonies on egg-based media, sometimes showing a wet surface rather than a dry one. HPLC analysis can be useful in the differentiation between *M. bovis* and *M. bovis* BCG. The growth of *M. bovis* on 7H11 agar can be improved if the medium is prepared without glycerol and contains 0.4% pyruvate (23). Despite the rare occurrence of members of the complex other than *M. tuberculosis* in the United States, it is necessary to confirm, for epidemiological and other reasons, whether an *M. tuberculosis* complex isolate is *M. tuberculosis* or *M. bovis*. Practically, a laboratory report that the isolate belongs to the *M. tuberculosis* complex is sufficient to justify immediate public health measures and to start therapy, which can be adjusted later in the rare occasions when the isolate is *M. bovis*. Two to three weeks is a reasonable period for identification of *M. tuberculosis* complex if specimens have been submitted to a laboratory that uses a liquid medium system (among others) for primary isolation and is properly equipped to perform DNA probe tests or HPLC analysis with a broth culture. Use of amplification techniques, such as the MTD test (*M. tuberculosis* direct test), (GenProbe, San Diego, Calif.) or a PCR test for *M. tuberculosis*, may shorten this period to a few days, but some additional procedures can help obtain, in very short periods, data indicating whether the growing culture is *M. tuberculosis* rather than one of the NTM. One such tool is examination of a smear made from broth to detect the cording typical of *M. tuberculosis* but not typical of other mycobacteria (except *M. kansasii*). However, the lack of cording does not necessarily exclude *M. tuberculosis*, since some strains produce cords only after prolonged incubation. These data cannot be used for precise bacteriological diagnosis but can help in making decisions about necessary preventive and treatment measures.

Nontuberculous Mycobacteria

More than 60 mycobacterial species other than *M. tuberculosis* can be found in specimens from humans. It is not the aim of this chapter to address the features of these organisms or the methods of deter-

Table 1. Differentiation among the members of the *M. tuberculosis* complex

Species	Result[a] in following test:						
	Niacin	Nitrate reduction	Catalase (68°C)	Pyrazinamidase	Urease	Tween hydrolysis 10d	Susceptibility to TCH
M. tuberculosis	Pos	Pos	Neg/Pos	Pos	Pos/Neg	Neg/Pos	Res
M. bovis (including BCG)	Neg	Neg	Neg	Neg	Pos/Neg	Neg/Pos	Susc
M. africanum	Pos/Neg	Neg	Neg	Pos	Pos	Neg	Variable
M. microti	Pos/Neg	Neg	Neg/Pos	Pos	Pos/Neg	Neg/Pos	Variable

[a]Pos, positive; neg, negative; res, resistant; susc, susceptible.

mining their species, descriptions of which can be found in specialized reviews (40, 111, 113).

Rapid Identification Methods

Techniques such as nucleic acid amplification and sequencing of 16S rDNA, which can be used for rapid identification of *M. tuberculosis* and NTM, are addressed elsewhere in this book. We present here a short description only of the procedures more commonly used in clinical laboratories: cell wall lipid (mycolic acid) analysis by HPLC and the use of DNA probes.

Cell wall lipid analysis

Three chromatographic methods have been proposed for the determination of mycobacterial species on the basis of their cell wall lipids: gas-liquid chromatography, HPLC, and thin-layer chromatography. Of these approaches, HPLC is now the most popular in clinical mycobacteriology (13, 14, 30, 33, 100). HPLC uses a liquid mobile phase at high pressure to carry a sample through a column packed with a particulate material-stationary phase, in which separation into components takes place (13–15). Mycolic acids extracted from saponified mycobacterial cells are converted to the *p*-bromophenacyl esters, and the characteristic mycolic acid pattern associated with each species is detected by chromatographic separation of the esters. The analysis is based on a comparison of retention time of the peaks and their height ratios. A recent review of HPLC in mycobacteriology describes 63 chromatographic patterns representative of 73 known mycobacterial species that may, as the authors stated, help laboratory personnel in the visual interpretation of such patterns for species determination (15).

The HPLC method was implemented by the CDC in many state laboratories in the 1990s. The major problem was that HPLC, which is based on UV spectrophotometry to separate the ester peaks, required a large harvest of bacteria. Subsequently, it was reported that a combination of HPLC with fluorescence detection made the method much more sensitive, so that the AFB-positive BACTEC broth cultures can be used instead of a large harvest from solid media for identification of *M. tuberculosis* and *M. avium* (51). This may decrease the turnaround time to 10 to 14 days, which makes the method comparable to the BACTEC NAP (*p*-nitro-α-acetylamino-β-hydroxypropiophenone; Becton Dickinson) and AccuProbe (GenProbe) tests. The sensitivity of this method for detection of mycobacteria directly in sputum specimens was suboptimal since it showed only 33.3 and 56.8% positivity for *M. avium* and *M. tuber-*

culosis, respectively, in AFB-positive specimens (51). However, when a characteristic HPLC pattern is observed in a specimen from sputum sediment, it is possible to report identification of mycobacteria belonging to these complexes. For more details on cell wall lipid analysis methods, see the reviews by Roberts et al. (84) and by Butler and Guthertz (15).

Nucleic acid probes

AccuProbe DNA hybridization tests are commonly used for identification of *M. tuberculosis* complex, *M. avium* complex, *M. avium*, *M. intracellulare*, *M. kansasii*, and *M. gordonae*. The test employs a chemiluminescent acridinium ester-labeled single-stranded DNA probe complementary to the rDNA for the target bacteria. Association of the two strands forms a stable hybrid. Chemiluminescence is developed by the addition of hydrogen peroxide and is measured in a luminometer (5). The test can be done with cultures grown on solid or in liquid media. With most clinical isolates, a minimum of 3 weeks on 7H11 agar plates and about 10 days in a liquid medium is required to achieve growth sufficient for this test. If the test with the *M. tuberculosis* probe is positive, the results are reported as *M. tuberculosis* complex because this probe does not distinguish between *M. tuberculosis* and other members of the complex. Such a report is sufficient for timely public health actions and appropriate treatment decisions. From a practical standpoint, this identification is almost final for patients in the United States because the probability of *M. bovis* and *M. africanum* infections is very low. Nevertheless, final identification to the species level is necessary for epidemiological reasons and because one of the first-line drugs, pyrazinamide, should not be included in the treatment regimen if the isolate is *M. bovis*. Because *M. africanum* and *M. tuberculosis* appear to have indistinguishable epidemiology and both generally are treatable by pyrazinamide, there may be no compelling reason to differentiate between these species on a routine basis. Differentiation between *M. tuberculosis* and *M. bovis* can be accomplished by the four tests mentioned previously—niacin production, nitrate reduction, pyrazinamide, and susceptibility to thiophe-2-carboxylic acid hydrazide (TCH) (Table 1)—or, if available, by molecular methods such as spoligotyping or genomic deletion analysis.

Amplification methods

A number of amplification methods, both in-house assays and commercial systems, have been developed for detection and identification of mycobacteria (particularly *M. tuberculosis*) directly in the patient's specimen (24, 27, 50, 73, 89, 91, 95, 96, 105). Three of these systems are most familiar to those working in clinical mycobacteriology laboratories: Amplicor MTB, a PCR assay by Roche Molecular Systems (Branchburg, N.J.); MTD (Gen-Probe); and ProbeTec Direct TB, a strand displacement amplification (SDA) test by Becton-Dickinson. Detailed descriptions of the amplification methods can be found in chapter 6 of this book. We would like to stress here that the amplification tests are found to be most useful for testing body fluids from sterile sites (especially cerebrospinal fluid) and for rapid differentiation between *M. tuberculosis* and NTM in smear-positive sputum specimens, so that necessary actions, including patient isolation and treatment, can be effectively limited to new tuberculosis patients. In cases of doubtful negative results with smear-negative sputum specimens, such testing can be repeated with broth cultures at the earliest possible detection of growth (22).

Nucleic acid sequencing

The rapidly progressing methodology of nucleic acid sequencing is very useful in the accurate identification of the NTM species, mostly on the basis of the 16S rDNA sequencing (47, 54, 55, 86). The details of this method can be found in chapter 6 of this book.

Conventional Identification Tests

M. tuberculosis colonies grow on 7H10 or 7H11 agar plates in 2 to 3 weeks during incubation at 35 to 37°C, while no growth appears at 25, 32, or 42°C. The buff-colored colonies are always nonpigmented, have a rough, dry surface and irregular edges, and often have a wrinkled surface. It is typical to find serpentine cording in smears made from a broth culture (Color Plate 3). Results of four tests may be used for final identification of *M. tuberculosis* and its differentiation from *M. bovis*: positive niacin production, positive nitrate reduction, resistance to 5 μg of the thiophene-2-carboxylic acid hydrazide (TCH) per ml incorporated into 7H11 agar, and positive pyrazinamidase test (Table 1). The results of these four tests are reversed for *M. bovis*.

A negative heat-stable catalase test and production of a <45-mm column of foam in the room temperature catalase test are also important for final identification, but they do not differentiate between *M. tuberculosis* and *M. bovis*. The niacin test is negative for some *M. tuberculosis* strains, especially those resistant to isoniazid. The same applies to the nitrate reduction test. The pyrazinamidase test with *M. tuberculosis* can be negative if the patient has

been treated with pyrazinamide (PZA) and resistance to this agent has developed. In addition, false-negative results with any of these tests may appear owing to the quite common deviation from the prescribed technique. Laboratories that perform the PZA susceptibility test (for example, in BACTEC-460) use this procedure first to differentiate between *M. tuberculosis* and *M. bovis* and perform other tests if the isolate is resistant to PZA.

Niacin test

Formerly the niacin test was relied on for identification of *M. tuberculosis* (53, 58, 115), but the advent of rapid methods has greatly diminished its value. It should be recognized that the niacin test can be positive with some mycobacterial species other than *M. tuberculosis*, such as *M. simiae*; some BCG strains; and some rapidly growing mycobacteria. Many laboratories use 3- to 4-week old cultures grown on Middlebrook 7H10 or 7H11 agar, and the test works well in most cases. However, some *M. tuberculosis* strains do not produce sufficient niacin on this medium for detection. The frequency of these false-negative results can be decreased if the agar medium is enriched with L-asparagine (0.25%) or its potassium salt (0.1%). False-negative results can be almost completely eliminated by using 6-week-old or older cultures on Löwenstein-Jensen medium inoculated with raw specimen. This can serve as a backup if results with the agar-grown culture after 3 weeks of cultivation are negative. The presence of some contaminants in the culture may cause false-positive results; therefore, it is necessary to confirm the purity of the culture by examining a smear stained by the Ziehl-Neelsen method.

Nitrate reduction test

The second most important test for identifying *M. tuberculosis*, and particularly for differentiating it from *M. bovis* if the isolate already has been identified as *M. tuberculosis* complex, is the nitrate reduction test (59, 76, 104). Besides *M. tuberculosis*, other species (*M. kansasii*, *M. szulgai*, *M. flavescens*, *M. fortuitum*, *M. terrae*, *M. triviale*, *M. phlei*, *M. smegmatis*, and *M. vaccae*) produce nitrate reductase. The test is negative with *M. bovis* but can be weakly positive with some BCG strains. Like the niacin test, the best results are obtained with a culture grown on egg-based medium at least 4 weeks old, but it can be done with a culture on agar medium if the growth is sufficient. Two techniques are commonly used, one with liquid reagents and another with commercially available paper strips (76).

Pyrazinamidase test

The pyrazinamidase test detects the presence of the enzyme that converts PZA to pyrazinoic acid (107). Pyrazinamidase can be found in cultures of *M. tuberculosis* strains susceptible to PZA, but PZA-resistant *M. tuberculosis* strains do not possess detectable amounts of the enzyme. All *M. bovis* strains including BCG are resistant to PZA; therefore, this drug is not used in therapy of *M. bovis* infection and the organism shows negative results in the pyrazinamidase test. This test, as well as the PZA susceptibility test (described in another section of this chapter), is useful for differentiation between *M. tuberculosis* and *M. bovis*. Positive results confirm *M. tuberculosis,* while a negative test suggests *M. bovis*. One must be alert to negative reactions with *M. tuberculosis* strains resistant to PZA that were isolated from patients previously treated with this drug. *M. africanum* is susceptible to PZA and is positive in the pyrazinamidase test. All NTM are resistant to PZA, but some of them are pyrazinamidase positive (*M. marinum, M. avium, M. intracellulare, M. xenopi, M. malmoense,* and *M. flavescens*), and some are negative (*M. kansasii, M. simiae, M. szulgai,* and *M. gastri*). Therefore, this test can be used for differentiation between some of these species, for example, between *M. kansasii* and *M. marinum*.

TCH susceptibility

The test for susceptibility to TCH (12, 103) is especially useful for differentiation between *M. bovis* and MDR strains of *M. tuberculosis*, since these strains can produce negative results in the three other differentiation tests described above. Only *M. bovis* strains (including BCG) are susceptible to 1.0 and 5.0 μg of TCH per ml incorporated into Middlebrook 7H10 or 7H11 agar medium. This test is performed in the same way as an indirect susceptibility test, and all mycobacterial species other than *M. bovis* produce growth in the presence of TCH that greatly exceeds the required 1% in comparison with that in the drug-free medium. Some strains of *M. bovis* may produce minimal growth in the presence of 1.0 μg of TCH per ml but no growth in the presence of 5.0 μg/ml.

Heat-stable catalase test

The heat-stable (68°C) catalase test (at pH 7.0) aids in the identification of *M. tuberculosis* complex (52) but plays no role in differentiating *M. tuberculosis* from *M. bovis*, since both species produce negative results. The test is also negative for *M. gastri* and *M. malmoense* and is useful for differentiating between these species and other slowly growing nonchromogenic mycobacteria.

DRUG SUSCEPTIBILITY TESTING FOR DETECTION OF INITIAL AND ACQUIRED DRUG RESISTANCE

The growing prevalence of MDR tuberculosis around the world places the importance of *M. tuberculosis* drug susceptibility testing (DST), especially for initial clinical isolates, in a new perspective. An alternative to the detection of MDR tuberculosis by a laboratory test is an empirical assumption based on the patient's failure to respond to the standard treatment regimen. Such an option lacks accuracy, and it can be dangerous and costly. It can be dangerous for individual patients, who may receive inappropriate treatment, and it is costly for society because of the prolonged period during which a patient infected with MDR tuberculosis is infectious. Management of patients infected with MDR tuberculosis, even if their numbers are still small, can be much more expensive than the cost of DST of the initial isolates from all new patients.

The DST system is most likely to be economically affordable if it is based on direct delivery of raw specimens to a central mycobacteriology laboratory that has a large operational volume, has well trained personnel, and is properly equipped (28, 39).

The main requirement for DST is the ability to make a distinction between susceptible and resistant *M. tuberculosis* strains. This distinction can be reliably achieved by a traditional strategy based on cultivation, because *M. tuberculosis* isolates from patients never before treated are quite uniform in the degree of their susceptibility, as evidenced by the relatively narrow ranges of the MICs of the conventional antituberculosis drugs (41, 42). The classical definition of a drug-resistant strain of *M. tuberculosis* is that it is significantly different, in its degree of susceptibility, from a wild-type strain that has never come into contact with the drug (16, 17). The drug concentrations used to distinguish between susceptible and resistant strains, the so-called "critical concentrations," should be somewhere between the highest MIC found among the wild-type strains and the lowest MIC found among the isolates considered resistant. Progress in molecular biology may provide a new definition of drug resistance but also may raise new questions to be addressed, especially considering that resistance to some drugs has more than one genetic mechanism responsible for low and high levels of resistance (98). It should also be taken into account that phenotypic differences in the degree of resistance may reflect differences in the proportions of resistant mutants in the bacterial population.

Different methods for *M. tuberculosis* drug susceptibility testing, as well as their advantages and disadvantages, have been discussed in detail in our previous review (39). Newer molecular biology-based methods for detection of mutations associated with drug resistance offer several advantages over the conventional phenotypic methods. Among them are (i) speed (results may be available in a matter of hours or days); (ii) better reproducibility, especially in cases of low-level resistance; and (iii) ability to work with poorly growing and/or mixed cultures. These methods are addressed in chapter 8.

Classical phenotypic methods, which involve culturing mycobacteria in the presence of drugs under standardized conditions to detect inhibition of growth, offer several advantages. These methods are less expensive, which makes them more affordable in resource-limited settings. Clinical trials performed in the past have established the clinical relevance of results obtained by phenotypic methods for some primary drugs in predicting treatment success or failure. Phenotypic methods allow the detection of drug resistance regardless of mechanism or molecular basis, which may be important in cases when mechanisms of drug resistance are not known and when present knowledge may change over time. In addition, phenotypic methods are not affected by some mutations that may not cause drug resistance.

DST methods based on mycobacterial cultivation on solid media, either egg or agar based, can be performed as direct or indirect tests. In the direct test, a set of drug-containing and drug-free media is inoculated directly with a concentrated specimen. An indirect test involves inoculation of the media with a pure culture and is classically performed with a bacterial suspension made from growth on solid media (Löwenstein-Jensen slant; 7H10 or 7H11 agar). A 7H9 broth culture can be used for the same purpose when it is grown up to the turbidity of a McFarland standard 1 (5 to 8 days), and two dilutions, 10^{-3} and 10^{-5}, are then used as inocula for agar plates with critical concentrations of drugs or drug-free control media. For 7H12 broth cultures as a source of the inoculum, dilutions of 10^{-2} and 10^{-4} can be used when the daily radiometric growth index reaches 800 or higher.

The advantage of the direct tests over the indirect tests is that the results are available sooner (within 3 weeks on agar plates) and better represent the patient's original bacterial population. If the results of the direct test are not valid because there is insufficient or excessive growth in drug-free controls or heavy contamination, the test must be repeated with a pure culture, i.e., as an indirect test.

Antimicrobial agents to be incorporated into culture medium should be obtained in pure forms from the manufacturer (not from the pharmacy). Appropriate stock solutions of the drugs should be made in accordance with the batch potency provided by the manufacturer. For example, if 25 ml of a stock solution of 10,000 µg/ml is needed and the drug has a potency of 940 mg/g (or 940 µg/mg), the following amount of drug powder is to be weighed and dissolved in 25 ml of the solvent: 10,000 µg/ml × 25 ml × 1 mg/940 µg = 265.96 mg. The diluent appropriate for each drug is indicated by the drug manufacturer or can be found listed in the Merck Index. For example, distilled water is recommended for isoniazid (INH), streptomycin, *p*-aminosalicylic acid (PAS), kanamycin, amikacin, capreomycin, ethambutol, ofloxacin, and PZA. Rifampin should be dissolved in methanol, dimethyl sulfoxide, or 95% ethanol. Ethionamide and thiacetazone can be dissolved in ethylene glycol (analytical grade) or in dimethyl sulfoxide. The stock solutions of the water-soluble drugs should be sterilized through a 0.45-µm-pore-size membrane filter. Aliquots of the stock solutions should be kept in special vials at either −70°C for up to 12 months or −20°C for not more than 2 months. When needed, one of these vials can be used to prepare the working solutions in sterile distilled water. After being thawed, the stock solution vial must not be refrozen. On the other hand, it has been reported that INH, ethambutol, ethionamide, and kanamycin are stable in the refrigerator in solutions for up to 1 year (32).

Testing on Solid Medium

Three methods were originally suggested by the WHO panel for starch-free Löwenstein-Jensen medium: the proportion method, the resistance ratio method, and the absolute-concentration method (16, 17). The main characteristics of these methods are summarized in our recent reviews (39, 42), and in this chapter we limit the description to the two methods most widely used in the United States. The first is the direct or indirect test using 7H10 or 7H11 agar. The disadvantage of this method is that cultivation on 7H10 or 7H11 agar requires an incubator that can provide 5 to 10% CO_2 and the plates should be sealed in CO_2-permeable polyethylene bags after inoculation. The advantage of performing tests on agar plates is that the final results can be reported within 3 weeks instead of 4 to 6 weeks or more, as required using Löwenstein-Jensen medium. The CDC recommends that the test be performed on 7H10 agar (52), with the drug concentrations shown in Table 2. The 7H10 or 7H11 agar medium is usually made from

Table 2. Critical concentrations for *M. tuberculosis* in different media

Drug	Critical concn (µg/ml) of drug in:			
	LJ[a] (proportion method)	7H10 agar	7H11 agar	BACTEC 7H12[b]
INH	0.2	0.2,1.0[c]	0.2,1.0[c]	0.1
Rifampin	40.0	1.0	1.0	0.5
Rifapentine		0.5	0.5	0.5
Streptomycin	4.0	2.0	2.0	4.0
PZA	100.0[d]			300.0[e]
Ethambutol	2.0	5.0	7.5	4.0
Ethionamide	20.0	5.0	10.0	2.5
Kanamycin	20.0	5.0	10.0	5.0
Amikacin			4.0	5.0
Capreomycin	20.0	10.0	10.0	5.0
Thiacetazone				3.0
PAS	0.5	2.0	8.0	
Cycloserine		20.0	60.0	
Ofloxacin			4.0	2.0
Ciprofloxacin			4.0	2.0

[a]LJ, Löwenstein-Jensen medium.
[b]Concentrations in use at the National Jewish Medical and Research Center.
[c]Values are for detecting low and high levels of resistance.
[d]At pH 5.5.
[e]At pH 6.0.

a commercially available Middlebrook 7H10 agar base. Laboratories which perform agar proportion drug susceptibility testing must be aware that significant lot-to-lot differences have been observed for oleate-albumin-dextrose-catalase (OADC). Parallel testing with each new lot of OADC is recommended before it is accepted for use. Each flask of the medium is used to prepare either a drug-free control or one of the drug-containing media. The appropriate working solutions of the drugs, made from an aliquot of the stock solution, are added to ensure the final concentrations indicated in Table 2. The contents of each flask are distributed to one of the quadrants in a set of sterile quadrant plates, about 5.0 ml per quadrant, one quadrant for drug-free medium and the other three for media containing drugs. Two plates (each with a drug-free quadrant) are necessary for a test with four first-line drugs, and four plates are needed for a test with 10 drugs. After a sterility check, the plates are stored protected from light in the refrigerator and must be used within 6 weeks of preparation.

For each strain, two identical sets of plates are used, one inoculated with 10^{-3} and the other with 10^{-5} dilutions of the bacterial suspension (if it is an indirect test), adjusted to the optical density of the McFarland standard no. 1, 0.1 ml per quadrant. The plates are incubated for 3 weeks at 35 to 37°C in an atmosphere of 10% CO_2. The results can be reported earlier if they show that the strain is "resistant." The percentage of resistant bacteria in the population is reported on the basis of comparison of the number of CFU on the drug-containing and drug-free quadrants. More details on this technique can be found in the CDC manual (52).

Another technique can be used when a small number of cultures have to be tested (31, 108). Drug-impregnated disks are placed aseptically into the centers of the quadrants of the plates, and exactly 5.0 ml of OADC-supplemented 7H10 agar is pipetted over each disk. The disks must remain submerged. The plates are left overnight at room temperature (5°C for ethambutol-containing plates) to allow the drugs to diffuse into the agar. The following commercially available disks can be used for this technique: INH, 1.0 µg/disk; streptomycin, 10.0 µg/disk; ethambutol, 25.0 µg/disk; rifampin, 5.0 µg/disk; PAS, 10.0 µg/disk; ethionamide, 25.0 µg/disk; and kanamycin, 30.0 µg/disk.

Indirect Test in Liquid Medium—BACTEC Method

New automated liquid medium systems (MB/BacT, MGIT-960, and ESP) have been introduced recently, but most of our experience has been accumulated from using the radiometric BACTEC-460 system. The BACTEC-460 system detects the presence of growing bacteria by measuring an increase in $^{14}CO_2$ (indicated as a growth index [GI]), and when growth is inhibited by the antimicrobial agent, susceptibility is detected by the inhibition of daily GI increases (42, 83, 90). The major advantage of this technique is the ability to detect growth and its inhibition earlier than by methods involving solid medium. In the National Jewish laboratory, an indirect DST in this system required an average of 9.3 days (37). The overall mean time for primary isolation plus indirect test was 18 days in a cooperative study by five institutions (83). The major disadvantage of the BACTEC system is the problem of disposal of a large volume of radioactive materials (12B vials), although of very low radioactivity. Another disadvantage is the cost, which is much higher than for tests with any of the solid media, although it is less expensive than the newer nonradioactive liquid-medium systems.

The BACTEC method has been used as a qualitative test with four first-line drugs: INH, rifampin, ethambutol, and streptomycin. An additional test with PZA requires special BACTEC medium (PZA vials) with a lower pH (6.0 versus 6.8 in 12B vials). The manufacturer has been changing over time the critical concentrations of some drugs to improve the outcome of the test: streptomycin from 4.0 to 2.0 μg/ml and ethambutol from 7.5 to 2.5 μg/ml. According to a number of reports, the new concentrations, especially ethambutol at 2.5 μg/ml, appear to be too low. However, revision of the recommended test concentration would require an expensive clinical trial and clearance by the U.S. Food and Drug Administration. Such a revision may not occur, since manufacturers are focused on the nonradioactive systems. In the meantime, based on our many years of experience with this system, we have been successfully using different drug concentrations (42), which are shown in Table 2. Another difference from the manufacturer's manual is the concentration of PZA: the National Jewish Research and Medical Center uses 300.0 instead of 100.0 μg/ml (45). In addition, as shown in Table 2, the National Jewish Laboratory has established critical concentrations for other drugs (second-line drugs) to be used in this system: ethionamide, kanamycin-amikacin, capreomycin, thiacetazone, ofloxacin-ciprofloxacin, and rifapentine (42, 44). Besides the qualitative test with one critical concentration, there is also an option for a quantitative test for MIC determination, which requires at least two additional concentrations of each drug (42).

To perform a test in the BACTEC-460 system, the appropriate working drug solutions (40-fold concentrates of the required final target concentrations) are added to the vials. Lyophilized primary drugs can be purchased from Becton Dickinson. The original 12B culture can be used undiluted as the inoculum, at 0.1 ml per vial, if the GI is between 300 and 800. The culture in the "seed vial" (4.0 ml) should be diluted by adding 2.0 ml of diluting fluid if the GI is 800 or higher. Two drug-free controls may be included: the first is inoculated with the same suspension as for the drug-containing vials, and the second is inoculated with a 1:100-diluted bacterial suspension (1:10 for the PZA test). As an alternative, only the 1:100 dilution control may be used to reduce cost. The curves of daily-recorded GIs in drug-containing vials are compared with those in two drug-free controls. It is assumed that the culture contains more than 1% resistant bacteria (10% in a test with PZA) if growth in the drug-containing vial progresses to a higher level than that in the 1:100 control (1:10 for PZA). On the other hand, the culture is designated "susceptible" if there are no significant daily GI increases in the presence of the critical drug concentration and the GI in the diluted control increases faster than that in the drug-containing vial. Even assuming that this technique has the ability to distinguish between fully susceptible isolates and those containing 1% (10% for PZA) or more resistant bacteria, this method cannot determine the actual proportion of resistant bacteria in a culture. Therefore, it is a misnomer to call this technique the "BACTEC proportion method," as it has been labeled in a number of publications. In addition, there is evidence that the BACTEC method may not be a reliable tool for detecting resistance in cultures containing less than 10% of drug-resistant bacteria (44). Drug susceptibility testing in the BACTEC system (or in newer liquid-medium systems) is reasonable if the same system is also used for the primary culture isolation. The total turnaround time of an indirect test with four drugs (including primary isolation) for most isolates is usually less than 3 weeks.

MGIT Indirect Test

The nonradioactive automated BACTEC 960 system with MGIT tubes from Becton Dickinson is another option for performing an indirect test in a liquid medium with five first-line drugs. This method has been approved by the Food and Drug Administration, and the drugs are used in the following critical concentrations: INH, 0.1 μg/ml; rifampin, 1.0 μg/ml; ethambutol, 5.0 μg/ml; streptomycin, 1.0 μg/ml; and PZA (at pH 5.9), 100.0 μg/ml. Comparison of this method with the BACTEC-460 system (11), as well as with the agar proportion method indicates that this new method is quite promising. Further studies in different laboratory settings with a large number of clinical isolates are required before this method is considered as reliable as the agar proportion method or the BACTEC-460 method.

Rapid Drug Susceptibility Methods

Even with the improvements on classical methods described above, drug susceptibility testing remains a bottleneck in the management of tuberculosis cases, and considerable research effort has been dedicated to finding ways to speed the process. These efforts have spawned some truly creative tests that take advantage of the latest technological advances in molecular biology, genome analysis, computerization, microfluidics, and robotics. Here we briefly describe examples of some such phenotypic methods which require bacterial growth but allow detection more rapidly by means other than conventional growth inhibition.

Mycobacteriophage-based tests

Mycobacteriophages have been incorporated in two methods, the luciferase reporter phage (LRP) assay and the FASTPlaque TB-RIF test (BioTec Laboratories, Ipswich, United Kingdom). LRPs are phages harboring the *fflux* reporter gene, which codes for the firefly luciferase, which in turn catalyzes a reaction that releases light in the presence of its substrate luciferin and ATP. LRPs are able to infect, replicate, and express their genome and the *fflux* gene only within viable mycobacterial cells. Luciferase activity can then be detected only if cellular ATP is present, allowing the detection of *M. tuberculosis* in clinical samples (10, 81). If a decontaminated clinical specimen or culture containing *M. tuberculosis* is pretreated with antibiotics and then infected with LRPs, light emission will be proportional to mycobacterial viability; hence, LRPs are promising candidates for drug susceptibility testing (18, 80, 82). Luciferase activity is detected by means of a luminometer or photographic film. The luminometer offers higher sensitivity and quantitative results (8, 10); Polaroid film offers an inexpensive, "low-tech" alternative that is called the Bronx box (82). In a recent prospective study conducted in a diagnostic laboratory in Mexico City, the LRP-NAP assay confirmed mycobacterial growth in 79 of 84 (94%) of the positive MGIT cultures and correctly identified *M. tuberculosis* complex in 70 of 72 (94%) of the cultures (8). When testing for drug susceptibility the LRP test was in 100% agreement with BACTEC-460 for rifampin, INH, and streptomycin; four discrepancies were found with ethambutol, all of which were resistant in the LRP test, and these were confirmed as false-resistant results when retested by the conventional agar proportion method. In another study testing INH and rifampin, the LRP test was in 100% agreement with the agar proportion method, with the time to final result being 94 h for the Bronx box and 54 h for the luminometer (36). Even using a more sensitive LRP (phAE142), detection, identification, and drug susceptibility testing requires amplification of the my-

cobacteria in the processed sputum pellets; however, these tests can be completed in a median of 12 days (10). One can envision that both formats would be useful, the Bronx box in clinical settings in the developing world and the luminometer in reference laboratories. Commercialization of this method is necessary before it can be put into a routine diagnostic setting.

The FASTPlaque test is similar in biological principle to the LRP test, except that wild-type mycobacteriophages are used (110). Proliferation of the phages in viable mycobacterial cells is detected by a plating procedure in which the phage-infected pathogen suspension is mixed with rapidly growing *M. smegmatis* cells, and phage released from lysed *M. tuberculosis* cells infect the *M. smegmatis* cells. Such infection events are detectable 1 day later as "plaques" on the lawn of *M. smegmatis* colonies. The procedure is obviously more laborious than LRP but does not require special equipment to detect light emission. In several studies, the FASTPlaque test demonstrated high correlation with BACTEC-460 for detection of rifampin susceptibility in *M. tuberculosis* cultures, and the results were available within 2 days after primary isolation (positive BACTEC cultures or growth on solid media) (1, 2, 56). FASTPlaque may be considered an alternative method for susceptibility testing in developing countries, where the prevalence of drug resistance is low and susceptibility tests are performed mainly for surveillance instead of patient management. A new generation of test has been developed for testing sputum specimens directly; however, its performance characteristics are not known. If future evaluations can confirm that the new direct FASTPlaque test reliably detects small numbers of organisms in clinical specimens, it will be the first commercial drug susceptibility test that is truly rapid and relies on microbiological techniques.

Microplate assays

In an effort to provide simple and inexpensive methods for detecting drug-resistant *M. tuberculosis*, several colorimetric assays have been developed which utilize oxidation-reduction indicators for detection of mycobacterial growth in the presence of antituberculosis drugs (9, 19, 29, 70, 71). These indicators include Alamar blue, resazurin, and tetrazolium. Briefly, the assay involves the addition of an indicator to microplates containing antimicrobials in increasing concentrations and pure cultures of isolates. After incubation for 5 to 7 days, the growth can be observed as a change in the color of the indicator due to reduction of the dye. MICs of each drug can be determined by this change of color in the wells. The main concern with this type of test is biosafety: indicator dye is added to the wells after 5 to 7 days of growth; however, modification of the test to use a closed screw cap tube format would avoid this problem. Another microplate assay, which has less biosafety risk, uses critical drug concentrations and measures growth by microscopic reading (20). For INH and rifampin, it shows 100% agreement with the agar proportion method (72) and 89% agreement with the Alamar blue assay (20). Detection of mycobacteria in the microscopic observation drug susceptibility assay is technically similar to microscopic examination of a smear, which could be an attractive alternative to solid media methods in laboratories where routine smear and culture are performed.

A GLANCE INTO THE FUTURE

The future of tuberculosis laboratories and their ability to play a significant role in National Tuberculosis Programs in countries with a high burden of tuberculosis will depend on their ability to detect drug-resistant bacteria in a timely manner while taking financial constraints into account. There are reasonable indications that the future development of rapid methods will be associated with progress in technologies classified in the literature as either molecular phenotypic or molecular genotypic (39, 96, 97). At present, laboratory services in low- and middle-income countries depend largely on the conventional, cultivation-based methods described in this chapter.

REFERENCES

1. Albert, H., A. Heydenrych, R. Mole, A. Trollip, and L. Blumberg. 2001. Evaluation of FASTPlaque TB-RIF™, a rapid, manual test for the determination of rifampicin resistance from *Mycobacterium tuberculosis* cultures. *Int. J. Tuberc. Lung Dis.* 5:906–911.
2. Albert, H., A. P. Trollip, R. J. Mole, J. B. Hatch, and L. Blumberg. 2002. Rapid indication of multidrug-resistant tuberculosis from liquid cultures using FASTPlaque TB-RIF™, a manual phage-based test. *Int. J. Tuberc. Lung Dis.* 6:523–528.
3. American Thoracic Society. 1974. Policy statement: quality of the laboratory for mycobacterial disease. *Am. Rev. Respir. Dis.* 110:376–377.
4. American Thoracic Society. 1983. Levels of laboratory services. *Am. Rev. Respir. Dis.* 128:213–215.
5. Arnold, L. J., P. W. Hammond, W. A. Wiese, and N. C. Nelson. 1989. Assay formats involving acridinium-ester-labeled DNA probes. *Clin. Chem.* 35:1588–1594.
6. Association of State and Territorial Public Health Directors and U.S. Department of Health and Human Services. 1995. *Mycobacterium tuberculosis: Assessing Your Laboratory.* Centers for Disease Control and Prevention, Atlanta, Ga.
7. Bailey, G. V. J., D. Savic, G. D. Gothi, V. B. Naidu, and S. S. Nair. 1967. Potential yield of pulmonary tuberculosis cases by direct microscopy of an acid-fast bacilli. *Rev. Infect. Dis.* 6:214–222.

8. Banaiee, N., S. Bobadilla-de-Valle, S. Bardarov, Jr., P. Riska, P. M. Small, A. Ponce-de-Leon, W. R. Jacobs, Jr., G. F. Hatfull, and J. Sifuentes-Osornio. 2001. Luciferase reporter mycobacteriophages for detection, identification and antibiotic susceptibility testing of *Mycobacterium tuberculosis* in Mexico. *J. Clin. Microbiol.* 39:3883–3888.
9. Banfi, E., G. Scialino, and C. Monti-Bragadin. 2003. Development of a microdilution method to evaluate mycobacterium tuberculosis drug susceptibility. *J. Antimicrob. Chemother.* 5:796–800.
10. Bardarov, S., Jr., H. Dou, K. D. Eisenach, N. Banaiee, S. Ya, J. Chan, W. R. Jacobs Jr., and P. F. Riska. 2003. Detection and drug-susceptibility testing of *M. tuberculosis* from sputum samples using luciferase reporter phage: comparison with the Mycobacteria Growth Indicator Tube (MGIT) system. *Diagn. Microbiol. Infect. Dis.* 45:53–61.
11. Bemer, P., F. Palicova, S. Rusch-Gerdes, H. Drugeon, and G. Pfyffer. 2002. Multicenter evaluation of fully automated BACTEC Mycobacteria Growth Indicator Tube 960 system for susceptibility testing of *Mycobacterium tuberculosis.* *J. Clin. Microbiol.* 40:150–154.
12. Bönicke, R. 1958. Die differenzierung humaner and boviner tuberkelterien mit hilfe von thiophen-2–carbonsaure-hydrazid. *Naturwissenschaften* 46:392–393.
13. Butler, W. R., and J. O. Kilburn. 1988. Identification of major slowly growing pathogenic mycobacteria and *Mycobacterium gordonae* by high-performance liquid chromatography of their mycolic acids. *J. Clin. Microbiol.* 26:50–53.
14. Butler, W. R., K. C. Jost, and J. O. Kilburn. 1991. Identification of mycobacteria by high-performance liquid chromatography. *J. Clin. Microbiol.* 29:2468–2472.
15. Butler, W. R., and L. S. Guthertz. 2001. Mycolic acid analysis by high-performance liquid chromatography for identification of *Mycobacterium* species. *Clin. Microbiol. Rev.* 14:704–726.
16. Canetti, G., W. Fox, A. Khomenko, H. T. Mahler, M. K. Menon, D. A. Mitchison, M. Rist, and M. A. Smelev. 1969. Advances in techniques of testing mycobacterial drug sensitivity and the use of sensitivity tests in tuberculosis control programs. *Bull. W. H. O.* 41:21–43.
17. Canetti, G., S. Froman, J. Grosset, P. Hauduroy, M. Langerova, H. T. Mahler, G. Meissner, D. A. Mitchison, and L. Sula. 1963. Mycobacteria: laboratory methods for testing drug sensitivity and resistance. *Bull. W. H. O.* 29:565–578.
18. Carriere, C., P. F. Riska, O. Zimhony, J. Kriakov, S. Bardarov, J. Burns, J. Chan, and W. R. Jacobs, Jr. 1997 Conditionally replicating luciferase reporter phages: improves sensitivity for rapid detection and assessment of drug susceptibility of mycobacterium tuberculosis. *J. Clin. Microbiol.* 35:3232–3239.
19. Caviedes, L., J. Delgado, and R. H. Gilman. 2002. Tetrazolium microplate assay as a rapid and inexpensive colorimetric method for determination of antibiotic susceptibility of *Mycobacterium tuberculosis.* *J. Clin. Microbiol.* 40:1873–1874.
20. Caviedes, L., T. Lee, R. H. Gilman, P. Sheen, E. Spellman, E. H. Lee, D. E. Berg, S. Montenegro-James, and the Tuberculosis Group in Peru. 2000. Rapid, efficient detection and drug susceptibility testing of *Mycobacterium tuberculosis* in sputum by microscopic observation of broth cultures. *J. Clin. Microbiol.* 38:1203–1208.
21. Cohn, M. L., R. F. Waggoner, and J. K. McClatchy. 1968. The 7H11 medium for the culture of mycobacteria. *Am. Rev. Respir. Dis.* 98:295–296.
22. Desmond, E., and K. Loretz. 2001. Use of the Gen-Probe amplified Mycobacterium Tuberculosis Direct Test for early de-

tection of *Mycobacterium tuberculosis* in BACTEC 12B medium. *J. Clin. Microbiol.* **39**:1993–1995.

23. **Dixon, D., and E. H. Gutherberg.** 1967. Isolation of tubercle bacilli from uncentrifuged sputum on pyruvic acid medium. *Am. Rev. Respir. Dis.* **96**:119–122.

24. **Eisenach, K. D., M. D. Sifford, M. D. Cave, J. H. Bates, and J. T. Crawford.** 1991. Detection of *Mycobacterium tuberculosis* in sputum samples using polymerase chain reaction. *Am. Rev. Respir. Dis.* **144**:1160–1163.

25. **Enarson, D. A.** 1995. The International Union Against Tuberculosis and Lung Disease. Model national tuberculosis programmes. *Tubercle Lung Dis.* **76**:95–99.

26. **Fleming, D. O., J. H. Richardson, J. J. Tulis, and D. Vesley** (ed.). 1995. *Laboratory Safety*, 2nd ed. ASM Press, Washington, D.C.

27. **Forbes, B. A., and K. E. S. Hicks.** 1993. Direct detection of *Mycobacterium tuberculosis* in respiratory specimens in a clinical laboratory by polymerase chain reaction. *J. Clin. Microbiol.* **31**:1688–1694

28. **Foulds, J., and R. O'Brien.** 1998. New tools of the diagnosis of tuberculosis: the perspective for developing countries. *Int. J. Tuberc. Lung Dis.* **3**:1–18.

29. **Franzblau, S. G., R. S. Gitzig, J. C. McLaughlin, P. Torres, G. Madico, A. Hernandez, M. T. Degnan, M. B. Cook, V. K. Quenzer, R. M. Ferguson, and R. H Gilman.** 1998. Rapid, Low-technology MIC determination with clinical *Mycobacterium tuberculosis* isolates by using the microplate Alamar Blue assay. *J. Clin. Microbiol.* **36**:362–366.

30. **Glickman, S. E., S. O. Kilburn, and W. R. Butler.** 1994. Rapid identification of mycolic acid patterns of mycobacteria by high-performance liquid chromatography using pattern recognition software and a *Mycobacterium* library. *J. Clin. Microbiol.* **32**:740–749.

31. **Griffith, D. E., H. L. Barrett, H. L. Bodily, and R. M. Wood.** 1967. Drug susceptibility tests for tuberculosis using drug impregnated discs. *Am. J. Clin. Pathol.* **47**:812–817.

32. **Griffith, M., and H. Bodily.** 1992. Stability of antimycobacterial drugs in susceptibility testing. *Antimicrob. Agents Chemother.* **36**:2398–2402.

33. **Guthertz, L. S., S. D. Lim, Y. Jang, and P. S. Duffey.** 1993. Curvilinear-gradient high-performance liquid chromatography for identification of mycobacteria. *J. Clin. Microbiol.* **31**:1876–1881.

34. **Hall, G. S.** 1996. Primary processing of specimens, isolation and cultivation of mycobacteria. *Clin. Lab. Med.* **16**:551–558.

35. **Harrington, J. M., and H. S. Shannon.** 1976. Incidence of tuberculosis, hepatitis, brucellosis, and shigellosis in British medical laboratory workers. *Br. Med. J.* **1**:759–762.

36. **Hazbon, M. H., N. Guarin, B. E. Ferro, A. L. Rodriguez, L. A. Labrada, R. Tovar, P. F. Riska, and W. R. Jacobs, Jr.** 2003. Photographic and luminometric detection of luciferase reporter phages for drug susceptibility testing of clinical *Mycobacterium tuberculosis* isolates. *J. Clin. Microbiol.* **41**:4865–4869.

37. **Heifets, L.** 1986. Rapid automated method (BACTEC system) in clinical mycobacteriology. *Semin. Respir. Med.* **1**:242–249.

38. **Heifets, L.** 2001. False diagnosis of tuberculosis. *Int. J. Tuberc. Lung Dis.* **5**:789–790.

39. **Heifets, L., and G. A. Cangelosi.** 1999. Drug susceptibility testing of *Mycobacterium tuberculosis*—a neglected problem at the turn of the century. *Int. J. Tuberc. Lung Dis.* **3**:1–18.

40. **Heifets, L., and P. A. Jenkins.** 1998. Speciation of mycobacteria in clinical laboratories, p. 308–350. *In* P. R. Gangadharam and P. Jenkins (ed.), *Mycobacteria, I. Basic Aspects.* Chapman and Hall, Thompson Science, New York, NY.

41. **Heifets, L.** 1996. Drug susceptibility testing in mycobacteriology. *Clin. Lab. Med.* **16**:641–656.

42. **Heifets, L.** 1991. Drug susceptibility tests in the management of chemotherapy of tuberculosis, p. 89–121. *In* L. B. Heifets (ed.), *Drug Susceptibility in the Chemotherapy of Mycobacterial Infections.* CRC Press, Inc., Boca Raton, Fl.

43. **Heifets, L., T. Lindler, T. Sanchez, D. Spencer, and J. Brennan.** 2000. Two liquid medium systems, Mycobacterial Growth Indicator Tube and MB Redox Tube, for *Mycobacterium tuberculosis* isolation from sputum specimens. *J. Clin. Microbiol.* **38**:1227–1230.

44. **Heifets, L., T. Sanchez, J. Vanderkolk, and V. Pham.** 1999. Development of rifapentine susceptibility tests for *Mycobacterium tuberculosis. Antimicrob. Agents Chemother.* **43**:25–28.

45. **Heifets, L. B.** 1999. Pyrazinamide, p. 668–676. *In* V. Yu, T. C. Merigan, and S. L. Barriere (ed.), *Antimicrobial Therapy and Vaccines.* The Williams & Wilkins Co., Baltimore, Md.

46. **Hoffner, S. E., M. Haile, and G. Kallenius.** 1992. A biphasic system for primary isolation of mycobactia compared to solid medium and broth culture. *J. Med. Microbiol.* **37**:332–334.

47. **Hultmann, T., S. Stahl, and E. Hornes.** 1980. Direct solid phase sequencing of genomic and plasmlid DNA using magnetic beads as support. *Nucleic Acids Res.* **17**:4939–4946.

48. **Isenberg, H. D.** (ed.). 1992. *Mycobacteriology*, 3.1.1–3.16.4. *In Clinical Microbiology Procedure Handbook.* ASM Press, Washington, D.C.

49. **Isenberg, H. D., R. F. D'Amato, L. Heifets, P. R. Murray, M. Scardamaglia, M. C. Jacobs, P. Alperstein, and A. Niles.** 1991. Collaborative feasibility study of a biphasic system (Roche Septi-Chek AFB) for rapid detection and isolation of mycobacteria. *J. Clin. Microbiol.* **29**:1719–22.

50. **Jonas, V., M. J. Alden, J. I. Curri, K. Kamisango, C. A. Knott, R. Lankford, J. M. Wolfe, and D. F. Moore.** 1993. Detection and identification of *Mycobacterium tuberculosis* directly from sputum sediments by amplification of rRNA. *J. Clin. Microbiol.* **31**:2410–2416.

51. **Jost, K. C., Jr., D. F. Dunbar, S. S. Barth, V. L. Headley, and L. B. Elliot.** 1995. Identification of *Mycobacterium tuberculosis* and *M. avium* complex directly from smear-positive sputum specimens and BACTEC 12B cultures by high-performance liquid chromatography with fluorescence detection and computer-driven pattern recognition models. *J. Clin. Microbiol.* **33**:1270–1277.

52. **Kent, P. T., and G. P. Kubica.** 1985. *Public Health Mycobacteriology: a Guide for the Level III Laboratory.* Centers for Disease Control and Prevention, Atlanta, Ga.

53. **Kilburn, J. O., and G. P. Kubica.** 1968. Reagent impregnated paper strips for detection of niacin. *Am. J. Clin. Pathol.* **50**:530–532.

54. **Kirschner, P., A. Meier, and E. C. Böttger.** 1993. Genotypic identification and detection of mycobacteria facing novel and uncultured pathogens, p. 173–190. *In* D. H. Persing, T. F. Smith, F. C. Tenover, and T. J. White (ed.), *Diagnostic Molecular Microbiology.* American Society for Microbiology, Washington, D.C.

55. **Kirschner, P., B. Springer, and U. Vogel.** 1993. Genotypic identification of mycobacteria by nucleic acid sequence determination: report of a two year experience in a clinical laboratory. *J. Clin. Microbiol.* **31**:2882–2889.

56. **Kisa, O., A. Albay, O. Bedir, O. Baylan, and L. Doganci.** 2003. Evaluation of FASTPlaqueTB-RIF™ for determination of rifampicin resistance in *Mycobacterium tuberculosis* complex isolates. *Int. J. Tuberc. Lung Dis.* **7**:284–288.

57. Kleeberg, H. H. 1985. A simple method for testing the drug susceptibility of *M. tuberculosis*, a report of an international collaborative study. *Bull. Int. Union Tuberc.* **60:**147–153.

58. Konno, K. 1956. New chemical method to differentiate human-type tubercle bacilli from other mycobacteria. *Science* **124:**985.

59. Kubica, G. P. 1964. A combined niacin-nitrate reduction test for use in the identification of mycobacteria. *Acta Tuberc. Scand.* **45:**161–167.

60. Kubica, G. P., W. E. Dye, M. L. Cohn, and G. Middlebrook. 1963. Sputum digestion and decontamination with N-acetyl-L-cysteine-sodium hydroxide for culture of mycobacteria. *Am. Rev. Respir. Dis.* **87:**775–779.

61. Kubica, G. P., W. M. Gross, J. E. Hawkins, A. Sommers, L. Vestal, and L. G. Wayne. 1975. Laboratory services for mycobacterial diseases. *Am. Rev. Respir. Dis.* **112:**773–787.

62. Kubica, G. P., A. J. Kauffmann, and W. E. Dye. 1964. Comments on the use of the new mucolytic agent N-acetyl-L-cysteine as a sputum digestant for the isolation of mycobacteria. *Am. Rev. Respir. Dis.* **89:**284–286.

63. Laszlo, A. 1996. Tuberculosis bacteriology laboratory services and incremental protocols for developing countries. *Clin. Lab. Med.* **16:**697–716.

64. McClatchy, J. K., R. F. Waggoner, W. Kanes, M. S. Cernich, and T. L. Bolton. 1976. Isolation of mycobacteria from clinical specimens by use of selective 7H11 medium. *Am. J. Clin. Pathol.* **65:**412–415.

65. Middlebrook, G., and M. L. Cohn. 1958. Bacteriology of tuberculosis: laboratory methods. *Am. J. Public Health* **48:**844–853.

66. Middlebrook, G., L. Cohn, W. E. Dye, W. F. Russell, and D. Levy. 1960. Microbiologic procedures of value in tuberculosis. *Acta Tuberc. Scand.* **38:**66–81.

67. Middlebrook, G., Z. Reggiardo, and W. D. Tigertt. 1977. Automatable radiometric detection of growth of *M. tuberculosis* in selective media. *Am. Rev. Respir. Dis.* **115:**1066–1069.

68. Nolte, F. S., and B. Metchock. 1995. *Mycobacterium*, p. 400–449. *In* P. R. Murray, E. J. Baron, M. A. Pfaller, F. C. Tenover, and R. H. Yolken (ed.), *Manual of Clinical Microbiology*. ASM Press, Washington, D.C.

69. Palomono, J. C. 2000. Novel rapid antimicrobial susceptibility tests for *M. tuberculosis*, p. 145–162. *In* I. Bastian and F. Portaels (ed.), *Multi-drug Resistant Tuberculosis*, Kluwer Academic Publishing, Dordrecht, The Netherlands.

70. Palomino, J. C., A. Martin, H. Camacho, J. Guerra, J. Swings, and F. Portaels. 2002. Resazurin microtiter assay plate: simple and inexpensive methods for detection of drug resistance in *Mycobacterium tuberculosis*. *Antimicrob. Agents Chemother.* **46:**2720–2722.

71. Palomino, J. C., and F. Portaels. 1999. Simple procedure for drug susceptibility testing of *Mycobacterium tuberculosis* using a commercial colorimetic assay. *Eur. J. Clin. Microbiol. Infect. Dis.* **18:**380–383.

72. Park, W. G., W. R. Bishai, R. E. Chaisson, and S. E. Dorman. 2002. Performance of the microscopic observation drug susceptibility assay in drug susceptibility testing for *Mycobacterium tuberculosis*. *J. Clin. Microbiol.* **40:**4750–4752.

73. Pfyffer, G. E., P. Kissling, R. Wirth, and R. Weber. 1994. Direct detection of *Mycobacterium tuberculosis* complex in respiratory specimens by a target-amplified test system. *J. Clin. Microbiol.* **32:**918–923.

74. Pike, R. M. 1976. Laboratory-associated infections: summary and analysis of 3,921 cases. *Health Lab. Sci.* **13:**105–114.

75. Pike, R. M., S. E. Sulkin, and M. L. Schulze. 1965. Continuing importance of laboratory-acquired infections. *Am. J. Public Health* **55:**190–199.

76. Quigley, H. S. and H. R. Elston. 1970. Nitrite strips for detection of nitrite reduction by mycobacteria. *Am. J. Clin. Pathol.* **53:**663–665.

77. Reid, D. D. 1957. Incidence of tuberculosis among workers in medical laboratories. *Br. Med. J.* **2:**10–14.

78. Richmond, J. Y., and R. W. Mckinney (ed.). 1993. *Biosafety in Microbiological and Biomedical Laboratories*, 3rd ed. Publication 93-8395. Centers for Disease Control, Atlanta, Ga.

79. Richmond, J. Y., R. C. Knudsen, and R. C. Good. 1996. Biosafety in the clinical mycobacteriology laboratory. *Clin. Lab. Med.* **6:**527–550.

80. Riska, P. F., and W. R. Jacobs, Jr. 1998. The use of luciferase-reporter phage for antibiotic-susceptibility testing of mycobacteria. *Methods Mol. Biol.* **101:**431–453.

81. Riska, P. F., W. R. Jacobs, Jr., B. R. Bloom, J. McKitrick, and J. Chan. 1997. Specific identification of *Mycobacterium tuberculosis* with the luciferase reporter mycobacteriophage: use of p-nitro-α-acetylamino-β-hydroxy propiophenone. *J. Clin. Microbiol.* **35:**3225–3231.

82. Riska, P. F., Y. Su, S. Bardarov, L. Freundlich, G. Sarkie, G. Hatfull, C. Carriere, V. Kumar, J. Chan, and W. R. Jacobs, Jr. 1999. Rapid film-based determination of antibiotic susceptibilities of *Mycobacterium tuberculosis* strains by using a luciferase reporter phage and the Bronx Box. *J. Clin. Microbiol.* **37:**1144–1149.

83. Roberts, G., N. L. Goodman, L. Heifets, H. W. Larsh, T. H. Lindner, J. K. McClatchy, M. R. McGinnis, S. H. Siddiqi, and P. Wright. 1983. Evaluation of the BACTEC radiometric method for recovery of mycobacteria and drug susceptibility testing of *Mycobacterium tuberculosis* from acid-fast smear-positive specimens. *J. Clin. Microbiol.* **18:**689–696.

84. Roberts, G. D., E. C. Böttger, and L. Stockman. 1996. Rapid methods for the identification of mycobacterial species. *Clin. Lab. Med.* **16:**603–616.

85. Roberts, G. D., E. W. Koneman, and Y. K. Kim. 1991. *Mycobacterium*, p. 304–339. *In* A. Balows, W. J. Hausles, K. L. Herrmann, H. D. Isenberg, and H. J. Shadomy (ed.), *Manual of Clinical Microbiology*, 5th ed. American Society for Microbiology, Washington, D.C.

86. Rogall, T., T. Flohr, and E. C. Böttger. 1990. Differentiation of *Mycobacterium* species by direct sequencing of amplified DNA. *J. Gen. Microbiol.* **136:**1915–1920.

87. Sanchez, T., J. Vanderkolk, S. Seay, and L. Heifets. 1994. Quantitation of mycobacteria in blood specimens from patients with AIDS. *Tubercle Lung Dis.* **75:**386–390.

88. Sewell, D. L., and R. B. Schifman. 1995. Quality assurance: quality improvement, quality control, and test validation, p. 55–85. *In* P. R. Murray, E. J. Baron, M. A. Pfaller, F. C. Tenover, and R. H. Yolken (ed.), *Manual of Clinical Microbiology*, 6th ed. ASM Press, Washington, D.C.

89. Shinnick, T. M., and V. Jonas. 1994. Molecular approach to the diagnosis of tuberculosis, p. 517–530. *In* B. R. Bloom, (ed.), *Tuberculosis: Pathogenesis, Protection, and Control*. ASM Press, Washington, D.C.

90. Siddiqi, S. H., J. P. Libonati, and G. Middlebrook. 1981. Evaluation of rapid radiometric method for drug susceptibility testing of *Mycobacterium tuberculosis*. *J. Clin. Microbiol.* **13:**908–912.

91. Sjobring, U., M. Mecklenburg, A. B. Andersen, and H. Miorner. 1990. Polymerase chain reaction for detection of *Mycobacterium tuberculosis*. *J. Clin. Microbiol.* **28:**2200–2204.

92. Skinholj, P. 1974. Occupational risks in Danish clinical chemical laboratories. II. Infections. *Scand. J. Clin. Lab. Investig.* **33:**27–29.

93. **Smithwick, R. W.** 1976. *Laboratory Manual for Acid Fast Microscopy.* Centers for Disease Control, Atlanta, Ga.

94. **Sommers, H. M., and J. K. McClatchy.** 1983. Cumitech 16, *Laboratory Diagnosis of the Mycobacterioses.* Josephine A. Morello, Coordinating ed. American Society for Microbiology, Washington, D.C.

95. **Spargo, C. A., P. D. Haaland, S. R. Jurgensen, D. D. Shank, and G. T. Walker.** 1993. Chemiluminescent detection of strand displacement amplified DNA from species comprising the *Mycobacterium tuberculosis* complex. *Mol. Cell. Probes* 7:395–404.

96. **Sritharan, V., and R. H. Barker, Jr.** 1991. A simple method for diagnosing *M. tuberculosis* infection in clinical samples using PCR. *Mol. Cell. Probes* 5:385–395.

97. **Takiff, H. E.** 2000. The molecular mechanisms of drug resistance in *M. tuberculosis*, p. 77–114. *In* I. Bastian and F. Portaels (ed.), *Multi-Drug Resistant Tuberculosis.* Kluwer Academic Publishing, Dordrecht, The Netherlands.

98. **Telenti, A.** 1997. Genetics of drug resistance in tuberculosis. *Clin. Chest Med.* 18:55–64.

99. **Tenover, F. C., J. T. Crawford, R. E. Heubner, L. J. Geiter, C. R. Horsburgh, and R. C. Good.** 1993. The resurgence of tuberculosis: is your laboratory ready? *J. Clin. Microbiol.* 31:767–770.

100. **Thibert, L., and S. Lapierre.** 1993. Routine application of high-performance liquid chromatography for identification of mycobacteria. *J. Clin. Microbiol.* 31:1759–1763.

101. **Tortoli, E., F. Mandler, and M. Bartolucci.** 1993. Multi-center evaluation of a biphasic culture system for recovery of mycobacteria from clinical specimens. *Eur. J. Clin. Microbiol. Infect. Dis.* 12:425–429.

102. **Vestal, A. L.** 1977. *Procedures for the Isolation and Identification of Mycobacteria.* HEW publication (CDC) 77-8230. Centers for Disease Control, Atlanta, Ga.

103. **Vestal, A. L., and G. P. Kubica.** 1967. Differential identification of mycobacteria. III. Use of thiacetazone, thiophen-2-carboxylic acid hydrozide and triphenyltetrazolim chloride. *Scand. J. Respir. Dis.* 48:142–148.

104. **Virtanen, S.** 1960. A study of nitrate reduction by mycobacteria. *Acta Tuberc. Scand. Suppl.* 48:111–119.

105. **Walker, G. T., M. C. Little, J. G. Nadeau, and D. D. Shank.** 1992. Isothermal *in vitro* amplification of DNA by a restriction enzyme/DNA polymerase system. *Proc. Natl. Acad. Sci. USA* 89:392–396.

106. **Warren, N. G., and J. R. Cord.** 1996. Activities and recommendations by the Association of State and Territorial Public Health Laboratory Directors. *Clin. Lab. Med.* 16:551–568.

107. **Wayne, L. G.** 1974. Simple pyrazinamide and urease tests for routine identification of mycobacteria. *Am. Rev. Respir. Dis.* 109:147–151.

108. **Wayne, L. G., and I. Krasnow.** 1966. Preparation of tuberculosis susceptibility testing medium by means of impregnated discs. *Am. J. Clin. Pathol.* 45:769–771.

109. **Welch, D. F., A. P. Guruswamy, S. J. Sides, C. H. Shaw, and M. J. R. Gilchrist.** 1993. Timely culture for mycobacteria which utilizes a microcolony method. *J. Clin. Microbiol.* 31:2178–2184.

110. **Wilson, S. M., Z. al-Suwaidi, R. McNerney, J. Porter, and F. Drobniewski.** 1997. Evaluation of a new rapid bacteriophage-based method for the drug susceptibility testing of *Mycobacterium tuberculosis. Nat. Med.* 3:465–468.

111. **Witebsky, F. G., and P. Kruczak-Filipov.** 1996. Identification of mycobacteria by conventional methods. *Clin. Lab. Med.* 16:569–602.

112. **Woods, G. L., and J. C. Ridderhof.** 1996. Quality assurance in the mycobacteriology laboratory. *Clin. Lab. Med.* 16:657–675.

113. **Woods, G. L., and J. A. Washington.** 1987. Mycobacteria other than *M. tuberculosis*: a review of microbiologic and clinical aspects. *Rev. Infect. Dis.* 9:275–294.

114. **Woods, G. L., and F. G. Witebsky.** 1995. College of American Pathologists mycobacteriology E Proficiency Testing Survey. Summary of participant performance, 1979–1992. *Arch. Pathol. Lab. Med.* 119:17–22.

115. **Young, W. D., Jr., A. Maslansky, M. S. Lefar, and D. P. Kronish.** 1970. Development of a paper strip test for detection of niacin produced by mycobacteria. *Appl. Microbiol.* 20:939–945.

Tuberculosis and the Tubercle Bacillus
Edited by Stewart T. Cole et al.
© 2005 ASM Press, Washington, D.C.

Chapter 5

Immune-Based Methods

SUMAN LAAL AND YASIR A. W. SKEIKY

Approximately 8 million new cases of tuberculosis (TB) are diagnosed every year; 90% of these patients live in developing countries, where microscopic examination of sputum samples for acid-fast bacilli (AFB) and occasionally chest X rays are the only diagnostic tools used. AFB microscopy is highly specific but has significant limitations in that it diagnoses only relatively advanced TB and the sensitivity varies among laboratories. In addition, the requirement for repeat patient visits to acquire three samples results in significant patient dropout rates. Finally, the test is tedious, requires functional equipment (microscopes and electrical power), misses paucibacillary patients (smear-negative and pediatric patients and those with extrapulmonary TB) and the risk of transmission to laboratory staff is high (27). In developed countries, TB diagnosis is based on microscopic detection of AFB and their culture and the use of nucleic acid amplification tests (AMPLICOR *Mycobacterium tuberculosis* Test, Roche Diagnostics Systems, Indianapolis, Ind.; and Amplified *Mycobacterium tuberculosis* Direct Test; GenProbe, San Diego, Calif.) for early confirmation of the presence of tubercle bacilli in cultures. Despite the use of multiple diagnostic techniques, it takes 3 to 5 days for a definitive diagnosis in smear-positive TB cases and several weeks for diagnosis of smear-negative TB cases. Moreover, approximately 20% of the TB patients determined to have TB based on clinical and/or radiological improvement while taking anti-TB medications have no positive bacteriological cultures for *M. tuberculosis* (8). Clearly, there is a need for improved diagnostic tests for active TB in both developing and developed countries. Moreover, since about 90% of new human immunodeficiency virus (HIV) infections occur in developing countries where TB is already endemic, there is an increasing need for diagnostic tests that can identify coinfected individuals with active incipi-

ent but subclinical TB prior to progression to bacteriology-positive clinical TB (29, 33, 34).

Considerable resources are spent on contact tracing, administration, and monitoring of preventive therapy in latently infected individuals in developed countries (8). The test currently used for the identification of latent *M. tuberculosis* infection is the skin reactivity to purified protein derivative (PPD). However, PPD contains >200 different mycobacterial antigens, many of which are shared by a large range of mycobacteria including the vaccine strain *M. bovis* BCG. As a result, PPD has poor specificity and fails to reliably distinguish between active disease, BCG vaccination, prior infection with *M. tuberculosis*, and cross-sensitization by nonpathogenic environmental mycobacteria. The utility of the PPD test is even lower for HIV-infected individuals with compromised cellular immunity. Thus, there is also an urgent need for diagnostic reagents that can identify both newly and latently infected individuals who are at high risk of developing active TB.

On infection with *M. tuberculosis*, antigen-specific humoral and cell-mediated immune responses are elicited in the host. This chapter reviews the recent advances toward the development of diagnostic tests for clinical and latent TB based on the identification of immunodominant antigens of *M. tuberculosis* and characterization of both the antibody and T-cell responses mounted by the host.

TESTS BASED ON DETECTION OF HUMORAL IMMUNE RESPONSES

Efforts to devise an antibody-detection based diagnostic test for active TB have been under way for decades, but despite the extensive work (as evidenced by a vast amount of published literature), no test with

Suman Laal • Department of Pathology, New York University School of Medicine, c/o VA Medical Center, 423 East 23rd Street, Rm. 18124N, New York, NY 10010. **Yasir A. W. Skeiky** • Aeras Global TB Vaccine Foundation, 7500 Old Georgetown Road, Suite 800, Bethesda, MD 20814.

adequate sensitivity and specificity has emerged. Only in recent years have the reasons for this failure and confusion become clear. In the absence of information about and understanding of gene regulation and expression by *M. tuberculosis* at different stages of disease progression in vivo, in most cases, the antigens used for developing serodiagnostic tests have been chosen based on criteria such as amenability to biochemical purification, presence in large quantities in culture filtrates (e.g., the 38-kDa protein [antigen 5] and antigens 85 A and B) (19, 20, 62), or immunodominance in animals immunized with preparations made from in vitro-grown killed bacteria (38-kDa protein, 14/16-kDa alpha-crystalline homologue protein, 19-kDa lipoprotein, 10-kDa heat shock protein, etc.) (9, 32). Of these, the 38-kDa protein is the only promising candidate antigen; however, the presence of anti-38 kDa antibodies primarily in patients with recurrent, chronic cavitary TB limits its utility in diagnostic assays (9, 21). This antigen, alone or in combination with other proteins, is the basis of almost all currently available commercial rapid tests, none of which perform with adequate sensitivity and specificity (58).

Despite the long history of failed attempts to develop accurate serodiagnosis, recent studies have permitted an understanding of the lacunae in the efforts made so far and provided a basis for the research and development needed to develop an immunodiagnostic test for TB. Considering that *M. tuberculosis* encodes ~4,000 proteins and alters the profile of genes expressed to adapt to the environment, it is to be expected that the bacterium expresses different genes and proteins during the different stages of infection and disease progression (15). Thus, differences in gene and protein expression are expected during initial infection, during replication in nonactivated alveolar macrophages, during dissemination to other organs, in granulomas, during breakdown of granulomas, during noncavitary stages of disease, and in cavitary lesions (52, 57, 63). In fact, studies have shown that the metabolic state of the bacteria differs even in different cavitary environments in the same host (48). Moreover, modulation of bacterial gene expression can occur in response to the immune responses that are elicited (52, 70). For these reasons, a test based on the detection of immune responses of the host must comprise bacterial antigens that are expressed during the various stages of disease progression in the host. However, few studies of serodiagnostics have focused on the identification of antigens that are expressed by the in vivo bacteria at the time when disease is manifest and are available to, and recognized by, the immune response, although such antigens would be the logical targets for development of a serodiagnostic test.

Challenges in Devising a Test for Active Tuberculosis

TB is a chronic disease, which progresses slowly (except in immunocompromised individuals) and can manifest as pulmonary or extrapulmonary disease. Even pulmonary TB is not a single-stage acute disease, and patients present with a spectrum of clinical, radiological, and bacterial indications. Thus, patients may have no pulmonary involvement or only inflammatory infiltration or may have progressed to different levels of cavitation and pulmonary damage. The local in situ environment in the lung is different at these different stages; the bacterial loads vary, being significantly higher in individuals with cavitary lesions where the opportunity to replicate extracellularly exists. As a result of the complex disease processes and the spectrum of pathological and bacteriological conditions presented by the patients, an ideal diagnostic test for TB must have the ability to identify different types of TB patients. Thus, the test must be able to diagnose smear-positive TB patients and identify TB patients with smear-negative pulmonary disease, other forms of paucibacillary disease, and coinfection with HIV.

Smear-positive TB

Smear-positive TB patients have high bacterial loads in their lungs and have already developed cavitary lesions, where the bacteria replicate extracellularly. In developing countries, patients tend to present to the health care facility with advanced cavities and heavy smear-positive sputum. In contrast, in developed countries patients generally present earlier, with fewer tubercle bacilli in the sputum and few or no cavities, and are diagnosed as smear positive because of access to more sophisticated and careful microscopy. Thus, even smear-positive patients from different geographical settings can represent different stages of TB.

Smear-negative pulmonary TB

Patients with smear-negative pulmonary TB have lower bacillary loads and generally lack cavitary lesions, and the ongoing bacterial replication is presumably intracellular.

Other forms of paucibacillary disease

Patients with other forms of paucibacillary disease include pediatric TB cases and patients with extrapulmonary TB (TB meningitis, skeletal TB, genitourinary TB, gastrointestinal TB, TB lymphadenitis, cutaneous TB, etc.) in whom the bacteria survive in completely different environments.

Coinfection with HIV

TB progresses rapidly in HIV-infected individuals, but the immune dysfunction and the poor or absent delayed-type hypersensitivity (DTH) responses preclude the formation of cavitary lesions. As a result, HIV-infected TB patients can have high bacillary loads in the lungs but still have normal chest X rays or show pulmonary infiltration and negative or paucibacillary sputum smears.

Test requirements

Besides providing a high sensitivity of diagnosis in various types of TB patients, the test has to be highly specific. Thus, the test would be based either on detection of M. tuberculosis specific antigens or on M. tuberculosis specific epitopes on cross-reactive antigens. Conversely, a test could be based on detection of host immune responses to specific antigens or to specific epitopes on cross-reactive antigens. In addition, since a major portion of the global TB burden is in resource-poor developing countries, the test must be rapid, low-cost, robust, stable, and amenable to large-scale production and must require minimal laboratory infrastructure and personnel training to have any impact on the epidemic.

Progress in the Development of Antibody Detection-Based Diagnostic Tests

In recent years, several new antigens of M. tuberculosis have been cloned and evaluated for their serodiagnostic potential (Tables 1 and 2). The proteins present in culture filtrates of M. tuberculosis replicating in bacteriological media have been extensively evaluated based on the presumption that the same antigens would also be expressed by the in vivo replicating bacteria (22, 45, 46, 63).

Based on the hypothesis that M. tuberculosis may express different genes and proteins in vivo and in vitro and that the profile of proteins may vary with the stage of the disease, an approach focusing on a systematic analysis of antigens of M. tuberculosis that elicit antibodies in TB patients at different stages of disease and in different classes of TB patients has been used by Laal et al. (41, 42, 63–65). Thus, profiles of culture filtrate proteins of M. tuberculosis that are recognized by serum antibodies from individuals who had latent infection or patients who were AFB

Table 1. Reactivity of smear-positive and smear-negative TB patients with recombinant antigens

Antigen	Alternative names	Rv no.	Smear-positive specimens		Smear-negative specimens		Source
			Specificity (%)	Sensitivity (%)	Specificity (%)	Sensitivity (%)	
ESAT-6		Rv3875	>95	27	>95	12	PHRI[a]
α-Crystallin	16 kDa, HSP, Acr, HSPX, 14 kDa Ag	Rv2031c	>95	36	>95	50	
MPT 63		Rv1926c	>95	22	>95	8	
19 kDa	LpqH	Rv3763	>95	32	>95	42	
MPT 64		Rv1980c	>95	9	>95	16	
MPT 51		Rv3803c	>95	18	>95	4	
MTC 28		Rv0040c	>95	23	>95	29	
Ag 85B	Alpha Ag, Ag6, MPB, MPT 59, FbpB	Rv1886c	>95	23	>95	12	
38 kDa	CIE Ag78, Pab, US-Japan Ag5, PhoS1	Rv0934	>95	36	>95	16	
KatG		Rv1908c	>95	18	>95	12	
M.tb 48[b]		Rv3881c	>95	32	>95	17	Corixa
38 kDa	CIE Ag78, Pab, US-Japan Ag5, PhoS1	Rv0934	>95	47	>95	24	
CFP-10	M. tb 11, MTSA-10	Rv1335	>95	28	>95	25	
M.tb 81	GlcB, 88-kDa Ag	Rv1837c	>95	58	>95	—	
TbF6			>95	70	>95	52	
81/88 kDa	GlcB, M.tb 81	Rv1837c	>95	76	>95	50	NYU/CSU
MPT 51		Rv3803c	>95	60	>95	57	
Ag 85C	MPT 45, FbpC	Rv0129c	>95	10	>95	0	
MPT 32	Apa, ModD, 45-kDa glycoprotein	Rv1860	>95	28	>95	0	

[a]PHRI, Public Health Research Institute TB Center, Newark, N.J.; Corixa, Corixa Corp. Seattle, Wash.; NYU, Department of Pathology, New York University School of Medicine, New York, N.Y.; CSU, Department of Microbiology, Immunology and Pathology, Mycobacterial Research Laboratories, Colorado State University, Ft. Collins, Colo.
[b]M.tb, M. tuberculosis.

Table 2. Reactivity of HIV-infected TB patients with recombinant antigens

Antigen	Specificity (%)	Sensitivity (%)
ESAT-6	>95	19
α-Crystallin	>95	12
MPT 63	>95	10
19 kDa	>95	10
MPT 64	>95	5
MPT 70	>95	10
MPT 51	>95	17
Ag 85B	>95	22
38 kDa	>95	30
KatG	>95	17
M.tb 81[a]	>95	92
M.tb 48	>95	44
38 kDa	>95	66
TbF6	>95	<47
81/88 kDa	>95	66
MPT 51	>95	75

[a]M.tb, *M. tuberculosis.*

smear positive or smear negative, with or without cavitary lesions, and with or without concurrent HIV infection were determined by two-dimensional mapping (63, 64). These studies have provided important insights into antigens expressed by *M. tuberculosis* in vivo during different stages of infection and disease progression with the following findings.

In PPD skin test-positive individuals with no evidence of active TB, antibody responses are directed primarily against 4 to 6 of the >100 proteins present in culture filtrates. In contrast, patients with advanced cavitary TB have antibodies directed against 24 to 26 of the >100 proteins. This suggests that even *M. tuberculosis* replicating extracellularly in vivo may not express many of the same proteins expressed by *M. tuberculosis* replicating extracellularly in bacteriological media. Alternatively, not all proteins expressed in vivo may be accessible to the immune system or may be immunodominant. Only about 12 of the 24 to 26 culture filtrate proteins were major targets recognized by antibodies from all classes of TB patients (cavitary or noncavitary, smear positive or smear negative, non-HIV or HIV-infected). Of these 12 commonly recognized antigens, 2 were the 81/88-kDa GlcB protein and MPT 51.

The profile of antigens recognized by antibodies correlated with the presence or absence of cavitary lesions; patients with cavitary lesions tended to have antibodies against 24 to 26 immunodominant culture filtrate antigens, while those without such lesions (non-HIV and HIV infected) had antibodies against only the subset of approximately 12 of the 26 antigens. The absence of anti-38-kDa antibodies in most HIV-infected TB patients is probably related to their

inability to develop cavitary lesions, rather than to dysfunctional B-cell responses (24, 41, 63, 73). In contrast, the smear status correlated with titers of antibodies, not with the profile of antigens recognized. Some differences in antigen profile recognition between individual patients is expected since antibody titers against individual antigens would vary in individuals, formation of immune complexes could inhibit detection of low titers of antibodies, and differences in the mycobacterial strains exist. Despite these variations, a remarkable homogeneity was observed in the repertoire of antigens recognized by different individual TB patients.

These results are encouraging because for the first time, a small set of *M. tuberculosis* proteins that are recognized by antibodies in patients at different stages of active TB and in patients with different forms of TB disease have been identified. A combination of such antigens, recognized by patients with noncavitary or cavitary TB and regardless of the presence of coinfection with HIV, would be a rational basis for a TB serodiagnostic test and is likely to provide a more sensitive assay than the use of the 38-kDa protein alone, which is recognized primarily by patients with cavitary disease (9, 21). Any test based on antigens that elicit antibodies only in a subset of patients or only at a particular stage of TB is likely to face limitations similar to those of the 38-kDa protein. In contrast, antigens like the 81/88-kDa GlcB protein and MPT 51, which are recognized by antibodies from a significant proportion (at least 50%) of the different types of TB patients (smear-positive, smear-negative and HIV-infected TB patients) will lead to higher sensitivities (Tables 1 and 2). Preliminary studies have shown that, together, these two antigens provide about 80% sensitivity in all three types of patients (S. Laal, data not shown).

Gennaro and colleagues cloned 10 culture filtrate proteins (CFP), which, when tested individually in different cohorts, showed a wide range in sensitivity with individual antigens (9 to 50%) and sensitivities of 46 to 75% with all antigens combined (13, 46, 47; S. Perry, A. Catanzaro, K. P. Lyashchenko, P. A. LoBue, A. Rendon, and M. L. Gennaro, *Tuberc. Past Present Future Conf.*, abstr. 87, p. 44, 2000). Approximately 16% of the *M. tuberculosis* genome has been estimated to encode proteins that are specific to *M. tuberculosis* (15), and comparative analysis of the *M. bovis* BCG and *M. tuberculosis* genomes has identified several regions (encoding ~100 proteins) that are present only in the latter species (7). Theoretically, these *M. tuberculosis*-specific proteins should be optimal targets for developing a diagnostic test for TB. However, when six such proteins encoded by the RD1 region of the *M. tuberculosis* genome were cloned, the antigens showed very low sensitivities (3 to

Table 3. *M. tuberculosis* T-cell antigens for use in diagnosis

Antigen	Alternative name	Rv designation	Reference
Mtb8.4	DPV	Rv1174c	17
Mtb9.8	MSL	Rv0287	Dillon et al., (unpublished)
Mtb9.9a– Mtb9.9e	MTI	Rv1793, Rv3619c, Rv1198, Rv1037c, Rv2346c	1
ESAT-6	ESAT-6	Rv3875	5
CFP-10(Mtb11)	MTSA-10	Rv3874	6, 22
α-Crystallin	Mtb16	Rv2031c	18
Ag85B	Ag85B	Rv1886c	56
MPT-64	MPT 64	Rv1980c	37
Mtb32	Ra35/Ra12	Rv0125	66
Mtb39a– Mtb39e	TbH9	Rv1196, Rv1361c, Rv3478	23
Mtb40	HTCC#1	Rv3616c	Skeiky et al., (unpublished)
Mtb41	MTCC#2	Rv0915c	67

16%) (11). It is not clear whether the lack of antibody recognition is due to low expression of these proteins by the in vivo bacteria, protein expression during only certain stages of in vivo replication, lack of recognition by the patient's immune system, or inability of the recombinant proteins to mimic the epitopes that are expressed by the native molecules (59, 60, 65). Possibly, *M. tuberculosis*-specific proteins may not exhibit the immunodominance required for inclusion in a diagnostic test.

Finally, a large number of *M. tuberculosis* proteins chosen on the basis of proteomic approaches and screening of expression libraries of H37Rv and H37Ra with sera from patients with extrapulmonary TB, patients with active pulmonary TB, and patients lacking anti-38-kDa antibodies and with rabbit antibodies raised against culture filtrate proteins have been cloned by investigators at Corixa Corp. (22, 31, 35, 45). Studies with these proteins resulted in the prioritization of three potential candidate proteins for inclusion in an immunodiagnostic assay (22, 31, 45). These are Mtb 81 (same as the 81/88-kDa GlcB protein), CFP 10, and Mtb 48. Interestingly, all three of these proteins were immunodominant when tested with human sera (22, 31, 42, 45). Of these, the 81/88-kDa GlcB antigen provided the highest sensitivity of antibody detection in the cohorts evaluated at Corixa (31). The high sensitivities obtained with the 81/88-kDa protein in cohorts tested by Laal et al. and scientists at Corixa emphasize the immunodominance of this protein in strains from different geographical locations (31, 41, 42, 65). Recently, investigators at Corixa cloned a genetically fused polyprotein, TbF6, which encodes portions of four antigens (38 kDa, CFP 10, Mtb 48, and Mtb 8) (35). TbF6 provided 70% sensitivity in smear-positive and 52% sensitivity in smear-negative TB patients but appeared to be poorly recognized by HIV-infected TB patients (35). The use of TbF6 with another protein, DPEP (MPT 32), led to antibody detection in about 80% of smear-positive, about 60% of smear-negative, and about 45% of HIV-infected TB patients; in the same cohort of HIV-infected TB patients, the majority (80%) had anti-81/88-kDa antibodies (35).

One important fact that has emerged from these studies is that in contrast to the antigen mixtures (culture filtrate proteins, PPD, whole-cell lysates, etc.), higher specificities are achieved with defined, purified recombinant proteins (Tables 1 and 2).

Serodiagnostic Test for Incipient, Subclinical Tuberculosis

Nearly 90% of HIV-infected individuals live in developing countries where TB is endemic. The immune dysfunction caused by progressive HIV infection results in high rates of reactivation of latent TB, an increased incidence of progression of infection to primary TB, and an accelerated course of disease progression. As a result, TB is the major opportunistic infection in these countries, with 50 to 70% of HIV-infected patients developing TB (4, 29, 33, 34, 53). Preventive TB therapy reduces the risk of TB in PPD-positive HIV-infected individuals, but the scarcity of resources in these countries makes it impossible to provide preventive therapy and to monitor adherence and adverse drug reactions in all HIV-infected individuals (30). Moreover, the detection of infection is currently based on the PPD skin test, which has little value in individuals with dysfunctional cellular immunity. As a result, TB in HIV-infected individuals is diagnosed only when clinical TB is identified by the sputum smear, by which time the patient is highly infectious. Concurrent TB, in turn, causes rapid progression of HIV infection (78). Tests that can identify HIV-infected individuals with active, subclinical infection with *M. tuberculosis*, who are at a high risk of progressing to clinical TB, would enable targeted intervention in these individuals. In turn, this could prevent progression to clinical TB, contribute to the interruption of transmission into communities, and retard the progression of HIV infection in patients unable to obtain antiretroviral therapy.

Early studies aimed at determining the integrity of humoral immune responses in HIV-infected individuals revealed that prior to the onset of AIDS, patients make significant amounts of high-affinity immunoglobulin G antibodies (36, 40). Since *M. tuberculosis* grows slowly in vivo and in vitro and since TB can develop early during the course of HIV progression, when the immune system is relatively intact, the presence of antimycobacterial antibodies in sera obtained prior to progression to bacteriology-proven disease was ascertained in a unique cohort of HIV-infected TB patients (41). These were HIV-infected individuals who were being monitored for CD4/CD8 T-cell numbers at the New York Veterans Administration hospital during the 1980s and early 1990s, and several of these individuals developed clinical TB. Since serial serum samples from all previous clinic visits by these HIV-infected TB patients had been saved, these specimens provided the opportunity to evaluate the retrospective sera obtained during subclinical TB for the presence of antibodies to antigens of *M. tuberculosis*. Using a combination of immunological, biochemical, and proteomic approaches, antibodies to the 81/88-kDa GlcB B protein were found to be present in the retrospective sera from about 74% of the HIV-infected TB patients (41). These antibodies were undetectable in the sera from non-TB HIV-infected individuals and from HIV-infected individuals with *M. avium* complex disease. These results suggest that the presence of anti-81/88-kDa antibodies in the sera of HIV-infected individuals may serve as surrogate markers to identify individuals at high risk of progression to clinical TB. Two-dimensional mapping of dominant culture filtrate proteins recognized by antibodies present in the subclinical TB sera has been accomplished recently by Laal et al. (unpublished data). The results revealed that antibodies to the subset of about 12 antigens recognized in patients at all other stages of TB (described above) were also present in the sera obtained several months before manifestation of clinical TB. Since 2 of these 12 proteins (GlcB and MPT 51) have now been cloned, evaluation of their utility for diagnosis of incipient, sub-clinical TB in different cohorts is in progress. Antibodies to another *M. tuberculosis* antigen, SL-IV, were also reported to be present in retrospective sera obtained 1 to 30 months before the manifestation of TB in HIV-infected individuals (50).

Clearly, significant progress has been made in recent years in identifying and studying the potential of new antigens of *M. tuberculosis* for serodiagnosis. The availability of the genome sequence and the new tools of genomics and proteomics will undoubtedly enhance the speed at which additional antigens that can further increase the sensitivity and specificity of diagnostic assays will be obtained. Most studies so far have focused on developing diagnoses for pulmonary TB; it is probable that additional antigens that are specifically associated with different types of extrapulmonary TB or with pediatric TB exist, and specific efforts to recognize such antigens are required. Also, the low cost and relative simplicity of dipstick or lateral-flow immunodiagnostic tests makes them attractive candidate formats for use in resource-limited developing countries and in settings where large numbers of individuals need to be tested. Development of rapid tests based on the new antigens will be a challenge for the diagnostic industry. Given sustained effort, the field is moving in the direction of finally achieving the perfect immunodiagnostic test that has eluded the efforts made in last several decades.

TESTS BASED ON DETECTION OF CELLULAR IMMUNE RESPONSES

Cellular immune responses elicited on infection with *M. tuberculosis* involve the generation of both CD4$^+$ and CD8$^+$ T-cell subsets. Compared to the more involved experimental protocol needed for determining CD8$^+$ T-cell responses, methods for the evaluation of CD4$^+$ T-cell recall are relatively simple, sensitive, and routine in most laboratories. Furthermore, because most *M. tuberculosis*-infected individuals mount a relatively strong CD4$^+$ T-cell response to a broad spectrum of *M. tuberculosis* antigens, efforts are under way to develop a CD4$^+$ T-cell based assay for use in diagnosing and monitoring the outcome of TB infection. Typically, such assays are performed using whole blood or purified peripheral blood mononuclear cells (PBMC) and stimulated in vitro with PPD, culture filtrate protein (CFP), or defined *M. tuberculosis* antigens. Responses are monitored by measurement of the stimulation indices and/or the production of gamma inerferon (IFN-γ). As with most other diagnostic tests, the selection of antigens should maintain a relatively high sensitivity without compromising the specificity of the assay.

Identification of CD4$^+$ T-Cell Antigens

Biochemical, proteomic and genomics approaches

Over the past decade, several approaches have been used for the identification of T-cell antigens of *M. tuberculosis* capable of stimulating CD4$^+$ T cells in infected individuals and experimentally infected animals. The earliest of these, brute-force biochemistry, led to the identification of several of the most abundant proteins (Ag85 complex, MPT 32, PhoS, DnaK, GroES, MPT 46, MPT 53, MPT 63, and the 19-kDa lipoprotein) found in the culture filtrate fraction (2, 56, 80). Indeed, some were shown to be immunogenic in infected guinea pigs and mice (28, 80).

A more refined biochemical approach (gel electrophoretic fractionation of culture filtrate proteins) was later employed, which, when coupled with the use of memory immune CD4$^+$ T cells from infected mice, resulted in the identification of a defined set of antigens in the low-molecular-mass range of 6 to 10 kDa (ESAT-6 family) and 26 to 34 kDa (Ag85B or MPT 59) (3, 69). However, while these approaches met with some success in identifying immunologically relevant antigens, they did not provide a comprehensive list of CD4$^+$ T-cell antigens encoded by the mycobacteria. In part, this may have been due to the emphasis on the culture filtrate fraction as the source of starting material coupled with the inherent difficulty of identifying antigens of low abundance. As it has turned out, we now know that some of the most immunogenic mycobacterial antigens are localized in subcellular compartments other than the culture filtrate fraction. In addition, the most potent T-cell antigens are not necessarily the most abundant.

The sequencing of the entire genome of *M. tuberculosis* (15) had an immediate impact on our understanding of the biology of this infectious agent and has facilitated the development of vaccine and diagnostic reagents to combat the disease. Notably, genomic information has facilitated the identification of previously unknown related families of genes, including promising vaccine and diagnostic candidates. Moreover, comparative genomics of pathogenic *M. bovis* and BCG (49) and comparative DNA microarray analysis of *M. tuberculosis* H37Rv and BCG (7) have led to the identification of three regions (RD1 to RD3) that are present in all strains of *M. tuberculosis* and pathogenic *M. bovis* strains but deleted in all BCG vaccine strains and most environmental mycobacteria. Interestingly, two of the better-characterized T-cell antigens with potential diagnostic utility (ESAT-6 and CFP-10) are encoded within the RD1 region. Because of their absence from BCG, these two proteins are of particular interest in the development of a specific diagnostic test to distinguish between infection and BCG vaccination.

Complementing the genetic information, proteomics has evolved into a powerful tool, and its successful implementation was demonstrated by the comparative proteome of *M. tuberculosis* and *M. bovis* BCG (39, 49, 74), the identification and subcellular localization of the *M. tuberculosis* proteins (18, 61, 71), and the identification of new proteins not predicted by genome scanning (38). Furthermore, the application of proteomics in defining T-cell antigens of *M. tuberculosis* has resulted in the identification of several immunogenic antigens capable of stimulating splenocyte cultures from *M. tuberculosis*-infected C57BL/6 mice and PBMC from individuals with TB (18).

Expression cloning

The expression cloning approach using CD4$^+$ T cells was only recently applied to the field of *M. tuberculosis* antigen discovery and has met with tremendous success. It has proven to be a rapid, simple, and sensitive technique for the identification of CD4$^+$ T-cell antigens, using as a starting material T cells from *M. tuberculosis*-infected donors or experimentally infected mice (1, 67). Its strength lies in the direct utilization of memory T cells to identify immunogenic sequences encoded by the mycobacterial genome. Most importantly, it does not incorporate any antigen or biochemical fractionation protocol but, rather, relies exclusively on the *Escherichia coli* host to generate polypeptides corresponding to the genomic sequence of *M. tuberculosis*. The successful implementation of this approach required the generation of a representative *M. tuberculosis* expression library in *E. coli*. Because of its relatively small genome size, the generation of randomly sheared genomic libraries in lambda vectors has the added advantage of identifying potentially all open reading frames without the concerns of variability in the type of medium or growth conditions used in producing the bacteria, the source of the infectious agent (in vivo or in vitro derived), or the transcriptional bias toward abundant mRNAs (44). In addition, the generation of T-cell lines by using autologous blood-derived dendritic cells infected with *M. tuberculosis* presumably reflects the process of natural infection and peptide processing and ensures that the antigens detected are available to the immune response during infection with *M. tuberculosis*.

Finally, even though serological expression cloning has been around for over a decade, until recently only a handful of predominant abundant antigens were identified. Recent successes in utilizing this approach have been due in part to the refinement of the technical steps involved in the process. For example, the use of serological screening as a complementary approach for the identification of T-cell antigens has led to the recent identification of two new candidate antigens, CFP-10 (Mtb11) and the Mtb39 family of proteins (22, 23). Both have been validated as potent T-cell antigens capable of eliciting robust proliferative responses and IFN-γ production from PBMC of infected donors (22, 23).

Using the combined serological and CD4$^+$ T-cell expression cloning approaches, about 100 T-cell antigens were initially identified by scientists at Corixa Corp. These antigens were subsequently ranked based on the criteria that any single antigen must (i) elicit a strong T-cell response (proliferation and IFN-γ production) with PBMC derived from PPD-positive donors, (ii) be recognized by a panel of ethnically diverse donors, and (iii) show low to no background reactivity on donor PBMC derived from healthy PPD-negative and presumed uninfected controls. Based on these criteria, 12 antigens were prioritized as lead candidates (Table 3). Included in this list are antigens previously identified by other investigators, including Ag85 and ESAT-6. Surprisingly, several of the most immunogenic human T-cell antigens discovered by expression cloning techniques were not previously reported or identified by the other approaches. Of these, Mtb39a to Mtb39c (PPE family of proteins) and Mtb9.9a to Mtb9.9e represent three and five highly homologous proteins, respectively, with >80% protein identity and comprising shared as well as unique T-cell epitopes (1, 23). Mtb41 was identified by the murine T-cell expression cloning approach, and it also belongs to the PPE family, but with limited homology to the Mtb39 proteins (23). Of the remaining four antigens, Mtb32 is a serine protease (66) while Mtb40 (Y. A. W. Skeiky, J. A. Guderian, P. J. Ovendale, S. G. Reed, and M. R. Alderson, unpublished data), Mtb9.8 (D. C. Dillon, D. Molash, L. Zhu, P. Ovendale, C. H. Day, Y. A. Skeiky, A. Campos-Nero, S. G. Reed, and M. R. Alderson, unpublished data), and Mtb8.4 (17), are apparently unique (with no known function), given the absence of homologous sequences in other organisms.

Interestingly, by performing immunoblot analyses with specific antibodies against the prioritized antigens, most of the newly identified candidates (Mtb39, Mtb40, Mtb41, Mtb9.9, and Mtb9.8) were found to be localized on the membrane or cell wall compartment (Skeiky et al., unpublished data). In addition, multiple banding patterns were observed for some of these proteins (Mtb39, Mtb40, and Mtb41), in agreement with the presence of related family members. Furthermore, most of the proteins that localized in the highly enriched membrane and cell wall fractions could not be detected in the whole-cell lysate, thereby supporting the notion that several of the highly immunogenic antigens represent a small fraction of M. tuberculosis proteins. Not surprisingly, these antigens escaped detection by the traditional biochemical purification approach.

CD4+ T-cell responses

Evaluation of recombinant M. tuberculosis proteins on a panel of donor PBMC from healthy infected PPD-positive individuals revealed that the responses to the defined single antigens were often similar in magnitude to those elicited by the complex mixture of proteins present in CFP (Color Plate 4). Using a stimulation index of 5 as a measure of positive response, the percentage of donors covered by any of the individual candidates ranged from 50 to 80%, while CFP was recognized by all donors. Included in this evaluation are two weakly recognized recombinant M. tuberculosis antigens, Mtb12 and Mtb14 (77). However, as with the PPD skin test, the specificity of CFP (and Ag85B) as a T-cell diagnostic antigen is evidently compromised by the relatively high background responses in about 50% of uninfected donors. Interestingly, several of the prioritized antigens were found to elicit robust responses in infected donors when evaluated in vitro at very low antigen concentrations (<0.1 μg/ml), thereby validating the notion that M. tuberculosis antigens expressed at low levels retain their ability to trigger potent immune responses.

Epitope mapping of some of these antigens revealed T-cell responses to multiple shared and unique epitopes. In the case of the Mtb9.9 family, despite the small size of their open reading frames (encoding 94 amino acids) and the very high amino acid homology (>90% identity), heterogeneity in the T-cell response to each of the antigens was also observed. For example, T cells from a donor may react with the full-length recombinant antigen or with peptides from one of the proteins but not with the corresponding sequences from another of the family members, differing by as little as 1 or 2 amino acids (1). Cumulatively, at least five different epitopes have been mapped for members of the Mtb9.9 family of proteins. Similarly, at least 10 peptides have been mapped for the open reading frames of Mtb40 and Mtb41 (Y. A. W. Skeiky and M. R. Alderson, unpublished data). Furthermore, multiple T-cell epitopes, scattered throughout the protein sequence of ESAT-6 and CFP-10, have also been identified. Interestingly, the predominant recognition epitope of ESAT-6 appears to be different among tuberculosis patients from four different geographical locations, suggesting a genetic influence of peptide recognition in terms of major histocompatibility complex restriction (55). As with the Mtb9.9 family of proteins, a recent study revealed that the fine specificity of the T-cell responses to three closely related ESAT-6 family members (TB10.4, TB10.3, and TB12.9) were markedly different, with minimal differences in the amino acid sequence translating to profound differences in their T-cell recognition (68). Because most donors mount a T-cell response to several antigens directed against both shared and unique epitopes, cumulative data suggest that infection of the outbred human population induces responses to a broad repertoire of mycobacterial antigens. Whether this is due to antigen-specific immunogenicity or redundancy of the immune response resulting from shared epitopes, the net result is reflected in the amplification of the robustness of the CD4$^+$ T-cell response. In parallel, evaluation of the IFN-γ production by these PBMC revealed a direct correlation between the proliferative responses and the secretion of this cytokine.

T-Cell Antigens and Diagnosis of TB Infection

As discussed above, important efforts have been made in identifying immunodominant mycobacterial antigens, with the objective of developing new vaccines and immunodiagnostic reagents. These well-characterized, immunologically relevant antigens have the potential to circumvent many of the disadvantages associated with the use of crude antigen preparations (such as in the case of PPD or CFP) of poorly defined specificity. For use in an immunodiagnostic assay, the antigen composition must not be part of any intended vaccine and should also be sensitive enough to detect infected individuals while maintaining sufficient specificity to distinguish between *M. tuberculosis* infection, BCG vaccination, and prior exposure to environmental mycobacteria. Given that the repertoire of human T-cell antigens induced by natural infection is directed toward several proteins, the development of a sensitive T-cell-based diagnostic assay would require a mix of antigens with sufficient complementation to detect most infected individuals. Several factors may contribute to the variability of the responses to any one antigen, and these may include mycobacterial load, antigen expression level of different *M. tuberculosis* strains, major histocompatibility complex restriction, and cytokine secretion profiles.

Of the prioritized antigens, ESAT-6 and CFP-10 have been the most extensively evaluated antigens for the development of a T-cell-based assay and have been shown to specifically distinguish between, on the one hand, patients with pulmonary disease resulting from *M. tuberculosis* infection and, on the other hand, those infected with *M. avium* complex and recipients of BCG vaccination (43). In addition, compared to the responses with complex antigens present in *M. tuberculosis* sonicate, PPD, or CFP, T-cell responses to ESAT-6 and CFP-10 have been reported to be highly sensitive and specific in discriminating between TB patients and noninfected individuals (5, 43, 75).

Perhaps the most useful diagnostic TB test would be one that can predict whether the response of donor PBMC to any particular antigen is indicative of a higher risk of developing TB and whether the patient is therefore likely to benefit from preventive antimycobacterial therapy. In this regard, in a 2-year follow-up study of healthy household contacts of TB patients in Ethiopia, a strong recognition of ESAT-6 was found to correlate with the subsequent development of active TB in 86% of the healthy responders (25). In contrast, PBMC from the majority of contacts, regardless of their clinical outcome (including those who remained healthy throughout the observation period), responded to a comparable magnitude upon stimulation with PPD. A recent report of a comprehensive multicenter longitudinal study in The Gambia and Ethiopia found that when healthy household contacts ($n = 96$) were divided into high-risk ESAT-6 responders ($n = 38$) and low-risk ESAT-6 nonresponders ($n = 58$), the high-risk contacts had elevated levels of mRNA for interleukin-4 (IL-4) and its splice variant, IL-4δ2 (R. Brookes, H. Fletcher, P. Hill, P. Owiafe, M. Holland, A. Fox, D. Jeffries, A. Hammond, R. Adegbola, M. Doherty, K. McAdam, and G. Rook, *Abstr. First Int. Conf. TB Vaccines World*, 2003; T. M. Doherty, A. Demissie, A. Aseffa, H. Fletcher, G. Rook, A. Zumla, R. Brookes, P. Owiafe, K. P. McAdam, and P. Andersen, *Abstr. First Int. Conf. TB Vaccines World*, 2003). In contrast, no such correlation was observed when the contacts were segregated on the basis of their responsiveness to antigens other than ESAT-6. Furthermore, the utility of ESAT-6 in the identification of latently infected individuals has been addressed in several studies of community controls in countries where the incidence of TB is high, exposure to environmental mycobacteria is widespread, and >90% of the population have been vaccinated with BCG. In The Gambia, for example, about 30% of the community controls were found to respond to ESAT-6, in agreement with estimates of the prevalence of *M. tuberculosis* infection in Africa (76).

In general, even though the T-cell responses to ESAT-6 and CFP-10 for detection of infection are less sensitive than those observed with PPD (~70 versus ~100%), the assays are consistently found to be more specific (100 versus 72%). Clearly, the use of these antigens, and in particular ESAT-6, as reagents for the identification of latent TB and markers for identifying contacts who would probably progress to active disease will have a significant impact on the control of TB. However, their utility, and that of other antigens that are overexpressed in latently infected individuals (e.g., α-crystalline antigen), will be of limited use as a diagnostic reagent in distinguishing between healthy infected individuals and active TB and in monitoring the successful completion of therapy. Thus, the identification and evaluation of additional candidates that could complement ESAT-6 and CFP-10 are currently being addressed (54), and evaluation of the antigens (Mtb9.9a to Mtb9.9e, Mtb9.8, the Mtb39 family, etc.) identified by T-cell expression cloning have just begun in field trials.

Preliminary data suggest that some of the new candidates hold promise for inclusion in a T-cell-based diagnostic assay.

Finally, advances have also been made in the development of assays for measuring IFN-γ. Blood tests based on the in vitro detection of IFN-γ released in response to mycobacterial antigens have been routinely performed on purified PBMC by using standard IFN-γ enzyme-linked immunosorbent assays. However, methods involving the purification of PBMC are time-consuming and require specialized skills. Recently, a new test, QuantiFERON-TB (QFT; manufactured by Cellestis Ltd., Melbourne, Australia), was developed for measuring IFN-γ production in whole-blood samples stimulated with PPD or any defined antigen. In a study evaluating the clinical utility of the whole-blood IFN-γ assay with the tuberculin skin test, the specificity and sensitivity of the QFT test were comparable to or better than those of the traditional PPD skin test in terms of its ability to detect latent TB infection, and the test was able to distinguish between exposure to nontuberculous mycobacteria, latent TB infection, and, to some extent, BCG vaccination (37, 51, 72). This assay has also been evaluated in several studies comparing PPD with defined *M. tuberculosis* antigens. In one such study, it was concluded that in contrast to PPD, the use of ESAT-6 and CFP-10 resulted in an increased specificity of the whole-blood test and hence in discrimination between responses due to BCG vaccination, atypical mycobacterial exposure, and TB infection (10). Therefore, combined with the use of defined and specific *M. tuberculosis* antigens, the QFT test has already been validated as representing a significant improvement over the traditionally used tuberculin PPD skin test.

Skin test diagnostics

In the search for new skin test antigens specific for the diagnosis of TB infection, several candidates have been evaluated in the guinea pig model. These include CFP-10 (MTSA-10), ESAT-6, MPT 64 and DPPD (14, 16, 26). Both ESAT-6 and MPT 64 were reported to elicit DTH skin test responses in a large percentage of outbred guinea pigs infected with *M. tuberculosis* but not in animals sensitized with *M. bovis* BCG or *M. avium* (26). Furthermore, the combined use of ESAT-6 and MPT64 resulted in a positive skin test response in all 18 *M. tuberculosis*-infected guinea pigs tested. Similarly, CFP-10 was shown to elicit positive DTH responses in guinea pigs infected with *M. tuberculosis* but not in animals immunized with *M. bovis* BCG or *M. avium* (14). However, while these antigens have shown promise as skin test diagnostic candidates in the guinea pig model, their clinical utility will have to be validated in human clinical trials. For example, a small-scale clinical study using MPT 64 and MPT 59 (Ag85B) concluded that neither of these two antigens had properties superior to those of tuberculin PPD and that MPT64 did not induce DTH reactions in the majority of infected individuals (79). Perhaps the most promising of the more recently characterized antigens is rDPPD. This antigen, shown to be specific for members of the *M. tuberculosis* complex, has been evaluated in experiments with both infected guinea pigs and humans. In the guinea pig model, a 2.0-μg dose of rDPPD elicited a strong DTH response in 12 of 12 *M. tuberculosis*-infected animals but not in the uninfected controls or animals sensitized with *M. bovis* BCG or nine different strains of nonpathogenic environmental mycobacteria (16). In marked contrast, regardless of the *Mycobacterium* strain used to sensitize the animals, a strong DTH response was observed in all groups tested with PPD. Furthermore, rDPPD was shown to elicit a positive DTH response in 24 of 26 patients with confirmed pulmonary TB but not in any of the 25 PPD-negative healthy individuals (12). As part of the same study, a small-scale clinical trial was performed with randomly selected healthy individuals in Salvador, Brazil. Of the 270 healthy individuals tested, 40% developed a positive skin test to rDPPD, compared to 70% who developed a positive skin test to PPD. The study also revealed that while PPD responses resulted in a skewed histogram, rDPPD revealed a bimodal histogram of skin test positivity indicative of a clear separation between positive and negative DTH reactions (12). The percentage of rDPPD-reactive donors is close to the estimates of the prevalence of TB in areas of endemic infection. It is therefore tempting to speculate that positive skin test reactivity to rDPPD represents a distinction between individuals sensitized to environmental mycobacteria and those infected with tubercle bacilli. However, this study did not address whether the skin test reactivity to rDPPD could distinguish between BCG vaccination and healthy individuals with latent TB. Such a differential diagnosis is undoubtedly of great importance, particularly for use in countries where BCG vaccination is routine. Additional trials designed to address this issue are being contemplated. However, until such studies are performed, the diagnostic utility of rDPPD as a specific skin test reagent in identifying *M. tuberculosis*-infected individuals could be useful in countries such as the United States where BCG vaccination is uncommon.

SUMMARY

Thus, new antigens that can provide sensitive and specific identification of individuals infected with *M.*

tuberculosis are on the horizon. These antigens will be especially useful in countries where targeted intervention will allow significant reduction of progression to clinical, infectious TB, resulting in the reduction of further transmission. If the promise of new antigens that may be able to distinguish a latent infection from active but subclinical infection materializes, it will have a great impact not only on early treatment but also in clinical evaluation of new vaccines. The accelerated pace of antigen discovery and evaluation appears to be on the threshold of providing better diagnosis than has been available for almost a century.

REFERENCES

1. Alderson, M. R., T. Bement, C. H. Day, L. Zhu, D. Molesh, Y. A. Skeiky, R. Coler, D. M. Lewinsohn, S. G. Reed, and D. C. Dillon. 2000. Expression cloning of an immunodominant family of *Mycobacterium tuberculosis* antigens using human CD4(+) T cells. *J. Exp. Med.* 191:551–560.

2. Andersen, A. B., and E. B. Hansen. 1989. Structure and mapping of antigenic domains of protein antigen b, a 38,000-molecular-weight protein of *Mycobacterium tuberculosis*. *Infect. Immun.* 57:2481–2488.

3. Andersen, P., A. B. Andersen, A. L. Sorensen, and S. Nagai. 1995. Recall of long-lived immunity to *Mycobacterium tuberculosis* infection in mice. *J. Imunnol.* 154:3359–3372.

4. Ansari, N. A., A. H. Kombe, T. A. Kenyon, N. M. Hone, J. W. Tappero, S. T. Nyirenda, N. J. Binkin, and S. B. Lucas. 2002. Pathology and causes of death in a group of 128 predominantly HIV-positive patients in Botswana, 1997–1998. *Int. J. Tuberc. Lung Dis.* 6:55–63.

5. Arend, S. M., P. Andersen, K. E. van Meijgaarden, R. L. Skjot, Y. W. Subronto, J. T. van Dissel, and T. H. Ottenhoff. 2000. Detection of active tuberculosis infection by T cell responses to early-secreted antigenic target 6-kDa protein and culture filtrate protein 10. *J. Infect. Dis.* 181:1850–1854.

6. Arend, S. M., A. Geluk, K. E. van Meijgaarden, J. T. van Dissel, M. Theisen, P. Andersen, and T. H. Ottenhoff. 2000. Antigenic equivalence of human T-cell responses to *Mycobacterium tuberculosis*-specific RD1-encoded protein antigens ESAT-6 and culture filtrate protein 10 and to mixtures of synthetic peptides. *Infect. Immun.* 68:3314–3321.

7. Behr, M. A., M. A. Wilson, W. P. Gill, H. Salamon, G. K. Schoolnik, S. Rane, and P. M. Small. 1999. Comparative genomics of BCG vaccines by whole-genome DNA microarray. *Science* 284:1520–1523.

8. Binkin, N. J., A. A. Vernon, P. M. Simone, E. McCray, B. I. Miller, C. W. Schieffelbein, and K. G. Castro. 1999. Tuberculosis prevention and control activities in the United States: an overview of the organization of tuberculosis services. *Int. J. Tuberc. Lung. Dis.* 3:663–674.

9. Bothamley, G. H., R. Rudd, F. Festenstein, and J. Ivanyi. 1992. Clinical value of the measurement of *Mycobacterium tuberculosis* specific antibody in pulmonary tuberculosis. *Thorax* 47:270–275.

10. Brock, I., M. E. Munk, A. Kok-Jensen, and P. Andersen. 2001. Performance of whole blood IFN-gamma test for tuberculosis diagnosis based on PPD or the specific antigens ESAT-6 and CFP-10. *Int. J. Tuberc. Lung Dis.* 5:462–467.

11. Brusasca, P. N., R. Colangeli, K. P. Lyashchenko, X. Zhao, M. Vogelstein, J. S. Spencer, D. N. McMurray, and M. L. Gennaro. 2001. Immunological characterization of antigens encoded by the RD1 region of the *Mycobacterium tuberculosis* genome. *Scand. J. Immunol.* 54:448–452.

12. Campos-Neto, A., V. Rodrigues-Junior, D. B. Pedral-Sampaio, E. M. Netto, P. J. Ovendale, R. N. Coler, Y. A. Skeiky, R. Badaro, and S. G. Reed. 2001. Evaluation of DPPD, a single recombinant *Mycobacterium tuberculosis* protein as an alternative antigen for the Mantoux test. *Tuberculosis* (Edinburgh) 81:353–358.

13. Colangeli, R., A. Antinori, A. Cingolani, L. Ortona, K. Lyashchenko, G. Fadda, and M. L. Gennaro. 1999. Humoral immune responses to multiple antigens of *Mycobacterium tuberculosis* in tuberculosis patients co-infected with the human immunodeficiency virus. *Int. J. Tuberc. Lung Dis.* 3:1127–1131.

14. Colangeli, R., J. S. Spencer, P. Bifani, A. Williams, K. Lyashchenko, M. A. Keen, P. J. Hill, J. Belisle, and M. L. Gennaro. 2000. MTSA-10, the product of the Rv3874 gene of *Mycobacterium tuberculosis*, elicits tuberculosis-specific, delayed-type hypersensitivity in guinea pigs. *Infect. Immun.* 68:990–993.

15. Cole, S. T., R. Brosch, J. Parkhill, T. Garnier, C. Churcher, D. Harris, S. V. Gordon, K. Eiglmeier, S. Gas, C. E. Barry III, F. Tekaia, K. Badcock, D. Basham, D. Brown, T. Chillingworth, R. Connor, R. Davies, K. Devlin, T. Feltwell, S. Gentles, N. Hamlin, S. Holroyd, T. Hornsby, K. Jagels, A. Krogh, J. McLean, S. Moule, L. Murphy, K. Oliver, J. Osborne, M. A. Quail, M. A. Rajandream, J. Rogers, S. Rutter, K. Seegar, J. Skelton, R. Squares, S. squares, J. E. Sulston, K. Taylor, S. Whitehead, and B. G. Barell. 1998. Deciphering the biology of *Mycobacterium tuberculosis* from the complete genome sequence. *Nature* 393:537–544.

16. Coler, R. N., Y. A. Skeiky, P. J. Ovendale, T. S. Vedvick, L. Gervassi, J. Guderian, S. Jen, S. G. Reed, and A. Campos-Neto. 2000. Cloning of a *Mycobacterium tuberculosis* gene encoding a purifed protein derivative protein that elicits strong tuberculosis-specific delayed-type hypersensitivity. *J. Infect. Dis.* 182:224–233.

17. Coler, R. N., Y. A. W. Skeiky, T. Vedvick, T. Bement, P. Ovendale, A. Campos-Neto, M. R. Alderson, and S. G. Reed. 1998. Moleular cloning and Immunologic reactivity of a novel low molecular mass antigen of *Mycobacterium tuberculosis*. *J. Immunol.* 161:2356–2364.

18. Covert, B. A., J. S. Spencer, I. M. Orme, and J. T. Belisle. 2001. The application of proteomics in defining the T cell antigens of *Mycobacterium tuberculosis*. *Proteomics* 1:574–586.

19. Daniel, T. M., and P. A. Anderson. 1978. The isolation by immunoabsorbent affinity chromatography and physiochemical characterization of *Mycobacterium tuberculosis* antigen. *Am. Rev. Respir. Dis.* 117:533–539.

20. Daniel, T. M., and B. W. Janicki. 1978. Mycobacterial antigens: a review of their isolation, chemistry and immunological properties. *Microbiol. Rev.* 42:84–113.

21. Daniel, T. M. 1996. Immunodiagnosis of tuberculosis, p. 223–231. *In* S. Garay (ed.), *Tuberculosis*. Little, Brown & Co. Inc., Boston, Mass.

22. Dillon, D. C., M. R. Alderson, C. H. Day, T. Bement, A. Campos-Neto, Y. A. Skeiky, T. Vedvick, R. Badaro, S. G. Reed, and R. Houghton. 2000. Molecular and immunological characterization of *Mycobacterium tuberculosis* CFP-10, an immunodiagnostic antigen missing in *Mycobacterium bovis* BCG. *J. Clin. Microbiol.* 38:3285–3290.

23. Dillon, D. C., M. R. Alderson, C. H. Day, D. Lewinsohn, R. Coler, T. Bement, A. Campos-Neto, Y. A. W. Sheiky, I. M. Orme, A. Roberts, S. Steen, W. Dalemans, R. Badaro, and S. G. Reed. 1999. Molecular characterization and human T-cell responses to a member of a novel *Mycobacterium tuberculosis* mtb39 gene family. *Infect. Immun.* 67:2941–2950.

24. DiPerri, G., A. Cazzadori, S. Vento, M. Malena, L. Bontempini, M. Lanzafame, B. Allegranzi, and E. Concia. 1996. Comparative histopathological study of pulmonary tuberculosis in human immunodeficiency virus-infected and non-infected patients. *Tubercle Lung Dis.* **77:**244–249.

25. Doherty, T. M., A. Demissie, J. Olobo, D. Wolday, S. Britton, T. Eguale, P. Ravn, and P. Andersen. 2002. Immune responses to the *Mycobacterium tuberculosis*-specific antigen ESAT-6 signal subclinical infection among contacts of tuberculosis patients. *J. Clin. Microbiol.* **40:**704–706.

26. Elhay, M. J., T. Oettinger, and P. Andersen. 1998. Delayed-type hypersensitivity responses to ESAT-6 and MPT64 from *Mycobacterium tuberculosis* in the guinea pig. *Infect. Immun.* **66:**3454–3456.

27. Foulds, J., and R. O'Brien. 1998. New tools for the diagnosis of tuberculosis: the perspective of developing countries. *Int. J. Tuberc. Lung Dis.* **2:**778–783.

28. Harboe, M., T. Oettinger, H. G. Wiker, I. Rosenkrands, and P. Andersen. 1996. Evidence for occurrence of the ESAT-6 protein in *Mycobacterium tuberculosis* and virulent *Mycobacterium bovis* and for its absence in *Mycobacterium bovis* BCG. *Infect. Immun.* **64:**16–22.

29. Harries, A. D., N. J. Hargreaves, J. Kemp, A. Jindani, D. A. Enarson, D. Maher, and F. M. Salaniponi. 2001. Deaths from tuberculosis in sub-Saharan African countries with a high prevalence of HIV-1. *Lancet* **357:**1519–1523.

30. Hawken, M. P. and D. W. Muhindi. 1999. Tuberculosis preventive therapy in HIV-infected persons: feasibility issues in developing countries. *Int. J. Tuberc. Lung Dis.* **3:**646–650.

31. Hendrickson, R. C., J. F. Douglass, L. D. Reynolds, P. D. McNeill, D. Carter, S. G. Reed, and R. L. Houghton. 2000. Mass spectrometric identification of *Mtb81*, a novel serological marker for tuberculosis. *J. Clin. Microbiol.* **38:**2354–2361.

32. Hewitt, A. R. M. Coates, D. A. Mitchinson, and J. Ivanyi. 1982. The use of murine monoclonal antibodies without purification of antigen in the serodiagnosis of tuberculosis. *J. Immunol. Methods* **55:**205–211.

33. Hira, S. K., A. S. R. Srinivasa Rao, and J. Thanekat. 1999. Evidence of AIDS-related mortality in Mumbai, India. *Lancet* **354:**1175–1176.

34. Holmes, C. B., E. Losina, R. P. Walensky, Y. Yazdanpanah, and K. A. Freedberg. 2003. Review of human immunodeficiency virus type 1-related opportunistic infections in sub-Saharan Africa. *Clin. Infect. Dis.* **36:**652–662.

35. Houghton, R. L., M. J. Lodes, D. C. Dillon, L. D. Reynolds, C. H. Day, P. D. McNeill, R. C. Hendrickson, Y. A. Skeiky, D. P. Sampaio, R. Badaro, K. P. Lyashchenko, and S. G. Reed. 2002. Use of multiepitope polyproteins in serodiagnosis of active tuberculosis. *Clin. Diagn. Lab. Immunol.* **9:**883–891.

36. Janoff, E. N., W. D. Hardy, P. D. Smith, and S. M. Wahl. 1991. Humoral recall responses in HIV infection. *J. Immunol.* **147:**2130–2135.

37. Johnson, P. D., R. L. Stuart, M. L. Grayson, D. Olden, A. Clancy, P. Ravn, P. Andersen, W. J. Britton, and J. S. Rothel. 1999. Tuberculin-purified protein derivative-, MPT-64-, and ESAT-6-stimulated gamma interferon responses in medical students before and after *Mycobacterium bovis* BCG vaccination and in patients with tuberculosis. *Clin. Diagn. Lab. Immunol.* **6:**934–937.

38. Jungblut, P. R., E. C. Muller, J. Mattow, and S. H. Kaufmann. 2001. Proteomics reveals open reading frames in *Mycobacterium tuberculosis* H37Rv not predicted by genomics. *Infect. Immun.* **69:**5905–5907.

39. Jungblut, P. R., U. E. Schaible, H. J. Mollenkopf, U. Zimny-Arndt, B. Raupach, J. Mattow, P. Halada, S. Lamer, K. Hagens, and S. H. Kaufmann. 1999. Comparative proteome analysis of *Mycobacterium tuberculosis* and *Mycobacterium bovis* BCG strains: towards functional genomics of microbial pathogens. *Mol. Microbiol.* **33:**1103–1117.

40. Kroon, F. P., J. T. Van Dissel, J. Labadie, A. M. Van Loon, and R. Van Furth. 1995. Antibody response to diphtheria, tetanus, and poliomyelitis vaccines in relation to the number of cd4⁺ T lymphocytes in adults infected with human immunodeficiency virus. *Clin. Infect. Dis.* **21:**1197–1203.

41. Laal, S., K. M. Samanich, M. G. Sonnenberg, J. T. Belisle, J. O'Leary, M. S. Simberkoff, and S. Zolla-Pazner. 1997. Surrogate marker of preclinical tuberculosis in human immunodeficiency virus infection: antibodies to an 88 kDa secreted antigen of *Mycobacterium tuberculosis*. *J. Infect. Dis.* **176:**133–143.

42. Laal, S., K. M. Samanich, M. G. Sonnenberg, S. Zolla-Pazner, J. M. Phadtare, and J. T. Belisle. 1996. Human humoral responses to antigens of *Mycobacterium tuberculosis*: immunodominance of high molecular weight antigens. *Clin. Diagn. Lab. Immunol.* **4:**49–56.

43. Lein, A. D., C. F. von Reyn, P. Ravn, C. R. Horsburgh, Jr., L. N. Alexander, and P. Andersen. 1999. Cellular immune responses to ESAT-6 discriminate between patients with pulmonary disease due to *Mycobacterium avium* complex and those with pulmonary disease due to *Mycobacterium tuberculosis*. *Clin. Diagn. Lab. Immunol.* **6:**606–609.

44. Lodes, M., D. C. Dillon, R. L. Houghton, and Y. A. Skeiky. 2003. *Expression Cloning*, 2nd ed. Humana Press, Totowa, N.J.

45. Lodes, M. J., D. C. Dillon, R. Mohamath, C. H. Day, D. R. Benson, L. D. Reynolds, P. McNeill, D. P. Sampaio, Y. A. Skeiky, R. Badaro, D. H. Persing, S. G. Reed, and R. L. Houghton. 2001. Serological expression cloning and immunological evaluation of MTB48, a novel *Mycobacterium tuberculosis* antigen. *J. Clin. Microbiol.* **39:**2485–2493.

46. Lyashchenko, K., R. Colangeli, M. Houde, H. Al Jahdali, D. Menzies, and M. Gennaro. 1998. Heterogeneous antibody responses in tuberculosis. *Infect. Immun.* **66:**3936–3940.

47. Lyashchenko, K. P., M. Singh, R. Colangeli, and M. L. Gennaro. 2000. A multi-antigen print immunoassay for the development of serological diagnosis of infectious diseases. *J. Immunol. Methods* **242:**91–100.

48. MacVandiviere, H., W. E. Loring, I. Melvin, and S. Willis. 1956. The treated pulmonary lesion and its tubercle bacillus. II. The death and resurrection. *Am. J. Med. Sci.* **1956** (July): 31–37.

49. Mahairas, G. G., P. J. Sabo, M. J. Hickey, D. C. Singh, and C. K. Stover. 1996. Molecular analysis of genetic differences between *Mycobacterium bovis* BCG and virulent *M. bovis*. *J. Bacteriol.* **178:**1274–1282.

50. Martin-Casabona, N., T. G. Fuente, F. Papa, J. R. Urgell, R. V. Pla, G. C. Grau, and I. R. Camps. 1992. Time course of anti-SL-IV immunoglobulin G antibodies in patients with tuberculosis and tuberculosis-associated AIDS. *J. Clin. Microbiol.* **30:**1089–1093.

51. Mazurek, G. H., P. A. LoBue, C. L. Daley, J. Bernardo, A. A. Lardizabal, W. R. Bishai, M. F. Iademarco, and J. S. Rothel. 2001. Comparison of a whole-blood interferon gamma assay with tuberculin skin testing for detecting latent *Mycobacterium tuberculosis* infection. *JAMA* **286:**1740–1747.

52. McKinney, J. D., K. Honer zu Bentrup, E. J. Munoz-Elias, A. Miczak, B. Chen, W. T. Chan, D. Swenson, J. C. Sacchettini, W. R. Jacobs, Jr., and D. G. Russell. 2000. Persistence of *Mycobacterium tuberculosis* in macrophages and mice requires the glyoxylate shunt enzyme isocitrate lyase. *Nature* **406:**735–738.

53. Misra, S. N., D. Sengupta, and S. K. Satpathy. 1998. AIDS in India: recent trends in opportunistic infections. *Southeast Asian J. Trop. Med. Public Health* **29:**373–376.

54. Mustafa, A. S., H. A. Amoudy, H. G. Wiker, A. T. Abal, P. Ravn, F. Oftung, and P. Andersen. 1998. Comparison of antigen-specific T cell responses of tuberculosis patients using complex or single antigens of *Mycobacterium tuberculosis*. *Scand. J. Immunol.* **48**:535–543.

55. Mustafa, A. S., F. Oftung, H. A. Amoudy, N. M. Madi, A. T. Abal, F. Shaban, I. Rosenkrands, and P. Andersen. 2000. Multiple epitopes from the *Mycobacterium tuberculosis* ESAT-6 antigen are recognized by antigen-specific human T cell lines. *Clin. Infect. Dis.* **30**(Suppl. 3):S201–S205.

56. Nagai, S., H. G. Wiker, M. Harboe, and M. Kinomoto. 1991. Isolation and partial characterization of major protein antigens in the culture fluid of *Mycobacterium tuberculosis*. *Infect. Immun.* **59**:372–382.

57. Pethe, K., S. Alonso, F. Biet, G. Delogu, M. J. Brennan, C. Locht, and F. D. Menozzi. 2001. The heparin-binding haemagglutinin of M. tuberculosis is required for extrapulmonary dissemination. *Nature* **412**:190–194.

58. Pottumarthy, S., V. C. Weels, and A. J. Morris. 2000. A comparison of seven tests for serological diagnosis of tuberculosis. *J. Clin. Microbiol.* **38**:2227–2231.

59. Roche, P. W., N. Winter, J. A. Triccas, C. G. Feng, and W. J. Britton. 1996. Expression of *Mycobacterium tuberculosis* MPT64 in recombinant *Mycobacterium smegmatis*: purification, immunogenicity and application of skin tests for tuberculosis. *Clin. Exp. Immunol.* **103**:226–232.

60. Romain, F., C. Horn, P. Pescher, A. Namane, M. Riviere, G. Puzo, O. Barzu, and G. Marchal. 1999. Deglycosylation of the 45/47-kilodalton antigen complex of *Mycobacterium tuberculosis* decreases its capacity to elicit in vivo or in vitro cellular immune responses. *Infect. Immun.* **67**:5567–5572.

61. Rosenkrands, I., K. Weldingh, S. Jacobsen, C. V. Hansen, W. Florio, I. Gianetri, and P. Andersen. 2000. Mapping and identification of *Mycobacterium tuberculosis* proteins by two-dimensional gel electrophoresis, microsequencing and immunodetection. *Electrophoresis* **21**:935–948.

62. Sada, E., L. E. Ferguson, and T. M. Daniel. 1990. An ELISA for the serodiagnosis of tuberculosis using a 30,000-Da native antigen of *Mycobacterium tuberculosis*. *J. Infect. Dis.* **162**:928–931.

63. Samanich, K., J. T. Belisle, and S. Laal. 2001. Homogeneity of antibody responses in tuberculosis patients. *Infect. Immun.* **69**:4600–4609.

64. Samanich, K. M., J. T. Belisle, M. G. Sonnenberg, M. A. Keen, S. Zolla-Pazner, and S. Laal. 1998. Delineation of human antibody responses to culture filtrate antigens of *Mycobacterium tuberculosis*. *J. Infect. Dis.* **178**:1534–1538.

65. Samanich, K. M., M. A. Keen, V. D. Vissa, J. D. Harder, J. S. Spencer, J. T. Belisle, S. Zolla-Pazner, and S. Laal. 2000. Serodiagnostic potential of culture filtrate antigens of *Mycobacterium tuberculosis*. *Clin. Diagn. Lab. Immunol.* **7**:662–668.

66. Skeiky, Y. A., M. J. Lodes, J. A. Guderian, R. Mohamath, T. Bement, M. R. Alderson, and S. G. Reed. 1999. Cloning, expression, and immunological evaluation of two putative secreted serine protease antigens of *Mycobacterium tuberculosis*. *Infect. Immun.* **67**:3998–4007.

67. Skeiky, Y. A., P. J. Ovendale, S. Jen, M. R. Alderson, D. C. Dillon, S. Smith, C. B. Wilson, I. M. Orme, S. G. Reed, and A. Campos-Neto. 2000. T cell expression cloning of a *Mycobacterium tuberculosis* gene encoding a protective antigen associ-

ated with the early control of infection. *J. Immunol.* **165**:7140–7149.

68. Skjot, R. L., I. Brock, S. M. Arend, M. E. Munk, M. Theisen, T. H. Ottenhoff, and P. Andersen. 2002. Epitope mapping of the immunodominant antigen TB10.4 and the two homologous proteins TB10.3 and TB12.9, which constitute a subfamily of the esat-6 gene family. *Infect. Immun.* **70**:5446–5453.

69. Skjot, R. L., T. Oettinger, I. Rosenkrands, P. Ravn, I. Brock, S. Jacobsen, and P. Andersen. 2000. Comparative evaluation of low-molecular-mass proteins from *Mycobacterium tuberculosis* identifies members of the ESAT-6 family as immunodominant T-cell antigens. *Infect. Immun.* **68**:214–220.

70. Smith, H. 1998. What happens to bacterial pathogens in vivo? *Trends Microbiol.* **6**:239–243.

71. Sonnenberg, M. G., and J. T. Belisle. 1997. Definition of *Mycobacterium tuberculosis* culture filtrate proteins by two-dimensional polyacrylamide gel electrophoresis, N-terminal amino acid sequencing and electrospray mass spectrometry. *Infect. Immun.* **65**:4515–4524.

72. Streeton, J. A., N. Desem, and S. L. Jones. 1998. Sensitivity and specificity of a gamma interferon blood test for tuberculosis infection. *Int. J. Tuberc. Lung Dis.* **2**:443–450.

73. Thybo, S., C. Richter, H. Wachmann, S. Y. Maselle, D. H. Mwakyusa, I. Mtoni, and A. B. Anderson. 1995. Humoral response to *Mycobacterium tuberculosis*-specific antigens in African tuberculosis patients with high prevalence of human immunodeficiency virus infection. *Tubercle Lung Dis.* **76**:149–155.

74. Urquhart, B. L., T. E. Atsalos, D. Roach, D. J. Basseal, B. Bjellqvist, W. L. Britton, and I. Humphery-Smith. 1997. 'Proteomic contigs' of *Mycobacterium tuberculosis* and *Mycobacterium bovis* (BCG) using novel immobilised pH gradients. *Electrophoresis* **18**:1384–1392.

75. van Pinxteren, L. A., P. Ravn, E. M. Agger, J. Pollock, and P. Andersen. 2000. Diagnosis of tuberculosis based on the two specific antigens ESAT-6 and CFP10. *Clin. Diagn. Lab. Immunol.* **7**:155–160.

76. Vekemans, J., C. Lienhardt, J. S. Sillah, J. G. Wheeler, G. P. Lahai, M. T. Doherty, T. Corrah, P. Andersen, K. P. McAdam, and A. Marchant. 2001. Tuberculosis contacts but not patients have higher gamma interferon responses to ESAT-6 than do community controls in The Gambia. *Infect. Immun.* **69**:6554–6557.

77. Webb, J. R., T. S. Vedvick, M. R. Alderson, J. A. Guderian, S. S. Jen, P. J. Ovendale, S. M. Johnson, S. G. Reed, and Y. A. Skeiky. 1998. Molecular cloning, expression, and immunogenicity of MTB12, a novel low-molecular-weight antigen secreted by *Mycobacterium tuberculosis*. *Infect. Immun.* **66**:4208–4214.

78. Whalen, C., C. R. Horsburg, D. Hom, C. Lahart, M. Simberkoff, and J. Ellner. 1995. Accelerated course of human immunodeficiency virus infection after tuberculosis. *Am. J. Respir. Crit. Care Med.* **151**:129–135.

79. Wilcke, J., B. Jensen, P. Ravn, A. Andersen, and K. Haslov. 1996. Clinical evaluation of MPT-64 and MPT-59, two protiens secreted from *Mycobacterium tuberculosis*, for skin test reagents. *Tubercle Lung Dis.* **77**:250–256.

80. Young, D. B., and T. R. Garbe. 1991. Lipoprotein antigens of *Mycobacteriun tuberculosis*. *Res. Microbiol.* **142**:55–65.

Tuberculosis and the Tubercle Bacillus
Edited by Stewart T. Cole et al.
© 2005 ASM Press, Washington, D.C.

Chapter 6

Molecular Diagnosis of Mycobacterial Infections

BETTY A. FORBES, GABY PFYFFER, AND KATHLEEN D. EISENACH

Clinical mycobacteriology laboratories play a key role in the control of the spread of tuberculosis (TB) through the timely detection, isolation, identification, and drug susceptibility testing of *Mycobacterium tuberculosis* isolates. The obvious demands for reliable and rapid means of diagnosing TB, as well as infections caused by nontuberculous mycobacteria (NTM), have generated a lot of interest in molecular biology-based assays that can directly detect the presence and drug resistance of the *M. tuberculosis* complex in clinical specimens. With the use of amplification systems, nucleic acid sequences can be detected directly in clinical specimens, offering better accuracy than acid-fast bacillus (AFB) smear and greater speed than culture. The applications of these assays are discussed, as well as their advantages, limitations, and, where appropriate, clinical utility.

DIRECT DETECTION IN CLINICAL SPECIMENS

A number of amplification methods that directly detect *M. tuberculosis* in respiratory and nonrespiratory clinical specimens include those developed in academic research laboratories or by industry. Discovery of PCR in 1986 made it possible to amplify target nucleic acid sequences, leading to the development of exquisitely sensitive and very rapid assays for detecting microorganisms directly in clinical specimens. Soon thereafter, alternative amplification techniques were developed which utilize different enzymes and strategies, such as amplification of target, probe, or signal; however, they are all based on reiterative reactions. Amplification targets include DNA and RNA, and those most frequently amplified in *M. tuberculosis* are the IS*6110* repetitive element, 16S ribosomal

DNA (rDNA), and 16S rRNA. Discussions of the various gene targets, amplification strategies, and methods for nucleic acid extraction and amplified-product detection are beyond the scope of this chapter; the reader is referred to relevant articles on these topics (23, 61).

Nucleic Acid Assay Performance

Numerous studies have been published on the ability of nucleic acid amplification assays (NAAs) to directly detect *M. tuberculosis* complex in clinical specimens. Drawing definitive conclusions regarding sensitivity, specificity, and predictive values from the myriad of studies is difficult, being complicated by various nucleic acid isolation procedures, mycobacterial gene targets for amplification, sample size inputs, cycling parameters, and patient populations. To date, the U.S. Food and Drug Administration (FDA) has approved only two commercial assays that directly detect *M. tuberculosis* complex in clinical specimens, the amplified *Mycobacterium tuberculosis* direct test (AMTD or MTD) (Gen-Probe, Inc., San Diego, Calif.) and the AMPLICOR *Mycobacterium tuberculosis* test (Roche Molecular Systems, Branchburg, N.J.). Although the discussions are focused on commercial assays available in the United States and abroad, similar issues are also germane to the in-house-developed ("home-brew") assays.

Most published studies report that the detection limit of NAAs is 5 to 100 CFU of mycobacteria when using dilutions of broth-grown organisms. However, when actual clinical specimens are tested and the results are compared with those of quantitative culture, the assay sensitivities are much lower. Decreased sensitivity with clinical specimens is most probably due to inhibitory substances in the specimen which

Betty A. Forbes • Department of Pathology, Medical College of Virginia, VCU Health System, Richmond, VA 23298-0210. Gaby Pfyffer • Department of Medical Microbiology, Kantonsspital, Lucerne 16 6000, Switzerland. Kathleen D. Eisenach • Mycobacteriology Research Laboratory, University of Arkansas for Medical Sciences and Central Arkansas Veterans Healthcare System, 4300 West 7th St., Little Rock, AR 72205.

interfere with the PCR or other amplification methods; however, other possibilities could be that organisms directly from humans are more resistant to lysis or more buoyant (more difficult to concentrate by centrifugation) than broth-grown organisms.

Respiratory specimens

Commercially available NAAs were initially evaluated as screening tests; i.e., all respiratory specimens were tested regardless of the suspected risk(s) for TB. Sensitivity and specificity were based on culture, the "gold standard," with clinical records used to evaluate discrepant results. When testing AFB smear-positive specimens, these assays performed well (sensitivity, 95 to 96%; specificity, 99 to 100%); however, with AFB smear-negative specimens, the sensitivities of NAAs were much lower (48 to 53%) (2). Some studies showed that there was a strong correlation between NAA sensitivity and the number of tested specimens for each patient (just as with culture), thus confirming that NAA performance is critically affected by the mycobacterial burden and its distribution in the sample (17, 62). Due to the poor sensitivity with AFB smear-negative specimens, the FDA approved the AMTD and AMPLICOR assays for use with only AFB smear-positive respiratory specimens. Subsequently, Gen-Probe, Inc., reformulated the AMTD assay to accommodate a larger volume of sample, which increased the assay's sensitivity. The enhanced, second-generation AMTD (AMTD2 or E-MTD) was approved by the FDA for testing both AFB smear-positive and smear-negative respiratory specimens. Moreover, the AMTD2 kit was cleared for testing nonrespiratory specimens.

Another issue identified early in the use of NAAs was that of false-positive results with samples from culture-negative patients who were receiving antituberculosis drugs (33). Nucleic acids are very stable and can be readily detected in clinical specimens that yield no organisms on culture. Thus, specimens from patients who have received antituberculosis drugs for 7 days or more or have been treated for TB within the last 12 months were excluded by the FDA from NAA testing.

Nonrespiratory specimens

The use of NAAs is particularly attractive for suspected cases of extrapulmonary TB since clinical diagnosis is often uncertain and the AFB smear and culture lack sensitivity. Both FDA-approved and other commercially available and home-brew assays have been tested extensively with nonrespiratory specimens, such as pleural fluids, gastric aspirates,

formalin-fixed paraffin-embedded tissues, fresh tissues, cerebrospinal fluids, and other sterile body fluids. Although promising, the performance of these assays has varied, with sensitivities ranging from 53.6 to 92.3% (3, 9, 10, 56, 57, 60, 66, 96). Clearly, several technical factors affect the performance of amplification tests. Several studies have shown that the inhibitory rate was significantly higher in extrapulmonary specimens (36, 44, 71), which would account, in part, for the lower sensitivities of the tests. On the other hand, other studies have detected few to no inhibitors in extrapulmonary specimens (27). Sensitivity appears to be dependent on the specimen type (some are more likely to contain inhibitory substances, e.g., pleural fluid), processing method, and, most importantly, specimen volume. For amplification assays to be of value with nonrespiratory specimens, more studies are needed to establish optimum sample volumes, processing and nucleic acid extraction methods based on specimen type, amplification parameters (such as nested PCR), and uniform criteria for interpretation of results (e.g., lowering the cutoff for a positive result).

Clinical Utility and Interpretation of Results

Conventional laboratory methods for the diagnosis of TB have notable limitations. First, although rapid, a sputum AFB smear has a reported sensitivity range of 22 to 78%. Moreover, the specificity of AFB smears can be a problem if specimens are obtained from individuals who are heavily colonized with or have chronic disease due to NTM. Similarly, sputum cultures are positive in a majority of patients if multiple specimens are obtained; however, the results for almost 30% of patients reported to have TB, including 22% of patients with pulmonary TB, are not culture confirmed. For isolation of *M. tuberculosis*, even with automated liquid-culture methods, the process may take 2 to 5 weeks. Yet, despite these limitations, NAAs cannot replace AFB smears or cultures. AFB smears provide an index of the degree of infectiousness, thereby facilitating informed decisions regarding public health measures. Cultures are essential for determining drug susceptibility profiles and, if indicated, strain genotyping.

As mentioned above, commercial amplification assays were initially evaluated as screening rather than diagnostic tests and their utility in clinical practice or public health settings was not investigated. Further evaluations with all commercially available NAAs have been carried out, and sensitivities, specificities, positive predictive values (PPVs), and negative predictive values (NPVs) were determined from the comparison to culture and clinical diagnosis; this is discussed in two excellent literature reviews (61, 96). To fully appreciate the accuracy of a test, the prevalence of the disease in that setting must be considered; in other words, the actual accuracy of the NAA depends on how common TB is in the population being tested. The clinical value of these tests depends largely on their PPVs and NPVs, and these vary considerably with the pretest probability of TB. Very few studies have evaluated amplification tests in the context of clinical risk assessments; however, several aspects of a multicenter trial conducted by Catanzaro et al. (13) have advanced these efforts. In this trial, they evaluated the performance of the AMTD2 assay with specimens from different patients stratified by level of clinical suspicion. Sensitivities of 83, 75, and 87% and corresponding specificities of 97, 100, and 100% for patients with low, intermediate, and high clinical suspicion, respectively, were reported. When stratified for these risk levels, the sensitivity and specificity of the AMTD2 were higher than those of the AFB smear. For the low-risk group (5% prior risk), both AFB smear and AMTD2 appeared useful for ruling out TB, with NPVs of 96% (AFB smear) to 99% (AMTD2). While neither test provided convincing evidence for ruling in disease at this level, the AMTD2 was potentially more useful, with a PPV of 59% compared with 36% for the AFB smear. Conversely, both tests were useful for ruling in disease for the high-clinical-suspicion group (87% prior risk), with PPVs of 94% for AFB smear and 100% for AMTD2. Only the AMTD2 would be useful in ruling out disease in this risk group (NPV of 91% for AMTD2 versus 37% for AFB smear). The AMTD2 appeared to offer greatest utility overall in the intermediate-clinical-suspicion group (29% risk), demonstrating a PPV of 100% (versus 30% for AFB smear) and an NPV of 91% (versus 71% for AFB smear). This clinically complex group included more cases of NTM infection, human immunodeficiency virus infection, and patients with risk factors such as contact exposure and positive skin tests than did the low- and high-suspicion groups. Hopefully, more rigorously controlled, fully blinded, head-to-head studies with careful documentation of the pretest risk of TB will be conducted to further elucidate which patients will benefit most from NAAs.

The results of patient-based evaluations underscore the need to individualize the use of amplification tests according to the clinical setting as well as interpret NAA results within the context of patient history, clinical findings, and other risk factors (7, 41). To assist laboratories and clinicians in this regard, guidelines for the use of these assays were proposed by the Centers for Disease Control and Prevention (15). In the algorithm, it is recommended that sputum specimens be collected on three separate days for AFB microscopy and culture. If AFB smears are positive and the NAA test is positive, the patient can be presumed to have TB without the need for additional NAA testing. If an AFP smear-positive specimen is NAA negative, a test for inhibitors should first be done. If no inhibitors are present, additional specimens (up to three) should be tested if NAA tests are repeatedly negative; if all NAA tests are negative, the patient is presumed to have NTM infection. If AFB smears are negative, an NAA test is performed on the first specimen collected; if the NAA test is positive or negative, additional specimens should be tested. The patient can be presumed to be noninfectious if all smear and NAA test results are negative. The clinician must rely on clinical judgment regarding the need for antituberculosis treatment and further diagnostic work-up because negative NAA results do not exclude the possibility of active pulmonary TB. Ultimately, the patient's response to therapy and culture results is used to confirm or refute a diagnosis of TB.

Given the additional expense of NAAs, their use with patients for whom the likelihood of TB is either very high or very low may represent an improper use of health care resources (5, 73). Amplification tests should be used when they are more likely to influence decisions regarding further diagnostic evaluation and antituberculosis therapy, such as cases when the likelihood of TB is neither very high nor very low. This particularly includes patients, most of whom are in the industrialized countries, for whom AFB smears are negative but the clinical suspicion is intermediate or high.

Specific Laboratory Issues

It is evident that molecular diagnostic assays have great potential to enhance our diagnostic capabilities; however, their results must be clearly interpreted within the clinical context, discussed above and in light of their performance characteristics demonstrated by the laboratory (95). In other words, a thorough understanding of the NAA parameters, including its procedural limitations, is critical for proper interpretation of results. Clearly, any NAA must be validated in terms of both its analytical and its clinical sensitivity and specificity prior to implementation. The laboratory must have appropriately designed workspace and equipment (e.g., positive-displacement pipettors with barrier tips, PCR/UV workstation, etc.) to physically control cross-contamination. In addition, staff must be properly trained in techniques to minimize cross-contamination of clinical specimens, DNA samples, and amplified product.

As with any laboratory test, the quality of the results is monitored by using appropriate controls. To monitor for inhibition, an internal control with a different molecular weight from the mycobacterial target but containing the upstream and downstream primer recognition sequences should be incorporated into each patient's sample reaction mixture. Thus, amplification of the internal control target indicates that there are no interfering substances. Neither of the FDA-approved assays has an internal control; however, they are included in the Roche COBAS AMPLICOR and Becton Dickinson ProbeTec Direct TB assays. If there is a question of inhibition with the other assays, a second reaction must be set up in which the patient sample is spiked with the known target nucleic acid and then amplified. Regardless of the format, a positive control for monitoring the efficiency of lysis and amplification (pooled smear-positive sputum) and a negative control for detecting contamination with nucleic acids or amplicon (master mix or water) must be run in parallel with patient samples. When an in-house-developed assay is used, a positive control should be included that is near the lower limits of detection for the assay. As with any other laboratory assay, if these controls do not perform as expected, the run must be repeated.

In addition to an internal quality control program, participation in an external quality control program for the direct detection of *M. tuberculosis*, such as that offered by the CDC, is highly desirable. The necessity for such participation was underscored by the study published by Noordhoek et al. (55), in which only 5 of 30 laboratories participating in a quality control study of NAA correctly identified the presence or absence of *M. tuberculosis* in all specimens.

Cost-effectiveness of NAAs is an important consideration. Since NAAs cannot currently replace conventional methods for the diagnosis and management of TB, an NAA is an additional test with associated high costs. Dowdy et al. (21) conducted a decision analysis to evaluate the cost-effectiveness of programs in which the AMTD was used to exclude *M. tuberculosis* complex as a cause of disease in smear-positive respiratory specimens. The marginal cost of the AMTD was estimated as $338 per smear-positive patient or $494 for early exclusion of TB based on negative AMTD results. By comparison, the cost of respiratory isolation and drugs averted by AMT testing was estimated at $201 per early exclusion. AMTD was therefore not cost-effective in this scenario. While routine NAA testing may not result in a lower financial cost for most individual hospitals, centralized reference laboratories may be able to implement NAAs in a cost-effective manner across a wide range of situations.

Non-FDA-Approved Commercial Amplification Tests

There are four commercial amplification tests that are widely used outside of the United States: COBAS AMPLICOR Mycobacterium system (Roche), LCx MTB assay (Abbott Laboratories, Abbott Park, Ill.), ProbeTec Direct TB (DTB) energy transfer (ET) system (Becton Dickinson Biosciences Microbiology Products, Sparks, Md.), and INNO-LiPA Rif. TB assay (Innogenetics NV, Zwijndrecht, Belgium).

The COBAS AMPLICOR system is an automated format of the AMPLICOR MTB PCR test. The whole process, with the exception of sample preparation, is automatically performed on this instrument. A distinct advantage is the inclusion of an internal control that is coamplified with each patient specimen tested. In addition to probes for *M. tuberculosis* complex, species-specific probes are available for *M. avium* and *M. intracellulare*, thus enabling the detection of common NTM. Results with the COBAS AMPLICOR MTB test are comparable to those of its manual version (62).

The LCx (ligase chain reaction) MTB assay detects the gene for the PAB protein, is based on probe amplification, and is recommended for respiratory specimens. Lack of sensitivity is the main shortcoming of the system; however, the assay was modified in the field to improve test sensitivity. Successful approaches included increasing the concentration of extracted target DNA and the number of amplification cycles, lowering cutoff values, and performing double washes of the sputum sediment to remove inhibitors. In 2002, the LCx MTB assay was withdrawn from the European market.

The ProbeTec Direct TB system is based on strand displacement amplification, which is an isothermal enzymatic process that amplifies DNA exponentially. Target sequences of the IS6110 and 16S rRNA gene are coamplified. Published sensitivities and specificities compared to liquid culture and clinical correlation are 60.7 to 100% and 98.9 to 100%, respectively (61). ProbeTec offers several advantages for clinical laboratories performing routine NAA tests. The most important one is the inclusion of an internal amplification control in the same well as the patient specimen. Initial specimen processing and amplification can be carried out in the same room, and all reagents can be stored at room temperature. Moreover, amplicon contamination is minimized, with the microwell being sealed and never opened after amplification. Sample preparation is labor-intensive; however, the assay is almost completely automated. Interestingly, when ProbeTec was compared to AMTD2, the sensitivities of the ProbeTec with extrapulmonary specimens and specimens from patients with conclusive TB diagnosis were significantly higher, and these differences were associated with the presence of inhibitory samples that the AMTD2, lacking an internal amplification control, could not detect (60).

The INNO-LiPA Rif. TB assay can detect the presence of both *M. tuberculosis* and its resistance to rifampin; it is discussed later in this chapter.

SPECIES IDENTIFICATION

Formats

Traditional methods for mycobacterial identification are based on growth parameters, biochemical characteristics, and the analysis of cell wall lipids; these methods are slow and cumbersome. Furthermore, results frequently vary among isolates of the same species and phenotypic patterns often overlap with those of different species such that identification is impossible. During the last two decades, mycobacteriology laboratories have realized important advances in mycobacterial identification through the application of molecular biology techniques. First, the introduction of radioisotope-labeled DNA probes and then acridinium ester-labeled DNA probes (AccuProbes; Gen-Probe, Inc.) greatly facilitated the identification of commonly isolated mycobacteria. Subsequently, commercially available and in-house-developed NAA tests were successfully used for the early identification of *M. tuberculosis* complex grown in liquid cultures (6, 37, 72). This approach not only significantly reduces the time to identification of *M. tuberculosis* in culture but also circumvents assay inhibition associated with clinical specimens such that sensitivities greater than 98% are achieved. Of note, a commercially available system in which the 16S-23S rRNA spacer region of mycobacterial species is amplified and then hybridized to a membrane strip containing probes to the eight most commonly isolated mycobacterial species (INNO-LiPA Mycobacteria; Innogenetics) has been successfully used to directly detect and identify mycobacteria in aliquots of positive MB/BacT Alert 3D, BACTEC 12B, and BACTEC MGIT cultures (47, 72, 77). A second commercial system, GenoType Mycobacterium (Hain Lifescience GmbH, Nehrin, Germany), using a similar format, has additional probes for *M. celatum*, *M. malmoense*, *M. peregrinum*, *M. phlei*, and two subgroups of *M. fortuitum*, expanding the coverage of species (43).

In recent years, the identification of NTM has become a challenge for clinical laboratories since there are currently more than 90 accepted species, coupled with an increasing recognition of the significant role of these organisms in a range of clinical presentations

(30). Direct sequencing of the hypervariable region of the 16S rDNA has become more and more important for identifying mycobacterial species when faced with growth-deficient mycobacteria and strains representing new species (59). The other common noncommercial approach is to PCR amplify a highly conserved gene and perform restriction enzyme analysis on the PCR product. Both 16S rRNA and *hsp65* genes have been successfully used for this purpose (12, 19, 26). All of the above methods are more rapid and accurate than conventional methods (76).

Laboratory Issues

Direct sequencing of the 16S rRNA gene is widely accepted for species identification; however, there are multiple problems with sequence repositories, such as base errors, ambiguous base designation, and incomplete sequences, which can lead to misleading results (91). To overcome some of these problems, Applied Biosystems (Foster City, Calif.) developed a quality-controlled database containing over 80 species of *Mycobacterium* (16, 31); the MicroSeq 500 16S rDNA Bacterial ID system includes all reagents required for amplifying and sequencing the full or partial 16S rRNA gene in addition to the software package (MicroSeq ID analysis software) for comparison with the database. As more sequencing has been done, it is obvious that standardization of the procedure and a quality-controlled database are essential for accurate identification. Data reveal that there are many undiscovered mycobacterial species in existence and that establishment of new species in situations where the 16S rDNA are very similar may be influenced by clinical relevance.

As an alternative to nucleotide sequencing, many laboratories use PCR amplification-restriction fragment length polymorphism analysis (RFLP) of the *hsp65* gene. With this method, RFLP patterns are distinctive for *M. tuberculosis*, *M. bovis*, *M. avium*, *M. intracellulare*, *M. kansasii*, and *M. gordonae*; however, analysis is becoming more cumbersome and challenging due to the growing number of *hsp65* alleles being described. Another complication arising from PCR-RFLP analysis is the lack of standardization of electrophoretic conditions, which makes comparison of data difficult from one laboratory to another (12).

Differentiation among Members of the *M. tuberculosis* Complex

The similarity of *M. tuberculosis*, *M. bovis*, *M. bovis* BCG, and *M. africanum* in clinical presentation and treatment of infections has resulted in the laboratory not differentiating these species of the complex. However, in certain situations it may be clinically relevant to confirm the identification of BCG, which is used as a vaccine against *M. tuberculosis*, as a recombinant vehicle for multivalent vaccines, and as a cancer immunotherapy. For epidemiologic purposes, it may be important to identify the source of infection, i.e., zoonotic (cattle and unpasteurized dairy products) versus human sources of TB; therefore, one may need to distinguish between *M. bovis* and *M. tuberculosis*. Furthermore, it may be useful to be able to identify the increasingly recognized *M. bovis* subspecies *caprae* and *M. tuberculosis* subspecies *canettii*.

Commercial molecular tests cannot differentiate these species because of the genetic identities of their 16S rRNA gene sequences. Likewise, other target loci that are useful for differentiating *M. tuberculosis* complex from NTM cannot discriminate the individual *M. tuberculosis* complex species due to genetic invariance. Comparative genomic analyses with the complete DNA sequence of *M. tuberculosis* H37Rv have provided information on regions of difference (RD 1 to RD 16) deleted in members of the *M. tuberculosis* complex other than *M. tuberculosis*. An algorithm developed using six RD regions and selected phenotypic tests (pyrazinamidase [PZA] susceptibility, thiophen-2-carboxylic acid hydrazide susceptibility, and O_2 tolerance) is a rapid and simple means of differentiating members of the *M. tuberculosis* complex (58). In addition, a novel PCR-based system using seven PCR primer pairs specific for various loci including 16S rRNA was shown to accurately identify members of the *M. tuberculosis* complex and clearly segregate these from NTM (35).

DETECTION OF RESISTANCE TO ANTITUBERCULOSIS DRUGS

Drugs administered in the therapy of TB mainly include compounds which inhibit cell wall synthesis (isoniazid [INH], ethambutol [EMB]), transcription (rifampin [RMP]), protein synthesis (streptomycin [SM] and other aminoglycosides), and nucleic acid synthesis (fluoroquinolones such as ofloxacin). PZA is also an important first-line drug; its cellular target and mechanism of action have yet to be determined. In the past few years, there has been considerable progress in the understanding of the mechanisms causing *M. tuberculosis* resistance to antituberculosis agents at the molecular level (see chapter 8). Resistance in *M. tuberculosis* is a result of mutations which seem to be conferred exclusively to chromosomal DNA and does not involve mobile genetic elements such as plasmids or transposons as seen in other bacteria. With more than two dozen genes known to date to be involved in resistance and with a large array of novel genotypic assays, the clinical mycobacteriology laboratory may approach rapid drug susceptibility testing from a new direction.

From Amplicons to Detection of Mutations— A Multistrategy Approach

Although many different genotypic assays are currently available for drug susceptibility testing, most are based on PCR amplification of a specific region of an *M. tuberculosis* gene (hot spot) followed by analysis of the PCR product for specific mutations associated with resistance to a particular drug. The presence or absence of mutations can be detected by several methods (Table 1), such as automated sequencing, gel electrophoresis (following single-strand conformation polymorphism [SSCP] or dideoxy fingerprinting), solid-phase hybridization (line probe assays, DNA arrays, or microchips), or hybridization in the liquid phase (heteroduplex analysis, mismatch cleaving assays, or molecular beacons); an extensive review of these methods can be found elsewhere (23).

Relevant mutations for resistance to most primary and some second-line antituberculosis drugs have been described. Resistance arises either from a mutation on a single gene or as a result of a complex single or multiple mutations (deletions, missense mutations, etc.) on different genes such as that for INH resistance.

Rifampin

Resistance to RMP, an important component of current TB treatment regimens, is associated with a short (81-bp) hot-spot region (codons 507 to 533) in the *rpoB* gene, which encodes the β-subunit of RNA polymerase (86). Of all RMP-resistant *M. tuberculosis* isolates analyzed so far, 90 to 98% have a mutation in this specific core region. While mutations occur in codons 531, 526, and 516 and generally result in high-level resistance and cross-resistance to other rifamycins, others, e.g., at codons 511, 518, and 522, result in low-level resistance and cross-resistance to certain rifamycins (see references in reference 99). A low level of resistance has also been reported to be associated with a few loci outside the hot spot in *rpoB*, e.g., L176F. As more RMP-resistant strains from around the world have been examined by sequencing, previously unreported mutations have been identified (65).

Due to the straightforward nature of RMP resistance and the fact that in most settings RMP resistance is a marker of multidrug-resistant TB, there are numerous data on RMP-resistant isolates from all parts of the world. While early studies were based mainly on PCR plus gene sequencing or PCR-SSCP, resistance is now frequently determined using a line probe assay that is commercially available (INNO LiPA Rif. TB assay). In this assay, a decontaminated specimen is used in a nested PCR and biotin is incorporated into the amplicon. The amplified biotinylated products are hybridized with a set of 10 oligonucleotides which are immobilized as parallel lines on a membrane strip. From the hybridization pattern obtained (colorimetric reaction as purple-brown lines), the presence or absence of mutations can easily be assessed. In addition to conjugate and *M. tuberculosis* control probes, there are five probes for wild-type *rpoB* sequences and four probes for the most frequently observed mutations (i.e., mutations occurring in 75% of the isolates tested thus far). With a turnaround time of <24 h, the test is easy and rapid to perform with smear-positive specimens and early stages of culture. Usually, results of the line probe assay correlate well with results obtained by conventional susceptibility testing (20, 69), automated gene sequencing (14), and RNA-RNA mismatch assays (49) (Table 1).

Other assays, including those based on nested PCR, single-tube PCR, and real-time PCR, work equally well in detecting point mutations on the *rpoB* gene, no matter whether PCR products were detected by enzyme-linked immunosorbent assays (ELISAs) (28), heteroduplex generator assays (70, 94), or molecular beacons (24). PCR and LCR on oligonucleotide microchips have also been successfully, though rarely, applied (45, 46, 79) (Table 1).

Isoniazid

Studies have identified INH resistance-associated mutations in the *katG, inhA, kasA,* and *ndh* genes and in the *oxyR-ahpC* intergenic regions. In contrast to RMP, the prevalence of the mutations conferring INH resistance varies. With the use of PCR-based methods (Table 1), alterations in the *katG* gene have been found in 22 to 64% of resistant strains analyzed, while mutations in the *inhA* gene and in the *ahpC* gene have been detected in 20 to 34% and 10% of the resistant strains, respectively (68, 99). However, recent studies showed that INH resistance is far more complex. For example, Ramaswamy et al. (64) sequenced 20 genes which may be implicated in INH resistance and found that 44.7% of the strains analyzed had a single-locus, resistance-associated mutation in either the *katG, mabA,* or *Rv1772* genes whereas the same proportion had resistance-associated

mutations in two or more genes. Overall, 76% had mutations in the *katG* gene. Mutations were also identified in the *fadE24, Rv1592c, Rv1772, Rv0340,* and *iniBAC* genes. Nevertheless, in those studies, phenotypically INH-resistant strains have been found in which none of the above mutations could be detected.

Another observation adding to the complexity of detecting INH resistance is that some *katG* mutations associated with INH resistance have been found in INH-susceptible strains (M.H. Hazbon, M. Varma, M. Bobadilla del Valle, L. Garcia, J. Sifuentes-Osomio, A. Ponce de Leon, M.D. Cave, and D. Alland, *Tuberc. Integrating Host Pathog. Biol. Keystone Symp.* abstr. 426, 2003), which emphasizes the importance of testing drug-susceptible strains along with drug resistant strains.

Ethambutol

The EMB resistance-determining region (ERDR) has been proposed as a mutational hot spot in the *embB* gene (87). The most common mutations are substitutions in the amino acid at position 306 of *embB*, which are associated with high-level resistance. They are seen in 48 to 62% of the strains analyzed so far. Rinder et al. (67) have recently described a PCR protocol targeting mutations in *embB* codon 306 directly from sputum samples within two working days. A multiplex allele-specific PCR assay to detect simultaneously mutations in the first and third bases of the *embB* codon 306ATG has been established (50). Strains have, however, also been reported for which the EMB MICs are <10 μg/ml and which do not have a mutation in the ERDR (1). In these strains, moderate resistance may result from EmbB overexpression or, conceivably, from mutations outside the ERDR.

Pyrazinamide

For PZA, mainly affecting semidormant, intracellular *M. tuberculosis* in an acidic environment (e.g., during the active process of inflammation), the only mechanism of resistance at the molecular level known so far involves mutations in the *pncA* gene, which are reported to occur at a frequency of 72 to 96% (68). If these occur, strains are defective for pyrazinamidase activity and, as a consequence, resistant to PZA. Hannan et al. (32) recently demonstrated that monoresistance to PZA not only is an intrinsic feature of *M. bovis* but also may occur in *M. tuberculosis*.

PCR followed by gene sequencing or SSCP of the *pncA* gene has been used by several groups. Hou et al. (34) reported on 35 PZA-resistant strains of *M. tuberculosis* from China, of which 91.4% had nu-

Table 1. Molecular biology techniques commonly used to detect of mutations causing *M. tuberculosis* resistance to antimicrobial agents

Drug	Cellular target or mechanism	Gene	Technique	Reference(s)[a]
RMP	Nucleic acids (inhibition of transcription)	*rpoB*	PCR-sequencing	54
				14
				49
				70
				98
		rpoB	n-PCR–sequencing	39
		rpoB	Single-tube heminested PCR/sequencing	93
		rpoB	PCR-SSCP	86
		rpoB	n-PCR–SSCP	38
		rpoB	PCR-ELISA	28
		rpoB	PCR-line probe assay (INNO-LiPA)	20
				89
				14
				49
				92
		rpoB	PCR-reverse line blot hybridization	53
		rpoB	PCR/double gradient-denaturing gradient gel electrophoresis	72a
		rpoB	Single-tube, PCR/molecular beacons	24
		rpoB	PCR-heteroduplex analysis	54
		rpoB	PCR-universal heteroduplex generator assay	94
				70
		rpoB	Allele-specific PCR assay	52
		rpoB	Real-time PCR-fluorescence	88
		rpoB	Real-time PCR-sequencing	29
		rpoB	Real-time PCR-biprobe analysis	22
		rpoB	Hybridization-PCR on microchip	45, 46
		rpoB	Hybridization-LCR on microchip	46
		rpoB	RNA-RNA mismatch assay	49
		rpoB	Branch migration inhibition/luminescence oxygen-channeling assay	42
INH	Cell wall (inhibition of mycolic acid synthesis, potential interference with DNA, as well as with lipid, carbohydrate, and NAD metabolism)	*katG* *mabA-inhA* 20 genes (*katG*; *mabA-inhA* regulon)	PCR-sequencing	4, 64
		katG	PCR-RFLP	54
				92
		katG	Multiplex allele-specific PCR assay	51
		katG	Real-time PCR-fluorescence	88
		katG	Real-time PCR-sequencing	29
EMB	Cell wall (inhibition of arabinogalactan biosynthesis)	*embB* *embB* *embB* *iniA* operon	PCR-sequencing	82
				1
				63
		embB	PCR-SSCP	82
		embB	PCR-gel electrophoresis	67
		embB	Multiplex allele-specific PCR assay	50

Continued on following page

Table 1. *Continued*

Drug	Cellular target or mechanism	Gene	Technique	Reference(s)[a]
PZA	Unknown	*pncA*	PCR-sequencing	8
				34
				25
		pncA *oxyR*		32
		pncA	PCR-SSCP	18
				34
		pncA *oxyR*	PCR-RFLP	32
		pncA	Branch migration inhibition/ uminescence-oxygen channeling assay	42
		pncA	PCR/in vitro transcription-translation system	84
SM	Protein synthesis (inhibition)	*rpsL* *rrs*	PCR-sequencing	80
		rpsL	PCR-RFLP	54
Fluoroquinolones	Nucleic acids (inhibition of DNA gyrase)	*gyrA*	PCR-sequencing	85
				97
		gyrA, gyrB		40
		gyrA	PCR-SSCP	78

[a]Selected references to studies published recently.

cleotide substitutions, insertions, or deletions. By using the same method, Endoh et al. (25) described a new deletion in that gene in Japanese strains. Sequence analysis of *pncA* in South African *M. tuberculosis* strains indicated, however, that 5 of 15 strains lacked pyrazinamidase activity although they carried a wild-type *pncA* sequence, suggesting alternative mechanisms for drug resistance (8). Similarly, Davies et al. (18) identified four isolates which were phenotypically resistant to PZA but which had active pyrazinamidase enzyme in the Wayne assay and a wild-type *pncA* gene on molecular analysis, thus rendering genotypic assessment of PZA resistance even more confusing and unreliable.

Streptomycin

Since the discovery of the more potent drugs INH and RMP, SM has become a less important therapeutic agent. Mutations in the *rpsL* and/or *rrs* gene(s) correlate with intermediate- or high-level resistance to SM in 52 to 59% and 8 to 21%, respectively, of the strains analyzed (68). Based on PCR plus gene sequencing and PCR-RFLP of the *rpsL* gene, the A-to-G transition in codon 43 is seen most frequently, while in the *rrs* gene an A-to-G base substitution at position 1400 remains the major type of mutation.

Fluoroquinolones

High-level resistance to fluoroquinolones, which are used as second-line drugs, is related to mutations in the quinolone resistance-determining region (QRDR) of the *gyrA* gene. These mutations have been found with a frequency of 75 to 94% (68). To date, all high-level-resistant strains of *M. tuberculosis* show mutations at codons 88, 90, 91, or 94 while low-level-resistant strains have no mutations at these loci, suggesting the use of alternate mechanisms (85, 97). A polymorphism in codon 95 of *gyrA*, found in approximately 15% of all *M. tuberculosis* strains (81), is, remarkably, not associated with increased resistance.

Current State-of-the-Art for Clinical Mycobacteriology Laboratories

The advantages of genotypic assessment of resistance are clear. Apart from short turnaround time and the potential for automation, considerably smaller numbers of viable bacteria are handled, thus decreasing the biohazard risk. However, aspects such as laboratory workflow, quality control/quality assurance, cost-effectiveness, and appropriate setting for implementation of such tests have not been addressed, mainly for two reasons. First, resistance to anti-TB drugs often involves changes at several possible loci within a gene or alterations in multiple genes, making testing very complex and cumbersome. Second, not all mechanisms of resistance have been identified. Therefore, a lack of mutations in the target gene(s) does not guarantee susceptibility of the organisms, implying that results generated by any of the molecular biology methods would have to be confirmed by phenotypic methods.

CONCLUDING REMARKS AND FUTURE DIRECTIONS

The application of molecular testing methods in the mycobacteriology laboratory has the potential to significantly improve our ability to detect M. tuberculosis directly in clinical specimens or cultures as well as to differentiate mycobacterial species and drug-resistant strains. The practical utility of direct amplification tests will be maximized only when clinicians select the appropriate patients for testing and interpret the results in the context of the clinical data. Using molecular methods for confirmation of species provides rapid and definitive results, and it would seem prudent to carry out this testing in larger reference laboratories, where it is likely to be cost-effective and where experienced technologists are dedicated to this type of work. While routine drug susceptibility testing by molecular methods may not be practical, in high-prevalence settings of multidrug-resistant TB a rapid direct test for RMP-resistant M. tuberculosis, such as the INNO-LiPA Rif. TB assay, would be a less expensive alternative to routine liquid culture and drug susceptibility testing and may be cost-effective in terms of patient management and treatment. Test expense is an issue in both industrialized and developing countries; however, selective testing enables cost savings mainly by allowing early detection and treatment of patients and appropriate use of isolation facilities. Formal, prospective trials should be conducted to compare the effect of early identification by NAA tests on patient care outcomes (treatment cure, completion of therapy, treatment failures and relapses, length of hospitalization, and death), implementation of infection control measures, and correlates of transmission. Hopefully, the outcome assessments of such trials will demonstrate that the use of amplification tests has a high cost-benefit ratio in particular settings.

As methods become more refined and automated, NAAs will become more amenable to the clinical mycobacteriology laboratory, and different formats will be available that are appropriate for specific applications and laboratory settings. As new technologies and instruments are developed, they are continually being applied to the detection and identification of mycobacteria as well as to the detection of drug resistance because of the advantages of speed and simplicity, i.e., real-time PCR, peptide nucleic acids, and microarrays (45, 46, 48, 75, 83, 90). To streamline testing, new strategies and formats employing various miniaturized instruments and innovative technologies are being developed that will enable all aspects of the assay—from specimen processing to readout—to be performed in one small device. Conceptually, it is possible to have mobile testing units for diagnosing TB under field conditions in the near future (74).

REFERENCES

1. Alcaide, F., G. E. Pfyffer, and A. Telenti. 1997. Role of embB in natural and acquired resistance to ethambutol in mycobacteria. Antimicrob. Agents Chemother. 41:2270–2273.
2. American Thoracic Society Workshop. 1997. Rapid diagnostic tests for tuberculosis. What is the appropriate use? Am. J. Respir. Crit. Care Med. 155:1804–1814.
3. Baker, C. A., C. P. Cartwright, D. N. Williams, S. M. Nelson, and P. K. Peterson. 2002. Early detection of central nervous system tuberculosis with the Gen-Probe nucleic acid amplification assay: utility in an inner city hospital. Clin. Infect. Dis. 35:339–342.
4. Bakonyte, D., A. Baranauskaite, J. Cicenaite, A. Sosnovskaja, and P. Stakenas. 2003. Molecular characterization of isoniazid-resistant Mycobacterium tuberculosis clinical isolates in Lithuania. Antimicrob. Agents Chemother. 47:2009–2011.
5. Barnes, P. F. 1997. Rapid diagnostic tests for tuberculosis: progress but no gold standard. Am. J. Respir. Crit. Care Med. 155:1497–1498.
6. Bergmann, J. S. and G. L. Woods. 1999. Enhanced Amplified Mycobacterium tuberculosis Direct Test for detection of Mycobacterium tuberculosis complex in positive BACTEC 12B broth cultures of respiratory specimens. J. Clin. Microbiol. 37:2099–2101.
7. Bergmann, J. S., G. Yuoh, G. Fish, and G. L. Woods. 1999. Clinical evaluation of the enhanced Gen-Probe Amplified Mycobacterium tuberculosis Direct Test for rapid diagnosis of tuberculosis in prison inmates. J. Clin. Microbiol. 37:1419–1425.
8. Bishop, K. S., L. Blumberg, P. Trollip, A. N. Smith, L. Roux, D. F. York, and P. Kiepela. 2001. Characterization of the pncA gene in Mycobacterium tuberculosis isolates from Gauteng, South Africa. Int. J. Tuberc. Lung Dis. 5:952–957.
9. Bonington, A., J. I. G. Strang, P. E. Klapper, S. V. Hood, W. Rubombora, M. Penny, R. Willers, and E. G. L. Wilkins. 1998. Use of Roche AMPLICOR Mycobacterium tuberculosis PCR in early diagnosis of tuberculous meningitis. J. Clin. Microbiol. 36:1251–1254.
10. Brown, T. J., E. G. Power, and G. L. French. 1999. Evaluation of three commercial detection systems for Mycobacterium tuberculosis where clinical diagnosis is difficult. Clin. Pathol. 52:193–197.
11. Brown-Elliott, B. A., D. E. Griffith, and R. J. Wallace, Jr. 2002. Diagnosis of nontuberculous mycobacterial infections. Clin. Lab. Med. 22:911–925.
12. Brunello, F., M. Ligozzi, E. Cristell, S. Bonora, E. Tortoli, and R. Fontana. 2001. Identification of 54 mycobacterial species

by PCR-restriction fragment length polymorphism analysis of the *hsp65* gene. *J. Clin. Microbiol.* **39**:2799–2806.

13. Catanzaro, A., S. Perry, J. E. Clarridge, S. Dunbar, S. Goodnight-White, P. A. LoBue, C. Peter, G. E. Pfyffer, M. Sierra, R. Weber, G. Woods, G. Mathews, V. Jones, K. Smith, and P. Della-Latta. 2000. The role of clinical suspicion in evaluating a new diagnostic test for active tuberculosis. *JAMA* **283**:639–645.

14. Cavusoglu, C., S. Hilmioglu, S. Guneri, and A. Bilgic. 2002. Characterization of *rpoB* mutations in rifampin-resistant clinical isolates of *Mycobacterium tuberculosis* from Turkey by DNA sequencing and line probe assay. *J. Clin. Microbiol.* **40**:4435–4438.

15. Centers for Disease Control and Prevention. 2000. Update: nucleic acid amplification tests for tuberculosis. *Morb. Mortal. Wkly. Rep.* **49**:593–594.

16. Cloud, J. L., H. Neal, R. Rosenberry, C. Y. Turenne, M. Jama, D. R. Hillyard, and K. C. Carroll. 2002. Identification of *Mycobacterium* spp. by using a commercial 16S ribosomal DNA sequencing kit and additional sequencing libraries. *J. Clin. Microbiol.* **40**:400–406.

17. Cohen, R. A., S. Muzzafar, D. Schwartz, S. Bashir, L. Luke, L. P. McGartland, and K. Kaul. 1998. Diagnosis of pulmonary tuberculosis using PCR assay on sputum collected within 24 hours of hospital admission. *Am. J. Respir. Crit. Care Med.* **156**:156–161.

18. Davies, A. P., O. J. Billington, T. D. McHugh, D. A. Mitchison, and S. H. Gillespie. 2000. Comparison of phenotypic and genotypic methods for pyrazinamide susceptibility testing with *Mycobacterium tuberculosis*. *J. Clin. Microbiol.* **38**:3686–3688.

19. De Baere, T., R. de Mendonca, G. Claeys, G. Verschraegen, W. Mijs, R. Verhelst, S. Rottiers, L. Van Simaey, C. De Ganck, and M. Vaneechoutte. 2002. Evaluation of amplified rDNA restriction analysis (ARDRA) for the identification of cultured mycobacteria in a diagnostic laboratory. *BMC Microbiol.* **2**:4.

20. De Beenhouwer, H., Z. Lhiang, G. Jannes, W. Mijs, L. Machtelinckx, R. Rossau, H. Traore, and F. Portaels. 1995. Rapid detection of rifampicin resistance in sputum and biopsy specimens from tuberculosis patients by PCR and line probe assay. *Tubercle Lung Dis.* **76**:425–430.

21. Dowdy, D. W., A. Maters, N. Parrish, C. Beyrer, and S. E. Dorman. 2003. Cost-effectiveness analysis of the Gen-Probe Amplified Mycobacterium tuberculosis Direct Test as used routinely on smear-positive respiratory specimens. *J. Clin. Microbiol.* **41**: 948–953.

22. Edwards, K. J., L. A. Metherell, M. Yates, and N. A. Saunders. 2001. Detection of *rpoB* mutations in *Mycobacterium tuberculosis* by biprobe analysis. *J. Clin. Microbiol.* **39**:3350–3352.

23. Eisenach, K. D. 1999. Molecular diagnostics, p. 161–179. *In* C. Ratledge and J. Dale (ed.), *Mycobacteria: Molecular Biology and Virulence.* Blackwell Science, Oxford, United Kingdom.

24. El-Hajj, H. H., S. A. Marras, S. Tyagi, F. R. Kramer, and D. Alland. 2001. Detection of rifampin resistance in *Mycobacterium tuberculosis* in a single tube with molecular beacons. *J. Clin. Microbiol.* **39**:4131–4137.

25. Endoh, T., A. Yagihashi, N. Uehara, D. Kobayashi, N. Tsuji, M. Nakamura, S. Hayashi, N. Fujii, and N. Watanabe. 2002. Pyrazinamide resistance associated with *pncA* gene mutations in *Mycobacterium tuberculosis*. *Epidemiol. Infect.* **128**:337–342.

26. Ergin, A., and G. Hascelik. 2004. Non tuberculous mycobacteria (NTM) in patients with underlying diseases: results obtained by using polymerase chain reaction-restriction enzyme analysis between 1997–2002. *New Microbiol.* **27**:49–53.

27. Gamboa, F., P. J. Cardona, J. M. Manterola, J. Lonca, L. Matas, E. Padilla, J. R. Manzano, and V. Ausina. 1998. Evaluation of a commercial probe assay for detection of rifampin resistance in *Mycobacterium tuberculosis* directly from respiratory and nonrespiratory clinical samples. *Eur. J. Clin. Microbiol. Infect. Dis.* **17**:189–192.

28. Garcia, L., M. Alonso-Sanz, M. J. Rebollo, J. C. Tercero, and F. Chaves. 2001. Mutations in the *rpoB* gene of rifampin-resistant *Mycobacterium tuberculosis* isolates in Spain and their rapid detection by PCR-enzyme-linked immunosorbent assay. *J. Clin. Microbiol.* **39**:1813–1818.

29. Garcia de Viedma, D., M. del Sol Diaz Infantes, F. Lasala, F. Chaves, L. Alcala, and E. Biouzal. 2002. New real-time PCR able to detect in a single tube multiple rifampin resistance mutations and high-level isoniazid resistance mutations in *Mycobacterium tuberculosis*. *J. Clin. Microbiol.* **40**:988–995.

30. Griffith, D. E., B. A. Brown-Elliott, and R. J. Wallace. 2002. Diagnosing nontuberculous mycobacterial lung disease. *Infect. Dis. Clin. North Am.* **16**:235–249.

31. Hall, L., K. A. Doerr, S. L. Wohlfiel, and G. D. Roberts. 2003. Evaluation of the MicroSeq system for identification of mycobacteria by 16S ribosomal DNA sequencing and its integration into a routine clinical mycobacteriology laboratory. *J. Clin. Microbiol.* **41**:1447–1453.

32. Hannan, M. M., E. P. Desmond, G. P. Morlock, G. H. Mazurek, and J. T. Crawford. 2001. Pyrazinamide-monoresistant *Mycobacterium tuberculosis* isolates in the United States. *J. Clin. Microbiol.* **39**:647–650.

33. Hellyer, T., T. W. Fletcher, J. H. Bates, W. W. Stead, G. L. Templeton, M. D. Cave, and K. D. Eisenach. 1996. Strand displacement amplification and the polymerase chain reaction for monitoring response to treatment in patients with pulmonary tuberculosis. *J. Infect. Dis.* **173**:934–941.

34. Hou, L., D. Osei-Hyiaman, Z. Zhang, B. Wang, A. Yang, and K. Kano. 2000. Molecular characterization of *pncA* gene mutations in *Mycobacterium tuberculosis* clinical isolates from China. *Epidemiol. Infect.* **124**:227–232.

35. Huard, R. C., L. C. de Oliveira Lazzarini, W. R. Butler, D. van Soolingen, and J. L. Ho. 2003. PCR-based method to differentiate the subspecies of the *Mycobacterium tuberculosis* complex on the basis of genomic deletions. *J. Clin. Microbiol.* **41**:1637–1650.

36. Johansen, I. S., V. O. Thomsen, A. Johansen, P. Andersen, and B. Lundgren. 2002. Evaluation of a new commercial assay for diagnosis of pulmonary and nonpulmonary tuberculosis. *Eur. J. Clin. Microbiol. Infect. Dis.* **21**:455–460.

37. Katila, M. L., P. Katila, and R. Erkinjuntti-Pekkanen. 2000. Accelerated detection of mycobacteria with MGIT 960 and COBAS AMPLICOR systems. *J. Clin. Microbiol.* **38**:960–964.

38. Kim, B. J., S. J. Kim, B. H. Park, M. A. Lyu, I. M. Park, G. H. Bai, S. J. Kim, C. Y. Cha, and Y. H. Kook. 1997. Mutations in the *rpoB* gene of *Mycobacterium tuberculosis* that interfere with PCR-single-strand conformation polymorphism analysis for rifampin susceptibility testing. *J. Clin. Microbiol.* **35**:492–494.

39. Kim, B. J., K. H. Lee, B. N. Park, S. J. Kim, E. M. Park, Y. G. Park, G. H. Bai, S. J. Kim, and Y. H. Kook. 2001. Detection of rifampin-resistant *Mycobacterium tuberculosis* in sputa by nested PCR-linked single-strand conformation polymorphism and DNA sequencing. *J. Clin. Microbiol.* **39**:2610–2617.

40. Lee, A. S., L. L. Tang, I. H. Lim, and S. Y. Wong. 2002. Characterization of pyrazinamide and ofloxacin resistance and drug resistant *Mycobacterium tuberculosis* isolates from Singapore. *Int. J. Tuberc. Lung Dis.* **6**:48–51.

41. Lim, T. K., A. Mukhopadhyay, A. Gough, K.-L. Khoo, S.-M. Khoo, K.-H. Lee, and G. Kumarasinghe. 2003. Role of clinical judgment in the amplification of a nucleic acid amplification

test for the rapid diagnosis of pulmonary tuberculosis. *Chest* 124:902–908.

42. Liu, Y. P., M. A. Behr, P. M. Small, and N. Kurn. 2000. Genotypic determination of *Mycobacterium tuberculosis* antibiotic resistance using a novel mutation detection method, the branch migration inhibition M. *tuberculosis* antibiotic resistance test. *J. Clin. Microbiol.* 38:3656–3662.

43. Mäkinen, J., A. Sarkola, M. Marjamäki, M. K. Viljanen, and H. Soini. 2002. Evaluation of GenoType and LiPA MYCOBACTERIA assays for identification of Finnish mycobacterial isolates. *J. Clin. Microbiol.* 40:3478–3481.

44. Maugein, J., J. Fourche, S. Vacher, C. Grimond, and C. Bebear. Evaluation of the BDProbeTec ET DTB assay(1) for direct detection of *Mycobacterium tuberculosis* complex from clinical samples. *Diagn. Microbiol. Infect. Dis.* 44:151–155.

45. Mikhailovich, V., S. Lapa, D. Gryadunov, A. Sobolev, B. Strizhkov, N. Chernyh, O. Skotnikova, O. Irtuganova, A. Moroz, V. Litvinov, M. Vladimirskii, M. Perelman, L. Chernousova, V. Erokhin, A. Zasedat, and A. Mirzabekov. 2001. Identification of rifampin-resistant *Mycobacterium tuberculosis* strains by hybridization, PCR, and ligase detection reaction on oligonucleotide microchips. *J. Clin. Microbiol.* 39:2531–2540.

46. Mikhailovich, V. M., S. A. Lapa, D. A. Gryadunov, B. N. Strizhkov, A. Y. Sobolev, O. I. Skotnikova, O. A. Irtuganova, A. M. Moroz, V. I. Litvinov, L. K. Shipina, M. A. Vladimirskii, L. N. Chernousova, V. V. Erokhin, and A. D. Mirzabekov. 2001. Detection of rifampicin-resistant *Mycobacterium tuberculosis* strains by hybridization and polymerase chain reaction on specialized TB-microchip. *Bull. Exp. Biol. Med.* 131:94–98.

47. Miller, N., S. Infante, and T. Cleary. 2000. Evaluation of the LiPA MYCOBACTERIA assay for identification of mycobacterial species from BACTEC 12B bottles. *J. Clin. Microbiol.* 38:1915–1919.

48. Miller, N., T. Cleary, G. Kraus, A. K. Young, G. Spruill, and H. J. Hnatyszyn. 2002. Rapid and specific detection of *Mycobacterium tuberculosis* from acid-fast bacillus smear-positive respiratory specimens and BacT/ALERT MP culture bottles by using fluorogenic probes and real-time PCR. *J. Clin. Microbiol.* 40:4143–4147.

49. Mokrousov, I., I. Filliol, E. Legrand, C. Sola, T. Otten, E. Vyshnevskaya, E. Limeschenko, B. Vyshnevskiy, O. Narvskaya, and N. Rastogi. 2002. Molecular characterization of multiple-drug-resistant *Mycobacterium tuberculosis* isolates from northwestern Russia and analysis of rifampin resistance using RNA/RNA mismatch analysis as compared to the line probe assay and sequencing of the *rpoB* gene. *Res. Microbiol.* 153:213–219.

50. Mokrousov, I., O. Narvskaya, E. Limeschenko, T. Otten, and B. Vishnevskiy. 2002. Detection of ethambutol-resistant *Mycobacterium tuberculosis* strains by muliplex allele-specific PCR assay targeting *embB306* mutations. *J. Clin. Microbiol.* 40:1617–1620.

51. Mokrousov, I., T. Otten, M. Filipenko, A. Vyazovaya, E. Chrapov, E. Limeschenko, L. Steklova, B. Vishnevskiy, and O. Narvskaya. 2002. Detection of isoniazid-resistant *Mycobacterium tuberculosis* strains by a multiplex allele-specific PCR assay targeting *katG* codon 315 variation. *J. Clin. Microbiol.* 40:2509–2512.

52. Mokrousov, I., T. Otten, B. Vyshnevskiy, and O. Narvskaya. 2003. Allele-specific *rpoB* PCR assays for detection of rifampin-resistant *Mycobacterium tuberculosis* in sputum smears. *Antimicrob. Agents Chemother.* 47:2231–2235.

53. Morcillo, N., M. Zumarraga, A. Alito, A. Dolmann, L. Schouls, A. Cataldi, K. Kemer, and D. van Soolingen. 2002. A low cost, home-made, reverse-line blot hybridization assay for

rapid detection of rifampicin resistance in *Mycobacterium tuberculosis. Int. J. Tuberc. Lung Dis.* 6:959–965.

54. Nachamkin, I., C. Kang, and M. P. Weinstein. 1997. Detection of resistance to isoniazid, rifampin, and streptomycin of clinical isolates of *Mycobacterium tuberculosis* by molecular methods. *Clin. Infect. Dis.* 24:894–900.

55. Noordhoek, G. T., J. D. A. van Embden, and A. H. Kolk. 1996. Reliability of nucleic acid amplification for detection of *Mycobacterium tuberculosis*: an international collaborative quality control study among 30 laboratories. *J. Clin. Microbiol.* 34:2522–2525.

56. O'Sullivan, C. E., D. R. Miller, P. S. Schneider, and G. D. Roberts. 2002. Evaluation of Gen-Probe Amplified *Mycobacterium tuberculosis* Direct Test by using respiratory and nonrespiratory specimens in a tertiary-care center laboratory. *J. Clin. Microbiol.* 40:1723–1727.

57. Park do, Y., J. Y. Kim, K. U. Choi, J. S. Lee, M. Y. Sol, and K. S. Suh. 2003. Comparison of polymerase chain reaction with histopathologic features for diagnosis of tuberculosis in formalin-fixed, paraffin-embedded histologic specimens. *Arch. Pathol. Lab. Med.* 127:326–330.

58. Parsons, L. M., R. Brosch, S. T. Cole, A. Somoskovi, A. Loder, G. Bretzel, D. Van Soolingen, Y. M. Hale, and M. Salfinger. 2002. Rapid and simple approach for identification of *Mycobacterium tuberculosis* complex isolates by PCR-based genomic deletion analysis. *J. Clin. Microbiol.* 40:2339–2345.

59. Pauls, R. J., C. Y. Turenne, J. N. Wolfe, and A. Kabani. 2003. A high proportion of novel mycobacteria species identified by 16S rDNA analysis among slowly growing AccuProbe-negative strains in a clinical setting. *Am. J. Clin. Pathol.* 120: 560–566.

60. Piersimoni, C., C. Scarparo, P. Piccoli, A. Rigon, G. Ruggiero, D. Nista, and S. Bornigia. 2002. Performance assessment of two commercial amplification assays for direct detection of *Mycobacterium tuberculosis* complex from respiratory and extrapulmonary specimens. *J. Clin. Microbiol.* 40:4138–4142.

61. Piersimoni, C. and C. Scarparo. 2003. Relevance of commercial amplification methods for direct detection of *Mycobacterium tuberculosis* complex in clinical specimens. *J. Clin. Microbiol.* 41:5355–5365.

62. Rajalahti, I., P. Vourinen, M. M. Nieminen, and A. Miettinen. 1998. Detection of *Mycobacterium tuberculosis* complex by the automated Roche Cobas Amplicor *Mycobacterium tuberculosis* test. *J. Clin. Microbiol.* 36:975–978.

63. Ramaswamy, S. V., A. G. Amin, S. Goksel, C. E. Stager, S. J. Dou, H. El Sahly, S. L. Moghazeh, B. N. Kreiswirth, and J. M. Musser. 2000. Molecular genetic analysis of nucleotide polymorphisms associated with ethambutol resistance in human isolates of *Mycobacterium tuberculosis. Antimicrob. Agents Chemother.* 44:326–336.

64. Ramaswamy, S. V., R. Reich, S.-J. Dou, L. Jasperse, X. Pan, A. Wanger, T. Quitugua, and E. A. Graviss. 2003. Single nucleotide polymorphisms in genes associated with isoniazid resistance in *Mycobacterium tuberculosis. Antimicrob. Agents Chemother.* 47:1241–1250.

65. Ramaswamy, S. V., S. J. Dou, A. Rendon, Z. Yang, M. D. Cave, and E. A. Graviss. 2004. Genotypic analysis of multidrug-resistant *Mycobacterium tuberculosis* isolates from Monterrey, Mexico. *J. Med. Microbiol.* 53:107–113.

66. Rimek, D., S. Tyagi, and R. Kappe. 2002. Performance of an IS6110-based PCR assay and the COBAS AMPLICOR MTB PCR system for detection of *Mycobacterium tuberculosis* complex DNA in human lymph node samples. *J. Clin. Microbiol.* 40:3089–3092.

67. Rinder, H., K. T. Mieskes, E. Tortoli, E. Richter, M. Casal, M.

Vaquero, E. Cambau, K. Feldmann, and T. Loscher. 2001. Detection of *embB* codon 306 mutations in ethambutol resistant *Mycobacterium tuberculosis* directly from sputum samples: a low-cost, rapid approach. *Mol. Cell. Probes* **15**:37–42.

68. Riska, P. F., W. R. Jacobs, Jr., and D. Alland. 2000. Molecular determinants of drug resistance in tuberculosis. *Int. J. Tuberc. Lung Dis.* **4**:S4–S10.

69. Rossau, R., H. Traore, H. De Beenhouwer, W. Mijs, G. Jannes, P. De Rijk, and F. Portaels. 1997. Evaluation of the INNO-LiPA Rif. TB assay, a reverse hybridization assay for the simultaneous detection of *Mycobacterium tuberculosis* complex and its relevance to rifampin. *Antimicrob. Agents Chemother.* **41**:2093–2098.

70. Saribas, Z., T. Kocagöz, A. Alp, and A. Günalp. 2003. Rapid detection of rifampin resistance in *Mycobacterium tuberculosis* isolates by heteroduplex analysis and determination of rifamycin cross-resistance in rifampin-resistant isolates. *J. Clin. Microbiol.* **41**:816–818.

71. Scarparo, C., P. Piccoli, A. Rigon, G. Ruggiero, M. Scagnelli, and C. Piersimoni. 2000. Comparison of enhanced Mycobacterium tuberculosis amplified direct test with COBAS AMPLICOR Mycobacterium tuberculosis assay for direct detection of *Mycobacterium tuberculosis* complex in respiratory and extrapulmonary specimens. *J. Clin. Microbiol.* **38**:1559–1562.

72. Scarparo, C., P. Piccoli, A. Rigon, G. Ruggiero, D. Nista, and C. Piersimoni. 2001. Direct identification of mycobacteria from MB/BacT Alert 3D bottles: comparative evaluation of two commercial probe assays. *J. Clin. Microbiol.* **39**:3222–3227.

72a. Scarpellini, P., S. Braglia, P. Carrera, M. Cedri, P. Chichero, A. Colombo, R. Crucianelli, A. Gori, M. Ferrari, and A. Lazzarin. 1999. Detection of rifampin resistance in *Mycobacterium tuberculosis* by double-gradient-denaturing gradient gel electrophoresis. *Antimicrob. Agents Chemother.* **43**:2550–2554.

73. Schluger, N. W. 2001. Changing approaches to the diagnosis of tuberculosis. *Am. J. Respir. Crit. Care Med.* **164**:2020–2024.

74. Schneegass, I., and Köhler, J. M. 2001. Flow-through polymerase chain reactions in chip thermocyclers. *Rev. Mol. Biotechnol.* **82**:101–121.

75. Shrestha, N. K., M. J. Tuohy, G. S. Hall, U. Reischl, S. M. Gordon, and G. W. Procop. 2003. Detection and differentiation of *Mycobacterium tuberculosis* and nontuberculous mycobacterial isolates by real-time PCR. *J. Clin. Microbiol.* **41**:5121–5126.

76. Somoskovi, A., J. Mester, Y. M. Hale, L.M. Parsons, and M. Salfinger. 2002. Laboratory diagnosis of nontuberculous mycobacteria. *Clin. Chest Med.* **23**:585–597.

77. Somoskovi, A., Q. Song, J. Mester, C. Tanner, Y. M. Hale, L. M. Parsons, and M. Salfinger. 2003. Use of molecular methods to identify the *Mycobacterium tuberculosis* complex (MTBC) and other mycobacterial species and to detect rifampin resistance in MTBC isolates following growth detection with the BACTEC MGIT 960 system. *J. Clin. Microbiol.* **41**:2822–2826.

78. Sougakoff, W., N. Lemaitre, E. Cambau, M. Szpytma, V. Revel, and V. Jarlier. 1997. Nonradioactive single-strand conformation polymorphism analysis for detection of fluoroquinolone resistance in mycobacteria. *Eur. J. Clin. Microbiol. Infect. Dis.* **16**:395–398.

79. Sougakoff, W., M. Rodrigue, C. Truffot-Pernot, M. Renard, N. Durin, M. Szpytma, R. Vachon, A. Troesch, and V. Jarlier. 2004. Use of a high-density DNA probe array for detecting mutations involved in rifampicin resistance in *Mycobacterium tuberculosis*. *Clin. Microbiol. Infect.* **10**:289–294.

80. Sreevatsan, S., X. Pan, K. E. Stockbauer, D. L. Williams, B. N. Kreiswirth, and J. M. Musser. 1996. Characterization of *rpsl* and *rrs* mutations in streptomycin-resistant *Mycobacterium tuberculosis* isolates from diverse geographic regions. *Antimicrob. Agents Chemother.* **40**:1024–1026.

81. Sreevatsan, S., X. Pan, K. E. Stockbauer, N. D. Connell, B. N. Kreiswirth, T. S. Whittam, and J. M. Musser. 1997. Restricted structural gene polymorphism in the *Mycobacterium tuberculosis* complex indicates evolutionarily recent global dissemination. *Proc. Natl. Acad. Sci. USA* **94**:9869–9874.

82. Sreevatsan S., K. E. Stockbauer, X. Pan, B. N. Kreiswirth, S. L. Moghazeh, W. R. Jacobs, Jr., A. Telenti, and J. M. Musser. 1997. Ethambutol resistance in *Mycobacterium tuberculosis*: critical role for *embB* mutations. *Antimicrob. Agents Chemother.* **41**:1677–1681.

83. Stender, H., K. Lund, K. H. Petersen, O. F. Rasmussen, P. Hongmanee, H. Miörner, and S. E. Godtfredsen. 1999. Fluorescence in situ hybridization assay using peptide nucleic acid probes for differentiation between tuberculous and nontuberculous *Mycobacterium* species in smears of *Mycobacterium* cultures. *J. Clin. Microbiol.* **37**:2760–2765.

84. Suzuki, Y., A. Suzuki, A. Tamaru, C. Katsukawa, and H. Oda. 2002. Rapid detection of pyrazinamide-resistant *Mycobacterium tuberculosis* by a PCR-based in vitro system. *J. Clin. Microbiol.* **40**:501–507.

85. Takiff, H. E., L. Salazar, C. Guerrero, W. Philipp, W. M. Huang, B. Kreiswirth, S. Cole, W. R. Jacobs, Jr., and A. Telenti. 1994. Cloning and nucleotide sequence of *Mycobacterium tuberculosis gyrA* and *gyrB* genes and detection of quinolone resistance mutations. *Antimicrob. Agents Chemother.* **38**:773–780.

86. Telenti, A., P. Imboden, F. Marchesi, D. Lowrie, S. Cole, M. J. Colston, L. Matter, K. Schopfer, and T. Bodmer. 1993. Detection of rifampin-resistant mutations in *Mycobacterium tuberculosis*. *Lancet* **341**:647–650.

87. Telenti, A., W. Philipp, S. Sreevatsan, C. Bernasconi, K. E. Stockbauer, B. Wieles, J. M. Musser, and W. R. Jacobs, Jr. 1997. The *emb* operon, a unique gene cluster of *Mycobacterium tuberculosis* involved in resistance to ethambutol. *Nat. Med.* **3**:567–570.

88. Torres, M. J., A. Craido, J. C. Palomares, and J. Aznar. 2000. Use of real-time PCR and fluorimetry for rapid detection of rifampin and isoniazid resistance-associated mutations in *Mycobacterium tuberculosis*. *J. Clin. Microbiol.* **38**:3194–3199.

89. Traore, H., K. Fissette, I. Bastian, M. Devleeschouwer, and F. Portaels. 2000. Detection of rifampin resistance in *Mycobacterium tuberculosis* isolates from diverse countries by commercial line probe assay as an initial indicator of multidrug resistance. *Int. J. Tuberc. Lung Dis.* **4**:481–484.

90. Troesch, A., H. Nguyen, C. G. Miyada, S. Desvarenne, T. R. Gingeras, P. M. Kaplan, P. Cros, and C. Mabilat. 1999. *Mycobacterium* species identification and rifampin resistance testing with high-density DNA probe arrays. *J. Clin. Microbiol.* **37**:49–55.

91. Turenne, C. Y., L. Tschetter, J. Wolfe, and A. Kabani. 2001. Necessity of quality-controlled 16S rRNA gene sequence databases: identifying nontuberculous *Mycobacterium* species. *J. Clin. Microbiol.* **39**:3637–3648.

92. Viader-Salvado, J. M., C. M. Luna-Aguirre, J. M. Reyes-Ruiz, R. Valdez-Leon, L. del Bosque-Moncayo Mde, R. Tijerina-Menchaca, and M. Guerrero-Olazaran. 2003. Frequency of mutations in *rpoB* and codons 315 and 463 of *katG* in rifampin-and/or idoniazid-resistant *Mycobacterium tuberculosis* isolates from northeast Mexico. *Microbiol. Drug Resist.* **9**:33–38.

93. Whelen, A. C., T. A. Felmlee, J. M. Hunt, D. L. Williams, G. D. Roberts, L. Stockman, and D. H. Persing. 1995. Direct

genotypic detection of *Mycobacterium tuberculosis* rifampin resistance in clinical specimens by using single-tube, hemi-nested PCR. *J. Clin. Microbiol.* **33**:556–561.

94. **Williams, D. L., L. Spring, T. P. Gillis, M. Salfinger, and D. H. Persing.** 1998. Evaluation of a polymerase chain reaction-based universal heteroduplex generator assay for direct detection of rifampin susceptibility of *Mycobacterium tuberculosis* from sputum specimens. *Clin. Infect. Dis.* **26**:446–450.

95. **Wolk, D., S. Mitchell, and R. Patel.** 2001. Principles of molecular biology testing methods. *Infect. Dis. Clin. North Am.* **15**:1157–1204.

96. **Woods, G. L.** 2001. Molecular techniques in mycobacterial detection. *Arch. Pathol. Lab. Med.* **125**: 122–126.

97. **Xu, C., B. N. Kreiswirth, S. Sreevatsan, J. M. Musser, and K. Drlica.** 1996. Fluoroquinolone resistance associated with specific gyrase mutations in clinical isolates of multidrug-resistant *Mycobacterium tuberculosis*. *J. Infect. Dis.* **174**:1127–1130.

98. **Yue, J., W. Shi, J. Xie, Y. Li, E. Zena, and H. Wang.** 2003. Mutations in the *rpoB* gene of multidrug-resistant *Mycobacterium tuberculosis* isolates from China. *J. Clin. Microbiol.* **41**:2209–2212.

99. **Zhang, Y., and A. Telenti.** 2000. Genetics of drug resistance in *Mycobacterium tuberculosis*, p. 235–254. *In* G. Hatfull and W. R. Jacobs (ed.), *Molecular Genetics of Mycobacteria*. ASM Press, Washington, D.C.

IV. CURRENT THERAPIES AND DRUG RESISTANCE

Chapter 7

Global Impact of Multidrug Resistance

MARCOS A. ESPINAL AND MAX SALFINGER

Multidrug-resistant tuberculosis (MDR-TB) is a form of TB caused by strains of *Mycobacterium tuberculosis* resistant to at least isoniazid and rifampin. MDR-TB exacerbates the already serious global TB problem; it is difficult to treat, and treatment requires drugs that are expensive, toxic, and less effective. Inadequately treated patients become chronic carriers and spread MDR-TB to their families and communities (102).

MDR-TB is, in most cases, the result of poor TB control, including lack (or misuse) of high-quality drugs, poor follow-up of patients receiving treatment, and outdated TB control strategies. Circulation and continuous transmission of MDR-TB strains also hamper control efforts. Because 95% of the global incidence of TB is generated in resource-limited countries (27) and because, for historical and economic reasons, the management and assessment of the magnitude of MDR-TB in high-income countries is different from that in resource-poor countries, this chapter assesses the global impact of MDR-TB from the dual perspective of high-income and resource-limited countries. It also addresses the laboratory services needed for diagnosis and management strategies and discusses the future of MDR-TB.

IMPACT OF MDR-TB IN HIGH-INCOME COUNTRIES

MDR-TB has been the focus of international attention since the late 1980s and early 1990s, when several outbreaks were reported in the industrialized world. These outbreaks, along with the human immunodeficiency virus (HIV)-AIDS pandemic, catalyzed the awakening of high-income countries to refocus interest on TB, which had been neglected for almost two decades. The origins of MDR-TB are closely linked to the introduction of chemotherapy for TB. Discoveries of streptomycin by Schatz, Bugie,

and Waksman (101) and *p*-aminosalicylic acid (PAS) by Lehmann (80) brought good news to the fight against TB, but they also marked the onset of drug resistance. Development of resistance was reported shortly after these drugs had been introduced (121). It is therefore crucial to revisit the history of drug-resistant TB in order to understand the essence of the problem, as the impact of today's situation may not be much different from that of yesteryear.

History of the Problem

In the 1950s and 1960s, MDR-TB was basically known as resistance of *M. tuberculosis* to isoniazid, streptomycin, and PAS, the most important anti-TB drugs of that time. Isoniazid and rifampin were introduced in 1952 (98) and 1966 (83), respectively. Rifampin, however, did not reach the market in high-income countries until the early 1970s. The work of the British Medical Research Council (BMRC) was landmark, and much of the knowledge of today is due to the Council's extensive work in the field (45). Since the early days of streptomycin, the BMRC has led the way by developing methods for measuring drug resistance, demonstrating that some strains of drug-resistant TB are not virulent in guinea pigs, and establishing the well-known principle of combination therapy to prevent the emergence of drug resistance. In the early 1960s, the World Health Organization (WHO) organized two meetings that led to the description of reliable criteria and techniques for testing mycobacteria for resistance to anti-TB drugs (14, 15). Finally, several clinical trials conducted by the BMRC, the U.S. Public Health Service, and the U.S. Armed Forces Study Unit, some of which were sponsored by the International Union Against TB and Lung Disease (IUATLD) and the WHO, were also ground-breaking, as most of them reported the development of drug resistance. For additional description

Marcos A. Espinal • Stop TB Partnership, World Health Organization, 1211 Geneva 27, Switzerland.   **Max Salfinger** • Department of Biomedical Sciences, School of Public Health, University at Albany, New York State Department of Health, Wadsworth Center, Albany, NY 12201-0509.

of these trials, the reader is referred to Iseman's *A Clinician's Guide to Tuberculosis* (65).

Following the introduction of anti-TB chemotherapy, surveys of resistance to anti-TB drugs, including large national samples, were conducted in several countries (3, 17, 44, 59, 61, 65, 113). These studies suggested low prevalences of primary drug resistance to streptomycin, isoniazid, or PAS. Monitoring of trends suggested the maintenance of stable levels of primary resistance between the 1950s and 1960s (18, 31, 86, 111). The main concern was the high prevalence of primary resistance to streptomycin demonstrated in some countries. This was attributed in great extent to the wide use of streptomycin as monotherapy in the early years of TB chemotherapy.

Acquired drug resistance also became the focus of attention during the 1950s and 1960s. Data available were suggesting a serious problem among previously treated cases. In 1957, Rist and Crofton, in a study conducted in 17 countries involving 4,341 *M. tuberculosis* strains from patients previously treated for TB, showed that 42% of the strains were resistant to at least one drug (96). Levels of resistance to isoniazid, streptomycin, and PAS were 31.5, 21.7, and 12.1%, respectively. The British TB Association conducted a study in 1960 to 1961 to assess the magnitude of acquired drug resistance in 38 chest clinics. Of 410 patients for whom drug susceptibility testing results were available, 81.7% had developed acquired resistance to one or more drugs. This study estimated that there were 3,500 patients in Great Britain excreting drug-resistant bacilli and at least 1,800 patients with bacilli resistant to the three standard drugs of the time (11). Likewise, other reports were also suggesting increases in acquired drug resistance (60), although the quality and scope of many of the reported studies were limited to some extent.

Despite the existence of drug-resistant TB since the introduction of chemotherapy (in many cases resistance to the three most important drugs), TB continued to decline in incidence in the industrialized world at a rate of 10 to 14% annually. Such a decline was suggesting that the positive impact of combined chemotherapy on the incidence of TB was outweighing the negative impact of drug-resistant TB. Furthermore, a 1969 review of the worldwide magnitude of drug-resistant TB concluded that "the peak infection period with drug-resistant strains may well be over in the affluent countries of the Western Hemisphere" (60).

By the early 1970s, parallel to the ongoing TB decline, interest in the disease was unfortunately also dwindling. Funding in several countries was curtailed, so that control and surveillance activities were severely reduced and sometimes even entirely closed down (62, 67). Even though rifampin was just being introduced into the fight against TB, the deadly combination of resistance to rifampin and isoniazid together was never envisaged as a future problem. Only a few high-income countries conducted surveillance of drug-resistant TB throughout the 1970s and 1980s. Periodic surveys done in the United States suggested stable or decreasing rates of resistance to anti-TB drugs (19, 20, 73). MDR-TB was rarely reported. Likewise, Japan also conducted periodic nationwide surveys of drug-resistant TB (58, 112). MDR-TB in all cases declined from 3.5% in 1977 to 2.4% in 1992. Furthermore, among new TB cases, the prevalence of MDR-TB constantly remained below 1%.

The New Tuberculosis

The advent of the HIV/AIDS epidemic in the 1980s, along with other factors, culminated in an increase in TB in the United States for the first time in many years, after a steady decline since the 1950s. Immigration from high-incidence countries, homelessness, and limited access to medical care due to cuts in public health programs were some of the other factors contributing either to the increase in TB or to a slowing of the decline in incidence in many high-income countries. Several outbreaks of MDR-TB among hospitalized HIV/AIDS patients, shelter residents, and correctional-facility inmates were documented in the United States and in parts of Europe in the late 1980s and early 1990s (8, 21, 43, 90, 95). These outbreaks were characterized by rapid progression to death, high case-fatality rates, high rates of tuberculin conversion among health care workers, and, in some cases, highly fit strains of *M. tuberculosis* (2). This emergency prompted the United States to conduct a survey of drug-resistant TB in 1991, which showed that MDR strains accounted for 3.5% (6% of the reported MDR-TB cases alone in New York City) of the *M. tuberculosis* strains isolated (5). U.S.-born adults aged 25 to 44 years and persons infected with HIV were the population groups most strongly affected.

Measures to address TB were again implemented in high-income countries. These included standards of rapid diagnosis and treatment, drug susceptibility testing for all culture-positive TB patients, requirement for quality assurance of recording and reporting, directly observed therapy and adherence-promoting strategies, and enhancement of infection control procedures in hospitals and other congregate settings. By the late 1980s and early 1990s, routine surveillance of drug-resistant TB was under way in several countries to monitor the effects of renewed TB control efforts on the problem of drug resistance (29, 30, 88, 97, 109). To date, the available data (including trends) consistently show a very low prevalence of MDR-TB among new TB cases in high-income countries (Color Plate 5), suggesting that MDR-TB is no longer a major public health problem in high-income countries. On the other hand, drug resistance among previously treated patients is at a high prevalence in several of these countries, similar to the situation in the 1950s and 1960s. However, the public health impact of drug resistance among previously treated patients is rather limited, since the proportion of such cases among all TB cases is fairly minimal.

The Case of Foreign-Born Populations

The decline of TB in high-income countries is slower among foreign-born than among native-born persons. Tuberculosis in foreign-born persons constitutes a substantial proportion of all TB cases (100). Migrants, refugees, and asylum seekers are in most cases from countries with a high prevalence of TB. Foreign-born persons usually reflect the public health situation of their country of origin, since the majority of them acquired *M. tuberculosis* years before emigrating. Drug resistance is also generally more common among foreign-born than among indigenous populations in high-income countries. In the Netherlands, the strains infecting 9% of indigenous and 18% of foreign-born TB patients were reported to have resistance to anti-TB drugs between 1993 and 1994 (76). Of 268 patients with drug resistance, 203 (76%) were foreign born. More importantly, of the 19 patients reported to be infected with MDR-TB, 15 were foreign born. In Switzerland, 14 patients with MDR-TB, 13 of them foreign born, were reported to the Swiss Federal Office of Public Health between 1995 and 1997 (57). In Australia, the country of origin was known for 76 of 82 TB patients reported to be infected with drug-resistant strains in 2000; of these, 70 (92.1%) had migrated from a total of 17 countries (81). Trends from Denmark reveal that MDR-TB was found in 15 TB patients between 1991 and 1998; of these, 14 were in foreign-born individuals (109). In the United Kingdom, although the proportion of MDR-TB isolates decreased significantly, from 1.3% in 1994 to 0.8% in 1999, 2% of the foreign-born individuals with TB had MDR-TB, compared to 1% of the native-born population (30). Similarly, in the United States, the proportion of MDR-TB has been declining; however, the decline has been greater among native-born than among foreign-born individuals. Of the 114 MDR-TB cases reported in 2001, 68% were in foreign-born persons (22).

In summary, it is now clear that in high-income countries, the majority of drug resistance and MDR-TB is occurring in foreign-born individuals. Fortunately, there is also evidence suggesting that trans-mission of *M. tuberculosis* from the foreign-born population to the indigenous one is minimal (92, 109). Immigrants usually tend to live and interact within their own communities in their host countries. Thus, transmission of *M. tuberculosis* tends to remain largely within such communities. Foreign-born persons constitute one of the population groups for whom enhanced control efforts should be prioritized in high-income countries.

Concluding Remarks

In high-income countries, MDR among new TB cases is not currently a major public health problem. Similar to the 1950s and 1960s, the public health impact of drug resistance and, more importantly, MDR in terms of offsetting the declining rates of TB in these countries has been very limited. The single great exception was severe outbreak of MDR-TB in the city of New York where millions of dollars were spent in order to bring it under control. On the other hand, there is no evidence that MDR-TB has turned into a major "superbug" with the capacity to replace drug-susceptible strains of *M. tuberculosis*. The rapid implementation of specific preventive and control measures in the early 1990s, following several outbreaks in high-income countries, has been a critical factor in further limiting the impact of MDR-TB in these countries. Despite such reassuring news, these countries have not shown complacency; they continue to monitor, prevent, and aggressively manage MDR-TB. Because of their nature, immigrants from countries with a high incidence of TB, the homeless, and persons in congregate settings are quite vulnerable to MDR-TB, requiring constant vigilance.

IMPACT OF MDR-TB IN RESOURCE-LIMITED COUNTRIES

Accurate and reliable information about the magnitude of drug-resistant TB from resource-limited countries (middle- and low-income countries) has been limited until recently. While information about the issue has been available since the early years of chemotherapy, in most cases it was considered to be of poor quality (25, 60, 72). Therefore, a thorough assessment of the impact of drug-resistant TB and, more importantly, MDR-TB, is not as straight forward in resource-limited countries as it is in the industrialized world.

History of the Problem

Studies conducted in resource-limited countries in the 1950s and 1960s, shortly after the introduction of anti-TB drugs, showed a high prevalence of primary resistance to isoniazid in Uganda (8.7%), Malawi (8%), Sudan (10%), Kenya (10%), and Algeria (15%) (60). Data from East Africa between 1953 and 1964 suggested worrying trends regarding primary resistance to isoniazid. In Madras, India, primary resistance to isoniazid increased from 3.8% in 1956 to 6.4% in 1963. Disturbing prevalences of primary resistance to isoniazid were also found in other Indian cities including Hyderabad, New Delhi, Bangalore, and Madanapalle. These studies also reported high prevalences of *M. tuberculosis* strains resistant to streptomycin and PAS. A common feature of these data was the higher prevalence of drug-resistant TB reported compared to that in high-income countries. Nevertheless, several methodological problems were pointed out, including the confounding of acquired resistance with primary resistance, the lack of representativeness of the sample sizes with regard to the populations surveyed, and the lack of standard criteria for the assessment of drug resistance (60).

Only a few resource-limited countries monitored trends on drug-resistant TB by using standard methods. Among these were Algeria, Chile, Korea, and Tanzania. Between 1965 and 1985, primary resistance to at least one drug decreased in Algeria from 15 to 6.3% and acquired resistance decreased from 81.9 to 35.7% (7). Such decreases were attributed to the implementation of TB control, including standardization of chemotherapy and rifampin-containing short-course chemotherapy. Nevertheless, the frequency of MDR-TB increased from 2.7% in 1975–1980 to 11% in 1981–1985. In the Republic of Korea, the frequency of any drug resistance increased from 36.3% in 1975 to 48% in 1980 (70). This was attributed to both an increase in case finding and neglect in ensuring the cure of newly diagnosed TB cases. Since the introduction of short-course chemotherapy and case-management procedures in the early 1980s, cure rates of new TB cases improved steadily, and drug resistance started to decrease once again. The frequency of combined MDR-TB decreased to 2.3% in 1998, after having increased from 1.7% in 1980 to 8.5% in 1985. MDR-TB among new patients decreased from 2.5% in 1985 to 1.9% in 1995 (69). In previously treated patients, MDR-TB increased from 1.2% in 1975 to 17.9% in 1995; however, this was the result of a decrease in the total number of previously treated patients, from 81 to 28. Such an effect is expected in the presence of an efficient TB control program that is able to reduce the pool of previously treated cases over time through the cure of newly untreated cases. In Tanzania, drug resistance also decreased, as a result of improvement in TB control (23). Chile has implemented the direct-observation-of-treatment strategy (DOTS) program for more than 30 years, and drug resistance there is not a major public health problem (114).

Algeria, Chile, Korea, and Tanzania were, however, exceptional cases. The majority of studies in resource-limited countries before the 1990s were not able to shed much light on the magnitude of the problem. Hospital-based surveys, small and selected samples, lack of laboratory quality control, and limited information about the type of drug resistance were some of the common methodological pitfalls. Two reviews of more than 150 published and unpublished studies, conducted between the 1960s and 1970s, concluded that the evidence from resource-limited countries was more difficult to interpret than that from the more resource-rich countries (71, 72). Notwithstanding the limitations, these reviews also pointed out that drug-resistant TB was ubiquitous and that isoniazid and streptomycin resistance was heterogeneously present throughout the world. Rifampin resistance was documented in only a few countries, probably because of the limited availability of this drug. As importantly, resistance to second-line drugs including capreomycin and ethionamide was also documented. Lack of treatment compliance, initiation of inappropriate treatment regimens, and unsupervised usage of drugs obtained without prescription were highlighted as the most important causes of resistance to anti-TB drugs. In a follow-up review of 63 studies conducted between 1985 and 1994, Cohn et al. suggested that the true global magnitude of the problem could not be determined from those studies because of several limitations of the data available (25). Nevertheless, the evidence assessed suggested the existence of a high prevalence of acquired MDR-TB in Bolivia, India, and Nepal, among others.

These uncertainties and limitations led the Third World Congress on TB in 1992 to conclude that there was little information about the global magnitude of MDR-TB and its impact on TB control (104). The majority of countries did not have in place proper surveillance methods for TB, including MDR-TB. In 1994, the international community launched the Global Project on Anti-TB Drug Resistance Surveillance, coordinated by the WHO and IUATLD, aimed at assessing the magnitude and trends of drug-resistant TB, especially in resource-limited countries.

Current Magnitude of the Problem: the WHO/IUATLD Global Project on Drug Resistance Surveillance

Evidence collected between 1994 and 2002, within the framework of the Global Project on Anti-TB Drug Resistance Surveillance and from other sources, has confirmed previous assertions that in resource-limited countries, drug-resistant TB, including MDR-TB, is ubiquitous. However, the magnitude of the problem is much lower than that of drug-susceptible TB. Reports from 64 countries and geographical sites suggest that the global median prevalence of MDR-TB is around 1%. There are, however, considerable data suggesting the presence of regional MDR-TB epidemics (Fig. 1). These regions include countries in Eastern Europe such as Estonia (14%), Latvia (9%), Lithuania (9%), Kazakhstan (10%), and Russia (the oblasts of Archangels [13%], Ivanovo [9%], and Tomsk [7%]) (38, 40, 93, 110, 118, 119). Trends from Estonia, Latvia, and areas of Russia have confirmed that MDR-TB is a severe problem and that specific control measures beyond routine TB control are needed to address it. The shift from a planned to a market economy, increasing poverty, collapse of the public health system, and continuation of outdated TB control measures have contributed to a reversal of the declining trends in TB in many of these countries. Until 1990, TB was declin-

ing in Eastern Europe at a rate of 5% per year; thereafter, it started to increase by 8% per year (120). This increase, together with the lack of infection control, standardization of treatment, and direct treatment supervision, created the basis for the generation of MDR-TB.

China and India, the countries with the highest TB incidence in the world, also have documented MDR-TB among new TB cases in some of their geographical areas (119). The situation in the rest of the world appears to be less serious, except for some countries in Africa and Latin America (32, 35). Sub-Saharan Africa is the highest reservoir of HIV infection. Fortunately, the available evidence suggests that the frequency of MDR-TB is below 1% in many of the countries severely hit by the HIV epidemic, including Botswana, Kenya, The Gambia, Uganda, and Zimbabwe (1, 10, 38, 50, 68). Efficient TB control, limited use of rifampin, and lack of access to health care by patients have been highlighted as potential factors responsible for such low rates of MDR-TB. On the other hand, Côte d'Ivoire has shown a worry-

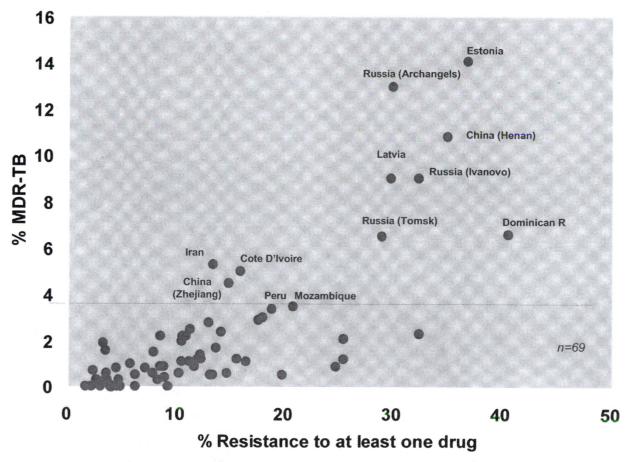

Figure 1. Correlation of MDR and resistance to any drug among new TB cases. The magnitude of MDR-TB strains correlates with the magnitude of TB strains with resistance to at least one drug. The majority of countries show low prevalence of both MDR-TB and TB resistant to at least one drug, with the exception of countries in Eastern Europe and other areas (70).

ing 5.3% rate of MDR-TB among new TB cases (32). However, HIV and MDR-TB were found not to be associated risk factors in this country. Poor TB control practices appear to be the main factor in the genesis of MDR-TB in Côte d'Ivoire.

According to international guidelines, MDR-TB is not a major problem in countries that have been implementing TB control for several years. Chile, Cuba, Hong Kong, the Republic of Korea, and Uruguay have all shown a low prevalence of MDR-TB, which is a good indication that efficient TB control prevents the onset and spread of MDR-TB. The case of Hong Kong is illustrative. In Hong Kong, since the introduction of short-course chemotherapy in 1987, primary TB and acquired MDR-TB have been declining at rates of 0.013 and 0.85% per year, respectively (66). This suggests that MDR-TB can be eliminated faster than can overall TB disease when control measures are effectively implemented, including judicious use of first- and second-line drugs.

Drug resistance in previously treated patients is a problem in several countries. Globally, the prevalence of resistance to at least one drug in 58 sites reporting data was 33% (range, 0 to 94%) and that of MDR-TB was 9% (range, 0 to 48%) (119). Some countries, however, show a high prevalence of MDR-TB as a result of the small number of previously treated cases. A high prevalence of drug resistance among previously treated patients may, paradoxically, be a reflection of years of successful management of TB. As new TB cases are treated and cured, the generation of previously treated cases decreases over time. Therefore, only few previously treated cases may be available: only those with drug resistance. Because of this paradox, the prevalence of drug resistance among previously treated patients is high, even when the absolute number is actually low.

Concluding Remarks

The recently held 2002 Fourth World Congress on TB concluded that, since the last congress in 1992, much progress has been achieved in defining the global burden of drug-resistant TB including MDR-TB (39). The available evidence shows that areas of Eastern Europe, Asia, and other parts of the world endure a problem with drug-resistant TB that deserves full attention and close monitoring. While the data collected point to the existence of local epidemics of MDR-TB, several countries, including some of those with the highest TB incidence, have provided no reliable information about the magnitude of their drug-resistant TB problem. Longitudinal trends from the 22 countries that generate 80% of the TB cases worldwide are urgently needed to make

consistent inferences. Thus, in the absence of longitudinal data for MDR-TB from many resource-limited countries, caution should be exercised if conclusions are to be suggested.

Fortuitously, it is also clear that most of the world is currently afflicted by a pandemic of drug-susceptible TB, which makes the handling of the problem of resistance a less difficult task to undertake. Drug-susceptible TB, and even some forms of drug-resistant TB, can be conquered by the implementation of basic TB control measures based on international guidelines.

Nevertheless, the overall impact of drug-resistant TB and MDR-TB on the TB control efforts in resource-limited countries cannot be judged purely on the basis of available numbers. The finding of MDR-TB at a low prevalence in a given country should not mean that the issue can be ignored or forgotten there. Continuous transmission of MDR-TB strains by even a small number of patients may develop into a serious problem if the issue is not addressed promptly. Ignored, it will mean more cases and higher costs to the health care system of an already impoverished country. MDR-TB is far more expensive and difficult to manage than either drug-susceptible TB or other types of resistant strains. Public health measures to control or reverse the problem, where dissemination has already occurred, can be extremely expensive and are often beyond the means of such countries. It is clear that MDR-TB, when found at high prevalence, completely disrupts TB control efforts. This situation was seen in New York City (46) and is currently seen in Estonia (74). Therefore, there is a critical need to find feasible and cost-effective approaches to tackle this problem in resource-limited countries.

COMPREHENSIVE LABORATORY SERVICES

Characteristics of Drug-Resistant *M. tuberculosis*

Members of the genus *Mycobacterium* share several means of natural or intrinsic drug resistance. A hydrophobic cell envelope that serves as a permeability barrier to many compounds (9) surrounds these organisms. Also, drug efflux systems and drug-modifying enzymes are present in *M. tuberculosis* complex (26, 75).

In vitro studies have demonstrated that, depending on the antibiotic, resistant mutants arise spontaneously at a rate of 1 in 10^3 to 10^8 organisms; isoniazid resistance arises at a rate of 1 in 10^6, and rifampin resistance arises at a rate of 1 in 10^8 (28). Resistance most probably occurs within cavitary lesions containing more than 10^8 organisms per lesion (16). Since mutations are not linked, the probability of a strain developing a spontaneous mutation conferring resistance to both isoniazid and rifampin is approximately 1 in 10^{14}. Thus, the presence of an organism spontaneously resistant to both isoniazid and rifampin is unlikely even in cavitary lesions and would be virtually impossible in areas of infiltration or granulomas, which contain only 10^2 to 10^3 bacilli (16). The model breaks down, however, when chemotherapy has been inadequate. In the circumstance of monotherapy, erratic drug ingestion, omission of one or more of the prescribed agents, suboptimal dosage, poor drug absorption, or an insufficient number of active agents in a regimen, a susceptible strain of *M. tuberculosis* may become resistant to multiple drugs within a matter of months. Remaining susceptible organisms in the population are eliminated, allowing the surviving, drug-resistant organisms to then comprise the entire population (64, 102).

Genetic studies have confirmed that mutations in genes encoding drug targets or drug-activating enzymes are responsible for resistance, and point mutations and/or deletions have been found for all first-line drugs (94, 106). Molecular epidemiologic studies in The Netherlands showed that isoniazid-resistant *M. tuberculosis* strains were less likely to be clustered than drug-susceptible strains (116), confirming an observation made by Middlebrook and Cohn in the 1950s that isoniazid-resistant strains are of low virulence (85) and are therefore less readily transmissible in humans. A subsequent study provided evidence that the mutation of the *katG* gene coding for amino acid 315 is not associated with reduced virulence (117). However, this mutation is very common and is associated with MDR strains. Other studies from South Africa and Mexico suggest that MDR-TB strains are less clustered than susceptible strains and therefore show a reduced capacity to spread and cause disease (47, 52). Although MDR-TB patients have active disease for extended periods, biological or social factors may limit the transmission of their MDR-TB strains.

Current Issues in the Diagnosis of Drug-Resistant TB

Proper specimen collection and expedited transport of specimens to the laboratory are the foundation of rapid, accurate microbiological diagnosis of TB. To ensure collection of the best possible specimen, the health care worker must be properly trained and the patient must receive clearly presented and fully understood instructions and be supervised during specimen collection. Unsupervised collection can result in an unacceptable specimen, as well as the possibility that the patient can substitute a specimen that is not his or her own.

Acid-fast bacillus (AFB) smear microscopy is an important tool in diagnosing highly infectious TB patients, although its sensitivity varies between 40 and 60%. In addition, AFB smear microscopy is used in patient management, especially in resource-limited countries, where a positive AFB smear after 2 to 3 months of treatment triggers the collection of a culture for *M. tuberculosis* and subsequent drug susceptibility testing. Therefore, it is important to recognize this method's potential for inaccurate results. Lan et al., in a study in Vietnam, demonstrated the importance of unblinded rereading of AFB smears as a quality assurance tool (77). Three sets of 750 slides were prepared: an unblinded set, an unblinded set in which 13% of negative slides were replaced by weakly positive slides purposely mislabeled as negative, and a blinded set. Findings suggested that rarely was a negative slide misread as positive. In contrast, in the unblinded arm, 2.9% of positive slides were misread as negative, compared with 18.7% in the blinded set and 11.3% in the unblinded set with mislabeled slides. Blinded rereading of systematically selected AFB slides is superior in the detection of deficiencies compared to nonblinded rereading; this conclusion has been confirmed by a recent study from India (103). The use of cold staining was identified as an additional source of faulty smear results (13).

The recent U.S. Institute of Medicine report on the quality of care, "*To Err Is Human,*" has provided an awakening for the health care system in this country. The report states that errors cause between 44,000 and 98,000 deaths every year in American hospitals (63). Already in 1994, Leape stated, "But it is apparent that the most fundamental change that will be needed if hospitals are to make meaningful progress in error reduction is a cultural one. Physicians and nurses need to accept the notion that error is part of the human condition, even among conscientious professionals with high standards. Errors must be accepted as evidence of system flaws not character flaws. Until and unless that happens," it seems that microbiologists, health care providers, and public health officers are taking the high error rate to heart and are publishing an ever-growing number of studies dealing with false laboratory results (79). Burman and Reeves reviewed the mechanisms of false-positive TB cultures and their frequency, clinical consequences, and laboratory characteristics. They found 14 large studies involving more than 100 patients. The median false-positive rate was 3.1% (interquartile range, 2.2 to 10.5%). However, much higher rates were seen when there was a major error in laboratory techniques or conditions (12). The impact of false-positive cultures may be reflected in unnecessary multidrug therapy, with its potential for adverse reactions; placement of the patient in respiratory isolation; manpower-intensive investigation of close contacts; and subjection of the patient to unnecessary diagnostic tests, including bronchoscopy, biopsies, and surgery. Among people with proven TB, the occurrence of false-positive cultures during or after treatment can result in an inappropriate diagnosis of treatment failure or relapse.

Cross-contamination of specimens in the laboratory has received the greatest attention in studies of false-positive cultures thus far. However, events before the arrival of a specimen in the laboratory can also cause false-positive results. As mentioned above, unsupervised sputum collection allows the patient to substitute a specimen that is not his or her own. The channels of the fiberoptic bronchoscope may be difficult to sterilize once contaminated with mycobacteria or residual DNA sequences of *M. tuberculosis*, which may lead to false-positive PCR results. Finally, mislabeling of specimens on the patients' ward and in the laboratory has been a documented cause of false-positive results.

Recently, the WHO/IUATLD Supranational Reference Laboratory Network published the results of five rounds of proficiency testing for drug susceptibility testing carried out between 1994 and 1998 (78). Only 14 of the 25 participating laboratories completed all five rounds. Media used for this testing included Löwenstein-Jensen (12 laboratories), Middlebrook 7H10 (1 laboratory), and the radiometric BACTEC 12B (1 laboratory). The sensitivity and specificity of the drug susceptibility testing were reliable for rifampin and isoniazid, with values ranging from 97 to 99%. Testing of streptomycin and ethambutol was less dependable, however, with values ranging from 90 to 93%. It is important to recognize that the test performances for the individual anti-TB drugs differ. Standardization of the critical concentrations of streptomycin and ethambutol to be used in the radiometric procedure has not been achieved without controversy (56). It is noteworthy that the recommended concentrations for streptomycin and ethambutol have undergone adjustments over time. These modifications have resulted in questions, particularly about whether the use of a 2.5-μg/ml concentration will provide accurate determination of resistance to ethambutol by using this method (82).

A study of 70 patients identified as having MDR-TB showed that after careful rereview of medical and laboratory records, pulmonary MDR-TB had been misdiagnosed in 9 (13%) of them (91). Several reasons for the erroneous results were found, including growth of an MDR-TB strain from an old tuberculous lesion in a patient who was never treated for TB and whose diagnosis predated anti-TB drugs,

documented contamination with *M. avium* complex, suspected cross-contamination, suspected specimen mislabeling, successful treatment using drugs to which the isolate was reportedly resistant, discrepant susceptibility test results on additional sputum specimens submitted by the patient, and lack of any clinical evidence of TB. This study underscores the fact that susceptibility test results alone are not sufficient to dictate the initiation of treatment for drug-resistant TB, and that careful clinical correlation is necessary in making the diagnosis of MDR-TB.

Standards of Laboratory Services

Since the mid-1980s and early 1990s, the TB laboratories in resource-rich countries have implemented newer technologies such as broth-based culture media for growth detection and susceptibility testing and rapid assays for identification of mycobacteria. This upgrade of TB laboratory practice was seen to be imperative after the onset of the new drug-resistant TB epidemic (especially in the United States), which demanded faster laboratory results (99, 107). Furthermore, good laboratory practice demands the implementation of a continuous quality improvement program covering test methods and procedures, verification and validation of new tests, adherence to a procedure manual, proper content and storage of records, competency of personnel, and the signing up of external proficiency testing. Clinical experience reminds us that no results are better than wrong results.

DOTS recommends AFB smear microscopy as a minimal diagnostic requirement. While there are existing guidelines about a proper quality assurance program for smear microscopy, there are no publications documenting the quality of the smear microscopy laboratory service throughout a high-burden country. However, when a case of drug-resistant TB within the DOTS-Plus program is suspected, efforts must be made to provide real-time culture, identification, and susceptibility testing, in addition to a documented smear microscopy service that has been verified to be functioning well. The implementation of such a comprehensive laboratory service constitutes a huge paradigm shift and will require an as yet unknown amount of additional resources, as well as synchronization with national TB control programs. This transformation stretches through several phases and requires several years to become established. The implementation of more complex and faster laboratory services will be hampered by the lack of trained technical personnel, as well as the lack of a system-wide external proficiency test program available to monitor the process at least twice yearly. Such a comprehensive program is much needed, especially for the work-up of sputum samples. In a recent publication (55), the Malawi National TB Control Programme assessed the entire process, from patient registration at the regional hospital to the arrival of the sputum specimen at the central reference laboratory to the reporting of culture and susceptibility testing results. This kind of system-wide thinking is required to identify where the biggest obstacles exist, in order to improve progress throughout the country.

MANAGEMENT OF PATIENTS WITH MDR-TB

Although treatment for patients with MDR-TB has been available in high-income countries for many years, this is not the case for resource-limited countries. The management of MDR-TB is complex, time-consuming, and demanding to both the patient and the provider. Thus, it is often recommended that such a task be undertaken only in hospitals equipped with appropriate isolation units, stringent infection control measures, multidisciplinary medical teams, and access to high-quality reference laboratories. In high-income countries these components are likely to be available, and treatment is tailored to use second-line and newer drugs according to the drug susceptibility profile of the patient's isolates. Costs, however, are estimated to run into thousands of dollars per patient, ranging from $60,000 in the Netherlands to $90,000 in the United Kingdom, to as high as $180,000 in the United States (48, 84, 89). Drugs, toxicity monitoring, in-patient and outpatient care, medical time and nursing, and facility charges are some of the factors to consider when evaluating costs. In addition to financial costs, there is the problem of lost productivity of the patient and, probably, of his or her family as well.

To manage MDR-TB in resource-limited countries, approaches that are feasible, balanced, and cost-effective must be integrated into current TB control efforts. Short-course chemotherapy, while very efficacious in the majority of TB cases, shows very poor results when administered to patients with MDR-TB and other drug-resistant infections (37). Nevertheless, to manage MDR-TB, it is highly necessary that basic TB control follows recommended international guidelines such as implementation of high-quality DOTS, which will cure the majority of drug susceptible TB cases and prevent the generation of new drug-resistant or MDR-TB cases. Areas of the world with a significant MDR-TB problem may need parallel implementation of DOTS and specific measures to manage MDR-TB (41).

Current efforts by the international community toward the introduction of MDR-TB management in resource-limited countries are very promising. The WHO and several partners launched DOTS-Plus in the late 1990s, a program which is currently under operational testing in several countries (36, 42). DOTS-Plus is built on the foundations of DOTS, the internationally recommended TB control strategy. Second-line drugs provided at concessional prices by the pharmaceutical industry are carefully introduced and monitored in the health care system and within the framework of TB control programs of resource-limited countries (53). Stringent technical protocols are followed under the umbrella of the Green Light Committee (Table 1) (54). To achieve the highest cure rate possible, DOTS-Plus allows countries the option of using either standardized or tailored treatment regimens, according to the particular health care infrastructure, feasibility, and technical and financial resources of the countries involved. Other important elements of DOTS-Plus include the availability of laboratories whose continuous quality improvement program is overseen by external laboratories, a high level of clinical expertise to manage drug toxicity, well-designed drug procurement and delivery plans, and implementation of patient compliance strategies. Preliminary evidence is suggesting that in such settings the management of MDR-TB may be feasible within program conditions (105) or through centers of excellence (87).

FUTURE OF MDR-TB

Theoretical and controversial estimates of the future evolution of MDR-TB have surfaced in the recent years. Much recent attention has focused on as-

Table 1. Green Light Committee—approved projects for MDR-TB management

Country	No. of patients[a]
Bolivia	11
Costa Rica	14
Estonia	200
Haiti	60
Latvia	350
Malawi	27
Mexico	127
Peru	1,845
Philippines	200
Russia (Archangels)	300
Russia (Kemerovo)	150
Russia (Orel)	240
Russia (Tomsk)	630
Russia (Ivanovo)	200
Uzbekistan	100
Total	**4,452**

[a]Number of patients approved for treatment as of December 2003.

sessing the global burden of MDR-TB and predicting the future threat posed by this pathogen. Despite this attention, a consensus has not yet been achieved on either the magnitude of the problem or its future trends. The future of MDR-TB will certainly depend on the relative and absolute fitness of *M. tuberculosis*, including drug-susceptible and drug-resistant strains. Fitness is influenced by the strains' genetics (or their abilities to develop critical mutations in genes leading to drug resistance) and the environments in which they occur (or treatment practices). Fitness is a composite measure of the ability of an organism to survive, reproduce, and be transmitted. It reflects the growth characteristics of an organism within its host, its ability to withstand within-host and between-host environmental stresses, and its capacity to disseminate and to set up residence in a new host. Some of these characteristics can be quantified in the laboratory, although their precise contributions to the empirical success of an organism in the "real world" may not be clear (24). Furthermore, there is evidence from several experimental systems that the initial fitness deficit associated with the development of resistance disappears with repeated multiplication (49). Several molecular and classical epidemiologic studies have suggested that isoniazid-resistant and MDR-TB *M. tuberculosis* strains are less clustered than susceptible strains and are therefore less able to spread readily (47, 52, 116). At the same time, other studies have shown different, even opposite results (74, 108, 117). Strains of the Beijing/W genotype family have been suggested to possess the potential to spread faster than others and to become associated with drug resistance (4, 51). Fortunately, such strains are thus far mainly pansusceptible to first-line drugs.

Recent estimates suggest that there were 273,000 new cases of MDR-TB worldwide (95% confidence intervals, 185,000 and 414,000) in 2000, or 3% of the global TB total (34). No estimates have been constructed regarding previously treated cases. One scenario for the future suggests that MDR-TB will remain a locally severe problem rather than a global one, provided that case management based on recommended guidelines is enforced and provided that MDR-TB strains are actually less fit than drug-susceptible ones (33, 34). Ensuring appropriate treatment and cure of new drug-susceptible TB cases will definitely prevent such cases from failing to respond to treatment and thus will lessen further selection for resistant strains. If, indeed, drug-resistant strains are and remain less fit than drug-susceptible strains, as suggested above, the prospect for a global pandemic of MDR-TB of the size of the drug-susceptible one is very small. Since short-course chemotherapy cures over 85% of pansusceptible cases and around 80%

of cases resistant to a single first-line drug (except for rifampin), enforcement of cure rates and increase in case detection should keep MDR-TB at a low rate in the long run. Certainly, the global data available point out that the great majority of TB cases are susceptible to first-line drugs; that isoniazid and rifampicin have not been lost as agents for treatment after several decades of steady use; and, finally, that long-term trends from several countries do not reveal a replacement of drug-susceptible strains by drug-resistant strains.

Others, however, have predicted a different scenario, suggesting that a large number of drug-resistant latent infections will surface over a long period (6). Some of the problems relating to such a scenario are that, first, latent infection may never turn into active disease and second, there is no current tool to determine whether latent infection is due to a drug-susceptible or a drug-resistant strain. Since most active TB cases are drug susceptible, we can postulate that the majority of existing latent infections are due to drug-susceptible strains. Furthermore, a recent review has basically dismissed attempts to predict the future of MDR-TB by concluding that the fitness estimates of drug-resistant *M. tuberculosis* strains are quite heterogeneous and that more knowledge about the effects of the mutations on bacterial survival, reproduction, and transmission are needed if we are to predict future trends of drug-resistant TB, including MDR-TB (24).

Whatever the future of MDR-TB, it is certain that containment of MDR-TB will depend on the efforts that individual countries and the international community are willing to expend in order to accelerate the implementation of TB control according to recognized and tested international guidelines that include judicious use of first- and second-line and newer anti-TB drugs. Upgrading of laboratory services, strengthening of surveillance, and introduction of new diagnostic tools and new anti-TB drugs in the next few years will also be key in expanding the prevention, detection, and management of MDR-TB beyond the current limitations.

REFERENCES

1. Adegbola, R. A., P. Hill, I. Baldeh, J. Otu, R. Sarr, J. Sillah, C. Lienhardt, T. Corrah, K. Manneh, F. Drobniewski, and K. P. W. McAdam. 2003. Surveillance of drug-resistant *Mycobacterium tuberculosis* in The Gambia. *Int. J. Tuberc. Lung Dis.* 7:306–311.

2. Agerton, T. B., S. E. Valway, R. J. Blinkhorn, K. L. Shilkret, R. Reves, W. W. Schluter, B. Gore, C. J. Pozsik, B. B. Plikaytis, C. Woodley, and I. M. Onorato. 1999. Spread of strain W, a highly drug-resistant strain of *Mycobacterium tuberculosis*, across the United States. *Clin. Infect. Dis.* 29:85–92.

3. **Armstrong, A. R.** 1966. The prevalence in Canada of drug resistant tubercle bacilli in newly discovered untreated patients with tuberculosis. *Can. Med. Assoc. J.* **94:**420–425.

4. **Bifani, P. J., B. Mathema, N. E. Kurepina, and B. Kreiswirth.** 2002. Global dissemination of the *Mycobacterium tuberculosis* W-Beijing family strains. *Trends Microbiol.* **10:**45–52.

5. **Bloch, A. B., G. M. Cauthen, I. M. Onorato, K. G. Dansbury, G. D. Kelly, C. R. Driver, and D. E. Snider.** 1994. Nationwide survey of drug-resistant tuberculosis in the United States. *JAMA* **271:**665–671.

6. **Blower, S. M., and J. L. G. Gerberding.** 1998. Understanding, predicting and controlling the emergence of drug-resistant tuberculosis: a theoretical framework. *J. Mol. Med.* **76:**624–636.

7. **Boulahbal, F., S. Khaled, and M. Tazir.** 1989. The interest of follow-up of resistance of the tubercle bacillus in the evaluation of a programme. *Bull. IUATLD* **64:**23–25.

8. **Bouvet, E.** 1993. Transmission nosocomiale de tuberculose multirésistante parmi les patients infectés par le VIH. *Bull. Epidémiol. Hebdom.* **45:**195–197.

9. **Brennan, P. J., and H. Nikaido.** 1995. The envelope of mycobacteria. *Annu. Rev. Biochem.* **64:**29–63.

10. **Bretzel, G., M. Aziz, U. Wendl-Richter, F. Adatu, T. Aisu, A. van Wijnen, and V. Sticht-Groh.** 1999. Anti-tuberculosis drug resistance surveillance in Uganda 1996–1997. *Int. J. Tuberc. Lung Dis.* **3:**810–815.

11. **British Tuberculosis Association.** 1963. Acquired drug-resistance in patients with pulmonary tuberculosis in Great Britain—a national survey, 1960–61. *Tubercle* (London) **44:**1–26.

12. **Burman, W. J., and R. R. Reves.** 2000. Review of false-positive cultures for *Mycobacterium tuberculosis* and recommendations for avoiding unnecessary treatment. *Clin. Infect. Dis.* **31:**1390–1395.

13. **Buzingo T., M. Sanders, J.-P. Masabo, S. Nyandwi, and A. Van Deun.** 2003. Systematic restaining of sputum smears for quality control is useful in Burundi. *Int. J. Tuberc. Lung Dis.* **7:**439–444.

13a. **Canadian Tuberculosis Laboratory Surveillance System.** 2003. *Tuberculosis: Drug Resistance in Canada,* p. 1–23. Health Canada, Ottawa, Canada.

14. **Canetti, G., S. Froman, J. Grosset, P. Hauduroy, M. Langerová, H. T. Mahler, G. Meissner, D. A. Mitchison, and L. Sula.** 1963. Mycobacteria: laboratory methods for testing drug sensitivity and resistance. *Bull. W. H. O.* **29:**565–578.

15. **Canetti G., W. Fox, A. Khomenko, H. T. Mahler, N. K. Menon, D. A. Mitchison, N. Rist, and N. A. Smelev.** 1969. Advances in techniques of testing mycobacterial drug sensitivity, and the use of sensitivity tests in tuberculosis control programs. *Bull. W. H. O.* **41:**21–43.

16. **Canetti, G.** 1955. The tubercle bacillus in the pulmonary tuberculous lesion, p. 29–85. *In* G. Canetti (ed.), *The Tubercle Bacillus.* Springer Publishing Co., New York, N.Y.

17. **Canetti, G., N. Rist, and J. Grosset.** 1964. Primary drug resistance in tuberculosis. *Am. Rev. Respir. Dis.* **90:**792–802.

18. **Canetti, G., P. H. Gay, and M. Le Lirzin.** 1972. Trends in the prevalence of primary drug resistance in pulmonary tuberculosis in France from 1962 to 1979: a national survey. *Tubercle* **53:**57–83.

19. **Centers for Disease Control.** 1980. Primary resistance to antituberculosis drugs—United States. *Morb. Mortal. Wkly. Rep.* **29:**345–346.

20. **Centers for Disease Control.** 1983. Primary resistance to antituberculosis drugs—United States. *Morb. Mortal. Wkly. Rep.* **32:**521–523.

21. **Centers for Disease Control.** 1992. Transmission of multidrug-resistant TB among immuno-compromised persons in a correctional system—New York, 1991. *Morb. Mortal. Wkly. Rep.* **41:**507–509.

22. **Centers for Disease Control and Prevention.** 2002. *Reported Tuberculosis in the United States, 2001.* U.S. Department of Health and Human Services, Centers for Disease Control and Prevention, Atlanta, Ga.

23. **Chonde, T. M.** 1989. The role of bacteriological services in the National Tuberculosis and Leprosy Programme in Tanzania. *Bull. Int. Union. Tuberc. Lung Dis.* **64:**37–39.

24. **Cohen, T., B. Sommers, and M. Murray.** 2003. The effect of drug resistance on the fitness of *Mycobacterium turberculosis. Lancet Infect. Dis.* **3:**13–21.

25. **Cohn, D., F. Bustreo, and M. C. Raviglione.** 1997. Drug resistant tuberculosis: review of the worldwide situation. *Clin. Infect. Dis.* **24:**s121–s130.

26. **Cole, S. T., R. Brosch, J. Parkhill, T. Garnier, C. Churcher, D. Harris, S. V. Gordon, K. Eiglmeier, S. Gas, C. E. Barry III, F. Tekaia, K. Badcock, D. Basham, D. Brown, T. Chillingworth, R. Conner, R. Davies, K. Devlin, T. Feltwell, S. Gentles, N. Hamlin, S. Holroyd, T. Hornsby, K. Jagels, A. Krogh, J. McLean, S. Moule, L. Murphy, K. Oliver, J. Osborne, M. A. Quail, M.-A. Rajandream, J. Rogers, S. Rutter, K. Seeger, J. Skelton, R. Squares, S. Squares, J. E. Sulston, K. Taylor, S. Whitehead, and B. G. Barrell.** 1998. Deciphering the biology of *Mycobacterium tuberculosis* from the complete genome sequence. *Nature* **393:**537–544.

27. **Corbett, E. L., C. J. Watt, N. Walker, D. Maher, B. G. Williams, M. C. Raviglione, and C. Dye.** 2003. The growing burden of tuberculosis—global trends and interactions with the HIV epidemic. *Arch. Intern. Med.* **163:**1009–1021.

28. **David, H. L.** 1970. Probability distribution of drug-resistant mutants of unselected population of *Mycobacterium tuberculosis. Appl. Microbiol. Biotechnol.* **20:**810–814.

29. **Dawson, D., D. F. Cheah, W. K. Chew, F. C. Havekort, R. Lumb, and A. S. Sievers.** 1995. Tuberculosis in Australia, 1989–1992: bacteriology confirmed cases and drug resistance. *Med. J. Aust.* **62:**287–290.

30. **Djuretic, T., J. Herbert, F. Drobniewski, M. Yates, E. G. Smith, J. G. Magee, R. Williams, P. Flanagan, B. Watt, A. Rayner, M. Crowe, M. V. Chadwick, A. M. Middleton, and J. M. Watson.** 2002. Antibiotic resistant tuberculosis in the United Kingdom: 1993–1999. *Thorax* **57:**477–482.

31. **Doster, B., G. J. Caras, and D. E. Snider.** 1976. A continuing survey of primary drug resistance in tuberculosis, 1961 to 1968. *Am. Rev. Respir. Dis.* **113:**419–425.

32. **Dosso, M., D. Bonard, P. Msellati, A. Bamba, C. Doulhourou, V. Vincent, M. Peyre, M. Traore, K. Koffi, and I. M. Coulibaly.** 1999. Primary resistance to antituberculosis drugs: a national survey conducted in Côte d'Ivoire in 1995–1996. *Int. J. Tuberc. Lung Dis.* **3:**805–809.

33. **Dye, C., and M. A. Espinal.** 2001. Will tuberculosis become resistant to all antibiotics? *Proc. R. Soc. London B. Ser.* **268:**45–52.

34. **Dye, C., M. A. Espinal, C. J. Watt, C. Mbiaga, and B. G. Williams.** 2002. Worldwide incidence of multidrug-resistant tuberculosis. *J. Infect. Dis.* **185:**1197–202.

35. **Espinal, M. A., J. Báez, G. Soriano, V. Garcia, A. Laszlo, A. L. Reingold, and S. Sanchez.** 1998. Drug-resistant tuberculosis in the Dominican Republic: results of a nationwide survey. *Int. J. Tuberc. Lung Dis.* **2:**490–498.

36. **Espinal, M. A., C. Dye, M. Raviglione, and A. Kochi.** 1999. Rational DOTS-Plus for the control of MDRTB. *Int. J. Tuberc. Lung Dis.* **3:**561–563.

37. **Espinal, M. A., S. J. Kim, P. G. Suarez, K. M. Kam, A. G. Khomenko, G. B. Migliori, J. Baéz, A. Kochi, C. Dye, and**

M. C. Raviglione. 2000. Standard short-course chemotherapy for drug-resistant tuberculosis: treatment outcome in 6 countries. *JAMA* 283:2537–2545.

38. Espinal, M. A., A. Laszlo, L. Simonsen, F. Boulahbal, S. J. Kim, A. Reniero, S. Hoffner, H. L. Rieder, N. Binkin, C. Dye, R. Williams, and M. C. Raviglione. 2001. Global trends in resistance to antituberculosis drugs. *N. Engl. J. Med.* 344:1294–1303.

39. Espinal, M. 2003. The global situation of MDR-TB. *Tuberculosis* 83:44–51.

40. EuroTB and the National Coordinators for Tuberculosis Surveillance in the WHO European Region. 2003. *Surveillance of Tuberculosis in Europe. Report on Tuberculosis Cases Notified in 2000*, p. 57–58. EuroTB/InVS, Saint-Maurice Cedex, France.

41. Farmer, P., J. Bayona, M. Becerra, J. Furin, C. Henry, H. Hiatt, J. Y. Kim, C. Mitnick, E. Nardell, and S. Shin. 1998. The dilemma of MDR-TB in the global era. *Int. J. Tuberc. Lung Dis.* 2:869–876.

42. Farmer, P., and J. Y. Kim. 1998. Community based approaches to the control of multidrug resistant tuberculosis: introducing "DOTS-Plus." *Br. Med. J.* 317S:671–674.

43. Fischl, M. A., R. B. Uttamchandani, G. L. Daikos, R. B. Poblete, J. N. Moreno, R. R. Reyes, A. M. Boota, L. M. Thompson, T. J. Cleary, and S. Lai. 1992. An outbreak of tuberculosis caused by multiple-drug resistant tubercle bacilli among patients with HIV infection. *Ann. Intern. Med.* 39:719–722.

44. Fox, W., A. Wiener, D. H. Mitchison, J. B. Selkon, and I. Sutherland. 1957. The prevalence of drug-resistant tubercle bacilli in untreated patients with pulmonary tuberculosis: a national survey, 1955–56. *Tubercle* 38:71–84.

45. Fox, W., G. A. Ellard, and D. A. Mitchison. 1999. Studies on the treatment of tuberculosis undertaken by the British Medical Research Council tuberculosis Units, 1946–1986, with relevant subsequent publications. *Int. J. Tuberc. Lung Dis.* 3:S231–S279.

46. Frieden, T. R., P. I. Fujiwara, R. M. Washko, and M. A. Hamburg. 1995. Tuberculosis in New York City—turning the tide. *N. Engl. J. Med.* 333:229–233.

47. Garcia-Garcia, M., A. Ponce-de-Leon, M. E. Jimenez-Corona, A. Jimenez-Corona, M. Palacios-Martinez, S. Balandrano-Campos, L. Ferreyra-Reyes, L. Juarez-Sandino, J. Sifuentes-Osornio, H. Olivera-Diaz, J. L. Valdespino-Gomez, and P. M. Small. 2000. Clinical consequences and transmissibility of drug-resistant tuberculosis in Southern Mexico. *Arch. Intern. Med.* 160:630–636.

48. Geerligs, W. A., R. van Altena, W. C. M. de Lange, D. van Soolingen, and T. S. van der Werf. 2000. Multidrug-resistant tuberculosis: long-term treatment outcome in The Netherlands. *Int. J. Tuberc. Lung Dis.* 4:758–764.

49. Gillespie, S. H. 2002. Evolution of drug resistance in *Mycobacterium tuberculosis*: clinical and molecular perspective. *Antimicrob. Agents Chemother.* 46:267–274.

50. Githui, W. A., E. S. Juma, J. van Gorkom, D. Kibuga, J. Odhiambo, and F. Drobniewski. 1998. Antituberculosis drug resistance surveillance in Kenya, 1995. *Int. J. Tuberc. Lung Dis.* 2:499–505.

51. Glynn, J. R., J. Whiteley, P. J. Bifani, K. Kremer, and D. van Soolingen. 2001. Worldwide occurrence of Beijing/W strains of *Mycobacterium tuberculosis*: a systematic review. *Emerg. Infect. Dis.* 8:843–849.

52. Godfrey-Faussett, P., P. Sonnenberg, S. C. Shearer, M. C. Bruce, C. Mee, L. Morris, and J. Murray. 2000. Tuberculosis control and molecular epidemiology in a South African gold-mining community. *Lancet* 356:1066–1071.

53. Gupta, R., J. Y. Kim, M. A. Espinal, J. M. Caudron, B. Pecoul, P. E. Farmer, and M. C. Raviglione. 2001. Responding to market failures in tuberculosis control. *Science* 293:1049–1051.

54. Gupta, R., J. P. Gegielski, M. A. Espinal, M. Henkens, J. Y. Kim, C. S. B. Lambregts-van Weezenbeek, J. W. Lee, M. C. Raviglione, P. G. Suarez, and F. Varaine. 2002. Increasing transparency for health—introducing the Green Light Committee. *Trop. Med. Int. Health* 7:970–976.

55. Harries A. D., J. Michongwe, T. E. Nyirenda, J. R. Kemp, S. B. Squire, A. R. Ramsay, P. Godfrey-Faussett, and F. M. Salaniponi. 2004. The use of a bus service for transporting sputum specimens to the central reference laboratory: effect on the routine tuberculosis culture service in Malawi. *Int. J. Tuberc. Lung Dis.* 8:1–7.

56. Heifets, L. B. 1991. *Drug Susceptibility Tests in the Management of Chemotherapy of Tuberculosis*, p. 89–121. CRC Press, Inc., Boca Raton, Fla.

57. Helbling P., P. A. Altpeter, G. E. Pfyffer, and J. P. Zellweger. 2000. Surveillance of antituberculosis drug resistance in Switzerland 1995–1997: the central link. *Eur. Respir. J.* 16:200–202.

58. Hirano, K., Y. Kazumi, C. Abe, T. Mori, M. Aoki, and T. Aoyagi. 1996. Resistance to antituberculosis drugs in Japan. *Tubercle Lung Dis.* 77:130–135.

59. Hobby, G. L., P. M. Johnson, T. F. Lenert, L. Crawford-Gagliardi, L. Greetham, T. Ivaska, A. Lapin, J. Maier, P. O'Malley, and C. Trembley. 1964. A continuing study of primary drug resistance in tuberculosis in a veteran population within the United States. I. *Am. Rev. Respir. Dis.* 89:337–341.

60. Horne, N. W. 1969. Drug-resistant tuberculosis: a review of the world situation. *Tubercle* 50(Suppl):S2–12.

61. Howells, G. 1969. Primary drug resistance in Australia in 1968. *Tubercle* 50:344–349.

62. Institute of Medicine. 2000. *Ending Neglect: the Elimination of Tuberculosis in the United States*. National Academy Press, Washington, D.C.

63. Institute of Medicine. 2000. *To Err Is Human—Building a Safer Health System* (L. T. Kohn, J. M. Corrigan, and M. S. Donaldson, ed.) National Academy Press, Washington, D.C.

64. Iseman, M. D. 1993. Treatment of multidrug-resistant tuberculosis. *N. Engl. J. Med.* 329:784–791.

65. Iseman, M. D. 2000. *A Clinician's Guide to Tuberculosis*. Lippincott, Williams & Wilkins, Philadelphia, Pa.

66. Kam, K. M., C. W. Yip, L. W. Tse, O. C. Leung, L. P. Sin, M. Y. Chan, and W. S. Wong. 2002. Trends in multidrug-resistant *Mycobacterium tuberculosis* in relation to sputum smear positivity in Hong Kong, 1989–1999. *Clin. Infect. Dis.* 34:324–329.

67. Keers, R.Y. 1978. *Pulmonary Tuberculosis: a Journey down the Centuries*. Balliere-Tindall, London, United Kingdom.

68. Kenyon, T. A., M. J. Mwasekaga, R. Huebner, D. Rumisha, N. Binkin, and E. Maganu. 1999. Low levels of drug resistance amidst rapidly increasing tuberculosis and human immunodeficiency virus co-epidemics in Botswana. *Int. J. Tuberc. Lung Dis.* 3:4–11.

69. Kim, S. J., G. H. Bai, and Y. P. Hong. 1997. Drug-resistant tuberculosis in Korea, 1994. *Int. J. Tuberc. Lung Dis.* 1:302–308.

70. Kim, S. J. 2002. Current problems of drug-resistant tuberculosis and its control. *Kekkaku* 77:735–740.

71. Kleeberg, H. H., and M. S. Boshoff. 1980. *A World Atlas of Initial Drug Resistance*. Scientific Committee on Bacteriology and Immunology of the International Union against Tuberculosis. Tuberculosis Research Institute of the South African Medical Research Council, Pretoria.

72. Kleeberg, H. H., and M. S. Olivier. 1984. *A World Atlas of Initial Drug Resistance,* 2nd ed. Tuberculosis Research Institute of the South African Medical Research Council, Pretoria.

73. Kopanoff, D. E., J. O. Kilburn, J. L. Classroth, D. E. Snider, L. S. Farer, and R. C. Good. 1978. A continuing survey of tuberculosis primary drug resistance in the United States: March 1975 to November 1977. *Am. Rev. Respir. Dis.* 118: 835–842.

74. Krunner, A., S. E. Hoffner, H. Sillastu, M. Danilovits, K. Levina, S. B. Svenson, S. Ghebremichael, T. Koivula, and G. Kallenius. 2001. Spread of drug-resistant pulmonary tuberculosis in Estonia. *J. Clin. Microbiol.* 39:3339–3345.

75. Kwon, H. H., H. Tomioka, and H. Saito. 1995. Distribution and characterization of beta-lactamases of mycobacteria and related organisms. *Tubercle Lung Dis.* 76:141–148.

76. Lambregts-van Weezenbeek, C. S. B., H. M. Jansen, J. Veen, N. J. D. Nagelkerke, M. M. G. G. Sebek, and D. van Soolingen. 1998. Origin and management of primary and acquired drug-resistant tuberculosis in The Netherlands: the truth behind the rates. *Int. J. Tuberc. Lung Dis.* 2:296–302.

77. Lan N. T. N., C. D. Wells, N. J. Binkin, J. E. Becerra, P. D. Linh, and N. V. Co. 1999. Quality control of smear microscopy for acid-fast bacilli: the case for blinded re-reading. *Int. J. Tuberc. Lung Dis.* 3:55–61.

78. Laszlo, A., M. Rahman, M. Espinal, and M. Raviglione. 2002. Quality assurance programme for drug susceptibility testing of *Mycobacterium tuberculosis* in the WHO/IUATLD Supranational Reference Laboratory Network: five rounds of proficiency testing, 1994–1998. *Int. J. Tuberc. Lung Dis.* 6:748–756.

79. Leape, L. L. 1994. Error in medicine. *JAMA* 272:1851–1857.

80. Lehmann, J. 1946. Para-aminosalicylic acid in the treatment of tuberculosis. *Lancet* i:15–16.

81. Lumb, R., I. Bastian, D. Dawson, C. Gilpin, F. Havekort, P. Howard, and A. Sievers. 2002. Tuberculosis in Australia: bacteriologically confirmed cases and drug resistance, 2000. *Commun. Dis. Intell.* 26:226–233.

81a. Lumb, R., I. Bastian, W. Chew, C. Gilpin, F. Haverkort, and A. Sievers. 2003. Tuberculosis in Australia: bacteriologically confirmed cases and drug resistance, 2002. *Commun. Dis. Intell.* 27:459–465.

82. Madison, B., B. Robinson-Dunn, I. George, W. Gross, H. Lipman, B. Metchock, A. Sloutsky, G. Washabaugh, G. Mazurek, and J. Ridderhof. 2002. Multicenter evaluation of ethambutol susceptibility testing of *Mycobacterium tuberculosis* by agar proportion and radiometric methods. *J. Clin. Microbiol.* 40:3976–3979.

83. Maggi, N., C. Pasqualucci, R. Ballotta, and P. Sensi. 1966. Rifampicin: a new orally active rifamycin. *Chemoterapia* 11:285–292.

84. Mahmoudi, A., and M. D. Iseman. 1993. Pitfalls in the care of patients with tuberculosis: common errors and their association with the acquisition of drug resistance. *JAMA* 270:65–68.

85. Middlebrook, G., and M. L. Cohn. 1954. Some observations on the pathogenicity of isoniazid-resistant variants of tubercle bacilli. *Science* 118:297–299.

86. Miller, A. B., R. Tall, W. Fox, M. J. Lefford, and D. A. Mitchison. 1966. Primary drug resistance in pulmonary tuberculosis in Great Britain: second national survey. *Tubercle* 47:92–108.

87. Mitnick, C., J. Bayona, E. Palacios, S. Shin, J. Furin, F. Alcántara, E. Sánchez, M. Sarria, M. Becerra, M. C. Smith-Fawzi, S. Kapiga, D. Neuberg, J. H. Maguire, J. Y. Kim, and P. Farmer. 2003. Community-based therapy for multidrug-resistant tuberculosis in Lima, Peru. *N. Engl. J. Med.* 348:119–128.

88. Moore, M., E. McCray, and I. M. Onorato. 2000. The epidemiology of multidrug-resistant tuberculosis in the United States and other established market economies, p. 17–28. *In* I. Bastian and F. Portaels (ed.), *Multidrug-Resistant Tuberculosis.* Kluwer Academic Publishers, Dordrecht, The Netherlands.

89. Moore-Gillon, J. 2001. Multidrug-resistant tuberculosis: this is the cost. *Ann. N. Y. Acad. Sci.* 953:233–240.

90. Moro, M. L., A. Gori, I. Errante, A. Infuso, F. Franzetti, L. Sodano, and E. Lemoli. 1998. An outbreak of multidrug-resistant tuberculosis involving HIV-infected patients of two hospitals in Milan, Italy. *AIDS* 12:1095–1102.

91. Nitta, A. T., P. T. Davidson, M. L. de Koning, and R. J. Kilman. 1996. Misdiagnosis of multi-drug resistant tuberculosis possibly due to laboratory-related errors. *JAMA* 276:1980–1983.

92. Ormerod, L. P., R. M. Green, N. Horsfield, and R. White. 2001. Drug resistance trends in *M. tuberculosis*: Blackburn 1990–1999. *Int. J. Tuberc. Lung Dis.* 5:903–905.

93. Pablos-Mendez, A., M. C. Raviglione, A. Laszlo, N. Binkin, H. L. Rieder, F. Bustreo, D. L. Cohn, C. S. B. Lambregts-van Weezenbeek, S. J. Kim, P. Chaulet, and P. Nunn. 1998. Global surveillance for antituberculosis-drug resistance, 1994–1997. *N. Engl. J. Med.* 338:1641–1649.

94. Parsons, L. M., A. Somoskovi, R. Urbanczik, and M. Salfinger. 2004. Laboratory diagnostic aspects of drug resistant tuberculosis. *Front. Biosci.* 9:2086–2105.

95. Public Health Laboratory Service/Communicable Disease Surveillance Centre. 1995. Outbreak of hospital-acquired multidrug resistant tuberculosis. *Commun. Dis. Rep. Wkly.* 5:161.

96. Rist, N., and J. Crofton. 1960. Drug resistance in hospitals and sanatoria. A report to the committee on laboratory methods and to the committee on antibiotics and chemotherapy of the International Union against Tuberculosis. *Bull. Int. Union Tuberc.* 30:3–39.

97. Robert, J., D. Trystram, C. Pernot-Truffot, and V. Jarlier. 2002. Surveillance de la tuberculose à bacilles multirésistants en France en 1998. *Bull. Epidemiol. Hebdom.* 16–17: 71–72.

98. Robitzek, E. H., and I. J. Selikoff. 1952. Hydrazine derivative of isonicotinic acid in the treatment of acute progressive caseous-pneumonic tuberculosis. A preliminary report. *Am. Rev. Tuberc.* 65:402–428.

99. Salfinger M., and G. E. Pfyffer. 1994. The new diagnostic mycobacteriology laboratory. *Eur. J. Clin. Microbiol. Infect. Dis.* 13:961–979.

100. Saraiya, M., and N. J. Binkin. 2000. Tuberculosis among immigrants, p. 661–693. *In* L. B. Reichman and E. S. Hershfield (ed.), *Tuberculosis, a Comprehensive International Approach,* 2nd ed. Marcel Dekker, Inc., New York, N.Y.

101. Schatz, A., E. Bugie, and S. A. Waksman. 1944. Streptomycin, a substance exhibiting antibiotic activity against gram-positive and gram-negative bacteria. *Proc. Soc. Exp. Biol. Med.* 55:66–69.

102. Seaworth, B. 2002. Multidrug resistant tuberculosis. *Inf. Dis. Clin. North. Am.* 16:73–105.

103. Selvakumar N., E. Prabhakaran, F. Rahman, N. A. Chandu, S. Srinivasan, T. Santha, L. S. Chauhan, and P. R. Narayanan. 2003. Blinded rechecking of sputum smears for acid-fast bacilli to ensure the quality and usefulness of restaining smears to assess fals-positive errors. *Int. J. Tuberc. Lung Dis.* 7:1077–1082.

104. Snider, D. E., and J. R. La Montagne. 1994. The neglected

global toberculosis problem: a report of the 1992 World Congress on Tuberculosis *J. Infect. Dis.* **169:**1189–1196.

105. Suarez, P. G., K. Floyd, J. Portocarrero, E. Alarcón, E. Rapiti, G. Ramos, C. Bonilla, I. Sabogal, I. Aranda, C. Dye, M. Raviglione, and M. A. Espinal. 2002. Feasibility and cost-effectiveness of standardised second-line drug treatment for chronic tuberculosis patients: a national cohort study in Peru. *Lancet* **359:**1980–1989.

106. Telenti, A., and F. C. Tenover. 2002. Genetic methods for detecting bacterial resistance genes, p. 239–264. *In* K. Lewis, A. A. Salyers, H. W. Taber, and R. G. Wax (ed.), *Bacterial Resistance to Antimicrobials*, p. 239–264. Marcel Dekker, Inc., New York, N.Y.

107. Tenover F. C., J. T. Crawford, R. E. Huebner, L. J. Geiter, C. R. Horsburgh, Jr., R. C. Good. 1993. The resurgence of tuberculosis: is your laboratory ready? *J. Clin. Microbiol.* **31:**767–770.

108. Texeira, L., M. D. Perkins, J. L. Johnson, R. Keller, M. Palaci, V. do Valle Dettoni, L. M. Canedo Rocha, S. Debanne, E. Talbot, and R. Dietze. 2001. Infection and disease among household contacts of patients with multidrug-resistant tuberculosis. *Int. J. Tuberc. Lung Dis.* **5:**321–328.

109. Thomsen, V. Ø., J. Bauer, T. Lillebaek, and S. Glismann. 2000. Results from 8 years of susceptibility testing of clinical *Mycobacterium tuberculosis* isolates in Denmark. *Eur. Respir. J.* **15:**203–208.

110. Toungoussova, O. S., D. A. Caugant, P. Sandven, A. O. Mariandyshev, and G. Bjune. 2002. Drug resistance of *Mycobacterium tuberculosis* strains isolated from patients with pulmonary tuberculosis in Archangels, Russia. *Int. J. Tuberc. Lung Dis.* **6:**406–414.

111. Tuberculosis Research Committee. 1975. A study on prevalence of resistance to major drugs among newly admitted pulmonary tuberculosis patients in 1972: comparison of results in 1972 with those in 1957, 1959, 1961, 1963, 1966, and 1969. *Kekkaku* **50:**1–8.

112. Tuberculosis Research Committee. 1991. A study on drug resistance of newly admitted pulmonary tuberculosis patients: prevalence of drug resistance according to the sensitivity test at local laboratories, and its trend over twenty-five years in Japan. *Kekkaku* **66:**367–373.

113. U.S. Public Health Service Cooperative Investigation. 1964. Prevalence of drug resistance in previously untreated patients. *Am. Rev. Respir. Dis.* **89:**327–331.

114. Valenzuela, M. T., P. Garcia, J. Ponce, R. Lepe, M. Velasco, and S. Piffardi. 1989. Drug resistance of *M. tuberculosis* in Chile: rates of initial resistance for 1986 and acquired resistance for 1985. *Bull. Int. Union Tuberc. Lung Dis.* **64:** 13–14.

115. Van Rie, A. R., M. Warren, M. Richardson, R. P. Gie, D. A. Enarson, N. Beyers, and P. D. Van Helden. 2000. Classification of drug-resistant tuberculosis in an epidemic area. *Lancet* **356:**22–25.

116. Van Soolingen, D., M. W. Borgdorff, P. E. W. de Haas, M. M. G. G. Sebek, J. Veen, M. Dessens, K. Kremer, and J. D. A. van Embden. 1999. Molecular epidemiology of tuberculosis in the Netherlands: a nationwide study from 1993 through 1997. *J. Infect. Dis.* **180:**726–736.

117. Van Soolingen, D., P. E. W. de Haas, H. R. van Door, E. Kuijper, H. Rinder, and M. W. Borgdorff. 2000. Muations at amino acid position 315 of the *katG* gene are associated with high-level resistance to isoniazid, other drug resistance, and successful transmission of *Mycobacterium tuberculosis* in The Netherlands. *J. Infect. Dis.* **182:**1788–1790.

118. World Health Organization. 1997. *Anti-Tuberculosis Drug Resistance in the World.* WHO/TB/97.229. World Health Organization, Geneva, Switzerland.

119. World Health Organization. 2000. *Anti-Tuberculosis Drug Resistance in the World: Prevalence and Trends.* Report no. 2. WHO/CDS/TB/2000.278. World Health Organization, Geneva, Switzerland.

120. World Health Organization. 2003. *Global Tuberculosis Control: Surveillance, Planning, Financing.* WHO report 2002. WHO/CDS/TB/2003.316. World Health Organization, Geneva, Switzerland.

121. Youmans, G. P., E. H. Williston, W. H. Feldman, and H. C. Hinshaw. 1946. Increase in resistance of tubercle bacilli to streptomycin: a preliminary report. *Proc. Staff Meet. Mayo Clin.* **21:**126–127.

Tuberculosis and the Tubercle Bacillus
Edited by Stewart T. Cole et al.
© 2005 ASM Press, Washington, D.C.

Chapter 8

Mechanisms of Drug Resistance in *Mycobacterium tuberculosis*

YING ZHANG, CATHERINE VILCHÈZE, AND WILLIAM R. JACOBS, JR.

INTRODUCTION

Drug Resistance in *M. tuberculosis*

Despite the declaration of tuberculosis (TB) as a global emergency by the World Health Organization 10 years ago, the global problem of TB has worsened due to increased drug resistance and the human immunodeficiency virus (HIV) pandemic (39). Drug resistance in TB is a particular problem because the lengthy therapy of at least 6 months makes patient compliance very difficult, which frequently creates drug-resistant strains of *Mycobacterium tuberculosis*. The WHO reports the presence of drug-resistant strains of *M. tuberculosis* in 72 countries, with frequencies ranging from 3 to 41% (230). Multidrug-resistant TB (MDR-TB) caused by *M. tuberculosis* strains resistant to two or more drugs, usually isoniazid (INH) and rifampin (RIF), caused several fatal outbreaks worldwide and is an increasing threat to global TB control programs (39). While drug-sensitive TB can be effectively treated with four drugs, INH, RIF, ethambutol (EMB), and pyrazinamide (PZA), in a 6-month regimen called short-course chemotherapy, treatment of a case of MDR-TB can exceed 2 years, thus increasing the costs and side effects significantly. In the absence of any new treatment and with the growing epidemic of HIV infection, which weakens the host immune system and allows easier transmission of TB and the drug-resistant form, there is increasing concern about the control of the disease. In view of the problem of drug-resistant TB and with the advent of modern molecular biology tools, there has been great interest in understanding the molecular mechanisms of drug resistance and drug action in *M. tuberculosis*. Tremendous progress has been made in this area in the last decade. This chapter provides an update on genes associated with drug resistance and our current understanding of mechanisms of drug resistance and drug action in *M. tuberculosis*.

The Phenotype of Drug Resistance

Resistance is a phenotype, the ability of a bacterial cell to survive the presence of a drug at a concentration that normally kills or inhibits growth. Resistance is caused by mutation and can be differentiated from tolerance, which is a conditional phenotype mediated by the physiological state of the bacilli. For example, *M. tuberculosis* cells are resistant to INH when the cells are in stationary phase (135). For this reason, drug susceptibility of *M. tuberculosis* is measured by testing cells in the exponential phase of growth. The phenotype of drug resistance is determined in liquid medium containing the drug, as in the BACTEC method (184), or in solid medium, as in agar plate dilution analysis in medium containing various concentrations of the drug. The MIC is thus defined as the minimum concentration of the drug which kills 99% of cells. The MIC of INH can vary dramatically depending on the strain and the mutation conferring INH resistance. *M. tuberculosis* is exquisitely sensitive to INH, with INH MICs in the range of 0.02 to 0.2 μg/ml. Resistance levels show two distinct phenotypic ranges. High-level resistance can occur in a single step at ranges between 10 and 100 μg/ml (200- to 2,000-fold above normal). Low-level resistance occurs at 0.25 to 2.0 μg/ml (5- to 100-fold above normal). As described later in this chapter, many of the genetic bases for these differences have been defined. However, it must be emphasized that the in vitro MIC does not necessarily reflect the drug concentration required to kill or inhibit tubercle bacilli in vivo. A pertinent example is PZA, which has a MIC of 100 μg/ml by the BACTEC method that is considerably higher than its effective concentration in vivo. Drug resistance in *M. tuberculosis* can be either intrinsic (or natural) or acquired. Intrinsic resistance refers to nonsusceptibility due to unique characteristics of *M. tuberculosis* such as its natural resistance to penicillin or clarithromycin.

Ying Zhang • Department of Molecular Microbiology and Immunology, Bloomberg School of Public Health, Johns Hopkins University, Baltimore, MD 21205. **William R. Jacobs, Jr., and Catherine Vilchèze** • Howard Hughes Medical Institute, Department of Microbiology and Immunology, Albert Einstein College of Medicine, New York, NY 10043.

Acquired resistance refers to susceptible *M. tuberculosis* becoming resistant to drugs as a result of mutations. In some rare situations, drug-resistant mycobacteria can become drug dependent; that is, they grow only in the presence of the drug. For example, streptomycin (SM)-dependent resistant *M. tuberculosis* strains have been found in some cases that have characteristic changes or mutations in the ribosome (75) (see the section on SM resistance [below]).

Identification of Genotypes Conferring Drug-Resistant Phenotypes

The emergence of drug resistance in bacteria is one of the easiest demonstrations of the "survival of the fittest" concept of Darwin's theory of evolution. From the time when drugs were first used to treat bacterial infections, drug resistance was observed (2). This is because the large number of bacterial cells in populations allows for the selection of mutants that are resistant to the drugs (96). Resistance is thus due to a change in the genotype resulting in a drug-resistant phenotype of a bacterium, which can be passed on to subsequent generations. This is in contrast to tolerance, or phenotypic resistance, another phenomenon that is common to *M. tuberculosis* and other bacterial species, in which changes in the metabolic or physiological status of the cell induce temporary drug resistance as seen in stationary-phase, starved, or dormant bacteria. Knowledge about the mutations conferring drug resistance not only leads to understanding of the mechanisms of drug resistance and drug action but also facilitates rapid detection of drug resistance by molecular means. To date, the definitive method for identification of mutations that confer drug resistance is the transfer of genes conferring drug resistance or drug susceptibility to, or from, drug-resistant strains. This represents the fulfillment of Koch's molecular postulate (49). For the broad-spectrum antibiotics, RIF, SM, and fluoroquinolones, the mechanisms of drug action and resistance had been elucidated previously by using genetically tractable organisms. Analogous mutations could thus be identified by DNA sequence analysis of drug-resistant strains of *M. tuberculosis*. However, the lack of gene transfer systems for mycobacteria had prevented the discovery of the drug-resistant alleles for any of the *Mycobacterium*-specific drugs. Thus, as of 1992, no drug resistance alleles had been identified for INH, ethionamide (ETH), EMB, PZA, or *p*-aminosalicylic acid (PAS). With the development of plasmid transformation systems for mycobacteria, for the first time it was possible to clone and transfer the minimal DNA fragment required to confer drug susceptibility. Using this system, tremendous progress has been made

in identifying mycobacterial drug resistance alleles, as summarized in Table 1.

It is important to note that the mutations that confer drug resistance can be either recessive or dominant with respect to the wild-type gene. The characteristic of recessive or dominant behavior is a direct consequence of the merodiploid state (i.e., the introduction of a wild-type or mutant allele into a strain with a mutated gene or the wild-type gene). Recessive mutations represent the loss of some function. For example, Middlebrook had isolated INH-resistant mutants of *M. tuberculosis* and showed that the majority of strains had lost their catalase peroxidase activity (128). Zhang et al. cloned a DNA fragment that encoded the catalase peroxidase gene and demonstrated that the transfer of this wild-type gene to an INH-resistant strain restored INH susceptibility (235). Thus, the mutations in the INH-resistant mutants were recessive to the wild-type gene. In contrast, the introduction of plasmids which caused overexpression of the wild-type *inhA* gene, by virtue of multicopy plasmids or strongly expressed promoters, led to a dominant phenotype with respect to the wild-type *inhA* allele in the recipient strain (12, 95) and to INH resistance. The transferred alleles for drug resistance are characterized in terms of recessive or dominant behavior with respect to the wild-type genes.

Drug Resistance Mechanisms

Bacteria can become resistant to antibiotics or antibacterial agents by a number of common strategies, including target modification, target overexpression, barrier mechanisms, drug-inactivating enzymes, inactivation of drug-activating enzymes, and drug extrusion mechanisms. The first strategy described for bacteria was that of mutations in the target, which cause either reduced drug binding or overexpression of the drug target. Similar mechanisms exist for both prokaryotic and eukaryotic cells with the drug trimethoprim or methotrexate and the gene encoding the target of dihydrofolate reductase.

Since drugs must enter bacterial cells to be active, bacteria can become resistant by preventing entry of the drug. Barrier mechanisms can be mediated by decreased uptake, such as that caused by the porin (PenB) mutation in *Neisseria gonorrhoeae*, resulting in resistance to β-lactams and tetracycline (58), or by increased removal of antibiotics from the cell, such as the enhanced efflux for tetracycline mediated by efflux proteins TetA to TetE, TetG, TetH, and TetZ (121). Although mycobacteria have porins (150), they have not been shown to be involved in clinical drug resistance. Resistance to fluoroquinolones is also known

Table 1. Mechanisms of drug action and resistance in mycobacteria

Drug[a]	MIC (µg/ml)	Gene(s) involved in resistance	Gene function	Role	Mechanism of action	Mutation frequency (%)	Allele type
Isoniazid	0.02–0.2	katG	Catalase-peroxidase	Prodrug conversion	Inhibition of mycolic acid biosynthesis and other multiple effects on DNA, lipids, carbohydrates, and NAD metabolism	20–80	Recessive
		inhA	Enoyl ACP reductase	Drug target		15–43	Dominant
		ndh	NADH dehydrogenase II	Modulator of INH activity		10	Recessive
		ahpC	Alkyl hydroperoxidase	Marker of resistance		10–15	Dominant
Rifampin	0.5–2	rpoB	RNA polymerase	Drug target	Inhibition of transcription	96	Dominant
Pyrazinamide	16–50 (pH5.5)	pncA	Nicotinamidase/pyrazinamidase	Prodrug conversion	Acidification of cytoplasm and de-energized membrane	72–97	Recessive
5-Chloro-pyrazinamide	8–32	fasI	FASI	Drug target	Inhibition of FASI	NA[b]	Dominant
Ethambutol	1–5	embCAB		Drug target	Inhibition of arabinogalactan synthesis	47–65	Dominant
Streptomycin	2–8	rpsL	S12 ribosomal protein	Drug target	Inhibition of protein synthesis	52–59	Recessive
		rrs	16S rRNA	Drug target		8–21	Dominant
Amikacin/ kanamycin	2–4	rrs	16S rRNA	Drug target	Inhibition of protein synthesis	76	Dominant
Quinolones	0.5–2.5	gyrA	DNA gyrase subunit A	Drug target	Inhibition of DNA gyrase	75–94	Dominant
		gyrB	DNA gyrase subunit B	Participates in drug binding?		In vitro	
Ethionamide	2.5–10	etaAlethA	Flavin monooxygenase	Prodrug conversion	Inhibition of mycolic acid biosynthesis	37	Recessive
		inhA		Drug target		56	

[a]Rifampin, aminoglycosides, and fluoroquinolones (underlined) are broad-spectrum antibiotics, whose mechanism of resistance in *M. tuberculosis* is the same as in other bacteria.
[b]NA, not available.

to be mediated by efflux pumps that block drug up-take (104). Another mechanism of resistance is that of drug inactivation mediated by drug-degrading or inactivating enzymes (e.g., cleavage of penicillin by β-lactamase). Typically, resistance mediated by drug-inactivating enzymes is present at much higher levels than the resistance mediated by target alterations. The common theme for all these mechanisms is that they confer the phenotype of resistance of the drug to the recipient cell.

Prodrug Activation: a Unique Mycobacterial Phenomenon

M. tuberculosis is unique to date among bacteria because three of its drugs require activation to be-come inhibitory. The drugs INH, ETH, and PZA all require activation for activity against *M. tuberculo-sis*, as discussed in subsequent sections. Thus, resis-tance can be mediated by mutations that eliminate the activation step. Such inactivation has been demon-strated for KatG (catalase-peroxidase) in INH resis-tance (235), PncA (nicotinamidase/pyrazinamidase) in PZA resistance (181), and EtaA/EthA (flavin adenine dinucleotide [FAD]-containing monooxygenase) in ETH resistance (15, 42, 53, 208). The *M. tuberculo-sis* genome contains single copies of *katG* and *pncA*, which cause INH and PZA resistance, respectively, when mutated. It is interesting that *M. tuberculosis* has over 60 homologues of the ETH activator EthA. These monooxygenase-like enzymes are involved in detoxification in other systems, but no other organism has as many such enzymes in their genome. Metro-nidazole and nitrofuran are nitro-substituted prodrugs whose activation relies on nitroreductases in anaero-bic bacteria. For example, resistance to metronida-zole in *Helicobacter pylori* has recently been shown to be caused by mutations in *rdxA*, encoding NADPH nitroreductase (60), or in *frxA*, encoding NAD(P)H flavin oxidoreductase (93). Although it has been known for some time that nitrofuran resistance in *Escherichia coli* is accompanied by loss of nitro-reductase enzyme (114), the genetic basis of nitrofu-ran resistance was identified more recently and was shown to be due to mutations in nitroreductase NfsA or NfsB, which is involved in activation of nitrofuran (220). It is noteworthy that the first molecular study to elucidate this type of resistance mechanism was that of KatG mutations in INH resistance (234, 235). Surprisingly, the mechanism of resistance due to loss of drug activating enzymes is not presented in most reviews or book chapters on this topic (160, 213). We would like to emphasize the importance of muta-tion in prodrug-activating enzymes as a new mecha-nism of drug resistance.

Defining a Drug Target

The first step in understanding the mechanism of drug action is to identify the drug target. At the out-set, it is useful to define the basic concept of a drug target, which we define as a substrate, typically an essential enzyme, to which a drug binds and inacti-vates, possibly leading to cell death. Genetically, drug targets are defined by two types of mutations in the gene encoding the target that either alter its structure or cause overexpression. Mutations that alter the tar-get prevent binding of the drug. Mutations that cause overexpression of the drug target mediate resistance by the excess copies titrating the drug, thereby reduc-ing the effective drug concentrations. For example, drugs that target essential metabolic pathways, such as the sulfonamides or trimethoprim, were found to bind to and inhibit the essential enzyme dihydro-pteroate synthase or dihydrofolate reductase, respec-tively. For both these cases, resistance is mediated by target overexpression or modification and the mutant alleles would confer a resistance phenotype dominant to the wild-type allele. Nevertheless, over-expression of a gene is not sufficient evidence to prove that a gene encodes a target. For example, a drug-inactivating enzyme such as the arylamine N-acetyltransferase Nat can confer INH resistance when overexpressed, but *nat* is not the target of INH (155). Target verification also requires that mutations in the structural gene causing target alteration be iden-tified. Thus, allelic exchange needs to be performed, in which a linked gene is cotransformed with a puta-tive drug resistance allele to provide an unselected marker, thereby ascertaining if the allele confers re-sistance by target modification. Such strategies have been used to demonstrate that alleles of *rpoB*, *gyrA*, or *rpsL* confer resistance to RIF, fluoroquinolones, or SM, respectively. In addition to these genetic tests, biochemical and X-ray crystallographic studies re-vealing drug binding and inhibition can further con-firm if an enzyme is a target. Defining a drug target is the key first step in elucidating the mechanism of ac-tion of a drug.

Mechanisms of Drug Action

Drugs can be either bacteriostatic or bacterici-dal. Once a drug enters and binds the target, the cell's metabolism is altered, which first leads to growth ar-rest and/or a cidal event. Bacteriostatic drugs simply inhibit a metabolic pathway and the cell stops grow-ing. In contrast, drugs that induce cell death are bac-tericidal. The anti-TB drug PAS is thought to inhibit dihydropteroate synthase, although the genetic basis for this has yet to be determined. The bacteriostatic activity of PAS on *M. tuberculosis* reduced its efficacy as an anti-TB agent as drug resistance rapidly emerged. Nevertheless, the introduction of PAS led to an important concept for modern chemotherapy, namely, that the use of two or more drugs in combating bacterial infections prevents the development of drug resistance. The addition of PAS to SM monotherapy greatly reduced the frequency of emergence of drug resistance (124). The use of two or more drugs for effectively treating mycobacterial infections remains a standard therapy for mycobacterial infections and, indeed, for treating other infections such as those caused by HIV and *H. pylori*. Despite these attempts, the improper use of drugs has led to the emergence of MDR-TB throughout the world today.

An example of a bactericidal drug is penicillin, which targets peptidoglycan biosynthesis, leading to lysis of actively growing cells. Penicillin is effective only on actively growing cells as the cell growth leads to the subsequent lysis of the bacterial cell (73). The discovery of penicillin by Fleming, and its application by Florey and Chain, were indeed landmarks in microbiology, since penicillin remains a highly effective bactericidal agent to this date.

SM, an antibacterial agent discovered by Schatz and Waksman in 1944, was hailed as the first broad-spectrum antibacterial and was even active against *M. tuberculosis* (178). This drug targets a specific ribosomal protein (S12 of the small ribosomal subunit encoded by the *rpsL* gene), thereby inhibiting protein biosynthesis. Inactivation of protein biosynthesis is a bactericidal event that leads to cell death, but, in contrast to penicillin, this does not trigger cell lysis.

Lack of R-Factor-Mediated Resistance

MDR was first detected in *Shigella* in 1955, when it was demonstrated that *Shigella* strains acquired resistance to numerous antibiotics such as sulfonamides, SM, ampicillin, chloramphenicol, and tetracycline through R plasmids (48, 215). Plasmids, transposons, or integrons are known to mediate drug resistance in various bacterial species (J. E. Davies, *Abstr. Ciba Found. Symp.*, abstr. 41a, p. 15–35, 1997; R. M. Hall, *Abstr. Ciba Found. Symp.*, abstr. 65a, p. 192–205, 1997) and in the fast-growing mycobacterium *M. fortuitum* but not in *M. tuberculosis* (110, 111). Instead, drug resistance in *M. tuberculosis* is caused by mutations in chromosomal genes (69). Typically, no single pleiotropic mutation mediates the MDR phenotype in *M. tuberculosis*, although coresistance to INH and ETH can occur with mutations in the target gene *inhA* (12, 142). Thus,

the MDR phenotype is caused by sequential accumulation of mutations in different genes involved in resistance to individual drugs as a result of inappropriate treatment or poor adherence. Mechanisms of resistance to TB-specific drugs, such as INH and PZA, are unique to *M. tuberculosis*. On the other hand, mechanisms of resistance to broad-spectrum antibiotics such as SM, RIF, and fluoroquinolones in *M. tuberculosis* are the same as in other bacteria. Mycobacteria are naturally resistant to many antibiotics due to a highly hydrophobic cell envelope acting as an effective permeability barrier (27, 80), drug efflux systems (e.g., the major facilitator family and numerous ABC transporters) (37), and hydrolytic enzymes (e.g., β-lactamases and aminoglycoside acetyltransferases) (37, 94). Most of this chapter deals with drug resistance caused by genetic mutations. However, because of the increasing awareness of the problem of phenotypic resistance, the last section of this review briefly discusses this topic. The chemical structures of the most commonly used antituberculous drugs are shown in Fig. 1.

MECHANISMS OF DRUG ACTION AND RESISTANCE

Isoniazid

Isoniazid (isonicotinic acid hydrazide, INH) is an important first-line TB drug, and was introduced in 1952 (18, 52, 151). INH is highly active against *M. tuberculosis*, with a MIC in the range of 0.02 to 0.2 μg/ml. It has a simple structure containing a pyridine ring and a hydrazide group, and both moieties are essential for its high activity against *M. tuberculosis*.

Mechanism of action

The mode of action of INH is highly complex. The discovery of INH as a potent TB drug arose from two independent observations that nicotinamide had certain activity against *M. tuberculosis* in guinea pigs and mice (35, 120), and that the sulfa drug thiosemicarbazones had activity against *M. tuberculosis* (151). Synthesis of nicotinamide analogs and reshuffling of chemical moieties of thiosemicarbazones led to the discovery of INH. Several early studies reported that INH affected DNA biosynthesis (56), NAD biosynthesis (16, 191), and NAD metabolism by incorporation into NAD through exchange with nicotinamide (233) or by activation of NAD glycohydrolase by removing its repressor leading to NAD depletion (16) as possible mechanisms of action. INH is active against growing tubercle bacilli but not resting bacilli (135, 176). Oxygen plays an important role in INH

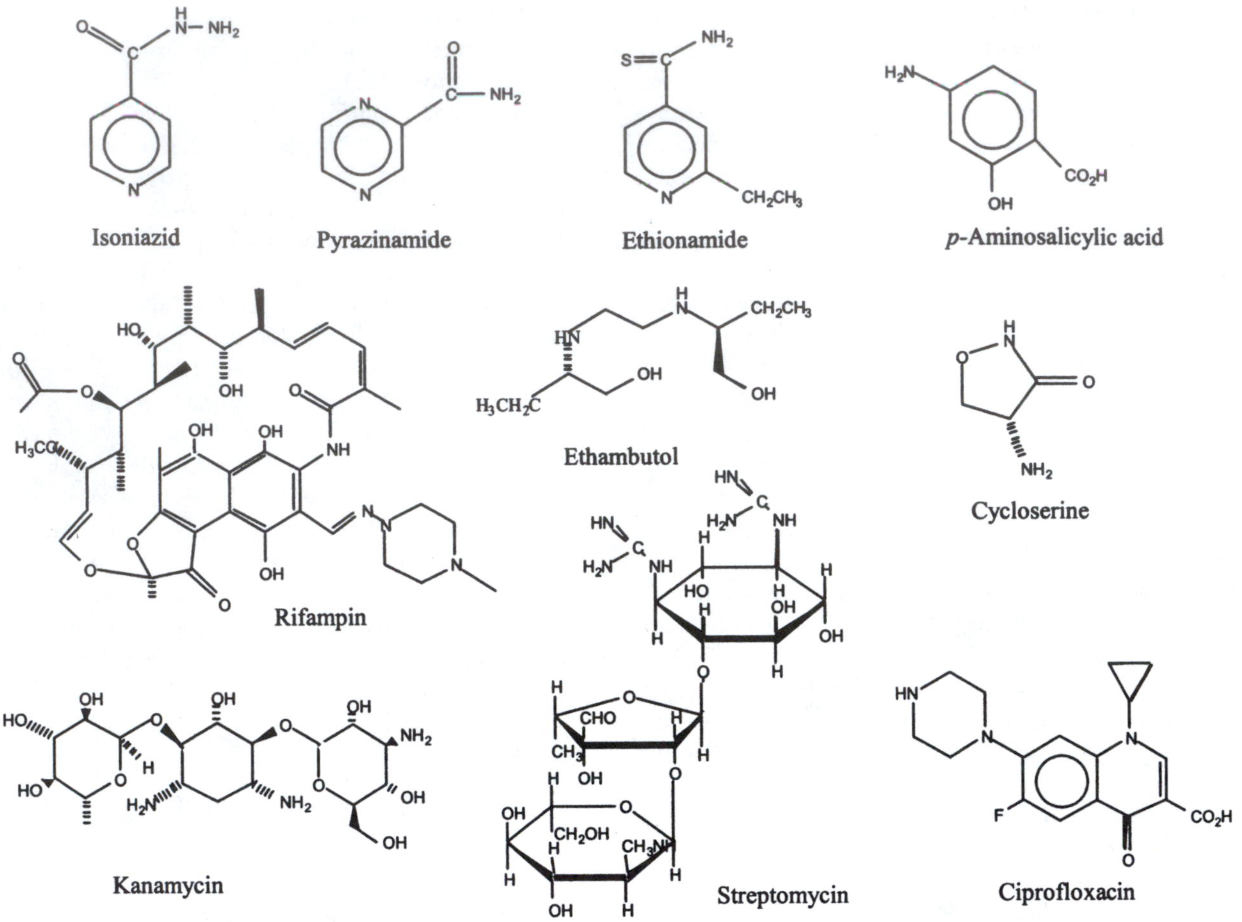

Figure 1. Structures of first-line and some second-line TB drugs.

action, since INH has no activity against *M. tuberculosis* under anaerobic conditions (135). The first report that INH inhibited the synthesis of mycolic acids, the long-chain (C_{70} to C_{90}) α-branched β-hydroxy fatty acids of the mycobacterial cell envelope, was published by Winder et al. (228). Takayama et al. extended this work (197) to demonstrate that the inhibition of mycolic acid synthesis led to a characteristic disruption of membranes and cell death (198). Furthermore, they demonstrated that INH treatment of *M. tuberculosis* led to the accumulation of a saturated C_{26} fatty acid and postulated that the enzyme that was inhibited was either a desaturase, a mycolic acid elongation enzyme, or a cyclopropanase (196).

Zhang et al. showed that INH was activated by the catalase-peroxidase KatG (235) to generate a range of reactive (oxygen and organic) species, which then attack multiple targets in the tubercle bacillus. One of these species, the isonicotinic acyl radical, was shown to attack the nicotinamide group of NAD^+ to form an INH-NAD adduct (172). A recent study showed that the isonicotinic acyl radical can form

different isomeric INH-NAD adducts, the open form and cyclic form (149, 223). Questions are raised about whether the open or cyclic form, or both, is the active species (29). The KatG-mediated INH activation can also be achieved with manganese (Mn^{2+}) (101). Mn^{2+} facilitates the INH activation by enhancing the production of the INH-NAD adduct by both wild-type and mutant KatG enzymes (216). Although *M. tuberculosis* KatG itself is sufficient for INH activation, *M. smegmatis* KatG cannot directly activate INH and requires Mn^{2+} for activation (216). This may provide a likely explanation for the relative nonsusceptibility of *M. smegmatis* to INH. In fact, the introduction of the *M. tuberculosis katG* gene into wild-type *M. smegmatis* increases the susceptibility of *M. smegmatis* to INH by 50-fold (47). Superoxide plays a role in KatG-mediated INH action (30, 214). Treatment of *M. tuberculosis* H37Rv strain or a strain carrying the S315T KatG mutation with plumbagin and clofazimine, two compounds capable of generating superoxide radicals, rendered the strains more susceptible to INH (30, 214).

Defining the precise target of action of INH required the development of plasmid transformation systems and led to the discovery of *inhA*, a gene from *M. tuberculosis* that conferred coresistance to INH and ETH when expressed in *M. smegmatis* (12). In these studies, a common missense mutation causing a substitution of an alanine for the serine at position 94 (S94A) was found in INH-resistant mutants of *M. bovis* and *M. smegmatis*. Mycolic acid biosynthetic assays from cell lysates from either the overexpressed *inhA* recombinants or the S94A mutant were resistant to INH inhibition compared to the parental strain. These studies led to the conclusion that *inhA* encoded the target for both INH and ETH.

The *inhA* gene encodes an NADH-specific enoyl-acyl carrier protein (ACP) reductase (165), part of the fatty acid synthase type II (FASII) system (109), and its three-dimensional structure was determined with NADH bound (45). The S94A mutant was shown to bind NADH five times less efficiently than the wild-type InhA protein did, and the X-ray crystallographic data revealed that replacing serine with alanine resulted in reduced hydrogen bonding of NADH to InhA (45). Quemard et al. were the first to demonstrate that KatG-activated radioactive INH bound to InhA but that this was inhibited by high concentrations of NADH (164). Johnsson and Schultz demonstrated that KatG-activated INH inhibited the InhA activity and that the S94A mutant was resistant to this inhibition (83). Basso et al. found that numerous InhA proteins from INH-resistant clinical isolates resisted KatG-activated INH inactivation and were all defective for NADH binding (14).

Mdluli et al. proposed that the β-ketoacyl-ACP synthase, KasA, also part of the FASII system, was the primary target of INH (123). They found that INH (1 μg/ml) induced two *M. tuberculosis* proteins involved in fatty acid and mycolic acid synthesis, the ACP AcpM and KasA, resulting in the formation of a complex containing KasA, AcpM, and INH (123). Since the inhibition of a β-ketoacyl-ACP synthase could explain the accumulation of a saturated C_{26} fatty acid on INH treatment of *M. tuberculosis*, as described by Takayama et al. (196), the authors concluded that KasA was the primary target of INH. Later, Kremer and colleagues showed that the KasA-AcpM-INH complex does not contain INH and that this complex is not induced by inhibition of KasA but is induced when InhA is inhibited (90). In the same study, the authors also demonstrated that activated INH does not inhibit purified KasA in vitro (90). Therefore, it remains to be demonstrated how the activated form of INH reacts with KasA or AcpM and if these interactions play any role in INH bactericidal activity.

Despite the efforts to establish that *inhA* encoded the primary target of INH, several significant questions remain unanswered. First, blocking enoyl reductase activity should result in the accumulation of a monounsaturated fatty acid, and yet several workers found the accumulation of a saturated C_{26} fatty acid on INH treatment of *M. tuberculosis* (123, 196). Second, transformation of *M. tuberculosis* with a multicopy plasmid library did not yield any clones that conferred resistance to INH or ETH (122). Third, it was unclear how a mutation that altered NADH binding had any relationship to INH resistance.

Vilchèze et al. hypothesized that the accumulation of a saturated C_{26} fatty acid did not result directly from a blockage of InhA but, rather, from the blockage of the FASII system resulting in accumulation of the end product of FASI (211). Mycobacteria, unlike most other bacteria, possess two different systems for generating fatty acids. Most bacteria make C_2 to C_{16} fatty acids by using the independent, ACP-based FASII system. In mycobacteria, FASII is used to extend C_{18} or C_{26} fatty acids to C_{56} while the eukaryote-like FASI system, first described by Bloch and coworkers (21, 28), makes C_2 to $C_{24/26}$ fatty acids. By isolating a temperature-sensitive mutation in *inhA*, Vilchèze et al. were able to demonstrate that thermal inactivation of InhA did result in the accumulation of a saturated FASI end product (211). Moreover, the thermal inactivation of InhA in *M. smegmatis* led to death kinetics and lysis that was very similar to that induced by INH (211). In addition to explaining the accumulation of a saturated FASI end product, this work established that inactivation of InhA was sufficient for cell lysis, fulfilling another drug target criterion.

The failure of the multicopy library to confer INH resistance on *M. tuberculosis*, observed by Mdluli et al. (122), was confirmed by E. Dubnau and W. R. Jacobs, Jr. (unpublished observation). However, the introduction of the same *M. tuberculosis* library into *M. smegmatis* yielded plasmids containing the *inhA* operon (12). Furthermore, the introduction of an *M. smegmatis* library into *M. bovis* BCG yielded an *inhA*-containing plasmid (12). The basis of this inconsistency was hypothesized to result from the *M. tuberculosis* *inhA* operon being tightly regulated in *M. tuberculosis* and *M. bovis* BCG. To address this possibility and to test if overexpressed *inhA* conferred resistance to INH and ETH in *M. tuberculosis*, the *inhA* gene from *M. tuberculosis* was fused to two independent promoters. Both resulting constructs conferred coresistance to INH and ETH in *M. tuberculosis*, *M. bovis* BCG, and *M. smegmatis* (95).

The relationship between INH and NADH was resolved with the surprising X-ray crystallographic visualization of an INH-NAD adduct in the InhA binding pocket (172). This result suggested that a mutant of InhA that was defective in binding NADH (like S94A) should also be defective (hence resistant) in binding the INH-NAD adduct. Moreover, it also suggested that activated ETH might also form a similar adduct to inhibit InhA. Evidence supporting this observation comes from the discovery that mutations in NADH dehydrogenase II which result in increased NADH/NAD$^+$ ratios mediate coresistance to INH and ETH (see below).

In summary, the current model for the mode of action of INH is as follows (Fig. 2). INH is a prodrug that requires activation by the *katG*-encoded catalase-peroxidase (KatG) (235). The active species, an isonicotinic acyl radical, attacks the nicotinamide group of NAD$^+$ to form a covalent INH-NAD adduct (172), which inhibits InhA, resulting in a blockage of FASII

activity. The blockage of FASII leads to accumulation of FASI end products. Unable to obtain mycolic acids required for the synthesis of the cell wall, the mycobacterial cells lyse.

Mechanisms of INH resistance

Loss of the *katG*-encoded catalase peroxidase. Middlebrook reported the isolation of spontaneous INH-resistant mutants of *M. tuberculosis* in the laboratory shortly after the discovery of the drug (129). Interestingly, he made the observation that INH-resistant isolates often lost catalase activity and also became attenuated for virulence in guinea pigs (128). The role of catalase in INH resistance remained unclear for many years, since not all INH-resistant strains lost catalase activity and since it was not known whether the loss of catalase was the cause of

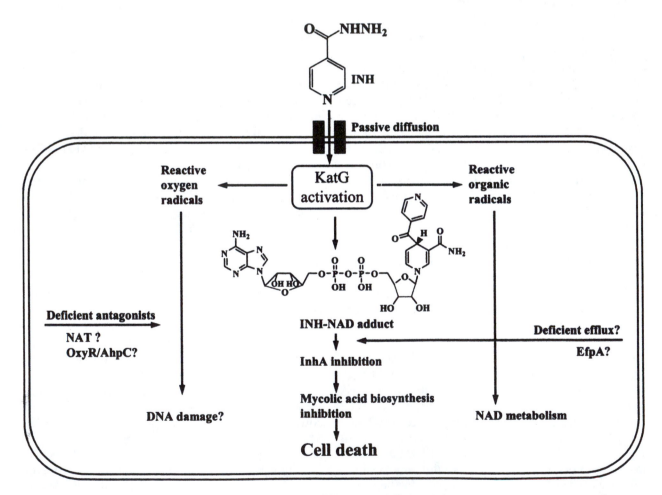

Figure 2. Mode of action of INH. INH enters tubercle bacilli by passive diffusion and is activated by KatG to a range of reactive species. These reactive species or radicals, which include both reactive oxygen species (hydrogen peroxide, superoxide, peroxynitrite, and hydroxyl radical) and organic radicals attack multiple targets, e.g., mycolic acid synthesis, DNA damage, and NAD metabolism in the cell. The isonicotinoyl acyl radical reacts with NAD$^+$ to form an INH-NAD adduct, which inhibits the enoyl-ACP reductase InhA of the FASII system. Inhibition of InhA results in mycolic acid biosynthesis inhibition and ultimately in cell lysis. Deficient efflux and insufficient antagonism of INH-derived radicals, such as a defective anti-oxidative defense, may underlie the unique susceptibility of *M. tuberculosis* to INH.

INH resistance or just an accompanying event. Winder hypothesized that the loss of catalase-peroxidase activity may indicate that the enzyme was an activator for INH (227). Later, Middlebrook's observation led to the cloning of the catalase-peroxidase gene (*katG*) and identification of *katG* mutations as the cause of INH resistance in *M. tuberculosis* by gene transfer (234, 235). Analysis of three INH-resistant strains in the original study (235) showed that *katG* deletions were found in two highly resistant strains. Subsequent studies have shown that *katG* point mutations are more frequent than deletions in INH-resistant strains (85). Restoration of INH susceptibility to KatG-defective, INH-resistant strains (with either *katG* deletion or point mutations) by transformation with a functional *katG* gene demonstrated that *katG* mutations caused INH resistance (234). Loss of KatG function due to mutations in *katG* reduces the ability of KatG to activate the prodrug INH, thus leading to INH resistance, and this represents a novel mechanism of drug resistance. Between 20 and 80% of INH-resistant *M. tuberculosis* strains contain a mutation in the *katG* gene, depending on the geographical region of the clinical isolates (1, 4, 69, 85, 86, 98, 138, 143, 144, 147, 158, 168, 169, 171, 203).

Among the various mutations in KatG, the S315T mutation is the most common, occurring in about 50 to 93% of INH-resistant clinical isolates carrying a *katG* mutation (1, 4, 11, 65, 68, 86, 113, 138, 158, 168, 171, 182). The KatG S315T mutation reduces the catalase and peroxidase activity by 50% (174, 218, 231) and is associated with relatively high levels of INH resistance (MIC, 5 to 10 µg/ml) (209). The S315T mutation affects the binding of INH to KatG, resulting in less activated INH (107, 217, 231). The KatG R463L substitution is found in *M. bovis*, *M. africanum*, and *M. microti* (54), but this enzyme is as capable at activating INH as is the wild-type KatG (82) and is generally considered to not contribute to INH resistance (85). The *katG* gene forms an operon with the upstream gene *furA* in various mycobacteria including *M. tuberculosis* (44, 153). FurA is a negative regulator of *katG*, and its removal causes overexpression of KatG and hypersensitivity to INH whereas overexpression of FurA reduces KatG expression (232). Mutations in *furA* may cause INH resistance through repression of KatG expression, but this has not been observed in INH-resistant strains. The *katG* gene is situated in a highly variable region of the genome (241) containing repetitive DNA, and this, in turn, may contribute to the high frequency of *katG* mutations in INH-resistant strains.

Overexpression or alterations in the INH target, InhA. When *inhA* was overexpressed from a multi-copy plasmid, the MIC of INH increased by 20- to 80-fold above the MICs of three independent *M. tuberculosis* strains (95). Mutations in INH-resistant clinical isolates of *M. tuberculosis* have been mapped to the promoter region and the *inhA* structural gene. These mutations occur in 15 to 43% of the INH-resistant *M. tuberculosis* strains and are usually associated with a low level of INH resistance (MIC, ≤1 µg/ml) (12, 14, 69, 85, 86, 98, 143–145, 158, 168, 171). A recent study, analyzing ETH-resistant *M. tuberculosis* isolates, revealed that 14 of 41 strains had promoter mutations in *inhA*, with no mutations in *katG* or *ethA* (142). All of these strains were coresistant to INH. These data are consistent with the premise that overexpression of *inhA* mediates coresistance to INH and ETH and that *inhA* encodes the target of INH and ETH.

In addition to overexpression of the InhA target, the same missense mutation, S94A, was found in the structural gene of *inhA* for an INH-resistant mutant of *M. smegmatis* and *M. bovis* (12). Allelic exchanges were performed with a kanamycin resistance gene linked to the *inhA* gene to prove that the S94A mutation was sufficient to mediate coresistance to INH and ETH. Interestingly, another recent study identified three clinical isolates of *M. tuberculosis* that possess the S94A mutation and all are coresistant to INH and ETH (142). In addition to this mutation, four independent I21T or I21V mutations in InhA were found, all of which confer coresistance to INH and ETH. Numerous additional studies have identified structural mutations in *inhA* as well (85, 86, 144, 168, 171, 182). Resistance to INH and ETH can be mediated by mutations that cause overexpression of *inhA* or cause alterations in the InhA protein.

Loss of NADH dehydrogenase II activity: a modulator of INH-NAD and ETH-NAD formation or binding. The NADH dehydrogenase type II gene, *ndh*, was shown to be involved in INH resistance by complementation of an INH-resistant, temperature-sensitive *M. smegmatis* mutant with a genomic library of *M. tuberculosis* (130). *ndh* mutations conferred coresistance to INH and ETH in *M. smegmatis* by lowering the rate of NADH oxidation. In a recent study, *ndh* mutations were detected in 8 (9.5%) of 84 INH-resistant *M. tuberculosis* clinical isolates, 7 of which had the same R268H mutation and 1 of which had the T110A mutation (98). The eight *M. tuberculosis* strains with *ndh* mutations were resistant to at least 0.1 µg of INH per ml, but the exact level of resistance was not reported. A more comprehensive study has been recently completed, demonstrating the analysis of 26 new *M. smegmatis* and *M. bovis* BCG *ndh* mutants. The mutations map over the entire length of the NdhII protein, and all result in diminished NdhII activity (C. Vilchèze, T. R. Weisbrod, B. Chen, L. Kremer, M. H. Hazbón, F. Wang, D. Alland, J. C. Sacchettini, and W. R. Jacobs, Jr., submitted for publication). Moreover, the measurement of NADH/NAD$^+$ ratios demonstrates a striking increase between the mutants and the parental strains. A recent study showed that an increased amount of NADH can protect InhA from the inhibition by the INH-NAD adduct (149) by either competing with the INH-NAD adduct for binding to the active site of InhA or promoting displacement of the INH-NAD adduct from InhA. Since all of the *ndh* strains are coresistant to INH and ETH, the data support the hypothesis that altered NADH/NAD$^+$ ratios would mediate resistance by competitively inhibiting the binding of the INH-NAD adduct. By analogy, the coresistance to both INH and ETH suggests the existence of an ETH-NAD inhibitor for InhA, although this remains to be demonstrated experimentally.

Another gene that also complemented the temperature sensitivity and INH resistance phenotype in *M. smegmatis ndh* mutants was *mdh*, which encodes a malate dehydrogenase (130). Mdh catalyzes the NADH-dependent interconversion of oxaloacetate and malate in the tricarboxylic acid cycle. Although *M. smegmatis* does not possess the *mdh* gene, it was postulated that Mdh allows the restoration of the Ndh enzymatic activity by combining with the *M. smegmatis* Mqo (malate:quinone oxidoreductase) enzyme (140). However, mutations in *mdh* have not yet been found in INH-resistant *M. tuberculosis* isolates.

Alterations and overexpression of KasA. Mdluli et al. first reported mutations in *kasA* in INH-resistant clinical isolates of *M. tuberculosis* but did not perform any gene transfer experiment to prove that these mutations confer the INH resistance phenotype (123). Subsequent studies have revealed that three of the four mutations in *kasA* reported by Mdluli et al. were found in INH-resistant as well as in INH-susceptible isolates (97, 168), suggesting that these mutations do not play any role in conferring INH resistance.

Slayden and Barry have reported that overexpression of *kasA* conferred low-level resistance to INH in *M. tuberculosis* (185). In addition, these studies showed that overexpressed *kasA* confers resistance to thiolactomycin, a drug which has been shown to inhibit both KasA and KasB in *M. bovis* BCG (89). In another study by Kremer et al., it was shown that while the overexpression of *kasA* did confer resistance to thiolactomycin, it did not increase resistance to INH in BCG (89). To address these discrepancies, the various *kasA* and *inhA* overexpression plasmids (89, 185) were transformed into *M. smegmatis, M. bovis*

BCG, and three different strains of *M. tuberculosis* and analyzed by four independent laboratories (95). The results consistently revealed that overexpression of *kasA* conferred no increased resistance to INH or ETH whereas overexpressed *InhA* increased resistance to INH and ETH by 20- to 80-fold (97). Further biochemical and structural studies are needed to elucidate the role of KasA in INH action and resistance.

Other genes potentially involved in INH resistance. Although most INH-resistant strains may be accounted for by mutations in the above genes, some catalase-positive low-level INH-resistant clinical isolates do not have mutations in *katG, inhA, ndh*, or *kasA* (86, 98, 158, 168, 203), indicating that additional, unknown genes may be involved in INH resistance. The *mdh* gene (130) and the INH-inducible genes with unknown functions identified in a microarray analysis (224) could be candidates. In fact, some of the genes identified by the array analysis have recently been shown to contain mutations in some INH-resistant clinical isolates (168), although the genetic transfer experiments that confirm their role in INH resistance remain to be performed. One candidate gene is the efflux protein EfpA, which was shown to be induced by INH (224). Although no mutation resulting in increased EfpA expression has yet been found to cause INH resistance, one recent study using sequential exposure of an INH-sensitive strain to increasing levels of INH seems to show induction of transient high-level resistance to INH through induction of a reserpine-sensitive efflux mechanism (212). In addition, the arylamine N-acetyltransferase (NAT) enzyme, which is present in humans as two isoforms, NAT1 and NAT2, and can acetylate arylamines and hydrazines and inactivate INH, could be a candidate. NAT homologs occur in *M. tuberculosis* and *M. smegmatis*, and the purified enzyme converts INH to N-acetyl-INH in vitro (155, 156, 207). Overexpression of *nat* from *M. tuberculosis* in *M. smegmatis* caused a three-fold increase in resistance to INH (155). An *M. smegmatis nat* knockout mutant had a slightly increased susceptibility to INH (156). Eighteen percent of clinical isolates of *M. tuberculosis* contained a single point mutation (G207R) in the *nat* gene (207). The NAT G207R mutation appeared to correlate with a very slight decrease in INH susceptibility, at 0.02 µg/ml in two strains that harbor the mutation compared with 0.005 µg/ml in the sensitive control strain H37Rv (207). It will be of interest to determine the level of *nat* gene expression and the intrinsic enzymatic activity of the NAT protein in *M. tuberculosis* in comparison with other less susceptible mycobacterial species, as well as to investigate the possibility that NAT overexpression due to promoter up-mutations might be involved in INH resistance in *M. tuberculosis*.

Rifampin

Mechanism of action

RIF is a broad-spectrum rifamycin derivative that interferes with RNA synthesis by binding to bacterial RNA polymerase, an oligomer consisting of a core enzyme, formed by four chains ($\alpha_2\beta\beta'$), that associates with the σ subunit to specifically initiate transcription from promoters. There is evidence positioning the RIF binding site shortly upstream of the catalytic center (146), in keeping with the model that RIF plugs the product exit channel (116). Analysis of RIF-resistant mutants has contributed to a more precise definition of a priming nucleotide site overlapping with a larger site holding the RNA product in the active center during elongation. RIF is active against growing tubercle bacilli and also stationary-phase bacilli with reduced metabolism. The activity against the latter bacterial population is thought to be important in shortening the duration of treatment (134).

Mechanism of resistance

In *M. tuberculosis*, resistance to RIF occurs at a frequency of 1 in 10^7 to 10^8 bacilli. As in other bacteria, mutations in a defined region of *rpoB* have been found in >95% of RIF-resistant clinical isolates of *M. tuberculosis* (204). Resistance to RIF in *M. leprae* follows the same mechanism (74). Although *rpoB* mutations have been found in RIF-resistant *M. avium* (222), many isolates from the *M. avium-intracellulare* complex present a significant level of natural resistance to RIF, probably due to decreased permeability (61, 79). The role of *rpoB* mutations in causing resistance has been confirmed by genetic transformation experiments (132, 221). Mutation in *rpoB* generally results in high-level resistance (MIC, >32 µg/ml) and cross-resistance to all rifamycins. However, specific mutations in codons 511, 516, 518, and 522 are associated with lower-level resistance to RIF and rifapentin but retained susceptibility to rifabutin and the new rifamycin KRM1648 (22, 137, 221). Low-level resistance (MIC, 4 µg/ml) has been associated with an L176F mutation in a separate region of RpoB (R. Rossau, W. Mijs, G. Jannes, K. de Smet, D. van Heuverswijn, H. Traore, and F. Portaels, *Abstr. 20th Annu. Conf. Eur. Soc. Mycobacteriol.*, abstr. OC27, 1999), corresponding to *E. coli* L146F, a codon mutated in 2% of RIF-resistant *E. coli* strains (81, 183). Ribosylation, a degradative mechanism of resistance to RIF, has been found in the rapidly growing mycobacteria such as *M. smegmatis, M. chelonae,*

M. flavescens, and *M. vaccae* (40, 163), but not in *M. tuberculosis.*

Pyrazinamide

PZA is an unconventional and paradoxical TB drug that has high in vivo activity but poor in vitro activity (236). The discovery of PZA followed independent observations made by Chorine and Huant, who found that nicotinamide had activity against mycobacteria in vivo in totally different settings (35, 78). This led to the subsequent discovery of not only PZA (108) but also INH (52). The nicotinamide activity on *M. tuberculosis* was rediscovered by McKenzie et al. at Lederle Laboratories (120), where analogs of nicotinamide were synthesized, and at Merck. PZA was found to be the most active agent (92, 108, 186). What is remarkable is that the screening was performed directly on infected mice without in vitro susceptibility testing. Luckily, with hindsight, it is now appreciated that if the screening had been performed first under normal culture conditions in vitro, PZA would never have been discovered. The discovery of PZA is a telling story that the current drug screening using growing bacteria under normal culture conditions has significant limitations. Not only was the discovery of PZA unconventional, but also its mode of action is unusual and has puzzled investigators for decades.

Despite its powerful in vivo sterilizing activity, as demonstrated by its ability to shorten chemotherapy both in animal models and in humans (13, 192), PZA has no activity in vitro under normal culture conditions (202), but is active only at acidic pH in vitro (119). Even then, PZA has a high MIC (50 to 100 µg/ml) at pH 5.5 to 6.0, and unlike other TB drugs (e.g., INH and RIF), PZA kills *M. tuberculosis* cells only slowly and incompletely over a period of 2 weeks (66). Unlike conventional antibiotics, which are active mainly against growing bacteria, PZA kills nongrowing tubercle bacilli more effectively than metabolically active growing bacilli (237). PZA can show bactericidal or bacteriostatic activity depending on the metabolic status of the tubercle bacilli, pH, and drug concentration (236). In vivo, PZA has an achievable peak concentration in serum of 30 µg/ml, which is lower than its MIC. The high in vivo activity but poor in vitro activity of PZA presumably reflects differences between these environments. Indeed, the discovery of the acid-pH requirement for PZA activity by McDermott and Tompsett in 1954 was based on this reasoning (119). We have recently found that the increased local iron concentrations during active inflammation and the hypoxic conditions present in granulomatous lesions enhance the activity of PZA (187, 212a), providing an additional explanation for the high in vivo activity and poor in vitro activity of PZA. The ability of PZA to shorten therapy is thought to be related to its bactericidal activity on a population of semidormant bacilli residing in an acidic environment (e.g., during inflammation) that are not effectively killed by other drugs (134). Besides acidic pH, various other factors such as metabolic status, age of the bacilli, albumin, inoculum size, and energy inhibitors (240) affect PZA activity (236, 237).

Mechanism of action

PZA is a prodrug that is converted to the active form, pyrazinoic acid (POA), by bacterial pyrazinamidase (PZase)/nicotinamidase (88, 181). Based on our recent studies (181, 238, 240, 242), we proposed the following model for the mode of action of PZA (Fig. 3): PZA enters the bacilli through passive diffusion and is converted into POA (a strong weak acid with pK_a of 2.9) by the cytoplasmic PZase. However, it is worth noting that PZA uptake and conversion to POA in *M. tuberculosis* are much slower than in the naturally resistant nontuberculous mycobacteria or *E. coli*, presumably due to higher PZase activity in other bacteria (238). POA is then excreted from the cell by passive diffusion and a weak efflux mechanism in *M. tuberculosis* (238). Once POA is outside the cell, if the extracellular pH is acidic, a small proportion of POA becomes the uncharged conjugate acid HPOA, which permeates through the membrane easily. However, acidic pH does not facilitate the uptake of PZA. The acid-facil-itated POA influx is stronger than the weak POA efflux, and this causes accumulation of POA in *M. tuberculosis* cells. The HPOA brings protons into the cell, and this could eventually cause cytoplasmic acidification, such that vital enzymes are inhibited, as a potential mechanism of POA action. In addition, HPOA could potentially deenergize the membrane by collapsing the proton motive force and affect membrane transport as a possible mechanism of POA action (239). At neutral or alkaline pH, little POA was found in the tubercle bacilli, because over 99.9% of POA was in the charged anionic form. This observation explains why PZA is active at acidic pH but not at neutral pH (202) and also explains the correlation between the MIC of PZA and low acid pH (175, 237). While the process of acid-facilitated uptake of a weak acid is nonspecific, the unique activity of PZA against *M. tuberculosis* appears to be related to a deficient POA efflux mechanism (238) that is unable to counteract the effect of acid-facilitated POA influx, which could lead to eventual acidification of the cytoplasm, deenergized membranes, and a generally poor ability to maintain membrane energetics, especially in nongrowing tubercle bacilli at acid pH. Indeed, we have recently obtained the following data that further support the above hypothesis (240, 242): (i) acidic pH decreases the membrane potential, and this is reduced further by POA; (ii) POA inhibits the transport of nutrients such as serine, methionine, and uracil in *M. tuberculosis* at acidic pH through disruption of the membrane potential; (iii) the activity of PZA or POA is significantly enhanced by energy in-

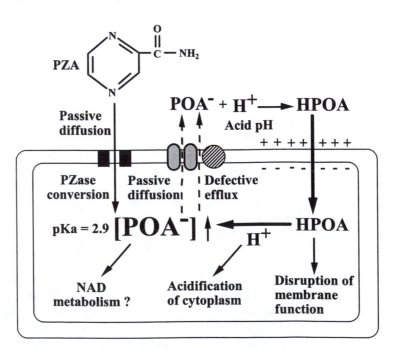

Figure 3. Mode of action of PZA.

hibitors such as DCCD (F1F0-ATPase inhibitor), rotenone (NADH dehydrogenase I-Complex I inhibitor), and azide (cytochrome *c* oxidase inhibitor) (240); (iv) PZA activity is significantly higher under hypoxic or anaerobic conditions than under atmospheric conditions with ambient oxygen (212a) (the preferential activity of PZA against tubercle bacilli under hypoxic conditions may result from low energy production); and (v) tubercle bacilli have a generally weak-acid-susceptible phenotype (240). Thus, the currently available data suggest that POA/PZA targets the membrane and affects membrane bioenergetics as a mechanism of action. In addition, this model explains best the various peculiar features of PZA, i.e., the requirement of acidic pH for activity, the preferential activity of PZA against old, nongrowing bacilli, and its higher activity under hypoxic conditions.

The target of PZA or POA has been suggested to be FASI in a study showing that PZA inhibits fatty acid biosynthesis in *M. tuberculosis* and from the finding that the multicopy *fas1* gene from *M. avium*, *M. bovis* BCG, or *M. tuberculosis* confers resistance to the PZA analog 5-chloropyrazinamide (5-Cl-PZA) in *M. smegmatis* (243). However, no mutations in FASI have been found in PZA-resistant *M. tuberculosis* strains. The proposition that FASI is the target of PZA in *M. tuberculosis* has recently been questioned. Boshoff et al. showed that while FASI is the target of 5-Cl-PZA, it is not the target of PZA (24). The available data do not support the presence of a specific cellular target for POA (239), although this possibility cannot be excluded. First, no POA-resistant mutants can be isolated (180). Furthermore, among clinical isolates of *M. tuberculosis* resistant to PZA, none are resistant to POA (Y. Zhang, unpublished data). However, it is unclear whether the inability to obtain a POA-resistant mutant is because the mutated target influences viability or because POA affects multiple cellular targets such that no specific mutant can be selected. Second, POA does not appear to bind to any cellular components in *M. tuberculosis* (Zhang, unpublished). Third, if there was a specific cellular target for POA, which is produced from PZA in the bacilli at both acidic pH and neutral pH (238), POA would have bound and shown an inhibitory effect even at neutral pH, which is not the case. The possibility remains that POA, as an analog of nicotinic acid, might be incorporated into NAD and affect NAD function, but preliminary results do not support this hypothesis (Zhang, unpublished).

Mechanism of resistance

M. tuberculosis strains are uniquely susceptible to PZA, which has an MIC of about 50 µg/ml at pH 5.5, whereas nontuberculous mycobacteria and other bacteria are intrinsically resistant to PZA; e.g., the MIC for *M. smegmatis* and *E. coli* is >2,000 µg/ml (23, 239). In *M. tuberculosis*, PZA susceptibility correlates with the presence of PZase activity. Like INH-resistant *M. tuberculosis* strains that lose catalase-peroxidase activity (128), *M. tuberculosis* strains lose PZase/nicotinamidase activity when they develop PZA resistance (88), and there is a good correlation between loss of PZase activity and PZA resistance (115, 133, 206). Defective PZase activity resulting from *pncA* mutations is the major mechanism for PZA resistance in *M. tuberculosis* (180), as confirmed by numerous other studies (71, 72, 77, 99, 102, 112, 127, 141, 154, 173, 189).

The *pncA* mutations identified are largely missense mutations causing amino acid substitutions and in some cases nucleotide insertions or deletions, nonsense mutations in the *pncA* structural gene, or nonsense mutations in the putative promoter region. A frequently occurring mutation at −11 (putative promoter region) was found in several studies (34, 99, 127, 154, 180, 189). The *pncA* mutations are highly diverse and are scattered along the gene with some degree of clustering that affects three regions (regions 3 to 17, 61 to 85, and 132 to 142) of the PncA protein (102, 180) that are likely to contain catalytic sites. The crystal structure of the *Pyrococcus horikoshii* PncA (37% identity to *M. tuberculosis* PncA) has provided some structural basis for understanding the *pncA* mutations in *M. tuberculosis* that cause PZA resistance (46), since the three regions where they cluster correspond to three of the four loops that contribute to the scaffold of the active site. Mutations at C138, D8, K96, D49, H51, and H71 modify the active-site triad and metal binding site. Residues F13, L19, H57 (position of the characteristic mutation of H57D in *M. bovis*), W68, G97, Y103, I113, A134, and H137 line the active site, and mutations at these positions are also predicted to cause loss of enzyme activity. Mutations at Q10, D12, S104, and T142 are predicted to disrupt the hydrogen-bonding interactions between the side-chain and main-chain atoms. Loss of PZase activity due to mutations at other sites can be attributed to potential perturbation of the active site or disruption of the protein core (46). These predictions need to be confirmed when the structure of the *M. tuberculosis* PncA is determined. The diverse nature of *pncA* mutations is unique to the PZA resis-tance, and other drug resistance genes usually do not show this degree of diversity. Although the basis for this is unclear, it is likely that since *pncA* is not an essential gene in *M. tuberculosis* (34), there is no selective pressure such that mutations can be tolerated anywhere in *pncA*.

Although most PZA-resistant *M. tuberculosis* strains have mutations in *pncA* (34, 180), there are some resistant strains that do not, and these include PZase-negative strains (34, 102, 112) with a high level of resistance. This indicates that mutations in an undefined *pncA* regulatory gene may be involved in PZA resistance. Another type of such strain has low-level resistance and positive PZase activity, presumably due to an alternative mechanism of resistance.

While acquired PZA resistance in susceptible *M. tuberculosis* is due to *pncA* mutations, the natural PZA resistance in other mycobacteria or bacteria is not due to *pncA* mutations, with the exception of *M. bovis,* a member of the *M. tuberculosis* complex. Strains of *M. bovis* including BCG are known to be naturally resistant to PZA and lack PZase, and these features are commonly used to distinguish *M. bovis* from *M. tuberculosis.* The natural PZA resistance in *M. bovis* and BCG is due to a single point mutation of C to G at nucleotide position 169 of the *pncA* gene, causing amino acid substitution H57D (181). This single point mutation is the cause of the defective PZase activity and natural resistance to PZA in *M. bovis* and BCG and can be a useful marker for rapid differentiation of *M. bovis* from *M. tuberculosis* (179). Thus, *M. bovis* can be considered a special case of PZA-resistant *M. tuberculosis.* In a similar manner, as a result of PZase activity being affected, *M. kansasii,* which is naturally resistant to PZA (MIC, 250 µg/ml), also has very weak PZase activity with positive nicotin-amidase activity (67). The natural PZA resistance in *M. kansasii* is due to reduced PZase activity, as shown by transformation studies with the *pncA* gene from *M. tuberculosis* or *M. avium* (193). However, the correlation between PZase activity and PZA susceptibility is not true for other naturally PZA-resistant mycobacterial species. For example, we have found that the natural PZA resistance in *M. smegmatis* is not due to defective PZase activity. On the contrary, *M. smegmatis* has two highly active PZase enzymes, PzaA (23) and PncA (63), and yet, it is highly resistant to PZA (MIC, >2,000 µg/ml) at acid pH (5.5) due to a highly active POA efflux mechanism. This efflux mechanism is also likely to be the cause of the intrinsic PZA resistance in many other bacterial species such as *M. avium, M. vaccae,* and *E. coli* (193, 238). In contrast, *M. tuberculosis* has a weak or deficient POA efflux mechanism as an underlying mechanism of its unique susceptibility to PZA and POA (238).

Ethambutol

Mechanism of action

EMB [(*S,S'*)-2,2′-(ethylenediimino)-di-1-butanol] inhibits the biosynthesis of arabinogalactan, the major polysaccharide of the mycobacterial cell wall (195). EMB interferes with the polymerization of cell wall arabinan of arabinogalactan and of lipo-arabinomannan (131) and induces the accumulation of β-D-arabinofuranosyl-*P*-decaprenol, an intermediate in arabinan biosynthesis (100, 229). Arabinosyl-transferase, an enzyme involved in the synthesis of arabinogalactan, has been proposed as the target of EMB (17). The enzyme is encoded by *embB,* which is part of an operon comprising the *embA* and *embB* genes in *M. avium* (17) and the *embC, embA,* and *embB* genes in other mycobacteria such as *M. smegmatis* (7, 205). The Emb proteins are about 65% identical to each other and are predicted to be integral membrane proteins with 12 transmembrane-spanning domains (205). However, the precise mechanism of how EMB inhibits EmbB is not known.

Mechanism of resistance

Mutations in the *embCAB* operon were identified in up to 65% of EMB-resistant clinical isolates of *M. tuberculosis.* Mutations at codon 306 of *embB* occur most frequently (167, 190, 205), but mutations at amino acid residues Asp328, Gly406, and Glu497 are also found (167, 190). The codon 306 region is highly conserved among the various Emb proteins and among different mycobacteria (7, 103, 205), although the EMB-resistant *M. leprae, M. chelonae,* and *M. abscessus* display variant amino acids at this position. Genetic transfer experiments involving these *emb* alleles supported the role of this region in determining natural resistance to EMB (7). However, a recent study from Russia has found that EmbB306 mutations were detected not only in 48.3% of EMB-resistant strains but also in 31.2% of EMB-susceptible strains (139), raising some doubts about the significance of *embB* mutations in EMB resistance. Additional mutations in the *embC-embA* intergenic region have been found in strains that also had resistance-associated amino acid substitutions in EmbA or EmbB (167), and these may play a secondary or compensatory role in resistance. An *embR* homologue, which is located 2 Mb from the *embCAB* locus in *M. tuberculosis* rather than immediately upstream of the *embAB* genes in *M. avium,* has recently been shown to contain mutations (a Q379R replacement and an A insertion at position 137 upstream of the *embR* start codon) associated with EMB resistance in *M. tuberculosis* (167). A mutation 24 bp upstream of the start codon of the *Rv0340* gene, which precedes the INH and EMB-inducible *iniBAC* operon (8), was associated with EMB resistance (167). Mutations in *rmlD* (S257P and T284L, or a G-to-T nucleotide change at position 71) and *rmlA2* (D152N), both of which are involved in modification of rhamnose, were found to be associated with EMB resistance (167). Despite more new genes being identified as involved in EMB resistance, about 24% of EMB-resistant *M. tuberculosis* strains do not have mutations in any of the genes described above (167). Further genetic and biochemical studies are needed to confirm the role of the above genes in EMB resistance.

Streptomycin

Mechanism of action

SM is an aminoglycoside antibiotic that primarily interferes with protein synthesis but has some other effects such as damage to the cell membrane (9), inhibition of respiration, and stimulation of RNA synthesis (55). In addition, SM can cause misreading or miscoding of the genetic code (41). The site of action of SM is the 30S subunit of the ribosome, specifically at ribosomal protein S12 and the 16S rRNA (57). In *E. coli*, SM binds the bases between positions 903 and 910 of 16S rRNA and interferes with protein S12 in the translation process (136). The knowledge of how SM kills bacteria is derived largely from numerous studies carried out primarily with *E. coli*. The mode of action of SM in *M. tuberculosis* is presumed to be the same as in *E. coli*, as shown by the presence of mutations in the same target, i.e., ribosomal S12 protein (encoded by *rpsL*) and 16S rRNA (encoded by *rrs*).

Mechanism of resistance

M. tuberculosis becomes resistant by mutating the target of SM in the ribosome. The principal site of mutation is the *rpsL* gene, encoding ribosomal protein S12 (51, 75, 84, 148, 188). As in *E. coli*, residues 42 and 88 are the most important in the development of SM resistance. In mycobacteria, rates of selection for potentially nonrestrictive and restrictive mutations may vary from in vitro to in vivo circumstances. While restrictive mutations are selected in vitro at rates similar to that for the nonrestrictive K42R, they are rarely observed in vivo (26). This suggests that such mutants are under a strong negative pressure and that compensatory mutations fail to retain those mutants in the global pool. A second mechanism of resistance in *M. tuberculosis* is in *rrs*, the gene encoding 16S rRNA. While most bacteria have multiple copies of *rrs*, *M. tuberculosis* and other slow-growing mycobacteria have a single copy whereas rapidly growing mycobacteria have two copies (25). Mutation in the loops of 16S rRNA, the highly conserved 530 loop and on the adjacent 915 region (51), that interact with the S12 protein constitute an easily se-

lected resistance site. An SM-dependent mutant of *M. tuberculosis* contained an insertion of cytosine in the 530 loop as a likely cause of its SM dependence (76). A previously described nucleotide change at position 491 of the *rrs* gene, in two clinical isolates resistant to SM (125, 188), is a polymorphism that is not associated with SM resistance (210).

Mutations in *rpsL* and *rrs* structures are identified in 50 and 20% of SM-resistant clinical isolates, respectively, and result in intermediate (MICs, 64 to 512 µg/ml) or high-level (MICs, >1,000 µg/ml) resistance. A third mechanism accounting for low-level resistance (MICs, 4 to 32 µg/ml) remains unidentified, but it may involve changes in drug uptake (38). Genes for aminoglycoside-modifying enzymes are present in the chromosome of *M. tuberculosis* and other mycobacteria (5, 37), but their role in resistance is not clear. The expression of the aminoglycoside 2'-N-acetyltransferase *aac(2')-Ic* and *aac(2')-Id* genes in *M. smegmatis* has been studied, and only *aac(2')-Id* is correlated with aminoglycoside resistance (5).

Resistance to Other Drugs

Studies with other bacteria (50) have shown the presence of quinolone resistance mutations in (i) the DNA gyrase (composed of subunits GyrA and GyrB), (ii) topoisomerase IV, and (iii) the cell membrane proteins that regulate the intracellular concentration of the drug by mediating drug permeability and efflux. Stepwise accumulation of mutations in several of these genes can result in high levels of resistance. In *M. tuberculosis*, *gyrA* mutations cause resistance to ciprofloxacin (200) and cross-resistance to other fluoroquinolones (e.g., ofloxacin) (32). Amino acid sequences in GyrA may determine the level of susceptibility to quinolones (62). Although recognized as contributing to resistance in *E. coli*, mutations in *gyrB* have been identified only in laboratory mutants of *M. tuberculosis* (87). Interestingly, the genome of *M. tuberculosis* does not contain a definitive topoisomerase IV homologue (ParC or GrlA) (37), which causes quinolone resistance when mutated in other bacteria. Although the efflux pump, LfrA, confers low-level quinolone resistance in *M. smegmatis* (106, 199), such a mechanism has not been demonstrated to cause quinolone resistance in *M. tuberculosis*.

Kanamycin and capreomycin, like SM, inhibit protein synthesis through modification of ribosomal structures at the 16S rRNA. Mutations at *rrs* position 1400 are associated with high-level resistance to kanamycin and amikacin (6, 194, 201). Cross-resistance may be observed between kanamycin and capreomycin or viomycin (6, 194, 201).

The mechanism of resistance to PAS is unknown. Interference with folic acid biosynthesis and inhibition of iron uptake have been proposed as two possible mechanisms of action for PAS (227).

ETH is also a prodrug and inhibits mycolic acid biosynthesis. Mutations in *inhA* confer cross-resistance to INH and ETH (12, 142). Two independent studies identified a gene, *etaA* (42), also called *ethA* (15), which encodes an enzyme involved in activation of ETH. EtaA is an FAD-containing enzyme that oxidizes ETH to the corresponding S oxide, which is further oxidized to 2-ethyl-4-amidopyridine, presumably via the unstable oxidized sulfinic acid intermediate (208). This flavoenzyme also oxidizes thiacetazone, thiobenzamide, isothionicotinamide, and probably other thioamide drugs (208). Mutations in EtaA were found in all MDR-TB strains examined, and these strains displayed cross-resistance to thiocarbonyl-containing drugs including thiacetazone and thiocarlide (42). A more recent study of ETH-resistant *M. tuberculosis* clinical isolates showed that 95% of the strains were also INH resistant and that the ETH-resistant and INH-resistant phenotypes in 51% of the strains were due solely to mutations in the *inhA* gene and/or its promoter region whereas mutations in *ethA* were found in 37% of the strains (142).

Cycloserine inhibits the synthesis of peptidoglycan by blocking the action of D-alanine racemase and D-alanine:alanine synthase. The D-alanine racemase enzyme, encoded by *alrA*, has been cloned from *M. smegmatis*, and its expression from a multicopy vector in *M. smegmatis* or *M. bovis* BCG results in resistance to D-cycloserine (31). Inactivation of *alrA* in *M. smegmatis* caused increased sensitivity to D-cycloserine (33). In a recent study, mutation in an open reading frame with homology to the *E. coli* penicillin binding protein 4 (PBP4) gene was found to cause D-cycloserine resistance in *M. smegmatis* (157). However, the genetic basis of cycloserine resistance in *M. tuberculosis* remains to be identified.

FITNESS AND VIRULENCE OF DRUG-RESISTANT ORGANISMS

Different fitness phenotypes of *M. tuberculosis*, as manifested in differences in replication kinetics, mutation rate, and infectivity, may translate into differences in virulence in vivo. The issue of diminished fitness in the presence of resistance mutations needs to be examined carefully because of the different degree of fitness or virulence even among drug-susceptible strains. Use of isogenic strains is essential in addressing the virulence of drug-resistant organisms in experimental-animal models of infection. However, this issue is even more complex in human infections, due to differences in both bacterial and host factors. The W-Beijing family strains are associated predominantly with the MDR phenotype, which prompted speculation that these strains may have a higher frequency of mutations (10, 91). Mutations were found in the putative mutator genes (*mutT2* and *Rv3908*) in some W-Beijing families of *M. tuberculosis* strains, which could potentially cause increased mutation frequency and better adaptability to stress conditions, leading to increased spread of such strains (166). However, in a separate study, drug-susceptible W-Beijing strains of *M. tuberculosis* were no more prone to develop RIF resistance than were non-W-Beijing strains (219). It would be of interest to determine if the mutator mutations contribute to a more fit in vivo phenotype and higher frequency of developing drug resistance in W-Beijing family strains. Future studies using isogenic mutator strains and genetic complementation are required to address these issues.

Resistance to INH is probably the only case where acquisition of drug resistance has been shown to affect the virulence of the bacilli. It is well known that INH-resistant strains often lose not only catalase activity but also virulence for guinea pigs (128). There is generally a good correlation between loss of catalase activity and attenuation of virulence in guinea pigs and the level of INH resistance (126, 227). Attenuation of virulence in INH-resistant, catalase-deficient strains is less easily demonstrated in the mouse model. With the identification of *katG*, encoding catalase-peroxidase (235), it was shown that reintroducing the *katG* gene restored not only INH susceptibility but also virulence for INH-resistant, catalase-deficient strains in a guinea pig model (105, 226). If a particular mutation in *katG* eliminates catalase-peroxidase activity, the mutation is expected to attenuate virulence. In contrast, if some enzyme activity is retained, it would still be virulent to some degree. For instance, an INH-resistant strain containing the frequently occurring S315T KatG mutation still produced active catalase-peroxidase and was virulent in the mouse model (162), whereas the P275T KatG mutation, which completely eliminates catalase-peroxidase activity, was not (162). In a recent study in Holland, INH-resistant strains with the S315T KatG mutation were found to cause secondary TB cases as often as INH-susceptible organisms did (209). The mechanism of INH resistance could influence the virulence of the organisms. INH-resistant strains with mutations in genes other than *katG*, such as *inhA* or *ndh*, are expected still to be fully virulent. For example, in a study with isogenic strains of *M. bovis,* loss of virulence for guinea pigs was associated with loss of KatG activity but not with mutations in *inhA* (226). While mutation in the promoter region of *ahpC,* leading to overexpression of AhpC, is important for restoring peroxide homeostasis in the KatG-deficient organism, it does not appear to contribute to increased virulence in mice (70). However, blocking the expression of AhpC by using the antisense-RNA strategy appeared to attenuate the virulence of *M. bovis* in the guinea pig model (225). This discrepancy could be due to the different animal models used.

Resistance to other TB drugs is usually not associated with loss of virulence for *M. tuberculosis* isolates. We have found active transmission of TB due to PZase-negative, PZA-monoresistant strains exhibiting the same characteristic *pncA* mutation (an 8-bp deletion and an R140S mutation) and almost identical IS*6110* profile in Quebec, Canada (34). Mutations in RpoB could modify the enzymatic activity and the fitness of *M. tuberculosis* in vitro (20). Competitive coculturing of a parental strain of *M. tuberculosis* with various isogenic *rpoB* mutants identified various patterns of mutation-specific loss of replicative fitness in culture, but results of in vivo studies are not yet available. The S351L mutation, the most prevalent substitution in RIF-resistant isolates, conferred the smallest reduction of replication efficiency in vitro, whereas bacilli with the less frequently encountered mutations H526Y, H526D, and H526R, displayed a more profound diminution of fitness. Analysis of SM-resistant *M. tuberculosis* clinical isolates suggests that the nonrestrictive (more fit) *rpsL* mutation, K42R, is much more prevalent than the restrictive mutations found in SM-resistant mutants in vitro (26). There is a need for molecular epidemiology studies that combine precise genetic characterization of drug-resistant strains and strain typing to investigate the issues of fitness and virulence of MDR-TB organisms. At present, most MDR-TB outbreaks have involved HIV-positive individuals. A real concern is that specific MDR-TB clones would become epidemic in the general population. The particularly successful strain W (Beijing family), which caused the MDR-TB outbreak in New York City and spread across the United States and abroad (3), is capable of causing active transmission of the disease in HIV-positive individuals. It is worth noting that strain W, which is resistant to INH (containing the common *katG* mutation S315T), still retains some catalase activity (19). It is likely that defective immune responses during HIV infection may underlie the transmission of the disease caused by this strain, which may be less easily transmitted in healthy individuals.

PHENOTYPIC RESISTANCE

Resistance in Stationary-Phase, Persistent, and Dormant Bacilli

Antibiotics usually act against actively growing bacteria but not against nongrowing forms. The lack of susceptibility of the nongrowing bacteria to antibiotics is due to changes in bacterial metabolism or physiological state and is therefore called phenotypic resistance. It is well known that when bacteria grow into the stationary phase they become nonsusceptible or phenotypically resistant to many antibiotics even though the bacteria are fully viable. Another type of phenotypic resistance, or drug tolerance, relates to the phenomenon of "persisters," a small number of surviving bacteria, from actively growing cultures, that are not killed after exposure to antibiotics. This is why the MIC is commonly defined as the lowest concentration of antibiotic that kills 99% of bacterial populations but never 100%. It remains to be determined if the very observation of persisters in the presence of antibiotics in vitro underlies mycobacterial persistence in vivo.

Phenotypic resistance is a major problem for antibiotic therapy, especially for TB. Nongrowing bacteria can be divided roughly into two different types depending on whether they grow immediately on subculture into a defined fresh medium. The nongrowing forms are a constant source of confusion for people who study bacterial persistence or dormancy. This confusion stems largely from the fact that very little is known about bacterial life-styles (especially those of the nongrowing bacteria), the definition of dormancy, and the definition of viability and death. It also stems partly from semantics. The term "persistent bacilli" often refers to in vivo-derived bacteria, and these can be either colony-forming or non-colony-forming bacteria, whereas "dormant bacilli" refers to bacteria that do not grow immediately on plates but can be resuscitated under certain specific conditions in liquid medium (with or without "resuscitation factors") to grow on plates. Despite this distinction, both persistent and dormant bacilli are phenotypically resistant to antibiotics.

The presence of dormant tubercle bacilli is best demonstrated in the Cornell mouse model (117), where mice infected with *M. tuberculosis* were treated with INH and PZA for 3 months. At the end of treatment, no bacilli could be demonstrated in the infected organs by colony formation on agar plates. However, 3 months after cessation of the chemotherapy, one-third of the mice relapsed with TB, and almost all mice relapsed if immunosuppressant steroids were given. The bacilli recovered from the relapsed mice were fully susceptible to INH or PZA, indicating that the dormant bacilli did not develop stable genetic drug resistance but were phenotypically resistant. These findings suggest that dormant bacilli present in the tissues were not dead, even though they failed to form colonies. The presence of persistent and dormant TB bacteria is one of the reasons for the lengthy duration of TB chemotherapy, since the current drugs are not effective in eliminating persistent or dormant bacilli. There has been considerable interest in the study of mycobacterial persistence and dormancy in recent years (59), with the aim of better understanding the mechanism behind this phenomenon and of devising therapeutic strategies targeting the persistent or dormant organisms.

Salicylate-Induced Resistance

Salicylate was first described to induce a multiple antibiotic resistance (Mar) phenotype in E. coli (170), and is now known to induce antibiotic resistance in a variety of bacteria (161). We have recently shown that salicylate also induces resistance to multiple antituberculosis drugs in vitro for both avirulent strain M. tuberculosis H37Ra and virulent strain M. tuberculosis H37Rv (177). In the presence of salicylate, the killing effect of INH, RIF, EMB, SM, and PAS was reduced, and when salicylate and the anti-TB agents were incorporated into plates, salicylate-induced resistance was more pronounced for PAS, SM, and EMB but was not apparent for INH and RIF. The decreased killing of bacteria by antibiotics, which causes an increased number of survivors in the presence of salicylate, has been shown to facilitate the emergence of genetically drug-resistant mutants of Staphylococcus aureus (64). It remains to be determined if salicylate could facilitate the emergence of drug-resistant M. tuberculosis mutants.

In E. coli, salicylate induces antibiotic resistance by binding to MarR and activating the transcription of marA and marB. MarAB regulates a range of genes to confer a Mar phenotype, including down-regulation of the OmpF porin expression via micF antisense RNA to limit the entry of antibiotics (36, 43) and switching on efflux pumps such as AcrAB to more effectively extrude antibiotics from the cells (152). In addition, salicylate induces antibiotic resistance through a Mar-independent pathway in E. coli, since a Mar deletion strain still showed resistance in the presence of salicylate (36). The mechanism of the salicylate-induced resistance in M. tuberculosis is unknown, although the bacillus may have a Mar-like regulatory mechanism, as in E. coli. Overexpression of E. coli marA on a multicopy plasmid in the fast-growing M. smegmatis mediates resistance to multiple antimycobacterial agents, indicating the presence of a mar-like regulatory system in this organism (118). However, this experiment has not been performed with M. tuberculosis. A MarA homolog (Rv1931) was reported to be present in the M. tuberculosis genome; however, the degree of similarity is quite low (118). Preliminary studies showed that the Rv1931 mRNA was not induced by salicylate (Zhang, unpublished), indicating that Rv1931 is unlikely to be responsible for the salicylate-induced drug resistance in M. tuberculosis. On the other hand, salicylate may reduce the permeability of the mycobacterial cell membrane as a mechanism for drug resistance in M. tuberculosis. A preliminary study using ^{14}C-labeled INH has suggested that the uptake of INH by M. tuberculosis H37Ra was reduced in the presence of salicylate (Zhang, unpublished). The possibility of involvement of efflux pumps in the salicylate-induced resistance in M. tuberculosis remains to be tested, and further studies are needed. Since salicylate is widely used in the prevention and treatment of diverse disease conditions at concentrations (159) that are known to induce resistance to various drugs in M. tuberculosis in vitro, it will be of interest to determine the effect of salicylate on the treatment of TB in animal models.

Acknowledgments. Y. Z. acknowledges support by NIH grants AI44063 and AI49485. W.R.J. acknowledges support by NIH grants AI43268 and AI26170.

REFERENCES

1. **Abal, A. T., S. Ahmad, and E. Mokaddas.** 2002. Variations in the occurrence of the S315T mutation within the katG gene in isoniazid-resistant clinical Mycobacterium tuberculosis isolates from Kuwait. Microb. Drug Resist. 8:99–105.
2. **Abraham, E. P., and E. Chain.** 1940. An enzyme from bacteria able to destroy penicillin. Nature 146:837.
3. **Agerton, T. B., S. E. Valway, R. J. Blinkhorn, K. L. Shilkret, R. Reves, W. W. Schluter, B. Gore, C. J. Pozsik, B. B. Plikaytis, C. Woodley, and I. M. Onorato.** 1999. Spread of strain W, a highly drug-resistant strain of Mycobacterium tuberculosis, across the United States. Clin. Infect. Dis. 29:85–95.
4. **Ahmad, S., E. Fares, G. F. Araj, T. D. Chugh, and A. S. Mustafa.** 2002. Prevalence of S315T mutation within the katG gene in isoniazid-resistant clinical Mycobacterium tuberculosis isolates from Dubai and Beirut. Int J. Tuberc. Lung Dis. 6:920–926.
5. **Ainsa, J. A., E. Perez, V. Pelicic, F. X. Berthet, B. Gicquel, and C. Martin.** 1997. Aminoglycoside 2'-N-acetyltransferase genes are universally present in mycobacteria: characterization of the aac(2')-Ic gene from Mycobacterium tuberculosis and the aac(2')-Id gene from Mycobacterium smegmatis. Mol. Microbiol. 24:431–441.
6. **Alangaden, G. J., B. N. Kreiswirth, A. Aouad, M. Khetarpal, F. R. Igno, S. L. Moghazeh, E. K. Manavathu, and S. A. Lerner.** 1998. Mechanism of resistance to amikacin and kanamycin in Mycobacterium tuberculosis. Antimicrob. Agents Chemother. 42:1295–1297.

7. Alcaide, F., G. E. Pfyffer, and A. Telenti. 1997. Role of *embB* in natural and acquired resistance to ethambutol in mycobacteria. *Antimicrob. Agents Chemother.* **41:**2270–2273.

8. Alland, D., I. Kramnik, T. R. Weisbrod, L. Otsubo, R. Cerny, L. P. Miller, W. R. Jacobs, Jr., and B. R. Bloom. 1998. Identification of differentially expressed mRNA in prokaryotic organisms by customized amplification libraries (DECAL): the effect of isoniazid on gene expression in *Mycobacterium tuberculosis. Proc. Natl. Acad. Sci. USA* **95:**13227–13232.

9. Anand, N., and B. D. Davis. 1960. Effect of streptomycin on *Escherichia coli. Nature* **185:**22–23.

10. Anh, D. D., M. W. Borgdorff, L. N. Van, N. T. Lan, T. van Gorkom, K. Kremer, and D. van Soolingen. 2000. *Mycobacterium tuberculosis* Beijing genotype emerging in Vietnam. *Emerg. Infect. Dis.* **6:**302–305.

11. Bakonyte, D., A. Baranauskaite, J. Cicenaite, A. Sosnovskaja, and P. Stakenas. 2003. Molecular characterization of isoniazid-resistant *Mycobacterium tuberculosis* clinical isolates in Lithuania. *Antimicrob. Agents Chemother.* **47:**2009–2011.

12. Banerjee, A., E. Dubnau, A. Quemard, V. Balasubramanian, K. S. Um, T. Wilson, D. Collins, G. de Lisle, and W. R. Jacobs, Jr. 1994. *inhA*, a gene encoding a target for isoniazid and ethionamide in *Mycobacterium tuberculosis. Science* **263:**227–230.

13. Bass, J. B., Jr., L. S. Farer, P. C. Hopewell, R. O'Brien, R. F. Jacobs, F. Ruben, D. E. Snider, Jr., and G. Thornton. 1994. Treatment of tuberculosis and tuberculosis infection in adults and children. American Thoracic Society and The Centers for Disease Control and Prevention. *Am. J. Respir. Crit. Care Med.* **149:**1359–1374.

14. Basso, L. A., R. Zheng, J. M. Musser, W. R. Jacobs, Jr., and J. S. Blanchard. 1998. Mechanisms of isoniazid resistance in *Mycobacterium tuberculosis*: enzymatic characterization of enoyl reductase mutants identified in isoniazid-resistant clinical isolates. *J. Infect. Dis.* **178:**769–775.

15. Baulard, A. R., J. C. Betts, J. Engohang-Ndong, S. Quan, R. A. McAdam, P. J. Brennan, C. Locht, and G. S. Besra. 2000. Activation of the pro-drug ethionamide is regulated in mycobacteria. *J. Biol. Chem.* **275:**28326–28331.

16. Bekierkunst, A. 1966. Nicotinamide-adenine dinucleotide in tubercle bacilli exposed to isoniazid. *Science* **152:**525–526.

17. Belanger, A. E., G. S. Besra, M. E. Ford, K. Mikusova, J. T. Belisle, P. J. Brennan, and J. M. Inamine. 1996. The *embAB* genes of *Mycobacterium avium* encode an arabinosyl transferase involved in cell wall arabinan biosynthesis that is the target for the antimycobacterial drug ethambutol. *Proc. Natl. Acad. Sci. USA* **93:**11919–11924.

18. Bernstein, J. W., A. Lott, B. A. Steinberg, and H. L. Yale. 1952. Chemotherapy of experimental tuberculosis. *Am. Rev. Tuberc.* **65:**357–374.

19. Bifani, P. J., B. B. Plikaytis, V. Kapur, K. Stockbauer, X. Pan, M. L. Lutfey, S. L. Moghazeh, W. Eisner, T. M. Daniel, M. H. Kaplan, J. T. Crawford, J. M. Musser, and B. N. Kreiswirth. 1996. Origin and interstate spread of a New York City multidrug-resistant *Mycobacterium tuberculosis* clone family. *JAMA* **275:**452–457.

20. Billington, O. J., T. D. McHugh, and S. H. Gillespie. 1999. Physiological cost of rifampin resistance induced in vitro in *Mycobacterium tuberculosis. Antimicrob. Agents Chemother.* **43:**1866–1869.

21. Bloch, K. 1977. Control mechanisms for fatty acid synthesis in *Mycobacterium smegmatis. Adv. Enzymol. Relat. Areas Mol. Biol.* **45:**1–84.

22. Bodmer, T., G. Zurcher, P. Imboden, and A. Telenti. 1995. Mutation position and type of substitution in the beta-subunit of the RNA polymerase influence in-vitro activity of rifamycins in rifampicin-resistant *Mycobacterium tuberculosis. J. Antimicrob. Chemother.* **35:**345–348.

23. Boshoff, H. I., and V. Mizrahi. 1998. Purification, gene cloning, targeted knockout, overexpression, and biochemical characterization of the major pyrazinamidase from *Mycobacterium smegmatis. J. Bacteriol.* **180:**5809–5814.

24. Boshoff, H. I., V. Mizrahi, and C. E. Barry, III. 2002. Effects of pyrazinamide on fatty acid synthesis by whole mycobacterial cells and purified fatty acid synthase I. *J. Bacteriol.* **184:**2167–2172.

25. Bottger, E. C. 1994. Resistance to drugs targeting protein synthesis in mycobacteria. *Trends Microbiol.* **2:**416–421.

26. Bottger, E. C., B. Springer, M. Pletschette, and P. Sander. 1998. Fitness of antibiotic-resistant microorganisms and compensatory mutations. *Nat. Med.* **4:**1343–1344.

27. Brennan, P. J., and H. Nikaido. 1995. The envelope of mycobacteria. *Annu. Rev. Biochem.* **64:**29–63.

28. Brindley, D. N., S. Matsumura, and K. Bloch. 1969. *Mycobacterium phlei* fatty acid synthase—a bacterial multienzyme complex. *Nature* **224:**666–669.

29. Broussy, S., Y. Coppel, M. Nguyen, J. Bernadou, and B. Meunier. 2003. ^{1}H and ^{13}C NMR characterization of hemiamidal isoniazid-NAD(H) adducts as possible inhibitors of InhA reductase of *Mycobacterium tuberculosis. Chemistry* **9:**2034–2038.

30. Bulatovic, V. M., N. L. Wengenack, J. R. Uhl, L. Hall, G. D. Roberts, F. R. Cockerill, III, and F. Rusnak. 2002. Oxidative stress increases susceptibility of *Mycobacterium tuberculosis* to isoniazid. *Antimicrob. Agents Chemother.* **46:**2765–2771.

31. Caceres, N. E., N. B. Harris, J. F. Wellehan, Z. Feng, V. Kapur, and R. G. Barletta. 1997. Overexpression of the D-alanine racemase gene confers resistance to D-cycloserine in *Mycobacterium smegmatis. J. Bacteriol.* **179:**5046–5055.

32. Cambau, E., W. Sougakoff, M. Besson, C. Truffot-Pernot, J. Grosset, and V. Jarlier. 1994. Selection of a *gyrA* mutant of *Mycobacterium tuberculosis* resistant to fluoroquinolones during treatment with ofloxacin. *J. Infect. Dis.* **170:**1351.

33. Chacon, O., Z. Feng, N. B. Harris, N. E. Caceres, L. G. Adams, and R. G. Barletta. 2002. *Mycobacterium smegmatis* D-alanine racemase mutants are not dependent on D-alanine for growth. *Antimicrob. Agents Chemother.* **46:**47–54.

34. Cheng, S. J., L. Thibert, T. Sanchez, L. Heifets, and Y. Zhang. 2000. *pncA* mutations as a major mechanism of pyrazinamide resistance in *Mycobacterium tuberculosis*: spread of a monoresistant strain in Quebec, Canada. *Antimicrob. Agents Chemother.* **44:**528–532.

35. Chorine, V. 1945. Action de l'amide nicotinique sur les bacilles du genre *Mycobacterium. C. R. Acad. Sci.* (Paris) **220:**150–151.

36. Cohen, S. P., S. B. Levy, J. Foulds, and J. L. Rosner. 1993. Salicylate induction of antibiotic resistance in *Escherichia coli*: activation of the *mar* operon and a *mar*-independent pathway. *J. Bacteriol.* **175:**7856–7862.

37. Cole, S. T., R. Brosch, J. Parkhill, T. Garnier, C. Churcher, D. Harris, S. V. Gordon, K. Eiglmeier, S. Gas, C. E. Barry, III, F. Tekaia, K. Badcock, D. Basham, D. Brown, T. Chillingworth, R. Connor, R. Davies, K. Devlin, T. Feltwell, S. Gentles, N. Hamlin, S. Holroyd, T. Hornsby, K. Jagels, A. Krogh, J. McLean, S. Moule, L. Murphy, K. Oliver, J. Osborne, M. A. Quail, M.-A. Rajandream, J. Rogers, S. Rutter, K. Seeger, J. Skelton, R. Squares, S. Squares, J. E. Sulston, K. Taylor, S. Whitehead, and B. G. Barrell. 1998.

Deciphering the biology of *Mycobacterium tuberculosis* from the complete genome sequence. *Nature* 393:537–544.

38. Cooksey, R. C., G. P. Morlock, A. McQueen, S. E. Glickman, and J. T. Crawford. 1996. Characterization of streptomycin resistance mechanisms among *Mycobacterium tuberculosis* isolates from patients in New York City. *Antimicrob. Agents Chemother.* 40:1186–1188.

39. Corbett, E. L., C. J. Watt, N. Walker, D. Maher, B. G. Williams, M. C. Raviglione, and C. Dye. 2003. The growing burden of tuberculosis: global trends and interactions with the HIV epidemic. *Arch. Intern. Med.* 163:1009–1021.

40. Dabbs, E. R., K. Yazawa, Y. Mikami, M. Miyaji, N. Morisaki, S. Iwasaki, and K. Furihata. 1995. Ribosylation by mycobacterial strains as a new mechanism of rifampin inactivation. *Antimicrob. Agents Chemother.* 39:1007–1009.

41. Davies, J., W. Gilbert, and L. Gorini. 1964. Streptomycin, suppression, and the Code. *Proc. Natl. Acad. Sci. USA* 51:883–890.

42. DeBarber, A. E., K. Mdluli, M. Bosman, L. G. Bekker, and C. E. Barry, III. 2000. Ethionamide activation and sensitivity in multidrug-resistant *Mycobacterium tuberculosis*. *Proc. Natl. Acad. Sci. USA* 97:9677–9682.

43. Delihas, N., and S. Forst. 2001. MicF: an antisense RNA gene involved in response of *Escherichia coli* to global stress factors. *J. Mol. Biol.* 313:1–12.

44. Deretic, V., J. Song, and E. Pagan-Ramos. 1997. Loss of *oxyR* in *Mycobacterium tuberculosis*. *Trends Microbiol.* 5:367–372.

45. Dessen, A., A. Quemard, J. S. Blanchard, W. R. Jacobs, Jr., and J. C. Sacchettini. 1995. Crystal structure and function of the isoniazid target of *Mycobacterium tuberculosis*. *Science* 267:1638–1641.

46. Du, X., W. Wang, R. Kim, H. Yakota, H. Nguyen, and S. H. Kim. 2001. Crystal structure and mechanism of catalysis of a pyrazinamidase from *Pyrococcus horikoshii*. *Biochemistry* 40:14166–14172.

47. Dubnau, E., S. Soares, T. J. Huang, and W. R. Jacobs, Jr. 1996. Overproduction of mycobacterial ribosomal protein S13 induces catalase/peroxidase activity and hypersensitivity to isoniazid in *Mycobacterium smegmatis*. *Gene* 170:17–22.

48. Falkow, S. 1975. *Infectious Multiple Drug Resistance*. Pion Ltd., London, United Kingdom.

49. Falkow, S. 1988. Molecular Koch's postulates applied to microbial pathogenicity. *Rev. Infect. Dis.* 10(Suppl. 2):S274–S276.

50. Ferrero, L., B. Cameron, and J. Crouzet. 1995. Analysis of *gyrA* and *grlA* mutations in stepwise-selected ciprofloxacin-resistant mutants of *Staphylococcus aureus*. *Antimicrob. Agents Chemother.* 39:1554–1558.

51. Finken, M., P. Kirschner, A. Meier, A. Wrede, and E. C. Bottger. 1993. Molecular basis of streptomycin resistance in *Mycobacterium tuberculosis*: alterations of the ribosomal protein S12 gene and point mutations within a functional 16S ribosomal RNA pseudoknot. *Mol. Microbiol.* 9:1239–1246.

52. Fox, H. H. 1952. The chemical approach to the control of tuberculosis. *Science* 116:129–134.

53. Fraaije, M. W., N. M. Kamerbeek, A. J. Heidekamp, R. Fortin, and D. B. Janssen. 2004. The prodrug activator EtaA from *Mycobacterium tuberculosis* is a Baeyer-Villiger monooxygenase. *J. Biol. Chem.* 279:3354–3360.

54. Frothingham, R., P. L. Strickland, G. Bretzel, S. Ramaswamy, J. M. Musser, and D. L. Williams. 1999. Phenotypic and genotypic characterization of *Mycobacterium africanum* isolates from West Africa. *J. Clin. Microbiol.* 37:1921–1926.

55. Gale, E. F., E. Cundliffe, P. E. Reynolds, M. Richmond, and M. J. Waring. 1981. *Antibiotic Inhibitors of Ribosome Function*, 2nd ed. John Wiley & Sons, Ltd., London, United Kingdom.

56. Gangadharam, P. R. J., F. M. Harold, and W. Schaefer. 1963. Selective inhibition of nucleic acid synthesis in *Mycobacterium tuberculosis* by isoniazid. *Nature* 198:712–714.

57. Garvin, R. T., D. K. Biswas, and L. Gorini. 1974. The effects of streptomycin or dihydrostreptomycin binding to 16S RNA or to 30S ribosomal subunits. *Proc. Natl. Acad. Sci. USA* 71:3814–3818.

58. Gill, M. J., S. Simjee, K. Al-Hattawi, B. D. Robertson, C. S. Easmon, and C. A. Ison. 1998. Gonococcal resistance to beta-lactams and tetracycline involves mutation in loop 3 of the porin encoded at the *penB* locus. *Antimicrob. Agents Chemother.* 42:2799–2803.

59. Gomez, J. E., and J. D. McKinney. 2004. *M. tuberculosis* persistence, latency, and drug tolerance. *Tuberculosis* (Edinburgh) 84:29–44.

60. Goodwin, A., D. Kersulyte, G. Sisson, S. J. Veldhuyzen van Zanten, D. E. Berg, and P. S. Hoffman. 1998. Metronidazole resistance in *Helicobacter pylori* is due to null mutations in a gene (*rdxA*) that encodes an oxygen-insensitive NADPH nitroreductase. *Mol. Microbiol.* 28:383–393.

61. Guerrero, C., L. Stockman, F. Marchesi, T. Bodmer, G. D. Roberts, and A. Telenti. 1994. Evaluation of the *rpoB* gene in rifampicin-susceptible and -resistant *Mycobacterium avium* and *Mycobacterium intracellulare*. *J. Antimicrob. Chemother.* 33:661–663.

62. Guillemin, I., V. Jarlier, and E. Cambau. 1998. Correlation between quinolone susceptibility patterns and sequences in the A and B subunits of DNA gyrase in mycobacteria. *Antimicrob. Agents Chemother.* 42:2084–2088.

63. Guo, M., Z. Sun, and Y. Zhang. 2000. *Mycobacterium smegmatis* has two pyrazinamidase enzymes, PncA and PzaA. *J. Bacteriol.* 182:3881–3884.

64. Gustafson, J. E., P. V. Candelaria, S. A. Fisher, J. P. Goodridge, T. M. Lichocik, T. M. McWilliams, C. T. Price, F. G. O'Brien, and W. B. Grubb. 1999. Growth in the presence of salicylate increases fluoroquinolone resistance in *Staphylococcus aureus*. *Antimicrob. Agents Chemother.* 43:990–992.

65. Haas, W. H., K. Schilke, J. Brand, B. Amthor, K. Weyer, P. B. Fourie, G. Bretzel, V. Sticht-Groh, and H. J. Bremer. 1997. Molecular analysis of *katG* gene mutations in strains of *Mycobacterium tuberculosis* complex from Africa. *Antimicrob. Agents Chemother.* 41:1601–1603.

66. Heifets, L. B., and P. J. Lindholm-Levy. 1990. Is pyrazinamide bactericidal against *Mycobacterium tuberculosis*? *Am. Rev. Respir. Dis.* 141:250–252.

67. Helbecque, D. M., V. Handzel, and L. Eidus. 1975. Simple amidase test for identification of mycobacteria. *J. Clin. Microbiol.* 1:50–53.

68. Heym, B., P. M. Alzari, N. Honore, and S. T. Cole. 1995. Missense mutations in the catalase-peroxidase gene, *katG*, are associated with isoniazid resistance in *Mycobacterium tuberculosis*. *Mol. Microbiol.* 15:235–245.

69. Heym, B., N. Honore, C. Truffot-Pernot, A. Banerjee, C. Schurra, W. R. Jacobs, Jr., J. D. van Embden, J. H. Grosset, and S. T. Cole. 1994. Implications of multidrug resistance for the future of short-course chemotherapy of tuberculosis: a molecular study. *Lancet* 344:293–298.

70. Heym, B., E. Stavropoulos, N. Honore, P. Domenech, B. Saint-Joanis, T. M. Wilson, D. M. Collins, M. J. Colston, and S. T. Cole. 1997. Effects of overexpression of the alkyl hydroperoxide reductase AhpC on the virulence and isoni-

azid resistance of *Mycobacterium tuberculosis*. *Infect. Immun.* **65**:1395–1401.

71. Hirano, K., M. Takahashi, Y. Kazumi, Y. Fukasawa, and C. Abe. 1997. Mutation in *pncA* is a major mechanism of pyrazinamide resistance in *Mycobacterium tuberculosis*. *Tubercle Lung Dis.* **78**:117–122.

72. Hoashi, S., H. Tai, and M. Tamari. 1999. *pncA* gene mutations in clinical isolates of tubercle bacillus by polymerase chain reaction-direct sequencing method: in relationship to pyrazinamide resistance. *Kekkaku* **74**:441–445.

73. Hobby, G. L., K. Meyer, and K. Chaffe. 1942. Observations on the mechanism of action of penicillin. *Proc. Soc. Exp. Biol. Med.* **50**:281.

74. Honore, N., and S. T. Cole. 1993. Molecular basis of rifampin resistance in *Mycobacterium leprae*. *Antimicrob. Agents Chemother.* **37**:414–418.

75. Honore, N., and S. T. Cole. 1994. Streptomycin resistance in mycobacteria. *Antimicrob. Agents Chemother.* **38**:238–242.

76. Honore, N., G. Marchal, and S. T. Cole. 1995. Novel mutation in 16S rRNA associated with streptomycin dependence in *Mycobacterium tuberculosis*. *Antimicrob. Agents Chemother.* **39**:769–770.

77. Hou, L., D. Osei-Hyiaman, Z. Zhang, B. Wang, A. Yang, and K. Kano. 2000. Molecular characterization of *pncA* gene mutations in *Mycobacterium tuberculosis* clinical isolates from China. *Epidemiol. Infect.* **124**:227–232.

78. Huant, E. 1945. Notes sur l'action de tres fortes doses d'amide nicotinique dans les lesions bacillaires. *Gaz. Hop.* **118**:259–260.

79. Hui, J., N. Gordon, and R. Kajioka. 1977. Permeability barrier to rifampin in mycobacteria. *Antimicrob. Agents Chemother.* **11**:773–779.

80. Jarlier, V., and H. Nikaido. 1990. Permeability barrier to hydrophilic solutes in *Mycobacterium chelonei*. *J. Bacteriol.* **172**:1418–1423.

81. Jin, D. J., and C. A. Gross. 1988. Mapping and sequencing of mutations in the *Escherichia coli rpoB* gene that lead to rifampicin resistance. *J. Mol. Biol.* **202**:45–58.

82. Johnsson, K., W. A. Froland, and P. G. Schultz. 1997. Overexpression, purification, and characterization of the catalase-peroxidase KatG from *Mycobacterium tuberculosis*. *J. Biol. Chem.* **272**:2834–2840.

83. Johnsson, K., and P. G. Schultz. 1994. Mechanistic studies of the oxidation of isoniazid by the catalase peroxidase from *Mycobacterium tuberculosis*. *J. Am. Chem. Soc.* **116**:7425–7426.

84. Kenney, T. J., and G. Churchward. 1994. Cloning and sequence analysis of the *rpsL* and *rpsG* genes of *Mycobacterium smegmatis* and characterization of mutations causing resistance to streptomycin. *J. Bacteriol.* **176**:6153–6156.

85. Kiepiela, P., K. S. Bishop, A. N. Smith, L. Roux, and D. F. York. 2000. Genomic mutations in the *katG*, *inhA* and *aphC* genes are useful for the prediction of isoniazid resistance in *Mycobacterium tuberculosis* isolates from Kwazulu Natal, South Africa. *Tubercle Lung Dis.* **80**:47–56.

86. Kim, S. Y., Y. J. Park, W. I. Kim, S. H. Lee, C. Ludgerus Chang, S. J. Kang, and C. S. Kang. 2003. Molecular analysis of isoniazid resistance in *Mycobacterium tuberculosis* isolates recovered from South Korea. *Diagn. Microbiol. Infect. Dis.* **47**:497–502.

87. Kocagoz, T., C. J. Hackbarth, I. Unsal, E. Y. Rosenberg, H. Nikaido, and H. F. Chambers. 1996. Gyrase mutations in laboratory-selected, fluoroquinolone-resistant mutants of *Mycobacterium tuberculosis* H37Ra. *Antimicrob. Agents Chemother.* **40**:1768–1774.

88. Konno, K., F. M. Feldmann, and W. McDermott. 1967. Pyrazinamide susceptibility and amidase activity of tubercle bacilli. *Am. Rev. Respir. Dis.* **95**:461–469.

89. Kremer, L., J. D. Douglas, A. R. Baulard, C. Morehouse, M. R. Guy, D. Alland, L. G. Dover, J. H. Lakey, W. R. Jacobs, Jr., P. J. Brennan, D. E. Minnikin, and G. S. Besra. 2000. Thiolactomycin and related analogues as novel antimycobacterial agents targeting KasA and KasB condensing enzymes in *Mycobacterium tuberculosis*. *J. Biol. Chem.* **275**:16857–16864.

90. Kremer, L., L. G. Dover, H. R. Morbidoni, C. Vilchèze, W. N. Maughan, A. Baulard, S. Tu, N. Honore, V. Deretic, J. C. Sacchettini, C. Locht, W. R. J. Jacobs, and G. Besra. 2003. Inhibition of InhA activity, but not KasA activity, induces formation of a KasA-containing complex in mycobacteria. *J. Biol. Chem.* **278**:20547–20554.

91. Kruuner, A., S. E. Hoffner, H. Sillastu, M. Danilovits, K. Levina, S. B. Svenson, S. Ghebremichael, T. Koivula, and G. Kallenius. 2001. Spread of drug-resistant pulmonary tuberculosis in Estonia. *J. Clin. Microbiol.* **39**:3339–3345.

92. Kushner, S., H. Dalalian, J. L. Sanjurjo, F. L. Bach, S. R. Safir, V. K. J. Smith, and J. H. Williams. 1952. Experimental chemotherapy of tuberculosis: the synthesis of pyrazinamides and related compounds. *J. Am. Chem. Soc.* **74**:3617–3621.

93. Kwon, D. H., M. Kato, F. A. El-Zaatari, M. S. Osato, and D. Y. Graham. 2000. Frame-shift mutations in NAD(P)H flavin oxidoreductase encoding gene (*frxA*) from metronidazole resistant *Helicobacter pylori* ATCC43504 and its involvement in metronidazole resistance. *FEMS Microbiol. Lett.* **188**:197–202.

94. Kwon, H. H., H. Tomioka, and H. Saito. 1995. Distribution and characterization of β-lactamases of mycobacteria and related organisms. *Tubercle Lung Dis.* **76**:141–148.

95. Larsen, M. H., C. Vilchèze, L. Kremer, G. S. Besra, L. Parsons, M. Salfinger, L. Heifets, M. H. Hazbon, D. Alland, J. C. Sacchettini, and W. R. Jacobs, Jr. 2002. Overexpression of *inhA*, but not *kasA*, confers resistance to isoniazid and ethionamide in *Mycobacterium smegmatis*, *M. bovis* BCG and *M. tuberculosis*. *Mol. Microbiol.* **46**:453–466.

96. Lederberg, J. 1952. Cell genetics and hereditary symbiosis. *Physiol. Rev.* **32**:403–430.

97. Lee, A. S., I. H. Lim, L. L. Tang, A. Telenti, and S. Y. Wong. 1999. Contribution of *kasA* analysis to detection of isoniazid-resistant *Mycobacterium tuberculosis* in Singapore. *Antimicrob. Agents Chemother.* **43**:2087–2089.

98. Lee, A. S., A. S. Teo, and S. Y. Wong. 2001. Novel mutations in *ndh* in isoniazid-resistant *Mycobacterium tuberculosis* isolates. *Antimicrob. Agents Chemother.* **45**:2157–2159.

99. Lee, K. W., J. M. Lee, and K. S. Jung. 2001. Characterization of *pncA* mutations of pyrazinamide-resistant *Mycobacterium tuberculosis* in Korea. *J. Korean Med. Sci.* **16**:537–43.

100. Lee, R. E., K. Mikusova, P. J. Brennan, and G. S. Besra. 1995. Synthesis of the arabinose donor beta-D-arabinofuranosyl-1-monophosphoryldecaprenol. Development of a basic arabinosyl-transferase assay, and identification of ethambutol as an arabinosyl transferase inhibitor. *J. Am. Chem. Soc.* **117**:11829–11832.

101. Lei, B., C. J. Wei, and S. C. Tu. 2000. Action mechanism of antitubercular isoniazid. Activation by *Mycobacterium tuberculosis* KatG, isolation, and characterization of *inhA* inhibitor. *J. Biol. Chem.* **275**:2520–2526.

102. Lemaitre, N., W. Sougakoff, C. Truffot-Pernot, and V. Jarlier. 1999. Characterization of new mutations in pyrazinamide-resistant strains of *Mycobacterium tuberculosis* and identification of conserved regions important for the catalytic

activity of the pyrazinamidase PncA. *Antimicrob. Agents Chemother.* 43:1761–1763.

103. Lety, M. A., S. Nair, P. Berche, and V. Escuyer. 1997. A single point mutation in the *embB* gene is responsible for resistance to ethambutol in *Mycobacterium smegmatis. Antimicrob. Agents Chemother.* 41:2629–2633.

104. Li, X. Z., and H. Nikaido. 2004. Efflux-mediated drug resistance in bacteria. *Drugs* 64:159–204.

105. Li, Z., C. Kelley, F. Collins, D. Rouse, and S. Morris. 1998. Expression of *katG* in *Mycobacterium tuberculosis* is associated with its growth and persistence in mice and guinea pigs. *J. Infect. Dis.* 177:1030–1035.

106. Liu, J., H. E. Takiff, and H. Nikaido. 1996. Active efflux of fluoroquinolones in *Mycobacterium smegmatis* mediated by LfrA, a multidrug efflux pump. *J. Bacteriol.* 178:3791–3795.

107. Lukat-Rodgers, G. S., N. L. Wengenack, F. Rusnak, and K. R. Rodgers. 2001. Carbon monoxide adducts of KatG and KatG(S315T) as probes of the heme site and isoniazid binding. *Biochemistry* 40:7149–7157.

108. Malone, L., A. Schurr, H. Lindh, D. McKenzie, J. S. Kiser, and J. H. Williams. 1952. The effect of pyrazinamide (Aldinamide) on experimental tuberculosis in mice. *Am. Rev. Respir. Dis.* 35:511–518.

109. Marrakchi, H., G. Laneelle, and A. Quemard. 2000. InhA, a target of the antituberculous drug isoniazid, is involved in a mycobacterial fatty acid elongation system, FAS-II. *Microbiology* 146:289–296.

110. Martin, C., M. Ranes, and B. Gicquel. 1990. *Plasmids, Antibiotic Resistance, and Mobile Elements in Mycobacteria.* Surrey University Press, Guildford, United Kingdom.

111. Martin, C., J. Timm, J. Rauzier, R. Gomez-Lus, J. Davies, and B. Gicquel. 1990. Transposition of an antibiotic resistance element in mycobacteria. *Nature* 345:739–743.

112. Marttila, H. J., M. Marjamaki, E. Vyshnevskaya, B. I. Vyshnevskiy, T. F. Otten, A. V. Vasilyef, and M. K. Viljanen. 1999. *pncA* mutations in pyrazinamide-resistant *Mycobacterium tuberculosis* isolates from northwestern Russia. *Antimicrob. Agents Chemother.* 43:1764–1766.

113. Marttila, H. J., H. Soini, E. Eerola, E. Vyshnevskaya, B. I. Vyshnevskiy, T. F. Otten, A. V. Vasilyef, and M. K. Viljanen. 1998. A Ser315Thr substitution in KatG is predominant in genetically heterogeneous multidrug-resistant *Mycobacterium tuberculosis* isolates originating from the St. Petersburg area in Russia. *Antimicrob. Agents Chemother.* 42: 2443–2445.

114. McCalla, D. R., A. Reuvers, and C. Kaiser. 1970. Mode of action of nitrofurazone. *J. Bacteriol.* 104:1126–1134.

115. McClatchy, J. K., A. Y. Tsang, and M. S. Cernich. 1981. Use of pyrazinamidase activity on *Mycobacterium tuberculosis* as a rapid method for determination of pyrazinamide susceptibility. *Antimicrob. Agents Chemother.* 20:556–557.

116. McClure, W. R., and C. L. Cech. 1978. On the mechanism of rifampicin inhibition of RNA synthesis. *J. Biol. Chem.* 253:8949–8956.

117. McCune, R. M., Jr., and R. Tompsett. 1956. Fate of *Mycobacterium tuberculosis* in mouse tissues as determined by the microbial enumeration technique. I. The persistence of drug-susceptible tubercle bacilli in the tissues despite prolonged antimicrobial therapy. *J. Exp. Med.* 104:737–762.

118. McDermott, P. F., D. G. White, I. Podglajen, M. N. Alekshun, and S. B. Levy. 1998. Multidrug resistance following expression of the *Escherichia coli marA* gene in *Mycobacterium smegmatis. J. Bacteriol.* 180:2995–2998.

119. McDermott, W., and R. Tompsett. 1954. Activation of pyrazinamide and nicotinamide in acidic environments in vitro. *Am. Rev. Tuberc.* 70:748–754.

120. McKenzie, D., L. Malone, S. Kushner, J. J. Oleson, and Y. Subbarow. 1948. The effect of nicotinic acid amide on experimental tuberculosis of white mice. *J. Lab. Clin. Med.* 33:1249–1253.

121. McMurry, L. M., and S. B. Levy. 2000. Tetracycline resistance in gram-positive bacteria, p. 660–677. *In* V. A. Fischetti, R. P. Novick, J. J. Ferretti, D. A. Portnoy, and J. I. Rood (ed.), *Gram-Positive Pathogens.* ASM Press, Washington, D.C.

122. Mdluli, K., D. R. Sherman, M. J. Hickey, B. N. Kreiswirth, S. Morris, C. K. Stover, and C. E. Barry, III. 1996. Biochemical and genetic data suggest that InhA is not the primary target for activated isoniazid in *Mycobacterium tuberculosis. J. Infect. Dis.* 174:1085–1090.

123. Mdluli, K., R. A. Slayden, Y. Zhu, S. Ramaswamy, X. Pan, D. Mead, D. D. Crane, J. M. Musser, and C. E. Barry, III. 1998. Inhibition of a *Mycobacterium tuberculosis* beta-ketoacyl ACP synthase by isoniazid. *Science* 280:1607–1610.

124. Medical Research Council. 1950. Treatment of pulmonary tuberculosis with streptomycin and *para*-aminosalicylic acid. *Br. Med. J.* 2:1037–1085.

125. Meier, A., P. Kirschner, F. C. Bange, U. Vogel, and E. C. Bottger. 1994. Genetic alterations in streptomycin-resistant *Mycobacterium tuberculosis*: mapping of mutations conferring resistance. *Antimicrob. Agents Chemother.* 38:228–233.

126. Meissner, G. 1964. *The Bacteriology of the Tubercle Bacillus.* Butterworths, London, United Kingdom.

127. Mestdagh, M., L. Realini, P. A. Fonteyne, R. Rossau, G. Jannes, W. Mijs, D. E. S. KA, F. Portaels, and E. Van den Eeckhout. 2000. Correlation of *pncA* sequence with pyrazinamide resistance level in BACTEC for 21 *Mycobacterium tuberculosis* clinical isolates. *Microb. Drug Resist.* 6:283–287.

128. Middlebrook, G. 1954. Isoniazid resistance and catalase activity of tubercle bacilli. *Am. Rev. Tuberc.* 69:471–472.

129. Middlebrook, G. 1952. Sterilization of tubercle bacilli by isonicotinic acid hydrazide and the incidence of variants resistant to the drug in vitro. *Am. Rev. Tuberc.* 65:765–767.

130. Miesel, L., T. R. Weisbrod, J. A. Marcinkeviciene, R. Bittman, and W. R. Jacobs, Jr. 1998. NADH dehydrogenase defects confer isoniazid resistance and conditional lethality in *Mycobacterium smegmatis. J. Bacteriol.* 180: 2459–2467.

131. Mikusova, K., R. A. Slayden, G. S. Besra, and P. J. Brennan. 1995. Biogenesis of the mycobacterial cell wall and the site of action of ethambutol. *Antimicrob. Agents Chemother.* 39:2484–2489.

132. Miller, L. P., J. T. Crawford, and T. M. Shinnick. 1994. The *rpoB* gene of *Mycobacterium tuberculosis. Antimicrob. Agents Chemother.* 38:805–811.

133. Miller, M. A., L. Thibert, F. Desjardins, S. H. Siddiqi, and A. Dascal. 1995. Testing of susceptibility of *Mycobacterium tuberculosis* to pyrazinamide: comparison of Bactec method with pyrazinamidase assay. *J. Clin. Microbiol.* 33:2468–2470.

134. Mitchison, D. A. 1985. The action of antituberculosis drugs in short-course chemotherapy. *Tubercle* 66:219–225.

135. Mitchison, D. A., and J. B. Selkon. 1956. The bactericidal activities of antituberculous drugs. *Am. Rev. Tuberc.* 74: 109–123.

136. Moazed, D., and H. F. Noller. 1987. Interaction of antibiotics with functional sites in 16S ribosomal RNA. *Nature* 327:389–394.

137. Moghazeh, S. L., X. Pan, T. Arain, C. K. Stover, J. M. Musser, and B. N. Kreiswirth. 1996. Comparative antimycobacterial activities of rifampin, rifapentine, and KRM-

1648 against a collection of rifampin-resistant *Mycobacterium tuberculosis* isolates with known *rpoB* mutations. *Antimicrob. Agents Chemother.* **40**:2655–2657.

138. **Mokrousov, I., O. Narvskaya, T. Otten, E. Limeschenko, L. Steklova, and B. Vyshnevskiy.** 2002. High prevalence of KatG Ser315Thr substitution among isoniazid-resistant *Mycobacterium tuberculosis* clinical isolates from northwestern Russia, 1996 to 2001. *Antimicrob. Agents Chemother.* **46:** 1417–1424.

139. **Mokrousov, I., T. Otten, B. Vyshnevskiy, and O. Narvskaya.** 2002. Detection of *embB306* mutations in ethambutol-susceptible clinical isolates of *Mycobacterium tuberculosis* from Northwestern Russia: implications for genotypic resistance testing. *J. Clin. Microbiol.* **40**:3810–3813.

140. **Molenaar, D., M. E. van der Rest, A. Drysch, and R. Yucel.** 2000. Functions of the membrane-associated and cytoplasmic malate dehydrogenases in the citric acid cycle of *Corynebacterium glutamicum. J. Bacteriol.* **182**:6884–6891.

141. **Morlock, G. P., J. T. Crawford, W. R. Butler, S. E. Brim, D. Sikes, G. H. Mazurek, C. L. Woodley, and R. C. Cooksey.** 2000. Phenotypic characterization of *pncA* mutants of *Mycobacterium tuberculosis. Antimicrob. Agents Chemother.* **44:** 2291–2295.

142. **Morlock, G. P., B. Metchock, D. Sikes, J. T. Crawford, and R. C. Cooksey.** 2003. *ethA, inhA,* and *katG* loci of ethionamide-resistant clinical *Mycobacterium tuberculosis* isolates. *Antimicrob. Agents Chemother.* **47**:3799–3805.

143. **Morris, S., G. H. Bai, P. Suffys, L. Portillo-Gomez, M. Fairchok, and D. Rouse.** 1995. Molecular mechanisms of multiple drug resistance in clinical isolates of *Mycobacterium tuberculosis. J. Infect. Dis.* **171**:954–960.

144. **Musser, J. M.** 1995. Antimicrobial agent resistance in mycobacteria: molecular genetic insights. *Clin. Microbiol. Rev.* **8:** 496–514.

145. **Musser, J. M., V. Kapur, D. L. Williams, B. N. Kreiswirth, D. van Soolingen, and J. D. van Embden.** 1996. Characterization of the catalase-peroxidase gene (*katG*) and *inhA* locus in isoniazid-resistant and -susceptible strains of *Mycobacterium tuberculosis* by automated DNA sequencing: restricted array of mutations associated with drug resistance. *J. Infect. Dis.* **173**:196–202.

146. **Mustaev, A., E. Zaychikov, K. Severinov, M. Kashlev, A. Polyakov, V. Nikiforov, and A. Goldfarb.** 1994. Topology of the RNA polymerase active center probed by chimeric rifampicin-nucleotide compounds. *Proc. Natl. Acad. Sci. USA* **91**:12036–12040.

147. **Nachamkin, I., C. Kang, and M. P. Weinstein.** 1997. Detection of resistance to isoniazid, rifampin, and streptomycin in clinical isolates of *Mycobacterium tuberculosis* by molecular methods. *Clin. Infect. Dis.* **24**:894–900.

148. **Nair, J., D. A. Rouse, G. H. Bai, and S. L. Morris.** 1993. The *rpsL* gene and streptomycin resistance in single and multiple drug-resistant strains of *Mycobacterium tuberculosis. Mol. Microbiol.* **10**:521–527.

149. **Nguyen, M., A. Quemard, S. Broussy, J. Bernadou, and B. Meunier.** 2002. Mn(III) pyrophosphate as an efficient tool for studying the mode of action of isoniazid on the InhA protein of *Mycobacterium tuberculosis. Antimicrob. Agents Chemother.* **46**:2137–2144.

150. **Niederweis, M.** 2003. Mycobacterial porins—new channel proteins in unique outer membranes. *Mol. Microbiol.* **49**:1167–1177.

151. **Offe, H. A., W. Siefken, and G. Domagk.** 1952. The tuberculostatic activity of hydrazine derivatives from pyridine carboxylic acids and carbonyl compounds. *Z. Naturforsch.* **7B**:462–468.

152. **Okusu, H., D. Ma, and H. Nikaido.** 1996. AcrAB efflux pump plays a major role in the antibiotic resistance phenotype of *Escherichia coli* multiple-antibiotic-resistance (Mar) mutants. *J. Bacteriol.* **178**:306–308.

153. **Pagan-Ramos, E., J. Song, M. McFalone, M. H. Mudd, and V. Deretic.** 1998. Oxidative stress response and characterization of the *oxyR-ahpC* and *furA-katG* loci in *Mycobacterium marinum. J. Bacteriol.* **180**:4856–4864.

154. **Park, S. K., J. Y. Lee, C. L. Chang, M. K. Lee, H. C. Son, C. M. Kim, H. J. Jang, H. K. Park, and S. H. Jeong.** 2001. *pncA* mutations in clinical *Mycobacterium tuberculosis* isolates from Korea. *BMC Infect. Dis.* **1**:4.

155. **Payton, M., R. Auty, R. Delgoda, M. Everett, and E. Sim.** 1999. Cloning and characterization of arylamine N-acetyltransferase genes from *Mycobacterium smegmatis* and *Mycobacterium tuberculosis:* increased expression results in isoniazid resistance. *J. Bacteriol.* **181**:1343–1347.

156. **Payton, M., C. Gifford, P. Schartau, C. Hagemeier, A. Mushtaq, S. Lucas, K. Pinter, and E. Sim.** 2001. Evidence towards the role of arylamine N-acetyltransferase in *Mycobacterium smegmatis* and development of a specific antiserum against the homologous enzyme of *Mycobacterium tuberculosis. Microbiology* **147**:3295–3302.

157. **Peteroy, M., A. Severin, F. Zhao, D. Rosner, U. Lopatin, H. Scherman, A. Belanger, B. Harvey, G. F. Hatfull, P. J. Brennan, and N. D. Connell.** 2000. Characterization of a *Mycobacterium smegmatis* mutant that is simultaneously resistant to D-cycloserine and vancomycin. *Antimicrob. Agents Chemother.* **44**:1701–1704.

158. **Piatek, A. S., A. Telenti, M. R. Murray, H. El-Hajj, W. R. Jacobs, Jr., F. R. Kramer, and D. Alland.** 2000. Genotypic analysis of *Mycobacterium tuberculosis* in two distinct populations using molecular beacons: implications for rapid susceptibility testing. *Antimicrob. Agents Chemother.* **44**:103–110.

159. **Plotz, P. H.** 1985. *Textbook of Rheumatology,* vol. 2. The W. B. Saunders Co., Philadelphia, Pa.

160. **Poole, K.** 2001. Overcoming antimicrobial resistance by targeting resistance mechanisms. *J. Pharm. Pharmacol.* **53:** 283–294.

161. **Price, C. T., I. R. Lee, and J. E. Gustafson.** 2000. The effects of salicylate on bacteria. *Int. J. Biochem. Cell Biol.* **32**:1029–1043.

162. **Pym, A. S., B. Saint-Joanis, and S. T. Cole.** 2002. Effect of *katG* mutations on the virulence of *Mycobacterium tuberculosis* and the implication for transmission in humans. *Infect. Immun.* **70**:4955–4960.

163. **Quan, S., H. Venter, and E. R. Dabbs.** 1997. Ribosylative inactivation of rifampin by *Mycobacterium smegmatis* is a principal contributor to its low susceptibility to this antibiotic. *Antimicrob. Agents Chemother.* **41**:2456–2460.

164. **Quemard, A., A. Dessen, M. Sugantino, W. R. Jacobs, Jr., J. C. Sacchettini, and J. S. Blanchard.** 1996. Binding of catalase-peroxidase-activated isoniazid to wild-type and mutant *Mycobacterium tuberculosis* enoyl-ACP reductases. *J. Am. Chem. Soc.* **118**:1561–1562.

165. **Quemard, A., J. C. Sacchettini, A. Dessen, C. Vilchèze, R. Bittman, W. R. Jacobs, Jr., and J. S. Blanchard.** 1995. Enzymatic characterization of the target for isoniazid in Mycobacterium tuberculosis. *Biochemistry* **34**:8235–8241.

166. **Rad, M. E., P. Bifani, C. Martin, K. Kremer, S. Samper, J. Rauzier, B. Kreiswirth, J. Blazquez, M. Jouan, D. van Soolingen, and B. Gicquel.** 2003. Mutations in putative mutator genes of *Mycobacterium tuberculosis* strains of the W-Beijing family. *Emerg. Infect. Dis.* **9**:838–845.

167. **Ramaswamy, S. V., A. G. Amin, S. Goksel, C. E. Stager, S. J. Dou, H. El Sahly, S. L. Moghazeh, B. N. Kreiswirth, and**

J. M. Musser. 2000. Molecular genetic analysis of nucleotide polymorphisms associated with ethambutol resistance in human isolates of *Mycobacterium tuberculosis*. *Antimicrob. Agents Chemother.* **44**:326–336.

168. Ramaswamy, S. V., R. Reich, S. J. Dou, L. Jasperse, X. Pan, A. Wanger, T. Quitugua, and E. A. Graviss. 2003. Single nucleotide polymorphisms in genes associated with isoniazid resistance in *Mycobacterium tuberculosis*. *Antimicrob. Agents Chemother.* **47**:1241–1250.

169. Riska, P. F., W. R. Jacobs, Jr., and D. Alland. 2000. Molecular determinants of drug resistance in tuberculosis. *Int. J. Tuberc. Lung Dis.* **4**:S4–S10.

170. Rosner, J. L. 1985. Nonheritable resistance to chloramphenicol and other antibiotics induced by salicylates and other chemotactic repellents in *Escherichia coli* K-12. *Proc. Natl. Acad. Sci. USA* **82**:8771–8774.

171. Rouse, D. A., Z. Li, G. H. Bai, and S. L. Morris. 1995. Characterization of the *katG* and *inhA* genes of isoniazid-resistant clinical isolates of *Mycobacterium tuberculosis*. *Antimicrob. Agents Chemother.* **39**:2472–2477.

172. Rozwarski, D. A., G. A. Grant, D. H. Barton, W. R. Jacobs, Jr., and J. C. Sacchettini. 1998. Modification of the NADH of the isoniazid target (InhA) from *Mycobacterium tuberculosis*. *Science* **279**:98–102.

173. Sachais, B. S., I. I. Nachamkindagger, J. K. Mills, and D. G. Leonard. 1998. Novel *pncA* mutations in pyrazinamide-resistant isolates of *Mycobacterium tuberculosis*. *Mol. Diagn.* **3**:229–231.

174. Saint-Joanis, B., H. Souchon, M. Wilming, K. Johnsson, P. M. Alzari, and S. T. Cole. 1999. Use of site-directed mutagenesis to probe the structure, function and isoniazid activation of the catalase/peroxidase, KatG, from *Mycobacterium tuberculosis*. *Biochem. J.* **338**:753–760.

175. Salfinger, M., and L. B. Heifets. 1988. Determination of pyrazinamide MICs for *Mycobacterium tuberculosis* at different pHs by the radiometric method. *Antimicrob. Agents Chemother.* **32**:1002–1004.

176. Schaefer, W. B. 1954. The effect of isoniazid on growing and resting tubercle bacilli. *Am. Rev. Tuberc.* **69**:125–127.

177. Schaller, A., Z. Sun, Y. Yang, A. Somoskovi, and Y. Zhang. 2002. Salicylate reduces susceptibility of *Mycobacterium tuberculosis* to multiple antituberculosis drugs. *Antimicrob. Agents Chemother.* **46**:2636–2639.

178. Schatz, A., and S. A. Waksman. 1944. Effect of streptomycin upon *Mycobacterium tuberculosis* and related organisms. *Proc. Soc. Exp. Biol. Med.* **67**:244–248.

179. Scorpio, A., D. Collins, D. Whipple, D. Cave, J. Bates, and Y. Zhang. 1997. Rapid differentiation of bovine and human tubercle bacilli based on a characteristic mutation in the bovine pyrazinamidase gene. *J. Clin. Microbiol.* **35**:106–110.

180. Scorpio, A., P. Lindholm-Levy, L. Heifets, R. Gilman, S. Siddiqi, M. Cynamon, and Y. Zhang. 1997. Characterization of *pncA* mutations in pyrazinamide-resistant *Mycobacterium tuberculosis*. *Antimicrob. Agents Chemother.* **41**:540–543.

181. Scorpio, A., and Y. Zhang. 1996. Mutations in *pncA*, a gene encoding pyrazinamidase/nicotinamidase, cause resistance to the antituberculous drug pyrazinamide in tubercle bacillus. *Nat. Med.* **2**:662–667.

182. Sechi, L. A., S. Zanetti, M. Sanguinetti, P. Molicotti, L. Romano, G. Leori, G. Delogu, S. Boccia, M. La Sorda, and G. Fadda. 2001. Molecular basis of rifampin and isoniazid resistance in *Mycobacterium bovis* strains isolated in Sardinia, Italy. *Antimicrob. Agents Chemother.* **45**:1645–1648.

183. Severinov, K., M. Soushko, A. Goldfarb, and V. Nikiforov. 1994. RifR mutations in the beginning of the *Escherichia coli rpoB* gene. *Mol. Gen. Genet.* **244**:120–126.

184. Siddiqui, S. H. 1992. *Antimicrobial Susceptibility Testing: Radiometric (BACTEC) Tests for Slowly Growing Mycobacteria*. ASM Press, Washington, D.C.

185. Slayden, R. A., and C. E. Barry. 2002. The role of KasA and KasB in the biosynthesis of meromycolic acids and isoniazid resistance in *Mycobacterium tuberculosis*. *Tuberculosis* (Edinburgh) **82**:149–160.

186. Solotorovsky, M., G. F.J., E. J. Ironson, E. J. Bugie, R. C. O'Neill, and K. Pfister III. 1952. Pyrazinoic acid amide—an agent active against experimental murine tuberculosis. *Soc. Exp. Biol. Med. Proc.* **79**:563–565.

187. Somoskovi, A., M. M. Wade, Z. Sun, and Y. Zhang. 2004. Iron enhances the antituberculous activity of pyrazinamide. *J. Antimicrob. Chemother.* **53**:192–196.

188. Sreevatsan, S., X. Pan, K. E. Stockbauer, D. L. Williams, B. N. Kreiswirth, and J. M. Musser. 1996. Characterization of *rpsL* and *rrs* mutations in streptomycin-resistant *Mycobacterium tuberculosis* isolates from diverse geographic localities. *Antimicrob. Agents Chemother.* **40**:1024–1026.

189. Sreevatsan, S., X. Pan, Y. Zhang, B. N. Kreiswirth, and J. M. Musser. 1997. Mutations associated with pyrazinamide resistance in *pncA* of *Mycobacterium tuberculosis* complex organisms. *Antimicrob. Agents Chemother.* **41**:636–640.

190. Sreevatsan, S., K. E. Stockbauer, X. Pan, B. N. Kreiswirth, S. L. Moghazeh, W. R. Jacobs, Jr., A. Telenti, and J. M. Musser. 1997. Ethambutol resistance in *Mycobacterium tuberculosis*: critical role of *embB* mutations. *Antimicrob. Agents Chemother.* **41**:1677–1681.

191. Sriprakash, K. S., and T. Ramakrishnan. 1969. Isoniazid and nicotinamide adenine dinucleotide synthesis in *M. tuberculosis*. *Indian J. Biochem.* **6**:49–50.

192. Steele, M. A., and R. M. Des Prez. 1988. The role of pyrazinamide in tuberculosis chemotherapy. *Chest* **94**:845–850.

193. Sun, Z., and Y. Zhang. 1999. Reduced pyrazinamidase activity and the natural resistance of *Mycobacterium kansasii* to the antituberculosis drug pyrazinamide. *Antimicrob. Agents Chemother.* **43**:537–542.

194. Suzuki, Y., C. Katsukawa, A. Tamaru, C. Abe, M. Makino, Y. Mizuguchi, and H. Taniguchi. 1998. Detection of kanamycin-resistant *Mycobacterium tuberculosis* by identifying mutations in the 16S rRNA gene. *J. Clin. Microbiol.* **36**:1220–1225.

195. Takayama, K., and J. O. Kilburn. 1989. Inhibition of synthesis of arabinogalactan by ethambutol in *Mycobacterium smegmatis*. *Antimicrob. Agents Chemother.* **33**:1493–1499.

196. Takayama, K., H. K. Schnoes, E. L. Armstrong, and R. W. Boyle. 1975. Site of inhibitory action of isoniazid in the synthesis of mycolic acids in *Mycobacterium tuberculosis*. *J. Lipid Res.* **16**:308–317.

197. Takayama, K., L. Wang, and H. L. David. 1972. Effect of isoniazid on the in vivo mycolic acid synthesis, cell growth, and viability of *Mycobacterium tuberculosis*. *Antimicrob. Agents Chemother.* **2**:29–35.

198. Takayama, K., L. Wang, and R. S. Merkal. 1973. Scanning electron microscopy of the H37Ra strain of *Mycobacterium tuberculosis* exposed to isoniazid. *Antimicrob. Agents Chemother.* **4**:62–65.

199. Takiff, H. E., M. Cimino, M. C. Musso, T. Weisbrod, R. Martinez, M. B. Delgado, L. Salazar, B. R. Bloom, and W. R. Jacobs, Jr. 1996. Efflux pump of the proton antiporter family confers low-level fluoroquinolone resistance in *Mycobacterium smegmatis*. *Proc. Natl. Acad. Sci. USA* **93**:362–366.

200. **Takiff, H. E., L. Salazar, C. Guerrero, W. Philipp, W. M. Huang, B. Kreiswirth, S. T. Cole, W. R. Jacobs, Jr., and A. Telenti.** 1994. Cloning and nucleotide sequence of *Mycobacterium tuberculosis gyrA* and *gyrB* genes and detection of quinolone resistance mutations. *Antimicrob. Agents Chemother.* **38:**773–780.

201. **Taniguchi, H., B. Chang, C. Abe, Y. Nikaido, Y. Mizuguchi, and S. I. Yoshida.** 1997. Molecular analysis of kanamycin and viomycin resistance in *Mycobacterium smegmatis* by use of the conjugation system. *J. Bacteriol.* **179:**4795–4801.

202. **Tarshis, M. S., and W. A. Weed, Jr.** 1953. Lack of significant in vitro sensitivity of *Mycobacterium tuberculosis* to pyrazinamide on three different solid media. *Am. Rev. Tuberc.* **67:** 391–395.

203. **Telenti, A., N. Honore, C. Bernasconi, J. March, A. Ortega, B. Heym, H. E. Takiff, and S. T. Cole.** 1997. Genotypic assessment of isoniazid and rifampin resistance in *Mycobacterium tuberculosis*: a blind study at reference laboratory level. *J. Clin. Microbiol.* **35:**719–723.

204. **Telenti, A., P. Imboden, F. Marchesi, D. Lowrie, S. Cole, M. J. Colston, L. Matter, K. Schopfer, and T. Bodmer.** 1993. Detection of rifampicin-resistance mutations in *Mycobacterium tuberculosis*. *Lancet* **341:**647–650.

205. **Telenti, A., W. J. Philipp, S. Sreevatsan, C. Bernasconi, K. E. Stockbauer, B. Wieles, J. M. Musser, and W. R. Jacobs, Jr.** 1997. The *emb* operon, a gene cluster of *Mycobacterium tuberculosis* involved in resistance to ethambutol. *Nat. Med.* **3:**567–570.

206. **Trivedi, S. S., and S. G. Desai.** 1987. Pyrazinamidase activity of *Mycobacterium tuberculosis*—a test of sensitivity to pyrazinamide. *Tubercle* **68:**221–224.

207. **Upton, A. M., A. Mushtaq, T. C. Victor, S. L. Sampson, J. Sandy, D. M. Smith, P. V. van Helden, and E. Sim.** 2001. Arylamine *N*-acetyltransferase of *Mycobacterium tuberculosis* is a polymorphic enzyme and a site of isoniazid metabolism. *Mol. Microbiol.* **42:**309–317.

208. **Vannelli, T. A., A. Dykman, and P. R. Ortiz de Montellano.** 2002. The antituberculosis drug ethionamide is activated by a flavoprotein monooxygenase. *J. Biol. Chem.* **277:**12824–12829.

209. **van Soolingen, D., P. E. de Haas, H. R. van Doorn, E. Kuijper, H. Rinder, and M. W. Borgdorff.** 2000. Mutations at amino acid position 315 of the *katG* gene are associated with high-level resistance to isoniazid, other drug resistance, and successful transmission of *Mycobacterium tuberculosis* in the Netherlands. *J. Infect. Dis.* **182:**1788–1790.

210. **Victor, T. C., A. van Rie, A. M. Jordaan, M. Richardson, G. D. van Der Spuy, N. Beyers, P. D. van Helden, and R. Warren.** 2001. Sequence polymorphism in the *rrs* gene of *Mycobacterium tuberculosis* is deeply rooted within an evolutionary clade and is not associated with streptomycin resistance. *J. Clin. Microbiol.* **39:**4184–4186.

211. **Vilchèze, C., H. R. Morbidoni, T. R. Weisbrod, H. Iwamoto, M. Kuo, J. C. Sacchettini, and W. R. Jacobs, Jr.** 2000. Inactivation of the *inhA*-encoded fatty acid synthase II (FASII) enoyl-acyl carrier protein reductase induces accumulation of the FASI end products and cell lysis of *Mycobacterium smegmatis*. *J. Bacteriol.* **182:**4059–4067.

212. **Viveiros, M., I. Portugal, R. Bettencourt, T. C. Victor, A. M. Jordaan, C. Leandro, D. Ordway, and L. Amaral.** 2002. Isoniazid-induced transient high-level resistance in *Mycobacterium tuberculosis*. *Antimicrob. Agents Chemother.* **46:** 2804–2810.

212a. **Wade, M. M., and Y. Zhang.** 2004. Anaerobic incubation conditions enhance pyrazinamide activity against *Mycobacterium tuberculosis*. *J. Med. Microbiol.* **53:**769–773.

213. **Walsh, C.** 2000. Molecular mechanisms that confer antibacterial drug resistance. *Nature* **406:**775–781.

214. **Wang, J. Y., R. M. Burger, and K. Drlica.** 1998. Role of superoxide in catalase-peroxidase-mediated isoniazid action against mycobacteria. *Antimicrob. Agents Chemother.* **42:** 709–711.

215. **Watanabe, T.** 1963. Infective heredity of multiple drug resistance in bacteria. *Bacteriol. Rev.* **27:**87–115.

216. **Wei, C. J., B. Lei, J. M. Musser, and S. C. Tu.** 2003. Isoniazid activation defects in recombinant *Mycobacterium tuberculosis* catalase-peroxidase (KatG) mutants evident in InhA inhibitor production. *Antimicrob. Agents Chemother.* **47:**670–675.

217. **Wengenack, N. L., S. Todorovic, L. Yu, and F. Rusnak.** 1998. Evidence for differential binding of isoniazid by *Mycobacterium tuberculosis* KatG and the isoniazid-resistant mutant KatG(S315T). *Biochemistry* **37:**15825–15834.

218. **Wengenack, N. L., J. R. Uhl, A. L. St Amand, A. J. Tomlinson, L. M. Benson, S. Naylor, B. C. Kline, F. R. Cockerill III, and F. Rusnak.** 1997. Recombinant *Mycobacterium tuberculosis* KatG(S315T) is a competent catalase-peroxidase with reduced activity toward isoniazid. *J. Infect. Dis.* **176:**722–727.

219. **Werngren, J., and S. E. Hoffner.** 2003. Drug-susceptible *Mycobacterium tuberculosis* Beijing genotype does not develop mutation-conferred resistance to rifampin at an elevated rate. *J. Clin. Microbiol.* **41:**1520–1524.

220. **Whiteway, J., P. Koziarz, J. Veall, N. Sandhu, P. Kumar, B. Hoecher, and I. B. Lambert.** 1998. Oxygen-insensitive nitroreductases: analysis of the roles of *nfsA* and *nfsB* in development of resistance to 5-nitrofuran derivatives in *Escherichia coli*. *J. Bacteriol.* **180:**5529–5539.

221. **Williams, D. L., L. Spring, L. Collins, L. P. Miller, L. B. Heifets, P. R. Gangadharam, and T. P. Gillis.** 1998. Contribution of *rpoB* mutations to development of rifamycin cross-resistance in *Mycobacterium tuberculosis*. *Antimicrob. Agents Chemother.* **42:**1853–1857.

222. **Williams, D. L., C. Waguespack, K. Eisenach, J. T. Crawford, F. Portaels, M. Salfinger, C. M. Nolan, C. Abe, V. Sticht-Groh, and T. P. Gillis.** 1994. Characterization of rifampin-resistance in pathogenic mycobacteria. *Antimicrob. Agents Chemother.* **38:**2380–2386.

223. **Wilming, M., and K. Johnsson.** 1999. Spontaneous formation of the bioactive form of the tuberculosis drug isoniazid. *Angew Chem. Int. Ed. Engl.* **38:**2588–2590.

224. **Wilson, M., J. DeRisi, H. H. Kristensen, P. Imboden, S. Rane, P. O. Brown, and G. K. Schoolnik.** 1999. Exploring drug-induced alterations in gene expression in *Mycobacterium tuberculosis* by microarray hybridization. *Proc. Natl. Acad. Sci. USA* **96:**12833–12838.

225. **Wilson, T., G. W. de Lisle, J. A. Marcinkeviciene, J. S. Blanchard, and D. M. Collins.** 1998. Antisense RNA to *ahpC*, an oxidative stress defence gene involved in isoniazid resistance, indicates that AhpC of *Mycobacterium bovis* has virulence properties. *Microbiology* **144:**2687–2695.

226. **Wilson, T. M., G. W. de Lisle, and D. M. Collins.** 1995. Effect of *inhA* and *katG* on isoniazid resistance and virulence of *Mycobacterium bovis*. *Mol. Microbiol.* **15:**1009–1015.

227. **Winder, F. G.** 1982. *Mode of Action of the Antimycobacterial Agents and Associated Aspects of the Molecular Biology of the Mycobacteria*. Academic Press Inc., New York, N.Y.

228. **Winder, F. G., P. Collins, and S. A. Rooney.** 1970. Effects of isoniazid on mycolic acid synthesis in *Mycobacterium tuberculosis* and on its cell envelope. *Biochem. J.* **117:**27P.

229. **Wolucka, B. A., M. R. McNeil, E. de Hoffmann, T. Chojnacki, and P. J. Brennan.** 1994. Recognition of the lipid intermediate for arabinogalactan/arabinomannan biosynthe-

sis and its relation to the mode of action of ethambutol on mycobacteria. *J. Biol. Chem.* **269:**23328–23335.

230. **World Health Organization.** 2000. *Anti-Tuberculosis Drug Resistance in the World.* Report no. 2. *Prevalence and Trends.* The WHO/IUATLD Global Project on Anti-Tuberculosis Drug Resistance Surveillance. Geneva, Switzerland.

231. **Yu, S., S. Girotto, C. Lee, and R. S. Magliozzo.** 2003. Reduced affinity for isoniazid in the S315T mutant of *Mycobacterium tuberculosis* KatG is a key factor in antibiotic resistance. *J. Biol. Chem.* **278:**14769–14775.

232. **Zahrt, T. C., J. Song, J. Siple, and V. Deretic.** 2001. Mycobacterial FurA is a negative regulator of catalase-peroxidase gene *katG. Mol. Microbiol.* **39:**1174–1185.

233. **Zatman, L. J., N. O. Kaplan, S. P. Colowick, and M. M. Ciotti.** 1954. Effect of isonicotinic acid hydrazide on diphosphopyridine nucleotidases. *J. Biol. Chem.* **209:**453–466.

234. **Zhang, Y., T. Garbe, and D. Young.** 1993. Transformation with *katG* restores isoniazid-sensitivity in *Mycobacterium tuberculosis* isolates resistant to a range of drug concentrations. *Mol. Microbiol.* **8:**521–524.

235. **Zhang, Y., B. Heym, B. Allen, D. Young, and S. Cole.** 1992. The catalase-peroxidase gene and isoniazid resistance of *Mycobacterium tuberculosis. Nature* **358:**591–593.

236. **Zhang, Y., and D. Mitchison.** 2003. The curious characteristics of pyrazinamide: a review. *Int. J. Tuberc. Lung Dis.* **7:**6–21.

237. **Zhang, Y., S. Permar, and Z. Sun.** 2002. Conditions that may affect the results of susceptibility testing of *Mycobacterium tuberculosis* to pyrazinamide. *J. Med. Microbiol.* **51:**42–49.

238. **Zhang, Y., A. Scorpio, H. Nikaido, and Z. Sun.** 1999. Role of acid pH and deficient efflux of pyrazinoic acid in unique susceptibility of *Mycobacterium tuberculosis* to pyrazinamide. *J. Bacteriol.* **181:**2044–2049.

239. **Zhang, Y., and A. Telenti.** 2000. *Genetics of Drug Resistance in* Mycobacterium tuberculosis. ASM Press, Washington, D.C.

240. **Zhang, Y., M. M. Wade, A. Scorpio, H. Zhang, and Z. Sun.** 2003. Mode of action of pyrazinamide: disruption of *Mycobacterium tuberculosis* membrane transport and energetics by pyrazinoic acid. *J. Antimicrob. Chemother.* **52:**790–795.

241. **Zhang, Y., and D. Young.** 1994. Strain variation in the *katG* region of *Mycobacterium tuberculosis. Mol. Microbiol.* **14:**301–308.

242. **Zhang, Y., H. Zhang, and Z. Sun.** 2003. Susceptibility of *Mycobacterium tuberculosis* to weak acids. *J. Antimicrob. Chemother.* **52:**56–60.

243. **Zimhony, O., J. S. Cox, J. T. Welch, C. Vilchèze, and W. R. Jacobs, Jr.** 2000. Pyrazinamide inhibits the eukaryotic-like fatty acid synthetase I (FASI) of *Mycobacterium tuberculosis. Nat. Med.* **6:**1043–1047.

THE ORGANISM *MYCOBACTERIUM TUBERCULOSIS*

V. GENOMICS

Chapter 9

Introduction to Functional Genomics of the *Mycobacterium tuberculosis* Complex

PRISCILLE BRODIN, CAROLINE DEMANGEL, AND STEWART T. COLE

The past decade has seen a giant step in the genomics of the *Mycobacterium tuberculosis* complex. The establishment of the genome sequence of *M. tuberculosis* H37Rv in 1998 paved the way for major breakthroughs in understanding the biology of tubercle bacilli in particular and mycobacteria in general (14). Until the 1990s, basic research on *M. tuberculosis* was greatly hampered by the slow growth of this organism, the lack of genetic tools, and the biohazard facilities necessary for its handling. The *M. tuberculosis* complex has been defined as a single species comprising five distinct members: *M. tuberculosis*, *M. bovis*, *M. africanum*, *M. canettii*, and *M. microti*. Of particular significance is the finding that all these members have very little genome variation, which makes comparative-genomics studies fairly straightforward (54).

This chapter starts with a description of the three complete genome sequences of *M. tuberculosis* H37Rv, *M. tuberculosis* CDC 1551, and *M. bovis* AF2122/97 and highlights the genomic differences between members of the *M. tuberculosis* complex. Emphasis is given to the comparison between the human pathogenic strains and the two vaccine strains, *M. bovis* bacille Calmette Guérin (BCG) and *M. microti*. In the second part, we focus on the application of functional genomic strategies, such as transcriptomics and transposon mutagenesis, to discover essential genes and to identify the function of the unknown open reading frames (ORFs). Finally, proteomics and structural genomics, approaches which have been made possible as a result of genomics, are discussed briefly.

GENOMICS AND COMPARATIVE GENOMICS

Characteristic Features of the *M. tuberculosis* Genome

Tremendous large-scale efforts have now led to the sequences of numerous genomes ranging from simple bacteria to complex organisms such as humans. The prokaryote world now accounts for more than 200 sequences, with the *Mycobacterium* genus being represented by 4 complete genome sequences, those of *M. tuberculosis* strains H37Rv and CDC 1551, *M. bovis* AF2122/97, and *M. leprae* (14, 15, 19, 21), while 10 others are currently being sequenced. This wealth of information can be downloaded from various websites (http://www.pasteur.fr/recherche/unites/Lgmb, http://www.sanger.ac.uk, and http://www.tigr.org).

The sequence of the first complete genome of *M. tuberculosis*, that of the paradigm laboratory strain H37Rv, comprises 4,411,532 bp. Its circular chromosome is about the size of that of *Escherichia coli* and is almost 10 times larger than the smallest bacterial one, that of *Mycoplasma genitalium* (58). Unlike *Helicobacter pylori*, the *M. tuberculosis* genome does not appear to carry a plasticity zone responsible for major chromosomal reorganization. It has a high G+C content of 65.6%, a parameter which is associated with an aerobic lifestyle (40). Unlike some environmental mycobacteria, no plasmid has yet been identified among the different members of the *M. tuberculosis* complex. A common feature, shared with most other bacteria, is the fact that virtually all of the DNA codes for proteins.

Priscille Brodin, Caroline Demangel, and Stewart T. Cole • Unité de Génétique Moléculaire Bactérienne, Institut Pasteur, 28 Rue du Docteur Roux, 75724 Paris Cedex 15, France.

Assignment of the ORFs was carried out by using a variety of bioinformatics routines, including codon usage, positional base preference, and database searches (14). All coding sequences were given a Rv number and, where appropriate, a systematic name. The last reannotation identified 4,043 genes thought to encode 3,993 proteins and 50 stable RNAs (11). Their sequences can be directly retrieved at http://genolist.pasteur.fr/TubercuList/. For the information to remain accurate, the database is constantly updated. Each ORF was assigned to a functional category, as shown in Fig. 1.

M. tuberculosis has the metabolic potential to adapt to aerobic and microaerophilic as well as anaerobic environments. It harbors complex gene regulatory systems with 13 sigma factors, 2 different signal transduction mechanisms comprising 11 two-component systems, and 11 Ser/Thr protein kinases, together with more than 100 other regulators. The most striking feature is the abundance of genes involved in lipid metabolism, 233 to date. Twenty cytochrome P-450 monooxygenases, which may modify lipids, are also present, whereas none is found in *E. coli*. Besides 56 insertion elements and 2 prophages, several large multigene families were uncovered (57). These include 167 genes for the unusual glycine-rich PE and PPE proteins, which occupy about 9% of the genome

and exhibit extensive sequence polymorphism; the 23-member *esx* family, encoding the ESAT-6 and CFP-10 proteins, strong T-cell antigens that exploit a novel protein secretion system for their export (41, 44, 53); and four large operons involved in mammalian cell entry (*mce*), which appear to encode effector molecules, expressed on the surface of *M. tuberculosis*, that are capable of eliciting plasma membrane perturbations in nonphagocytic mammalian cells (12). Finally, a set of 15 *mmpL* genes encodes large membrane proteins, belonging to the RND superfamily (57), which are probably all involved in (glyco)lipid export and may contribute to virulence (10, 16, 17).

Much of the genome sequence still remains to be explored. At present, only 52% of the predicted ORFs can be assigned a function (11). A combination of new bioinformatics tools and experimental data are now required to improve the genome annotation. For example, the crystal structure of Rv3853 revealed that neither this protein nor its orthologs in other bacteria are methyltransferases as suggested by the initial annotation carried out by genome comparison (29). Besides, the number and length of ORFs may change as more and more data emerge from complementary techniques such as proteomics (30).

More recently, the genome of a clinical strain of *M. tuberculosis*, CDC 1551, was sequenced (19).

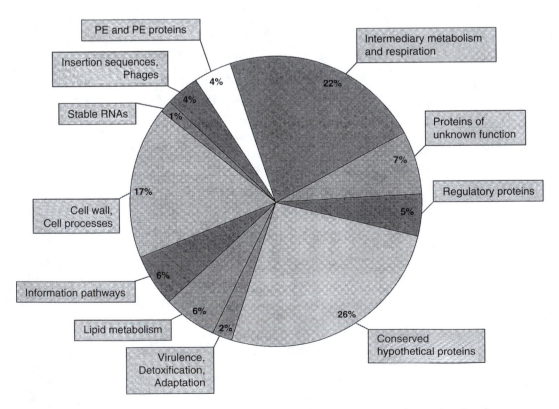

Figure 1. Distribution of the 4,043 genes in *M. tuberculosis* H37Rv according to their function.

This isolate appeared to be highly infectious in humans (60), capable of inducing greater immunoreactivity but displaying comparable growth rate in mice relative to *M. tuberculosis* H37Rv (35). Despite having suffered fewer passages, the genome of CDC 1551 was shown to be highly similar to that of *M. tuberculosis* H37Rv. As notable differences, CDC 1551 harbors 86 insertions or deletions greater than 10 bp (InDels) and 1,075 single-nucleotide polymorphisms (SNPs) relative to H37Rv. Of the nucleotide substitutions that occur in coding regions, 579 are nonsynonymous and induce amino acid changes. Some of the SNPs were previously described, like the GyrA-95 and the KatG-463 polymorphisms, whereas the newly identified ones may prove useful for deeper phylogenetic analysis (19). Among them, SNP-2904 and SNP-4090, localized in the genes encoding the carbon starvation protein A and a putative transcriptional regulator, respectively, are highly polymorphic. Regarding the larger deletions, 26 occur in coding regions whereas 11 are intergenic. The insertions introduced 17 complete ORFs, half of which have a known function, like the adenylate cyclase (MT1360), a glycosyltransferase (MT1800), an oxidoreductase (MT1801) and paralogs of *moaA* (MT3426) and *moaB* (MT3427). It is also worth noting a change in the 5' end of a phospholipase C gene and a transport protein, with 12 membrane-spanning segments, which may be potentially involved in mycobacterial virulence.

Another important feature is that almost half of the InDels involve genes encoding PPE or PE-PGRS family proteins (see chapter 33) (1, 6). Heterogeneity in these protein families appears to be frequent among other members of the *M. tuberculosis* complex, as discussed later for the *M. bovis* genome. The analysis of the CDC 1551 genome did not enable any obvious conclusion to be drawn regarding the peculiar phenotype of this strain relative to the reference one. These genomic data also confirm the fact that the *M. tuberculosis* genome sequence is highly conserved and raises the issue that differences among isolates are now more likely to be found through subtle global analysis of the biosynthesis, metabolic, or information pathways.

Another comparative-genomics approach undertaken was to compare *M. tuberculosis* with other human pathogens such as *M. leprae*, *M. avium*, and *M. ulcerans*. Of particular note, the *M. leprae* genome, at 3.27 Mb, is more than 1 Mb smaller than that of *M. tuberculosis* (15) and also contains numerous pseudogenes. This genome downsizing and gene decay have eliminated entire metabolic pathways together with their regulatory functions, especially those involved in catabolism. Since only 1,605 protein-

encoding genes remain in *M. leprae*, comparison of the two genomes generates new, testable hypotheses regarding which genes are essential for the survival of *M. tuberculosis*.

Comparison of *M. bovis* with *M. tuberculosis* Provides Clues for a New Evolutionary Scenario but Not for Host Spectrum

M. bovis, the bovine tubercle bacillus, has the broadest host tropism, and this includes humans. The genome sequence of the fully virulent strain AF2122/97, isolated in 1997 from a diseased cow in Great Britain, revealed a sequence identity greater than 99.95% relative to *M. tuberculosis* (21). At 4,345,492 bp, the bovine genome is ~60 kb smaller. Besides, with one exception, no genes appear to be present solely in *M. bovis*, which suggests that the host range is probably not due to the presence of a specific set of genes but, rather, to differential gene expression or to altered surface components. The variations between *M. tuberculosis* and *M. bovis* reside either in large genomic deletions named regions of difference (RD) or in SNPs. No obvious translocations, duplications, or inversions were found. The 11 RDs, ranging from 1 to 12.7 kb, were initially identified by using arrays and hybridization-based methods (2, 23, 24). Only one region, called TbD1, is present in *M. bovis* but absent from the majority of *M. tuberculosis* strains (8). Detailed sequence comparison revealed that there are 2,437 SNPs between *M. bovis* and *M. tuberculosis* H37Rv, which represents about 1 SNP every 2 kb, whereas comparison of the two *M. tuberculosis* sequences showed that SNPs occurred once every 4 kb (21).

The greatest variation between *M. bovis* and *M. tuberculosis* has been identified among cell wall components and secreted proteins. First, about 60% of the genes encoding PE-PGRS and PPE proteins suffered from in-frame insertions or deletions whereas the other gene families in the rest of the genome were essentially untouched. Second, a number of genes involved in the synthesis and export of polyketides (*pks* and *mmpSL* genes) differ. Third, regarding the known T-cell antigens, six genes of the ESAT-6 family are partially or fully absent from *M. bovis*. Concerning the serodominant antigens, MPB70 and MPB83 appear to be overexpressed in comparison to *M. tuberculosis*, possibly as a result of regulatory mutations.

Comparative genomics has also led to revision of the scheme for the evolution of the *M. tuberculosis* complex. It has long been postulated that the human tubercle bacillus evolved from the bovine one. A recent study by Brosch et al. refuted this hypothesis by demonstrating that several RDs can be considered with certainty as reliable evolutionary markers (8). Indeed, RD9 is absent from all strains of the evolutionary lineage represented by *M. africanum*, *M. microti*, and *M. bovis* whereas it is present in *M. tuberculosis* and *M. canettii*. In contrast, TbD1 is absent from most *M. tuberculosis* strains, especially those associated with current epidemics, yet present among all other members of the complex. Together, these results, combined with the absence of RD1, RD4, RD7, RD8, and RD10 from *M. tuberculosis*, showed that *M. tuberculosis* probably did not evolve from *M. bovis* but, instead, that *M. bovis* and *M. tuberculosis* are derived from a common ancestor that more closely resembled a human pathogen such as *M. canetti*. It is worth noting that InDels are appropriate markers for the molecular typing of the different isolates and extend and complement the current spoligotyping system (42).

Finding Virulence Factors of *M. tuberculosis* through the Features of the Attenuated and Vaccine Strains

Comparative genomics of the attenuated strain *M. tuberculosis* H37Ra, a close relative of H37Rv, identified several regions absent from the virulent strain, termed RvD1 to RvD5, that result from IS*6110*-mediated deletion events (9) but failed to uncover the genomic basis for the attenuation of this strain. Since it is likely that point mutations play a key role, the genome sequence of H37Ra would be of great help.

Besides H37Ra, genomic analysis has been undertaken with two other species that are avirulent in humans and have been used extensively as vaccines against tuberculosis, *M. microti* and *M. bovis* BCG. *M. microti* is naturally attenuated and was originally isolated from voles in the United Kingdom in the 1930s. Two live vaccines derived from the initial vole isolates were used by the British Medical Research Council in the United Kingdom and in Czechoslovakia in the 1960s. The second, and most widely used, vaccine is the bacille de Calmette et Guérin (BCG), which was obtained after multiple passages of the parental *M. bovis* strain on potato medium enriched with ox bile. Recently, the reasons for the attenuation of both *M. microti* and BCG were partially elucidated at the genomic level by comparing the distribution of RD loci between virulent and attenuated species (2, 23). For instance, RD1, RD2, and RD3 are confined to *M. bovis* BCG (34) whereas a further three regions, called MiD, were shown to be specific for *M. microti* strain OV254 relative to H37Rv (7). However, by functional genomics, only one deletion that is common to both *M. microti* and

BCG, but not identical, was shown to be responsible for attenuation.

The RD1^{bcg} deletion removes all or part of nine ORFs from Rv3871 to Rv3879, while, in *M. microti*, an overlapping deletion occurred in the RD1 locus and removed ORF Rv3864 to Rv3876 from all tested strains (7). Comparison of the RD1^{mic} and RD1^{bcg} regions revealed that four proteins, PE35, PPE68, CFP-10, and ESAT-6, are absent from the vaccine strains while present in the virulent strains. To assess their role in virulence, this 12.7-kb region was reintroduced into either *M. bovis* BCG or *M. microti* OV254 by using an integrating cosmid encompassing the entire RD1 (43). The resulting recombinants, named BCG::RD1 or *M. microti*::RD1 "knock-ins," were much more virulent than their parental strain in immunodeficient mice and induced severe splenomegaly. In contrast, an RD1 "knockout" mutant of *M. tuberculosis* H37Rv was strikingly less virulent than the wild type in immunocompetent animals and behaved similarly to the BCG control (28, 33). In immunocompetent mice, the BCG::RD1 knock-in was more persistent whereas no strong phenotype was observed for the BCG recombinants expressing other RDs such as RD3, RD4, RD5, RD7, or RD9. Together, these results show that RD1 is involved in pathogenicity and that its loss was indeed a major event in the attenuation process of BCG, although the full virulence of *M. bovis* or *M. tuberculosis* was not totally restored by complementation of BCG with RD1 alone. This implies that the virulence of *M. tuberculosis* is not mediated by a pathogenicity island, as in *Shigella* or *Yersinia*, but results from combinatorial effects. Thus, together with RD1, other RDs or point mutations are surely at play and remain to be found in *M. bovis* BCG. The ongoing assembly of the complete genome sequences of the avirulent members of the *M. tuberculosis* complex may bring new insight into potential virulence factors, although clues about pathogenicity are more likely to be found downstream, at either the transcriptome or proteome level.

To this effect, a recent comparison of the proteome of the virulent *M. tuberculosis* H37Rv and Erdmann strains with that of *M. bovis* BCG strains Chicago and Copenhagen resulted in the identification of 27 different proteins specifically absent from the attenuated strains (36). Whereas 8 of them are products of genes localized in the RDs, 19 proteins were not predicted by comparative genomics experiments. To fully understand the role of the identified transcriptome and proteome products, new genetic approaches have been undertaken and are detailed below.

TRANSCRIPTOMICS

The availability of the complete genome sequence of *M. tuberculosis,* combined with major progress in transcriptome technology, has led to the identification of a number of virulence genes. Gene expression analysis usually assumes that bacteria upregulate virulence factors only when functionally needed, a reasonable hypothesis considering that gene expression is tightly regulated in bacteria. Pinpointing clusters of genes that are coexpressed or cosuppressed under specific conditions has also been used to identify possible virulence genes, through "guilt by association." Typically, expression analysis compares the levels of RNA transcripts in two pools of bacteria grown under different conditions by hybridization to DNA chips or microarrays.

The first gene expression studies were performed with in vitro-grown organisms, with environmental or physiological conditions mimicking infection, on account of the small quantities of pure bacterial RNA that can be extracted from infected hosts. Of particular interest is the identification of an *M. tuberculosis* cluster of genes regulated under hypoxic conditions by Sherman et al. (51). Using a whole-genome array, the authors identified a set of more than 100 genes with altered expression at reduced oxygen tensions. Among them was the *acr* gene, encoding α-crystallin, a well-characterized virulence factor required for *M. tuberculosis* growth in macrophages (62), and an operon apparently regulating *acr* expression. Since several lines of evidence have linked *M. tuberculosis* growth inhibition with hypoxic conditions, these genes may be required for the establishment of latent states during tuberculosis. Shi et al. elegantly confirmed the up-regulation of *acr* expression in mouse lungs infected with *M. tuberculosis* (52). In this work, real-time PCR was used to enumerate copies of bacterial mRNAs specific for six genes, known to be induced by hypoxia or up-regulated in actively multiplying bacteria. In parallel with *acr* up-regulated expression, the authors observed that the genes for superoxide dismutase (*sodA* and *sodC*) and fibronectin binding protein B (*fbpB*) were down-regulated, defining a transcription signature for the transition of *M. tuberculosis* from growth to latency.

Using selective capture of transcribed sequences, genes expressed by *M. tuberculosis* in response to phagocytosis by macrophages were identified (25). These included genes encoding the alternative sigma factors (*sigE* and *sigH*), isocitrate lyase, a class I penicillin binding protein (*ponA*), a polyketide synthase (*pks2*), the UvrABC endonuclease, a cation transporter (*ctpV*), and several proteins of unknown function, as well as, once again, the *mce1* virulence operon.

More recently, an elegant microarray-based analysis of the *M. tuberculosis* transcriptome identified genes that are differentially expressed in naive and activated macrophage phagosomes, and the findings indicate that the intraphagosmal environment is rich in lipids, poor in iron and carbohydrates, and a strong source of oxidative and nitrosative stress (50). These gene expression-profiling studies provide new insights into the mechanisms employed by *M. tuberculosis* to survive the hostile intracellular environment and are valuable for the design of rational antimycobacterial treatments.

Promoters that are specifically activated in host cells or live animals have also been successfully identified by the differential fluorescence induction technique. Using differential fluorescence induction, genes induced in frogs chronically infected by *M. marinum* were selected (45). Two independent promoters were found to be activated in *M. marinum*-infected macrophages and in granulomas from infected frogs. Importantly, the downstream genes were homologous to two *M. tuberculosis* proteins of the PE-PGRS family. Mutants with insertions in those two genes had a decreased capacity to replicate within cultured macrophages and to persist in granulomas. Some PE-PGRS proteins have been shown to be surface proteins (1), but their function remains unclear (6, 14). This report demonstrates the direct implication of two PE-PGRS protein members in pathogenesis in *M. marinum*. Independent work based on transposon mutagenesis suggests that the PE-PGRS gene family is particularly rich in genes required for viability (32); assuming that this mutagenesis technique was not prone to positional bias, these results would extend this finding to mycobacterial survival in vivo.

MUTAGENESIS STUDIES

Knowledge of the *M. tuberculosis* genome sequence has allowed the rational design of a number of attenuated *M. tuberculosis* mutants by inactivation of genes involved in essential metabolic pathways using gene replacement technology (see chapter 12). These include mutants auxotrophic for several amino acids or mutants with altered nitrogen or iron metabolism, and are attenuated for growth in mice to various extents (see reference 27 for a review). Mutations in *icl* (encoding isocitrate lyase, a critical enzyme of the glyoxylate shunt required for fatty acid metabolism) did not affect bacterial growth during the acute phase of infection but limited the persistence of bacilli after establishment of acquired immunity by the host (38). The construction and characterization of defined mutants provide important clues to understanding the mechanisms used by *M. tuberculosis* to escape the immune system. However, the inactivation of genes one by one is a lengthy process, and so it was important to develop novel approaches to the high-throughput identification of virulence genes. These methods are generally based on a three-step process starting with high-density transposon mutagenesis followed by screening for mutants and finally by mapping or sequencing the insertion sites of the nonlethal mutations.

Transposons Tn*5367*, Tn*5368*, and Tn*5370*, which are derived from mycobacterial insertion sequences, can be efficiently delivered to the *M. tuberculosis* complex members. By combining the production of random mutant libraries with the identification of mutants with decreased virulence (26), signature-tagged mutagenesis has led to the isolation of a set of virulence-associated genes, almost all involved in lipid metabolism (10, 17). Using a different approach, McAdam et al. (37) have generated a defined library of *M. tuberculosis* mutants by insertional mutagenesis using the Tn*5370* transposon. Preliminary analysis of the mutants revealed that only a limited number of ORFs (351 ORFs) were actually mutated, probably as a result of the transposon showing insertion site bias. Then, screening of selected mutants for attenuated virulence using mice with severe combined immunodeficiency (the SCID mouse model) led to a number of clones with insertions in genes of known or unknown function, which were good candidates for further investigation. Three of them, inactivating Rv1891c, Rv3404c, and, more interestingly, Rv1290c, which encodes an integral membrane protein, were significantly attenuated.

An important breakthrough came when it was shown that the mariner transposon-based element, Himar1, which requires only the dinucleotide TA as its insertion site, could transpose efficiently in mycobacteria (47). This genetic tool, in conjunction with the use of microarrays, resulted in a powerful technique for the high-throughput identification of essential genes called TraSH (for "transposon site hybridization"). TraSH utilizes a transposon containing two outward-facing T7 RNA polymerase promoters, allowing the in vitro transcription of a labeled RNA complementary to the chromosomal DNA flanking each insertion site. TraSH appears particularly well suited to the identification of genes required for growth under one condition but not another. It has been used successfully to identify genes involved in optimal growth of *M. tuberculosis* (48, 49). These genes, although required for mycobacterial growth in vitro, are also likely to be important in vivo, and represent potential targets for antimycobacterial drugs that could be easily evaluated. Interestingly, 78% of

these genes have been retained in the much smaller genome of *M. leprae*, despite its extensive reductive evolution (15), and this indicates their likely importance in both organisms. *M. leprae* replicates remarkably slowly in vivo and has not been cultured in vitro despite numerous attempts; it is possible that the loss of some of the pathways identified as enhancing the growth of *M. tuberculosis* may account for this (48, 49).

Using *M. marinum* as a model for pathogenic aspects of tuberculosis, Gao et al. (20) have isolated by mariner-based mutagenesis a locus involved in the intracellular survival of *M. tuberculosis*, whereas Lamichhane et al. (32) used the same strategy to generate a library of defined *M. tuberculosis* mutants. Then, by combining the knowledge of TA-containing ORFs with a list of experimentally defined essential genes, the authors used a statistical approach to predict essential genes in the whole genome. The study concluded that only 35% of the *M. tuberculosis* ORFs are likely to be essential for simple viability and proposed a list of putative essential genes representing valuable tools for comparative functional genomics and therapeutic target design.

Stewart et al. (56) have combined targeted mutagenesis with whole-genome expression profiling using microarrays to investigate the heat shock response in *M. tuberculosis*. Heat shock proteins not only are expressed in response to increased ambient temperature but also are induced in both host and pathogen during infectious processes. In fact, partial disruption of heat shock regulation in *M. tuberculosis* was found to impair the ability of the bacteria to establish a chronic infection (55). Interestingly, this study demonstrated that a transcriptional repressor of heat shock genes controls the expression of an *acr* homolog in *M. tuberculosis*. Using a comparable approach, Dahl et al. (18) showed that inactivation of Rel_{Mtb} induces a general alteration of *M. tuberculosis* transcription and decreases substantially the capacity of the bacilli to adapt to starvation. Rel_{Mtb} is an enzyme controlling the intracellular level of hyperphosphorylated guanine nucleotides, which are signaling molecules produced in nutrient-limited environments. As demonstrated by microarray analysis, loss of Rel_{Mtb} was associated with major metabolic shifts, alterations in the expression of known virulence factors (macrophage cell entry *mce1* operon, *icl*, and PE-PGRS proteins) and of the major antigens, the antigen 85 gene complex and ESAT-6. Since Rel_{Mtb} mutants are defective for persistence in vivo and since bacilli extracted from granulomas show starvation symptoms, these results strongly suggest that nutrient deprivation is a critical element of disease containment by the host.

PROTEOMICS

The complete set of proteins from a given organism is referred to as the proteome; like the transcriptome, this is dynamic and can vary as a function of the growth conditions or environmental changes. Since chapter 16 presents a detailed description of the proteome, our selection is limited to a few biologically interesting examples. The classical proteome approach comprises protein separation by two-dimensional gel electrophoresis (2-DE) and spot identification by mass spectrometry or any biochemical or chemical cleavage techniques such as Edman degradation or enzymatic proteolysis. For each spot, the peptide sequences and/or masses determined experimentally are compared with peptide mass maps created by in silico cleavage of the predicted proteins in the *M. tuberculosis* database. This technique identified six *M. tuberculosis* proteins, with an average size of 10 kDa, that were not initially predicted by genomics (30). Proteomics has the potential to detect very subtle differences, for example posttranslational modifications such as methylation, glycosylation, and also proteolytic maturation. In addition, the analysis can focus on a given cellular fraction of the mycobacteria, like, for example, the secretome (referring to the secreted proteins), or on specific protein subsets like the kinome, corresponding to all the phosphorylated proteins. In each case, the proteome is strongly influenced by bacterial growth conditions such as the media, the pH, and the aerobic status.

Several mycobacterial proteome databases have been established and can be easily accessed via the Internet (Fig. 2). The first report of proteomics of whole-cell extracts and culture supernatants of *M. tuberculosis* H37Rv led to approximately 1,800 and 800 protein spots, respectively (31). It is worth remembering that a single protein could generate multiple spots on 2-DE. This analysis resulted in the identification of 1,300 protein species and proved useful in defining co- and posttranslational protein modifications, which could not be detected by a simple genomic or transcriptome analysis. Subsequently, with coupled mass spectrometry and immunodetection, Rosenkrands et al. were able to identify up to 49 culture filtrate proteins and 118 from whole-cell lysate, which were further classified according to their function (46). Surprisingly, to date, no proteome projects have been able to identify members belonging to the PE and PPE multigene families. This is perhaps due to their intrinsic properties of being membrane-bound proteins or to the paucity of Lys and Arg residues, the target of trypsin, the protease used to generate the peptides for MS analysis (1, 6).

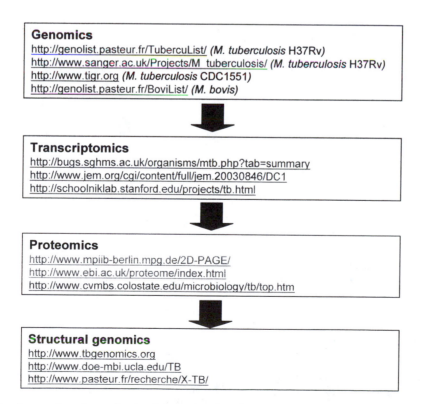

Genomics
http://genolist.pasteur.fr/Tuberculist/ *(M. tuberculosis* H37Rv)
http://www.sanger.ac.uk/Projects/M_tuberculosis/ *(M. tuberculosis* H37Rv)
http://www.tigr.org *(M. tuberculosis* CDC1551)
http://genolist.pasteur.fr/BoviList/ *(M. bovis)*

Transcriptomics
http://bugs.sghms.ac.uk/organisms/mtb.php?tab=summary
http://www.jem.org/cgi/content/full/jem.20030846/DC1
http://schoolniklab.stanford.edu/projects/tb.html

Proteomics
http://www.mpiib-berlin.mpg.de/2D-PAGE/
http://www.ebi.ac.uk/proteome/index.html
http://www.cvmbs.colostate.edu/microbiology/tb/top.htm

Structural genomics
http://www.tbgenomics.org
http://www.doe-mbi.ucla.edu/TB
http://www.pasteur.fr/recherche/X-TB/

Figure 2. Functional genomics scheme showing information flow from the genome to applications. The URLs of useful websites are indicated.

Another type of approach is comparative proteomics, where differences either between *M. tuberculosis* complex strains or between growth conditions can be monitored. First, the proteome of the *M. tuberculosis* strains H37Rv and Erdman was compared with that of BCG strains (31, 36). Among the 25 mobility variants between *M. tuberculosis* H37Rv and BCG Chicago, 6 were absent from the BCG proteome and 8 resulted from amino acid changes or posttranslational modification. Second, 2-DE gel comparisons combined with in silico analysis of the genome sequences were carried out for *M. tuberculosis* strains H37Rv and CDC 1551 (3). In this study, only 17 differences were uncovered between *M. tuberculosis* H37Rv and CDC 1551 out of approximately 1,750 distinct spots characterized (3). Mobility variants of the transcriptional regulator MoxR (Rv1479) and an alcohol dehydrogenase Rv0927c were seen in CDC 1551 culture, whereas alkyl hydroperoxide reductase chain C (AhpC) and HisA were overexpressed in H37Rv relative to CDC 1551. Bioinformatics comparisons of the proteome provided the explanation for MoxR, since a single-base change in the *moxR* sequence induced a change in the pI and M_r values of the corresponding protein. As for HisA, its absence resulted from a mutation in the upstream gene, *hisH*. Neither analysis of the genome nor analysis of the proteome of CDC 1551 enabled any obvious conclusion to be drawn regarding its peculiar phenotype relative to the reference strain.

Furthermore, Betts et al. identified a set of proteins differentially expressed during growth under nutrient starvation (4). Six proteins (Rv0351, Rv1860, Rv2462, Rv2557, Rv2558, and 16-kDa α-crystallin [Acr]) were identified as differentially expressed under these conditions. Another study focused on the mycobacterial proteome in vivo. Analysis of BCG-infected THP-1 macrophages showed increased expression inside macrophages of six mycobacterial proteins (16-kDa α-crystallin [Acr]), GroEL-1, GroEL-2, Rv2623, InhA, and elongation factor Tu) (39). Interestingly, although more than 500 gene transcripts were shown to be up- or down-regulated, only a few differences were observed at the proteome level, highlighting the need for better protein solubilization and quantitation techniques and for complementary approaches such as structural genomics.

STRUCTURAL GENOMICS

The goal of structural genomics is to apply high-throughput technologies to generate large amounts of recombinant proteins of *M. tuberculosis* for structure determination. Knowledge of the three-dimensional structure not only facilitates targeted research such as the rational design of inhibitors and drugs but also can catalyze discovery. For instance, functional information is lacking for as many as 40% of the proteins of *M. tuberculosis* since their sequences show no significant similarity to those of proteins with known functions. However, during evolution, the structures of proteins are generally much better conserved than their sequences; in consequence, comparison of new structures with those present in the Protein Data Bank can reveal common folds and organization that in turn provide potential information about the biological function that can be tested by experimentation. Examples of this approach are given elsewhere in this volume (chapter 11).

SOME APPLICATIONS

Genomic analysis of *M. tuberculosis* has provided us with a rich source of information about the pathogen, and while this new knowledge is resulting in a better understanding of the molecular basis of pathogenesis and elucidation of the biology of the tubercle bacilli, it is the application of functional genomics to problems of public health that is now required. There has been progress in three main areas: the development of diagnostic tests, the identification of novel drug targets and drug discovery, and vaccine development. Genomics has contributed directly to the improved detection of drug-resistant strains of *M. tuberculosis*, and a variety of rapid molecular biology-based drug susceptibility tests now exist (59). Likewise, various rapid methods to type clinical isolates to the species or strain level are finding growing application in clinical microbiology (42). The diagnosis of the disease itself is also benefiting from better definition of the antigens produced by the bacillus and their interaction with the cell-mediated immune system. For example, a powerful test has been developed for detecting antigen-specific production of gamma interferon in cattle infected with *M. bovis* (61), and similar tests will soon be available for evaluation in humans.

Extensive efforts have been made to identify and characterize essential proteins in *M. tuberculosis* that could serve as novel drug targets, and the combined application of comparative genomics and saturation transposon mutagenesis has resulted in major progress toward this goal (13, 32, 48, 49). Structural genomics is generating templates for rational drug design, and a variety of functional genomics techniques are facilitating the elucidation of the mechanism of action of new lead compounds. This is illustrated well by a recent study in which microarrays were used successfully to derive transcriptional signatures for new and old drugs (5), and transcriptomics will probably find application in monitoring the response of patients to chemotherapy by identifying gene expression profiles that predict recovery, nonresponsiveness, or relapse. In turn, this information will help shorten the drug development time line.

Genomics is also underpinning vaccine development programs by defining the complete set of antigens in the organism and providing the means for their discovery, production, and manipulation. The three main areas of vaccine development, i.e., subunit vaccines, live attenuated vaccines, and nucleic acid vaccines, are all benefiting greatly from our knowledge of the genome sequence of *M. tuberculosis*. For instance, secreted or surface-exposed proteins are widely regarded as good candidates for extensive immunological exploration owing to their early contact with the innate and acquired immune systems. Many of these proteins are currently being investigated following their identification by bioinformatics (22).

Developing a better vaccine, however, is likely to be the most challenging of all the prophylactic and therapeutic applications. Comparative genomics has provided insight into the coevolution of tubercle bacilli and their mammalian hosts, and one finding of some concern is the great diversity in the sequences of the PE and PPE proteins between strains. If these proteins serve as variable surface antigens, as seems increasingly likely, and thereby affect interactions with host cells and phagocytes, development of a more effective vaccine than BCG may be truly challenging.

Acknowledgments. We thank the Institut Pasteur, the European Community (QLRT-2001-02018), and the Association Française Raoul Follereau for financial support.

REFERENCES

1. Banu, S., N. Honore, B. Saint-Joanis, D. Philpott, M. C. Prevost, and S. T. Cole. 2002. Are the PE-PGRS proteins of *Mycobacterium tuberculosis* variable surface antigens? *Mol. Microbiol.* 44:9–19.

2. Behr, M. A., M. A. Wilson, W. P. Gill, H. Salamon, G. K. Schoolnik, S. Rane, and P. M. Small. 1999. Comparative genomics of BCG vaccines by whole-genome DNA microarray. *Science* 284:1520–1523.

3. Betts, J. C., P. Dodson, S. Quan, A. P. Lewis, P. J. Thomas, K. Duncan, and R. A. McAdam. 2000. Comparison of the proteome of *Mycobacterium tuberculosis* strain H37Rv with clinical isolate CDC 1551. *Microbiology* 146:3205–3216.

4. Betts, J. C., P. T. Lukey, L. C. Robb, R. A. McAdam, and K. Duncan. 2002. Evaluation of a nutrient starvation model of *Mycobacterium tuberculosis* persistence by gene and protein expression profiling. *Mol. Microbiol.* 43:717–731.

5. Betts, J. C., A. McLaren, M. G. Lennon, F. M. Kelly, P. T. Lukey, S. Blakemore, and K. Duncan. 2003. Signature gene expression profiles discriminate between isoniazid-, thiolactomycin-, and triclosan-treated *Mycobacterium tuberculosis*. *Antimicrob. Agents Chemother.* 47:2903–2913.

6. Brennan, M. J., G. Delogu, Y. Chen, S. Bardarov, J. Kriakov, M. Alavi, and W. R. Jacobs, Jr. 2001. Evidence that mycobacterial PE_PGRS proteins are cell surface constituents that influence interactions with other cells. *Infect. Immun.* 69:7326–7333.

7. Brodin, P., K. Eiglmeier, M. Marmiesse, A. Billault, T. Garnier, S. Niemann, S. T. Cole, and R. Brosch. 2002. Bacterial artificial chromosome-based comparative genomic analysis identifies *Mycobacterium microti* as a natural ESAT-6 deletion mutant. *Infect. Immun.* 70:5568–5578.

8. Brosch, R., S. V. Gordon, M. Marmiesse, P. Brodin, C. Buchrieser, K. Eiglmeier, T. Garnier, C. Gutierrez, G. Hewinson, K. Kremer, L. M. Parsons, A. S. Pym, S. Samper, D. van Soolingen, and S. T. Cole. 2002. A new evolutionary scenario for the *Mycobacterium tuberculosis* complex. *Proc. Natl. Acad. Sci. USA* 99:3684–3689.

9. Brosch, R., W. J. Philipp, E. Stavropoulos, M. J. Colston, S. T. Cole, and S. V. Gordon. 1999. Genomic analysis reveals variation between *Mycobacterium tuberculosis* H37Rv and the attenuated *M. tuberculosis* H37Ra strain. *Infect. Immun.* 67:5768–5774.

10. Camacho, L. R., D. Ensergueix, E. Perez, B. Gicquel, and C. Guilhot. 1999. Identification of a virulence gene cluster of *Mycobacterium tuberculosis* by signature-tagged transposon mutagenesis. *Mol. Microbiol.* 34:257–267.

11. Camus, J. C., M. J. Pryor, C. Medigue, and S. T. Cole. 2002. Re-annotation of the genome sequence of *Mycobacterium tuberculosis* H37Rv. *Microbiology* 148:2967–2973.

12. Chitale, S., S. Ehrt, I. Kawamura, T. Fujimura, N. Shimono, N. Anand, S. Lu, L. Cohen-Gould, and L. W. Riley. 2001. Recombinant *Mycobacterium tuberculosis* protein associated with mammalian cell entry. *Cell. Microbiol.* 3:247–254.

13. Cole, S. T. 2002. Comparative mycobacterial genomics as a tool for drug target and antigen discovery. *Eur. Respir. J.* 20: 78S–86S.

14. Cole, S. T., R. Brosch, J. Parkhill, T. Garnier, C. Churcher, D. Harris, S. V. Gordon, K. Eiglmeier, S. Gas, C. E. Barry, III, F. Tekaia, K. Badcock, D. Basham, D. Brown, T. Chillingworth, R. Connor, R. Davies, K. Devlin, T. Feltwell, S. Gentles, N. Hamlin, S. Holroyd, T. Hornsby, K. Jagels, A. Krogh, J. McLean, S. Moule, L. Murphy, K. Oliver, J. Osborne, M. A. Quail, M.-A. Rajandream, J. Rogers, S. Rutter, K. Seager, J. Skelton, R. Squares, S. Squares, J. E. Sulston, K. Taylor, S. Whitehead, and B. G. Barrell. 1998. Deciphering the biology of *Mycobacterium tuberculosis* from the complete genome sequence. *Nature* 393:537–544.

15. Cole, S. T., K. Eiglmeier, J. Parkhill, K. D. James, N. R. Thomson, P. R. Wheeler, N. Honore, T. Garnier, C. Churcher, D. Harris, K. Mungall, D. Basham, D. Brown, T. Chillingworth, R. Connor, R. M. Davies, K. Devlin, S. Duthoy, T. Feltwell, A. Fraser, N. Hamlin, S. Holroyd, T. Hornsby, K. Jagels, C. Lacroix, J. MacLean, S. Moule, L. Murphy, K. Oliver, M. A. Quail, M. A. Rajandream, K. M. Rutherford, S. Rutter, K. Seeger, S. Simon, M. Simmonds, J. Skelton, R. Squares, S. Squares, K. Stevens, K. Taylor, S. Whitehead, J. R. Woodward, and B. G. Barrell. 2001. Massive gene decay in the leprosy bacillus. *Nature* 409:1007–1011.

16. Converse, S., J. D. Mougous, M. D. Leavell, J. A. Leary, C. R. Bertozzi, and J. S. Cox. 2003. MmpL8 is required for sulfolipid-1 biosynthesis and *Mycobacterium tuberculosis* virulence. *Proc. Natl. Acad. Sci. USA* 100:6121–6126.

17. Cox, J. S., B. Chen, M. McNeil, and W. R. Jacobs, Jr. 1999. Complex lipid determines tissue-specific replication of *Mycobacterium tuberculosis* in mice. *Nature* 402:79–83.

18. Dahl, J. L., C. N. Kraus, H. I. Boshoff, B. Doan, K. Foley, D. Avarbock, G. Kaplan, V. Mizrahi, H. Rubin, and C. E. Barry

III. 2003. The role of RelMtb-mediated adaptation to stationary phase in long-term persistence of *Mycobacterium tuberculosis* in mice. *Proc. Natl. Acad. Sci. USA* **100**:10026–10031.

19. Fleischmann, R. D., D. Alland, J. A. Eisen, L. Carpenter, O. White, J. Peterson, R. DeBoy, R. Dodson, M. Gwinn, D. Haft, E. Hickey, J. F. Kolonay, W. C. Nelson, L. A. Umayam, M. Ermolaeva, S. L. Salzberg, A. Delcher, T. Utterback, J. Weidman, H. Khouri, J. Gill, A. Mikula, W. Bishai, W. R. Jacobs, Jr., J. C. Venter, and C. M. Fraser. 2002. Whole-genome comparison of *Mycobacterium tuberculosis* clinical and laboratory strains. *J. Bacteriol.* **184**:5479–5490.

20. Gao, L. Y., R. Groger, J. S. Cox, S. M. Beverley, E. H. Lawson, and E. J. Brown. 2003. Transposon mutagenesis of *Mycobacterium marinum* identifies a locus linking pigmentation and intracellular survival. *Infect. Immun.* **71**:922–929.

21. Garnier, T., K. Eiglmeier, J. C. Camus, N. Medina, H. Mansoor, M. Pryor, S. Duthoy, S. Grondin, C. Lacroix, C. Monsempe, S. Simon, B. Harris, R. Atkin, J. Doggett, R. Mayes, L. Keating, P. R. Wheeler, J. Parkhill, B. G. Barrell, S. T. Cole, S. V. Gordon, and R. G. Hewinson. 2003. The complete genome sequence of *Mycobacterium bovis*. *Proc. Natl. Acad. Sci. USA* **100**:7877–7882.

22. Gomez, M., S. Johnson, and M. L. Gennaro. 2000. Identification of secreted proteins of *Mycobacterium tuberculosis* by a bioinformatic approach. *Infect. Immun.* **68**:2323–2327.

23. Gordon, S. V., R. Brosch, A. Billault, T. Garnier, K. Eiglmeier, and S. T. Cole. 1999. Identification of variable regions in the genomes of tubercle bacilli using bacterial artificial chromosome arrays. *Mol. Microbiol.* **32**:643–655.

24. Gordon, S. V., K. Eiglmeier, T. Garnier, R. Brosch, J. Parkhill, B. Barrell, S. T. Cole, and R. G. Hewinson. 2001. Genomics of *Mycobacterium bovis*. *Tuberculosis* (Edinburgh) **81**:157–163.

25. Graham, J. E., and J. E. Clark-Curtiss. 1999. Identification of *Mycobacterium tuberculosis* RNAs synthesized in response to phagocytosis by human macrophages by selective capture of transcribed sequences (SCOTS). *Proc. Natl. Acad. Sci. USA* **96**:11554–11559.

26. Hensel, M., J. E. Shea, C. Gleeson, M. D. Jones, E. Dalton, and D. W. Holden. 1995. Simultaneous identification of bacterial virulence genes by negative selection. *Science* **269**:400–403.

27. Hingley-Wilson, S. M., V. K. Sambandamurthy, and W. R. Jacobs, Jr. 2003. Survival perspectives from the world's most successful pathogen, *Mycobacterium tuberculosis*. *Nat. Immunol.* **4**:949–955.

28. Hsu, T., S. M. Hingley-Wilson, B. Chen, M. Chen, A. Z. Dai, P. M. Morin, C. B. Marks, J. Padiyar, C. Goulding, M. Gingery, D. Eisenberg, R. G. Russell, S. C. Derrick, F. M. Collins, S. L. Morris, C. H. King, and W. R. Jacobs, Jr. 2003. The primary mechanism of attenuation of bacillus Calmette-Guérin is a loss of secreted lytic function required for invasion of lung interstitial tissue. *Proc. Natl. Acad. Sci. USA* **100**:12420–12425.

29. Johnston, J. M., V. L. Arcus, C. J. Morton, M. W. Parker, and E. N. Baker. 2003. Crystal structure of a putative methyltransferase from *Mycobacterium tuberculosis* misannotation of a genome clarified by protein structural analysis. *J. Bacteriol.* **185**:4057–4065.

30. Jungblut, P. R., E. C. Muller, J. Mattow, and S. H. Kaufmann. 2001. Proteomics reveals open reading frames in *Mycobacterium tuberculosis* H37Rv not predicted by genomics. *Infect. Immun.* **69**:5905–5907.

31. Jungblut, P. R., U. E. Schaible, H. J. Mollenkopf, U. Zimny-Arndt, B. Raupach, J. Mattow, P. Halada, S. Lamer, K. Hagens, and S. H. Kaufmann. 1999. Comparative proteome analysis of *Mycobacterium tuberculosis* and *Mycobacterium bovis* BCG strains: towards functional genomics of microbial pathogens. *Mol. Microbiol.* **33**:1103–1117.

32. Lamichhane, G., M. Zignol, N. J. Blades, D. E. Geiman, A. Dougherty, J. Grosset, K. W. Broman, and W. R. Bishai. 2003. A postgenomic method for predicting essential genes at subsaturation levels of mutagenesis: application to *Mycobacterium tuberculosis*. *Proc. Natl. Acad. Sci. USA* **100**:7213–7218.

33. Lewis, K. N., R. Liao, K. M. Guinn, M. J. Hickey, S. Smith, M. A. Behr, and D. R. Sherman. 2003. Deletion of RD1 from *Mycobacterium tuberculosis* mimics bacille Calmette-Guérin attenuation. *J. Infect. Dis.* **187**:117–123.

34. Mahairas, G. G., P. J. Sabo, M. J. Hickey, D. C. Singh, and C. K. Stover. 1996. Molecular analysis of genetic differences between *Mycobacterium bovis* BCG and virulent *M. bovis*. *J. Bacteriol.* **178**:1274–1282.

35. Manca, C., L. Tsenova, C. E. Barry III, A. Bergtold, S. Freeman, P. A. Haslett, J. M. Musser, V. H. Freedman, and G. Kaplan. 1999. *Mycobacterium tuberculosis* CDC1551 induces a more vigorous host response in vivo and in vitro, but is not more virulent than other clinical isolates. *J. Immunol.* **162**:6740–6746.

36. Mattow, J., P. R. Jungblut, U. E. Schaible, H. J. Mollenkopf, S. Lamer, U. Zimny-Arndt, K. Hagens, E. C. Muller, and S. H. Kaufmann. 2001. Identification of proteins from *Mycobacterium tuberculosis* missing in attenuated *Mycobacterium bovis* BCG strains. *Electrophoresis* **22**:2936–2946.

37. McAdam, R. A., S. Quan, D. A. Smith, S. Bardarov, J. C. Betts, F. C. Cook, E. U. Hooker, A. P. Lewis, P. Woollard, M. J. Everett, P. T. Lukey, G. J. Bancroft, W. R. Jacobs, Jr., and K. Duncan. 2002. Characterization of a *Mycobacterium tuberculosis* H37Rv transposon library reveals insertions in 351 ORFs and mutants with altered virulence. *Microbiology* **148**:2975–2986.

38. McKinney, J. D., K. Honer zu Bentrup, E. J. Munoz-Elias, A. Miczak, B. Chen, W. T. Chan, D. Swenson, J. C. Sacchettini, W. R. Jacobs, Jr., and D. G. Russell. 2000. Persistence of *Mycobacterium tuberculosis* in macrophages and mice requires the glyoxylate shunt enzyme isocitrate lyase. *Nature* **406**:735–738.

39. Monahan, I. M., J. Betts, D. K. Banerjee, and P. D. Butcher. 2001. Differential expression of mycobacterial proteins following phagocytosis by macrophages. *Microbiology* **147**:459–471.

40. Naya, H., H. Romero, A. Zavala, B. Alvarez, and H. Musto. 2002. Aerobiosis increases the genomic guanine plus cytosine content (GC%) in prokaryotes. *J. Mol. Evol.* **55**:260–264.

41. Pallen, M. J. 2002. The ESAT-6/WXG100 superfamily—and a new Gram-positive secretion system? *Trends Microbiol.* **10**:209–212.

42. Parsons, L. M., R. Brosch, S. T. Cole, A. Somoskovi, A. Loder, G. Bretzel, D. Van Soolingen, Y. M. Hale, and M. Salfinger. 2002. Rapid and simple approach for identification of *Mycobacterium tuberculosis* complex isolates by PCR-based genomic deletion analysis. *J. Clin. Microbiol.* **40**:2339–2345.

43. Pym, A. S., P. Brodin, R. Brosch, M. Huerre, and S. T. Cole. 2002. Loss of RD1 contributed to the attenuation of the live tuberculosis vaccines *Mycobacterium bovis* BCG and *Mycobacterium microti*. *Mol. Microbiol.* **46**:709–717.

44. Pym, A. S., P. Brodin, L. Majlessi, R. Brosch, C. Demangel, A. Williams, K. E. Griffiths, G. Marchal, C. Leclerc, and S. T. Cole. 2003. Recombinant BCG exporting ESAT-6 confers enhanced protection against tuberculosis. *Nat. Med.* **9**:533–539.

45. Ramakrishnan, L., N. A. Federspiel, and S. Falkow. 2000. Granuloma-specific expression of *Mycobacterium* virulence proteins from the glycine-rich PE-PGRS family. *Science* 288:1436–1439.

46. Rosenkrands, I., A. King, K. Weldingh, M. Moniatte, E. Moertz, and P. Andersen. 2000. Towards the proteome of *Mycobacterium tuberculosis*. *Electrophoresis* 21:3740–3756.

47. Rubin, E. J., B. J. Akerley, V. N. Novik, D. J. Lampe, R. N. Husson, and J. J. Mekalanos. 1999. In vivo transposition of mariner-based elements in enteric bacteria and mycobacteria. *Proc. Natl. Acad. Sci. USA* 96:1645–1650.

48. Sassetti, C. M., D. H. Boyd, and E. J. Rubin. 2001. Comprehensive identification of conditionally essential genes in mycobacteria. *Proc. Natl. Acad. Sci. USA* 98:12712–12717.

49. Sassetti, C. M., D. H. Boyd, and E. J. Rubin. 2003. Genes required for mycobacterial growth defined by high density mutagenesis. *Mol. Microbiol.* 48:77–84.

50. Schnappinger, D., S. Ehrt, M. I. Voskuil, Y. Liu, J. A. Mangan, I. M. Monahan, G. Dolganov, B. Efron, P. D. Butcher, C. Nathan, and G. K. Schoolnik. 2003. Transcriptional adaptation of *Mycobacterium tuberculosis* within macrophages: insights into the phagosomal environment. *J. Exp. Med.* 198:693–704.

51. Sherman, D. R., M. Voskuil, D. Schnappinger, R. Liao, M. I. Harrell, and G. K. Schoolnik. 2001. Regulation of the *Mycobacterium tuberculosis* hypoxic response gene encoding alpha-crystallin. *Proc. Natl. Acad. Sci. USA* 98:7534–7539.

52. Shi, L., Y. J. Jung, S. Tyagi, M. L. Gennaro, and R. J. North. 2003. Expression of Th1-mediated immunity in mouse lungs induces a *Mycobacterium tuberculosis* transcription pattern characteristic of nonreplicating persistence. *Proc. Natl. Acad. Sci. USA* 100:241–246.

53. Sorensen, A. L., S. Nagai, G. Houen, P. Andersen, and A. B. Andersen. 1995. Purification and characterization of a low-molecular-mass T-cell antigen secreted by *Mycobacterium tuberculosis*. *Infect. Immun.* 63:1710–1717.

54. Sreevatsan, S., X. Pan, K. E. Stockbauer, N. D. Connell, B. N. Kreiswirth, T. S. Whittam, and J. M. Musser. 1997. Restricted structural gene polymorphism in the *Mycobacterium tuberculosis* complex indicates evolutionarily recent global dissemination. *Proc. Natl. Acad. Sci. USA* 94:9869–9874.

55. Stewart, G. R., V. A. Snewin, G. Walzl, T. Hussell, P. Tormay, P. O'Gaora, M. Goyal, J. Betts, I. N. Brown, and D. B. Young. 2001. Overexpression of heat-shock proteins reduces survival of *Mycobacterium tuberculosis* in the chronic phase of infection. *Nat. Med.* 7:732–737.

56. Stewart, G. R., L. Wernisch, R. Stabler, J. A. Mangan, J. Hinds, K. G. Laing, D. B. Young, and P. D. Butcher. 2002. Dissection of the heat-shock response in *Mycobacterium tuberculosis* using mutants and microarrays. *Microbiology* 148:3129–3138.

57. Tekaia, F., S. V. Gordon, T. Garnier, R. Brosch, B. G. Barrell, and S. T. Cole. 1999. Analysis of the proteome of *Mycobacterium tuberculosis* in silico. *Tubercle Lung Dis.* 79:329–342.

58. Thomson, N., M. Sebaihia, M. Holden, A. Cerdeno-Tarraga, and J. Parkhill. 2001. Size matters? *Trends Microbiol.* 9:359.

59. Troesch, A., H. Nguyen, C. G. Miyada, S. Desvarenne, T. Gingeras, P. Kaplan, P. Cros, and C. Mabilat. 1999. *Mycobacterium* species identification and rifampin resistance testing with high-density DNA probe arrays. *J. Clin. Microbiol.* 49–55.

60. Valway, S. E., M. P. Sanchez, T. F. Shinnick, I. Orme, T. Agerton, D. Hoy, J. S. Jones, H. Westmoreland, and I. M. Onorato. 1998. An outbreak involving extensive transmission of a virulent strain of *Mycobacterium tuberculosis*. *N. Engl. J. Med.* 338:633–639.

61. Wood, P. R., and S. L. Jones. 2001. BOVIGAM: an in vitro cellular diagnostic test for bovine tuberculosis. *Tuberculosis* (Edinburgh) 81:147–155.

62. Yuan, Y., D. D. Crane, R. M. Simpson, Y. Q. Zhu, M. J. Hickey, D. R. Sherman, and C. E. Barry III. 1998. The 16-kDa alpha-crystallin (Acr) protein of *Mycobacterium tuberculosis* is required for growth in macrophages. *Proc. Natl. Acad. Sci. USA* 95:9578–9583.

Chapter 10

Comparative Genomics and Evolution of *Mycobacterium bovis* BCG

ROLAND BROSCH AND MARCEL A. BEHR

BCG, the live attenuated strain of *Mycobacterium bovis* obtained by Albert Calmette and Camille Guérin at the Institut Pasteur of Lille between 1906 and 1919, is one of the world's most widely used vaccines and the only anti-tuberculosis (anti-TB) vaccine that is still used on a large scale. BCG was obtained from a virulent culture of *M. bovis*, the agent of bovine TB, through 230 passages on potato slices soaked in ox bile and glycerol. Calmette and Guérin reported that during these passages, which each lasted for 3 weeks, the bacteria gradually lost their capacity to cause disease in various animal models (14), leading finally to the attempt to use it as vaccine for the prevention of TB in humans.

BCG is one of the six vaccines of the Expanded Program of Immunization of the World Health Organization. Only the Netherlands and the United States have never recommended universal BCG vaccination. Some countries such as Sweden or the Czech Republic have now moved to this policy. In most other parts of the world, routine BCG vaccination is applied with different policies that can be divided in three groups: BCG administration only at birth (or first contact with health services) (recommended by the Expanded Program of Immunization and the Global TB Program), BCG once in childhood, or repeated/booster BCG. Currently, an estimated 118 million doses of BCG are administered each year (18).

Since 1921, more than three billion doses of BCG have been administered worldwide, with a remarkably low incidence of major side effects in immunocompetent individuals. BCG is thought to be highly effective against disseminated forms of TB in children (80%), such as miliary TB and tuberculous meningitis (18), although most of the data supporting this protection are derived from observational and case-control studies. BCG vaccination has also been shown to protect against leprosy in a controlled trial (38). However, the protection conferred by BCG vaccination against pulmonary TB in adults, representing the majority of the disease burden, has been highly variable in clinical trials, ranging from 0 to 80% depending on the population, the country, and the BCG substrain used.

Although vaccines more effective than BCG are needed, BCG vaccination will probably continue for at least the next decade(s) on a worldwide scale until controlled long-term vaccine trials prove that novel anti-TB vaccines offer better protection. Moreover, of all the novel vaccines being developed, it is noteworthy that the only candidates that have performed better than BCG in animal models have been modified forms of BCG vaccines (27, 40). As such, molecular and immunological characterization of the presently used BCG vaccine strains continues to be an important research topic, not only to elucidate the genetic basis for the attenuation of BCG but also to learn more about the genetic background of diverse BCG substrains that may be involved in the variable protective efficacy. Recent advances in the field of mycobacterial genetics, genomics, comparative genomics, and related techniques have supplied an enormous amount of new information, which is summarized and discussed in this chapter.

HISTORY OF BCG SUBSTRAINS

From the 1920s, after BCG had been proven to be attenuated and safe by Calmette and Guérin, cultures of BCG strains were sent out from the Pasteur Institute to different laboratories throughout the world, where these cultures were further propagated and used for vaccine production. Lyophilization of vaccine lots became available in the latter half of the 20th century, exposing different BCG daughter strains to some 1,000 additional passages of in vitro evolution in different

Roland Brosch • Unité de Génétique Moléculaire Bactérienne, Institut Pasteur, 28 rue du Docteur Roux, 75724 Paris Cedex 15, France. **Marcel A. Behr** • Division of Infectious Diseases and Medical Microbiology, McGill University Health Centre, A5-156, Montreal General Hospital, 1650 Cedar Ave., Montreal, QC H3G 1A4 Canada.

laboratories. This means that BCG does not refer to a cloned strain but, rather, to a family of different BCG seed strains (substrains) used in BCG manufacture that have probably acquired particular genomic modifications during passaging in the various laboratories.

Detailed investigation of the records of when and to which laboratories BCG cultures were sent has enabled the reconstruction of the history of the different BCG daughter strains. Although BCG vaccines have been produced in a wide variety of countries (e.g., Australia, Bulgaria, Mexico, and Romania), a representative subset is generally selected for genetic studies of BCG strains and is based on strains used in clinical trials or currently in wide use in vaccination programs. Reviews of the history of these strains have been published by different groups, and they have shown agreement of the proposed provenance of these strains (3, 37). The natural historical division that usually arises from these genealogic trees is between "early strains" obtained in the 1920s (BCG Russia, BCG Brazil, BCG Tokyo, BCG Sweden, and BCG Birkhaug) and "late strains" obtained from the Pasteur Institute in 1931 or later (outlined in Fig. 1). Among these late strains, some BCG stocks were derived indirectly, i.e., via a different vaccine producer, so that one can describe a Danish group (BCG Danish and its derivatives BCG Prague and BCG Glaxo) and a Canadian group (BCG Frappier and its derivative BCG Connaught). The subdivisions into BCG families permit verification of genetic studies but are not known to correlate with potentially important vaccine phenotypes. In contrast, the distinction between early strains and late strains coincides with reports of ongoing attenuation of BCG in the late 1920s (16, 50) and is correlated with severely reduced production of the antigenic proteins MPB70, MPB83, and MPB64 in late strains (52). Unfortunately, the relevance of these differences among BCG substrains in terms of protective efficacy in humans is unknown, since randomized clinical trials of BCG vaccination have not employed any of the early strains.

BCG AS A MEMBER OF THE M. TUBERCULOSIS COMPLEX

As stated above, M. bovis BCG is an attenuated member of the M. tuberculosis complex, a tightly knit group of slow-growing mycobacteria comprising M. tuberculosis, the causative agent of the vast majority of human TB cases; Mycobacterium canetti and Mycobacterium africanum, both agents of human tuberculosis in sub-Saharan Africa; Mycobacterium microti, an agent of tuberculosis in voles; and M. bovis, which infects a wide variety of mammalian species including humans. The members of the complex have great genetic similarity, seen by homology at the DNA level of greater than 99.9%. However, some particular phenotypic characteristics, including different host preferences, have led researchers to maintain the traditional species names of these bacteria. In two recent studies, the evolutionary position of

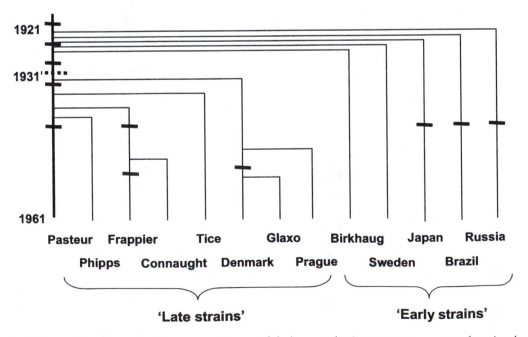

Figure 1. BCG genealogy. The vertical axis represents time, and the horizontal axis represents movement of vaccines between laboratories. Solid lines indicate deletions, and the dotted line indicates an SNP in *mmaA3*.

M. bovis BCG relative to the other members of the *M. tuberculosis* complex has been redefined (10, 34). The studies were based on the results of previous comparative genomic analyses, which demonstrated that there are at least 18 regions of difference (RD1 to RD18) in the size range of 0.3 bp to 12.7 kb, coding for over 120 genes that are present in *M. tuberculosis* H37Rv but absent from BCG strains (2, 21, 42). Specific PCR and sequence analyses of these RD regions, among members of the *M. tuberculosis* complex, showed that most of the RD regions absent from BCG were also missing from other strains of *M. bovis*, indicating that some of these variable regions reflect the evolutionary divergence of *M. tuberculosis* and *M. bovis* rather than being genomic modifications that were introduced during the attenuation process of BCG. As one example, Fig. 2 shows the gene content of the RD9 region, which was found in all *M. tuberculosis* and *M. canetti* strains but absent from *M. africanum*, *M. microti*, *M. bovis*, seal isolates, and *M. bovis* BCG. The segment is predicted to include two complete genes, Rv2073c and Rv2074, as well as the 5′ end of *cobL*. In silico comparison of the CobL sequence from *M. tuberculosis* with public databases revealed that CobL is highly conserved among a wide variety of bacteria. The interruption of CobL indicates that the RD9 polymorphism is most probably due to the deletion of a 2-kb fragment from

the common ancestor of *M. africanum*, *M. microti*, *M. bovis*, and *M. bovis* BCG rather than to the insertion of genes Rv2073c and Rv2074 into *M. tuberculosis*. This was confirmed by sequence analysis of the interruption sites of *cobL* in these species, which showed that the junction sequences of the RD9 region were identical. These findings were of particular importance for the interpretation of the evolution of the members of the *M. tuberculosis* complex, since they allowed us to define a direction for the evolutionary processes that have shaped the various lineages (13). Since the situation with most of the other RD regions that are absent from *M. bovis* and BCG is similar to that of RD9, i.e., the deletions have interrupted genes which are still intact in *M. tuberculosis* and *M. canetti*, it was possible to propose a new evolutionary scheme for the members of the *M. tuberculosis* complex (Fig. 3). This scheme, which was based on the presence or absence of 20 variable regions in a representative set of 100 strains from the *M. tuberculosis* complex (10), was confirmed in a separate study that also employed RD markers on a different set of strains (34). Moreover, a study employing multilocus sequence typing found similar phylogenetic relationships among strains of the *M. tuberculosis* complex to that proposed on the basis of deletion-based analysis (23). Taken together, these studies suggest that the agent of bovine TB, *M. bovis*, is not the ancestor of

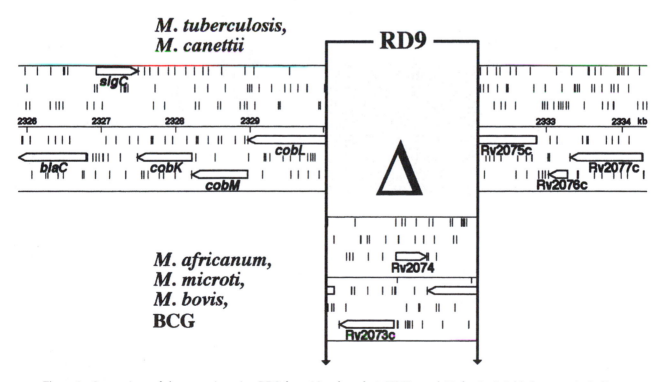

Figure 2. Comparison of the genomic region RD9 from *M. tuberculosis* H37Rv and *M. bovis*. A 2-kb fragment including highly conserved parts of *cobL* is absent from BCG, *M. bovis*, *M. microti*, and *M. africanum* strains but is present in *M. tuberculosis* and *M. canetti*.

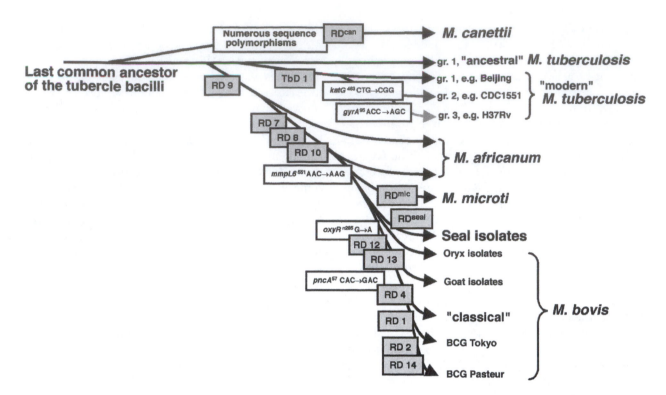

Figure 3. Evolutionary scheme of the *M. tuberculosis* complex, indicating that *M. bovis* BCG has lost numerous regions of difference, several of which are in common with other strains of the complex. Adapted from reference 10 with permission.

the human TB agent, *M. tuberculosis*, as was thought for a long time (24, 49). From these recent studies, it appears that the common ancestor of the *M. tuberculosis* complex resembled *M. tuberculosis* or *M. canetti* more closely than it resembled *M. bovis*. Final confirmation that the genome of *M. bovis* has indeed undergone several deletion processes relative to that of *M. tuberculosis* comes from the complete genome sequence of *M. bovis* (20), showing that the genome of *M. bovis* strain AF2122/97 is 66 kb smaller than the genome of *M. tuberculosis* H37Rv and, with one exception (*M. tuberculosis*-specific deleted region 1 [TbD1]), does not contain extra DNA that is not present in *M. tuberculosis* strains. Because the progenitor of BCG was a fully virulent bovine isolate of *M. bovis*, many of the genetic particularities of *M. bovis* revealed by the complete genome sequence of *M. bovis* AF2122/97 (20) also apply to BCG. Some of these features are discussed in the following paragraph.

BCG AND ITS GENETIC ROOTS FROM *M. BOVIS*

Since the original *M. bovis* culture supplied by Nocard, which was used by Calmette and Guérin as a starting culture for their passaging experiment, which led to BCG, was lost during the First World War, we have to restrict the genetic analysis of the closest ancestor of BCG to other *M. bovis* strains. For this purpose, the bovine isolate *M. bovis* AF2122/97, whose complete genome sequence was recently determined, offers an attractive alternative as a reference for BCG analyses.

The comparison of *M. bovis* AF2122/97 and *M. tuberculosis* H37Rv revealed 2,437 single-nucleotide polymorphisms (SNPs), whereas *M. bovis* AF2122/97 differed from *M. tuberculosis* CDC 1551, the second *M. tuberculosis* strain whose genome sequence has been entirely determined (19), by 2,423 SNPs. These numbers indicate that between *M. bovis* and *M. tuberculosis*, on average 1 nucleotide substitution per 1.8 kb of sequence can be found. Some of these point mutations have previously been shown to be responsible for a distinctive characteristic of the bovine bacillus. For example, a point mutation in the *pncA* gene in *M. bovis* confers resistance to the key anti-TB drug pyrazinamide and prevents the accumulation of niacin that is seen in *M. tuberculosis* (7, 44). BCG strains exhibit the same pyrazinamide resistance, as a result of the inherited *pncA* SNP from *M. bovis*. In their analysis, Garnier and colleagues have compared 2,504 selected coding sequences (CDS) of identical length across the genomes of *M. bovis* AF2122/97, *M. tuberculosis* H37Rv, and *M. tuberculosis* CDC 1551 and have found that 1,629 and

1,656 *M. bovis* CDS were identical in *M. tuberculosis* H37Rv and CDC 1551, respectively, whereas 2,082 CDS showed no difference between the two *M. tuberculosis* strains. Across these 2,504 CDS, *M. bovis* showed 506 synonymous and 769 nonsynonymous SNPs compared with *M. tuberculosis* H37Rv and showed 506 synonymous and 800 nonsynonymous SNPs against *M. tuberculosis* CDC 1551. By comparison, the two *M. tuberculosis* strains showed 339 nonsynonymous and 241 synonymous SNPs, respectively. These data confirm the high conservation of genes within the members of the *M. tuberculosis* complex but also indicate that *M. bovis* is more distant from *M. tuberculosis* than are the two sequenced *M. tuberculosis* strains from each other (20).

The greatest degree of sequence variation between the human and bovine bacilli was found in genes encoding cell wall and secreted proteins. For example, the genes encoding the lipoproteins LppO, LpqT, LpqG, and LprM were deleted or frameshifted in *M. bovis*. Similarly, the *rpfA* gene, one of a five-member family encoding secreted proteins that promote the resuscitation of dormant or nongrowing bacilli (36), showed an in-frame deletion of 240 bp in *M. bovis*. Another family of secreted proteins that showed extensive variation between *M. bovis* and *M. tuberculosis* includes the early secreted antigenic target of 6 kDa (ESAT-6). This small protein, originally described as a potent T-cell antigen secreted by *M. tuberculosis* (46), belongs to a >20-member family that contains several other T-cell antigens (6, 45). Six ESAT-6 proteins, encoded by Rv2346c, Rv2347c, Rv3619c, Rv3620c, Rv3890c (Mb3919c), and Rv3905c (Mb3935c) in *M. tuberculosis*, were missing or altered in *M. bovis* AF2122/97. The consequences of their loss are difficult to predict, although they may impact on antigen load either singly or in combination. These observations are also particularly relevant for BCG strains, since they lack, in addition to the other ESAT-6 family members missing from *M. bovis* AF2122/97, the genes for ESAT-6 and CFP-10, due to the RD1 deletion (described in detail below).

Extensive sequence polymorphism has also been observed for the large gene families encoding the PE and PPE proteins. Members of each family share a conserved NH_2-terminal domain of ~110 and 180 amino acid residues, with the characteristic motifs proline-glutamic acid or proline-proline-glutamic acid at positions 8 and 9 or 8 to 10, respectively. The N-terminal domain is generally followed by a C-terminal extension that is often of highly repetitive sequence. Although they were initially of unknown function, there is now a considerable body of evidence to suggest that at least some of these proteins are surface exposed and play a role in adhesion and immune modulation (1, 8). Between *M. bovis* AF2122/97 and *M. tuberculosis* H37Rv, there are blocks of sequence variation in genes encoding 29 different PE-PGRS and 28 PPE proteins resulting from in-frame insertions and deletions, whereas others are frameshifted. More than 60% of these proteins differ, and it seems that these proteins provide a source of variation on which selective pressures may act.

These examples clearly show that in spite of the conserved genome organization and the limited sequence polymorphism observed in housekeeping genes (47), in some aspects *M. bovis* differs quite extensively from *M. tuberculosis*, with these differences also applying to BCG.

Furthermore, the existence of a variety of contemporary BCG strains provides opportunities to logically deduce the genetics of the original BCG strain. For instance, BCG strains obtained before 1926 (BCG Russia, BCG Moreau, and BCG Tokyo) all have an IS*6110* element at bp 851592 of the *M. tuberculosis* H37Rv genome, unlike other BCG strains, where the sequence at this locus is identical to that of *M. tuberculosis* and *M. bovis* (35). One can reason that it is much more likely that the BCG strain of the early 1920s contained this second IS element, since the alternative explanation would be that on three different continents, a transpositional duplication of IS*6110* occurred at precisely the same locus. Therefore, based on the availability of a number of different BCG strains and the genomic sequences of *M. tuberculosis* H37Rv and *M. bovis* AF2122/97, it is now possible to describe the genomic evolution of BCG strains in various vaccine laboratories.

MOLECULAR EVOLUTION OF BCG SUBSTRAINS

As described above, BCG is not a clonal organism, and several substrains exist that may have accumulated individual genetic modifications due to long-term passaging in different laboratories and vaccine production facilities. Using the historical records about when and where BCG strains were distributed, together with information about genetic particularities of certain BCG substrains, reconstruction of the short-term evolution of BCG strains can be established. By employing techniques of comparative genome analyses, such as subtractive hybridization, the microarray technique, or bacterial artificial chromosome (BAC)-based hybridization, it was shown that several BCG daughter strains indeed have accumulated additional genomic modifications which apparently were not present in the original culture obtained by Calmette and Guérin (2, 12, 32). However, before the individual particularities of certain BCG substrains are described, it should be mentioned that in spite of its billion-fold application, none of the BCG substrains have ever reverted to the virulent form of *M. bovis*. This finding suggests that during the attenuation process of BCG, one or more irreversible genetic changes, such as deletions, have occurred in the genome of the original BCG culture that have permanently disabled BCG from causing disease in immunocompetent hosts. With the huge amount of genomic and array data that have been generated in the last few years for the members of the *M. tuberculosis* complex, including BCG strains (2, 10, 21, 28, 35, 42), it is now possible to differentiate between genetic characteristics that are specific to all BCG substrains but absent from other *M. bovis* strains and to identify genetic variations that are specific for only certain BCG substrains. Whereas the former may be directly involved in the attenuation of BCG, the latter may account for variation in protective efficacy and overattenuation of certain BCG substrains. For the genomic characteristics that apply for all BCG substrains and are shown to be implicated in virulence, the example of the RD1 region is discussed in a separate paragraph below. The variations that were observed for only certain substrains of BCG consist of deletions, duplications, and point mutations.

With prototype sequence information, along with comparative genomic tools such as subtractive hybridization, BAC libraries, and DNA microarrays, the discovery of genomic deletions has been greatly facilitated. Since these are arguably the easiest source of genomic variability to uncover, it is perhaps not surprising that 10 genomic deletions in BCG have been uncovered that date to a time after its first introduction. With the exception of the deletion of an IS6110 element from an intergenic region, the remaining nine deletions interfere with coding frames in the same manner as described above for RD9, providing a list of genes that appear to have been dispensable during prolonged growth in vitro. This list of deleted regions in presented in Table 1.

Of genes contained in BCG deletions, a number stand out as candidates for the ongoing attenuation of BCG strains in the laboratory. Rv3405c, annotated as a possible transcriptional regulator, has been independently deleted from two different BCG strains. Rv1773, also annotated as a probable transcriptional regulatory protein, has been deleted from the BCG Pasteur strain alone. Rv1985c, annotated as a probable transcriptional regulatory protein (probably from the LysR family), is deleted from all late strains. Finally, Rv1189, otherwise known as *sigI* (possible alternative RNA polymerase sigma factor SigI), is missing from all BCG strains obtained after 1933. The loss of regulatory genes from a number of different BCG strains argues that in the monotonous conditions of laboratory growth, the capacity to alter genetic expression may be less important and therefore genes encoding these functions can be deleted.

Comparative genomics has also uncovered two large tandem duplications of 29 and 36 kb (DU1 and DU2) in BCG Pasteur (12, 13). These seem to have arisen independently, since their presence and/or their size varies among the different BCG substrains. While DU1 appears to be restricted to BCG Pasteur, DU2 has been detected in all BCG substrains tested so far (R. Brosch, unpublished observations). Interestingly, DU1 comprises the *oriC* locus, indicating that BCG Pasteur is diploid for *oriC*, and several genes involved in replication (12, 13). For DU2, we know that the tandem duplication resulted in diploidy for 30 genes, including *sigH*, a sigma factor implicated in the heat shock response (17). Gene duplications are a common evolutionary response in bacteria exposed to

Table 1. Genomic deletions in certain BCG substrains

Deleted sequence	Deleted from	Start point	End point	Length (bp)	Affected ORFs
RD08	BCG Frappier and Connaught	378269	381696	3,428	Rv0309 to Rv0312
nRD18	BCG Pasteur, Phipps, Frappier, Connaught, and Tice	1332920	1334466	1,547	Rv1189 to Rv1191
IS6110	All BCG strains except Russia, Moreau, and Sweden	851592	851592		NA[a]
RD14	BCG Pasteur	1998225	2007297	9,073	Rv1766 to Rv1773c
RD Denmark/Glaxo	BCG Denmark and Glaxo	2052590	2053316	726	Rv1810 to Rv1811
RD02	BCG Pasteur, Phipps, Frappier, Connaught, Tice, Denmark, Glaxo, and Prague	2221057	2231845	10,788	Rv1978 to Rv1988
RD16	BCG Moreau	3817365	3824973	7,608	Rv3400 to Rv3405c
RD Japan	BCG Japan	3825022	3825043	22	Rv3405c
RD Frappier	BCG Frappier	3914224	3916195	1,971	Rv3495c to Rv3497c
RD Russia	BCG Russia	4140085	4141688	1,603	Rv3697c to Rv3698

[a]NA, not applicable.

different selection pressures in the laboratory and presumably in nature (31, 41), since they provide a means for increasing gene dosage and for generating novel functions from potential gene fusion events at duplication end points and represent a source of redundant DNA for divergence. Thus, the duplication events seen in BCG Pasteur may reflect a common adaptation mechanism of mycobacteria to cope with environmental stress, and they could influence the immunogenicity of a certain vaccine strain.

From the complete genome sequence of BCG Pasteur will come a fuller appreciation of the frequency of other genetic events during the evolution of BCG strains, such as small deletions and SNPs. One approach to quantifying the importance of these events involves sequencing a random selection of genes across the BCG strain panel; however, to date, this has not yielded any SNPs in five genes tested (M. A. Behr, unpublished data). Therefore, pending information from BCG Pasteur to guide the search for SNPs, a targeted approach, looking for SNPs associated with defined phenotypes is a preferable strategy. Such an example presented itself based on the known phenotypic variability in the production of mycolic acid subsets among BCG strains (33). Given that the *mmaA3* gene had been proposed to be responsible for the generation of the methoxy family of mycolic acids (53), the inability of late strains to make methoxymycolates could be hypothesized to result from genetic differences in their *mmaA3* sequence. On sequencing this gene across the panel of 13 defined BCG strains, it was observed that a guanine-to-adenine replacement at bp 293 of the gene correlated exactly with the inability to produce methoxymycolates and could be timed to the years 1927 to 1931 (Behr et al., 2000). By introducing this mutant form of *mmaA3* into *M. smegmatis*, it was possible to verify that ablation of methoxymycolate synthesis occurs with this mutation. More recently, the wild-type sequence of *mmaA3* has been complemented into BCG Danish and BCG Pasteur, and this has confirmed that methoxymycolate synthesis could be restored in BCG strains (A. Belley, T. D. Pietrantonio, M. Girard, E. Schurr, J. Liu, D. Sherman, and M. Behr, Keystone Symp., Tuberculosis: Integrating Host Pathog. Biol., abstr. 207, 2003). The impact of this altered mycolic acid profile on various in vitro and in vivo parameters is currently being studied.

ATTENUATION AND PROTECTIVE ANTIGENS OF BCG

By elucidating the genomic differences between the virulent and avirulent members of the *M. tuberculosis* complex, comparative genomics has the potential to define mycobacterial virulence determinants specific for humans and other host range-determining factors that may have an important impact on vaccine design (2, 11, 21, 32). At the time of writing, the only genomic region that was identified by comparative and functional studies as being implicated in the attenuation of BCG is the region RD1. This region of difference, 10.7 kb in size, was originally identified by subtractive hybridization as being absent from BCG but present in wild-type *M. bovis* strains (32). This observation was in agreement with the finding that BCG strains, unlike *M. tuberculosis* and virulent *M. bovis* strains, did not secrete the early secreted antigenic target of 6 kDa encoded in the RD1 region (25). Since preliminary complementation experiments of BCG with the RD1 region from *M. bovis* did not result in increased virulence of the recombinant BCG strain in mice (32), the hypothesis that RD1 could be involved in the attenuation of BCG remained unconfirmed for several years. The first experimental evidence that the loss of the RD1 locus did contribute to the attenuation of BCG was gained only very recently by two independent but complementary approaches.

In one, BCG Pasteur was complemented with an integrative cosmid clone containing the RD1 region and large flanking portions of the deleted region. This recombinant BCG strain was more virulent in mice with severe combined immune deficiency (SCID mice) than was the BCG vector control strain. The same recombinant BCG strain was found to persist to a greater degree in the organs of immunocompetent mice but induced considerably less pathology than did *M. tuberculosis* H37Rv (39). Since the complementation of RD1 only partially restored attributes that might correspond to virulence, these data suggested that the RD1 deletion in BCG may represent only one step of a multifactorial attenuation cascade in BCG, either during the derivation of BCG (1908 to 1919) or during subsequent passage of BCG Pasteur (1921 to 1961). The second approach, which showed that deletion of RD1 results in a decrease of virulence, was based on *M. tuberculosis* RD1 knockout mutants in which the 10.7-kb RD1 fragment was excised (30). In this experiment, the RD1 deletion mutant generally had comparable growth in macrophage cell lines and C57BL/6 mice to that observed with BCG Russia, and a histopathologic study also found that the RD1 knockout was closer to BCG than to H37Rv. These data suggested that the deletion of RD1 might be sufficient to explain the attenuation of BCG between 1908 and 1919. Even assuming that the phenotypic impact of these two modes of study is equivalent, the discrepant results could be explained by what is known about BCG attenuation, since BCG Pasteur is known to be separated by at least six genetic events (deletion of IS6110, RD2, nRD18, RD14; SNP in *mmaA3*; and duplication DU1) from the original BCG strain of 1921.

Notable for a live attenuated vaccine is the fact that the RD1 region contains the *esxAB* genes, encoding ESAT-6 and CFP10, two strongly immunogenic proteins which are found in early culture filtrates of *M. tuberculosis* but not in BCG cultures (6, 25, 45, 46). *M. microti* strains, which were used as anti-TB vaccines in the 1960s in Great Britain and Czechoslovakia (26, 51), have also been shown to fail to make these proteins, owing to a 14-kb deletion in the RD1 region of these strains (9). This means that all vaccine strains that have been employed on a large scale in the history of prevention of human TB were missing the important T-cell antigens ESAT-6 and CFP10. This raises the question whether reintegration of these antigens into modified BCG vaccines could enhance their protective efficacy. The first experimental evidence to address this was recently obtained (40). Recombinant BCG vaccines expressing ESAT-6 and CFP-10 protect better against generalized TB infections in mice and guinea pigs, although no significant improvement was observed in the lungs, the primary site of infection. Importantly, appropriate immune recognition of ESAT-6 and CFP10 was seen only when the two antigens were properly exported via a dedicated secretion apparatus, encoded by the genes situated next to *esxAB* at the RD1 locus (40). The RD1 region therefore represents one of the most interesting genomic regions of the tubercle bacillus, since it seems to be simultaneously involved in enhanced virulence in the immunocompromised host and in improved protection in the immunocompetent host, making it a very interesting target for drug development and vaccine design. This fact is also reflected by the numerous scientific articles that have appeared very recently on this subject, confirming the above-mentioned results (22, 28, 43, 48). Development of a recombinant BCG vaccine that finds a balance between these two opposing effects is one of the challenges of future TB research.

CONCLUSION AND PERSPECTIVES

The situation in mycobacterial research has considerably changed in the last few years due to the information contained in the whole-genome sequence of *M. tuberculosis* H37Rv (15). Since its publication, three other mycobacterial whole-genome sequences have been determined and seven others are at different stages of completion (for an overview, consult http://www.pasteur.fr/recherche/unites/Lgmb/Overview-Genome-Projects.html). The genome sequence of BCG Pasteur is in the finishing phase at the time of this writing; once obtained, it will certainly allow more detailed information about the genomic features that gave rise to one of the most often used live vaccines in human history. Together with the advances in mycobacterial genetics, these data should then allow the construction of improved vaccine candidates that combine the safety of BCG with higher immunogenicity, leading to better protection against pulmonary TB in high-risk populations that did not respond properly to "standard" BCG vaccination. A more efficient anti-TB vaccine seems to be one of the few possible public health interventions that would really have a major impact on the improvement of the worldwide TB situation.

Acknowledgments. We gratefully acknowledge the financial support of the Institut Pasteur (PTR35 and PTR110), the Association Française Raoul Follereau, and the European Union (QLRT-2000-02018).

REFERENCES

1. Banu, S., N. Honore, B. Saint-Joanis, D. Philpott, M. C. Prevost, and S. T. Cole. 2002. Are the PE-PGRS proteins of *Mycobacterium tuberculosis* variable surface antigens? *Mol. Microbiol.* 44:9–19.
2. Behr, M. A., M. A. Wilson, W. P. Gill, H. Salamon, G. K. Schoolnik, S. Rane, and P. M. Small. 1999. Comparative genomics of BCG vaccines by whole-genome DNA microarray. *Science* 284:1520–1523.
3. Behr, M. A., and P. M. Small. 1999. A historical and molecular phylogeny of BCG strains. *Vaccine* 17:915–922.
4. Behr, M. A., and P. M. Small. 1997. Has BCG attenuated to impotence? *Nature* 389:133–134.
5. Behr, M. A., B. G. Schroeder, J. N. Brinkman, R. A Slayden, and C. E. Barry III. 2000. A point mutation in the *mma3* gene is responsible for impaired methoxymycolic acid production in *Mycobacterium bovis* BCG strains obtained after 1927. *J. Bacteriol.* 182:3394–3399.
6. Berthet, F.-X., P. B. Rasmusse, I. Rosenkrands, P. Andersen, and B. Gicquel. 1998. A *Mycobacterium tuberculosis* operon encoding ESAT-6 and a novel low-molecular-mass culture filtrate protein (CFP-10). *Microbiology* 144:3195–3203.
7. Boshoff, H. I., V. Mizrahi, and C. E. Barry III. 2002. Effects of pyrazinamide on fatty acid synthesis by whole mycobacterial cells and purified fatty acid synthase I. *J. Bacteriol.* 184:2167–2172.
8. Brennan, M. J., and G. Delogu. 2001. The PE multigene family: a 'molecular mantra' for mycobacteria. *Trends Microbiol.* 10:246–249.
9. Brodin, P., K. Eiglmeier, M. Marmiesse, A. Billault, T. Garnier, S. Niemann, S. T. Cole, and R. Brosch. 2002. Bacterial artificial chromosome-based comparative genomic analysis identifies *Mycobacterium microti* as a natural ESAT-6 deletion mutant. *Infect. Immun.* 70:5568–5578.
10. Brosch, R., S. V. Gordon, M. Marmiesse, P. Brodin, C. Buchrieser, K. Eiglmeier, T. Garnier, C. Gutierrez, G. Hewinson, K. Kremer, L. M. Parsons, A. S. Pym, S. Samper, D. van Soolingen, and S. T. Cole. 2002. A new evolutionary scenario for the *Mycobacterium tuberculosis* complex. *Proc. Natl. Acad. Sci. USA* 99:3684–3689.

11. Brosch, R., S. V. Gordon, A. Billault, T. Garnier, K. Eiglmeier, C. Soravito, B. G. Barrell, and S. T. Cole. 1998. Use of a *Mycobacterium tuberculosis* H37Rv bacterial artificial chromosome library for genome mapping, sequencing, and comparative genomics. *Infect. Immun.* 66:2221–2229.

12. Brosch, R., S. V. Gordon, C. Buchrieser, A. S. Pym, T. Garnier, and S. T. Cole. 2000. Comparative genomics uncovers large tandem chromosomal duplications in *Mycobacterium bovis* BCG Pasteur. *Yeast (Comp. Funct. Genomics)* 17:111–123.

13. Brosch, R., A. S. Pym, S. V. Gordon, and S. T. Cole. 2001. The evolution of mycobacterial pathogenicity: clues from comparative genomics. *Trends Microbiol.* 9:452–458.

14. Calmette, A., and C. Guérin. 1920. Nouvelles recherches experimentales sur la vaccination des bovides contre la tuberculose. *Ann. Inst. Pasteur* 34:553–560.

15. Cole, S. T., R. Brosch, J. Parkhill, T. Garnier, C. Churcher, D. Harris, S. V. Gordon, K. Eiglmeier, S. Gas, C. E. Barry III, F. Tekaia, K. Badcock, D. Basham, D. Brown, T. Chillingworth, R. Connor, R. Davies, K. Devlin, T. Feltwell, S. Gentles, N. Hamlin, S. Holroyd, T. Hornsby, K. Jagels, A. Krogh, J. McLean, S. Moule, L. Murphy, K. Oliver, J. Osborne, M. A. Quail, M. A. Rajandream, J. Rogers, S. Rutter, K. Soeger, J. Skelton, R. Squares, S. Squares, J. E. Sulston, K. Taylor, S. Whitehead, and B. G. Barrell. 1998. Deciphering the biology of *Mycobacterium tuberculosis* from the complete genome sequence. *Nature* 393:537–544.

16. Dreyer, G., and R. L. Vollum. 1931. Mutation and pathogenicity experiments with BCG. *Lancet* i:9–14.

17. Fernandes, N. D., Q. L. Wu, D. Kong, X. Puyang, S. Garg, and R. N. Husson. 1999. A mycobacterial extracytoplasmic sigma factor involved in survival following heat shock and oxidative stress. *J. Bacteriol.* 181:4266–4274

18. Fine, P. E. M., I. A. M. Carneiro, J. B. Milstein, and C. J. Clements. 1999. *Issues Relating to the Use of BCG in Immunization Programmes. A Discussion Document.* WHO/V&B/99.23. Department of Vaccines and Biologicals, World Health Organization, Geneva, Switzerland.

19. Fleischmann, R. D., D. Alland, J. A. Eisen, L. Carpenter, O. White, J. Peterson, R. DeBoy, R. Dodson, M. Gwinn, D. Haft, E. Hickey, J. F. Kolonay, W. C. Nelson, L. A. Umayam, M. Ermolaeva, S. L. Salzberg, A. Delcher, T. Utterback, J. Weidman, H. Khouri, J. Gill, A. Mikula, W. Bishai, W. R. Jacobs, Jr., J. C. Venter, and C. M. Fraser. 2002. Whole-genome comparison of *Mycobacterium tuberculosis* clinical and laboratory strains. *J. Bacteriol.* 184:5479–5490.

20. Garnier, T., K. Eiglmeier, J. C. Camus, N. Medina, H. Mansoor, M. Pryor, S. Duthoy, S. Grondin, C. Lacroix, C. Monsempe, S. Simon, B. Harris, R. Atkin, J. Doggett, R. Mayes, L. Keating, P. R. Wheeler, J. Parkhill, B. G. Barrell, S. T. Cole, S.V. Gordon, and R. G. Hewinson. 2003. The complete genome sequence of *Mycobacterium bovis*. *Proc. Natl. Acad. Sci. USA* 100:7877–7882

21. Gordon, S. V., R. Brosch, A. Billault, T. Garnier, K. Eiglmeier, and S. T. Cole. 1999. Identification of variable regions in the genomes of tubercle bacilli using bacterial artificial chromosome arrays. *Mol. Microbiol.* 32:643–655.

22. Guinn, K. I., M. J. Hickey, S. K. Mathur, K. L. Zakel, J. E. Grotzke, D. M. Lewinsohn, S. Smith, and D. R. Sherman. 2004. Individual RD1-region genes are required for export of ESAT-6/CFP-10 and for virulence of *Mycobacterium tuberculosis*. *Mol. Microbiol.* 51:359–370.

23. Gutacker, M. M., J. C. Smoot, C. A. Migliaccio, S. M. Ricklefs, S. Hua, D. V. Cousins, E. A. Graviss, E. Shashkina, B. N. Kreiswirth, and J. M. Musser. 2002. Genome-wide analysis of synonymous single nucleotide polymorphisms in *Mycobacterium tuberculosis* complex organisms. Resolution of genetic relationships among closely related microbial strains. *Genetics* 162:1533–1543.

24 Haas, F., and S. S. Haas. 1996. The origins of *Mycobacterium tuberculosis* and the notion of its contagiousness, p. 3–19. *In* W. N. Rom and S. Garay (ed.), *Tuberculosis*. Little, Brown & Co., Boston, Mass.

25. Harboe, M., T. Oettinger, H. G. Wiker, I. Rosenkrands, and P. Andersen. 1996. Evidence for occurrence of the ESAT-6 protein in *Mycobacterium tuberculosis* and virulent *Mycobacterium bovis* and for its absence in *Mycobacterium bovis* BCG. *Infect. Immun.* 64:16–22.

26. Hart, P. D. A., and I. Sutherland. 1977. BCG and vole bacillus vaccines in the prevention of tuberculosis in adolescence and early adult life. *Br. Med. J.* 2:293–295.

27. Horwitz, M. A., G. Harth, B. J. Dillon, and S. Maslesa-Galic. 2000. Recombinant bacillus Calmette-Guerin (BCG) vaccines expressing the *Mycobacterium tuberculosis* 30-kDa major secretory protein induce greater protective immunity against tuberculosis than conventional BCG vaccines in a highly susceptible animal model. *Proc. Natl. Acad. Sci. USA* 97:13853–13858.

28. Hsu, T., S. M. Hingley-Wilson, B. Chen, M. Chen, A. Z. Dai, P. M. Morin, C. B. Marks, J. Padiyar, C. Goulding, M. Gingery, D. Eisenberg, R. G. Russell, S. C. Derrick, F. M. Collins, S. L. Morris, C. H. King, and W. R. Jacobs, Jr. 2003. The primary mechanism of attenuation of bacillus Calmette-Guerin is a loss of secreted lytic function required for invasion of lung interstitial tissue. *Proc. Natl. Acad. Sci. USA* 100:12420–12425.

29. Kato-Maeda, M., J. T. Rhee, T. R. Gingeras, H. Salamon, J. Drenkow, N. Smittipat, and P. M. Small. 2001. Comparing genomes within the species *Mycobacterium tuberculosis*. *Genome Res.* 11:547–554.

30. Lewis, K. N., R. Liao, K. M. Guinn, M. J. Hickey, S. Smith, M. A. Behr, and D. R. Sherman. 2003. Deletion of RD1 from *Mycobacterium tuberculosis* mimics bacille Calmette-Guérin attenuation. *J. Infect. Dis.* 187:117–123.

31. Lupski, J. R., J. R. Roth, and G. M. Weinstock. 1996. Chromosomal duplications in bacteria, fruit flies, and humans. *Am. J. Hum. Genet.* 58:21–27

32. Mahairas, G. G., P. J. Sabo, M. J. Hickey, D. C. Singh, and C. K. Stover. 1996. Molecular analysis of genetic differences between *Mycobacterium bovis* BCG and virulent *M. bovis*. *J. Bacteriol.* 178:1274–1282.

33. Minnikin, D. E, S. M. Minnikin, G. Dobson, M. Goodfellow, F. Portaels, L. van den Breen, and D. Sesardic. 1983. Mycolic acid patterns of four vaccine strains of *Mycobacterium bovis* BCG. *J. Gen. Microbiol.* 129:889–891.

34. Mostowy, S., D. Cousins, J. Brinkman, A. Aranaz, and M. A. Behr. 2002. Genomic deletions suggest a phylogeny for the *Mycobacterium tuberculosis* complex. *J. Infect. Dis.* 186:74–80.

35. Mostowy, S., A. G. Tsolaki, P. M Small, and M. A. Behr. 2003. The in vitro evolution of BCG vaccines. *Vaccine* 21:4270–4274.

36. Mukamolova, G. V., O. A Turapov, D. I. Young, A. S. Kaprelyants, D. B. Kell, and M. Young. 2002. A family of autocrine growth factors in *Mycobacterium tuberculosis*. *Mol. Microbiol.* 46:623–635.

37. Oettinger, T., M. Jorgensen, A. Ladefoged, K. Haslov, and P. Andersen. 1999. Development of the *Mycobacterium bovis* BCG vaccine: review of the historical and biochemical evidence for a genealogical tree. *Tubercle Lung Dis.* 79:243–250.

38. Ponnighaus, J. M., P. E. Fine, J. A. Sterne, R. J. Wilson, E. Msosa, P. J. Gruer, P. A. Jenkins, S. B. Lucas, N. G. Liomba, and L. Bliss. 1992. Efficacy of BCG vaccine against leprosy and tuberculosis in northern Malawi. *Lancet* 339:636–639.

39. **Pym, A. S., P. Brodin, R. Brosch, M. Huerre, and S. T. Cole.** 2002. Loss of RD1 contributed to the attenuation of the live tuberculosis vaccines *Mycobacterium bovis* BCG and *Mycobacterium microti*. *Mol. Microbiol.* **46:**709–717.

40. **Pym, A. S., P. Brodin, L. Majlessi, R. Brosch, C. Demangel, A. Williams, K. E. Griffiths, G. Marchal, C. Leclerc, and S. T. Cole.** 2003. Recombinant BCG exporting ESAT-6 confers enhanced protection against tuberculosis. *Nat. Med.* **9:**533–539.

41. **Riehle, M. M., A. F. Benett, and A. D. Lang.** 2001. Genetic architecture of thermal adaptation in *Escherichia coli*. *Proc. Natl. Acad. Sci. USA* **98:**525–530

42. **Salamon, H., M. Kato-Maeda, P. M. Small, J. Drenkow, and T. R. Gingeras.** 2000. Detection of deleted genomic DNA using a semiautomated computational analysis of GeneChip data. *Genome Res.* **10:**2044–2054.

43. **Sassetti, C. M., and E. J. Rubin.** 2003. Genetic requirements for mycobacterial survival during infection. *Proc. Natl. Acad. Sci. USA* **100:**12989–12994.

44. **Scorpio, A., and Y. Zhang.** 1996. Mutations in *pncA*, a gene encoding pyrazinamidase/nicotinamidase, cause resistance to the antituberculous drug pyrazinamide in tubercle bacillus. *Nat. Med.* **2:**662–667.

45. **Skjot, R. L. V., T. Oettinger, I. Rosenkrands, P. Ravn, I. Brock, S. Jacobsen, and P. Andersen.** 2000. Comparative evaluation of low-molecular-mass proteins from *Mycobacterium tuberculosis* identifies members of the ESAT-6 family as immunodominant T-cell antigens. *Infect. Immun.* **68:**214–220.

46. **Sorensen, A. L., S. Nagai, G. Houen, P. Andersen, and A. Andersen.** 1995. Purification and characterization of a low molecular mass T-cell antigen secreted by *Mycobacterium tuberculosis*. *Infect. Immun.* **63:**1710–1717.

47. **Sreevatsan, S., X. Pan, K. E. Stockbauer, N. D. Connell, B. N. Kreiswirth, T. S. Whittam, and J. M. Musser.** 1997. Restricted structural gene polymorphism in the *Mycobacterium tuberculosis* complex indicates evolutionarily recent global dissemination. *Proc. Natl. Acad. Sci. USA* **94:**9869–9874.

48. **Stanley, S. A., S. Raghavan, W. W. Hwang, and J. S. Cox.** 2003. Acute infection and macrophage subversion by *Mycobacterium tuberculosis* require a specialized secretion system. *Proc. Natl. Acad. Sci. USA* **100:**13001–13006.

49. **Stead, W. W.** 1997. The origin and erratic global spread of tuberculosis. How the past explains the present and is the key to the future. *Clin. Chest Med.* **18:**65–77.

50. **Streng, K. O.** 1940. Etude des caracteres d'attennuation du bacille BCG suivant le nombre de passages de ce germe sur pomme de terre a la bile de boeuf. *Ann. Inst. Pasteur* **64:**196–202.

51. **Sula, L., and I. Radkovsky.** 1976. Protective effects of *M. microti* vaccine against tuberculosis. *J. Hyg. Epidemiol. Microbiol. Immunol.* **20:**1–6.

52. **Wiker, H. G., S. Nagai, R. G. Hewinson, W. P. Russell, and M. Harboe.** 1996. Heterogenous expression of the related MPB70 and MPB83 proteins distinguish various substrains of *Mycobacterium bovis* BCG and *Mycobacterium tuberculosis* H37Rv. *Scand. J. Immunol.* **43:**374–380.

53. **Yuan, Y., D. D. Crane, R. M. Simpson, Y. Zhu, M. J. Hickey, D. R. Sherman, and C. E. Barry III.** 1998. The 16-kDa α-crystallin (Acr) protein of *Mycobacterium tuberculosis* is required for growth in macrophages. *Proc. Natl. Acad. Sci. USA* **95:**9578–9583.

Tuberculosis and the Tubercle Bacillus
Edited by Stewart T. Cole et al.
© 2005 ASM Press, Washington, D.C.

Chapter 11

TB or Not TB: a Structural Genomics Mission?

CELIA W. GOULDING, DEBNATH PAL, AND DAVID EISENBERG

Tuberculosis structural genomics is the large-scale determination of protein structures from the bacterium *Mycobacterium tuberculosis* with the goal of elucidating its biology and pathogenicity and providing a structural foundation for drug discovery. The *M. tuberculosis* Structural Genomics Consortium consists of more than 200 structural biologists from around the world, who have agreed to work together to eradicate one of the world's deadliest infectious diseases, TB. In this chapter we describe the experimental path from gene to protein structure, the public TB Structural Genomics Consortium Database, and the structures that have been determined thus far and their biological relevance.

TOWARD STRUCTURAL GENOMICS

Structural genomics is the determination and analysis of protein structures on a genome-wide scale, proceeding from knowledge of the genome sequence to knowledge of the three-dimensional structure. One of the goals of structural genomics is to determine example structures for new protein families, so that three-dimensional structural models may be constructed with no structural information. Another goal is functional annotation of proteins with no known function by analysis of their atomic structures. A third goal is to construct protein-protein interaction networks of an entire genome. Lastly, for structural genomics projects to fulfill their goals, the process must be automated for high throughput. Hence, robots are being developed to automate individual steps of the path from gene to protein structure.

The TB Structural Genomics Consortium (http://www.doe-mbi.ucla.edu/TB) is devoted to facilitating and coordinating the determination and analysis of structures of proteins from *M. tuberculosis* (108). Consortium members work with other researchers to identify potential protein drug targets and other proteins that play important biological roles. Structural information about these proteins forms the basis for rational anti-TB drug design as well as shedding light on mechanistic aspects of these proteins. Two previous reviews have been published summarizing some of the structures solved by the consortium which are implicated as drug targets and of biological interest (39, 109), and Table 1 lists other structures that were not generated by the consortium. All PDB ID codes not in Color Plate 6 are listed in the appendix.

OUTLINE OF STRUCTURE PRODUCTION

The general experimental path for structure production is outlined in Fig. 1. The individual steps are discussed briefly below and in greater detail elsewhere (41). The gene of interest is cloned into an *Escherichia coli* expression vector with a cleavable N- or C-terminal protein tag to facilitate purification. Protein expression and solubility trials are then performed in an attempt to obtain milligram amounts of soluble protein. If the protein is insoluble, various solubilization strategies are tried. These include varying the buffers or tags, performing coexpression with chaperones, and refolding the insoluble protein. If the protein remains insoluble, the following options may be used: (i) directed evolution for point mutations to improve solubility (114, 115), (ii) coexpression of the desired protein with its predicted *M. tuberculosis* protein partner (105), and (iii) changing the expression system from *E. coli* to *M. smegmatis* (24).

Once suitable conditions have been found, expression is scaled up and the optimal purification scheme is adopted. This usually involves affinity chromatography, since most of the expressed proteins are tagged, followed by quality control procedures

Celia W. Goulding, Debnath Pal, and David Eisenberg • UCLA-DOE Institute of Genomics and Proteomics, P.O. Box 951570, Los Angeles, CA 90095-1570.

Table 1. Information about *M. tuberculosis* protein structures determined by consortium nonmembers prior to 1998

Protein or gene name	Rv no.	Reference	PDB code	Function
FabH	Rv0533c	95	1hzp	β-Ketoacyl-acyl carrier protein synthase III
MshD	Rv0819	111	1ozp	Mycothiol synthase
PstS-1	Rv0934	113	1pc3	Phosphate-binding protein
MscL	Rv0985c	14	1msl	Gated mechanosensitive channel
Hemoglobin N	Rv1542c	72	1idr	NO detoxification
ADPRase	Rv1700	60	1mk1	Nudix hydrolase
AcpM	Rv2244	120	1klp	Meromycolate extension acyl carrier protein
AhpD	Rv2429	11	1knc	Thioredoxin-like antioxidant defense
NDP kinase	Rv2445c	16	1k44	Nucleoside diphosphate kinase
Hemoglobin O	Rv2470	73	1ngk	Possible defense protein
Dhqase	Rv2537c	29	1h05	3-Dehydroquinase
MtSK	Rv2539c	43	1l4u	Shikimate kinase
IdeR	Rv2711	30	1b1b	Iron-dependent regulator
DHFR	Rv2763c	64	1dg8	Dihydrofolate reductase
DHPR	Rv2773c	18	1c3v	Dihydrodipicolinate reductase
PpsC	Rv2933	To be published (Gogos A)	1pqw	Phenolphthiocerol synthesis
TMP kinase	Rv3247c	65	1g3u	Thymidylate kinase
Pnp	Rv3307	99	1g2o	Purine-nucleoside phosphorylase
DHPS	Rv3608c	5	1eye	Dihydropteroate synthase
Fe-SOD	Rv3846	21	1gn4	Iron superoxide dismutase

such as mass spectrometry and circular dichroism. If necessary, tags are removed, although it is thought that the maltose-binding protein tag may organize within a crystal even with another protein fused to it. With this method, not only does one obtain a well-ordered crystal from packing of the maltose-binding protein but also one may obtain phases of the diffracted X-rays by using the maltose-binding protein as a probe in molecular replacement (101). Protein crystallization, an empirical art, is then undertaken to obtain single, well-diffracting crystals. The structure may be determined by molecular replacement if the protein target is a homolog of a protein of known structure (usually with greater than 40% sequence identity). If the protein structure is predicted to be novel, then heavy-metal phasing is required. This requires either a selenomethionine derivative of the target protein for the multiple-wavelength anomalous diffraction method of phase determination, soaking protein crystals in a solution of a heavy atom for multiple-wavelength anomalous diffraction, or traditional isomorphous replacement.

Technological advances have led to increased automation of these procedures; in particular, cloning, crystallization trials, crystal identification, crystal placement, and data collection are being automated (91, 92). Even interpretation of the electron density is being automated (83). The main bottlenecks in the automation process are protein production (since each protein has a unique sequence), solubility, and crystallization (again due to the effect of the protein sequence in determining the optimal solution for producing diffraction-quality crystals).

DATABASE, TARGETING, AND BOTTLENECKS

The TB Structural Genomics Database (http://www.doe-mbi.ucla.edu/TB) contains data for all 3,999 genes from the genome (12, 20) organized into three sections: (i) bioinformatics, (ii) targeting, and (iii) experimental information. The bioinformatics information is available for all the genes, while targeting and experimental data are recorded only when a consortium member makes an entry. The bioinformatics section contains the physicochemical properties, genomic and proteomic information, details of proteolysis sites, signal peptides, and transmembrane helices. The database provides further links to all homologous sequences available in the NR (Nonredundant; http://www.ncbi.nlm.nih.gov), PDB (Protein Data Bank; http://www.rcsb.org/pdb) and OMIM (On Mendelian Inheritance in Man; http://www.ncbi.nlm.nih.gov/entrez/query.fcgi?db=OMIM) databases through BLAST searches (2) (http://www.ncbi.nlm.nih.gov/BLAST); links to other programs which predict functional and structural information, such as PFAM (7) (http://pfam.wustl.edu/), HMM (27) (http://hmmer.wustl.edu/), CATH domains (82) (http://www.biochem.ucl.ac.uk/bsm/cath/), and DASEY (68) (http://fold.doe-mbi.ucla.edu/); and links to the related websites EBI (http://www.ebi.ac.uk), Sanger (http://www.sanger.ac.uk), Pedant (http://pedant.gsf.de), and Tuberculist (http://genolist.pasteur.fr).

The section on targeting facilitates communication among scientists within the consortium with the purpose of avoiding overlap of effort. Figure 2a sum-

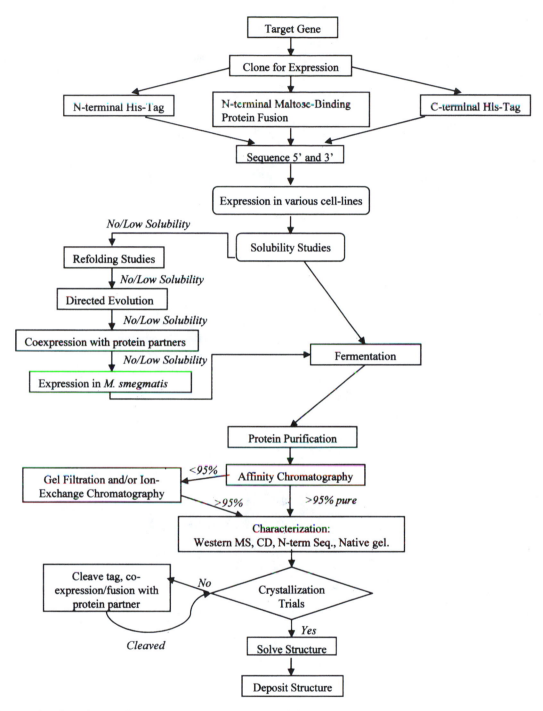

Figure 1. Flowchart showing the most common experimental path for the determination of structures by members of the TB Structural Genomics Consortium, although many variations of this path are taken in practice.

marizes the progress of the consortium. From 3,999 potential targets, representing every open reading frame (ORF) in the *M. tuberculosis* genome, 1,431 ORF have been targeted and 1,181 are active. To date, 40 structures are being or have been refined and deposited in the PDB. Given the low ratio for the number of structures so far solved per ORF targeted, it is instructive to look into the current bottlenecks of

the project. Any process with no bottleneck resembles an exponential curve in the initial stages, which is illustrated by the regression exponential fit (Fig. 2a). Interestingly, a closer look at the individual data points shows that some of the stages (namely, Cloning II, Expression, and Solubility I) are located on the top of the curve while others (such as Purification and Solubility II) are on the bottom. The bottlenecks may

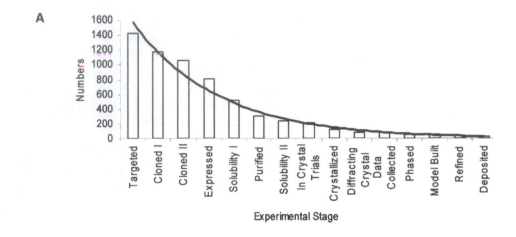

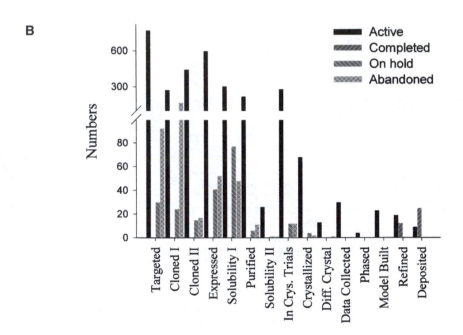

Figure 2. (A) The number of *M. tuberculosis* proteins (*y* axis) that have reached each experimental stage (*x* axis). The curve represents an exponential fit of the form $y = 2113.2 \exp(-0.2963x)$; $r^2 = 0.9834$. (B) Number of experiments conducted for all *M. tuberculosis* proteins at each given experimental stage.

be inferred by pinpointing the stages which cross the exponential curve from above the curve to below the curve. This suggests that "Expression and Solubility" and "Crystallization" are the largest bottlenecks.

Figure 2b shows the status of all experiments performed by consortium members. Examination of the figure shows that "Expressed" and "In Crystal Trials" stages are the most active stages in the protein production and protein crystallography steps, respectively. This could be interpreted as showing that experimental stages with low success rates remain active for the longest duration. Appreciable numbers of "On

hold" and "Abandoned" proteins indicate the great complexity of particular problems faced by the scientists working on these proteins. This inference is valid, assuming that the scientists are equally persis-tent in the success of their experiments.

The third section of the database contains experimental data from consortium members, high-throughput data collected automatically from the large-scale facilities for protein production and crystallization, together with protocols and observations classified by using unique identifiers based on the mmCIF dictionary (117) from the PDB. The data are stored in the database as tables and can be exported as text/XML. Examples of raw high-throughput crystallization data can be found at the TBSGC website (http://www.doe-mbi.ucla.edu/TB/DB/XTAL/llnl), and all data described in this section are freely available from the TB Consortium website (http://www.doe-mbi.ucla.edu/TB).

STRUCTURES OF *M. TUBERCULOSIS* PROTEINS SOLVED TO DATE

Secreted and Unusual Cell Wall Proteins of *M. tuberculosis*

Proteins are secreted by *M. tuberculosis* in response to environmental changes, for example, to protect against oxidative damage or to colonize a host successfully. Some of these proteins play biological roles in the cell envelope, whereas others act as virulence factors. Additionally, secretion of proteins by intracellular pathogens, such as *M. tuberculosis*, plays a central role in determining pathways of antigen presentation and recognition by effector T cells involved in protective immunity. Described below are structures and functions of secreted proteins, of proteins involved in the secretion and signaling systems, and of a set of proteins that are involved in the synthesis of cell wall components.

Secreted Proteins

Antigen 85B and 85C—Rv1886c and Rv0129c. The antigen 85 complex comprises three closely related enzymes, antigen 85A (Ag85A) (31 kDa), Ag85B (30 kDa), and Ag85C (31.5 kDa). These secreted proteins are both antigenic and involved in cell wall maintenance (118). They are the most abundant secreted proteins of tubercle bacilli cultivated in vitro (49) and are found inside human mononuclear phagocytes (61). Proteins of the Ag85 complex elicit protective immunity in animal models, making the Ag85 complex an attractive vaccine candidate (54) and drug candidate. Ag85 proteins have mycolyltransferase activity and catalyze the transfer of the fatty acid mycolate from one trehalose monomycolate molecule to another, resulting in the formation of trehalose dimycolate and free trehalose and helping to build the mycobacterial cell wall (22).

The structure of Ag85C was the first of the complex to be solved (88), revealing a single-domain, monomeric protein with an α/β-hydrolase fold (Color Plate 6a). The elongated active site pocket is a negatively charged cavity binding trehalose with a carbohydrate-binding motif. Also in the vicinity of the active site is a catalytic triad contributing the nucleophile for the mycolyl transfer reaction. The Ag85 complex stimulates the uptake of mycobacteria by human macrophages and has been implicated in interaction with the gelatin-binding site of human fibronectin. Each Ag85 protein contains a fibronectin-binding sequence located on an exposed surface.

The structure of Ag85B (4) is closely similar to that of Ag85C, as was expected from the 73% sequence similarity, but the bound ligands gave a clue about potential drug binding (Color Plate 6b). The trehalose-bound structure of Ag85B revealed that two molecules of trehalose are bound per monomer (4). The two molecules were located at opposite ends of the active site, one representing the liberated trehalose and the other representing the incoming trehalose monomycolate. The presence of dual trehalose sites in Ag85B suggests that a potential drug, consisting of two trehalose molecules joined by a linker, should inhibit the mycolyltransferase reaction.

Glutamine synthetase (GlnA)—Rv2220. Glutamine synthetase (GS) is a secreted protein which is released during the early stages of infection (46) and is thought to be necessary for the synthesis of poly-(L-glutamine-L-glutamate) chains (53), which form a large component of the cell wall. GS is essential for mycobacterial growth in both human macrophages and animal models (110) and is therefore an excellent drug target (47, 48). GS consists of two dodecamers in the asymmetric unit (Color Plate 6c), with their sixfold and twofold axes parallel to one another (34). Each subunit can be described as a "bi-funnel" in which ATP and glutamate bind at opposite ends, with a metal ion bound at one end of the bi-funnel. *M. tuberculosis* GS is an example of prokaryotic type I GS, whereas human GS is type II. Type I and II GS are different since type I is a dodecamer (1) and type II is possibly a seven- or eight-subunit oligomer (50), although the mechanism of action appears to be the same for both proteins (28). When the structure of a type II GS is solved, comparison of type I and II GS structures may lead to structure-based design of drugs to inhibit *M. tuberculosis* but not human GS.

MPT53 (DsbE)—Rv2878c. MPT53 (DsbE) is a secreted protein (78) that is conserved in tubercle bacilli (57). DsbE is an oxidoreductase which functions differently from its gram-negative bacterial homologs. It has a thioredoxin-like fold with its two active-site cysteines in the reduced form (Color Plate 6d) (40). Structural and functional analysis of DsbE suggests that it has a similar function to *E. coli* DsbA, which catalyzes the oxidation of reduced, unfolded secreted proteins to form disulfide bonds (40). It has been predicted that >60% of the 161 predicted secreted proteins of *M. tuberculosis* contain at least one disulfide bond (P. Mallick, personal communication). Hence, DsbE may be involved in virulence, since ~60% of secreted proteins require DsbE to ensure correct disulfide bond formation and folding.

MPT70 (MPB70)—Rv2875. The secreted antigen MPT70 and its homolog MPT83 (63% sequence identical) are highly immunogenic during the infection of mice (51). The structure of MPB70, the *M. bovis* ortholog of MPT70, has been solved by nuclear magnetic resonance spectroscopy and reveals a complex and novel bacterial fold (13). MPB70 (MPT70) is mainly an antiparallel seven-stranded β-barrel with eight α-helices that pack together on one side (Color Plate 6e). One side of the barrel is solvent exposed, whereas the other is decorated with four α-helices; the remaining four helices are positioned in a U-shaped arrangement at the top of the β-barrel. The N-terminal helix is anchored to the β-barrel by a disulfide bond. MPB70 has similar topology to the third and fourth FAS1 domains from eukaryotic fasciclin 1 (19). FAS1-containing extracellular matrix proteins (e.g., fasciclin 1) appear to bridge interactions between the cell surface and extracellular matrix (8) which implies that MPT70 and MPT83 bind to one or more cell surface host proteins, inducing changes in host cell behavior. It has been suggested that MPT70 and MPT83 may form a ring structure by internal disulfide bonding (59), in which case DsbE (Rv2878c) and its potential redox partner DsbD (Rv2874) may play a role in the formation of the internal disulfide bridges (40).

MPT63—Rv1926c. Rv1926c is a major secreted protein of unknown function, which is specific for mycobacteria (119, 124) and stimulates humoral immune responses in guinea pigs infected with *M. tuberculosis* (69). The structure of Rv1926c is an antiparallel β-sandwich (Color Plate 6f) with structural similarity to cell surface-binding proteins (e.g., arrestin, adaptin, and invasin), some of which are involved in endocytosis (42). Structural similarity implicates Rv1926c (MPT63) in possible host-bacterium interactions.

Rv0203—unknown function. Rv0203 is a predicted secreted protein of *M. tuberculosis*. Although the structure is at low resolution, one can see that it is mainly α-helical (Color Plate 6g). The monomer has two long α-helices and two short α-helices that dimerize to form a structure which resembles a catcher's mitt and then forms a tetramer which is cage-like (C. W. Goulding, unpublished data). Sedimentation analysis shows that Rv0203 is in equilibrium between dimer and tetramer in solution.

Secretion mechanism

SecA1—Rv3240c. In mycobacteria, one of the major secretion mechanisms is the type II, *sec*-dependent pathway catalyzed by a multiprotein translocase, which recognizes the signal sequence of a preprotein and uses ATP binding and hydrolysis as the driving force for transport (74). SecA plays a central role in the export pathway. In *M. tuberculosis*, there are two SecA homologs, which is unusual among bacterial species but appears to be common in actinobacteria (10). SecA1 is encoded by an essential gene and is equivalent to *E. coli* SecA (96). SecA2 is not essential, although it is required for full virulence (10). The crystal structure of SecA1 reveals two domains, a motor domain and a translocation domain (Color Plate 6h) (96). The motor domain contains two α/β-sheets, which resemble the DEAD motor ATPases; the two sheets are referred to as nucleotide-binding domains. The highly porous translocation domain is composed of the substrate specificity domain (preprotein-binding domain) and the helical core domain (consisting of four helices). SecA1 forms a dimer, which is predicted to interact with the SecYEG pore and function as a "molecular ratchet" that utilizes ATP hydrolysis for physical movement of the preprotein.

Extracellular to intracellular signaling mechanism

PknB (serine/threonine protein kinase)—Rv0014c. There are 11 serine/threonine protein kinases in *M. tuberculosis* (20); they belong to the eukaryotic kinase superfamily (45). PknB is thought to regulate cell division and growth, and the structure of its N-terminal kinase domain has been solved (Color Plate 6i) (80, 125). The intracellular kinase domain is followed by a transmembrane domain and then an extracellular domain that contains repeats which have similarity to the targeting domain of penicillin-binding proteins (PASTA domain) (125). The intracellular kinase domain complexed with ATP-γ-S adopts the characteristic two-lobed structure of eukaryotic serine/threonine kinases (56). Hence, we have an example of a transmembrane serine/threonine protein kinase that probably plays a role in signal transduction pathways within *M. tuberculosis* in response to environmental changes that lead to oligomerization.

Proteins Involved in the Synthesis of Cell Wall Components

Cyclopropane and inositol 1-phosphate synthases

CcmA1 (Rv3392c), CcmA2 (Rv0503c) and PcaA (Rv0470c). Cyclopropane synthases introduce a cyclopropane ring, at either the distal or proximal position of mycolic acids, which are critical to the structure and function of the cell envelope (33, 126). The cyclopropane synthase, encoded by *pcaA*, has been identified as a persistence factor (35, 102). The structures of three cyclopropane synthases, including PcaA, have been solved (also CcmA1 and CcmA2, [Color Plates 6j–l]). They show a seven-strand α/β-fold, similar to other methyltransferases, with a conserved interaction site for *S*-adenosyl-L-methionine (SAM) and a hydrophobic lipid-binding pocket (55). The ternary complexes reveal electron density that may represent a bicarbonate ion, which supports a methyltransferase mechanism via a carbocation. CcmA2 and PcaA both act at the proximal position, producing *cis* and *trans* cyclopropane rings, respectively (33, 35). Their structures are extremely similar. CcmA1 acts at the distal position (126). Structural comparison of CcmA1 with CcmA2 and PcaA shows that there is one differing region, which is a conserved basic/hydrophobic region that has been shifted in CcmA1 compared to CcmA2 and PcaA (55). It is hypothesized that this is the region where the cyclopropane synthase protein partner (AcpM) binds and presents the acyl chain of acyl-AcpM. Hence, acyl-AcpM may bind closer to the active site of CcmA2 and PcaA, favoring the reaction at the proximal position, whereas acyl-AcpM would sit further away from the active site to favor the reaction at the distal position (55). In conclusion, the study of three cyclopropane synthases has answered questions about the mechanism of cyclopropanation. Also, the structures of this diverse family of cyclopropane synthases are surprisingly similar, which may lead to the design of an inhibitor that could block all cyclopropanation reactions.

Ino1—Rv0046c. Inositol 1-phosphate synthase (Ino1) is a key enzyme in phosphatidylinositol synthesis. Phosphatidylinositol is a key precursor of many *M. tuberculosis* glycolipid cell wall components. The structure of Ino1 has been determined and comprises two domains connected by two hinge regions. Domain I has a Rossmann fold (NADH cofactor), and domain II contains residues which form the interface of the tetramer (79). Interestingly, a zinc ion bridges the nicotinamide ring of NAD^+ to the proteins, which raises the question whether the zinc is structural or functional.

InhA and protein partners

InhA—Rv1484. NADH-dependent enoyl-acyl carrier protein reductase (InhA) participates in FAS-II fatty acid biosynthesis, which produces mycolic acids. Inactivation of InhA alone is sufficient to inhibit mycolic acid biosynthesis and induce cell lysis (112), and isoniazid (INH) specifically targets InhA (6). The structure of InhA was solved in complex with NADH (26), leading to the conclusion that INH interacts with NADH. When the structure of the InhA-NADH-INH complex was solved, it was observed that INH was covalently bound to NADH in the presence of a divalent metal, hence inhibiting InhA (89, 90). Further drug design against InhA is under way.

NadC—Rv1595. Quinolinic acid phosphoribosyltransferase (QAPRTase) (NadC) catalyzes a key step in the de novo biosynthetic pathway of NAD. This is an important drug target because the anti-TB drug INH covalently modifies NAD and, in turn, the INH-NAD adduct inhibits mycolic acid synthesis, hence killing *M. tuberculosis*. The structure of apo-QAPRTase, with its substrate, products, and inhibitors bound, shows conformational changes which elucidate the catalytic mechanism (97).

Cytochrome P450 and partner proteins

CYP51 (Rv0764c) and CYP121 (Rv2276)—P450 proteins. Cytochrome P450s are *b*-heme-containing enzymes that bind and reduce molecular oxygen, mostly leading to monooxygenation of substrate and production of a molecule of water. They usually play oxidative roles in lipid metabolism and hence are potential anti-TB drug targets (76). Two P450 structures have been determined, CYP51 (84) and CYP121 (63). CYP121 is a novel P450 structure, including mixed heme conformations and putative proton relay pathways from the protein surface to the heme. Further investigation of the P450 mechanism with a potential redox partner, FprA (see below), is under way.

FprA—Rv3106c. FprA is an oxidoreductase that catalyzes the transfer of reducing equivalents from NADPH to a protein acceptor. The structures of both the oxidized and reduced forms of FprA have been solved (9) and revealed a homodimer with a flavin adenine dinucleotide domain and an NADPH domain exhibiting dinucleotide-binding fold topology. Interestingly, the FprA-$NADP^+$ complex shows that the $NADP^+$ nicotinamide ring exhibits the unusual *cis* conformation and that $NADP^+$ is covalently modified. FprA is a paralog of adrenodoxin reductase and therefore may be involved either with iron metabolism or with cytochrome P450 reductase activity.

Metabolic Pathways

Glyoxylate shunt pathway

Iso-citrate lyase (Icl)—Rv0467 and malate synthase (GlnB)—Rv1837. The glyoxylate shunt pathway, known to be essential for bacterial survival in activated macrophages and for persistent infection (52, 70), is induced when β-oxidation of fatty acids is used to generate energy and a carbon source. There are two enzymes involved in this process, iso-citrate lyase, which converts isocitrate to succinate and glyoxylate, and malate synthase, which forms malate by the addition of acetyl coenzyme A (acetyl-CoA) to glyoxylate. Isocitrate lyase is a tetramer with inter-subunit domain swapping and a large conformational change in the active-site loop on substrate binding (98). The monomer is an eight-α/β-barrel structure, with helix 8 interacting with the other monomers. The α/β-barrel domain-swapping phenomenon is also observed in the *M. tuberculosis* PanB structure. The structures of isocitrate lyase bound to two inhibitors were also solved and provide a blueprint for drug design. The structure of malate synthase (GlnB) demonstrates that it is a three-domain protein (100). Domain I is an eight-α/β-TIM barrel, the C-terminal domain II is mostly helical, and domain III which is inserted into the TIM barrel is β-strand rich. This β-insert is usual in the malate synthase G superfamily (66), and the fold which is more reminiscent of *M. tuberculosis* GlnB is pyruvate kinase. The active site is located at the interface of the TIM barrel and domain II, which is a long cavity. The structure of the complex of GlnB with Mg^{2+}-malate-CoA shows that the Mg^{2+} ion is coordinated to the base of the active site tunnel, followed by malate and then CoA, which protrudes slightly from the active site. The structure of GlnB complexed with cofactors and products also provides a promising starting point for the design of drugs active against GlnB.

Pantanoate acid synthesis and lysine biosynthesis

An auxotrophic mutant of *M. tuberculosis* defective in the de novo biosynthesis of pantothenate (Δ*panC/panD*) is highly attenuated in immunocompromised mice (94) but able to protect immunocompetent mice against virulent *M. tuberculosis* when used as a vaccine. Hence, pantothenate is essential for the virulence of *M. tuberculosis*. Lysine is required in protein biosynthesis and is essential for bacterial viability and development. It has been shown that the *lysA* gene is also essential for *M. tuberculosis* survival in an immunodeficient-mouse model (52, 81). Neither the pantothenate pathway nor LysA exists in higher mammals, and so these enzymes are attractive anti-TB drug targets, although one should bear in mind that some bacteria acquire pantothenate from their surroundings.

PanB (Rv2225) and PanC (Rv3602c). PanB is the first committed step in the biosynthesis of panthothenate, which is also a precursor to CoA. PanB, or ketopantoate hydroxymethyltransferase (KPHMT), converts α-ketoisovalerate to ketopantoate by a one-carbon transfer from a folate cofactor. PanB is a decamer formed from two pentameric rings stacked together; domain swapping is used to create a dimer of pentamers interface (15). The active site is situated at the top of the α/β-barrel due to the clustering of conserved residues within this region, where the substrate α-ketoisovalerate may bind. Also, at the top of the barrel, an Mg^{2+} ion is coordinated to conserved residues which may be the divalent metal ion which has been reported for activity (85). PanC (pantothenate synthetase) is involved in the last step of the pantothenate biosynthetic pathway. PanC catalyzes the ATP-dependent conversion of pantoate and β-alanine to form pantothenate. It is a dimer, with each subunit consisting of two domains (116) The N-terminal domain forms a typical Rossmann fold, with a central six-strand parallel β-sheet flanked by α-helices. The C-terminal domain forms a hinged lid over the active site cavity on the N-terminal domain. It has two layers, a three-strand antiparallel β-sheet with two α-helices layered on one side. Crystal structures of PanC with an ATP derivative, pantoate, and an intermediate analog, pantoyl adenylate, were also solved, giving clues to potential inhibitors of the PanC (116). Finally, the structure of PanE, an intermediate enzyme in the biosynthetic pathway, could provide insights into substrate pre-sentation and potential interactions between the proteins within the pantothenate pathway.

LysA—Rv1293c. The *lysA* gene encodes *meso*-diaminopimelate decarboxylase, the enzyme catalyzing the final step in the lysine biosynthetic pathway in which *meso*-diaminopimelic acid is converted to L-lysine, utilizing pyridoxal-5′-phosphate (PLP). The LysA structure has two domains; the central domain is an α/β-barrel, and the second domain consists of the N and C termini, which form a mixed β-sheet flanked by α-helices (36). PLP binds to the α/β-barrel, and the substrate/product is bound between the two domains, although the binding is mainly by the residues from the β-sheet domain. A suggested inhibitor of LysA is α-difluoromethyl ornithine, which would form an external aldimine linkage with PLP, which is covalently bound to Cys360, thus irreversibly blocking the substrate-binding site (36).

Metabolic proteins which are regulated

FolB—Rv3607c. The folate biosynthetic pathway is an essential pathway in all bacteria, whereas humans can both synthesize folate and obtain it from their diet. Sulfonamides are known antibacterial drugs which inhibit two enzymes (7,8-dihydropteroate synthase and dihydrofolate reductase) in this pathway; the structures of both enzymes have been determined (5, 64). Recently, the structure of *M. tuberculosis* FolB (7,8-dihydroneopterin aldolase), which catalyzes the second step in the pathway, has been solved with and without bound substrate (C. W. Goulding, M. I. Apostol, M. R. Sawaya, M. Philips, A. Parseghian, and D. Eisenberg, unpublished data). FolB without substrate is a tetramer, whereas in the presence of substrate *M. tuberculosis* FolB is octameric. The tetramer is a 16-strand β-barrel decorated with α-helices, and the octamer is a dimer of tetramers with a substrate molecule bound between each monomer. The transition between tetrameric and octomeric states requires a subtle conformational change, which appears to occur on substrate binding. This implies that FolB is a regulated enzyme, which could be due to its substrate, 7,8-dihydroneopterin, being utilized as an antioxidant.

HisG—Rv2121c. In the first designated step in histidine biosynthesis, N-1-(5'-phosphoribosyl)-ATP transferase (ATP-PRTase, HisG) catalyzes the condensation of ATP with 5'-phosphoribosyl 1'-pyrophosphate in the presence of a divalent metal (3). The structure of ATP-PRTase reveals an elongated molecule containing three domains, each of which contains a five- to six-strand β-sheet surrounded by different numbers of α-helices (17). Domains I and II form the catalytic core, while the feedback inhibitor histidine binds to domain III. ATP-PRTase exists as a dimer in its active form, where the interactions are mainly through domains I and II. Comparison of the structures of apo-ATP-PRTase and AMP:histidine-ATP-PRTase reveals that histidine is the allosteric regulator, since it appears to stabilize the inactive hexameric form (interactions are mainly through domain III) and hinders substrate binding.

Essential Housekeeping Proteins

RecA—Rv2737c. RecA plays an important role in recombinational repair, homologous recombination, and induction of the SOS response. RecA is a ubiquitous protein present in all organisms (87). Its activity requires the formation of a helical nucleoprotein filament, which results in binding of both Mg^{2+}-ATP and single-stranded DNA (31). Interestingly, the active form of the *M. tuberculosis* RecA enzyme is generated by a splicing mechanism (25). The structure of RecA has three distinct domains; the first domain is a long α-helix, the second has the nucleoside triphosphate hydrolase fold which contains the P-loop, and the third is an eight-strand β-sheet surrounded by α-helices (23). The monomers of RecA form helical filaments with a deep groove capable of binding DNA. The interactions between monomers are between the α-helix in domain I and some of the residues of domain II. The filamentous structure aggregates into bundles, probably a storage form of inactivated enzyme. Since RecA plays a central role in several processes for survival, it may be a good drug target. The initial focus for drug design might be on the DNA-binding groove, which is deeper than that of the ATP binding to the P-loop as seen in *E. coli* RecA (103, 104).

dUTPase—Rv2697c. dUTP pyrophosphatase is essential for depleting potentially toxic concentrations of dUTP in the cell. Because dUTP can be readily incorporated into DNA by DNA polymerases, its accumulation in the genetic material would overwhelm the DNA repair system, leading to multiple DNA strand breaks and, eventually, to cell death. Inhibition of dUTPase might also be a means to slow the growth of *M. tuberculosis*. However, comparison of the structure of *M. tuberculosis* dUTPase (M. R. Sawaya, S. Chan, B. Segelke, T. Lekin, H. Krupka, B.-S. Rho, C. M. Naranjo, Y. C. Rogers, C.-Y. Kim, U. Cho, M. S. Park, G. S. Waldo, I. Pashkov, D. Cascio, T. O. Yeates, J. L. Perry, T. C. Terwilliger, and D. Eisenberg, unpublished data) with that of the human dUTPase reveals only a modest increase in the breadth and width of the dUTP-binding pocket, hence making drug design a challenge. Surprisingly, the *M. tuberculosis* dUTPase appears to be evolutionarily equidistant from its human and *E. coli* orthologs. This evidence suggests that the human and *M. tuberculosis* enzymes have more similarity than would ordinarily be expected between a prokaryotic and a eukaryotic enzyme. The structure of *M. tuberculosis* dUTPase, complexed with the nonhydrolyzable inhibitor, α,β-imido-dUTP, suggests a revised mechanism of pyrophosphorolysis.

NusA (Rv2841c) and NusB (Rv2533c). Both prokaryotes and eukaryotes regulate RNA transcription through suppression of termination signals in the RNA secondary structure by using Nus proteins, which are part of a multiprotein assembly. NusA has RNA-binding properties, and *E. coli* NusA binds to RNA polymerase (67). NusA is a four-domain protein; the N-terminal domain resembles an ATP-binding protein, and the C-terminal segment consists of an S1 ribosomal domain followed by two K-homology domains (38). The S1 and K-homology domains interact to form an extensive RNA-binding structure. The C-terminal domain is flexibly linked to the N-terminal RNA polymerase-binding domain, which facilitates the simultaneous interaction of NusA with both the nascent RNA transcript and RNA polymerase. The structure of *M. tuberculosis* NusB has also been determined (37) and reveals a wedge-shaped seven-α-helix monomer. *M. tuberculosis* NusB also forms a dimer, whereas *E. coli* NusB is a monomer (62). A possible site of interaction with the box A RNA and phosphate-binding site are identified. It would be interesting to determine the other *M. tuberculosis* Nus structures in order to attempt to predict interactions between the Nus proteins, RNA, and RNA polymerase.

MsrA—Rv0137c. MsrA (methionine sulfoxide reductase A) repairs oxidative damage to methionine residues as a result of the action of reactive oxygen and nitrogen species; hence, it acts as a primary defense against oxidative damage (75). Structural analysis of *M. tuberculosis* MsrA shows that there only two reactive cysteines (107) and that a methionine residue is bound at the active site of a neighboring molecule. This gives insight into the protein-bound methionine sulfoxide recognition and repair.

Ssb—Rv0054. Ssb is a single-stranded DNA-binding protein which protects the transiently formed single-stranded DNA from nuclease and chemical attacks; it is therefore required for bacterial survival (77). The structure of *M. tuberculosis* Ssb exhibits a DNA fold and forms a tetramer (93). *M. tuberculosis* Ssb has a unique dimeric interface, which makes the oligomerized protein more stable than its human homolog (121). The structural variations between the human and *M. tuberculosis* Ssb structures may permit the design of drugs that target the *M. tuberculosis* Ssb specifically without targeting its human homolog.

Cpn10 (GroES)—Rv3418. Chaperone-10 (GroES; 10 kDa) is implicated as a virulence factor (32) and acts in concert with chaperone-60 (GroEL), of which *M. tuberculosis* has two forms. These proteins catalyze protein folding. The crystal structure of GroES has been determined by two separate groups (86, 106). It is a dimer of dome-shaped heptamers which forms a spherical cage-like structure. The two heptamers are held together by flexible loops extending outward from the base, and the cavity of the tetradecamer is hydrophilic. The base loops are essential for complexing with GroEL, and the crystal structure of the GroEL-GroES complex would be most informative.

Cytosolic Proteins of Unknown Function

FabG3—Rv2002. Rv2002 is a 250-residue protein belonging to the short-chain dehydrogenase/reductase family because it contains the characteristic dinucleotide binding motif. It has been annotated as FabG3, a homologue of β-ketoacyl acyl carrier protein reductase. The structure reveals four identical monomers which form a tetramer, each with a Rossmann fold domain. A ternary complex was crystallized with androsterone and NADH (122). This work suggests that the Rv2002 gene product is a unique member of the short-chain dehydrogenase/reductase family and may be involved in steroid metabolism.

MenG—Rv3853. Menaquinone (vitamin K) is an essential vitamin that is an obligatory component of the anaerobic electron transfer pathways that operate not only in strict anaerobes but also in aerobic bacteria (71). MenG is the final step of the biosynthetic pathway of vitamin K, in which it supposedly methylates demethylated menaquinone. The structure of MenG suggests that it is not a SAM-dependent methyltransferase, since it does not have the characteristic fold or the conserved binding pocket (58). The structure of Rv3853 is more consistent with the phosphohistidine transferase domain of pyruvate phosphate dikinase, and there is a potential histidine-binding site. However, further investigation is required.

Methyltransferase—Rv2118c. Rv2118c belongs to a group of conserved hypothetical proteins. The crystal structure, complexed with SAM, shows that the protein has two domains (44). The C-terminal domain binds the cofactor SAM, and the smaller N-terminal domain has a β-fold which is not found in other bacterial proteins. From sequence alignments, Rv2118c is proposed to be a tRNA methyltransferase.

Citrate lyase, β-chain—Rv2498c. Citrate lyase is usually a large (550-kDa) complex formed by six copies of each α, β, and γ subunit. *M. tuberculosis* does not possess the α or γ subunits; therefore, the activity of this protein needs to be determined. The structure of Rv2498c is an eight-α,β-barrel structure which has both dimer and trimer contacts. At the interface of the trimer, the diphosphate group of ATP, ADP, and GTP binds to the arginines in the structure (C. W. Goulding, unpublished data).

SUMMARY

In this chapter we have summarized the results of the TB Structural Genomics Consortium after its first two and three-quarter years of existence. The structures that have been described cover many biological functions both inside and outside of the *M. tuberculosis* cell, and many of them have potential as drug targets or vaccine candidates. During the next few years, the TB Structural Genomics Consortium will endeavor to determine many more structures, including membrane protein structures, in the hope that protein complexes, machines, and biological pathways may be constructed that shed light on the biology of *M. tuberculosis*. Structural and functional information determined through this effort is likely to enable the development of new drugs to cure tuberculosis.

APPENDIX

PDB ID codes for structures in this chapter not in Color Plate 6

PDB Code	Rv no.	Protein
1gr0	Rv0046	Ino1
1bvr	Rv1484	InhA
1qpr	Rv1595	NadC
1ea1	Rv0764c	CYP51
1n40	Rv2276	CYP121
1lqu	Rv3106c	FprA
1f8i	Rv0467	Icl
1ni8	Rv1837c	GlnB
1oyo	Rv2225	PanB
1n2e	Rv3602c	PanC
1hkv	Rv1293c	LysA
1nbu	Rv3607c	FolB
1nh7	Rv2121c	HisG
1g18	Rv2737c	RecA
1mq7	Rv2697c	dUTPase
1k0r	Rv2841c	NusA
1eyv	Rv2533c	NusB
1nwa	Rv0137c	MsrA
1ju2	Rv3418c	Ssb
1nfq	Rv2002	FabG3
1nxj	Rv3853	MenG
1i9g	Rv2118c	MeTr
	Rv2498c	CitE

Acknowledgments. We thank Thomas C. Terwilliger, Los Alamos National Laboratory, Principal Investigator of the TB Structural Genomics Consortium, who offers constant guidance and encouragement, and the many members of the consortium who have determined the structures. Full details of the consortium can be found at http://www.doe-mbi.ucla.edu/TB. Support for this project comes from NIGMS and NIAID grants for the consortium effort.

REFERENCES

1. Almassy, R. J., C. A. Janson, R. Hamlin, N. H. Xuong, and D. Eisenberg. 1986. Novel subunit-subunit interactions in the structure of glutamine synthetase. *Nature* 323:304–309.

2. Altschul, S. F., T. L. Madden, A. A. Schaffer, J. Zhang, Z. Zhang, W. Miller, and D. J. Lipman. 1997. Gapped BLAST and PSI-BLAST: a new generation of protein database search programs. *Nucleic Acids Res.* 25:3389–3402.

3. Ames, B. N., R. G. Martin, and B. J. Garry. 1961. The first step of histidine biosynthesis. *J. Biol. Chem.* 236:2019–2026.

4. Anderson, D. H., G. Harth, M. A. Horwitz, and D. Eisenberg. 2001. An interfacial mechanism and a class of inhibitors inferred from two crystal structures of the *Mycobacterium tuberculosis* 30 kDa major secretory protein (Antigen 85B), a mycolyl transferase. *J. Mol. Biol.* 307:671–681.

5. Baca, A. M., R. Sirawaraporn, S. Turley, W. Sirawaraporn, and W. G. Hol. 2000. Crystal structure of *Mycobacterium tuberculosis* 7,8-dihydropteroate synthase in complex with pterin monophosphate: new insight into the enzymatic mechanism and sulfa-drug action. *J. Mol. Biol.* 302:1193–1212.

6. Banerjee, A., E. Dubnau, A. Quemard, V. Balasubramanian, K. S. Um, T. Wilson, D. Collins, G. de Lisle, and W. R. Jacobs, Jr. 1994. *inhA*, a gene encoding a target for isoniazid and ethionamide in *Mycobacterium tuberculosis*. *Science* 263:227–230.

7. Bateman, A., and D. H. Haft. 2002. HMM-based databases in InterPro. *Brief Bioinform.* 3:236–245.

8. Billings, P. C., J. C. Whitbeck, C. S. Adams, W. R. Abrams, A. J. Cohen, B. N. Engelsberg, P. S. Howard, and J. Rosenbloom. 2002. The transforming growth factor-beta-inducible matrix protein (beta)ig-h3 interacts with fibronectin. *J. Biol. Chem.* 277:28003–28009.

9. Bossi, R. T., A. Aliverti, D. Raimondi, F. Fischer, G. Zanetti, D. Ferrari, N. Tahallah, C. S. Maier, A. J. Heck, M. Rizzi, and A. Mattevi. 2002. A covalent modification of NADP⁺ revealed by the atomic resolution structure of FprA, a *Mycobacterium tuberculosis* oxidoreductase. *Biochemistry* 41:8807–8818.

10. Braunstein, M., A. M. Brown, S. Kurtz, and W. R. Jacobs, Jr. 2001. Two nonredundant SecA homologues function in mycobacteria. *J. Bacteriol.* 183:6979–6990.

11. Bryk, R., C. D. Lima, H. Erdjument-Bromage, P. Tempst, and C. Nathan. 2002. Metabolic enzymes of mycobacteria linked to antioxidant defense by a thioredoxin-like protein. *Science* 295:1073–1077.

12. Camus, J. C., M. J. Pryor, C. Medigue, and S. T. Cole. 2002. Re-annotation of the genome sequence of *Mycobacterium tuberculosis* H37Rv. *Microbiology* 148:2967–2973.

13. Carr, M. D., M. J. Bloemink, E. Dentten, A. O. Whelan, S. V. Gordon, G. Kelly, T. A. Frenkiel, R. G. Hewinson, and R. A. Williamson. 2003. Solution structure of the *Mycobacterium tuberculosis* complex protein MPB70: from tuberculosis pathogenesis to inherited human corneal disease. *J. Biol. Chem.* 278:43736–43743.

14. Chang, G., R. H. Spencer, A. T. Lee, M. T. Barclay, and D. C. Rees. 1998. Structure of the MscL homolog from *Mycobacterium tuberculosis*: a gated mechanosensitive ion channel. *Science* 282:2220–2226.

15. Chaudhuri, B. N., M. R. Sawaya, C. Y. Kim, G. S. Waldo, M. S. Park, T. C. Terwilliger, and T. O. Yeates. 2003. The crystal structure of the first enzyme in the pantothenate biosynthetic pathway, ketopantoate hydroxymethyltransferase, from *M. tuberculosis*. *Structure* 11:753–764.

16. Chen, Y., S. Morera, J. Mocan, I. Lascu, and J. Janin. 2002. X-ray structure of *Mycobacterium tuberculosis* nucleoside diphosphate kinase. *Proteins* 47:556–557.

17. Cho, Y., V. Sharma, and J. C. Sacchettini. 2003. Crystal structure of ATP phosphoribosyltransferase from *Mycobacterium tuberculosis*. *J. Biol. Chem.* 278:8333–8339.

18. Cirilli, M., R. Zheng, G. Scapin, and J. S. Blanchard. 2003.

The three-dimensional structures of the *Mycobacterium tuberculosis* dihydrodipicolinate reductase-NADH-2,6-PDC and -NADPH-2,6-PDC complexes. Structural and mutagenic analysis of relaxed nucleotide specificity. *Biochemistry* 42:10644–10650.

19. Clout, N. J., D. Tisi, and E. Hohenester. 2003. Novel fold revealed by the structure of a FAS1 domain pair from the insect cell adhesion molecule fasciclin I. *Structure* 11:197–203.

20. Cole, S. T., R. Brosch, J. Parkhill, T. Garnier, C. Churcher, D. Harris, S. V. Gordon, K. Eiglmeier, S. Gas, C. E. Barry III, F. Tekaia, K. Badcock, D. Basham, D. Brown, T. Chillingworth, R. Connor, R. Davies, K. Devlin, T. Feltwell, S. Gentles, N. Hamlin, S. Holroyd, T. Hornsby, K. Jagels, A. Krogh, J. McLean, S. Moule, L. Murphy, K. Oliver, J. Osborne, M. A. Quail, M.-A. Rajandream, J. Rogers, S. Rutter, K. Soeger, J. Skelton, R. Squares, S. Squares, J. E. Sulston, K. Taylor, S. Whitehead, and B. G. Barrell. 1998. Deciphering the biology of *Mycobacterium tuberculosis* from the complete genome sequence. *Nature* 393:537–544.

21. Cooper, J. B., K. McIntyre, M. O. Badasso, S. P. Wood, Y. Zhang, T. R. Garbe, and D. Young. 1995. X-ray structure analysis of the iron-dependent superoxide dismutase from *Mycobacterium tuberculosis* at 2.0 Ångstroms resolution reveals novel dimer-dimer interactions. *J. Mol. Biol.* 246:531–544.

22. Daffe, M. 2000. The mycobacterial antigens 85 complex—from structure to function and beyond. *Trends Microbiol.* 8:438–440.

23. Datta, S., N. Ganesh, N. R. Chandra, K. Muniyappa, and M. Vijayan. 2003. Structural studies on MtRecA-nucleotide complexes: insights into DNA and nucleotide binding and the structural signature of NTP recognition. *Proteins* 50:474–485.

24. Daugelat, S., J. Kowall, J. Mattow, D. Bumann, R. Winter, R. Hurwitz, and S. H. Kaufmann. 2003. The RD1 proteins of *Mycobacterium tuberculosis*: expression in *Mycobacterium smegmatis* and biochemical characterization. *Microbes Infect.* 5:1082–1095.

25. Davis, E. O., S. G. Sedgwick, and M. J. Colston. 1991. Novel structure of the *recA* locus of *Mycobacterium tuberculosis* implies processing of the gene product. *J. Bacteriol.* 173:5653–5662.

26. Dessen, A., A. Quemard, J. S. Blanchard, W. R. Jacobs, Jr., and J. C. Sacchettini. 1995. Crystal structure and function of the isoniazid target of *Mycobacterium tuberculosis*. *Science* 267:1638–1641.

27. Durbin, R., and S. Dear. 1998. Base qualities help sequencing software. *Genome Res.* 8:161–162.

28. Eisenberg, D., H. S. Gill, G. M. Pfluegl, and S. H. Rotstein. 2000. Structure-function relationships of glutamine synthetases. *Biochim. Biophys. Acta* 1477:122–145.

29. Evans, L. D., A. W. Roszak, L. J. Noble, D. A. Robinson, P. A. Chalk, J. L. Matthews, J. R. Coggins, N. C. Price, and A. J. Lapthorn. 2002. Specificity of substrate recognition by type II dehydroquinases as revealed by binding of polyanions. *FEBS Lett.* 530:24–30.

30. Feese, M. D., B. P. Ingason, J. Goranson-Siekierke, R. K. Holmes, and W. G. Hol. 2001. Crystal structure of the iron-dependent regulator from *Mycobacterium tuberculosis* at 2.0-Å resolution reveals the Src homology domain 3-like fold and metal binding function of the third domain. *J. Biol. Chem.* 276:5959–5966.

31. Flory, J., S. S. Tsang, and K. Muniyappa. 1984. Isolation and visualization of active presynaptic filaments of recA protein and single-stranded DNA. *Proc. Natl. Acad. Sci. USA* 81:7026–7030.

32. Galli, G., P. Ghezzi, P. Mascagni, F. Marcucci, and M. Fratelli. 1996. *Mycobacterium tuberculosis* heat shock protein 10 in-

creases both proliferation and death in mouse P19 teratocarcinoma cells. *In Vitro Cell. Dev. Biol. Anim.* 32:446–450.

33. George, K. M., Y. Yuan, D. R. Sherman, and C. E. Barry III. 1995. The biosynthesis of cyclopropanated mycolic acids in *Mycobacterium tuberculosis*. Identification and functional analysis of CMAS-2. *J. Biol. Chem.* 270:27292–27298.

34. Gill, H. S., G. M. Pfluegl, and D. Eisenberg. 2002. Multicopy crystallographic refinement of a relaxed glutamine synthetase from *Mycobacterium tuberculosis* highlights flexible loops in the enzymatic mechanism and its regulation. *Biochemistry* 41:9863–9872.

35. Glickman, M. S., J. S. Cox, and W. R. Jacobs, Jr. 2000. A novel mycolic acid cyclopropane synthetase is required for cording, persistence, and virulence of *Mycobacterium tuberculosis*. *Mol. Cell.* 5:717–727.

36. Gokulan, K., B. Rupp, M. S. Pavelka, Jr., W. R. Jacobs, Jr., and J. C. Sacchettini. 2003. Crystal structure of *Mycobacterium tuberculosis* diaminopimelate decarboxylase, an essential enzyme in bacterial lysine biosynthesis. *J. Biol. Chem.* 278:18588–18596.

37. Gopal, B., L. F. Haire, R. A. Cox, M. Jo Colston, S. Major, J. A. Brannigan, S. J. Smerdon, and G. Dodson. 2000. The crystal structure of NusB from *Mycobacterium tuberculosis*. *Nat. Struct. Biol.* 7:475–478.

38. Gopal, B., L. F. Haire, S. J. Gamblin, E. J. Dodson, A. N. Lane, K. G. Papavinasasundaram, M. J. Colston, and G. Dodson. 2001. Crystal structure of the transcription elongation/anti-termination factor NusA from *Mycobacterium tuberculosis* at 1.7 A resolution. *J. Mol. Biol.* 314:1087–1095.

39. Goulding, C. W., M. Apostol, D. H. Anderson, H. S. Gill, C. V. Smith, M. R. Kuo, J. K. Yang, G. S. Waldo, S. W. Suh, R. Chauhan, A. Kale, N. Bachhawat, S. C. Mande, J. M. Johnston, J. S. Lott, E. N. Baker, V. L. Arcus, D. Leys, K. J. McLean, A. W. Munro, J. Berendzen, V. Sharma, M. S. Park, D. Eisenberg, J. Sacchettini, T. Alber, B. Rupp, W. Jacobs, Jr., and T. C. Terwilliger. 2002. The TB structural genomics consortium: providing a structural foundation for drug discovery. *Curr. Drug Targets Infect. Disord.* 2:121–141.

40. Goulding, C. W., S. Gleiter, M. I. Apostol, A. Parseghian, J. Bardwell, M. L. Gennaro, and D. Eisenberg. 2004. Gram-positive DsbE proteins function differently from gram-negative DsbE homologs: a structure to function analysis of DsbE from *Mycobacterium tuberculosis*. *J. Biol. Chem.* 279:3516–3524.

41. Goulding, C. W., and L. Jeanne Perry. 2003. Protein production in *Escherichia coli* for structural studies by X-ray crystallography. *J. Struct. Biol.* 142:133–143.

42. Goulding, C. W., A. Parseghian, M. R. Sawaya, D. Cascio, M. I. Apostol, M. L. Gennaro, and D. Eisenberg. 2002. Crystal structure of a major secreted protein of *Mycobacterium tuberculosis*-MPT63 at 1.5-Å resolution. *Protein Sci.* 11:2887–2893.

43. Gu, Y., L. Reshetnikova, Y. Li, Y. Wu, H. Yan, S. Singh, and X. Ji. 2002. Crystal structure of shikimate kinase from *Mycobacterium tuberculosis* reveals the dynamic role of the LID domain in catalysis. *J. Mol. Biol.* 319:779–789.

44. Gupta, A., P. H. Kumar, T. K. Dineshkumar, U. Varshney, and H. S. Subramanya. 2001. Crystal structure of Rv2118c: an AdoMet-dependent methyltransferase from *Mycobacterium tuberculosis* H37Rv. *J. Mol. Biol.* 312:381–391.

45. Hanks, S. K., and T. Hunter. 1995. Protein kinases 6. The eukaryotic protein kinase superfamily: kinase (catalytic) domain structure and classification. *FASEB J.* 9:576–596.

46. Harth, G., D. L. Clemens, and M. A. Horwitz. 1994. Glutamine synthetase of *Mycobacterium tuberculosis*: extracellular release and characterization of its enzymatic activity. *Proc. Natl. Acad. Sci. USA* 91:9342–9346.

47. Harth, G., and M. A. Horwitz. 2003. Inhibition of *Mycobacterium tuberculosis* glutamine synthetase as a novel antibiotic strategy against tuberculosis: demonstration of efficacy in vivo. *Infect. Immun.* **71**:456–464.

48. Harth, G., and M. A. Horwitz. 1999. An inhibitor of exported *Mycobacterium tuberculosis* glutamine synthetase selectively blocks the growth of pathogenic mycobacteria in axenic culture and in human monocytes: extracellular proteins as potential novel drug targets. *J. Exp. Med.* **189**:1425–1436.

49. Harth, G., B. Y. Lee, J. Wang, D. L. Clemens, and M. A. Horwitz. 1996. Novel insights into the genetics, biochemistry, and immunocytochemistry of the 30-kilodalton major extracellular protein of *Mycobacterium tuberculosis. Infect. Immun.* **64**:3038–3047.

50. Haschemeyer, R. H. 1968. Electron microscopy of enzymes. *Trans. N.Y. Acad. Sci.* **30**:875–891.

51. Hewinson, R. G., S. L. Michell, W. P. Russell, R. A. McAdam, and W. R. Jacobs, Jr. 1996. Molecular characterization of MPT83: a seroreactive antigen of *Mycobacterium tuberculosis* with homology to MPT70. *Scand. J. Immunol.* **43**:490–499.

52. Hingley-Wilson, S. M., V. K. Sambandamurthy, and W. R. Jacobs, Jr. 2003. Survival perspectives from the world's most successful pathogen, *Mycobacterium tuberculosis. Nat. Immunol.* **4**:949–955.

53. Hirschfield, G. R., M. McNeil, and P. J. Brennan. 1990. Peptidoglycan-associated polypeptides of *Mycobacterium tuberculosis. J. Bacteriol.* **172**:1005–1013.

54. Horwitz, M. A., G. Harth, B. J. Dillon, and S. Maslesa-Galic. 2000. Recombinant bacillus Calmette-Guérin (BCG) vaccines expressing the *Mycobacterium tuberculosis* 30-kDa major secretory protein induce greater protective immunity against tuberculosis than conventional BCG vaccines in a highly susceptible animal model. *Proc. Natl. Acad. Sci. USA* **97**:13853–13858.

55. Huang, C.-C., C. V. Smith, M. S. Glickman, W. R. Jacobs, Jr., and J. C. Sacchettini. 2002. Crystal structures of mycolic acid cyclopropane synthases from *M. tuberculosis. J. Biol. Chem.* **277**:11559–11569.

56. Huse, M., and J. Kuriyan. 2002. The conformational plasticity of protein kinases. *Cell* **109**:275–282.

57. Johnson, S., P. Brusasca, K. Lyashchenko, J. S. Spencer, H. G. Wiker, P. Bifani, E. Shashkina, B. Kreiswirth, M. Harboe, N. Schluger, M. Gomez, and M. L. Gennaro. 2001. Characterization of the secreted MPT53 antigen of *Mycobacterium tuberculosis. Infect. Immun.* **69**:5936–5939.

58. Johnston, J. M., V. L. Arcus, C. J. Morton, M. W. Parker, and E. N. Baker. 2003. Crystal structure of a putative methyltransferase from *Mycobacterium tuberculosis*: misannotation of a genome clarified by protein structural analysis. *J. Bacteriol.* **185**:4057–4065.

59. Juarez, M. D., A. Torres, and C. Espitia. 2001. Characterization of the *Mycobacterium tuberculosis* region containing the *mpt83* and *mpt70* genes. *FEMS Microbiol. Lett.* **203**:95–102.

60. Kang, L. W., S. B. Gabelli, J. E. Cunningham, S. F. O'Handley, and L. M. Amzel. 2003. Structure and mechanism of MT-ADPRase, a nudix hydrolase from *Mycobacterium tuberculosis. Structure* **11**:1015–1023.

61. Lee, B. Y., and M. A. Horwitz. 1995. Identification of macrophage and stress-induced proteins of *Mycobacterium tuberculosis. J. Clin. Investig.* **96**:245–249.

62. Legault, P., J. Li, J. Mogridge, L. E. Kay, and J. Greenblatt. 1998. NMR structure of the bacteriophage lambda N peptide/boxB RNA complex: recognition of a GNRA fold by an arginine-rich motif. *Cell* **93**:289–299.

63. Leys, D., C. G. Mowat, K. J. McLean, A. Richmond, S. K. Chapman, M. D. Walkinshaw, and A. W. Munro. 2003. Atomic structure of *Mycobacterium tuberculosis* CYP121 to 1.06 Å reveals novel features of cytochrome P450. *J. Biol. Chem.* **278**:5141–5147.

64. Li, R., R. Sirawaraporn, P. Chitnumsub, W. Sirawaraporn, J. Wooden, F. Athappilly, S. Turley, and W. G. Hol. 2000. Three-dimensional structure of *M. tuberculosis* dihydrofolate reductase reveals opportunities for the design of novel tuberculosis drugs. *J. Mol. Biol.* **295**:307–323.

65. Li de la Sierra, I., H. Munier-Lehmann, A. M. Gilles, O. Barzu, and M. Delarue. 2001. X-ray structure of TMP kinase from *Mycobacterium tuberculosis* complexed with TMP at 1.95 Å resolution. *J. Mol. Biol.* **311**:87–100.

66. Lo Conte, L., S. E. Brenner, T. J. Hubbard, C. Chothia, and A. G. Murzin. 2002. SCOP database in 2002: refinements accommodate structural genomics. *Nucleic Acids Res.* **30**:264–267.

67. Mah, T. F., K. Kuznedelov, A. Mushegian, K. Severinov, and J. Greenblatt. 2000. The alpha subunit of E. coli RNA polymerase activates RNA binding by NusA. *Genes Dev.* **14**:2664–2675.

68. Mallick, P., R. Weiss, and D. Eisenberg. 2002. The directional atomic solvation energy: an atom-based potential for the assignment of protein sequences to known folds. *Proc. Natl. Acad. Sci. USA* **99**:16041–16046.

69. Manca, C., K. Lyashchenko, H. G. Wiker, D. Usai, R. Colangeli, and M. L. Gennaro. 1997. Molecular cloning, purification, and serological characterization of MPT63, a novel antigen secreted by *Mycobacterium tuberculosis. Infect. Immun.* **65**:16–23.

70. McKinney, J. D., K. Honer zu Bentrup, E. J. Munoz-Elias, A. Miczak, B. Chen, W. T. Chan, D. Swenson, J. C. Sacchettini, W. R. Jacobs, Jr., and D. G. Russell. 2000. Persistence of *Mycobacterium tuberculosis* in macrophages and mice requires the glyoxylate shunt enzyme isocitrate lyase. *Nature* **406**:735–738.

71. Meganathan, R. 2001. Biosynthesis of menaquinone (vitamin K2) and ubiquinone (coenzyme Q): a perspective on enzymatic mechanisms. *Vitam. Horm.* **61**:173–218.

72. Milani, M., A. Pesce, Y. Ouellet, P. Ascenzi, M. Guertin, and M. Bolognesi. 2001. *Mycobacterium tuberculosis* hemoglobin N displays a protein tunnel suited for O_2 diffusion to the heme. *EMBO J.* **20**:3902–3909.

73. Milani, M., P. Y. Savard, H. Ouellet, P. Ascenzi, M. Guertin, and M. Bolognesi. 2003. A TyrCD1/TrpG8 hydrogen bond network and a TyrB10TyrCD1 covalent link shape the heme distal site of *Mycobacterium tuberculosis* hemoglobin O. *Proc. Natl. Acad. Sci. USA* **100**:5766–5771.

74. Mori, H., and K. Ito. 2001. The Sec protein-translocation pathway. *Trends Microbiol.* **9**:494–500.

75. Moskovitz, J., S. Bar-Noy, W. M. Williams, J. Requena, B. S. Berlett, and E. R. Stadtman. 2001. Methionine sulfoxide reductase (MsrA) is a regulator of antioxidant defense and lifespan in mammals. *Proc. Natl. Acad. Sci. USA* **98**:12920–12925.

76. Munro, A. W., K. J. McLean, K. R. Marshall, A. J. Warman, G. Lewis, O. Roitel, M. J. Sutcliffe, C. A. Kemp, S. Modi, N. S. Scrutton, and D. Leys. 2003. Cytochromes P450: novel drug targets in the war against multidrug-resistant *Mycobacterium tuberculosis. Biochem. Soc. Trans.* **31**:625–630.

77. Mushegian, A. R., and E. V. Koonin. 1996. A minimal gene set for cellular life derived by comparison of complete bacterial genomes. *Proc. Natl. Acad. Sci. USA* **93**:10268–10273.

78. Nagai, S., H. G. Wiker, M. Harboe, and M. Kinomoto. 1991. Isolation and partial characterization of major protein antigens in the culture fluid of *Mycobacterium tuberculosis. Infect. Immun.* **59**:372–382.

79. Norman, R. A., M. S. McAlister, J. Murray-Rust, F. Mova-hedzadeh, N. G. Stoker, and N. Q. McDonald. 2002. Crystal structure of inositol 1-phosphate synthase from *Mycobacterium tuberculosis*, a key enzyme in phosphatidylinositol synthesis. *Structure* 10:393–402.

80. Ortiz-Lombardia, M., F. Pompeo, B. Boitel, and P. M. Alzari. 2003. Crystal structure of the catalytic domain of the PknB serine/threonine kinase from *Mycobacterium tuberculosis. J. Biol. Chem.* 278:13094–13100.

81. Pavelka, M. S., Jr., B. Chen, C. L. Kelley, F. M. Collins, and W. R. Jacobs, Jr. 2003. Vaccine efficacy of a lysine auxotroph of *Mycobacterium tuberculosis. Infect. Immun.* 71:4190–4192.

82. Pearl, F. M., D. Lee, J. E. Bray, I. Sillitoe, A. E. Todd, A. P. Harrison, J. M. Thornton, and C. A. Orengo. 2000. Assigning genomic sequences to CATH. *Nucleic Acids Res.* 28: 277–282.

83. Perrakis, A., R. Morris, and V. S. Lamzin. 1999. Automated protein model building combined with iterative structure refinement. *Nat. Struct. Biol.* 6:458–463.

84. Podust, L. M., T. L. Poulos, and M. R. Waterman. 2001. Crystal structure of cytochrome P450 14alpha-sterol demethylase (CYP51) from *Mycobacterium tuberculosis* in complex with azole inhibitors. *Proc. Natl. Acad. Sci. USA* 98: 3068–3073.

85. Powers, S. G., and E. E. Snell. 1976. Ketopantoate hydroxy-methyltransferase. II. Physical, catalytic, and regulatory properties. *J. Biol. Chem.* 251:3786–3793.

86. Roberts, M. M., A. R. Coker, G. Fossati, P. Mascagni, A. R. Coates, and S. P. Wood. 2003. *Mycobacterium tuberculosis* chaperonin 10 heptamers self-associate through their biologically active loops. *J. Bacteriol.* 185:4172–4185.

87. Roca, A. I., and M. M. Cox. 1997. RecA protein: structure, function, and role in recombinational DNA repair. *Prog. Nucleic Acid Res. Mol. Biol.* 56:129–223.

88. Ronning, D. R., T. Klabunde, G. S. Besra, V. D. Vissa, J. T. Belisle, and J. C. Sacchettini. 2000. Crystal structure of the secreted form of antigen 85C reveals potential targets for mycobacterial drugs and vaccines. *Nat. Struct. Biol.* 7:141–146.

89. Rozwarski, D. A., G. A. Grant, D. H. Barton, W. R. Jacobs, Jr., and J. C. Sacchettini. 1998. Modification of the NADH of the isoniazid target (InhA) from *Mycobacterium tuberculosis. Science* 279:98–102.

90. Rozwarski, D. A., C. Vilcheze, M. Sugantino, R. Bittman, and J. C. Sacchettini. 1999. Crystal structure of the *Mycobacterium tuberculosis* enoyl-ACP reductase, InhA, in complex with NAD^+ and a C_{16} fatty acyl substrate. *J. Biol. Chem.* 274:15582–15589.

91. Rupp, B. 2003. High-throughput crystallography at an affordable cost: the TB Structural Genomics Consortium Crystallization Facility. *Acc. Chem. Res.* 36:173–181.

92. Rupp, B., B. W. Segelke, H. I. Krupka, T. Lekin, J. Schafer, A. Zemla, D. Toppani, G. Snell, and T. Earnest. 2002. The TB structural genomics consortium crystallization facility: towards automation from protein to electron density. *Acta Crystallogr. Ser. D* 58:1514–1518.

93. Saikrishnan, K., J. Jeyakanthan, J. Venkatesh, N. Acharya, K. Sekar, U. Varshney, and M. Vijayan. 2003. Structure of *Mycobacterium tuberculosis* single-stranded DNA-binding protein. Variability in quaternary structure and its implications. *J. Mol. Biol.* 331:385–393.

94. Sambandamurthy, V. K., X. Wang, B. Chen, R. G. Russell, S. Derrick, F. M. Collins, S. L. Morris, and W. R. Jacobs, Jr. 2002. A pantothenate auxotroph of *Mycobacterium tuberculosis* is highly attenuated and protects mice against tuberculosis. *Nat. Med.* 8:1171–1174.

95. Scarsdale, J. N., G. Kazanina, X. He, K. A. Reynolds, and H. T. Wright. 2001. Crystal structure of the *Mycobacterium tuberculosis* beta-ketoacyl-acyl carrier protein synthase III. *J. Biol. Chem.* 276:20516–205122.

96. Sharma, V., A. Arockiasamy, D. R. Ronning, C. G. Savva, A. Holzenburg, M. Braunstein, W. R. Jacobs, Jr., and J. C. Sacchettini. 2003. Crystal structure of *Mycobacterium tuberculosis* SecA, a preprotein translocating ATPase. *Proc. Natl. Acad. Sci. USA* 100:2243–2248.

97. Sharma, V., C. Grubmeyer, and J. C. Sacchettini. 1998. Crystal structure of quinolinic acid phosphoribosyltransferase from *Mycobacterium tuberculosis*: a potential TB drug target. *Structure* 6:1587–1599.

98. Sharma, V., S. Sharma, K. Hoener zu Bentrup, J. D. McKinney, D. G. Russell, W. R. Jacobs, Jr., and J. C. Sacchettini. 2000. Structure of isocitrate lyase, a persistence factor of *Mycobacterium tuberculosis. Nat. Struct. Biol.* 7:663–668.

99. Shi, W., L. A. Basso, D. S. Santos, P. C. Tyler, R. H. Furneaux, J. S. Blanchard, S. C. Almo, and V. L. Schramm. 2001. Structures of purine nucleoside phosphorylase from *Mycobacterium tuberculosis* in complexes with immucillin-H and its pieces. *Biochemistry* 40:8204–8215.

100. Smith, C. V., C. C. Huang, A. Miczak, D. G. Russell, J. C. Sacchettini, and K. Honer zu Bentrup. 2003. Biochemical and structural studies of malate synthase from *Mycobacterium tuberculosis. J. Biol. Chem.* 278:1735–1743.

101. Smyth, D. R., M. K. Mrozkiewicz, W. J. McGrath, P. Listwan, and B. Kobe. 2003. Crystal structures of fusion proteins with large-affinity tags. *Protein Sci.* 12:1313–1322.

102. Stewart, G., B. Robertson, and D. Young. 2003. Tuberculosis: a problem with persistence. *Nat. Rev. Microbiol.* 1:97–105.

103. Story, R. M., and T. A. Steitz. 1992. Structure of the recA protein-ADP complex. *Nature* 355:374–376.

104. Story, R. M., I. T. Weber, and T. A. Steitz. 1992. The structure of the *E. coli* recA protein monomer and polymer. *Nature* 355:318–325.

105. Strong, M., P. Mallick, M. Pellegrini, M. J. Thompson, and D. Eisenberg. 2003. Inference of protein function and protein linkages in *Mycobacterium tuberculosis* based on prokaryotic genome organization: a combined computational approach. *Genome Biol.* 4:R59.

106. Taneja, B., and S. C. Mande. 2002. Structure of *Mycobacterium tuberculosis* chaperonin-10 at 3.5 Å resolution. *Acta Crystallogr. Ser D* 58:260–266.

107. Taylor, A. B., D. M. Benglis, Jr., S. Dhandayuthapani, and P. J. Hart. 2003. Structure of *Mycobacterium tuberculosis* methionine sulfoxide reductase A in complex with protein-bound methionine. *J. Bacteriol.* 185:4119–4126.

108. Terwilliger, T. C. 2002. Structural genomics: foundation for the future of biology? *Sci. World J.* 2:5–6.

109. Terwilliger, T. C., M. S. Park, G. S. Waldo, J. Berendzen, L. W. Hung, C. Y. Kim, C. V. Smith, J. C. Sacchettini, M. Bellinzoni, R. Bossi, E. De Rossi, A. Mattevi, A. Milano, G. Riccardi, M. Rizzi, M. M. Roberts, A. R. Coker, G. Fossati, P. Mascagni, A. R. Coates, S. P. Wood, C. W. Goulding, M. I. Apostol, D. H. Anderson, H. S. Gill, D. S. Eisenberg, B. Taneja, S. Mande, E. Pohl, V. Lamzin, P. Tucker, M. Wilmanns, C. Colovos, W. Meyer-Klaucke, A. W. Munro, K. J. McLean, K. R. Marshall, D. Leys, J. K. Yang, H. J. Yoon, B. I. Lee, M. G. Lee, J. E. Kwak, B. W. Han, J. Y. Lee, S. H. Baek, S. W. Suh, M. M. Komen, V. L. Arcus, E. N. Baker, J. S. Lott, W. Jacobs, Jr., T. Alber, and B. Rupp. 2003. The TB structural genomics consortium: a resource for *Mycobacterium tuberculosis* biology. *Tuberculosis* (Edinburgh) 83:223–249.

110. Tullius, M. V., G. Harth, and M. A. Horwitz. 2003. Glutamine synthetase GlnA1 is essential for growth of *Mycobac-*

terium tuberculosis in human THP-1 macrophages and guinea pigs. *Infect. Immun.* **71**:3927–3936.

111. **Vetting, M. W., S. L. Roderick, M. Yu, and J. S. Blanchard.** 2003. Crystal structure of mycothiol synthase (Rv0819) from *Mycobacterium tuberculosis* shows structural homology to the GNAT family of N-acetyltransferases. *Protein Sci.* **12**:1954–1959.

112. **Vilcheze, C., H. R. Morbidoni, T. R. Weisbrod, H. Iwamoto, M. Kuo, J. C. Sacchettini, and W. R. Jacobs, Jr.** 2000. Inactivation of the inhA-encoded fatty acid synthase II (FASII) enoyl-acyl carrier protein reductase induces accumulation of the FASI end products and cell lysis of *Mycobacterium smegmatis*. *J. Bacteriol.* **182**:4059–4067.

113. **Vyas, N. K., M. N. Vyas, and F. A. Quiocho.** 2003. Crystal structure of *M. tuberculosis* ABC phosphate transport receptor: specificity and charge compensation dominated by ion-dipole interactions. *Structure* **11**:765–774.

114. **Waldo, G. S.** 2003. Genetic screens and directed evolution for protein solubility. *Curr. Opin. Chem. Biol.* **7**:33–38.

115. **Waldo, G. S., B. M. Standish, J. Berendzen, and T. C. Terwilliger.** 1999. Rapid protein-folding assay using green fluorescent protein. *Nat. Biotechnol.* **17**:691–695.

116. **Wang, S., and D. Eisenberg.** 2003. Crystal structures of a pantothenate synthetase from *M. tuberculosis* and its complexes with substrates and a reaction intermediate. *Protein Sci.* **12**:1097–1108.

117. **Westbrook, J. D., and P. M. Fitzgerald.** 2003. The PDB format, mmCIF, and other data formats. *Methods Biochem. Anal.* **44**:161–179.

118. **Wiker, H. G., and M. Harboe.** 1992. The antigen 85 complex: a major secretion product of *Mycobacterium tuberculosis*. *Microbiol Rev.* **56**:648–661.

119. **Wiker, H. G., M. Harboe, and S. Nagai.** 1991. A localization index for distinction between extracellular and intracellular antigens of *Mycobacterium tuberculosis*. *J. Gen. Microbiol.* **137**:875–884.

120. **Wong, H. C., G. Liu, Y. M. Zhang, C. O. Rock, and J. Zheng.** 2002. The solution structure of acyl carrier protein from *Mycobacterium tuberculosis*. *J. Biol. Chem.* **277**: 15874–15880.

121. **Yang, C., U. Curth, C. Urbanke, and C. Kang.** 1997. Crystal structure of human mitochondrial single-stranded DNA binding protein at 2.4 Å resolution. *Nat. Struct. Biol.* **4**:153–157.

122. **Yang, J. K., M. S. Park, G. S. Waldo, and S. W. Suh.** 2003. Directed evolution approach to a structural genomics project: Rv2002 from *Mycobacterium tuberculosis*. *Proc. Natl. Acad. Sci. USA* **100**:455–460.

123. **Yeats, C., R. D. Finn, and A. Bateman.** 2002. The PASTA domain: a beta-lactam-binding domain. *Trends Biochem. Sci.* **27**:438.

124. **Young, D., T. Garbe, R. Lathigra, C. Abou-Zeid, and Y. Zhang.** 1991. Characterization of prominent protein antigens from mycobacteria. *Bull. Int. Union Tuberc. Lung Dis.* **66**: 47–51.

125. **Young, T. A., B. Delagoutte, J. A. Endrizzi, A. M. Falick, and T. Alber.** 2003. Structure of *Mycobacterium tuberculosis* PknB supports a universal activation mechanism for Ser/Thr protein kinases. *Nat. Struct. Biol.* **10**:168–174.

126. **Yuan, Y., R. E. Lee, G. S. Besra, J. T. Belisle, and C. E. Barry III.** 1995. Identification of a gene involved in the biosynthesis of cyclopropanated mycolic acids in *Mycobacterium tuberculosis*. *Proc. Natl. Acad. Sci. USA* **92**:6630–6634.

VI. GENETICS

Tuberculosis and the Tubercle Bacillus
Edited by Stewart T. Cole et al.
© 2005 ASM Press, Washington, D.C.

Chapter 12

Gene Replacement Systems[†]

Neil G. Stoker, P. Sander, and J. M. Reyrat

With the completion of the *Mycobacterium tuberculosis* genome sequence (14), the focus of research has turned to functional characterization of genes, and, in particular, identification of virulence factors (13, 61). There are currently 3,995 predicted protein-coding genes, of which only 52% have some predicted function (11).

Isolation of defined isogenic mutants is a powerful approach for investigating cause-effect relationships and thus of determining function. Targeted gene inactivation is a hypothesis-driven approach to mutagenesis that allows the generation of specific mutants, irrespective of whether the gene itself confers a recognizable phenotype under the conditions tested. It offers complete control over the nature of the mutation introduced but is relatively labor-intensive. It is complementary to random transposon mutagenesis technologies (6, 10, 15, 47), where people may screen for genes whose inactivation produces a particular phenotype; the mutagenesis is rapid, but there is no control over mutations introduced, and significant effort may be involved in characterizing the lesions. Sequence-characterized transposon libraries (35) and the microarray-based TraSH methodology (58, 60) offer a hybrid between the two.

The basic tools of a mycobacterial genetic system were in place by 1990 (25). However, while targeted knockout mutants of the fast-growing *Mycobacterium smegmatis* were readily obtained (22), initial attempts to achieve homologous recombination in the *M. tuberculosis* complex resulted in failure (27) or partial success with a single-crossover event (1). The difficulty was attributed to a high level of illegitimate recombination and/or a low level of homologous recombination. One potential culprit was the unusual structure of the *M. tuberculosis* RecA,

which carries an intein (17). However, further research indicated that RecA of *M. tuberculosis* is fully functional with respect to promoting DNA repair mechanisms as well as with respect to promoting homologous recombination (18, 38). The inability to identify double-crossover events was a major impediment in the study of *M. tuberculosis* pathogenicity. We describe here the approaches that have been used to develop efficient allelic replacement systems in this pathogen.

THE EARLY DAYS OF THE SUICIDE STRATEGY

The first mutant of the *M. tuberculosis* complex made through allelic replacement was a *Mycobacterium bovis* BCG mutant, created using the *ureC* gene as a target (53). This mutant was obtained simply by electroporating a suicide vector containing the *ureC* gene disrupted by a kanamycin resistance marker. Urease is an excellent genetic marker, since it allows simple and rapid screening of the recombinants. Using the urea-indole test, several dozen recombinants could be screened, which facilitated the identification of rare genetic events. Four percent of the kanamycin-resistant colonies scored as urease negative, and it was demonstrated by PCR and Southern blotting that these were genuine mutants where allelic replacement had taken place. Shortly afterward a similar strategy was successfully used by Azad et al. (3) to inactivate the *mas* gene, encoding mycocerosic acid synthase. The frequency of mutants obtained (2 of 38) was similar to the frequency at the urease locus.

During the same period and using a suicide plasmid, Marklund et al. used *Mycobacterium intracellulare*

Neil G. Stoker • Department of Pathology & Infectious Diseases, Royal Veterinary College, Royal College Street, London NW1 0TU, United Kingdom. **P. Sander** • Institut für Medizinische Mikrobiologie, Universität Zürich, Gloriastr. 30/32, CH-8028 Zürich, Switzerland. **J. M. Reyrat** • Faculté de Médecine Necker-Enfants Malades, INSERM U570, 156 rue de Vaugirard, 75730 Paris Cedex 15, France.

[†]During the preparation of this chapter, Stoyan Bardarov, who made a major contribution to mycobacterial genetic research, sadly died. We would like to dedicate this chapter to his memory.

as an alternate model to show gene replacement through homologous recombination (34). Using a two-step strategy, they obtained efficient integration of the plasmid through a single crossover. One of these strains was then subcultured, and colonies were tested for antibiotic sensitivity until the loss of the vector through a second crossover was indicated.

Balasubramanian et al. (4) took advantage of suicide linear cosmids, approximately 40 to 50 kb in length, as recombination substrates to inactivate the *leuD* gene in *M. tuberculosis*. Using these long linear substrates, they obtained leucine auxotrophs at a frequency of 6% of the total kanamycin-resistant clones; no mutants were obtained when short linear recombination substrates were used.

It was shown by Hinds et al. (21) that the frequency of homologous recombination using suicide plasmids could be enhanced by treating the plasmid DNA with UV or alkali, and this was used successfully to make a mutant of *M. tuberculosis* lacking the hemolysin *tlyA*. Further use of this method led to the construction of several auxotrophic mutants (39). This work also demonstrated that there were great differences in efficiency depending on the gene locus. Rigorous characterization of the nonmutants showed that none was caused by illegitimate recombination but, rather, that they were obtained from single-crossover events or from spontaneous antibiotic resistance. Resistance to aminoglycosides is relatively frequent in *M. tuberculosis* because there is only one rRNA operon (57).

EXPLOITING SHUTTLE VECTORS

A major factor in the small number of mutants obtained using suicide plasmids was the efficiency of transformation. This difficulty is avoided by using replicating plasmids, although there is the new problem of ensuring plasmid loss. It was shown by Norman et al. (36) that intramolecular homologous recombination could be obtained using a shuttle plasmid. The shuttle plasmid (pUS950) contained two overlapping fragments of the Tn*903* kanamycin phosphotransferase gene (*aph*) separated by a functional hygromycin resistance gene. This plasmid allows for positive selection of homologous recombination between the two *aph* fragments, resulting in kanamycin resistance and the loss of hygromycin resistance. In *M. bovis* BCG, as many as 10^{-3} of cells were Kan^R Hyg^S, showing that homologous recombination had taken place. These experiments were, however, limited to plasmid intramolecular homologous recombination. A replicating plasmid carrying the *aacBC* gene interrupted by *aph* was made and introduced into *M. bovis*

BCG. Mutant-specific PCR showed that allelic replacement had taken place, but the authors were never able to isolate a clonal population of the mutant, either because of the deleterious effect of the mutation or because of the persistence of the plasmid.

Single-crossover events can disrupt genes, if appropriate constructs are made. A strategy based on a shuttle plasmid carrying a promoterless *aph* gene was developed by Baulard et al. (7), where insertion into the target gene allowed *aph* expression. This STORE system (selection technique of recombination events) was used to interrupt various genes in both fast- and slow-growing mycobacteria.

DEVELOPMENT OF MARKERS FOR COUNTERSELECTION AND SCREENING

A major breakthrough was the use of counterselectable markers in mycobacteria. These are dominant selectable markers which, under appropriate growth conditions, promote the death of the microorganism harboring them (54, 66). Thus, it is possible to select against bacteria that still carry the plasmid vector, whether replicating or integrated (Fig. 1).

The first counterselectable marker to be described in mycobacteria was streptomycin sensitivity (55). This system takes advantage of the fact that the S12 ribosomal protein is the target of streptomycin. Mutations in the *rpsL* gene, which encodes this protein, are responsible for resistance to high concentrations of streptomycin. However, mutation is recessive in a merodiploid strain (31). When both the wild-type and mutant alleles of the *rpsL* gene are expressed in the same strain, the strain is sensitive to streptomycin, possibly because of error-prone translation by wild-type ribosomes. It is necessary to start with a streptomycin-resistant strain, so that introduction of a plasmid carrying the *rpsL* gene confers streptomycin sensitivity. Loss of the plasmid (for example, following allelic replacement) restores resistance. This method was first shown to be effective for *M. smegmatis*, using *pyrF* as a model (55), and then for the *M. tuberculosis* complex. A variety of genes, including *recA*, *ompATb*, and *ahpC*, were interrupted using this method (52, 56, 62). The powerful streptomycin selection provides an efficient tool to generate knockout mutants for basic science. The fact that it gives rise to mutants resistant to streptomycin, an antibiotic which is used in some chemotherapeutic regimens, is a limitation to applications such as the construction of attenuated strains for use as live-vaccine candidates.

An alternative system that was applied, which can be used with any strain, was based on the *Bacil-*

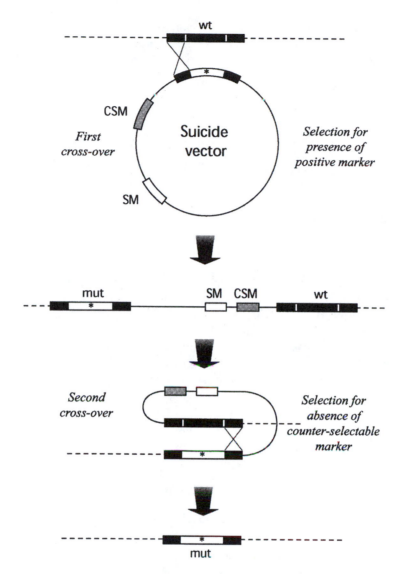

Figure 1. Two-step strategy for allelic replacement. Positive selection of allelic exchange mutants in a two-step selection strategy, using a counterselectable marker, is shown. CSM, counterselectable marker; SM, selectable marker; wt, wild-type allele; mut, mutated allele. Adapted from reference 54 with permission.

lus subtilis sacB gene encoding levansucrase. In its natural gram-positive environment, *sacB* expression is harmless to the bacterium. However, cloning of *sacB* in *Escherichia coli* or other gram-negative bacteria leads to the death of the transformed bacteria in the presence of sucrose. It has been proposed that the accumulation of levans (high-molecular-weight fructose polymers synthesized by the levansucrase) in the periplasm of gram-negative bacteria might be toxic. The expression of the *sacB* gene was shown to be lethal to corynebacteria but not to streptomycetes, organisms that, as with mycobacteria, belong to the order *Actinomycetales* (26). Interestingly, the counterselective property of *sacB* was shown to be effective with both rapidly and slowly growing mycobacteria in the presence of sucrose (48). It has been hypothe-

sized that the mechanism of toxicity in the corynebacteria and mycobacteria is due to the accumulation of levans in the "pseudo" periplasmic space delimited by the hydrophobic plasma membrane and mycolic acid layers. This *sacB* counterselectable marker was used to introduce an unmarked mutation in *M. smegmatis*, with the *pyrF* gene as a model (49), and has since been used widely (2, 8, 44, 46, 51).

The *pyrF* gene has been used not only as a model target gene but also as a selectable and counterselectable marker (28). The *pyrF* gene can be selected for in medium lacking uracil and can be selected against in medium containing 5′-fluoroorotic acid and uracil. The *pyrF* gene converts the 5′-fluoroorotic acid into a toxic nucleotide analog that irreversibly inactivates the essential enzyme thymidilate synthetase (9).

Another counterselectable marker that has been proposed is *katG*, encoding the catalase-peroxidase that activates isoniazid (36). The authors designed a shuttle vector which allows positive selection for plasmid loss when used with host strains in which the *katG* catalase-peroxidase has been deleted, leading to recessive resistance to isoniazid. Plasmid-carrying cells are isoniazid resistant and can be selected against. This system was present on the plasmid used to inactivate *aacBC* described above. However, using this system, the authors were never able to isolate a plasmid-free derivative, and hence a clonal population of the *aac* mutant was never obtained (36).

Markers that can be screened for are also effective tools for identifying mutants. They have been used in conjunction with *sacB*, due to the high frequency of spontaneous sucrose resistance (38, 46). The *xylE* gene from *Pseudomonas putida* encodes a catechol 2,3-dioxygenase that produces a bright yellow color when colonies are sprayed with catechol; it was first used in mycobacteria to measure promoter activity (16). It was combined with the *sacB*(Ts) replicon to distinguish genuine allelic exchange from false positives (caused, for example, by sucrose-resistance in cells carrying single-crossovers) (47). Similarly, the *lacZ* gene, widely used in bacterial genetics, has been used to differentiate cells that still carry plasmids from those that are plasmid free (39, 44) (Color Plate 7).

CONTROLLING LOSS OF REPLICATING PLASMIDS

A major drawback when using replicating plasmids was that it was necessary to isolate plasmid-free cells. To induce efficient plasmid loss at will, a thermosensitive replicon was isolated (20). This replicated at 32 but not at 39°C. When it was combined with *sacB*, the counterselection efficiency increased from 2.5×10^{-4} in the presence of only sucrose to 5×10^{-7} at the nonpermissive temperature and in the presence of sucrose (47). This system has proved to be efficient for site-directed mutagenesis, as demonstrated with the *purC* gene, where 100% of the selected clones were allelic-exchange mutants, whereas no mutants had been obtained using a suicide vector.

An alternative method for controlling plasmid loss was recently described (45), where two incompatible plasmids, one of which carries the gene of interest interrupted by an antibiotic resistance gene, are introduced into the mycobacterium. These plasmids coexist in the presence of selection for both of them but segregate rapidly in the absence of selection. After growth in selective medium to allow recombina-

tion to take place, antibiotics are removed and growth is continued. Cells are plated on the antibiotic within the targeted gene, and *lacZ* mutant colonies picked. Using the *pyrF* gene in *M. smegmatis*, up to 15% of colonies were white, and allelic replacement had taken place in all of them. This technology is applicable to the *M. tuberculosis* complex, since plasmid loss has been shown to occur on removal of selection.

BACTERIOPHAGE SYSTEMS

All the work described above relies on the use of plasmids. Bacteriophage systems are alternative vectors; their extraordinary efficiency of infection makes them ideal delivery systems. Bardarov et al. (6) constructed phasmids, which replicate as plasmids in *E. coli* and as phages in mycobacteria. They then isolated thermosensitive derivatives that enable efficient delivery of a transposon into both fast- and slow-growing mycobacteria. This was developed into an efficient gene replacement system (5). The target gene of interest is interrupted with a selectable marker and cloned into a cosmid vector in *E. coli*. This construct is cloned into a mycobacteriophage vector and packaged by transducing *M. smegmatis*. A high-titer stock can then be prepared to infect *M. tuberculosis*, and mutants are isolated at high frequency. The efficiency of the final step enables the same mutation to be easily introduced into multiple strains. In this way, a mutation was introduced into three strains of *M. bovis* BCG and three strains of *M. tuberculosis*.

MARKED AND UNMARKED MUTANTS

Marked mutants, in which an antibiotic resistance gene is used to interrupt the gene of interest, are the most straightforward to make. They have the advantage that they can be easily differentiated from the wild-type strain, and they may be the mutants of choice in certain situations, for example, where mutations are deleterious and mutants are difficult to isolate from mixed populations, or where it is important to differentiate strains such as in competitive growth situations or in protection experiments. However, it is often desirable to introduce unmarked mutations, for example, to avoid polar effects on downstream genes, to allow multiple mutations, or to introduce subtle mutations.

Making unmarked mutations requires a two-step strategy, where antibiotic resistance is used to select for the first crossover. This strain is then propagated, and the second crossover is isolated through counterselection and/or screening against the plasmid vector. This strategy has enabled the construction of unmarked mutants of both rapid and slow growers (44, 46, 49). It has also allowed the construction of the first double unmarked *M. tuberculosis* (*tlyA plcABC*) mutant (44). Although potentially slower than isolation of one-step mutants, this method is more reproducible, since each step is controlled and operator input is minimized; thus, it may be the method of choice even for making marked mutants. Using the counterselectable property of the *sacB* gene present on a mycobacterial suicidal plasmid, Pavelka and Jacobs constructed an unmarked deletion mutation in *M. smegmatis*, *M. bovis* BCG, and *M. tuberculosis* (46). Comparison of the recombination frequency suggests that the homologous recombination machinery of the three species is equally efficient.

The phage-based system described above creates only marked mutants. However, the use of site-specific recombination systems such as the γδ-resolvase can be used to excise the antibiotic resistance after the mutant has been isolated, whether made using a phage or a plasmid (5, 33).

COMPLEMENTATION

It is generally accepted that complementation of a mutant is a useful control to confirm that the phenotypes observed are due to the mutation. For example, second-site mutations may be introduced during the mutagenesis process, and a phenotype may be due to this second mutation. A range of replicating and integrating plasmids are available for this purpose (12).

However, there are occasions when complementation is not straightforward. The assumption is that introduction of a normal copy of the gene will restore the phenotype. One problem is the provision of a suitable promoter; the promoter to a gene may be several genes upstream and may be uncharacterized, so that the choice of which complementing fragment to use is not certain. Provision of a heterologous promoter can lead to artifacts due to copy number, or inappropriate expression levels or patterns. An *hspR* mutation was successfully complemented by using a single integrated copy of the gene using its own promoter (65), yet constructs using heterologous promoters were not viable (64). Thus, restoration of function may be partial or absent even when extraneous mutations have not occurred. Alternative solutions are to make the mutant twice and demonstrate that the phenotype is shared or to reconstruct a wild-type gene from the mutant one and to cross it back in by allelic replacement.

DEMONSTRATING THAT A GENE IS ESSENTIAL

It is possible to construct a mutant only when the candidate gene is not essential for growth under the conditions used. This situation may be suggested by failure to obtain a mutant, but there may be other explanations. To demonstrate essentiality, it is necessary to compare gene loss in a normal strain with loss in a strain in which an extra copy of the gene is present. This can be done by showing that homologous recombination leading to gene inactivation occurs only in the presence of a second copy of the gene. The gene duplicate may be obtained through the use of a replicative or integrating plasmid carrying the second copy of the gene. This method was used to conclusively demonstrate the essentiality of several genes involved in cell wall synthesis in *M. smegmatis* (23, 29, 37) and of the *glnE* and *aroK* genes in *M. tuberculosis* (41, 43).

One potential problem with the method described above is the necessity to show that the lack of mutants obtained is statistically significant and is not a chance effect. It may be difficult in some situations to obtain sufficient numbers of mutants of the merodiploid for significance. This difficulty can be avoided by making the merodiploid using the temperature-sensitive plasmid and comparing survival at high and low temperatures. Alternatively, if the merodiploid is made by using an integrating plasmid based on the phage L5 *int* gene, excision of the plasmid can be efficiently induced by introduction of a plasmid carrying the L5 excisionase gene *xis* (32). Efficient excision by the integrase gene could also be demonstrated when using a counterselectable marker (63). Comparison of survival in the presence and absence of the *xis* gene demonstrates whether the gene is essential (40). These methods also allow essentiality to be tested under different growth conditions. Other transposon-based methods provide evidence for gene essentiality on a genome-wide level (30, 58, 59). These provide an invaluable resource but do not provide definitive proof of essentiality; to do this, a method involving complementation is required.

CONSTRUCTION OF CONDITIONAL-LETHAL MUTANTS

Even when the gene studied is essential, studying the phenotype of a conditional mutant can be useful because it can help to unravel the function of the gene. Two complementary approaches have been described to study such a phenomenon. One system relies on the use of a conditional antisense mutagenesis system (42), which is based on the use of a strong inducible promoter to which is fused the gene of interest in order to produce the antisense message. The promoter corresponds to a 2.3-kpb region upstream of the acetamidase gene from *M. smegmatis*, which was shown to be upregulated by acetamide. This system was developed using the *hisD* gene as a model, and it was shown that, on induction by acetamide, the bacteria phenotypically became histidine auxotrophs. Auxotrophy was not observed under noninduced conditions. The other method is based on the utilization of a thermosensitive rescue plasmid. In this method, the bacterium contains both an inactivated chromosomal copy of the gene and a functional copy of the gene carried on a thermosensitive rescue plasmid. This method was used with the *pimA* gene as a target (23, 29, 37). The ability of this conditional mutant to synthesize phosphatidylinositol monomannoside and derived higher phosphatidylinositol mannosides was dependent on the growth temperature; the mutant was unable to grow at nonpermissive temperatures, demonstrating that PimA is essential for the growth of mycobacteria. This strategy has proven to be useful to analyze the physiology of the bacterium before death (23).

CONCLUSION

In conclusion, many genetic tools are now available for studying mycobacteria. It is possible to select directly for allelic exchange in a single-step strategy or to construct an unmarked mutation in a two-step strategy. The time when people thought that members of the *M. tuberculosis* complex were refractory to allelic exchange, possibly because of the unusual structure of the *recA* gene, is now a distant memory (17). It is now possible to construct any mutants of *M. tuberculosis* (19, 24, 50), provided that the gene is not essential, which will undoubtedly help us to unravel the virulence properties of the tubercle bacillus.

Acknowledgments. J.-M. R. is funded by an Avenir program of INSERM. We thank Tanya Parish and Vladimir Pelicic for helpful discussions. This work was supported in part by the Swiss National Science Foundation (Project *Mycobacterium tuberculosis*—mechanisms of virulence).

REFERENCES

1. Aldovini, A., R. N. Husson, and R. A. Young. 1993. The *uraA* locus and homologous recombination in *Mycobacterium bovis* BCG. *J. Bacteriol.* **175**:7282–7289.
2. Azad, A. K., T. D. Sirakova, N. D. Fernandes, and P. E. Kolattukudy. 1997. Gene knockout reveals a novel gene cluster for the synthesis of a class of cell wall lipids unique to pathogenic mycobacteria. *J. Biol. Chem.* **272**:16741–16745.
3. Azad, A. K., T. D. Sirakova, L. M. Rogers, and P. E. Kolattukudy. 1996. Targeted replacement of the mycocerosic acid synthase gene in *Mycobacterium bovis* BCG produces a mutant that lacks mycosides. *Proc. Natl. Acad. Sci. USA* **93**:4787–4792.
4. Balasubramanian, V., M. S. Pavelka, Jr., S. S. Bardarov, J. Martin, T. R. Weisbrod, R. A. McAdam, B. R. Bloom, and W. R. Jacobs, Jr. 1996. Allelic exchange in *Mycobacterium tuberculosis* with long linear recombination substrates. *J. Bacteriol.* **178**:273–279.
5. Bardarov, S., S. Bardarov, Jr., M. S. Pavelka, Jr., V. Sambandamurthy, M. Larsen, J. Tufariello, J. Chan, G. Hatfull, and W. R. Jacobs, Jr. 2002. Specialized transduction: an efficient method for generating marked and unmarked targeted gene disruptions in *Mycobacterium tuberculosis*, *M. bovis* BCG and *M. smegmatis*. *Microbiology* **148**:3007–3017.
6. Bardarov, S., J. Kriakov, C. Carriere, S. Yu, C. Vaamonde, R. A. McAdam, B. R. Bloom, G. F. Hatfull, and W. R. Jacobs, Jr. 1997. Conditionally replicating mycobacteriophages: a system for transposon delivery to *Mycobacterium tuberculosis*. *Proc. Natl. Acad. Sci. USA* **94**:10961–10966.
7. Baulard, A., L. Kremer, and C. Locht. 1996. Efficient homologous recombination in fast-growing and slow-growing mycobacteria. *J. Bacteriol.* **178**:3091–3098.
8. Berthet, F. X., M. Lagranderie, P. Gounon, C. Laurent-Winter, D. Ensergueix, P. Chavarot, F. Thouron, E. Maranghi, V. Pelicic, D. Portnoi, G. Marchal, and B. Gicquel. 1998. Attenuation of virulence by disruption of the *Mycobacterium tuberculosis erp* gene. *Science* **282**:759–762.
9. Boeke, J. D., F. LaCroute, and G. R. Fink. 1984. A positive selection for mutants lacking orotidine-5′-phosphate decarboxylase activity in yeast: 5-fluoroorotic acid resistance. *Mol. Gen. Genet.* **197**:345–346.
10. Camacho, L. R., D. Ensergueix, E. Perez, B. Gicquel, and C. Guilhot. 1999. Identification of a virulence gene cluster of *Mycobacterium tuberculosis* by signature-tagged transposon mutagenesis. *Mol. Microbiol.* **34**:257–267.
11. Camus, J. C., M. J. Pryor, C. Medigue, and S. T. Cole. 2002. Re-annotation of the genome sequence of *Mycobacterium tuberculosis* H37Rv. *Microbiology* **148**:2967–2973.
12. Casali, N., and S. Ehrt. 2001. Plasmid vectors, p. 1–17. *In* T. Parish and N. G. Stoker (ed.), *Mycobacterium tuberculosis Protocols*. Humana Press, Inc., Totowa, N.J.
13. Clark-Curtiss, J. E., and S. E. Haydel. 2003. Molecular genetics of *Mycobacterium tuberculosis* pathogenesis. *Annu. Rev. Microbiol.* **57**:517–549.
14. Cole, S. T., R. Brosch, J. Parkhill, T. Garnier, C. Churcher, D. Harris, S. V. Gordon, K. Eiglmeier, S. Gas, C. E. Barry, III, F. Tekaia, K. Badcock, D. Basham, D. Brown, T. Chillingworth, R. Connor, R. Davies, K. Devlin, T. Feltwell, S. Gentles, N. Hamlin, S. Holroyd, T. Hornsby, K. Jagels, and B. G. Barrell. 1998. Deciphering the biology of *Mycobacterium tuberculosis* from the complete genome sequence. *Nature* **393**:537–544.
15. Cox, J. S., B. Chen, M. McNeil, and W. R. Jacobs, Jr. 1999. Complex lipid determines tissue-specific replication of *Mycobacterium tuberculosis* in mice. *Nature* **402**:79–83.
16. Curcic, R., S. Dhandayuthapani, and V. Deretic. 1994. Gene expression in mycobacteria: transcriptional fusions based on *xylE* and analysis of the promoter region of the response regulator *mtrA* from *Mycobacterium tuberculosis*. *Mol. Microbiol.* **13**:1057–1064.
17. Davis, E. O., P. J. Jenner, P. C. Brooks, M. J. Colston, and S. G. Sedgwick. 1992. Protein splicing in the maturation of *M. tuberculosis recA* protein: a mechanism for tolerating a novel class of intervening sequence. *Cell* **71**:201–210.

18. Frischkorn, K., P. Sander, M. Scholz, K. Teschner, T. Prammananan, and E. C. Bottger. 1998. Investigation of mycobacterial *recA* function: protein introns in the RecA of pathogenic mycobacteria do not affect competency for homologous recombination. *Mol. Microbiol.* 29:1203–1214.

19. Glickman, M. S., and W. R. Jacobs, Jr. 2001. Microbial pathogenesis of *Mycobacterium tuberculosis*: dawn of a discipline. *Cell* 104:477–485.

20. Guilhot, C., B. Gicquel, and C. Martin. 1992. Temperature-sensitive mutants of the *Mycobacterium* plasmid pAL5000. *FEMS Microbiol. Lett.* 77:181–186.

21. Hinds, J., E. Mahenthiralingam, K. E. Kempsell, K. Duncan, R. W. Stokes, T. Parish, and N. G. Stoker. 1999. Enhanced gene replacement in mycobacteria. *Microbiology* 145:519–527.

22. Husson, R. N., B. E. James, and R. A. Young. 1990. Gene replacement and expression of foreign DNA in mycobacteria. *J. Bacteriol.* 172:519–524.

23. Jackson, M., D. C. Crick, and P. J. Brennan. 2000. Phosphatidylinositol is an essential phospholipid of mycobacteria. *J. Biol. Chem.* 275:30092–30099.

24. Jacobs, W. R., Jr. 2000. *Mycobacterium tuberculosis*: a once genetically intractable organism, p. 1–16. *In* G. F. Hatfull and W. R. Jacobs, Jr. (ed.), *Molecular Genetics of Mycobacteria*. ASM Press, Washington, D.C.

25. Jacobs, W. R., Jr., G. V. Kalpana, J. D. Cirillo, L. Pascopella, S. B. Snapper, R. A. Udani, W. Jones, R. G. Barletta, and B. R. Bloom. 1991. Genetic systems for mycobacteria. *Methods Enzymol.* 204:537–555.

26. Jager, W., A. Schafer, A. Puhler, G. Labes, and W. Wohlleben. 1992. Expression of the *Bacillus subtilis sacB* gene leads to sucrose sensitivity in the gram-positive bacterium *Corynebacterium glutamicum* but not in *Streptomyces lividans*. *J. Bacteriol.* 174:5462–5465.

27. Kalpana, G. V., B. R. Bloom, and W. R. Jacobs, Jr. 1991. Insertional mutagenesis and illegitimate recombination in mycobacteria. *Proc. Natl. Acad. Sci. USA* 88:5433–5437.

28. Knipfer, N., A. Seth, and T. E. Shrader. 1997. Unmarked gene integration into the chromosome of *Mycobacterium smegmatis* via precise replacement of the *pyrF* gene. *Plasmid* 37:129–140.

29. Kordulakova, J., M. Gilleron, K. Mikusova, G. Puzo, P. J. Brennan, B. Gicquel, and M. Jackson. 2002. Definition of the first mannosylation step in phosphatidylinositol mannoside synthesis. PimA is essential for growth of mycobacteria. *J. Biol. Chem.* 277:31335–31344.

30. Lamichhane, G., M. Zignol, N. J. Blades, D. E. Geiman, A. Dougherty, J. Grosset, K. W. Broman, and W. R. Bishai. 2003. A postgenomic method for predicting essential genes at subsaturation levels of mutagenesis: application to *Mycobacterium tuberculosis*. *Proc. Natl. Acad. Sci. USA* 100:7213–7218.

31. Lederberg, J. 1951. Streptomycin resistance: a genetically recessive mutation. *J. Bacteriol.* 61:549–550.

32. Lewis, J. A., and G. F. Hatfull. 2000. Identification and characterization of mycobacteriophage L5 excisionase. *Mol. Microbiol.* 35:350–360.

33. Malaga, W., E. Perez, and C. Guilhot. 2003. Production of unmarked mutations in mycobacteria using site-specific recombination. *FEMS Microbiol. Lett.* 219:261–268.

34. Marklund, B. I., D. P. Speert, and R. W. Stokes. 1995. Gene replacement through homologous recombination in *Mycobacterium intracellulare*. *J. Bacteriol.* 177:6100–6105.

35. McAdam, R. A., S. Quan, D. A. Smith, S. Bardarov, J. C. Betts, F. C. Cook, E. U. Hooker, A. P. Lewis, P. Woollard, M. J. Everett, P. T. Lukey, G. J. Bancroft, W. R. Jacobs, Jr.,

and K. Duncan. 2002. Characterization of a *Mycobacterium tuberculosis* H37Rv transposon library reveals insertions in 351 ORFs and mutants with altered virulence. *Microbiology* 148:2975–2986.

36. Norman, E., O. A. Dellagostin, J. McFadden, and J. W. Dale. 1995. Gene replacement by homologous recombination in *Mycobacterium bovis* BCG. *Mol. Microbiol.* 16:755–760.

37. Pan, F., M. Jackson, Y. Ma, and M. McNeil. 2001. Cell wall core galactofuran synthesis is essential for growth of mycobacteria. *J. Bacteriol.* 183:3991–3998.

38. Papavinasasundaram, K. G., M. J. Colston, and E. O. Davis. 1998. Construction and complementation of a *recA* deletion mutant of *Mycobacterium smegmatis* reveals that the intein in *Mycobacterium tuberculosis recA* does not affect RecA function. *Mol. Microbiol.* 30:525–534.

39. Parish, T., B. G. Gordhan, R. A. McAdam, K. Duncan, V. Mizrahi, and N. G. Stoker. 1999. Production of mutants in amino acid biosynthesis genes of *Mycobacterium tuberculosis* by homologous recombination. *Microbiology* 145:3497–3503.

40. Parish, T., J. Lewis, and N. G. Stoker. 2001. Use of the mycobacteriophage L5 excisionase in *Mycobacterium tuberculosis* to demonstrate gene essentiality. *Tuberculosis* 81:359–364.

41. Parish, T., and N. G. Stoker. 2002. The common aromatic amino acid biosynthesis pathway is essential in *Mycobacterium tuberculosis*. *Microbiology* 148:3069–3077.

42. Parish, T., and N. G. Stoker. 1997. Development and use of a conditional antisense mutagenesis system in mycobacteria. *FEMS Microbiol. Lett.* 154:151–157.

43. Parish, T., and N. G. Stoker. 2000. *glnE* is an essential gene in *Mycobacterium tuberculosis*. *J. Bacteriol.* 182:5715–5720.

44. Parish, T., and N. G. Stoker. 2000. Use of a flexible cassette method to generate a double unmarked *Mycobacterium tuberculosis tlyA plcABC* mutant by gene replacement. *Microbiology* 146:1969–1975.

45. Pashley, C. A., T. Parish, R. A. McAdam, K. Duncan, and N. G. Stoker. 2003. Gene replacement in mycobacteria by using incompatible plasmids. *Appl. Environ. Microbiol.* 69:517–523.

46. Pavelka, M. S., Jr., and W. R. Jacobs, Jr. 1999. Comparison of the construction of unmarked deletion mutations in *Mycobacterium smegmatis*, *Mycobacterium bovis* bacillus Calmette-Guérin, and *Mycobacterium tuberculosis* H37Rv by allelic exchange. *J. Bacteriol.* 181:4780–4789.

47. Pelicic, V., M. Jackson, J. M. Reyrat, W. R. Jacobs, Jr., B. Gicquel, and C. Guilhot. 1997. Efficient allelic exchange and transposon mutagenesis in *Mycobacterium tuberculosis*. *Proc. Natl. Acad. Sci. USA* 94:10955–10960.

48. Pelicic, V., J. M. Reyrat, and B. Gicquel. 1996. Expression of the *Bacillus subtilis sacB* gene confers sucrose sensitivity on mycobacteria. *J. Bacteriol.* 178:1197–1199.

49. Pelicic, V., J. M. Reyrat, and B. Gicquel. 1996. Generation of unmarked directed mutations in mycobacteria, using sucrose counter-selectable suicide vectors. *Mol. Microbiol.* 20:919–925.

50. Pelicic, V., J. M. Reyrat, and B. Gicquel. 1998. Genetic advances for studying *Mycobacterium tuberculosis* pathogenicity. *Mol. Microbiol.* 28:413–420.

51. Ramakrishnan, L., H. T. Tran, N. A. Federspiel, and S. Falkow. 1997. A *crtB* homolog essential for photochromogenicity in *Mycobacterium marinum*: isolation, characterization, and gene disruption via homologous recombination. *J. Bacteriol.* 179:5862–5865.

52. Raynaud, C., K. G. Papavinasasundaram, R. A. Speight, B. Springer, P. Sander, E. C. Bottger, M. J. Colston, and P. Draper. 2002. The functions of OmpATb, a pore-forming

protein of *Mycobacterium tuberculosis*. *Mol. Microbiol.* **46:**191–201.

53. Reyrat, J. M., F. X. Berthet, and B. Gicquel. 1995. The urease locus of *Mycobacterium tuberculosis* and its utilization for the demonstration of allelic exchange in *Mycobacterium bovis* bacillus Calmette-Guerin. *Proc. Natl. Acad. Sci. USA* **92:** 8768–8772.

54. Reyrat, J. M., V. Pelicic, B. Gicquel, and R. Rappuoli. 1998. Counterselectable markers: untapped tools for bacterial genetics and pathogenesis. *Infect. Immun.* **66:**4011–4017.

55. Sander, P., A. Meier, and E. C. Bottger. 1995. rpsL⁺: a dominant selectable marker for gene replacement in mycobacteria. *Mol. Microbiol.* **16:**991–1000.

56. Sander, P., K. G. Papavinasasundaram, T. Dick, E. Stavropoulos, K. Ellrott, B. Springer, M. J. Colston, and E. C. Bottger. 2001. *Mycobacterium bovis* BCG *recA* deletion mutant shows increased susceptibility to DNA-damaging agents but wildtype survival in a mouse infection model. *Infect. Immun.* **69:**3562–3568.

57. Sander, P., T. Prammananan, and E. C. Bottger. 1996. Introducing mutations into a chromosomal rRNA gene using a genetically modified eubacterial host with a single rRNA operon. *Mol. Microbiol.* **22:**841–848.

58. Sassetti, C. M., D. H. Boyd, and E. J. Rubin. 2001. Comprehensive identification of conditionally essential genes in mycobacteria. *Proc. Natl. Acad. Sci. USA* **98:**12712–12717.

59. Sassetti, C. M., D. H. Boyd, and E. J. Rubin. 2003. Genes required for mycobacterial growth defined by high density mutagenesis. *Mol. Microbiol.* **48:**77–84.

60. Sassetti, C. M., and E. J. Rubin. 2003. Genetic requirements for mycobacterial survival during infection. *Proc. Natl. Acad. Sci. USA* **100:**12989–12994.

61. Smith, I. 2003. *Mycobacterium tuberculosis* pathogenesis and molecular determinants of virulence. *Clin. Microbiol. Rev.* **16:**463–496.

62. Springer, B., S. Master, P. Sander, T. Zahrt, M. McFalone, J. Song, K. G. Papavinasasundaram, M. J. Colston, E. Boettger, and V. Deretic. 2001. Silencing of oxidative stress response in *Mycobacterium tuberculosis*: expression patterns of *ahpC* in virulent and avirulent strains and effect of *ahpC* inactivation. *Infect. Immun.* **69:**5967–5973.

63. Springer, B., P. Sander, L. Sedlacek, K. Ellrott, and E. C. Bottger. 2001. Instability and site-specific excision of integration-proficient mycobacteriophage L5 plasmids: development of stably maintained integrative vectors. *Int. J. Med. Microbiol.* **290:**669–675.

64. Stewart, G. R., V. A. Snewin, G. Walzl, T. Hussell, P. Tormay, P. O'Gaora, M. Goyal, J. Betts, I. N. Brown, and D. B. Young. 2001. Overexpression of heatshock proteins reduces survival of *Mycobacterium tuberculosis* in the chronic phase of infection. *Nat. Med.* **7:**732–737.

65. Stewart, G. R., L. Wernisch, R. Stabler, J. A. Mangan, J. Hinds, K. G. Laing, D. B. Young, and P. D. Butcher. 2002. Dissection of the heat-shock response in *Mycobacterium tuberculosis* using mutants and microarrays. *Microbiology* **148:**3129–3138.

66. Stibitz, S. 1994. Use of conditionally counterselectable suicide vectors for allelic exchange. *Methods Enzymol.* **235:**458–465.

Tuberculosis and the Tubercle Bacillus
Edited by Stewart T. Cole et al.
© 2005 ASM Press, Washington, D.C.

Chapter 13

Repetitive DNA in the *Mycobacterium tuberculosis* Complex

STEPHEN V. GORDON AND PHILIP SUPPLY

Repetitive DNA is universally present in bacterial and eukaryotic genomes, with two major classes usually distinguished: interspersed repeats, such as mobile genetic elements, and tandem repeats (TRs). Repetitive DNA sequences can promote genetic variation by a variety of mechanisms, sometimes with a high degree of sophistication. This genetic variation can be associated with a diverse set of phenotypes, ranging from subtle changes in certain genetic traits to major modifications in physiology, differentiation, and cellular organization. Although many repetitive-DNA sequences, especially mobile and extragenic elements, were thought to be primarily parasitic, recent work suggests that coadaptations between them and host genomes may occur. These coadaptations could lead to a "domestication" of such elements, which could carry out specialized and beneficial functions for their hosts (41). Moreover, some of these repetitive elements are remarkably species or phylum specific, which suggests that "infection" by these elements coincides with speciation events and is involved in evolutionary changes (55). Their association with genetic variation also means that many repetitive sequences are valuable molecular markers for studying epidemiological and evolutionary relationships.

The deciphering of the *Mycobacterium tuberculosis* genome revealed a richness of sequences that fall into either of the two major classes but also the existence of some nonclassical repetitive elements that transcend this division (16, 31, 80). This chapter (i) describes these different types of sequences, (ii) discusses their relative impacts on *M. tuberculosis* genetic variation and related functions, and finally (iii) addresses their exploitation for molecular epidemiology, evolution, and population genetics.

TANDEM REPEATS

TRs are by definition made up of monomeric units repeated periodically, with the contiguous units arranged in a "head-to-tail" configuration. Conventionally, TR tracts are referred to as satellites, minisatellites, and microsatellites when monomers are in the ranges of, roughly, hundreds of base pairs, 10 to 100 bp, and 1 to 10 bp, respectively (61, 83, 84). This classification is based on distinctive properties in sequence structure and destabilization mechanisms. Many of these tracts show variability in their repeat numbers and are therefore also termed variable number tandem repeat (VNTR) loci (61). While the ubiquitous presence of TRs has been identified in higher organisms for decades (7, 20), recognition of their widespread distribution and contribution to genetic variation in many bacterial species has only recently emerged following the accumulation of genome data (47, 58, 80, 87).

Using the Tandem Repeat Finder program (4), the number of TR regions in *M. tuberculosis* is estimated to be at least 200 to 300 (47, 94), depending notably on the threshold of sequence conservation between the monomers. The following two sections describe the major classes of TR in *M. tuberculosis*.

Polymorphic GC-Rich Repetitive Sequences and Major Polymorphic Tandem Repeats

For *M. tuberculosis*, the first identification of microsatellite TRs and of polymorphic minisatellite TRs corresponded to the polymorphic GC-rich repetitive sequence (PGRS) and the major polymorphic tandem repeat (MPTR) (34, 67, 70). These sequences

Stephen V. Gordon • TB Research, Veterinary Laboratories Agency (Weybridge), New Haw Addlestone, Surrey KT15 3NB, United Kingdom.   **Philip Supply** • Laboratoire des Mécanismes Moléculaires de la Pathogenèse Bactérienne, INSERM U447, Institut Pasteur de Lille, F-59019 Lille Cedex, France.

were identified through hybridization of genomic libraries with probes containing repetitive sequences. It is now clear that the MPTR and PGRS form part of the PE and PPE genes that encode two of the major protein families in the *M. tuberculosis* complex (16). Specific PE-PGRS genes have a microsatellite structure that shows variation across strains (16). As such, it is intriguing that *M. tuberculosis* does not appear to possess *mutS*, since loss of MutS function has been linked to increased microsatellite instability (3, 56). The MPTR loci present a minisatellite (10-bp) repeat separated by 5-bp spacers (34). The identification of a polymorphic minisatellite upstream of the *katG* gene, intergenic to the PPE-MPTR Rv1917c, was first reported by Zhang and Young (95). This locus has also been designated exact tandem repeat A (ETR-A) by Frothingham and Meeker-O'Connell (28). This latter report also detailed five other loci, ETR-B to ETR-F, two of them corresponding to MIRUs (ETR-D and ETR-E [see below]). The positions on the *M. tuberculosis* H37Rv chromosome of 46 polymorphic microsatellites and minisatellites, including the loci described above and below, are shown in Fig. 1.

Mycobacterial Interspersed Repetitive Units

Mycobacterial interspersed repetitive units (MIRUs) are homologous sequences dispersed throughout the genomes of *Mycobacterium* complex strains, as well as of *Mycobacterium leprae*, where they were originally named REP. They are classified into three major subfamilies, defined by their length and sequence organization (79). Their size ranges from 46 to 101 bp, with 65 MIRU copies present in 41 loci of *M. tuberculosis* H37Rv. MIRUs differ from other known repetitive sequences by their structural features, insertion sites, and coding capacity, as well as their dual status of interspersed and VNTR sequences.

MIRUs display no significant homology to other bacterial repetitive sequences outside the *Mycobacterium* genus; in contrast to many other repeat elements, they do not contain obvious palindromic structures. Many MIRUs encompass intercistronic regions within putative operons. The genes flanking MIRUs cover a wide spectrum of unrelated functional categories (lipid, nucleic acid, and protein biosynthesis or degradation; energy production; or regulatory functions). In about half of the cases, MIRUs are made of small open reading frames (ORFs) oriented in the same translational direction as the contiguous cistrons and are found overlapping termination and initiation codons of adjacent genes. Such partial ORF overlaps are typical of translationally coupled genes (54). Moreover, most sequence deletions found in two subfamilies of MIRUs preserve the reading frame, since they are multiples of 3 nucleotides. These observations suggest that MIRU ORFs are translated under the control of the upstream genes. Experimental results based on analysis of the *senX3-regX3* MIRU-VNTR locus using various reporter gene constructs

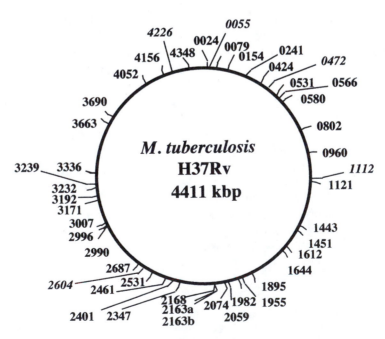

Figure 1. Positions of 46 VNTR repeat loci on the *M. tuberculosis* H37Rv chromosome. Arabic numbers designate positions in kilobase pairs. Numbers in italics and in plain style correspond to microsatellites (repeat units with a length of 10 bp or less) and minisatellites (repeat units with a length of more than 10 bp), respectively. See the text for references.

indicate that these ORFs are translated (P. Supply, unpublished data). On the other hand, among the different ORF-containing MIRUs, the amino acid sequences do not appear to be more highly conserved than the nucleotide sequences, indicating no tendency for conserved nucleotide variations. In addition, MIRU-encoded peptide sequences are no more highly conserved within one mycobacterial species than between species. Thus, the corresponding peptides may serve several different functions; alternatively, the primary sequences of MIRU-encoded peptides may not be crucial for their function. In support of the second hypothesis, genetic analyses suggest that translation of MIRU ORFs can modulate expression of the downstream genes (Supply et al., unpublished). Several MIRUs, as well as members of other families of dispersed repetitive sequences (see below), are also found within predicted coding regions.

A PCR scan and sequence analysis of the 41 MIRU loci in 31 *M. tuberculosis* complex strains revealed that 12 of them (included in Fig. 1) contain MIRUs organized in TRs, which vary in copy number among strains (80). Most of these VNTR loci contain repeats with minor sequence variations between them, as seen in higher-eukaryote minisatellites. Interestingly, the repeat variants in the MIRU-VNTR loci are distributed nonrandomly, since identical repeats are clustered in blocks of contiguous units. Strain-to-strain variation at these loci nearly always consists of simple additions or deletions in blocks of identical repeats. Such preferential changes in identical sequence tracts are consistent with the strong requirement for perfect repeat sequence conservation in replication slippage-driven changes (23). Such a requirement can also be inferred from comparison of VNTR with non-VNTR loci over the 41 MIRU sites, which indicates that the presence of at least two identical or nearly identical TRs is necessary and sufficient to generate variability (80). This condition for TR variability is supported a contrario by *M. leprae* genome analysis, where 20 sites containing MIRUs were detected, but only as single copies and not as TRs. Four of these loci were conserved between *M. leprae* and *M. tuberculosis*, with the latter organism containing multiple MIRUs. PCR and sequence analysis indicated the presence of only single MIRU copies in all loci investigated in geographically diverse *M. leprae* strains (15).

Analysis of the 12 MIRU-VNTR loci in genealogically distant *Mycobacterium bovis* BCG strains revealed that only one locus (locus 4) is polymorphic, with variable numbers of perfectly identical repeats among these strains, while the 11 other loci are monomorphic. Phylogenetic reconstruction of the changes in one VNTR locus among BCG strains indicates that VNTR events were generated by single-step additions and deletions of repeat units during cultivation of BCG daughter strains (80). Such single-step changes are a hallmark of replication slippage (84). VNTR changes in classic microsatellites are driven by replication slippage and inefficient mismatch repair in bacterial, yeast, or mammalian cells. However, depending on the organism and cell types, minisatellites can be destabilized by different mechanisms involving recombination or replication-dependent phenomena (10, 23, 49).

Three other families of interspersed tandemly repeated sequences, with repeat unit sizes falling into the same range as MIRUs, have been identified in the *M. tuberculosis* complex genomes. Most of these sequences also correspond to VNTR loci (included in Fig. 1). As with MIRU-VNTRs, marked differences in allelic diversities are found when these different loci are compared. Some of them are intergenic, while others with repeat units with lengths that are multiples of 3 nucleotides are found in frame within coding regions of various genes, including some members of the PPE family (48, 69, 75–77). For *leuA*, encoding α-isopropylmalate synthase and containing such an in-frame VNTR minisatellite, experimental data have suggested that the VNTR polymorphism resulted in a polymorphic protein (13).

INTERSPERSED REPEATS

A range of interspersed repeated sequences are present in the genomes of *M. tuberculosis* complex members, including gene duplications, short sequence repeats, and mobile genetic elements. In the class of gene duplication events, over 50% of genes in *M. tuberculosis* have arisen by duplication, with the PE and PPE gene families being a striking example of this trend (16, 85). In addition to their dispersal on the genome, these families contain TRs that show allelic variation across strains of the complex (see above).

IS Elements

Insertion sequences can be grouped into families on the basis of their genetic structure, similarity between encoded transposase enzymes, and fate of the target sites (52). Analysis of the *M. tuberculosis* H37Rv genome revealed 56 loci with similarity to IS elements, occupying approximately 77 kb (16, 31). These elements can be classified into the major IS families such as IS3, IS5, or IS21 (Table 1). A novel IS grouping, the IS1535 family, was originally identified that contained six seemingly intact elements and one pseudogene. However, with the increased number of available genome sequences from other bacteria, it is

Table 1. IS elements in *M. tuberculosis* H37Rv

Element (copy no.)	IS family[a]	Comments
IS6110 (16) IS1540 (1) IS1604 (1)	IS3	IS1604 shows low similarity to other IS3 members, so its grouping is tentative.
IS1560 (2) IS-like (2)	IS5	One copy of IS1560 is defective.
IS1532 (1) IS1533 (1) IS1534 (1)	IS21	These IS elements show variable presence or absence across *M. tuberculosis* isolates. IS1532 is part of RD6.
IS1603 (1)	IS30	
IS1547 (2) IS1558 (2) IS1607 (1) IS1608' (2)	IS110	One copy of IS1558 is truncated, while the short length of IS608' suggests a defective IS.
IS1081 (6) IS1552' (1) IS1553 (1) IS1554 (1)	IS256	IS1554 contains the IS256 characteristic "mutator family" motif.
IS1535 (1) IS1536 (1) IS1537 (1) IS1538 (1) IS1539 (1) IS1602 (1) IS1605' (1)	IS605	Originally placed in their own family, these IS elements are members of the IS605 family along with IS200 (*Salmonella enterica* serovar Typhimurium) and/or IS605 (*Helicobacter pylori*).
IS1555 (1) IS1557 (3) IS1561' (1) IS1606' (1)	ISL3	One copy of IS1557 is truncated. IS1561' is deleted from *M. microti* OV254.
IS1556 (1)	Unknown	Low similarity to IS3 transposases.

[a]As defined in reference 52.

now apparent that the IS1535 group forms part of the IS605 family (as defined in the IS Finder database; http://www.is.biotoul.fr/is.html) and should not be considered separate.

The most abundant IS element in the genome of *M. tuberculosis* is IS6110, an IS3 family member that varies from 0 to >25 copies (86). This divergence in copy number between *M. tuberculosis* isolates is the basis of the IS6110-based molecular typing system. Other IS elements show limited variation, with only IS1532, IS1533, IS1534, and IS1561' absent across a panel of *M. tuberculosis* complex strains tested (31). However, it is currently not clear whether loss of these elements was due to transposition of the elements. Indeed, in the case of IS1532, this element was deleted as part of RD6 (32).

Le Dantec et al. (46) have uncovered evidence for IS-mediated horizontal transfer between myco-

bacteria through work on the pCLP linear plasmid from *Mycobacterium celatum*. Sequence analysis of pCLP disclosed a region with 85% DNA identity to Rv2812 (IS1604) and Rv2813 of *M. tuberculosis*, two ORFs adjacent to the DR locus. The presence of IS1604, along with the ability of pCLP to replicate in the *M. tuberculosis* complex, suggests a mechanism for DNA exchange. However, horizontal transfer is not a significant force in shaping the *M. tuberculosis* genome (82).

REP13E12 Family

The genomes of the *M. tuberculosis* complex contain a family of seven repeats, the REP13E12 family, ranging in size from 1.3 to 1.4 kb and so called after the annotation of the first element on cosmid MTCY13E12 (31). The family has some parallels with mobile elements, such as synthesis of the protein by a possible translational frameshifting mechanism. Intriguingly, Davis et al. have shown that transcription of REP13E12 genes shows induction in response to DNA damage, with each of the elements preceded by a consensus SOS box that suggests regulation by LexA (21). Whether the increased level of transcription induced transposition was not reported. At least four of these elements also contain attachment sites for the ΦRv1 prophage-like element (5) (see below). It is therefore tempting to speculate that induction of REP13E12 in response to DNA damage may also induce the integrated prophage elements.

Prophage

Two prophage-like elements, ΦRv1 and ΦRv2, are present on the *M. tuberculosis* H37Rv genome (16). The presence and position of these prophages are variable across sequenced members of the *M. tuberculosis* complex, with ΦRv2 deleted in with *M. bovis* AF2122/97, with *M. bovis* BCG missing both prophages, and with *M. tuberculosis* CDC1551 having ΦRv2 integrated at a different locus from H37Rv (16, 27, 29, 51). Indeed, ΦRv1 was originally identified as RD3, a deletion from the genome of *M. bovis* BCG (51). The variation in integration sites of ΦRv2 is due to its attachment site being repeated in at least four members of the REP13E12 family. Bibb and Hatfull have shown that ΦRv1 encodes an active-site-specific recombination system and that the element is fully competent to integrate and excise (5).

The deletion of both ΦRv1 and ΦRv2 from the genome of *M. bovis* BCG is intriguing, since it is unclear whether the *M. bovis* progenitor strain naturally lacked these two phages or whether they were lost during in vitro passage. To date, our investigations have not identified an *M. bovis* strain that lacks both phages (S. V. Gordon, unpublished data), so it is possible that at least one phage was lost during in vitro passage. The loss of prophage could have effects on the virulence of the organisms, as has been noted in the effects of lamboid prophage on the virulence of members of the *Enterobacteriaceae*. Complementation of *M. bovis* BCG with RD3 did not, however, increase the virulence of the recombinant (68).

CRISPR Sequences

A number of groups have undertaken systematic analysis of short sequence repeats in prokaryotic genomes, with Schouls and colleagues introducing the clustered regularly interspaced short palindromic repeats (CRISPR) terminology (38, 57). These loci are characterized by direct repeats that vary in size from 27 to 37 bp and that are interspaced by similarly sized nonrepetitive sequences. The direct-repeat (DR) locus of *M. tuberculosis* complex strains, which is composed of multiple 36-bp DR copies interspersed by unique sequences called spacers, represents such a CRISPR sequence (39). Furthermore, the genes flanking the DR locus, Rv2817 and Rv2816, represent CRISPR-associated genes *cas1* and *cas2*, respectively. While the function of the DR locus remains cryptic, Jansen et al. reported deletion of this locus from *M. tuberculosis* (38); hence, it is not essential for in vitro growth. The DR locus is the basis for spacer oligonucleotide typing (spoligotyping), by which a barcode can be generated for *M. tuberculosis* complex isolates that differ in the presence or absence of spacers and adjacent repeats (39).

FUNCTIONAL CONSEQUENCES

Although they are often considered to be parasite or junk DNA, recent studies suggested that interspersed repetitive sequences play a role in the evolution of their host genomes (60, 63), including the creation of new protein sequences and functions (64). Higher mutability of microsatellite loci in pathogenic bacteria has been proposed to provide bacterial populations with sufficient evolutionary flexibility to adapt to environmental change in situations where classical regulation of gene expression is not efficient (58, 87). Consistent with this notion, changes in VNTR copy numbers often affect the expression of genes involved in adaptive responses (37, 65, 88, 93). Disruption of coding sequences by IS insertion is also an obvious example of the impact that mobile elements can have on an organism. Several observations suggest that MIRUs and other interspersed repetitive

sequences play a role in the evolution and diversification of functions in mycobacteria.

Genome Plasticity

IS elements can provoke a variety of chromosomal rearrangements. Integration or excision of an IS element can generate deletions of regions flanking the target site, while homologous recombination between IS elements can lead to deletion of the intervening sequence (Fig. 2). A case in point is seen in the variation between the *M. tuberculosis* strains H37Rv and H37Ra. A combination of restriction mapping, pulsed-field gel electrophoresis, and sequencing identified a deletion from the genome of *M. tuberculosis* H37Rv, termed RvD2, which had been catalyzed by an IS6110 homologous recombination event (9). Sequencing of the corresponding region in *M. tuberculosis* H37Ra allowed the identification of the original genome arrangement, with two directly repeated copies of IS6110 flanking the RvD2 locus. Examination of IS6110 copies in *M. tuberculosis* that lacked 3-bp DRs, combined with in silico comparison to the genome of *M. bovis*, allowed the identification of three more IS-mediated deletion events from H37Rv, although in these cases the antecedent genome arrangement could not be deduced (9). It is notable that one of these, RvD3, is located close to the RvD2 locus, suggesting that this region may be prone to deletion events. Indeed, Ho et al. (36) identified extensive variation in a 20-kb segment encompassing the RvD2 locus in a collection of *M. tuberculosis* clinical isolates, with IS6110 gene disruption and deletion events apparent. Evidence of IS-mediated deletions has also been uncovered in *M. microti*, where three deletions were shown to be due to IS6110 recombination (8). One of these deletions, MiD1, is adjacent to the DR region and is in part responsible for the characteristic spoligotype pattern of *M. microti*.

Analysis of the *M. tuberculosis* H37Rv genome revealed that disruption of coding sequences by IS elements was uncommon in this strain (31, 66). Rearrangement at RvD2 led to disrupted remnants of *plcD* (Rv1755c), a phospholipase C homologue, and Rv1758, a possible cutinase, while an IS6110 interrupted Rv2353c, a PPE protein. A copy of IS1081 was inserted into the molybdopterin biosynthesis operon located at Mb ~3.48, but it is not clear whether this disrupted the operon. However, mapping of IS6110 insertion sites across *M. tuberculosis* isolates has revealed that disruption of ORFs by IS6110 is a relatively common event, with van Helden and colleagues reporting that 60% of mapped IS6110 insertions occurred within coding regions against 33% in intergenic locations (71). It is therefore possible that transposition

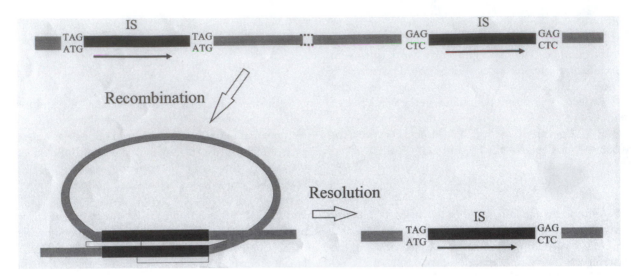

Figure 2. IS-mediated deletion mechanism. Two IS elements are shown in the same orientation, flanked by 3-bp DRs. Homologous recombination between the IS elements leads to looping out and deletion of the intervening sequence. The remaining IS element now appears without direct repeats. Homologous recombination between proximal IS elements appears to be a major force in shaping the genomes of the *M. tuberculosis* complex.

of IS exerts significant phenotypic variation across *M. tuberculosis* strains.

Hot spots for insertion of IS elements are apparent on the genome. Fang and colleagues (24, 25) identified a preferential insertion locus for IS6110, the *ipl* locus, which is itself contained within IS1547, present in two copies on the *M. tuberculosis* genome. They furthermore identified deletions affecting the *ipl* loci due to homologous recombination between adjacent IS6110 elements (26). A range of preferential integration loci for IS6110 have subsequently been identified, including the intergenic *dnaA-dnaN* region and the RvD2 locus (36, 44, 71, 92). The DR region is an IS hot spot, with the *M. tuberculosis* H37Rv genome showing insertions of IS6110 and proximal copies of IS604 and IS1555 (16, 71). Van Helden and colleagues (92, 72) have examined the impact of IS6110 insertion on the evolution of the DR region in *M. tuberculosis* and have shown some surprising differences to other reports. Using molecular typing data to identify predicted ancestors and daughter strains, they identified deletions that appeared to have been caused by IS6110 elements orientated in opposite directions (72). Normally, this orientation would result in the inversion of the intervening DNA sequence rather than in deletion. The mechanism for the generation of these deletions in the DR region remains unclear.

The genome of *M. leprae* offers an interesting parallel to evolution of the *M. tuberculosis* complex. The *M. leprae* genome contains at least four families of repetitive DNA, contributing approximately 2% to the total genome size. These sequences are designated RLEP (37 copies), REPLEP (15 copies), LEPREP (8 copies), and LEPRPT (5 copies) (17). Furthermore, there are 26 transposase pseudogenes but apparently no functional IS. The LEPREP sequences are pseudogenes with similarity to transposases and the maturases of class II introns, enzymes that catalyse DNA transposition. This suggests a once-functional system for replication of the sequence through the genome. Most strikingly, recombination between sequence repeats has been a major force in shaping the *M. leprae* genome. Comparison with *M. tuberculosis* revealed that breakpoints in synteny between the genomes are occupied by repetitive elements. It is possible that recombination of repetitive elements led to deletion of the intervening DNA segments. This is similar to the IS6110-mediated deletion mechanism in *M. tuberculosis* described above. While homologous recombination functions may no longer be active in *M. leprae* due to mutation of genes for the RecBCD complex, it is probable that this system functioned in the past to catalyze recombination events.

MIRUs: Dynamics of Intragenomic Dissemination

In addition to their association with intergenic minisatellites, which is rarely observed in bacteria (47), the presence of homologous repetitive sequences such as MIRUs in multiple VNTR and non-VNTR loci inevitably raises questions about the means and dynamics of their dispersion in mycobacterial genomes. The dissemination of repeated sequences has been proposed to be based on either gene conversion or mobilization via transposition or site-specific recombination (30, 35). Sequence analyses of *M. tuberculosis* MIRU loci versus orthologous sites in other mycobacteria devoid of MIRUs suggest that MIRUs may disseminate by insertion into ATGA sites involved in translational coupling in polycistronic operons. Examination of several sites, such as those shown in Fig. 3 and in reference 79, indicated that the ATGA motif which served as the apparent target for insertion is duplicated at the extremities of the MIRU in *M. tuberculosis*. In these cases, the duplication corresponds to the overlapping stop and start codons of two contiguous genes (encoding the SenX3 histidine kinase and the RegX3 response regulator from a two-component signal transduction system in the example shown in Fig. 3), which is compatible with a mobilization mechanism such as transposition, involving duplication of flanking base pairs at the target site. However, since MIRU ORFs are so short, proteins essential for mobilization must be provided in *trans*.

Analysis of the 41 chromosomal sites containing MIRUs in H37Rv in >50 other strains of *M. tuberculosis*, *M. africanum*, and *M. bovis* from diverse geographic origins indicated the systematic presence of at least one MIRU copy in all sites of the latter isolates (80; Supply et al., unpublished). In contrast, several orthologous sites of more distant mycobacterial species,

such as *M. canetti* or species outside the *M. tuberculosis* complex, are devoid of any MIRU copy (Fig. 3 in this chapter; Fig. 2 in reference 79; Supply et al., unpublished). These results indicate that MIRUs were integrated into the 41 chromosomal sites before the divergence of *M. tuberculosis*, *M. africanum*, and *M. bovis* and that insertion-excision events are scarce or nonexistent over this evolutionary scale but, rather, occur over longer periods concomitantly with speciation events.

The observation of generally slow evolutionary changes of MIRU-VNTR and other VNTRs (see also below), combined with their insertion into translational coupling sites or into coding regions of unrelated genes, suggests specialized roles for these polymorphic sequences in adaptive evolution of the bacterial population. These roles might be particularly important, given the otherwise high conservation of the genome sequence and the clonal nature of the species (78, 82). Such roles are consistent with the concept of coadaptations between initially parasitic repetitive sequences and host genomes (41). By their insertion into translational coupling sites, MIRU(-VNTR)s can partially hijack the expression potential of target operons for their own coding sequence. In this respect, it is interesting that many MIRUs contain a sequence at their 3' end

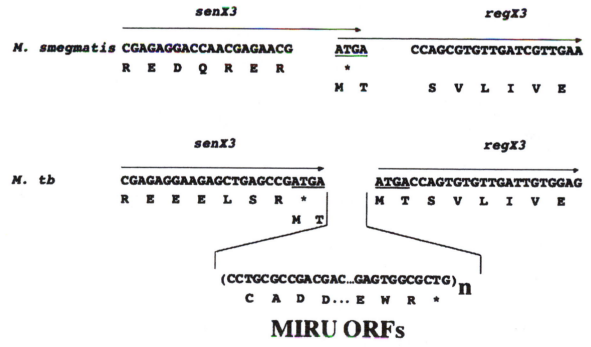

MIRU ORFs

Figure 3. DNA sequence alignment of orthologous intergenic regions in *M. smegmatis* and *M. tuberculosis* H37Rv, indicating the position of the MIRU in the *M. tuberculosis* sequence. The sequences of the *senX3* and *regX3* genes (*rv0490* and *rv0491* in H37Rv, respectively) and their encoded products are shown. Duplicated nucleotides surrounding the MIRU insertion site are underlined. The stars correspond to stop codons. The "n" symbol indicates the presence of VNTRs in this locus. Translational coupling sites are apparent targets for MIRU insertion. This insertion predictably places the MIRU ORF under translational control of the upstream genes.

that is somewhat complementary to the 3' end of the 16S rRNA and could therefore possibly control the translational initiation of MIRU-downstream genes.

It is also possible that MIRUs exert no particular function and may therefore be considered as selfish DNA, as suggested for other repeated DNA sequences (35). In this regard, the localization of MIRUs between translationally coupled genes places their ORFs under the transcriptional and translational control of the upstream genes of the target operons, suggesting that their expression might play some role in MIRU dissemination or replication. In this case, the expected effect of MIRU insertions on the translation of the downstream genes would be fortuitous.

APPLICATIONS

The association of repetitive sequences with genetic variation makes them valuable molecular markers for studying bacterial populations. In the *M. tuberculosis* complex, IS6110 restriction fragment length polymorphism (RFLP) is the current "gold standard" for molecular epidemiological studies. This method has been used for over a decade and has proven its value in a range of epidemiological settings (6, 14, 18, 74, 90). However, for use with strains with a low copy number of IS6110, this technique has obvious limitations. Spoligotyping, based on variation at the DR locus, has also been widely used, in particular for *M. bovis* since this strain contains only one or two copies of IS6110. At the Veterinary Laboratories Agency, spoligotyping is currently the method of choice for routine molecular typing of *M. bovis*, with the current database (July 2003) containing spoligotypes of >22,000 *M. bovis* isolates (unpublished). The application of molecular methods to the epidemiology of tuberculosis has been reviewed elsewhere (11, 59, 89), but the application of MIRU-VNTRs and other VNTRS has received less attention; we therefore focus on them for the rest of this section.

VNTR genotyping is based on changes in the number of repetitive sequences in microsatellites or minisatellites. It is a universal tool to study various aspects of evolution, ranging from pedigree to evolutionarily distant phylogenetic relationships, for humans and virtually all higher eukaryote species. VNTR sequences have progressively emerged as powerful markers for genotyping of many bacterial species, especially for genetically homogeneous pathogens such as *Bacillus anthracis* (40, 47), *Yersinia pestis* (1, 42, 47), and the *M. tuberculosis* complex members (see below). These methods rely on PCR amplification with primers specific for the flanking regions of the VNTRs and on the determination of the sizes of the amplicons,

from which the numbers of the amplified VNTR copies are calculated by comparison with reference alleles of known sizes and VNTR contents. VNTR alleles for each of the different target loci are then combined in a numerical genotype, which is a simple and portable format adequate to study the global molecular epidemiology of infectious agents.

Different sets of VNTR loci have been described for the typing of *M. tuberculosis* complex strains (28, 33, 47, 50, 62, 69, 75–77, 80). The first set which was used at significant scale for *M. tuberculosis* typing included five loci, called ETR-A to ETR-E (28). This set has been successfully used as a secondary typing method in addition to IS6110 RFLP or to spoligotyping, in outbreak investigations, in population-based studies, or to detect laboratory contaminations. However, the polymorphism of these loci is much too low to accurately discriminate different clones (43). Another system based on 12 MIRU-VNTR loci is applicable for reliable genotyping and molecular epidemiology studies of *M. tuberculosis* (19, 45, 53, 81). MIRU-VNTR genotyping can be performed using simple agarose gel electrophoresis or with a high-capacity genotyping system, based on the analysis of multiplex PCRs on a fluorescence-based DNA analyzer. This typing method is appropriate for all *M. tuberculosis* isolates, including those with a few or without IS6110 copies, and provides a resolution close to that of IS6110 RFLP to differentiate unrelated strains (53, 81).

The performance of MIRU-VNTR typing for *M. tuberculosis* molecular epidemiology has been evaluated in different epidemiological settings, in comparison with those of the current standard method based on IS6110 RFLP. *M. tuberculosis* strains with identical IS6110 RFLP profiles, isolated from different patients, are generally considered to be clonal and to correspond to recent transmission events. Consistently, strains identified in outbreaks most often display the same IS6110 RFLP patterns, and population-based studies have revealed that clustering is associated with identified risk factors for transmission (12, 22). Virtually all epidemiologically linked isolates tested, resulting from transmission or relapses, isolation from different anatomical sites from the same patient, or laboratory cross-contaminations, displayed identical MIRU-VNTR genotypes (45, 53, 73). Consistent with the analysis of the *M. bovis* BCG vaccine phylogeny (80), these results indicate that the MIRU-VNTRs are remarkably stable over time and are useful for tracking key events in epidemiological investigations.

In these studies, most strains with identical IS6110 RFLP patterns also displayed identical MIRU-VNTR genotypes. However, a few isolates with identical MIRU-VNTR types had slightly distinct IS6110 RFLP patterns, although some of these were clearly epidemiologically linked. Gain or loss of one IS6110 copy in isolates from patients in case clusters has been reported in several other studies, with more extensive changes in IS6110 RFLP observed in strains that apparently underwent clonal expansion in the New York area within a few years (6). Conversely, some isolates with no known epidemiological links featuring identical fingerprints with high or low IS6110 copy numbers were found to be discriminated by MIRU-VNTRs or other VNTRs (45; Supply, unpublished). These results might reflect variations of the IS6110 RFLP evolution rate among different strains, due to the effects of the local genomic context of specific IS6110 insertion sites on the transposition rate (2, 91, 92). Therefore, the equations "nonidentical IS6110 RFLP = unrelated case" and "identical IS6110 RFLP = recently related case" are not always true. In contrast to the diversity of IS6110 insertion sites, the nature of the loci containing the VNTR targets is identical regardless of which strain is analyzed. Therefore, the rate of change of these VNTRs might be globally less influenced by the surrounding genetic context among different strains, i.e., these markers might thus function as more regular molecular clocks than IS6110-RFLP. Taken together, these results suggest that VNTR typing may be particularly appropriate for long-term epidemiological analyses and may be used to reevaluate previously estimated degrees of transmission in populations.

MIRU-VNTRs have proven to be useful tools for investigating the population structure of *M. tuberculosis*. The restricted sequence polymorphism of *M. tuberculosis* gene sequences (78) precludes population studies using multilocus sequence typing or multilocus enzyme electrophoresis. However, highly significant linkage disequilibrium could be shown among the 12 MIRU-VNTR loci in a sample of 209 *M. tuberculosis* isolates, representative of the genetic diversity in Cape Town, South Africa (82). This strong linkage between multilocus markers not only discloses a clonal evolution of *M. tuberculosis* in this local setting but also, in light of previous results (53), strongly suggests that the entire species has a clonal population structure.

CONCLUSIONS

Repetitive DNA plays a central role in the biology of the *M. tuberculosis* complex. IS-mediated mutagenesis through gene disruption or deletion events is evident and is likely to have a range of phenotypic effects on the host. Also, changes in intragenic micro-

satellites and minisatellites may be a mechanism of antigenic variation, while intergenic MIRUs could alter the expression of flanking genes. Further research should seek to clarify the strength of such effects. Finally, variation of repetitive DNA sequences is key to the molecular epidemiological tools that have had such a dramatic impact on our understanding of *M. tuberculosis* population structure and evolution. Continued analysis of repetitive DNA will allow us to tease out more fully the dynamics of the *M. tuberculosis* genome.

REFERENCES

1. **Adair, D. M., P. L. Worsham, K. K. Hill, A. M. Klevytska, P. J. Jackson, A. M. Friedlander, and P. Keim.** 2000. Diversity in a variable-number tandem repeat from *Yersinia pestis*. *J. Clin. Microbiol.* **38:**1516–1519.
2. **Alito, A., N. Morcillo, S. Scipioni, A. Dolmann, M. I. Romano, A. Cataldi, and D. van Soolingen.** 1999. The IS6110 restriction fragment length polymorphism in particular multidrug-resistant *Mycobacterium tuberculosis* strains may evolve too fast for reliable use in outbreak investigation. *J. Clin. Microbiol.* **37:**788–791.
3. **Bayliss, C. D., T. van de Ven, and E. R. Moxon.** 2002. Mutations in *polI* but not *mutSLH* destabilize *Haemophilus influenzae* tetranucleotide repeats. *EMBO J.* **21:**1465–1476.
4. **Benson, G.** 1999. Tandem repeats finder: a program to analyze DNA sequences. *Nucleic Acids Res.* **27:**573–580.
5. **Bibb, L. A., and G. F. Hatfull.** 2002. Integration and excision of the *Mycobacterium tuberculosis* prophage-like element, phiRv1. *Mol. Microbiol.* **45:**1515–1526.
6. **Bifani, P. J., B. B. Plikaytis, V. Kapur, K. Stockbauer, X. Pan, M. L. Lutfey, S. L. Moghazeh, W. Eisner, T. M. Daniel, M. H. Kaplan, J. T. Crawford, J. M. Musser, and B. N. Kreiswirth.** 1996. Origin and interstate spread of a New York City multidrug-resistant *Mycobacterium tuberculosis* clone family. *JAMA* **275:**452–457.
7. **Britten, R. J., and D. E. Kohne.** 1968. Repeated sequences in DNA. Hundreds of thousands of copies of DNA sequences have been incorporated into the genomes of higher organisms. *Science* **161:**529–540.
8. **Brodin, P., K. Eiglmeier, M. Marmiesse, A. Billault, T. Garnier, S. Niemann, S. T. Cole, and R. Brosch.** 2002. Bacterial artificial chromosome-based comparative genomic analysis identifies *Mycobacterium microti* as a natural ESAT-6 deletion mutant. *Infect. Immun.* **70:**5568–5578.
9. **Brosch, R., W. J. Philipp, E. Stavropoulos, M. J. Colston, S. T. Cole, and S. V. Gordon.** 1999. Genomic analysis reveals variation between *Mycobacterium tuberculosis* H37Rv and the attenuated *M. tuberculosis* H37Ra strain. *Infect. Immun.* **67:**5768–5774.
10. **Buard, J., A. Collick, J. Brown, and A. J. Jeffreys.** 2000. Somatic versus germline mutation processes at minisatellite CEB1 (D2S90) in humans and transgenic mice. *Genomics* **65:**95–103.
11. **Burgos, M. V., and A. S. Pym.** 2002. Molecular epidemiology of tuberculosis. *Eur. Respir. J. Suppl.* **36:**54s–65s.
12. **Cave, M. D., K. D. Eisenach, G. Templeton, M. Salfinger, G. Mazurek, J. H. Bates, and J. T. Crawford.** 1994. Stability of DNA fingerprint pattern produced with IS6110 in strains of *Mycobacterium tuberculosis*. *J. Clin. Microbiol.* **32:**262–266.

13. Chanchaem, W., and P. Palittapongarnpim. 2002. A variable number of tandem repeats result in polymorphic alphaisopropylmalate synthase in *Mycobacterium tuberculosis*. *Tuberculosis* (Edinburgh) 82:1–6.

14. Chevrel-Dellagi, D., A. Abderrahman, R. Haltiti, H. Koubaji, B. Gicquel, and K. Dellagi. 1993. Large-scale DNA fingerprinting of *Mycobacterium tuberculosis* strains as a tool for epidemiological studies of tuberculosis. *J. Clin. Microbiol.* 31:2446–2450.

15. Cole, S. T., P. Supply, and N. Honore. 2001a. Repetitive sequences in *Mycobacterium leprae* and their impact on genome plasticity. *Lepr. Rev.* 72:449–461.

16. Cole, S. T., R. Brosch, J. Parkhill, T. Garnier, C. Churcher, D. Harris, S. V. Gordon, K. Eiglmeier, S. Gas, C. E. Barry III, F. Tekaia, K. Badcock, D. Basham, D. Brown, T. Chillingworth, R. Connor, R. Davies, K. Devlin, T. Feltwell, S. Gentles, N. Hamlin, S. Holroyd, T. Hornsby, K. Jagels, A. Krogh, J. McLean, S. Moule, L. Murphy, K. Oliver, J. Osborne, M. A. Quail, M.-A. Rajandream, J. Rogers, S. Rutter, K. Seeger, J. Skelton, R. Squares, S. Squares, J. G. Sulston, K. Taylor, S. Whitehead, and B. G. Barrell. 1998. Deciphering the biology of *Mycobacterium tuberculosis* from the complete genome sequence. *Nature* 393:537–544.

17. Cole, S. T., K. Eiglmeier, J. Parkhill, K. D. James, N. R. Thomson, P. R. Wheeler, N. Honore, T. Garnier, C. Churcher, D. Harris, K. Mungall, D. Basham, D. Brown, T. Chillingworth, R. Connor, R. M. Davies, K. Devlin, S. Duthoy, T. Feltwell, A. Fraser, N. Hamlin, S. Holroyd, T. Hornsby, K. Jagels, C. Lacroix, J. Maclean, S. Moule, L. Murphy, K. Oliver, M. A. Quail, M. A. Rajandream, K. M. Rutherford, S. Rutter, K. Seeger, S. Simon, M. Simmonds, J. Skelton, R. Squares, S. Squares, K. Stevens, K. Taylor, S. Whitehead, J. R. Woodward, and B. G. Barrell. 2001. Massive gene decay in the leprosy bacillus. *Nature* 409:1007–1011.

18. Cowan, L. S., and J. T. Crawford. 2002. Genotype analysis of *Mycobacterium tuberculosis* isolates from a sentinel surveillance population. *Emerg. Infect. Dis.* 8:1294–1302.

19. Cowan, L. S., L. Mosher, L. Diem, J. P. Massey, and J. T. Crawford. 2002. Variable-number tandem repeat typing of *Mycobacterium tuberculosis* isolates with low copy numbers of IS*6110* by using mycobacterial interspersed repetitive units. *J. Clin. Microbiol.* 40:1592–1602.

20. Cox, R., and S. M. Mirkin. 1997. Characteristic enrichment of DNA repeats in different genomes. *Proc. Natl. Acad. Sci. USA* 94:5237–5242.

21. Davis, E. O., E. M. Dullaghan, and L. Rand. 2002. Definition of the mycobacterial SOS box and use to identify LexA-regulated genes in *Mycobacterium tuberculosis*. *J. Bacteriol.* 184:3287–3295.

22. de Boer, A. S., M. W. Borgdorff, P. E. de Haas, N. J. Nagelkerke, J. D. van Embden, and D. van Soolingen. 1999. Analysis of rate of change of IS*6110* RFLP patterns of *Mycobacterium tuberculosis* based on serial patient isolates. *J. Infect. Dis.* 180:1238–1244.

23. Ellegren, H. 2000. Heterogeneous mutation processes in human microsatellite DNA sequences. *Nat. Genet.* 24:400–402.

24. Fang, Z., and K. J. Forbes. 1997. A *Mycobacterium tuberculosis* IS*6110* preferential locus (*ipl*) for insertion into the genome. *J. Clin. Microbiol.* 35:479–481.

25. Fang, Z., C. Doig, N. Morrison, B. Watt, and K. J. Forbes. 1999. Characterization of IS*1547*, a new member of the IS*900* family in the *Mycobacterium tuberculosis* complex, and its association with IS*6110*. *J. Bacteriol.* 181:1021–1024.

26. Fang, Z., C. Doig, D. T. Kenna, N. Smittipat, P. Palittapongarnpim, B. Watt, and K. J. Forbes. 1999. IS*6110*-mediated

deletions of wild-type chromosomes of *Mycobacterium tuberculosis*. *J. Bacteriol.* 181:1014–1020.

27. Fleischmann, R. D., D. Alland, J. A. Eisen, L. Carpenter, O. White, J. Peterson, R. DeBoy, R. Dodson, M. Gwinn, D. Haft, E. Hickey, J. F. Kolonay, W. C. Nelson, L. A. Umayam, M. Ermolaeva, S. L. Salzberg, A. Delcher, T. Utterback, J. Weidman, H. Khouri, J. Gill, A. Mikula, W. Bishai, W. R. Jacobs, Jr., J. C. Venter, and C. M. Fraser. 2002. Whole-genome comparison of *Mycobacterium tuberculosis* clinical and laboratory strains. *J. Bacteriol.* 184:5479–5490.

28. Frothingham, R., and W. A. Meeker-O'Connell. 1998. Genetic diversity in the *Mycobacterium tuberculosis* complex based on variable numbers of tandem DNA repeats. *Microbiology* 144:1189–1196.

29. Garnier, T., K. Eiglmeier, J. C. Camus, N. Medina, H. Mansoor, M. Pryor, S. Duthoy, S. Grondin, C. Lacroix, C. Monsempe, S. Simon, B. Harris, R. Atkin, J. Doggett, R. Mayes, L. Keating, P. R. Wheeler, J. Parkhill, B. G. Barrell, S. T. Cole, S. V. Gordon, and R. G. Hewinson. 2003. The complete genome sequence of *Mycobacterium bovis*. *Proc. Natl. Acad. Sci. USA* 100:7877–7882.

30. Gilson, E., D. Perrin, W. Saurin, and M. Hofnung. 1987. Species specificity of bacterial palindromic units. *J. Mol. Evol.* 25:371–373.

31. Gordon, S. V., B. Heym, J. Parkhill, B. Barrell, and S. T. Cole. 1999. New insertion sequences and a novel repeated sequence in the genome of *Mycobacterium tuberculosis* H37Rv. *Microbiology* 145:881–892.

32. Gordon, S. V., R. Brosch, A. Billault, T. Garnier, K. Eiglmeier, and S. T. Cole. 1999. Identification of variable regions in the genomes of tubercle bacilli using bacterial artificial chromosome arrays. *Mol. Microbiol.* 32:643–655.

33. Goyal, M., D. Young, Y. Zhang, P. A. Jenkins, and R. J. Shaw. 1994. PCR amplification of variable sequence upstream of *katG* gene to subdivide strains of *Mycobacterium tuberculosis* complex. *J. Clin. Microbiol.* 32:3070–3071.

34. Hermans, P. W., D. van Soolingen, and J. D. van Embden. 1992. Characterization of a major polymorphic tandem repeat in *Mycobacterium tuberculosis* and its potential use in the epidemiology of *Mycobacterium kansasii* and *Mycobacterium gordonae*. *J. Bacteriol.* 174:4157–4165.

35. Higgins, C. F., R. S. McLaren, and S. F. Newbury. 1988. Repetitive extragenic palindromic sequences, mRNA stability and gene expression: evolution by gene conversion? A review. *Gene* 72:3–14.

36. Ho, T. B., B. D. Robertson, G. M. Taylor, R. J. Shaw, and D. B. Young. 2000. Comparison of *Mycobacterium tuberculosis* genomes reveals frequent deletions in a 20 kb variable region in clinical isolates. *Yeast* 17:272–282.

37. Hood, D. W., M. E. Deadman, M. P. Jennings, M. Bisercic, R. D. Fleischmann, J. C. Venter, and E. R. Moxon. 1996. DNA repeats identify novel virulence genes in *Haemophilus influenzae*. *Proc. Natl. Acad. Sci. USA* 93:11121–11125.

38. Jansen, R., J. D. van Embden, W. Gaastra, and L. M. Schouls. (2002). Identification of genes that are associated with DNA repeats in prokaryotes. *Mol. Microbiol.* 43:1565–1575.

39. Kamerbeek, J., L. Schouls, A. Kolk, M. van Agterveld, D. van Soolingen, S. Kuijper, A. Bunschoten, H. Molhuizen, R. Shaw, M. Goyal, and J. van Embden. (1997). Simultaneous detection and strain differentiation of *Mycobacterium tuberculosis* for diagnosis and epidemiology. *J. Clin. Microbiol.* 35:907–914.

40. Keim, P., L. B. Price, A. M. Klevytska, K. L. Smith, J. M. Schupp, R. Okinaka, P. J. Jackson, and M. E. Hugh-Jones. 2000. Multiple-locus variable-number tandem repeat analysis reveals genetic relationships within *Bacillus anthracis*. *J. Bacteriol.* 182:2928–2936.

41. Kidwell, M. G., and D. Lisch. 1997. Transposable elements as sources of variation in animals and plants. *Proc. Natl. Acad. Sci. USA* **94:**7704–7711.

42. Klevytska, A. M., L. B. Price, J. M. Schupp, P. L. Worsham, J. Wong, and P. Keim. 2001. Identification and characterization of variable-number tandem repeats in the *Yersinia pestis* genome. *J. Clin. Microbiol.* **39:**3179–3185.

43. Kremer, K., D. van Soolingen, R. Frothingham, W. H. Haas, P. W. Hermans, C. Martin, P. Palittapongarnpim, B. B. Plikaytis, L. W. Riley, M. A. Yakrus, J. M. Musser, and J. D. van Embden. 1999. Comparison of methods based on different molecular epidemiological markers for typing of *Mycobacterium tuberculosis* complex strains: interlaboratory study of discriminatory power and reproducibility. *J. Clin. Microbiol.* **37:**2607–2618.

44. Kurepina, N. E., S. Sreevatsan, B. B. Plikaytis, P. J. Bifani, N. D. Connell, R. J. Donnelly, D. van Soolingen, J. M. Musser, and B. N. Kreiswirth. 1998. Characterization of the phylogenetic distribution and chrmosomal insertion sites of five IS*6110* elements in *Mycobacterium tuberculois:* nonrandom integration in the *dnaA-dnaN* region. *Tubercle Lung Dis.* **79:**31–42.

45. Kwara, A., R. Schiro, L. S. Cowan, N. E. Hyslop, M. F. Wiser, S. Roahen Harrison, P. Kissinger, L. Diem, and J. T. Crawford. 2003. Evaluation of the epidemiologic utility of secondary typing methods for differentiation of *Mycobacterium tuberculosis* isolates. *J. Clin. Microbiol.* **41:**2683–2685.

46. Le Dantec, C., N. Winter, B. Gicquel, V. Vincent, and M. Picardeau. 2001. Genomic sequence and transcriptional analysis of a 23-kilobase mycobacterial linear plasmid: evidence for horizontal transfer and identification of plasmid maintenance systems. *J. Bacteriol.* **183:**2157–2164.

47. Le Fleche, P., Y. Hauck, L. Onteniente, A. Prieur, F. Denoeud, V. Ramisse, P. Sylvestre, G. Benson, F. Ramisse, and G. Vergnaud. 2001. A tandem repeats database for bacterial genomes: application to the genotyping of *Yersinia pestis* and *Bacillus anthracis. BMC Microbiol* **1:**2.

48. Le Fleche, P., M. Fabre, F. Denoeud, J. L. Koeck, and G. Vergnaud. (2002). High resolution, on-line identification of strains from the *Mycobacterium tuberculosis* complex based on tandem repeat typing. *BMC Microbiol.* **2:**37.

49. Lopes, J., H. Debrauwere, J. Buard, and A. Nicolas. 2002. Instability of the human minisatellite CEB1 in *rad27Δ* and *dna2-1* replication-deficient yeast cells. *EMBO J.* **21:**3201–3211.

50. Magdalena, J., P. Supply, and C. Locht. 1998. Specific differentiation between *Mycobacterium bovis* BCG and virulent strains of the *Mycobacterium tuberculosis* complex. *J. Clin. Microbiol.* **36:**2471–2476.

51. Mahairas, G. G., P. J. Sabo, M. J. Hickey, D. C. Singh, and C. K. Stover. 1996. Molecular analysis of genetic differences between *Mycobacterium bovis* BCG and virulent *M. bovis. J. Bacteriol.* **178:**1274–1282.

52. Mahillon, J., and M. Chandler. 1998. Insertion sequences. *Microbiol. Mol. Biol. Rev.* **62:**725–774.

53. Mazars, E., S. Lesjean, A. L. Banuls, M. Gilbert, V. Vincent, B. Gicquel, M. Tibayrenc, C. Locht, and P. Supply. 2001. High-resolution minisatellite-based typing as a portable approach to global analysis of *Mycobacterium tuberculosis* molecular epidemiology. *Proc. Natl. Acad. Sci. USA* **98:**1901–1906.

54. McCarthy, J. E., and C. Gualerzi. 1990. Translational control of prokaryotic gene expression. *Trends Genet.* **6:**78–85.

55. McFadden, J., and G. Knowles. 1997. Escape from evolutionary stasis by transposon-mediated deleterious mutations. *J. Theor. Biol.* **186:**441–447.

56. Mizrahi, V., and S. J. Andersen. 1998. DNA repair in *Mycobacterium tuberculosis.* What have we learnt from the genome sequence? *Mol. Microbiol.* **29:**1331–1339.

57. Mojica, F. J., C. Diez-Villasenor, E. Soria, and G. Juez. 2000. Biological significance of a family of regularly spaced repeats in the genomes of Archaea, Bacteria and mitochondria. *Mol. Microbiol.* **36.**244–246.

58. Moxon, E. R., P. B. Rainey, M. A. Nowak, and R. E. Lenski. 1994. Adaptive evolution of highly mutable loci in pathogenic bacteria. *Curr. Biol.* **4:**24–33.

59. Murray, M., and E. Nardell. 2002. Molecular epidemiology of tuberculosis: achievements and challenges to current knowledge. *Bull. W. H. O.* **80:**477–482.

60. Nadir, E., H. Margalit, T. Gallily, and S. A. Ben-Sasson. 1996. Microsatellite spreading in the human genome: evolutionary mechanisms and structural implications. *Proc. Natl. Acad. Sci. USA* **93:**6470–6475.

61. Nakamura, Y., M. Leppert, P. O'Connell, R. Wolff, T. Holm, M. Culver, C. Martin, E. Fujimoto, M. Hoff, E. Kumlin, et al. 1987. Variable number of tandem repeat (VNTR) markers for human gene mapping. *Science* **235:**1616–1622.

62. Namwat, W., P. Luangsuk, and P. Palittapongarnpim. 1998. The genetic diversity of *Mycobacterium tuberculosis* strains in Thailand studied by amplification of DNA segments containing direct repetitive sequences. *Int. J. Tuberc. Lung Dis.* **2:**153–159.

63. Nowak, R. 1994. Mining treasures from "junk DNA." *Science* **263:**608–610.

64. Ogata, H., S. Audic, V. Barbe, F. Artiguenave, P. E. Fournier, D. Raoult, and J. M. Claverie. 2000. Selfish DNA in protein-coding genes of *Rickettsia. Science* **290:**347–350.

65. Peak, I. R., M. P. Jennings, D. W. Hood, M. Bisercic, and E. R. Moxon. 1996. Tetrameric repeat units associated with virulence factor phase variation in *Haemophilus* also occur in *Neisseria* spp. and *Moraxella catarrhalis. FEMS Microbiol. Lett.* **137:**109–114.

66. Philipp, W. J., S. Poulet, K. Eiglmeier, L. Pascopella, V. Balasubramanian, B. Heym, S. Bergh, B. R. Bloom, W. R. Jacobs, Jr. and S. T. Cole. 1996. An integrated map of the genome of the tubercle bacillus, *Mycobacterium tuberculosis* H37Rv, and comparison with *Mycobacterium leprae. Proc. Natl. Acad. Sci. USA* **93:**3132–3137.

67. Poulet, S., and S. T. Cole. 1995. Characterization of the highly abundant polymorphic GC-rich-repetitive sequence (PGRS) present in *Mycobacterium tuberculosis. Arch. Microbiol.* **163:**87–95.

68. Pym, A. S., P. Brodin, R. Brosch, M. Huerre, and S. T. Cole. 2002. Loss of RD1 contributed to the attenuation of the live tuberculosis vaccines *Mycobacterium bovis* BCG and *Mycobacterium microti. Mol. Microbiol.* **46:**709–717.

69. Roring, S., A. Scott, D. Brittain, I. Walker, G. Hewinson, S. Neill, and R. Skuce. 2002. Development of variable-number tandem repeat typing of *Mycobacterium bovis:* comparison of results with those obtained by using existing exact tandem repeats and spoligotyping. *J. Clin. Microbiol.* **40:**2126–2133.

70. Ross, B. C., K. Raios, K. Jackson, and B. Dwyer. 1992. Molecular cloning of a highly repeated DNA element from *Mycobacterium tuberculosis* and its use as an epidemiological tool. *J. Clin. Microbiol.* **30:**942–946.

71. Sampson, S., R. Warren, M. Richardson, G. van der Spuy, and P. van Helden. 2001. IS*6110* insertions in *Mycobacterium tuberculosis:* predominantly into coding regions. *J. Clin. Microbiol.* **39:**3423–3424.

72. Sampson, S. L., R. M. Warren, M. Richardson, T. C. Victor, A. M. Jordaan, G. D. van der Spuy, and P. D. van Helden. 2003. IS*6110*-mediated deletion polymorphism in the direct

repeat region of clinical isolates of *Mycobacterium tuberculosis*. *J. Bacteriol.* **185**:2856–2866.

73. Savine, E., R. M. Warren, G. D. van der Spuy, N. Beyers, P. D. van Helden, C. Locht, and P. Supply. 2002. Stability of variable-number tandem repeats of mycobacterial interspersed repetitive units from 12 loci in serial isolates of *Mycobacterium tuberculosis*. *J. Clin. Microbiol.* **40**:4561–4566.

74. Siddiqi, N., M. Shamim, A. Amin, D. S. Chauhan, R. Das, K. Srivastava, D. Singh, V. D. Sharma, V. M. Katoch, S. K. Sharma, M. Hanief, and S. E. Hasnain. 2001. Typing of drug resistant isolates of *Mycobacterium tuberculosis* from India using the IS*6110* element reveals substantive polymorphism. *Infect. Genet. Evol.* **1**:109–116.

75. Skuce, R. A., T. P. McCorry, J. F. McCarroll, S. M. Roring, A. N. Scott, D. Brittain, S. L. Hughes, R. G. Hewinson, and S. D. Neill. 2002. Discrimination of *Mycobacterium tuberculosis* complex bacteria using novel VNTR-PCR targets. *Microbiology* **148**:519–528.

76. Smittipat, N., and P. Palittapongarnpim. 2000. Identification of possible loci of variable number of tandem repeats in *Mycobacterium tuberculosis*. *Tubercle Lung Dis.* **80**:69–74.

77. Spurgiesz, R. C., T. N. Quitugua, K. L. Smith, J. Schupp, E. G. Palmer, R. A. Cox, and P. Kiem. 2003. Molecular typing of *Mycobacterium tuberculosis* by using nine novel variable-number tandem repeats across the Beijing family and low-copy-number IS*6110* isolates. *J. Clin. Microbiol.* **41**:4224–4230.

78. Sreevatsan, S., X. Pan, K. E. Stockbauer, N. D. Connell, B. N. Kreiswirth, T. S. Whittam, and J. M. Musser. 1997. Restricted structural gene polymorphism in the *Mycobacterium tuberculosis* complex indicates evolutionarily recent global dissemination. *Proc. Natl. Acad. Sci. USA* **94**:9869–9874.

79. Supply, P., J. Magdalena, S. Himpens, and C. Locht. (1997). Identification of novel intergenic repetitive units in a mycobacterial two-component system operon. *Mol. Microbiol.* **26**:991–1003.

80. Supply, P., E. Mazars, S. Lesjean, V. Vincent, B. Gicquel, and C. Locht. 2000. Variable human minisatellite-like regions in the *Mycobacterium tuberculosis* genome. *Mol. Microbiol.* **36**:762–771.

81. Supply, P., S. Lesjean, E. Savine, K. Kremer, D. van Soolingen, and C. Locht. 2001. Automated high-throughput genotyping for study of global epidemiology of *Mycobacterium tuberculosis* based on mycobacterial interspersed repetitive units. *J. Clin. Microbiol.* **39**:3563–3571.

82. Supply, P., R. M. Warren, A. L. Banuls, S. Lesjean, G. D. Van Der Spuy, L. A. Lewis, M. Tibayrenc, P. D. Van Helden, and C. Locht. 2003. Linkage disequilibrium between minisatellite loci supports clonal evolution of *Mycobacterium tuberculosis* in a high tuberculosis incidence area. *Mol. Microbiol.* **47**:529–538.

83. Tautz, D., and M. Renz. 1984. Simple sequences are ubiquitous repetitive components of eukaryotic genomes. *Nucleic Acids Res.* **12**:4127–4138.

84. Tautz, D., and C. Schlotterer. 1994. Simple sequences. *Curr. Opin. Genet. Dev.* **4**:832–837.

85. Tekaia, F., S. V. Gordon, T. Garnier, R. Brosch, B. G. Barrell, S. T. Cole. 1999. Analysis of the proteome of *Mycobacterium tuberculosis* in silico. *Tubercle Lung Dis.* **79**:329–342.

86. Thierry, D., A. Brisson-Noel, V. Vincent-Levy-Frebault, S. Nguyen, J. L. Guesdon, and B. Gicquel. 1990. Characterization of a *Mycobacterium tuberculosis* insertion sequence, IS*6110*, and its application in diagnosis. *J. Clin. Microbiol.* **28**:2668–2673.

87. van Belkum, A., S. Scherer, L. van Alphen, and H. Verbrugh. 1998. Short-sequence DNA repeats in prokaryotic genomes. *Microbiol. Mol. Biol. Rev.* **62**:275–293.

88. van Belkum, A., S. Scherer, W. van Leeuwen, D. Willemse, L. van Alphen, and H. Verbrugh. 1997. Variable number of tandem repeats in clinical strains of *Haemophilus influenzae*. *Infect. Immun.* **65**:5017–5027.

89. Van Soolingen, D. 2001. Molecular epidemiology of tuberculosis and other mycobacterial infections: main methodologies and achievements. *J. Intern. Med.* **249**:1–26.

90. van Soolingen, D., L. Qian, P. E. de Haas, J. T. Douglas, H. Traore, F. Portaels, H. Z. Qing, D. Enkhsaikan, P. Nymadawa, and J. D. van Embden. 1995. Predominance of a single genotype of *Mycobacterium tuberculosis* in countries of east Asia. *J. Clin. Microbiol.* **33**:3234–3238.

91. Wall, S., K. Ghanekar, J. McFadden, and J. W. Dale. 1999. Context-sensitive transposition of IS*6110* in mycobacteria. *Microbiology* **145**:3169–3176.

92. Warren, R. M., S. L. Sampson, M. Richardson, G. D. Van Der Spuy, C. J. Lombard, T. C. Victor, and P. D. van Helden. 2000. Mapping of IS*6110* flanking regions in clinical isolates of *Mycobacterium tuberculosis* demonstrates genome plasticity. *Mol. Microbiol.* **37**:1405–1416.

93. Weiser, J. N., J. M. Love, and E. R. Moxon. 1989. The molecular mechanism of phase variation of *H. influenzae* lipopolysaccharide. *Cell* **59**:657–665.

94. Yeramian, E., and H. Buc. 1999. Tandem repeats in complete bacterial genome sequences: sequence and structural analyses for comparative studies. *Res. Microbiol.* **150**:745–754.

95. Zhang, Y., and D. Young. 1994. Strain variation in the *katG* region of *Mycobacterium tuberculosis*. *Mol. Microbiol.* **14**:301–308.

Chapter 14

Mycobacteriophages and Tuberculosis

GRAHAM F. HATFULL

Mycobacteriophages have been central players in the understanding and control of tuberculosis for more than 50 years (31, 32, 62). The first mycobacteriophages were described in the 1950s, and more than 250 isolates have been described since then (33). Much of the early interest lay in the use of mycobacteriophages in the typing of clinical isolates (phage typing), taking advantage of specific host ranges that are characteristic of individual phages (19, 28, 44). Subsequently, the use of mycobacteriophages as genetic tools was explored, with identification of I3 as a generalized transducing phage of *Mycobacterium smegmatis* (79) and phages TM4 and D29 for the development of efficient transformation methods (40, 42). As the entire mycobacterial genetic system acquired greater sophistication, mycobacteriophages played ever more central roles, being used as delivery systems for reporter genes and transposons (5, 39), mediators of efficient gene replacement (4), sources of integration-proficient vectors (25, 56, 78, 84), and systems for studying mycobacterial gene expression (10, 27, 43, 57). Mycobacteriophages have also been useful for gaining insights into the biology of their hosts through the study of the mechanisms of absorption and resistance and the process of phage-mediated lysis (6, 9, 26, 27, 49).

Over the past 10 years, there has been considerable progress in the study of mycobacteriophage genomics, providing insights into the genetic diversity of mycobacteriophages, the evolutionary mechanisms that generate this diversity, and the role that phages play in the evolution of their mycobacterial hosts (23, 24, 34, 63, 70). These studies suggest that the mycobacteriophage population is both large and diverse and that these viruses are conveyors of a variety of genes that can influence the physiology of their hosts. While these studies are in their infancy, they promise many new insights into the biology of *Mycobacterium tuberculosis*.

There have been several reviews of mycobacteriophages in recent years, and the reader is directed to these for further information (31–33, 62). In this chapter, I focus on a discussion of recent developments in mycobacteriophage research with an emphasis on how these have advanced our understanding of tuberculosis.

MYCOBACTERIOPHAGE ECOLOGY

Where are mycobacteriophages? This issue has not been studied exhaustively, but in general—like all bacteriophages—they are present in locations where their hosts can also be found. Since the genus *Mycobacterium* encompasses a large number of species that occupy a plethora of environmental localities, the distribution of mycobacteria appears to be widespread. Mycobacteriophages have been isolated from rather exotic locations, such as the zebra pits at the Bronx zoo and the grounds of the tuberculosis hospital in Chenai, but they can be isolated from most soil and compost samples (70). It is noteworthy that the host range of these phages is unpredictable. A mycobacteriophage isolated from a soil sample is likely to be able to infect saprophytic species such as *M. smegmatis* but may also infect slow-growing strains such as *M. tuberculosis* and *Mycobacterium bovis* BCG.

MYCOBACTERIOPHAGE MORPHOLOGIES

Electron microscopic studies have revealed a number of different morphologies exhibited by mycobacteriophages (Fig. 1). Most mycobacteriophages analyzed to date belong to the morphological class *Siphoviridae*, with a long, flexible tail (130 to 265 nm in length) attached to an isometric, icosahedral head (~60 nm in diameter) that contains the DNA. Examples are L5, D29, DS6A, TM4, Bxb1, Bxz2, Che8,

Graham F. Hatfull • Pittsburgh Bacteriophage Institute and Department of Biological Sciences, University of Pittsburgh, 4249 5th Ave., Pittsburgh, PA 15260.

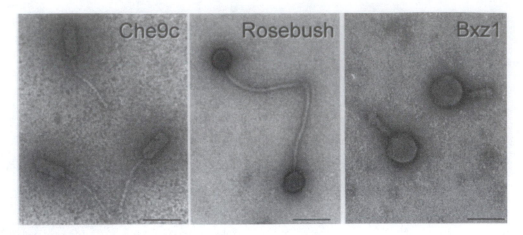

Figure 1. Mycobacteriophage morphologies. Three distinct types of mycobacteriophage virions morphologies are shown. Che9c and Rosebush are members of the *Siphoviridae* and have long, flexible tails but differently shaped heads. Most mycobacteriophages have isometric heads like Rosebush, whereas phages Che9c and Corndog (not shown) have prolate heads. Bxz1 is a member of the *Myoviridae* and has a somewhat larger head than Rosebush and a contractile tail.

Che9d, Cjw1, Omega, Rosebush, and Barnyard (70) (Fig. 1). There are two interesting additional examples that represent variations of this class. Mycobacteriophages Che9c and Corndog are also members of the *Siphoviridae* but have notably prolate heads with a length-to-width ratio of approximately 3:1 and 6:1, respectively (Fig. 1). Two mycobacteriophages—I3 and Bxz1—are morphologically classified as *Myoviridae*, having a contractile tail and an isometric, icosahedral head (~80 nm in diameter). As discussed below, these morphologies offer some insights into their biology but contribute little to our understanding of their genetic relationships. There are, for example, pairs of mycobacteriophages classified as *Siphoviridae* that share fewer genes than one mycobacteriophage member of the *Siphoviridae* shares with one of the *Myoviridae* (70).

GENOMIC DIVERSITY OF MYCOBACTERIOPHAGES

Currently, the complete genome sequences of 14 mycobacteriophages have been determined (Barnyard, Bxb1, Bxz1, Bxz2, Che8, Che9c, Che9d, Cjw1, Corndog, D29, L5, Omega, Rosebush, and TM4) (Table 1), and partial sequences for phages Ms6, FRAT1, I3, and DS6A (25, 27, 29, 70, 80, 81) have been determined. While the host ranges have not been fully explored for all these phages, approximately half of them infect both slow- and fast-growing mycobacteria. The first of these to be sequenced was the temperate phage L5, which was shown to have a genome 52,297 bp in length and an overall genome architecture reminiscent of phage lambda

and its relatives (34). However, L5 has no nucleic acid sequence similarity to the lambdoid phage and no closely related proteins, although the integrases are clearly both members of the tyrosine recombinase family (see below). The second phage sequenced was D29, which—in spite of having a host range distinct from that of L5, being lytic rather than temperate, and clearly isolated independently—has high similarity to L5 at the DNA level (23). The next two phages sequenced, TM4 and Bxb1, also have many proteins related to proteins of L5 and D29 (and Bxb1, L5, and D29 also have some DNA sequence similarity) (24, 63). Taken alone, these findings might be taken to suggest that the mycobacteriophage population is rather restricted in its diversity, occupied by isolates that may be distinct but have many common genes.

The sequence determination of another 10 mycobacteriophage genomes showed that this would be a false conclusion (70) (Table 1). Of these, one (Bxz2) does share many genes with the L5-D29-Bxb1 group, but most of the others do not. Some of the phages share very few genes with these phages, and Barnyard, for example, has no genes in common with the L5-D29-Bxb1-Bxz2 group at a BLAST score cutoff E value of 10^{-20} (at an E value cutoff of 10^{-4} they share two to four gene products). This suggests that this population of phages is actually quite broad and that many new phages distinct from those already isolated remain to be discovered.

The overall diversity of the mycobacteriophage population can also be examined by assessing the proportion of gene products that are unique and do not match any other mycobacteriophage genes. The group of 14 mycobacteriophages contains 1,659

Table 1. Mycobacteriophage genome features

Phage	Genome size (bp)	G+C	No. of tRNAs	No. of ORFs[b]	Avg. ORF size (bp)	No. of novel genes[c]	Other phages[b] Total no. (% of ORFs)	Other phages[b] Mphage only (% of total)[d]	Other phages[b] Non-Mphage (% also Mphage)[e]	Other phages[b] Non-Mphage only (% ORFs)[f]	Other organisms Total no. (% of ORFs)	Other organisms No. with no phage match[g]
L5	52,297	62.3	3	87	601	14	73 (84)	55 (75)	18 (100)	0 (0)	12	0
D29	49,136	63.5	5	77	638	10	67 (87)	49 (73)	18 (100)	0 (0)	14	0
TM4	52,797	68.1	0	92	574	53	38 (41)	26 (68)	12 (100)	0 (0)	8	0
Bxb1	50,550	63.7	0	86	588	29	54 (62)	44 (81)	10 (100)	0 (0)	9	1
Bxz1	156,102	64.8	26	225	694	164	54 (24)	38 (70)	16 (44)	9 (4)	20	7
Che8	59,471	61.3	0	112	531	20	91 (81)	82 (90)	9 (67)	3 (2.7)	10	1
Bxz2	50,913	64.2	3	86	599	22	64 (74)	49 (77)	15 (100)	0 (0)	11	0
Cjw1	75,931	63.1	1	141	546	77	62 (44)	47 (76)	15 (67)	5 (3.5)	15	1
Corndog	69,777	65.4	0	122	572	63	53 (43)	45 (85)	8 (100)	0 (0)	13	7
Che9c	57,050	65.4	0	84	671	39	39 (46)	26 (67)	13 (54)	6 (7.1)	12	5
Omega	110,857	61.4	2	237	466	134	98 (41)	76 (78)	22 (82)	4 (1.6)	20	3
Che9d	56,276	60.9	0	111	507	38	73 (66)	58 (79)	15 (93)	1 (0.09)	12	0
Barnyard	70,797	57.3	0	109	650	93	14 (13)	10 (71)	4 (50)	2 (1.8)	11	2
Rosebush	67,480	69.0	0	90	750	65	19 (21)	14 (73)	5 (20)	4 (4.4)	10	6
Total	979,434		40	1,659		821 (49.5%)	799 (48)	618 (77)	180 (81)	34 (2)	177 (82%e)	33 (2%)
Average	69,960	63.6	2.9	118.5	599	58.6						

[a]No database match at a BLAST E value cutoff of 10^{-4}.
[b]Regardless of matches to genes in other organisms. Mphage, mycobacteriophage.
[c]Defined as BLAST score hits with an E value of 10^{-4} or better or above 30% amino acid sequence identity.
[d]Excluding genes that match phages other than mycobacteriophages.
[e]Total numbers of genes shared with phages other than mycobacteriophages. Percentages of those that are also in other mycobacteriophages are shown in parentheses.
[f]Excluding all genes that match other mycobacteriophages.
[g]Excluding all genes that match any other phage gene.
[b]ORF, open reading frame.

genes, approximately half of which are related to other genes, but most of these (~90%) match other mycobacteriophage genes (70). However, approximately half of all of the genes (821 genes) are novel (i.e., do not match any other genes), which is more than all of the novel genes in the *M. tuberculosis* genome! Since the total bacteriophage population is extremely large (estimated at 10^{31} particles), these data suggest that bacteriophages probably represent the largest unexplored reservoir of biological sequence information (70).

GENOME LENGTH

It is sometimes stated that the average genome size for double-stranded DNA dsDNA tailed phages is about 50 kbp, perhaps based largely on the well-characterized and much utilized phage lambda. Since the first four mycobacteriophages sequenced were within a narrow range around 50 kbp (49.1 to 52.8 kbp), this seemed also to be true for mycobacteriophages. However, as more phages were analyzed, it became clear that these lie at the lower end of a spectrum that spans from 49.1 (D29) to 156.1 (Bxz1) kbp and the average length is 70 kbp (Table 1) (70).

The determinants of phage genome length are unknown, although capsid size must play a significant role. However, typically only 20 to 25 kbp of genetic information (~25 genes) is required to encode the functions needed to build a particle with an icosahedral head and a flexible tail. It is not clear why some mycobacteriophages have as many as 237 genes (phage Omega) when others can make do with as few as 77 genes (D29). One intriguing possibility is that genome size is determined by factors other than a strict requirement for gene function, such as fulfilling requirements for DNA packaging. If so, then many genes are simply along for the ride, with phages acting as natural cloning vehicles. Such an explanation has important implications for understanding the evolution of bacterial hosts including *M. tuberculosis*, since mycobacteriophages may be the conduits for frequent exchange of genetic information. Nevertheless, there are alternative explanations that suppose that genome length does indeed reflect selection of a specific set of gene functions. For example, the phages may have very different host ranges, and different sets of genes could be required to infect different hosts or combination of hosts.

Curiously, when all of the currently sequenced double-stranded DNA phage genomes less than 100 kbp long are examined, there is an apparent correlation between genome length and the G+C content, with larger genomes having higher G+C contents

(70). The reason for this is not obvious, although we note that the relatively large genomes of mycobacteriophages correlate with a high average G+C content (64%). Groups of phages that have lower G+C content have smaller genomes, and it is noteworthy that even the largest of the Dairy phages (phages infecting *Lactococcus*, *Lactobacillus*, and lactic streptococci) is smaller than the smallest of the mycobacteriophages! While the basis of this correlation is not understood, it does add weight to the argument that selective forces other than gene function may play a role in the determination of genome length and genetic content of bacteriophages.

GENOME MOSAICISM

One of the most evident features of these mycobacteriophage genomes is their pervasive mosaicism (70), a common feature of phage genomes (12, 35, 45, 54). This becomes obvious through comparative analysis of the genomes and examination of how individual genes are related to each other. An example of this mosaicism is shown in Fig. 2. In this illustration, seven Omega genes in the interval from genes 159 to 171 have homologues in other mycobacteriophage genomes. However, these do not correspond to a contiguous series of genes present elsewhere but represent individual modules, each with a unique relationship. Thus, Omega gp162 and gp163 are related to noncontiguous genes in Cjw1, Omega gp164 is related to TM4 gp57, Omega gp166 is related to Omega gp67 and Bxb1 gp60, and Omega gp159 and gp170 are related to Rosebush gp69 and Che8 gp85, respectively (Fig. 2). This mosaicism is found in other phage genomes but is particularly pervasive in the mycobacteriophages; it is notable in that the mosaic elements are frequently single genes rather than large sets of genes. Thus, each of the mycobacteriophages contains a genome that is a unique assemblage of these individual modules. This individualistic feature of these phage genomes justified the nonsystematic nomenclature that we have adopted for newly identified mycobacteriophages.

MECHANISMS OF PHAGE EVOLUTION

How are the mycobacteriophage genomes formed into these mosaic assemblages? First, homologous recombination must play a significant role since recombination between common genes generates different combinations of modules (12). Since related genes may not necessarily lie within colinear segments of genomes, this can also lead to either increases or de-

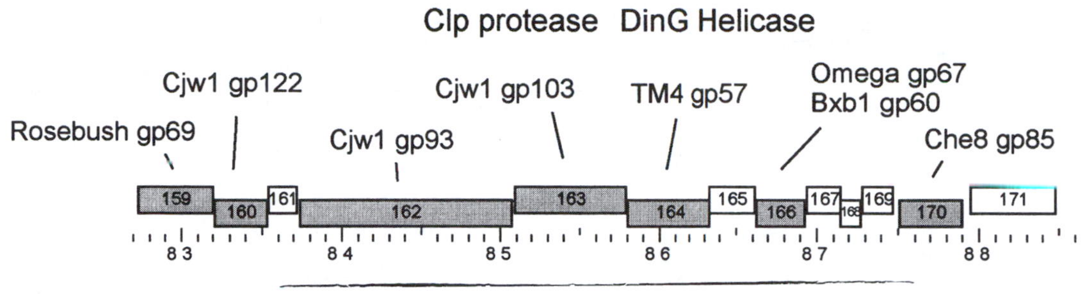

Clp protease   DinG Helicase

Figure 2. Mosaicism in mycobacteriophage genomes. A segment of the Omega genome coding genes *159* to *171* is shown with homologues found in other mycobacteriophages indicated. Six of the genes (*161, 165, 167, 168, 169* and *171*) have no homologues. Omega gp163 and gp164 are a Clp protease and a DinG helicase, respectively, as shown, but the functions of the other genes are not known. The genome is characteristically mosaic, with individual genes representing modules that are present in other phage genomes.

creases in genome size. However, it is less clear how homologous recombination can generate new mosaic boundaries.

Frequently, mosaic boundaries correspond to the beginning and ends of genes (11, 12, 14, 36, 45, 96). It was suggested previously that mosaicism could arise by homologous recombination between short boundary sequences located at gene junctions which could serve as targets for homologous recombination (96). Boundary-like sequences have been found in several *Escherichia coli* phages (14, 83) but are not obviously present in the mycobacteriophages, and it seems unlikely that this is the general mechanism used for generating mosaicism. An alternative explanation is that illegitimate recombination—exchange with little regard to sequence similarity—plays a major role (12). Such sequence-independent exchange events are expected to occur at relatively low frequency and to normally create genomic trash that is nonfunctional. However, when one or more events do give rise to viable viral recombinants, these carry new mosaic boundaries where the recombination events occurred. These boundaries will commonly be close to the ends of genes since this is less likely to interrupt their functions. Evidence to support this mode of evolution is provided by several examples where mycobacteriophage genomes have small segments of nucleotide sequence identity (or near identity) that must have arisen from relatively recent recombination events (70). The boundaries between identical and nonidentical sequences do not correspond precisely to gene boundaries, suggesting that they arose illegitimately, but also alter the extreme 3' ends of several genes. A closer examination of related genes in the mycobacteriophages suggests that these illegitimate events give rise to extensive "fraying" of the 3' ends of genes.

Who participates in this orgy of exchange events? It is tempting to think that recombination oc-

curs commonly between two coinfecting phages, much as it would in a laboratory phage cross. However, in nature this is expected to be a fairly infrequent occurrence, and recombination between an infecting phage and the host chromosome is probably more common. Moreover, while homologous recombination events may occur between an infecting phage genome and a resident prophage, illegitimate recombination may involve any part of the host genome, thus providing a mechanism for the ready acquisition of host genes by mycobacteriophages.

M. TUBERCULOSIS GENES IN MYCOBACTERIOPHAGES

In light of the above discussion of mechanisms of phage evolution, we might expect there to be many genes in mycobacteriophage genomes that are related to genes present in the genome of *M. tuberculosis* and other mycobacterial hosts. This does indeed appear to be true, and within the 14 completely sequenced mycobacteriophage genomes there are the homologues of over 70 *M. tuberculosis* genes (Table 2); about one-third of these are found in more than one of the mycobacteriophages (70).

Which types of *M. tuberculosis* genes are present? First, and not unexpectedly, some of these correspond to the genes encoded by the two prophage-like elements, φRv1 and φRv2 (see below) (15); there are 10 genes in this class. Many of the genes (28 genes) are of unknown function. A significant proportion of these genes are involved in DNA metabolism, although their products encompass a variety of functions including subunits of both DNA polymerase I and polymerase III, an assortment of primases and helicases, single-stranded DNA binding protein, and XerD and RecA recombinases; it is not difficult to

Table 2. TB gene homologues in mycobacteriophages[a]

M. tuberculosis protein	Function[b]	Phage (protein)	E-value
Rv0002 (DnaN)	Pol III Beta	Corndog (gp84)	10^{-4}
Rv0024	Unknown	Bxz1 (gp133)	2×10^{-19}
Rv0054 (SSB)	ssDNA binding	Cjw1 (gp102)	3×10^{-40}
Rv0058 (DnaB)	Helicase	Cjw1 (gp82)	3×10^{-53}
		Bxz1 (gp193)	3×10^{-6}
Rv0220 (LipC)	Esterase	Omega (gp105)	9×10^{-49}
Rv0320	Unknown	TM4 (gp17)	10^{-17}
Rv0344c (lpqJ)	Lipoprotein	Che9c (gp38)	2×10^{-17}
Rv0357c (PurA)	Adenylsuccinate synthetase	Bxz1 (gp250)	6×10^{-25}
Rv0399c (lpqK)	Dicarboxypeptidase	Cjw1 (gp27)	2×10^{-14}
		Bxb1 (gp30)	2×10^{-8}
		Che8 (gp20)	2×10^{-15}
		Corndog (gp62)	3×10^{-13}
		Omega (gp39)	7×10^{-16}
		Bxz1 (169)	8×10^{-17}
Rv0430	Unknown	Che9c (gp42)	2×10^{-9}
Rv0570 (NrdZ)	Ribonucleotide reductase	L5 (gp50)	7×10^{-24}
		D29 (gp50)	6×10^{-21}
		Bxz2 (gp50)	2×10^{-23}
Rv0861c	Unknown	Rosebush (gp50)	7×10^{-7}
Rv0867c	Cytokine	Barnyard (gp33)	7×10^{-21}
Rv0907	Unknown	Bxz1 (169)	3×10^{-10}
Rv0937	Unknown	Corndog (gp87)	6×10^{-35}
		Omega (gp206)	2×10^{-71}
Rv1009	Cytokine	Barnyard (gp33)	2×10^{-22}
Rv1054	Int related	Omega (gp85)	1×10^{-9}
Rv1055	Int related	Omega (gp85)	6×10^{-12}
Rv1115	Unknown	Cjw1 (gp22)	10^{-7}
		Che9c (gp15)	0.001
		Barnyard (gp33)	7×10^{-5}
		Rosebush (gp29)	0.003
Rv1271c	Unknown	Che8 (gp61)	7×10^{-6}
Rv1291c	Unknown	Che8 (gp61)	3×10^{-4}
Rv1299 (PrfA)	Peptide chain release factor 1	Bxb1 (gp200)	10^{-7}
Rv1367c	Unknown	Cjw1 (gp27)	3×10^{-5}
		Che8 (gp20)	6×10^{-6}
		Bxz1 (gp169)	2×10^{-5}
		Omega (gp39)	1×10^{-5}
Rv1399c (LipH)	Lipase	Omega (gp105)	10^{-11}
Rv1400c (LipI)	Lipase	Omega (gp105)	10^{-9}
Rv1426c (LipO)		Omega (gp105)	8×10^{-37}
Rv1547 (DnaE1)	DNA Pol III alpha	Bxz1 (gp199)	10^{-97}
		Barnyard (gp80)	3×10^{-80}
Rv1576c	phiRv1 capsid	Che9c (6)	10^{-53}
Rv1577c	phiRv1 protease	Che9c (5)	0.05
Rv1578c	phiRv1 terminase	Cjw1 (gp5)	0.005
Rv1582	phiRv1 primase/helicase	TM4 (gp70)	6×10^{-58}
		Barnyard (gp108)	2×10^{-24}
Rv1586c	phiRv1 integrase	Bxb1 (gp35)	4×10^{-10}
		Bxz2 (gp34)	8×10^{-9}
Rv1615	Unknown	Che9c (gp39)	4×10^{-5}
Rv1629 (Pol I)	DNA Pol	L5 (gp44)	4×10^{-22}
		D29 (gp44)	2×10^{-23}
		Bxb1 (gp41)	2×10^{-16}
		Bxz2 (gp44)	4×10^{-24}
		Rosebush (gp56)	6×10^{-9}
Rv1701 (XerD)	Recombination	Cjw1 (gp53)	4×10^{-8}
Rv1728c	Unknown	TM4 (gp17)	9×10^{-22}
		Bxz1 (gp95)	0.004

Continued on following page

Table 2. *Continued*

M. tuberculosis protein	Function[b]	Phage (protein)	E-value
Rv1730	Unknown	Cjw1 (gp27)	5×10^{-10}
		Bxb1 (gp30)	3×10^{-6}
		Che8 (gp20)	2×10^{-8}
		Corndog (gp62)	0.01
		Omega (gp39)	3×10^{-8}
		Bxz1 (gp169)	5×10^{-7}
Rv1884c	Cytokine	Barnyard (gp33)	2×10^{-15}
Rv1922	Unknown	Cjw1 (gp27)	3×10^{-13}
		Che8 (gp20)	10^{-11}
		Corndog (gp62)	4×10^{-7}
		Omega (gp39)	10^{-11}
		Bxz1 (gp169)	4×10^{-15}
Rv2017	DNA binding HTH	Che9c (gp32)	0.002
Rv2101 (HelZ)	Helicase	Barnyard (gp65)	7×10^{-21}
Rv2119	Unknown	L5 (gp69)	5×10^{-5}
		D20 (gp69)	4×10^{-7}
		Bxb1 (gp62)	0.02
		Bxz2 (gp69)	10^{-6}
Rv2176 (PknL)	Kinase	Bxz1 (gp247)	0.01
Rv2179c	Unknown	Che8 (gp101)	4×10^{-24}
Rv2284 (LipM)	Esterase	Omega (gp105)	10^{-40}
Rv2309c	Int related	Omega (gp85)	2×10^{-23}
Rv2343c (DnaG)	DNA Primase	L5 (gp58)	3×10^{-5}
		D29 (gp58)	3×10^{-6}
		Bxz2 (gp58)	9×10^{-7}
Rv2389c	Cytokine	Barnyard (gp33)	1×10^{-17}
Rv2450c	Cytokine	Barnyard (gp33)	4×10^{-16}
Rv2461c (ClpP)	Protease	Cjw1 (gp103)	0.02
		Omega (gp163)	7×10^{-5}
Rv2469c	HNH endonuclease	Che8 (gp112)	0.001
Rv2485c (LipQ)	Esterase	Omega (gp105)	9×10^{-39}
Rv2650c	PhiRv2 protein	Che9c (6)	2×10^{-54}
Rv2651c	PhiRv2 protein	Che9c (5)	0.01
Rv2652c	PhiRv2 protein	Cjw1 (gp5)	0.001
Rv2657c	PhiRv2 excise	L5 (gp36)	2×10^{-7}
		D29 (gp36)	2×10^{-7}
Rv2659c	Int related	Omega (gp85)	2×10^{-12}
Rv2715	Haloperoxidase	D29 (gp59.2)	6×10^{-6}
		Bxz2 (gp61)	10^{-6}
Rv2721c	Unknown	Barnyard (gp39)	6×10^{-5}
Rv2734	ATP transporter	Che9c (gp68)	5×10^{-52}
Rv2737c (RecA)	Recombination	Cjw1 (gp117)	3×10^{-93}
		Bxz1 (gp201)	10^{-22}
Rv2748c (FtsK)	Cell division	Omega (gp203)	10^{-108}
Rv2754c	Unknown	L5 (gp48)	2×10^{-44}
		D29 (gp48)	8×10^{-43}
		Bxz2 (gp48)	4×10^{-44}
RV2970c (LipN)	Lipase/esterase	Omega (gp105)	9×10^{-7}
Rv3053c (NrdH)	Glutaredoxin	Cjw1 (gp37)	3×10^{-9}
		TM4 (gp67)	2×10^{-5}
		Corndog (gp56)	4×10^{-4}
		L5 (gp56)	5×10^{-6}
		D29 (gp56)	4×10^{-6}
		Bxb1 (gp56)	3×10^{-6}
Rv3090	Unknown	Bxz1 (gp29)	2×10^{-61}
Rv3105c (PrfB)	Peptide chain release factor 2	Bxb1 (gp200)	2×10^{-7}
Rv3125c (PPE protein)	Unknown	Rosebush (gp29)	0.029
Rv3201c	UvrD helicase	Bxz2 (gp72)	0.004
Rv3202c	Unknown	Bxz2 (gp69)	4×10^{-5}

Continued on following page

Table 2. *Continued*

M. tuberculosis protein	Function[b]	Phage (protein)	E-value
Rv3219 (WhiB1),	Regulation	Cjw1 (gp95)	9×10^{-12}
Rv3260c (WhiB2)		TM4 (gp49)	10^{-15}
		Che8 (gp62)	2×10^{-11}
		Che8 (gp65)	4×10^{-20}
		Omega (gp139)	9×10^{-5}
Rv3333c	Unknown	Che8 (gp61)	0.001
Rv3427c	Unknown (DnaC?)	Bxz1 (gp192)	0.002
Rv3437	Unknown	Bxz2 (gp33)	10^{-5}
Rv3447c	Unknown	Omega (gp203)	10^{-15}
Rv3482	Unknown	Bxz2 (gp33)	10^{-6}
		Che9c (gp39)	2×10^{-5}
Rv3514	Glycine-rich protein	Bxz1 (gp94)	3×10^{-15}
Rv3532 (PPE protein)	Unknown	Che9c (gp35)	0.012
Rv3585 (RadA)	DNA repair	Rosebush (gp54)	0.023
Rv3594	Unknown	TM4 (gp29)	6×10^{-37}
		Corndog (gp69)	10^{-77}
		Bxz1 (gp126)	9×10^{-39}
		Barnyard (gp33)	7×10^{-33}
Rv3597c (Lsr2)	Unknown	Cjw1 (gp39)	5×10^{-13}
		Corndog (gp61)	5×10^{-12}
Rv3609c (FolE)	GTP cyclohydrolase	Rosebush (gp6)	1×10^{-27}
Rv3610c (FtsH)	Cell division	Corndog (gp96)	10^{-13}
Rv3751	Int related	Omega (gp85)	3×10^{-11}
Rv3766	Lysis	Cjw1 (gp32)	6×10^{-38}
Rv3811 (Csp)	Unknown	Barnyard (gp39)	1×10^{-5}
Rv3894c	Unknown	Omega (gp203)	5×10^{-10}
Rv3915 (CwlM)	Amidase	Che9c (gp25)	0.004

[a]*M. tuberculosis* genes with homologues in mycobacteriophages are listed in order of gene number. Since some mycobacterio-phage genes match more than one *M. tuberculosis* gene, some phage genes appear more than once.
[b]Pol, polymerase; ssDNA, single-stranded DNA; HTH, helix-turn-helix; HNH, HNH endonuclease; PPE, PPE family.

imagine the roles that these could play in phage life cycles. However, other genes correspond to functions that are not commonly found in phage genomes, and their role is less clear. For example, there are myco-bacteriophage homologues of *M. tuberculosis* es-terase, peptide chain release factor, lipase, Clp pro-tease, haloperoxidase, the cell division proteins FtsH and FtsK, glutaredoxin, WhiB regulatory proteins, repair enzyme RadA, kinases, the immunodominant antigen, and the GTP cyclohydrolase, FolE (Table 2). Since many of these genes are thought to play impor-tant roles in the physiology of *M. tuberculosis*, this raises the possibility that the mycobacteriophages could influence the biology of their hosts in a variety of interesting ways (see below).

OTHER UNUSUAL GENES IN MYCOBACTERIOPHAGE GENOMES

The 14 sequenced mycobacteriophages also en-code some unexpected genes that are not present in *M. tuberculosis* (70). Perhaps the most notable of these is Bxb1 gp220, which encodes a homologue of

the human Ro protein. In humans, this protein is a major target of the immune system in autoimmune diseases such as lupus, and disruption of the gene in mice leads to an autoimmune phenotype (30, 61, 100). The gene is found in mammals, flies, and worms but is absent from yeast (at least from *Saccha-romyces cerevisiae*) and rare in bacteria. The two bacterial species in which it has been identified are *Deinococcus radiodurans* and, interestingly, *M. smeg-matis* (13). The role of the protein is unclear, although *D. radiodurans* mutants with mutations in this pro-tein become more sensitive to UV irradiation and *Caenorhabditis elegans* mutants are defective in dauer formation (52). In *Xenopus*, the Ro ribonucleo-protein particle appears to be involved in the process-ing of 5S rRNA (90).

PROPHAGE-LIKE ELEMENTS, ΦRv1 AND ΦRv2

The sequenced *M. tuberculosis* genomes of strains H37Rv and CDC 1551 both carry two prophage-like elements, designated ΦRv1 and ΦRv2 (15, 21). Both of these elements are only about 10 kbp long—considerably shorter than a typical prophage—and thus unlikely to encode sufficient functions to generate viral particles similar to any of the characterized mycobacteriophages. The two elements are quite different in nucleotide sequence but contain similar genes (as indicated by similarity between gene products) in similar orders. Both φRv1 and φRv2 appear to have genes encoding capsid proteins and an associated protease involved in capsid assembly, suggesting that they might be able to form virus-like particles; neither element encodes tail genes (31). The biological role of these elements is unclear in that there are no compelling reports of virus-like particles being released from strains of *M. tuberculosis* or any indication of generalized transduction similar to that reported for *Methanococcus*, *Spirulina*, and *Rhodococcus* (7, 17, 37, 38, 53). A role in pathogenesis of *M. tuberculosis* cannot be excluded, and all or most clinical strains appear to contain at least one of the two elements; however, there are few genes with unaccounted functions that could play such a role. It is notable that both elements are absent from BCG (60).

The two elements differ in that they encode quite different systems for integration and excision. At the right end of φRv2, a gene encodes an integrase of the tyrosine recombinase family, and the element is clearly inserted into a host tRNA gene—a common feature of such integration systems. Nearby, a second gene encodes a small, basic protein with sequence similarity to the recombination directionality factor of phage L5, which presumably controls the directionality of φRv2 site-specific recombination (58). The observation that this element encodes an active site-specific recombination system (our unpublished observations) is consistent with the interpretation that it is not simply a defective prophage but encodes fully active functions.

φRv1 contains a site-specific recombinase in the same relative location as φRv2, but it is clearly a member of the serine recombinase family and is completely unrelated at the sequence level to its counterpart in φRv2. An initial indication that this integration system is active was provided by the observation that it is inserted into two separate chromosomal locations in the sequenced *M. tuberculosis* strains, H37Rv and CDC 1551 (21). The genes in the two strains are slightly different from each other, but biochemical studies have confirmed that the H37Rv φRv1 integrase is fully active in vivo and in vitro (8). This integration system differs from other such systems in that the host attachment site (*attB*) is located within a redundant repetitive element (REP13E12) that is present seven times in the *M. tuberculosis* genome (8). Analysis of the integration reaction in BCG (which lacks φRv1) shows that four of these elements contain a functional *attB* site, including those occupied by φRv1 in H37Rv and CDC 1551 (8).

In general, it is not known how the directionality of recombination is controlled in the serine integrase systems (93). In φRv1, a gene located colinear to the recombination directionality factor in φRv2 appears to also act as a directionality factor, in that it strongly confers the ability of the φRv1 integrase to excise the integrated element (8). It is not known how this protein functions, but it is small and basic like its φRv2 counterpart, and the two proteins have weak sequence similarity. Thus, although the two recombination systems are entirely unrelated and function with quite distinct mechanisms, the two directionality factors may act in similar ways.

TAPE MEASURE PROTEINS AS SIGNALING MOLECULES?

Thirteen of the mycobacteriophages with completely sequenced genomes have flexible, noncontractile tails. It has been shown that the length of such tails in other phage systems is determined by an assembly protein—the tape measure protein (Tmp), which forms an extended structure on which the major tail subunit protein assembles (47). This leads to a curious relationship between the genome and the virion particle, since the length of the *tmp* gene correlates with the length of the tail. Since most of the mycobacteriophage tails are quite long (130 to 265 nm), the *tmp* genes are usually quite easy to identify because they are often the longest gene in the genome (70). The length of these *tmp* genes correlates well with the tail lengths, and discrepancies probably result from posttranslational processing of the Tmp protein. The role of the Tmp protein in phage infection is unclear, although since it occupies the lumen of the tail through which the DNA must pass in the process of injection, the Tmp protein must be ejected and is likely to end up in the cytoplasm of the host cell.

Examination of mycobacteriophage Tmp proteins reveals the presence of small sequence motifs that are related to *M. tuberculosis* proteins (70). These motifs are short (80 to 100 amino acids) and are typically positioned about two-thirds of the way along the protein. It is therefore of interest how these sequence motifs function and what properties they confer on the phage particles. Motifs have been identified in nine of the completely sequenced genomes, and these appear to fall into three classes; motifs 1, 2, and 3. Eight of the phages contain just a single motif, while one (Barnyard) contains both motifs 1 and 2 (70).

A clue to the possible function of these motifs comes from sequence comparisons of motif 1. This motif is clearly related to a family of proteins with five members in *M. tuberculosis*, three members in *Streptomyces coelicolor*, and at least one member in *Micrococcus luteus* and *Rhodococcus rhodochrous* (48, 65, 66, 91, 101). In *Micrococcus luteus*, the motif is part of a small secreted protein called resuscitation-promoting factor (Rpf) since it has the ability to stimulate dormant, nongrowing *Micrococcus luteus* cells into full growth (65). Furthermore, *Micrococcus luteus* Rpf can also promote the growth of *M. smegmatis* and *M. tuberculosis*, suggesting that the mycobacterial proteins play similar roles (66). The five Rpf-related proteins in *M. tuberculosis* are of different lengths and may be processed at their C-termini as proposed for *Micrococcus luteus* Rpf. They also contain a variety of different N-terminal sequences, indicating that some may be secreted while others remain cell wall associated.

On reflection, it makes sense that bacteriophages would encode such signaling motifs in their Tmp proteins. It is likely that the majority of host cells encountered by phages in the environment are nongrowing, and this represents a problem for the virus since infection of a dormant cell is unlikely to be productive. It would therefore represent a significant advantage for a phage to carry its own alarm clock, which could tell the host to enter an active growth state and thus support the infection. The positioning of the signal in the Tmp protein seems to make good sense, since this is a component of the mature viral particle and therefore does not require gene expression in the host cell. Moreover, since the Tmp protein must be intimately associated with the cell wall and membrane during infection, it is ideally placed to interact with putative Rpf-associated signaling receptors that are presumably localized at the exterior of the cell.

These observations raise the question whether the other motifs (motifs 2 and 3) also play roles in cellular signaling in *M. tuberculosis*. Motif 3 is related to two small putatively secreted proteins, Rv0320 and Rv1728c, both of which are of unknown function; five mycobacteriophages encode related motifs within their Tmp proteins (70). Four phages have Tmp proteins containing motif 2, which is related to *M. tuberculosis* protein Rv1115. Rv1115 also has the features of a small secreted protein, although its role is also unknown. However, given the putative role of motif 1, we suggest that motifs 2 and 3 function similarly, perhaps by activating separate signaling pathways. The finding of these motifs illustrates two central points in the analysis of mycobacteriophages—that they are rich sources of new biological insights with

broad implications, and that they generate new avenues of exploration in our understanding of the biology of *M. tuberculosis*.

DO PHAGES CONTRIBUTE TO MYCOBACTERIAL PATHOGENESIS?

There are a growing number of bacterial pathogens in which bacteriophages clearly play central roles in the virulence of their hosts; these include *Vibrio cholerae*, *Clostridium botulinum*, *Salmonella enterica* serovar Typhimurium, and *Escherichia coli* (64, 97, 98). The question then arises whether phages play any role in the pathogenicity of *M. tuberculosis*. The simple answer appears to be that they do not, since the complete genome sequencings of two *M. tuberculosis* strains—one of which was a recent clinical isolate (CDC 1551)—do not show the presence of any prophages other than the two prophage-like elements ϕRv1 and ϕRv2 discussed above. Nevertheless, analysis of mycobacteriophage genomes suggests that some further discussion of this issue is warranted.

As described above, the 14 completely sequenced mycobacteriophage genomes reveal a number of genes that are unexpected in that they have not previously been seen within phage genomes (70). The role of such genes in phage growth is unclear, although since they are not shared by all of the phages, they are unlikely to play essential roles. It therefore seems more likely that they act to alter the properties of the host cell, either during a productive lytic cycle or by lysogenic conversion by temperate phages. One example is represented by Cjw1 gene *39* and Omega gene *61*, both of which are related to the *lsr2* gene of *M. tuberculosis*. The functional role of Lsr2 in *M. tuberculosis* is not known, but it is a major antigen that is recognized by both the cellular and humoral immune systems (51, 67). Lsr2-like proteins are also present in a number of other bacteria including *M. leprae*, *Rhodococcus equi*, *Thermobifida fusca*, *Streptomyces avermitilis*, and *S. coelicolor*. The finding of the Lsr2 homologues in two mycobacteriophages suggests that phages may have played an important role in the dissemination of this gene among these bacterial strains.

A second example is provided by a group of genes located to the left of the structural genes in mycobacteriophage Rosebush (Fig. 3). Four of these genes have not been seen in phage genomes previously, but all four are homologues of previously characterized proteins. Two of these, Rosebush gp6 and gp4, encode the enzymes GTP cyclohydrolase and 6-pyruvoyltetrahydropterin synthase, respectively. GTP cyclohydrolase catalyzes the first step in folate biosynthesis and converts GTP to 2-amino-4-hydroxy-6(D-*erythro*-1,2,3-trihydroxypropyl)dihydropteridine-P3. Rosebush gp4 (6-pyruvoyltetrahydropterin synthase) can convert this intermediate into 6(R)-pyruvoyltetrahydropterin, which is a direct precursor in the synthesis of 6(R)-5,6,7,8-tetrahydrobiopterin. However, Rosebush does not encode the enzyme sepiapterin reductase, which catalyzes the last step in the process. This pathway is of interest, since tetrahydropterin plays an important role as a cofactor in a variety of key metabolic processes, most notably as a cofactor for nitric oxide synthase, a central player in the cellular defense against *M. tuberculosis* invasion; it is also implicated in aspects of the immune response including interleukin-2-induced T-cell proliferation (85, 89). It thus becomes clear that mycobacteriophages carry genes that could profoundly influence the interaction of *M. tuberculosis* and related bacteria with their host cells.

There are two important implications in the finding of these potential virulence genes in mycobacteriophages. First, we cannot exclude the possibility that mycobacteriophages do play direct roles in determining the physiology—and perhaps the virulence—of mycobacterial pathogens other than *M. tuberculosis*. A variety of other mycobacterial pathogens are known, and in the absence of a complete genome sequence or extensive genetic characterization, it is not

possible to know the role that phages may play. Alternatively, these phages may provide physiological advantages to bacterial hosts that enjoy saprophytic life-styles.

A second intriguing consequence is the idea that mycobacteriophages could play an important role in the future development of *M. tuberculosis* as a yet more dangerous pathogen. *M. tuberculosis* has clearly been very successful in the pathogenic style that it has adopted, since it has infected one-third of the human population. Nevertheless, it is not difficult to imagine that relatively minor genetic alterations of the organism could lead to a pathogen that is even more hazardous, being easily disseminated, multidrug resistant, and with a high incidence of disease symptoms. Such an organism might not enjoy evolutionary longevity due to a propensity to exhaust its host, but it could have devastating consequences for the human population. Indeed, strains of *M. tuberculosis* have already been identified which are either multidrug resistant, appear to be highly disseminated, or yield high rates of disease (20, 82, 92). Therefore, the notion of the conversion of a current *M. tuberculosis* strain into a superbug is not perhaps so farfetched. Our current understanding of bacterial genomics shows that large proportions of bacterial chromosomes are acquired by horizontal genetic exchange and that bacteriophages are driving forces in bacterial evolution (55).

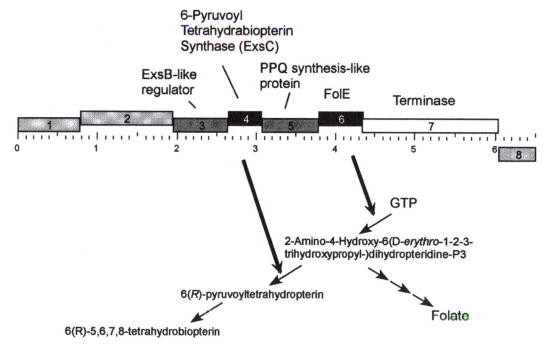

Figure 3. Rosebush genes involved in tetrahydrobiopterin biosynthesis. Rosebush genes *1* to *6* are located immediately to the left of the structural genes, with gene *7* encoding a putative terminase. Genes *1*, *2*, and *8* are of unknown function, and the functions of genes *3* to *6* are indicated. Rosebush gp4 and gp6 are involved in the biochemical pathway (shown below the diagram), which converts GTP to the cofactor 6(R)-5,6,7,8-tetrahydrobiopterin, an essential cofactor for nitric oxide synthase.

Since the study of mycobacteriophage genomes reveals the presence of genes that could profoundly influence *M. tuberculosis* virulence, the possibility that these could be acquired by *M. tuberculosis* and enhance its lethality cannot be excluded. Further examination of the mycobacteriophage population is needed to determine the full repertoire of virulence genes that are being mobilized by these viruses.

MYCOBACTERIOPHAGES AS DELIVERY VEHICLES

A notable characteristic of bacteriophages is the efficiency with which they can infect their bacterial hosts. For example, if an excess of phage particles are added to a bacterial culture, there is a high probability that every bacterial cell will be infected (40). This ability to deliver genetic material with such high efficiency is a very powerful feature that can be exploited for a variety of genetic and clinical tools.

Two primary genetic tools that take advantage of these features are the use of mycobacteriophages for the delivery of transposons and for gene replacement (4, 5, 87, 88). Transposon mutagenesis is a standard approach to the isolation of mutants that are physically marked and genetically stable. However, transposition frequencies are typically low and introduction of transposons by transformation combines two very inefficient processes, giving rise to few mutant progeny. An alternative possibility is the use of conditionally replicating plasmids as delivery vehicles, but although these can work well (73), it is often not easy to avoid the isolation of sibling mutants that originate from a rather small number of transposition events. The delivery of transposons by bacteriophages eliminates these problems by providing an efficient delivery system while also ensuring that each infection yields an independent insertion. However, for phages to be useful as such, it is important that infection does not result in death of the host, and phage mutants have been isolated that replicate conditionally, typically at 30°C but not at 37°C (5). Phage transposon delivery systems have now been described for several different transposons, using phages such as TM4 and D29 that infect both fast- and slow-growing mycobacteria (5).

A second genetic tool is the use of phages for gene replacement in *M. tuberculosis* (4). In numerous other organisms, gene replacement can be accomplished quite readily by electroporation with plasmid or other DNA constructs containing homologous segments to the chromosome and selection of an appropriate marker. However, for reasons that are still obscure, such approaches typically result in a high proportion of illegitimate integration events when applied to *M. tuberculosis* (1, 46). These problems can be alleviated somewhat by using conditionally replicating plasmids combined with counterselectable genetic markers (73–76). Phages are particularly effective tools for gene replacement, since a very high proportion of progeny correspond to the desired gene replacement mutant (4).

Mycobacteriophages are also excellent tools for the delivery of reporter genes to mycobacteria, which can then be used to monitor the physiological status of the organism. For example, recombinant phages have been described that carry the firefly luciferase gene, which causes the bacteria to emit light when a luciferin substrate is provided (39, 86). The efficiency of delivery, coupled with the specificity of the phages for their hosts, provides the features necessary to use this for clinical microbiology. Since the reporter gene must be expressed from live, growing bacteria, this assay can be readily adapted for the purposes of empirical determination of the drug susceptibility profiles of clinical isolates of *M. tuberculosis* (39). The accuracy of this method is at least as good as that of other available approaches, and the method has the advantage of providing the information simply and rapidly (2, 3). It is noteworthy that alternative applications that use nonrecombinant phages but that monitor phage replication have also been described (18, 99).

Investigators may be discouraged from using phage-based delivery tools for mycobacterial genetics due to the perceived complexity of constructing the necessary recombinant phages. However, these processes have been greatly simplified by the development of shuttle phasmids, chimeric molecules that replicate as viruses in mycobacteria and as large plasmids in *E. coli* (22, 41, 69, 94). Once shuttle phasmids have been generated in the appropriate genetic background, their further manipulation is usually straightforward. For example, shuttle phasmid pAE87 is a derivative of phage TM4 in which an *E. coli* cosmid has been inserted into the right arm. This phasmid can be readily propagated in *E. coli* and also can be packaged into phage lambda particles. The cosmid moiety is flanked by unique restriction sites and can therefore be readily substituted with cosmids carrying DNA segments of interest. For example, the cosmid pYUB584 carries a drug resistance marker flanked by a small polylinker on each side (4). To conduct a gene replacement experiment, it is just necessary to PCR amplify the chromosomal segments (~500 bp) to the immediate left and right of the gene to be replaced and clone these segments such that they flank the drug resistance marker. This cosmid can then be inserted into the shuttle plasmid by restriction, ligation, in vitro lambda packaging, and recovery in *E. coli*. DNA isolated from

E. coli can then be introduced into *M. smegmatis* by electroporation, phage plaques can be recovered, and a phage stock can be used to infect *M. tuberculosis*. As discussed above, provided that the gene is nonessential, more than 95% of the drug-resistant colonies recovered are of the desired genotype.

OTHER PHAGE-DERIVED TOOLS FOR *M. TUBERCULOSIS* GENETICS

Generalized Transduction

Generalized transduction is an important tool in bacterial genetics since it provides a simple means of generating isogenic strains and thus correlating genotypes and phenotypes with confidence. Mycobacteriophages I3 and Bxz1 both act as generalized transducing phages for *M. smegmatis*, although neither infects *M. tuberculosis* (77; unpublished observations). Isolation of a phage that does transduce *M. tuberculosis* is clearly important, not only as a general tool for tuberculosis genetics but also specifically for moving genetic markers associated with antibiotic resistance into a clean genetic background, where the role of these mutations can be evaluated.

Integration-Proficient Vectors

Integration-proficient vectors are those that use phage- or plasmid-derived integration systems to support stable transformation. These plasmids do not have origins for extrachromosomal replication and depend on successful integration in mycobacteria for propagation. Since the integration systems typically have a strong directional character—such that integration and excision have distinct requirements—the transformants have a high degree of genetic stability (56). Integration is typically efficient, yielding transformation frequencies that are as high as or higher than those with extrachromosomal plasmids. The efficient transformation, genetic stability, and ability to generate single-copy recombinants are attractive features for mycobacterial genetic manipulation. A higher degree of genetic stability can be obtained by providing the integrase gene on a separate plasmid from which it is transiently expressed and then lost, avoiding low levels of excise-independent integrase-dependent excision (77, 95). Integrated plasmids can be excised by providing the excise protein that is required for efficient excisive recombination (59, 68). Integration-proficient vectors have been derived from a variety of phages including L5, D29, FRAT1, Ms6, and Bxb1 (25, 50, 56, 78, 84). It is noteworthy that biochemical investigation of these processes also provides insight into the role of mycobacterial proteins such as the mycobacterial integration host factor (mIHF) (71, 72).

Immunity Selection

The ability of lysogenic strains to confer immunity to phage superinfection provides a useful alternative to the use of antibiotic markers for genetic selection. Superinfection immunity frequently requires just a single gene encoding the phage repressor, along with its expression signals. Thus, plasmids carrying the repressor gene can be selected for by challenge with a homoimmune phage in which its own repressor functions have been removed (16). In practice, this is straightforward, since the requirements are the phage repressor gene—which can be readily cloned—and clear-plaque mutants of the phage, which can also be identified quite easily. However, the only phage system for which this approach has been utilized is phage L5 (16). Other temperate phages have been isolated, and analogous selectable markers with different immune specificities could be developed.

CONCLUDING REMARKS

The study of mycobacteriophages has clearly progressed significantly over the past few years, especially with advances in bacteriophage genomics. Mycobacteriophages continue to shed new light on the biology of their mycobacterial hosts, including *M. tuberculosis*, and provide tools for mycobacterial genetic manipulation. However, these advances have raised many new questions that deserve our attention. For example, genomic approaches indicate that the diversity of the mycobacteriophage population is high, and further studies in this area will be helpful for exploring these questions. Mycobacteriophages are evidently replete with genes of known functions, and the study of these genes may well uncover additional interesting manners in which bacteriophages interact or modify their hosts. This enriched genetic landscape also presents many potential tools that can be developed to further enhance the available genetic systems. We can expect mycobacteriophages to play prominent roles in future studies aimed at understanding *M. tuberculosis* in the postgenomic era.

REFERENCES

1. Aldovini, A., R. N. Husson, and R. A. Young. 1993. The *uraA* locus and homologous recombination in *Mycobacterium bovis* BCG. *J. Bacteriol.* **175:**7282–7289.
2. Banaiee, N., M. Bobadilla-Del-Valle, S. Bardarov, Jr., P. F. Riska, P. M. Small, A. Ponce-De-Leon, W. R. Jacobs, Jr., G. F. Hatfull, and J. Sifuentes-Osornio. 2001. Luciferase reporter mycobacteriophages for detection, identification, and antibi-

otic susceptibility testing of *Mycobacterium tuberculosis* in Mexico. *J. Clin. Microbiol.* **39**:3883–3888.

3. **Banaiee, N., M. Bobadilla-del-Valle, P. F. Riska, S. Bardarov, Jr., P. M. Small, A. Ponce-de-Leon, W. R. Jacobs, Jr., G. F. Hatfull, and J. Sifuentes-Osornio.** 2003. Rapid identification and susceptibility testing of *Mycobacterium tuberculosis* from MGIT cultures with luciferase reporter mycobacteriophages. *J. Med. Microbiol.* **52**:557–561.

4. **Bardarov, S., S. Bardarov, Jr., M. S. Pavelka, Jr., V. Samban-damurthy, M. Larsen, J. Tufariello, J. Chan, G. Hatfull, and W. R. Jacobs, Jr.** 2002. Specialized transduction: an efficient method for generating marked and unmarked targeted gene disruptions in *Mycobacterium tuberculosis*, *M. bovis* BCG and *M. smegmatis*. *Microbiology* **148**:3007–3017.

5. **Bardarov, S., J. Kriakov, C. Carriere, S. Yu, C. Vaamonde, R. A. McAdam, B. R. Bloom, G. F. Hatfull, and W. R. Jacobs, Jr.** 1997. Conditionally replicating mycobacteriophages: a system for transposon delivery to *Mycobacterium tuberculosis*. *Proc. Natl. Acad. Sci. USA* **94**:10961–10966.

6. **Barsom, E. K., and G. F. Hatfull.** 1996. Characterization of *Mycobacterium smegmatis* gene that confers resistance to phages L5 and D29 when overexpressed. *Mol. Microbiol.* **21**:159–170.

7. **Bertani, G.** 1999. Transduction-like gene transfer in the methanogen *Methanococcus voltae*. *J. Bacteriol.* **181**:2992–3002.

8. **Bibb, L. A., and G. F. Hatfull.** 2002. Integration and excision of the *Mycobacterium tuberculosis* prophage-like element, phiRv1. *Mol. Microbiol.* **45**:1515–1526.

9. **Bisso, G., G. Castelnuovo, M. G. Nardelli, G. Orefici, G. Arancia, G. Laneelle, C. Asselineau, and J. Asselineau.** 1976. A study on the receptor for a mycobacteriophage : phage phlei. *Biochimie* **58**:87–97.

10. **Brown, K. L., G. J. Sarkis, C. Wadsworth, and G. F. Hatfull.** 1997. Transcriptional silencing by the mycobacteriophage L5 repressor. *EMBO J.* **16**:5914–5921.

11. **Brussow, H.** 2001. Phages of dairy bacteria. *Annu. Rev. Microbiol.* **55**:283–303.

12. **Brussow, H., and R. W. Hendrix.** 2002. Phage genomics: small is beautiful. *Cell* **108**:13–16.

13. **Chen, X., A. M. Quinn, and S. L. Wolin.** 2000. Ro ribonucleoproteins contribute to the resistance of *Deinococcus radiodurans* to ultraviolet irradiation. *Genes Dev.* **14**:777–782.

14. **Clark, A. J., W. Inwood, T. Cloutier, and T. S. Dhillon.** 2001. Nucleotide sequence of coliphage HK620 and the evolution of lambdoid phages. *J. Mol. Biol.* **311**:657–679.

15. **Cole, S. T., R. Brosch, J. Parkhill, T. Garnier, C. Churcher, D. Harris, S. V. Gordon, K. Eiglmeier, S. Gas, C. E. Barry III, F. Tekaia, K. Badcock, D. Basham, D. Brown, T. Chillingworth, R. Connor, R. Davies, K. Devlin, T. Feltwell, S. Gentles, N. Hamlin, S. Holroyd, T. Hornsby, K. Jagels, A. Krogh, J. McLean, S. Moule, L. Murphy, K. Oliver, J. Osborne, M. A. Quail, M.-A. Rajandream, J. Rogers, S. Rutter, K. Seeger, J. Skelton, R. Squares, S. Squares, J. E. Sulston, K. Taylor, S. Whitehead, and B. G. Barrell.** 1998. Deciphering the biology of *Mycobacterium tuberculosis* from the complete genome sequence. *Nature* **393**:537–544.

16. **Donnelly-Wu, M. K., W. R. Jacobs, Jr., and G. F. Hatfull.** 1993. Superinfection immunity of mycobacteriophage L5: applications for genetic transformation of mycobacteria. *Mol. Microbiol.* **7**:407–417.

17. **Eiserling, F., A. Pushkin, M. Gingery, and G. Bertani.** 1999. Bacteriophage-like particles associated with the gene transfer agent of *Methanococcus voltae* PS. *J. Gen. Virol.* **80**:3305–3308.

18. **Eltringham, I. J., S. M. Wilson, and F. A. Drobniewski.** 1999. Evaluation of a bacteriophage-based assay (phage amplified biologically assay) as a rapid screen for resistance to isoniazid, ethambutol, streptomycin, pyrazinamide, and ciprofloxacin among clinical isolates of *Mycobacterium tuberculosis*. *J. Clin. Microbiol.* **37**:3528–3532.

19. **Engel, H. W.** 1978. Mycobacteriophages and phage typing. *Ann. Microbiol.* (Paris) **129**:75–90.

20. **Espinal, M. A.** 2003. The global situation of MDR-TB. *Tuberculosis* (Edinburgh) **83**:44–51.

21. **Fleischmann, R. D., D. Alland, J. A. Eisen, L. Carpenter, O. White, J. Peterson, R. DeBoy, R. Dodson, M. Gwinn, D. Haft, E. Hickey, J. F. Kolonay, W. C. Nelson, L. A. Umayam, M. Ermolaeva, S. L. Salzberg, A. Delcher, T. Utterback, J. Weidman, H. Khouri, J. Gill, A. Mikula, W. Bishai, W. R. Jacobs, Jr., J. C. Venter, and C. M. Fraser.** 2002. Whole-genome comparison of *Mycobacterium tuberculosis* clinical and laboratory strains. *J. Bacteriol.* **184**:5479–5490.

22. **Foley-Thomas, E. M., D. L. Whipple, L. E. Bermudez, and R. G. Barletta.** 1995. Phage infection, transfection and transformation of *Mycobacterium avium* complex and *Mycobacterium paratuberculosis*. *Microbiology* **141**:1173–1181.

23. **Ford, M. E., G. J. Sarkis, A. E. Belanger, R. W. Hendrix, and G. F. Hatfull.** 1998. Genome structure of mycobacteriophage D29: implications for phage evolution. *J. Mol. Biol.* **279**:143–164.

24. **Ford, M. E., C. Stenstrom, R. W. Hendrix, and G. F. Hatfull.** 1998. Mycobacteriophage TM4: genome structure and gene expression. *Tubercle Lung Dis.* **79**:63–73.

25. **Freitas-Vieira, A., E. Anes, and J. Moniz-Pereira.** 1998. The site-specific recombination locus of mycobacteriophage Ms6 determines DNA integration at the tRNA(Ala) gene of *Mycobacterium* spp. *Microbiology* **144**:3397–3406.

26. **Furuchi, A., and T. Tokunaga.** 1972. Nature of the receptor substance of *Mycobacterium smegmatis* for D4 bacteriophage adsorption. *J. Bacteriol.* **111**:404–411.

27. **Garcia, M., M. Pimentel, and J. Moniz-Pereira.** 2002. Expression of Mycobacteriophage Ms6 lysis genes is driven by two sigma(70)-like promoters and is dependent on a transcription termination signal present in the leader RNA. *J. Bacteriol.* **184**:3034–3043.

28. **Good, R. C., and T. D. Mastro.** 1989. The modern mycobacteriology laboratory. How it can help the clinician. *Clin. Chest Med.* **10**:315–322.

29. **Haeseleer, F., J. F. Pollet, A. Bollen, and P. Jacobs.** 1992. Molecular cloning and sequencing of the attachment site and integrase gene of the temperate mycobacteriophage FRAT1. *Nucleic Acids Res.* **20**:1420.

30. **Harley, J. B., R. H. Scofield, and M. Reichlin.** 1992. Anti-Ro in Sjogren's syndrome and systemic lupus erythematosus. *Rheum. Dis. Clin. North Am.* **18**:337–358.

31. **Hatfull, G. F.** 2000. Molecular genetics of mycobacteriophages, p. 37–54. *In* G. F. Hatfull and W. R. Jacobs, Jr. (ed.), *Molecular Genetics of the Mycobacteria.* ASM Press, Washington, D.C.

32. **Hatfull, G. F.** 1999. Mycobacteriophages, p. 38–58. *In* C. Ratledge and J. Dale (ed.), *Mycobacteria: Molecular Biology and Virulence.* Chapman and Hall, London, United Kindom.

33. **Hatfull, G. F., and W. R. Jacobs, Jr.** 1994. Mycobacteriophages: cornerstones of mycobacterial research, p. 165–183. *In* B. R. Bloom (ed.), *Tuberculosis: Pathogenesis, Protection, and Control.* ASM Press, Washington, D.C.

34. **Hatfull, G. F., and G. J. Sarkis.** 1993. DNA sequence, structure and gene expression of mycobacteriophage L5: a phage system for mycobacterial genetics. *Mol. Microbiol.* **7**:395–405.

35. **Hendrix, R. W., M. C. Smith, R. N. Burns, M. E. Ford, and G. F. Hatfull.** 1999. Evolutionary relationships among diverse

bacteriophages and prophages: all the world's a phage. *Proc. Natl. Acad. Sci. USA* **96:**2192–2197.

36. **Highton, P. J., Y. Chang, and R. J. Myers.** 1990. Evidence for the exchange of segments between genomes during the evolution of lambdoid bacteriophages. *Mol. Microbiol.* **4:**1329–1340.

37. **Humphrey, S. B., T. B. Stanton, and N. S. Jensen.** 1995. Mitomycin C induction of bacteriophages from *Serpulina hyodysenteriae* and *Serpulina innocens. FEMS Microbiol. Lett.* **134:**97–101.

38. **Humphrey, S. B., T. B. Stanton, N. S. Jensen, and R. L. Zuerner.** 1997. Purification and characterization of VSH-1, a generalized transducing bacteriophage of *Serpulina hyodysenteriae. J. Bacteriol.* **179:**323–329.

39. **Jacobs, W. R., Jr., R. G. Barletta, R. Udani, J. Chan, G. Kalkut, G. Sosne, T. Kieser, G. J. Sarkis, G. F. Hatfull, and B. R. Bloom.** 1993. Rapid assessment of drug susceptibilities of *Mycobacterium tuberculosis* by means of luciferase reporter phages. *Science* **260:**819–822.

40. **Jacobs, W. R., Jr., S. B. Snapper, L. Lugosi, A. Jekkel, R. E. Melton, T. Kieser, and B. R. Bloom.** 1989. Development of genetic systems for the mycobacteria. *Acta Leprol.* **7:**203–207.

41. **Jacobs, W. R., Jr., S. B. Snapper, M. Tuckman, and B. R. Bloom.** 1989. Mycobacteriophage vector systems. *Rev. Infect. Dis.* **11**(Suppl. 2):S404–S410.

42. **Jacobs, W. R., Jr., M. Tuckman, and B. R. Bloom.** 1987. Introduction of foreign DNA into mycobacteria using a shuttle phasmid. *Nature* **327:**532–535.

43. **Jain, S., and G. F. Hatfull.** 2000. Transcriptional regulation and immunity in mycobacteriophage Bxb1. *Mol. Microbiol.* **38:**971–985.

44. **Jones, W. D., Jr.** 1988. Bacteriophage typing of *Mycobacterium tuberculosis* cultures from incidents of suspected laboratory cross-contamination. *Tubercle* **69:**43–66.

45. **Juhala, R. J., M. E. Ford, R. L. Duda, A. Youlton, G. F. Hatfull, and R. W. Hendrix.** 2000. Genomic sequences of bacteriophages HK97 and HK022: pervasive genetic mosaicism in the lambdoid bacteriophages. *J. Mol. Biol.* **299:**27–51.

46. **Kalpana, G. V., B. R. Bloom, and W. R. Jacobs, Jr.** 1991. Insertional mutagenesis and illegitimate recombination in mycobacteria. *Proc. Natl. Acad. Sci. USA* **88:**5433–5437.

47. **Katsura, I., and R. W. Hendrix.** 1984. Length determination in bacteriophage lambda tails. *Cell* **39:**691–698.

48. **Kell, D. B., and M. Young.** 2000. Bacterial dormancy and culturability: the role of autocrine growth factors. *Curr. Opin. Microbiol.* **3:**238–243.

49. **Khoo, K. H., R. Suzuki, A. Dell, H. R. Morris, M. R. McNeil, P. J. Brennan, and G. S. Besra.** 1996. Chemistry of the lyxose-containing mycobacteriophage receptors of *Mycobacterium phlei/Mycobacterium smegmatis. Biochemistry* **35:**11812–11819.

50. **Kim, A., P. Ghosh, M. A. Aaron, L. A. Bibb, S. Jain, and G. F. Hatfull.** 2003. Mycobacteriophage Bxb1 integrates into the *Mycobacterium smegmatis groEL1* gene. *Mol. Microbiol.* **50:**463–473.

51. **Laal, S., Y. D. Sharma, H. K. Prasad, A. Murtaza, S. Singh, S. Tangri, R. S. Misra, and I. Nath.** 1991. Recombinant fusion protein identified by lepromatous sera mimics native *Mycobacterium leprae* in T-cell responses across the leprosy spectrum. *Proc. Natl. Acad. Sci. USA* **88:**1054–1058.

52. **Labbe, J. C., J. Burgess, L. A. Rokeach, and S. Hekimi.** 2000. ROP-1, an RNA quality-control pathway component, affects *Caenorhabditis elegans* dauer formation. *Proc. Natl. Acad. Sci. USA* **97:**13233–13238.

53. **Lang, A. S., and J. T. Beatty.** 2000. Genetic analysis of a bacterial genetic exchange element: the gene transfer agent of *Rhodobacter capsulatus. Proc. Natl. Acad. Sci. USA* **97:**859–864.

54. **Lawrence, J. G., G. F. Hatfull, and R. W. Hendrix.** 2002. Imbroglios of viral taxonomy: genetic exchange and failings of phenetic approaches. *J. Bacteriol.* **184:**4891–4905.

55. **Lawrence, J. G., R. W. Hendrix, and S. Casjens.** 2001. Where are the pseudogenes in bacterial genomes? *Trends Microbiol.* **9:**535–540.

56. **Lee, M. H., L. Pascopella, W. R. Jacobs, Jr., and G. F. Hatfull.** 1991. Site-specific integration of mycobacteriophage L5: integration-proficient vectors for *Mycobacterium smegmatis, Mycobacterium tuberculosis,* and bacille Calmette-Guérin. *Proc. Natl. Acad. Sci. USA* **88:**3111–3115.

57. **Levin, M. E., and G. F. Hatfull.** 1993. *Mycobacterium smegmatis* RNA polymerase: DNA supercoiling, action of rifampicin and mechanism of rifampicin resistance. *Mol. Microbiol.* **8:**277–285.

58. **Lewis, J. A., and G. F. Hatfull.** 2001. Control of directionality in integrase-mediated recombination: examination of recombination directionality factors (RDFs) including Xis and Cox proteins. *Nucleic Acids Res.* **29:**2205–2216.

59. **Lewis, J. A., and G. F. Hatfull.** 2003. Control of directionality in L5 integrase-mediated site-specific recombination. *J. Mol. Biol.* **326:**805–821.

60. **Mahairas, G. G., P. J. Sabo, M. J. Hickey, D. C. Singh, and C. K. Stover.** 1996. Molecular analysis of genetic differences between *Mycobacterium bovis* BCG and virulent *M. bovis. J. Bacteriol.* **178:**1274–1282.

61. **McCauliffe, D. P., F. A. Lux, T. S. Lieu, I. Sanz, J. Hanke, M. M. Newkirk, M. J. Siciliano, R. D. Sontheimer, and J. D. Capra.** 1989. Ro/SS-A and the pathogenic significance of its antibodies. *J. Autoimmun.* **2:**375–381.

62. **McNerney, R.** 1999. TB: the return of the phage. A review of fifty years of mycobacteriophage research. *Int. J. Tuberc. Lung Dis.* **3:**179–184.

63. **Mediavilla, J., S. Jain, J. Kriakov, M. E. Ford, R. L. Duda, W. R. Jacobs, Jr., R. W. Hendrix, and G. F. Hatfull.** 2000. Genome organization and characterization of mycobacteriophage Bxb1. *Mol. Microbiol.* **38:**955–970.

64. **Mekalanos, J. J., E. J. Rubin, and M. K. Waldor.** 1997. Cholera: molecular basis for emergence and pathogenesis. *FEMS Immunol. Med. Microbiol.* **18:**241–248.

65. **Mukamolova, G. V., A. S. Kaprelyants, D. I. Young, M. Young, and D. B. Kell.** 1998. A bacterial cytokine. *Proc. Natl. Acad. Sci. USA* **95:**8916–8921.

66. **Mukamolova, G. V., O. A. Turapov, D. I. Young, A. S. Kaprelyants, D. B. Kell, and M. Young.** 2002. A family of autocrine growth factors in *Mycobacterium tuberculosis. Mol. Microbiol.* **46:**623–635.

67. **Oftung, F., A. S. Mustafa, and H. G. Wiker.** 2000. Extensive sequence homology between the *Mycobacterium leprae* LSR (12 kDa) antigen and its *Mycobacterium tuberculosis* counterpart. *FEMS Immunol. Med. Microbiol.* **27:**87–89.

68. **Parish, T., J. Lewis, and N. G. Stoker.** 2001. Use of the mycobacteriophage L5 excisionase in *Mycobacterium tuberculosis* to demonstrate gene essentiality. *Tuberculosis* (Edinburgh) **81:**359–364.

69. **Pearson, R. E., S. Jurgensen, G. J. Sarkis, G. F. Hatfull, and W. R. Jacobs, Jr.** 1996. Construction of D29 shuttle phasmids and luciferase reporter phages for detection of mycobacteria. *Gene* **183:**129–136.

70. **Pedulla, M. L., M. E. Ford, J. M. Houtz, T. Karthikeyan, C. Wadsworth, J. A. Lewis, D. Jacobs-Sera, J. Falbo, J. Gross, N. R. Pannunzio, W. Brucker, V. Kumar, J. Kandasamy, L. Keenan, S. Bardarov, J. Kriakov, J. G. Lawrence, W. R. Jacobs, R. W. Hendrix, and G. F. Hatfull.** 2003. Origins of highly mosaic mycobacteriophage genomes. *Cell* **113:**171–182.

71. **Pedulla, M. L., and G. F. Hatfull.** 1998. Characterization of

the mIHF gene of *Mycobacterium smegmatis*. *J. Bacteriol.* **180**:5473–5477.

72. Pedulla, M. L., M. H. Lee, D. C. Lever, and G. F. Hatfull. 1996. A novel host factor for integration of mycobacteriophage L5. *Proc. Natl. Acad. Sci. USA* **93**:15411–15416.

73. Pelicic, V., M. Jackson, J. M. Reyrat, W. R. Jacobs, Jr., B. Gicquel, and C. Guilhot. 1997. Efficient allelic exchange and transposon mutagenesis in *Mycobacterium tuberculosis*. *Proc. Natl. Acad. Sci. USA* **94**:10955–10960.

74. Pelicic, V., J. M. Reyrat, and B. Gicquel. 1996. Expression of the *Bacillus subtilis sacB* gene confers sucrose sensitivity on mycobacteria. *J. Bacteriol.* **178**:1197–1199.

75. Pelicic, V., J. M. Reyrat, and B. Gicquel. 1996. Generation of unmarked directed mutations in mycobacteria, using sucrose counter-selectable suicide vectors. *Mol. Microbiol.* **20**:919–925.

76. Pelicic, V., J. M. Reyrat, and B. Gicquel. 1996. Positive selection of allelic exchange mutants in *Mycobacterium bovis* BCG. *FEMS Microbiol. Lett.* **144**:161–166.

77. Peña, C. E., M. H. Lee, M. L. Pedulla, and G. F. Hatfull. 1997. Characterization of the mycobacteriophage L5 attachment site, *attP. J. Mol. Biol.* **266**:76–92.

78. Peña, C. E., J. Stoner, and G. F. Hatfull. 1998. Mycobacteriophage D29 integrase-mediated recombination: specificity of mycobacteriophage integration. *Gene* **225**:143–151.

79. Raj, C. V., and T. Ramakrishnan. 1970. Transduction in *Mycobacterium smegmatis*. *Nature* **228**:280–281.

80. Ramesh, G., and K. P. Gopinathan. 1995. Cloning and characterization of mycobacteriophage I3 promoters. *Indian J. Biochem. Biophys.* **32**:361–367.

81. Ramesh, G. R., and K. P. Gopinathan. 1994. Structural proteins of mycobacteriophage I3: cloning, expression and sequence analysis of a gene encoding a 70-kDa structural protein. *Gene* **143**:95–100.

82. Raviglione, M. C. 2003. The TB epidemic from 1992 to 2002. *Tuberculosis* (Edinburgh) **83**:4–14.

83. Recktenwald, J., and H. Schmidt. 2002. The nucleotide sequence of Shiga toxin (Stx) 2e-encoding phage phiP27 is not related to other Stx phage genomes, but the modular genetic structure is conserved. *Infect. Immun.* **70**:1896–1908.

84. Ribeiro, G., M. Viveiros, H. L. David, and J. V. Costa. 1997. Mycobacteriophage D29 contains an integration system similar to that of the temperate mycobacteriophage L5. *Microbiology* **143**:2701–2708.

85. Roman, L. J., P. Martasek, and B. S. Masters. 2002. Intrinsic and extrinsic modulation of nitric oxide synthase activity. *Chem. Rev.* **102**:1179–1190.

86. Sarkis, G. J., W. R. Jacobs, Jr., and G. F. Hatfull. 1995. L5 luciferase reporter mycobacteriophages: a sensitive tool for the detection and assay of live mycobacteria. *Mol. Microbiol.* **15**:1055–1067.

87. Sassetti, C. M., D. H. Boyd, and E. J. Rubin. 2001. Comprehensive identification of conditionally essential genes in mycobacteria. *Proc. Natl. Acad. Sci. USA* **98**:12712–12717.

88. Sassetti, C. M., D. H. Boyd, and E. J. Rubin. 2003. Genes required for mycobacterial growth defined by high density mutagenesis. *Mol. Microbiol.* **48**:77–84.

89. Scanga, C. A., V. P. Mohan, K. Tanaka, D. Alland, J. L. Flynn, and J. Chan. 2001. The inducible nitric oxide synthase locus confers protection against aerogenic challenge of both clinical and laboratory strains of *Mycobacterium tuberculosis* in mice. *Infect. Immun.* **69**:7711–7717.

90. Shi, H., C. A. O'Brien, D. J. Van Horn, and S. L. Wolin. 1996. A misfolded form of 5S rRNA is complexed with the Ro and La autoantigens. *RNA* **2**:769–784.

91. Shleeva, M. O., K. Bagramyan, M. V. Telkov, G. V. Mukamolova, M. Young, D. B. Kell, and A. S. Kaprelyants. 2002. Formation and resuscitation of "non-culturable" cells of *Rhodococcus rhodochrous* and *Mycobacterium tuberculosis* in prolonged stationary phase. *Microbiology* **148**:1581–1591.

92. Smith, I. 2003. Mycobacterium tuberculosis pathogenesis and molecular determinants of virulence. *Clin. Microbiol. Rev.* **16**:463–496.

93. Smith, M. C., and H. M. Thorpe. 2002. Diversity in the serine recombinases. *Mol. Microbiol.* **44**:299–307.

94. Snapper, S. B., L. Lugosi, A. Jekkel, R. E. Melton, T. Kieser, B. R. Bloom, and W. R. Jacobs, Jr. 1988. Lysogeny and transformation in mycobacteria: stable expression of foreign genes. *Proc. Natl. Acad. Sci. USA* **85**:6987–6991.

95. Springer, B., P. Sander, L. Sedlacek, K. Ellrott, and E. C. Bottger. 2001. Instability and site-specific excision of integration-proficient mycobacteriophage L5 plasmids: development of stably maintained integrative vectors. *Int. J. Med. Microbiol.* **290**:669–675.

96. Susskind, M. M., and D. Botstein. 1978. Molecular genetics of bacteriophage P22. *Microbiol Rev.* **42**:385–413.

97. Wagner, P. L., and M. K. Waldor. 2002. Bacteriophage control of bacterial virulence. *Infect. Immun.* **70**:3985–3993.

98. Waldor, M. K. 1998. Bacteriophage biology and bacterial virulence. *Trends Microbiol.* **6**:295–297.

99. Wilson, S. M., Z. al-Suwaidi, R. McNerney, J. Porter, and F. Drobniewski. 1997. Evaluation of a new rapid bacteriophage-based method for the drug susceptibility testing of *Mycobacterium tuberculosis*. *Nat. Med.* **3**:465–468.

100. Xue, D., H. Shi, J. D. Smith, X. Chen, D. A. Noe, T. Cedervall, D. D. Yang, E. Eynon, D. E. Brash, M. Kashgarian, R. A. Flavell, and S. L. Wolin. 2003. A lupus-like syndrome develops in mice lacking the Ro 60-kDa protein, a major lupus autoantigen. *Proc. Natl. Acad. Sci. USA* **100**:7503–7508.

101. Zhu, W., B. B. Plikaytis, and T. M. Shinnick. 2003. Resuscitation factors from mycobacteria: homologs of *Micrococcus luteus* proteins. *Tuberculosis* (Edinburgh) **83**:261–269.

Tuberculosis and the Tubercle Bacillus
Edited by Stewart T. Cole et al.
© 2005 ASM Press, Washington, D.C.

Chapter 15

Control of Mycobacterial Transcription

ISSAR SMITH, WILLIAM R. BISHAI, AND VALAKUNJA NAGARAJA

All living organisms must respond to changes in the environment in which they exist. This is true for free-living organisms like the nonpathogenic mycobacterial saprophytes *Mycobacterium smegmatis* and *M. phlei*, as well as pathogens in the *M. tuberculosis* and *M. avium-intracellulare* families and *M. leprae*. Cells usually respond to changing conditions by synthesizing new proteins that allow them to survive in the new environment. In bacteria, these response mechanisms are primarily at the transcriptional level of gene expression, although posttranscriptional processes also play significant roles. To better prevent and treat mycobacterial diseases, it is essential to understand how these bacteria regulate responses to their environments. It is especially important to learn about the transcriptional mechanisms used by pathogenic mycobacteria during the infectious process. A review of research in these areas was published in 2000 (24). Since then, much new information has appeared that permits an updating of hypotheses and speculations that were presented at that time. As in the previous review and because of space limitations, this chapter is limited to the controlling elements of mycobacterial transcriptional initiation. However, DNA conformation, transcriptional elongation, and termination are important events in the synthesis of RNAs from DNA templates, and there are recent articles that discuss these important areas in mycobacteria (36, 68).

REGULATION OF MYCOBACTERIAL TRANSCRIPTION

Transcriptional initiation can be divided into several steps, starting with the initial binding of RNA polymerase (RNAP) to the upstream regulatory region of the gene being transcribed. This is followed by the formation of the open complex, binding of the initiating nucleotide, ternary complex formation, etc. These steps are controlled by *cis* elements and *trans*-acting factors. The former are sequences in the DNA that are found directly upstream of the gene's coding sequences and include the promoters and other regulatory sequences. In addition to the RNAP holo-enzymes that bind to specific promoters and catalyze the synthesis of RNA, there are other *trans*-acting regulatory proteins that bind to specific sequences in the promoter regions and modulate transcription initiation in a positive (activation) or negative (repression) manner.

Mycobacterial Promoters

Promoter consensus sequences

The occurrence of multiple σ factors in *M. tuberculosis*, as discussed later in this chapter, suggests the presence of varied promoter sequences and structures. In addition, the high G+C content of mycobacterial genomes might be expected to contribute to variations in the sequence of these elements and possibly spacer distances, making it difficult to define consensus sequences. This problem is found in the related actinomycete *Streptomyces coelicolor,* which also has a high genomic G+C content (66). Earlier studies formulated consensus promoter sequences that diverge to different extents from the *Escherichia coli* paradigm (reviewed in reference 24 and references therein); however, these consensus sequences were obtained from both predicted and experimentally mapped promoters. A more recent approach to deriving a consensus for mycobacterial promoter architecture used only the experimentally mapped transcription start sites of 80 genes. In this study, a consensus matrix was generated for putative −35 and −10 hexamers based on the frequency of occurrence

Issar Smith • TB Center, Public Health Research Institute, International Center for Public Health, Newark, NJ 07103-3535.
William R. Bishai • Center for Tuberculosis Research, Johns Hopkins University School of Medicine, Baltimore, MD 21231-1001.
Valakunja Nagaraja • Department of Microbiology and Cell Biology, Indian Institute of Science, Bangalore, India 560012.

of different bases at each position (Fig. 1) (67). This analysis, combined with earlier studies, has led to the following conclusions. First, many promoters, 69 of 80, have *E. coli* σ^{70}-like −10 elements. Presumably, these are likely candidates for σ^A recognition, as discussed later in this chapter. Second, the extended −10 element, the TGn sequence, is recognized by the mycobacterial transcription machinery (1, 39, 53, 65). This sequence is found at nucleotide positions −16 to −14 relative to the transcription start site of certain prokaryotic promoters that usually do not have conserved −35 sequences. The promoter region of the *M. smegmatis rpsL* gene harbors both an extended −10 TGn element and a consensus −35-like sequence. Results obtained with mutations and deletions created in the −35 region of this promoter indicate that the presence of one of these elements is essential and that of the two, the extended −10 region is more important (39). Third, there is greater heterogeneity at the −35 region, reflecting a higher GC content, and in many cases there is no identifiable −35 element. Fourth, a large majority of mycobacterial promoters do not function in *E. coli*, even though many of these have sequences that resemble the *E. coli* consensus. This indicates that additional and as yet unknown features of some of these predicted mycobacterial σ^A promoters limit their function to mycobacteria. A suggestion about these unknown elements comes from experiments in which the region upstream of the −10 element was replaced with random DNA fragments. These studies indicate that there are important contacts between the polymerase and promoter in this region, although a consensus sequence is not obvious (1).

The 11 promoters in the remaining group of consensus sequences, defined as "SigGC" promoters, are likely to be unique to mycobacteria. This point is discussed later, in the sections describing the consensus promoter sequences and their recognition by RNAPs containing alternative σ factors.

Single versus multiple and overlapping promoters

Since the genomes of bacteria are compact, the probability of finding two promoters close to each other is quite high. Many genes are also driven by multiple promoters, and this is frequently based on cellular requirements. From the analysis of compiled promoter sequences, it appears that stable RNA (rRNA, tRNA, etc.) genes and other housekeeping genes (constitutively expressed genes) possess a major promoter having a σ^{70} type of promoter structure that is presumably recognized by σ^A-RNAP. The additional promoters found in some of the rRNA (*rrn*) operons (25) or the *gyr* locus of *M. tuberculosis* (67) do not have σ^{70}-like sequences, indicating the possi-

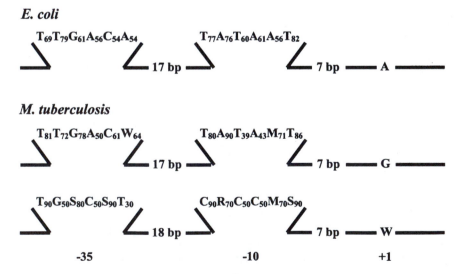

Figure 1. Mycobacterial promoter consensus sequences. This figure shows a compilation of 80 mycobacterial promoter sequences in which the transcriptional initiation nucleotides have been determined. The −10 and −35 recognition sequences refer to the 6-nucleotide sequences that interact, respectively, with regions 4.2 and 1.4 of σ factors. The most frequently occurring bases at each position are listed, and the number in the subscript gives the frequency of occurrence. R, W, S, and M have the same meaning as in Table 1; i.e., R denotes A or G, S denotes C or G, M denotes A or C, and W denotes A or T; +1 indicates the transcription-initiating nucleotide. Two classes of mycobacterial promoters were identified. The first class, comprising 69 promoters, illustrated in the second line from the top, shows consensus sequences resembling those of *E. coli*, which are shown in the top line. The second class of mycobacterial promoters, with 11 examples, shows a high G+C content, and its consensus sequences are presented in the bottom line.

ble usage of alternate σ factors for recognition. While there is no absolute correlation between the number of *rrn* cistrons and growth rate in mycobacteria (59), there appears to be some correlation with regard to promoter strength and utilization. Both *M. smegmatis* and *M. tuberculosis* contain only one copy of functional initiator tRNAs (9). The initiator tRNA promoter of *M. smegmatis* appears to be twofold stronger than the corresponding *M. tuberculosis* promoter both in *M. smegmatis* and in *M. tuberculosis*. In the case of multiple promoter-driven operons, such as the two *rrn* operons in *M. smegmatis*, the promoter efficiency is reported to vary with growth (25).

There are several cases where mycobacterial promoters are closely linked or overlapping and in some cases are transcribed in opposite directions. In addition to polycistronic mRNAs, the use of divergent promoters under a common regulatory circuit appears to be an efficient way of economizing genomic space in bacteria. Overlapping promoter architecture found in many genes is also a part of the cellular regulatory strategy (49). In such situations, polymerase occupancy at one promoter would prevent binding at the other site, leading to interesting regulatory consequences. For instance, the transcriptional organization of the *gyr* locus is quite different in *M. smegmatis* and *M. tuberculosis*, even though the genomic organization of *gyrB* closely followed by *gyrA* is identical in both species (67). *M. smegmatis* uses a single promoter, P*gyrB*, located upstream of *gyrB* that is polycistronic, including *gyrA* in the transcript, while *M. tuberculosis* uses multiple promoters. One such promoter, P*gyrB*$_1$, is identical to the *M. smegmatis* P*gyrB* and is also polycistronic. There is also a P*gyrA* promoter, upstream of *gyrA*, that is 70-fold weaker than P*gyrB*$_1$. Therefore, it is unlikely to contribute greatly to the steady-state levels of the GyrA protein. This weak promoter is likely to utilize an alternative σ factor. In addition, there is another promoter, P$_R$, that overlaps P*gyrB* and is divergently transcribed. The binding of RNAP to P$_R$ would be expected to prevent RNAP binding to P*gyrB*$_1$ and its transcription in the opposite orientation. Thus, P$_R$ may have a regulatory function since there is no apparent gene downstream of this promoter.

In addition to using alternative σ factors to transcribe multiple and overlapping promoters, mycobacteria use regulatory proteins for the same purpose. The *M. tuberculosis* IdeR protein, a DNA binding protein when activated by an electrostatic interaction with Fe^{2+}, represses two divergently transcribed genes, *hisE* and *irg2*, by binding to a unique sequence in the intergenic region (56), and a similar situation is observed in the IdeR repression of the *mbt* operon (20). A more complex example of divergent tran-

scriptional regulation by IdeR occurs in the *M. tuberculosis bfrA-bfd* genomic region. These genes are differentially controlled by the binding of this protein to a specific sequence in the intergenic space: *bfd* is repressed by IdeR:Fe^{2+} while the divergent transcription of the major *bfrA* promoter, P *bfrA*$_{High}$, encoding the iron storage protein bacterioferritin, is activated by this event. To further complicate matters, *bfrA* has another promoter, P*bfrA*$_{Low}$, 100 bp upstream of P*bfrA*$_{High}$, that is repressed by IdeR:Fe^{2+} binding (20). It is speculated that a function of P*bfrA*$_{Low}$ is to maintain minimal levels of bacterioferritin even when intracellular iron concentrations are limiting.

REGULATORY PROTEINS CONTROLLING TRANSCRIPTION INITIATION

The RNAPs from *M. tuberculosis* (28) and *M. smegmatis* (53) show an overall subunit composition in the core polymerase, i.e., the β, β', and two α proteins, that is identical to that found in *E. coli* and other prokaryotes. Genome-sequencing studies have revealed, as expected, that these subunits also show extensive conservation among different mycobacteria and other prokaryotes. Analysis of the *M. tuberculosis* H37Rv and CDC 1551 sequenced genomes has shown that there are approximately 200 proteins that are annotated as transcriptional regulators (6, 17), but less than 50 of these have been characterized to any extent. In the following section, the discussion is limited largely to the regulators whose function and/or mechanism of action is known. In other bacterial pathogens, transcription factors participate in adaptive responses necessary for virulence. σ factors regulate genes required for the pathogenicity of several bacterial pathogens (reviewed in reference 22 and references therein). Other regulatory proteins play an essential role in virulence, e.g., several response regulators (reviewed in reference 52 and references therein), including *M. tuberculosis*, and these are reviewed in chapter 22 of this book.

Mycobacterial σ Factors

σ factors play a major role in the early steps of prokaryotic transcription as they direct RNAP holoenzyme binding to cognate promoter sites and thereby confer specificity of transcription initiation (31). The use of alternative σ factors is one of the strategies used by bacteria to induce the expression of response genes under conditions requiring adaptation. The genome sequences of *M. tuberculosis* H37Rv and CDC 1551 indicate that there are 13 σ factor genes, which are named alphabetically, *sigA* through *sigM*

(6, 17). σ^A and σ^B belong to the family of bacterial σ factors containing the principal and highly related accessory σ factors. σ^F belongs to a branch of stress response and sporulation control σ factors. The other 10 σ factors belong to the extracytoplasmic function (ECF) category, which mainly controls cell envelope synthesis, secretory functions, and periplasmic proteins (31). All 13 σ factors are essentially conserved in *M. bovis* and therefore appear to have a critical function in the cell. However, deletions of many of them appear to be tolerated under laboratory conditions, with the strains only showing hypersensitivity to certain stresses. Interestingly, *M. smegmatis* seems to do without some of these functions, since BLAST searches of its genome indicate that *sigC*, *sigI*, and *sigK* are missing. The real surprise comes from the *M. leprae* genome (7). The genome contains for only 1,600 genes, about one-third of the average gene content in other slow-growing mycobacteria. Concomitant with this general decay in the genome of *M. leprae*, it retains unmutated genes for only four σ factors, σ^A, σ^B, σ^C, and σ^E. *sigI* and *sigL* are missing, and the genes for the other seven σ factors are pseudogenes. An important observation arising from these studies is that the different genomes belonging to the genus *Mycobacterium* encode a varied number of σ subunits, presumably reflecting the different environments faced by the members of this genus.

The relative expression levels of 10 of the 13 *M. tuberculosis* σ-factor genes were measured in vitro during exponential growth and under stress due to detergent, heat, cold, hydrogen peroxide, or low pH. All of the *sig* genes were expressed, although the levels were quite different, and individual gene responses to the stresses varied widely (41). The results with specific *sig* genes are discussed later in this chapter. In another study, the response of *M. tuberculosis* to nutrient starvation in vitro was evaluated using DNA array technology, and significant induction of *sigB*, *sigD*, *sigE*, and *sigF* expression was found (4). Using a cDNA enrichment method, another group found that mRNAs corresponding to *sigA*, *sigB*, *sigE*, *sigF*, and *sigH* were present 18 h after macrophage infection, and mRNAs for *sigA*, *sigF* (weak), and *sigH* were detectable after 48 h (26). This work suggested a significant role for alternative σ factors σ^E, σ^F, and σ^H in macrophage survival and virulence, as discussed later in this section.

Individual mycobacterial σ factors: role in physiology, stress response, and virulence

σ^A (Rv2703). The *sigA* genes of *M. smegmatis* and *M. tuberculosis* were postulated as encoding the principal σ factors in these organisms on the basis of

their primary amino acid sequence similarity to σ^A, the principal factor of *Streptomyces* spp., as well as their similarity to each other (13, 53). Moreover, *sigA* was shown to be essential in *M. smegmatis* (23) and in *M. tuberculosis* (J. Timm and I. Smith, unpublished results). Subsequently, several analyses assessed *M. tuberculosis sigA* gene expression under a variety of conditions and found that *sigA* was relatively stable during exponential growth of *M. tuberculosis* in vitro (23, 33) and in macrophages (14). According to the mycobacterial promoter consensus sequences discussed above (Fig. 1), RNAP containing σ^A should recognize promoters resembling the canonical *E. coli* one. In agreement with this hypothesis, purified σ^A-RNAP transcribed the *M. smegmatis rrnB* gene whose promoter is similar to the *E. coli*-like consensus sequence (Fig. 1; Table 1) (53) (G. Nair and I. Smith, unpublished results). Also transcribed by this RNAP holoenzyme was the *Bacillus subtilis* P*sinR* promoter, which does not have a recognizable -35 sequence but has the extended -10 sequence discussed above (Table 1) (53).

σ^A was the first mycobacterial sigma factor to be associated with a virulence defect in animal models. An *M. tuberculosis sigA*-containing DNA fragment restored guinea pig virulence to the attenuated *M. bovis* strain TMC403 that contains a missense mutation (R515H) in the *sigA* (*rpoV*) gene (8). This mutation is adjacent to region 4.2, which interacts with the promoter consensus -35 region, and mutations affecting the transcription of specific genes have been found in the same region adjacent to region 4.2 in the major σ factors of *E. coli* and *B. subtilis*. These mutations, which have no effect on general viability are postulated to prevent interaction between the major σ factor and several positive activators (19). Thus, the results with the *sigA* R515H mutation suggested that there is an activator protein that interacts with σ^A to transcribe *M. bovis* genes that are essential for pathogenicity. As discussed below, the WhiB3 protein is a likely candidate (63).

σ^B(Rv2710). *M. smegmatis*, *M. tuberculosis*, and *M. leprae*, as well as other mycobacteria, contain the *sigB* gene, which encodes a σ factor that is very similar to σ^A (13, 53). The expression of *sigB* is highly responsive to a number of stress conditions including detergent, diamide, and temperature stress (41, 42) and stationary-phase growth (33). *sigB* is not essential in *M. smegmatis* and *M. tuberculosis* H37Rv, and its loss does not affect *M. tuberculosis* growth in macrophages or mice (P. Fontan et al., unpublished results; R. Manganelli et al., unpublished results) (the effects of this mutation on mortality and tissue histopathology caused by *M. tuberculosis* during

Table 1. Binding sites for mycobacterial transcriptional regulatory proteins[a]

Regulator	Function	DNA recognition sequences and binding sites
		DNA recognition sequences
		(−35 spacer −10)
σ factors		
σ[A]	Major σ factor for housekeeping and virulence genes	TTGACW-spacer-TATAMT (consensus)
		TTGATC-spacer-TAACTT (P*rrnB*)
		-------- (TGC)-TATAAT (P*sinR*)
σ[B]	σ factor for stress response genes	Consensus not yet known
		-------- (TGC)-TATAAT (P*sinR*)
σ[F]	σ factor controlling late-growth genes and virulence	GGTTTC-spacer-GGGTAT (consensus)
		GGTTTC-spacer-GGGTAT (P*usfX*)
σ[C]	ECF σ factor for stress response and virulence	SSSAAT-spacer-CGTSSS (consensus)
σ[E]	ECF σ factor for stress response and virulence	nGGRMC-spacer-SGTTg (consensus)
		GGGAAC-spacer-CGTTA (P*sigB*)
σ[H]	ECF σ factor for oxidative stress response, heat shock, and virulence	SGGAAC-spacer-SGTTS (consensus)
		GGGAAC-spacer-CGTTAA (P*sigB*)
σ[L]	ECF σ factor of unknown function	Consensus not yet known
		GGGAAC-spacer-CGTTAA (P*sigB*)
		DNA binding sites
Other regulators		
RegX	RR[b] activator of unknown function	Consensus not yet known
		ATGGAACGGTAACCGAACAGCTGTGGCGTAG (P*regX*)
TcrR	RR activator of unknown function; affects virulence	Consensus not yet known
		ATAAGCGACATTTGAAAAATTTATGAAT (P*trcR*)
DosR	RR activator of hypoxia response genes; affects virulence	TTSGGGACTWWAGTCCCSAA (consensus)
		ACAGGGTCAATGGTCCCCAA (P*hspX*, dist. site)
		TCGGGGACTTCTGTCCCTAG (P*hspX*, prox. site)
IdeR	Repressor of iron uptake genes and activator of iron storage genes	TTAGGTTAGSCTAACCTAA (consensus)
		TTAGGGCAGCCTGTGCTAA (P*mbtB*)
		TTAGTGGAGTCTAGCCTAA (P*bfrA*, dist. site)
HspR	Repressor of heat shock response genes	AnTTGAGCGnnnnnGACTCAnCnTnG (consensus)
HcrA	Repressor of heat shock response genes	TnCTnGCACTCGnAngnGAGTGCTA (consensus)
LexA	Repressor of SOS response (DNA damage) genes	TCGAACnnnnGTTCGA (consensus)
		TCGAACACATGTTTGA (P*lexA*)
EthR	Repressor of ethionamide resistance genes	GTGTCGATAGTGTCGACATCTCGTTGACGGCCTCGACATTACGTTGA TTAGCGTGG (P*ethA*)

[a] The binding sites for several *M. tuberculosis* regulatory proteins are listed in this table. In the first group are σ factors, and the −10 and −35 recognition sequences refer to the 6-nucleotide sequences that interact, respectively, with regions 4.2 and 1.4 of σ factors. These sequences were determined by actual biochemical transcription studies with holoenzymes containing the σ factors and individual genes, and the consensus promoter sequences were determined in DNA array analyses and related experiments. The sequences for the other regulators have been demonstrated by DNA binding, and consensus sequences were determined from the results of DNA array experiments. All references for the data shown in this table are in the text. In certain cases, a consensus sequence has not yet been determined.

[b] RR signifies a response regulator. Symbols in the sequences, i.e., R, W, S, M, have the following meaning: R denotes A or G, S denotes C or G, M denotes A or C and W denotes A or T. A small "g" indicates that a G residue is found more frequently at this position than other nucleotides, and a small "n" means that there is no nucleotide preference at this position.

mouse infections have not been determined yet, but these experiments are currently being performed). Expression of *sigB* is dependent on several other sigma factors, including σ[E], which is necessary for full expression during exponential growth and detergent stress (43), and σ[H], which is required for the induction of *sigB* expression observed after diamide treatment and heat shock (38, 42, 55). Consistent with these observations, *sigB* is transcribed with RNAP holoenzymes containing σ[E] and σ[H] (Table 1) (S. Rodrigue et al., unpublished results), as discussed below. These results suggest that σ[B] may serve as a common mediator of generalized adaptive response pathways in mycobacteria, a role similar to that of

RpoS in *E. coli* and σ^B in *B. subtilis*. The 1.4 and 4.2 regions of σ^B, domains of σ factors that interact, respectively, with the -10 and -35 regions of promoters, are identical to those of σ^A (13, 53), suggesting that σ^B-RNAP and σ^A-RNAP recognize similar promoter sequences. In agreement with this hypothesis is the recent observation that mycobacterial RNAP core enzyme reconstituted with σ^B transcribes the -10 extended P*sinR* promoter, discussed above (Table 1) (Rodrigue et al., unpublished). DNA array analyses comparing the global transcription profile of wild-type *M. tuberculosis* H37Rv and the *sigB* mutant grown under different stress conditions indicate that σ^B plays a role in positively regulating heat shock response genes and *ideR*, encoding the iron regulator IdeR (Fontan et al., unpublished).

σ^F (**Rv3286c**). The *M. tuberculosis* σ^F was originally identified in *M. tuberculosis* (12), and sequence comparisons indicated that it was a homologue of alternative σ factors from *B. subtilis* (σ^B and σ^F) and *Streptomyces coelicolor* (σ^F), associated with both stress responses and sporulation (11). *sigF* expression was induced by entry into stationary phase as well as by other stresses, most notably cold shock and certain antibiotics (12, 45). An analysis of the upstream region of *sigF* showed that *usfX*, the gene directly preceding *sigF*, contains a promoter sequence that is recognized by σ^F-RNAP and that is the same promoter that is used when *M. tuberculosis* is grown in vitro (Table 1) (3). DNA array analyses comparing gene expression in wild-type *M. tuberculosis* and a *sigF* mutant at different stages of growth have now shown that many genes requiring a functional σ^F have a similar promoter sequence (Table 1) (D. Geiman et al., unpublished experiments). The *M. tuberculosis sigF* gene has been mutated, resulting in a strain with no detectable defect in ability to survive in macrophages but with reduced lethality for mice (5). *usfX*, directly upstream of *sigF*, was earlier reported to encode a protein that was similar to known anti-sigma factors and had anti-σ^F activity (11, 22). It has recently been shown that purified UsfX inhibited the in vitro transcription of a σ^F-dependent promoter by a protein-sequestering mechanism (3), consistent with known anti-σ factors from other species (34). Two additional gene products, Rv1365c and Rv3687c, were shown to bind to UsfX, disrupting the UsfX-σ^F complex and thus behaving like anti-anti-σ factors found in other bacteria (34). This study also suggested that the ability of these proteins to bind to UsfX and thus to release active σ^F may be dependent on redox levels (Rv1365c) or phosphorylation (Rv3687c). These findings, along with others discussed later in this section, underscore the fact that a significant de-

gree of posttranslational regulation of sigma factor activity is observed in mycobacteria.

σ^C (**Rv2069**). *sigC* is the most strongly transcribed of the *M. tuberculosis* σ-factor genes during in vitro growth in rich medium (41). When the gene was disrupted in *M. tuberculosis*, the mutant was more susceptible than the wild type to diamide and hydrogen peroxide stress but showed no survival defect in macrophages compared with the wild type (R. Sun et al., unpublished experiments). In mice, the *sigC* mutant was able to proliferate and survive in lungs at levels nearly identical to those observed with wild-type *M. tuberculosis*; however, the mutant did not produce severe tissue pathology, and in time-to-death analyses it was not lethal for mice infected by either the aerosol or intravenous routes. As assessed by microarray analysis, *M. tuberculosis* σ^C controls a broad array of biosynthetic genes, including those for the synthesis of cofactors, cell wall components, fatty acids, phospholipids, and energy metabolism, along with certain stress response genes, e.g., the α-crystallin-encoding gene *hspX*, and genes encoding surface antigens such as antigen 85C (*fbpC*) and lipoprotein Mpt83 (Sun et al., unpublished). These workers also derived a putative consensus sequence for σ^C-RNAP (Table 1).

σ^E (**Rv1221**). A mutant *M. smegmatis sigE* strain was constructed and found to be more susceptible than the wild type to heat, sodium dodecyl sulfate (SDS), acid, and oxidative stresses (70). A *sigE* mutant of *M. tuberculosis* was found to be more sensitive to heat, SDS, and oxidative stress than was the wild type (43). The *M. tuberculosis* mutant was also attenuated in its ability to survive within human and murine macrophages and mice (Manganelli et al., unpublished). DNA microarray analyses identified 38 genes which were transcribed less abundantly in the *M. tuberculosis sigE* mutant than in the wild type, and some of these were genes involved in fatty acid degradation and the classical heat shock response. A promoter consensus sequence for σ^E-RNAP was also derived from these experiments (Table 1). Significantly, the *M. tuberculosis sigE* was required for induction of *sigB* expression during exponential (unstressed) growth and after exposure to certain stress conditions such as SDS treatment, indicating a hierarchy between these two σ factors. σ^E-RNAP transcribes *sigB*, and the same initiating nucleotide is observed in these studies as when cells are growing in broth (Rodrigue et al., unpublished results). As demonstrated for σ^F, σ^E activity is inhibited by the binding of a specific anti-σ factor, RseA (Rv1222) (Rodrigue et al., unpublished).

σ^H (Rv3223c). A *sigH* mutant of *M. smegmatis* was constructed and found to be more susceptible than the wild type to cumene hydroperoxide stress (16). The same group (55) and two others (38, 42) made *M. tuberculosis sigH* mutants that were susceptible to heat and various oxidative stresses. *sigH* mutants exhibit wild-type survival in macrophages (42) and mice (38). However, like the *M. tuberculosis sigC* mutant, a *sigH* mutant did not elicit the same degree of tissue pathology as wild-type *M. tuberculosis* and, as a result, was much less lethal than the wild type in time-to-death analyses (38). By a combination of techniques, including in vitro transcription and DNA array global expression studies, the three groups identified σ^H-dependent genes, including some encoding proteins like thioredoxin and thioredoxin reductase, which are part of the oxidative stress response, as well as *sigB* and *sigH* itself. These independent studies derived a consensus promoter sequence for *M. tuberculosis* σ^H-dependent genes, as illustrated in Table 1. Biochemical studies have shown that *sigB* is transcribed by σ^H-RNAP and utilizes the same promoter and initiation nucleotide as σ^E-RNAP, which is the one used by *M. tuberculosis* growing in broth (Rodrigue et al., unpublished). σ^H activity is also inhibited by the binding of an anti-σ factor, RshA (Rv3221A) (Rodrigue et al., unpublished). This is identical to the situation for *S. coelicolor*, where the activity of σ^R, an ECF σ factor that is an ortholog of σ^H and has similar functions (50), is prevented by the binding of the oxidation-sensitive RsrA anti-σ factor that is homologous to RshA (37).

Surprisingly, RNAP containing another ECF σ factor, σ^L also transcribes the same promoter of *sigB*, and its activity is controlled by an anti-σ factor, RslA (Rv0736) (Rodrigue et al., unpublished). As discussed above, mycobacteria must need σ^B under different stress conditions, and adequate levels of this transcription factor presumably are maintained by the transcription of *sigB* by RNAPs containing different ECF σ factors. However, as discussed above, the activity of these σ factors is ordinarily inhibited by the binding of specific anti-σ factors. Presumably, a specific stress condition disrupts the inhibitory binding of one of the anti-σ factors to its cognate σ factor, which frees the specific ECF σ factor and allows transcription of *sigB* under that condition; e.g., SDS disrupts RseA binding to σ^E, and diamide or heat disrupts RshA binding to σ^H. The stress response in which σ^L plays a role is not known, and it is not clear which condition disrupts the binding of σ^L to its anti-σ-factor RslA. Experiments elucidating the role of σ^L in *M. tuberculosis* physiology and virulence are under way.

Two-Component Response Regulators

Bacteria use other regulatory proteins, in addition to alternative σ factors, that change RNAP promoter specificity in response to external signals. A major class consists of the two-component response regulators, which are activated for their role as direct-acting transcriptional regulators by an environmentally responsive cognate histidine kinase, as discussed elsewhere in this book (see chapter 22). This section discusses the two-component systems in which the signal leading to a response is known and/or the molecular mechanism of the response regulator function has been described. The other *M. tuberculosis* two-component systems and the role of these regulators in virulence is described in chapter 22.

DosR (Rv3133c). DosR, also known as DevR, has been studied in *M. smegmatis*, *M. bovis* BCG, and *M. tuberculosis* (reviewed in reference 51 and references therein). It is required for the expression of a regulon containing approximately 50 genes that is induced during hypoxia or anoxia during hypoxia-induced dormancy or persistence (51) and during nitric oxide stress (M. Voskiul et al., personal communication). Its genetic determinant is directly upstream of the gene encoding a histidine kinase, DosS. Among the DosR-requiring genes induced under these conditions are *hxpX*, encoding the α-crystalline chaperone-like protein; *narX* and *narK2*, annotated as encoding, respectively, a fused nitrate reductase and a nitrite extrusion protein; and *fdxA*, encoding ferredoxin, a protein involved in alternative respiratory pathways. DosR binds to a consensus sequence (Table 1) directly upstream of the promoter region of some of the genes, including *hspX*, that require DosR for their induction under the conditions mentioned above (51). There are two binding sites for DosR in the *hspX* promoter region, one at nucleotides −110 to −91 and the second at nucleotides −53 to −34 relative to the transcription start site. Mutational analyses indicate that both sites are important for the induction of *hxpX* expression, with the downstream site being essential. These data strongly suggest that DosR is an activator of *hspX*, presumably by interacting with the two DosR binding sites, which in turn facilitates the binding of RNAP to the *hspX* promoter.

TrcR (Rv1033c). The structural gene encoding *M. tuberculosis* TrcR is directly upstream of a gene (Rv1032c) encoding a histidine kinase, TrcS, and the latter can directly phosphorylate TrcR (30). Physiological studies using an *E. coli* surrogate expression system indicate that TrcR positively autoregulates its own expression. Molecular studies have shown that phosphorylated TrcR binds to the *trcR* promoter region (29). Mutational analyses of this interaction and DNase footprinting have identified an AT-rich sequence that is essential for TrcR binding and *trcR* regulation (Table 1). The environmental stress to which the TrcR-TrcS system responds is not currently known. In a recent study comparing the global transcription profile of an *M. tuberculosis trcS* mutant with wild-type H37Rv growing exponentially, 14 genes showed overexpression in the *trcS* strain and 36 showed lower expression in this mutant (69). Interestingly, *trcR* was not found in this latter group, an unexpected result considering the results discussed above, which indicated that TrcR positively autoregulates *trcR* (29).

PhoP (Rv0757). The *M. tuberculosis* response regulator PhoP, whose structural gene is directly upstream of one encoding a histidine kinase, PhoR, shows high similarity to the *Salmonella enterica* serovar Typhimurium PhoP response regulator, which senses Mg^{2+} starvation and controls the expression of virulence genes (27). Experiments in vitro have shown that an *M. tuberculosis* H37Rv *phoP* mutant grows poorly in low-Mg^{2+}-containing media, indicating that *M. tuberculosis* PhoP responds to Mg^{2+} starvation similarly to *S. enterica* serovar Typhimurium PhoP (S. Walters and I. Smith, unpublished observations). It is thought that PhoR senses Mg^{2+} depletion in the same way as the *Salmonella* ortholog, PhoQ, does. In addition, mutant cells have an altered, rounded shape and show differences in levels of lipoarabinomannan derivatives compared to the wild type (40). Importantly, *M. tuberculosis phoP* mutants are severely attenuated for growth in macrophages and mice (52) (Walters and Smith, unpublished). Genes requiring PhoP for their expression during growth in broth have been identified by DNA array transcription analyses, and among these 85 genes are those encoding proteins involved in lipid metabolism, cell wall synthesis, membrane transport, and oxidative stress response (Walters and Smith, unpublished). However, the binding of PhoP to these genes has not been demonstrated yet, and it is not known which, if any, of them are direct targets for this response regulator. A similar number of genes show higher expression in the *phoP* mutant, and the observation that many of these are also induced under hypoxic conditions and other stresses suggests that the absence of PhoP is, in itself, a severe stress condition. Current experiments are attempting to find which of the genes controlled by PhoP are necessary for virulence.

KdpE (Rv1028c). Genes annotated as being part of the *M. tuberculosis* K^+ uptake machinery are induced by low K^+ levels (64). The two-component system KdpE (reponse regulator)-KdpD (histidine kinase) is thought to control K^+ acquisition components in *M. tuberculosis* as related proteins do in other bacteria. An analysis of the interactions between KdpD, KdpE, and other initially unknown proteins was performed using yeast two-hybrid and three-hybrid systems and surface plasmon resonance assays (64). These elegant studies showed that the sensing domain of KdpD interacted with its histidine kinase domain, as well as with KdpE and with two membrane proteins, LprF and LprJ. Overexpression of the last two proteins increased the expression of the low-K^+-induced *kdpFABC*; mutation of these proteins modulated the expression of this regulon. These results suggest that LprJ, LprF, KdpD, and KdpE form a complex that plays a role in transducing the signal elicited by low K^+ levels. This leads to higher expression of components of the K^+ acquisition machinery, which presumably occurs by the binding of activated KdpE to promoters of regulons like *kdpFABC*. Direct interactions of KdpE with putative target promoters have not yet been demonstrated.

RegX (Rv0491). In a reversal of the usual genetic structure for two-component systems, the gene for the *M. tuberculosis* histidine kinase SenX3 (Rv0490) is directly upstream of the one for the response regulator RegX3. Biochemical experiments have shown that SenX3 can autophosphorylate itself and then transfer this phosphate to RegX3. RegX3 binds to the DNA region directly upstream of *senX3* (Table 1), and overexpression of *senX3-regX3* in *M. smegmatis* increases *senX3* promoter activity (32). These results suggest that phosphorylated RegX3 activates the expression of the *senX3-regX3* operon. It is not known which environmental stress SenX3 and RegX3 respond to or which other genes they control.

Other Transcriptional Regulators

IdeR (Rv2711). IdeR, a member of the DtxR-IdeR-SirR family, is the major, direct-acting regulator of iron acquisition and storage in mycobacterial species and is an essential protein (57). Proteins in this family of transcriptional regulators function as DNA binding proteins, and they usually repress genes for iron or manganese acquisition when activated by the electrostatic binding of the corresponding divalent metal. IdeR is unique among metalloregulatory DNA binding proteins because it has dual functions: it is a repressor of iron acquisition genes, i.e., those encoding enzymes that function in the siderophore biosynthetic pathway, as well as receptors for siderophore:Fe^{3+} uptake; IdeR is also an activator of *bfrA* and *bfrB*, which encode the iron storage proteins bacterioferritin and ferritin, respectively. The binding sites, or "iron boxes," involved in these two functions are very similar to the consensus IdeR binding sequence that was determined in biochemical and DNA array studies (Table 1) (20, 58). The iron boxes for genes that are repressed by IdeR-Fe^{2+} are all centered in the +1 to −10 region of the promoter and are expected to block RNAP binding, while the IdeR-Fe^{2+} binding sites in *bfrA* and *bfrB* are all upstream of the −35 region of the promoter. This strongly suggests that IdeR bound to these latter sites stimulates transcription by facilitating the binding of RNAP to the promoter or by contacting and activating already bound RNAP. Biochemical transcription studies to elucidate the mechanisms of transcriptional activation and repression by IdeR are under way.

In addition to IdeR, analysis of the *M. tuberculosis* genome reveals the presence of a gene, *sirR* (Rv2788), encoding a protein that belongs to the DtxR-IdeR-SirR family, but its function has not been characterized. In addition, *M. tuberculosis* has two genes, *furA* (Rv1909c) and *furB* (Rv2359), that encode proteins of the Fur family. Members of this group are widely found in gram-positive and gram-negative bacteria, and they function as repressors of iron acquisition and in some cases are required for the oxidative stress response (18), similar to the role of IdeR in mycobacterial physiology (57). The mycobacterial *furA* gene is found upstream of *katG*, encoding the mycobacterial catalase-peroxidase. Both genes are induced after oxidative stress and in macrophages (44, 46), but each gene has a unique promoter. In addition, *M. tuberculosis* FurA seems to negatively regulate *katG* expression since *furA* mutants overexpress *katG* (54, 71), but direct interaction between FurA and the *katG* promoter has not been shown yet. FurB remains uncharacterized, and an *M. tuberculosis furB* mutant shows normal growth in human macrophages and mice (G. M. Rodriguez and I. Smith, unpublished results).

HspR (Rv0353)/HcrA (Rv3734c). HspR and HcrA are discussed together here because both proteins are repressors of genes that are induced after heat shock in *M. tuberculosis*. Orthologs of these two proteins that also control heat shock genes are found in gram-positive bacteria. DNA array analyses comparing wild-type *M. tuberculosis* H37Rv with *hspR* and *hcrA* mutants identified the regulons controlled by HspR and HcrA (Table 1) (62). It was shown that HspR represses genes in the *hsp70* (*dnaK*) regulon while HcrA is a repressor of *hsp60* (*groEL*) and other

heat shock response genes. Sequences upstream of these genes were analyzed, and the genes controlled by HspR were found to have a HAIR sequence, identified as the HspR binding element in other bacteria. HrcA-repressed genes had a CIRCE element, likewise shown in other bacteria to be the binding sequence for HcrA. Interestingly, an *M. tuberculosis hspR* mutant was attenuated for virulence during mouse infections, even though it showed elevated expression of *hsp70* and other heat shock genes (61). It was postulated that the higher levels of heat shock proteins like Hsp70 in the *hspR* mutant may increase bacterial signaling to host immunosurveillance systems during infections, leading to greater bacterial killing.

LexA (Rv2720). LexA is a repressor of genes that are induced after DNA damage that define the SOS response in most bacteria. Among these genes are *recA* and *lexA* itself. A motif similar to the *B. subtilis* LexA binding site was identified upsteam of the *lexA* and *recA* genes in mycobacteria (15, 47). DNA binding studies, coupled with mutational analysis and DNA array experiments, have further refined the LexA binding sequence (Table 1) and have identified 15 DNA damage-inducible genes that are most probably regulated by LexA (10).

EthR (Rv3855). EthR is an *M. tuberculosis* repressor involved in controlling genes that determine resistance to the second-line antimycobacterial prodrug ethionamide. Ethionamide resistance usually results from inactivation of *ethA*, which encodes a monooxygenase that activates the prodrug ethionamide. Gene reporter experiments have shown that EthR overexpression represses *ethA* promoter activity (2), and biochemical studies have shown that EthR, a protein in the TetR family of transcriptional regulators, represses *ethA* by directly binding, in the form of an octamer, to the *ethA-ethR* intergenic region (Table 1) (J. Engohang-Ndong and A. Baulard, personal communication).

WhiB3 (Rv3416). WhiB3 is one of a family of seven *M. tuberculosis* proteins that resemble *Streptomyces* WhiB proteins, which are essential for sporulation (60). A yeast two-hybrid search identified this protein as one that interacts with the 4.2 domain of the wild-type *M. tuberculosis* σ^A protein but not that of the R515H-mutated one (63). As mentioned above, the R515H mutation in σ^A attenuates *M. bovis*, and this suggested that the mutation prevents the expression of a gene(s) needed for bacterial pathogenicity (8). The interaction of WhiB3 with σ^A is important for virulence since inactivation of *whiB3* in

M. bovis produces a strain with the same attenuated virulence phenotype in a guinea pig model, as seen in *M. bovis* with the R515H mutation. Interestingly, the *whiB3* mutation affected *M. bovis* pathogenicity more severely than the equivalent mutation did in *M. tuberculosis,* using the same animal model (63). The reason for this difference in the virulence phenotypes of mutant strains in these closely related bacteria is not known. Also, the genes essential for virulence that require WhiB3 interaction with σ^A-RNAP for their transcription are not known. Hopefully these will be identified in the near future with the new technologies available. Little else is known about WhiB3 except for the observations that *whiB3* is constitutively expressed in *M. tuberculosis* (48) and that a *whiB3* mutation in *M. smegmatis* has no apparent phenotype (35). Of the other mycobacterial *whiB* genes, only *whiB2* has been studied. A *whiB2* mutation in *M. smegmatis* affects septation and cell division (21), while a promoter trap search identified the *M. tuberculosis whiB2* as being expressed at higher levels during mouse infections (E. Dubnau et al., unpublished observations).

CONCLUSIONS AND PROSPECTS

An organism's response to its external environment is a key factor in its survival and, for a pathogen, is required for its ability to grow in a host and cause disease. Bacteria have evolved many mechanisms to deal with environmental stresses such as heat shock, oxidative stress, and nutrient limitation. These responses usually involve the elevated expression of genes that encode enzymes and other proteins that confer resistance to these conditions. It is not surprising that bacterial pathogens such as *M. tuberculosis* utilize many of the same mechanisms for the differential expression of genes required for pathogenicity. Among these are alternative σ factors that confer specificity to the RNA biosynthetic machinery, as well as other transcriptional factors, such as two-component response regulators, that modulate the expression of virulence genes. As discussed in this chapter and others in this book, the absence of some σ factors and other regulatory proteins causes a decrease in the virulence of *M. tuberculosis*. These results lead to several important and complementary questions. First, which mechanisms control the function of these regulatory proteins so that the virulence-determining genes they control are expressed correctly during infection? Second, which genes controlled by each regulator are essential for virulence? Third, and most important, what is the function of the essential virulence genes? In some cases, partial answers are available. For example, the activity of some σ factors necessary for virulence is prevented by their binding to anti-σ factors. In at least one case, that of σ^H, the mechanism is known since the cognate anti-σ factor is altered by oxidative stress, which prevents its binding to σ^H. It is also known that PhoP, a two-component response regulator, responds to Mg^{2+} starvation. The use of DNA arrays to study global transcription patterns in regulatory mutants and wild-type *M. tuberculosis* has enabled researchers to enumerate the genes controlled by these regulators, and the results have allowed the identification of putative consensus binding sequences in the promoters of these genes. In vitro and biochemical experiments can then be used to distinguish between the genes that are directly or indirectly controlled by the specific regulator. Several laboratories are now doing DNA array analyses of *M. tuberculosis* growing in macrophages. When these assays are performed with wild-type strains and regulatory mutants, the patterns of gene expression will give a clearer idea of which genes controlled by a particular regulator are essential for virulence, at least in macrophage models. The specific functions of the proteins encoded by the genes identified in these experiments will then have to be determined by biochemical means. The ultimate question would then be the following: are these genes and the proteins they encode essential for virulence, and, if so, how? The new technologies available for the genetic manipulation of *M. tuberculosis* and for measuring its virulence, as described elsewhere in this book, will be invaluable for these studies.

Acknowledgments. I.S. thanks the members of the Smith laboratory and his collaborators, Riccardo Manganelli (University of Padua, Padua, Italy) and Luc Gaudreau, Jocelyn Beaucher, and Sebastien Roderigue (University of Sherbrooke, Quebec, Canada); V.N. thanks his team members Sugopa Sengupta and Rich Gupta for their assistance. Work from our laboratories cited in this review was supported by NIH grants AI-44856, HL-64544, and Hl-68513 (awarded to I.S.), NIH grants AI-36973, AI-37856, and AI-51668 (awarded to W.R.B.) and the Indian Council of Medical Research, Council of Scientific and Industrial Research, Government of India (awarded to V.N.). We thank our colleagues in the TB research community who sent unpublished material for this review. Because of space considerations, review articles are cited whenever possible, and individual papers are noted only when they substantiated a specific point. Thus, some published studies were not identified, and the authors apologize to those colleagues whose important work was not directly referenced.

REFERENCES

1. **Bashyam, M. D., and A. K. Tyagi.** 1998. Identification and analysis of "extended −10" promoters from mycobacteria. *J. Bacteriol.* 180:2568–2573.
2. **Baulard, A. R., J. C. Betts, J. Engohang-Ndong, S. Quan, R. A. McAdam, P. J. Brennan, C. Locht, and G. S. Besra.** 2000.

Activation of the pro-drug ethionamide is regulated in mycobacteria. *J. Biol. Chem.* 275:28326–28331.

3. **Beaucher, J., S. Rodrigue, P. E. Jacques, I. Smith, R. Brzezinski, and L. Gaudreau.** 2002. Novel *Mycobacterium tuberculosis* anti-sigma factor antagonists control sigma F activity by distinct mechanisms. *Mol. Microbiol.* 45:1527–1540.

4. **Betts, J. C., P. T. Lukey, L. C. Robb, R. A. McAdam, and K. Duncan.** 2002. Evaluation of a nutrient starvation model of *Mycobacterium tuberculosis* persistence by gene and protein expression profiling. *Mol. Microbiol.* 43:717–731.

5. **Chen, P., R. E. Ruiz, Q. Li, R. F. Silver, and W. R. Bishai.** 2000. Construction and characterization of a *Mycobacterium tuberculosis* mutant lacking the alternate sigma factor gene, sigma F. *Infect. Immun.* 68:5575–5580.

6. **Cole, S. T., R. Brosch, J. Parkhill, T. Garnier, C. Churcher, D. Harris, S. V. Gordon, K. Eigenmeir, S. Gas, C. E. Barry III, F. Tekala, K. Badcock, D. Basham, D. Brown, T. Chillingworth, R. Conner, R. Davies, K. Devlin, T. Feltwell, S. Gentles, N. Hamlin, S. Holroyd, T. Hornsby, K. Jagels, A. Krogh, J. McLean, S. Moule, L. Murphy, K. Oliver, J. Osborne, M. A. Quail, M.-A. Rajandream, J. Rogers, S. Rutter, K. Seegar, J. Skelton, R. Squares, J. E. Sulston, K. Taylor, S. Whitehead, and B. G. Burrell.** 1998. Deciphering the biology of *Mycobacterium tuberculosis* from the complete genome sequence. *Nature* 393:537–544.

7. **Cole, S. T., K. Eiglmeier, J. Parkhill, K. D. James, N. R. Thomson, P. R. Wheeler, N. Honore, T. Garnier, C. Churcher, D. Harris, K. Mungall, D. Basham, D. Brown, T. Chillingworth, R. Connor, R. M. Davies, K. Devlin, S. Duthoy, T. Feltwell, A. Fraser, N. Hamlin, S. Holroyd, T. Hornsby, K. Jagels, C. Lacroix, J. Maclean, S. Moule, L. Murphy, K. Oliver, M. A. Quail, M. A. Rajandream, K. M. Rutherford, S. Rutter, K. Seeger, S. Simon, M. Simmonds, J. Skelton, R. Squares, S. Squares, K. Stevens, K. Taylor, S. Whitehead, J. R. Woodward, and B. G. Barrell.** 2001. Massive gene decay in the leprosy bacillus. *Nature* 409:1007–1011.

8. **Collins, D. M., R. P. Kawakami, G. W. de Lisle, L. Pascopella, B. R. Bloom, and W. R. Jacobs, Jr.** 1995. Mutation of the principal sigma factor causes loss of virulence in a strain of the *Mycobacterium tuberculosis* complex. *Proc. Natl. Acad. Sci. USA* 92:8036–8040.

9. **Dastur, A., P. Kumar, S. Ramesh, M. Vasanthakrishna, and U. Varshney.** 2002. Analysis of the initiator tRNA genes from a slow- and a fast-growing *Mycobacterium. Arch. Microbiol.* 178:288–296.

10. **Davis, E. O., E. M. Dullaghan, and L. Rand.** 2002. Definition of the mycobacterial SOS box and use to identify LexA-regulated genes in *Mycobacterium tuberculosis. J. Bacteriol.* 184:3287–3295.

11. **DeMaio, J., Y. Zhang, C. Ko, and W. R. Bishai.** 1997. *Mycobacterium tuberculosis sigF* is part of a gene cluster with similarities to the *Bacillus subtilis sigF* and *sigB* operons. *Tubercle Lung Dis.* 78:3–12.

12. **DeMaio, J., Y. Zhang, C. Ko, D. B. Young, and W. R. Bishai.** 1996. A stationary-phase stress-response sigma factor from *Mycobacterium tuberculosis. Proc. Natl. Acad. Sci. USA* 93:2790–2794.

13. **Doukhan, L., M. Predich, G. Nair, O. Dussurget, I. Mandic-Mulec, S. T. Cole, D. R. Smith, and I. Smith.** 1995. Genomic organization of the mycobacterial sigma gene cluster. *Gene* 165:67–70.

14. **Dubnau, E., P. Fontan, R. Manganelli, S. Soares-Appel, and I. Smith.** 2002. *Mycobacterium tuberculosis* genes induced during infection of human macrophages. *Infect. Immun.* 70:2787–2795.

15. **Durbach, S. I., S. J. Andersen, and V. Mizrahi.** 1997. SOS induction in mycobacteria: analysis of the DNA-binding activity

of LexA-like repressor and its role in DNA damage induction of the *recA* gene from *Mycobacterium smegmatis. Mol. Microbiol.* 26:643–653.

16. **Fernandes, N. D., Q.-L. Wu, D. Kong, X. Puyang, S. Garg, and R. N. Husson.** 1999. A mycobacterial extracytoplasmic sigma factor involved in survival following heat shock and oxidative stress. *J. Bacteriol.* 181:4266–4274.

17. **Fleischmann, R. D., D. Alland, J. A. Eisen, L. Carpenter, O. White, J. Peterson, R. DeBoy, R. Dodson, M. Gwinn, D. Haft, E. Hickey, J. F. Kolonay, W. C. Nelson, L. A. Umayam, M. Ermolaeva, S. L. Salzberg, A. Delcher, T. Utterback, J. Weidman, H. Khouri, J. Gill, A. Mikula, W. Bishai, W. R. Jacobs, Jr., J. C. Venter, and C. M. Fraser.** 2002. Whole-genome comparison of *Mycobacterium tuberculosis* clinical and laboratory strains. *J. Bacteriol.* 184:5479–5490.

18. **Fuangthong, M., A. F. Herbig, N. Bsat, and J. D. Helmann.** 2002. Regulation of the *Bacillus subtilis fur* and *perR* genes by PerR: not all members of the PerR regulon are peroxide inducible. *J. Bacteriol.* 184:3276–3286.

19. **Gardella, T., H. Moyle, and M. M. Susskind.** 1989. A mutant *Escherichia coli* sigma 70 subunit of RNA polymerase with altered promoter specificity. *J. Mol. Biol.* 206:579–590.

20. **Gold, B., G. M. Rodriguez, S. A. Marras, M. Pentecost, and I. Smith.** 2001. The *Mycobacterium tuberculosis* IdeR is a dual functional regulator that controls transcription of genes involved in iron acquisition, iron storage and survival in macrophages. *Mol. Microbiol.* 42:851–865.

21. **Gomez, J. E., and W. R. Bishai.** 2000. *whmD* is an essential mycobacterial gene required for proper septation and cell division. *Proc. Natl. Acad. Sci. USA* 97:8554–8559.

22. **Gomez, J. E., J.-M. Chen, and W. R. Bishai.** 1997. Sigma factors of *Mycobacterium tuberculosis. Tubercle Lung Dis.* 78:175–183.

23. **Gomez, M., G. Nair, L. Doukhan, and I. Smith.** 1998. *sigA* is an essential gene in *Mycobacterium smegmatis. Mol. Microbiol.* 29:617–628.

24. **Gomez, M., and I. Smith.** 2000. Determinants of mycobacterial gene expression, p. 111–129. *In* G. F. Hatfull and W. R. Jacobs, Jr. (ed.), *Molecular Genetics of Mycobacteria.* ASM Press, Washington, D.C.

25. **Gonzalez-y-Merchand, J. A., M. J. Colston, and R. A. Cox.** 1998. Roles of multiple promoters in transcription of ribosomal DNA: effects of growth conditions on precursor rRNA synthesis in mycobacteria. *J. Bacteriol.* 180:5756–5761.

26. **Graham, J. E., and J. E. Clark-Curtiss.** 1999. Identification of *Mycobacterium tuberculosis* RNAs synthesized in response to phagocytosis by human macrophages by selective capture of transcribed sequences (SCOTS). *Proc. Natl. Acad. Sci. USA* 96:11554–11559.

27. **Groisman, E. A.** 2001. The pleiotropic two-component regulatory system PhoP-PhoQ. *J. Bacteriol.* 183:1835–1842.

28. **Harshey, R. M., and T. Ramakrishnan.** 1976. Purification and properties of DNA-dependent RNA polymerase from *Mycobacterium tuberculosis* H37Rv. *Biochim. Biophys. Acta* 432:49–59.

29. **Haydel, S. E., W. H. Benjamin, Jr., N. E. Dunlap, and J. E. Clark-Curtiss.** 2002. Expression, autoregulation, and DNA binding properties of the *Mycobacterium tuberculosis* TrcR response regulator. *J. Bacteriol.* 184:2192–2203.

30. **Haydel, S. E., N. E. Dunlap, and W. H. Benjamin, Jr.** 1999. In vitro evidence of two-component system phosphorylation between the *Mycobacterium tuberculosis* TrcR/TrcS proteins. *Microb. Pathog.* 26:195–206.

31. **Helmann, J. D.** 2002. The extracytoplasmic function (ECF) sigma factors. *Adv. Microb. Pathog.* 46:47–110.

32. **Himpens, S., C. Locht, and P. Supply.** 2000. Molecular char-

acterization of the mycobacterial SenX3-RegX3 two-component system: evidence for autoregulation. *Microbiology* **146**: 3091–3098.

33. Hu, Y., and A. R. M. Coates. 1999. Transcrption of two sigma 70 homologue genes, *sigA* and *sigB*, in stationary-phase *Mycobacterium tuberculosis*. *J. Bacteriol.* **181**:499–476.

34. Hughes, K. T., and K. Mathee. 1998. The anti-sigma factors. *Annu. Rev. Microbiol.* **52**:231–286.

35. Hutter, B., and T. Dick. 1999. Molecular genetic characterisation of WhiB3, a mycobacterial homologue of a *Streptomyces* sporulation factor. *Res. Microbiol.* **150**:295–301.

36. Kalate, R. N., B. D. Kulkarni, and V. Nagaraja. 2002. Analysis of DNA curvature distribution in mycobacterial promoters using theoretical models. *Biophys. Chem.* **99**:77–97.

37. Kang, J. G., M. S. Paget, Y. J. Seok, M. Y. Hahn, J. B. Bae, J. S. Hahn, C. Kleanthous, M. J. Buttner, and J. H. Roe. 1999. RsrA, an anti-sigma factor regulated by redox change. *EMBO J.* **18**:4292–4298.

38. Kaushal, D., B. G. Schroeder, S. Tyagi, T. Yoshimatsu, C. Scott, C. Ko, L. Carpenter, J. Mehrotra, Y. C. Manabe, R. D. Fleischmann, and W. R. Bishai. 2002. Reduced immunopathology and mortality despite tissue persistence in a *Mycobacterium tuberculosis* mutant lacking alternative sigma factor, SigH. *Proc. Natl. Acad. Sci. USA* **99**:8330–8335.

39. Kenney, T. J., and G. Churchward. 1996. Genetic analysis of the *Mycobacterium smegmatis rpsL* promoter. *J. Bacteriol.* **178**:3564–3571.

40. Ludwiczak, P., M. Gilleron, Y. Bordat, C. Martin, B. Gicquel, and G. Puzo. 2002. *Mycobacterium tuberculosis phoP* mutant: lipoarabinomannan molecular structure. *Microbiology* **148**:3029–3037.

41. Manganelli, R., E. Dubnau, S. Tyagi, F. M. Kramer, and I. Smith. 1999. Differential expression of 10 sigma factor genes in *Mycobacterium tuberculosis*. *Mol. Microbiol.* **31**:715–724.

42. Manganelli, R., M. I. Voskuil, G. K. Schoolnik, E. Dubnau, M. Gomez, and I. Smith. 2002. Role of the extracytoplasmic-function sigma factor sigma H in *Mycobacterium tuberculosis* global gene expression. *Mol. Microbiol.* **45**:365–374.

43. Manganelli, R., M. I. Voskuil, G. K. Schoolnik, and I. Smith. 2001. The *Mycobacterium tuberculosis* ECF sigma factor sigma E: role in global gene expression and survival in macrophages. *Mol. Microbiol.* **41**:423–437.

44. Master, S., T. C. Zahrt, J. Song, and V. Deretic. 2001. Mapping of *Mycobacterium tuberculosis katG* promoters and their differential expression in infected macrophages. *J. Bacteriol.* **183**:4033–4039.

45. Michele, T. M., C. Ko, and W. R. Bishai. 1999. Exposure to antibiotics induces expression of the *Mycobacterium tuberculosis sigF* gene: implications for chemotherapy against mycobacterial persistors. *Antimicrob. Agents Chemother.* **43**:218–225.

46. Milano, A., F. Forti, C. Sala, G. Riccardi, and D. Ghisotti. 2001. Transcriptional regulation of *furA* and *katG* upon oxidative stress in *Mycobacterium smegmatis*. *J. Bacteriol.* **183**:6801–6806.

47. Movahedzadeh, F., M. J. Colston, and E. O. Davis. 1997. Characterization of *Mycobacterium tuberculosis* LexA: recognition of a Cheo (*Bacillus*-type SOS) box. *Microbiology* **143**:929–936.

48. Mulder, N. J., H. Zappe, and L. M. Steyn. 1999. Characterization of a *Mycobacterium tuberculosis* homologue of the *Streptomyces coelicolor whiB* gene. *Tubercle Lung Dis.* **79**:299–308.

49. Nagaraja, V. 1993. Control of transcriptional initiation. *J. Biosci.* **18**:13–25.

50. Paget, M. S., V. Molle, G. Cohen, Y. Aharonowitz, and M. J.

Buttner. 2001. Defining the disulphide stress response in *Streptomyces coelicolor* A3(2): identification of the sigma R regulon. *Mol. Microbiol.* **42**:1007–1020.

51. Park, H. D., K. M. Guinn, M. I. Harrell, R. Liao, M. I. Voskuil, M. Tompa, G. K. Schoolnik, and D. R. Sherman. 2003. Rv3133c/dosR is a transcription factor that mediates the hypoxic response of *Mycobacterium tuberculosis*. *Mol. Microbiol.* **48**:833–843.

52. Perez, E., S. Samper, Y. Bordas, C. Guilhot, B. Gicquel, and C. Martin. 2001. An essential role for *phoP* in *Mycobacterium tuberculosis* virulence. *Mol. Microbiol.* **41**:179–187.

53. Predich, M., L. Doukhan, G. Nair, and I. Smith. 1995. Characterization of RNA polymerase and two σ factor genes from *Mycobacterium smegmatis*. *Mol. Microbiol.* **15**:355–366.

54. Pym, A. S., P. Domenech, N. Honore, J. Song, V. Deretic, and S. T. Cole. 2001. Regulation of catalase-peroxidase (KatG) expression, isoniazid sensitivity and virulence by *furA* of *Mycobacterium tuberculosis*. *Mol. Microbiol.* **40**:879–889.

55. Raman, S., T. Song, X. Puyang, S. Bardarov, W. R. Jacobs, Jr., and R. N. Husson. 2001. The alternative sigma factor SigH regulates major components of oxidative and heat stress responses in *Mycobacterium tuberculosis*. *J. Bacteriol.* **183**: 6119–6125.

56. Rodriguez, G. M., B. Gold, M. Gomez, O. Dussurget, and I. Smith. 1999. Identification and characterization of two divergently transcribed iron regulated genes in *Mycobacterium tuberculosis*. *Tubercle Lung Dis.* **79**:287–298.

57. Rodriguez, G. M., and I. Smith. 2003. Mechanisms of iron regulation in mycobacteria: role in physiology and virulence. *Mol. Microbiol.* **47**:1485–1494.

58. Rodriguez, G. M., M. I. Voskuil, B. Gold, G. K. Schoolnik, and I. Smith. 2002. *ideR*, an essential gene in *Mycobacterium tuberculosis*: role of IdeR in iron-dependent gene expression, iron metabolism, and oxidative stress response. *Infect. Immun.* **70**:3371–3381.

59. Sander, P., T. Prammananan, and E. Bottger. 1996. Introducing mutations into a chromosomal rRNA gene using a genetically modified eubacterial host with a single rRNA operon. *Mol. Microbiol.* **22**:841–848.

60. Soliveri, J. A., J. Gomez, W. R. Bishai, and K. F. Chater. 2000. Multiple paralogous genes related to the *Streptomyces coelicolor* developmental regulatory gene *whiB* are present in *Streptomyces* and other actinomycetes. *Microbiology* **146**: 333–343.

61. Stewart, G. R., V. A. Snewin, G. Walzl, T. Hussell, P. Tormay, P. O'Gaora, M. Goyal, J. Betts, I. N. Brown, and D. B. Young. 2001. Overexpression of heat-shock proteins reduces survival of *Mycobacterium tuberculosis* in the chronic phase of infection. *Nat. Med.* **7**:732–737.

62. Stewart, G. R., L. Wernisch, R. Stabler, J. A. Mangan, J. Hinds, K. G. Laing, D. B. Young, and P. D. Butcher. 2002. Dissection of the heat-shock response in *Mycobacterium tuberculosis* using mutants and microarrays. *Microbiology* **148**:3129–3138.

63. Steyn, A. J., D. M. Collins, M. K. Hondalus, W. R. Jacobs, Jr., R. P. Kawakami, and B. R. Bloom. 2002. *Mycobacterium tuberculosis* WhiB3 interacts with RpoV to affect host survival but is dispensable for *in vivo* growth. *Proc. Natl. Acad. Sci. USA* **99**:3147–3152.

64. Steyn, A. J., J. Joseph, and B. R. Bloom. 2003. Interaction of the sensor module of *Mycobacterium tuberculosis* H37Rv KdpD with members of the Lpr family. *Mol. Microbiol.* **47**:1075–1089.

65. Stolt, P., Q. Zhang, and S. Ehlers. 1999. Identification of promoter elements in mycobacteria: mutational analysis of a highly symmetric dual promoter directing the expression of

replication genes of the *Mycobacterium* plasmid pAL5000. *Nucleic Acids Res.* **27:**396–402.

66. **Strohl, W. R.** 1992. Compilation and analysis of DNA sequences associated with apparent streptomycete promoters. *Nucleic Acids Res.* **20:**961–974.

67. **Unniraman, S., M. Chatterji, and V. Nagaraja.** 2002. DNA gyrase genes in *Mycobacterium tuberculosis*: a single operon driven by multiple promoters. *J. Bacteriol.* **184:**5449–5456.

68. **Unniraman, S., R. Prakash, and V. Nagaraja.** 2002. Conserved economics of transcription termination in eubacteria. *Nucleic Acids Res.* **30:**675–684.

69. **Wernisch, L., S. L. Kendall, S. Soneji, A. Wietzorrek, T. Parish, J. Hinds, P. D. Butcher, and N. G. Stoker.** 2003. Analysis of whole-genome microarray replicates using mixed models. *Bioinformatics* **19:**53–61.

70. **Wu, Q. L., D. Kong, K. Lam, and R. N. Husson.** 1997. A mycobacterial extracytoplasmic function sigma factor involved in survival following stress. *J. Bacteriol.* **179:**2922–2929.

71. **Zahrt, T. C., J. Song, J. Siple, and V. Deretic.** 2001. Mycobacterial FurA is a negative regulator of catalase-peroxidase gene *katG*. *Mol. Microbiol.* **39:**1174–1185.

VII. CELL STRUCTURE

Chapter 16

The Proteome of *Mycobacterium tuberculosis*

JOHN T. BELISLE, MIRIAM BRAUNSTEIN, IDA ROSENKRANDS, AND PETER ANDERSEN

It could be argued that analysis of the *Mycobacterium tuberculosis* proteome began with the production of tuberculin as a diagnostic reagent (107) and enrichment of the protein component of this material to generate purified protein derivative (PPD) (180). In fact, these preparations were the first protein extracts of *M. tuberculosis* evaluated for a specific biological property. In studies addressing the biochemical and immunological properties of PPD and culture filtrate proteins of *M. tuberculosis*, Affronti and Seibert (3) set the stage for protein research in tuberculosis over the next several decades. A retrospective look at this early work reveals that the field was driven by the immunology of the disease and the quest to identify the immunogenic proteins of the bacterium. Multiple studies conducted during the 1970s and 1980s employed a reductionist approach to identify the major immunogen(s) of *M. tuberculosis* and to provide some form of molecular identity to such proteins through antibody reactivity or N-terminal sequencing. These efforts were clearly successful in their goals and established the identity of several immunogenic proteins, including the antigen 85 (Ag85) complex, antigen 5 (PstS1), MPT64, GroES, GroEL, and MPT32, and to this day these are still considered major antigens of *M. tuberculosis* (for reviews, see references 4 and 221). Although defining protein antigens remained a focus during the 1990s, research efforts also expanded to include defining the physiological function of *M. tuberculosis* proteins. Such undertakings were motivated by the following needs: (i) to elucidate antituberculosis drug targets and mechanisms of drug resistance (11, 226); (ii) to define new drug targets (17); and (iii) to assess the contribution of individual gene products to pathogenicity (126). The ability to define the function of individual *M. tuberculosis* proteins was greatly facilitated by the establishment of genetic manipulation techniques for *M. tuberculosis* and other *Mycobacterium* spp. (100).

Several proteome-scale research endeavors were initiated well before the completion of the *M. tuberculosis* genome (9, 114, 133, 186). In particular, the work of Andersen and Heron (9) demonstrated that the purification and immunological assessment of a single protein based on antibody reactivity or its relative abundance could be replaced by relatively high-throughput immunological screens on defined fractions of a complex protein subset. However, the importance of the *M. tuberculosis* genome sequence (43) cannot be downplayed. It has accelerated investigations of the *M. tuberculosis* proteome in the sense of defining important antigens and the function of proteins. As described in the sections below, proteomic and genomic techniques are being widely applied to the study of *M. tuberculosis* and are providing key information regarding immune recognition, metabolic pathways, protein localization, and global regulation. However, it is important to recognize that defining protein function still requires detailed analysis of the protein in question and that proteomic or genomic data at best should be viewed as a guide for the design of subsequent experimentation.

The ultimate goal of studying the proteome of *M. tuberculosis* is to identify the many proteins that comprise the bacillus and to understand how they behave in concert with each other. This is a highly ambitious goal because the complexity of a bacterial proteome is not defined only by the number of predicted proteins but also includes factors such as differential expression, protein stability, protein modifications, and distinct subcellular localization. The objective of this chapter is to provide an overview of our current understanding of the *M. tuberculosis* proteome, including unique aspects, and a description of the approaches being applied.

John T. Belisle • Mycobacteria Research Laboratories, Department of Microbiology, Immunology, and Pathology, Colorado State University, Fort Collins, CO 80523. **Miriam Braunstein** • Department of Microbiology, University of North Carolina, Chapel Hill, NC 27599. **Ida Rosenkrands and Peter Andersen** • Department of Immunology, Statens Serum Institut, Copenhagen, Denmark.

IN SILICO PREDICTION OF THE M. TUBERCULOSIS PROTEOME

The original annotation of the *M. tuberculosis* H37Rv genome predicted 3,924 protein-coding sequences, 40% of which were assigned a function based on database comparisons (43). A recent reannotation of this genome increased the number of protein-coding sequences to 3,995 and provided functional predictions for 52% of the gene products (37). The increased number of predicted open reading frames (ORFs) resulted from decreasing the minimal predicted gene length, checking of codon usage, and inclusion of gene products that were identified via proteomic methods. In silico analyses of *M. tuberculosis* genome data provide information on the biochemical characteristics of the proteome beyond ORF annotation, and such information can be critical when designing and interpreting proteomic experiments. Using the original annotation, Urquhart et al. (199) determined that the pI of proteins ranged from 3.33 to 13.15. Over 60% of the predicted proteins have a pI of 7 or less (193), and there is a bimodal pI distribution with a major peak at pH 7 and a smaller peak at pH 11 (199). Approximately 40% of the predicted proteins of *M. tuberculosis* have a pI of 8 or greater, a range that is notoriously difficult to resolve by two-dimensional polyacrylamide gel electrophoresis (2-D PAGE). This latter fact is underscored in a comparison of the predicted proteome to the *M. tuberculosis* proteins resolved by 2-D PAGE, where very few proteins are observed in the range from pH 9 to 12 (199). In silico analyses of the proteome also reveal that the distribution of amino acids varies significantly from that in other bacteria (193). Specifically, Ala and Gly are the most abundant amino acids while Lys, Glu, Asn, Ile, Phe, and Tyr are less abundant, and there is an increased frequency of Arg, Ala, and Trp. The shift in overall amino acid composition of the predicted proteome can be largely explained by the high G+C content of the genome. However, evaluation of individual proteins uncovered a significant influence on the overall amino acid composition by two large multimember protein families (193). Specifically, the PE proteins, with their abundance of Gly residues, and the PPE proteins, with their abundance of Asn residues, fall outside of the normal amino acid composition exhibited by the majority of *M. tuberculosis* proteins. It is also interesting that nearly 20% of the predicted *M. tuberculosis* proteins lack a Cys residue. This is of particular importance to proteomic analyses employing isotope-coded affinity-tagged technologies that rely on modification of Cys residues.

PROTEOMIC STUDIES

Early Approach

Almost 20 years before the completion of the genome sequence and designation of each gene product with a specific Rv number (43), efforts were taken to apply a systematic approach for identification and nomenclature of *M. tuberculosis* proteins. The first attempt was based on the crossed-immunoelectrophoresis (CIE) technique, and with a polyvalent antibody preparation, reference systems were established for *M. bovis* BCG and *M. tuberculosis* (42, 208). At that time, the resolving power of CIE was considered quite high, and the technique had the ability to provide the partial identity of the three members of the Ag85 complex (209). Despite these advantages, the CIE method was not widely used, although some of the antigen names originating from this reference system are still in use (e.g., Ag84 and the Ag85 complex). Another early method to identify and catalogue *M. tuberculosis* proteins was based on mobility in nondenaturing PAGE. Sadamu Nagai introduced the term MPT (denoting a protein purified from *M. tuberculosis*) or MPB (protein purified from *M. bovis*) with a number referring to the protein's relative mobility by nondenaturing PAGE (132). For a number of proteins, the MPT designation is still used (e.g., MPT63, MPT64, and MPT83).

Pre-dating routine N-terminal sequence analysis and mass spectrometry (MS), monoclonal antibodies (MAbs) were widely applied for protein identification. Through the efforts of numerous laboratories, and coordinated by the World Health Organization (WHO) (105), a large panel of MAbs were generated against *M. tuberculosis* antigens and their reactivities were described in detail (5, 47, 97, 106, 118, 201, 202). Samples of most of these MAbs were collected and distributed by the WHO MAb bank as a valuable resource for protein identification (105), and many are still available through the National Institute for Allergy and Infectious Diseases contract for tuberculosis research reagents (http://www.cvmbs.colostate.edu/microbiology/tb/top.htm).

Modern Proteomic Analyses and Database Development

The application of more comprehensive proteomics techniques to *M. tuberculosis* was pioneered by Sadamu Nagai (133). These studies combined 2-D electrophoresis with N-terminal sequence analysis and established a 2-D map of the proteins secreted into culture medium (culture filtrate proteins); the 12 most abundant *M. tuberculosis* proteins were identified, and their positions were mapped. This work was a major achievement, leading to a substantial increase in the number of *M. tuberculosis* proteins identified at that time. Continuation of this work led to a more complete identification of the proteins in 2-D maps (covering approximately 40 proteins) through the use of the standard panel of MAbs combined with N-terminal sequence analysis or liquid chromatography-MS (165, 186). Today, MAbs and N-terminal sequence analysis have largely been replaced by MS and peptide mass fingerprinting. However, for proteins not well resolved by 2-D PAGE (e.g., the 19-kDa lipoprotein) (220), detection via MAbs remains a useful approach. Until recently, none of the 167 predicted members of the PE and PPE protein families were identified in proteome projects (163). The reason for this is unknown, but it may be due to the unusual amino acid composition of these proteins (193). In this regard, the first PPE protein was mapped in a lysate of *M. tuberculosis* with monospecific polyclonal antiserum, whereas attempts to identify the spot by matrix-assisted laser desorption ionization (MALDI)-MS were unsuccessful (140). This further underscores the importance of antibodies, even today, in evaluating the *M. tuberculosis* proteome.

In most proteome projects, only the cellular proteins are studied. However, the presence of T-cell antigens such as Ag85B (Rv1886c), MPT64 (Rv1980c), and ESAT-6 (Rv3875) in extracellular extracts of *M. tuberculosis* has led to detailed proteomic mapping of culture filtrate as well as cellular proteins (103, 163, 165). The most extensive of these studies utilized a large-gel format and highly sensitive MALDI-MS peptide mass fingerprinting to map and identify approximately 1,800 cellular proteins (from evaluation of the whole-cell lysate) and 800 culture filtrate proteins (103). The culture filtrate proteins yield fewer 2-D spots and form a unique pattern compared to the cellular proteins.

The overall complexity of the cellular-protein 2-D profiles can be a challenge to protein resolution. One way to address this issue is through the generation of cell wall and cytosolic subcellular fractionations prior to 2-D PAGE, with each of these subcellular fractions producing unique profiles (165). Increased 2-D gel resolution can also be obtained by using a narrow pH range and selecting the percentage in the second-dimension gel according to the mass range of interest. By this approach, Mattow et al. (122) focused on acidic, low-mass proteins from *M. tuberculosis* and succeeded in identifying 50 different proteins in the pH range from 4 to 6 and mass range from 6 to 15 kDa. The power of these proteomic studies is highlighted by the fact that seven ORFs not predicted in the H37Rv genome project were identified (102,

165). Each of these were small proteins (7 to 11 kDa), which are difficult to predict during genomic annotation (199). Furthermore, data from one proteome study suggest alternative start codons for four proteins as a result of N-terminal sequence analysis (165).

The wealth of information contained in proteomic maps is far above what can be placed in a typical research publication. Thus, to ensure the usefulness of such data for the research community, proteomic databases have been established. To date, two mycobacterial proteome databases exist, both available through the WORLD-2-DPAGE server (http://us.expasy.org/ch2d/2d-index.html). The Berlin database (http://www.mpiib-berlin.mpg.de/2D-PAGE) is an interactive database (130) with 2-D PAGE images of *M. tuberculosis* and *M. bovis* BCG cellular and culture supernatant proteins (103). The Copenhagen database (http://www.ssi.dk/graphics/html/tbimmun/Protein_database/protein_database.htm) displays 2-D gel images of *M. tuberculosis* cellular, culture filtrate, cytosol, and cell wall proteins (163, 165). Recently, two databases were developed for the in silico analyses of annotated genomes. The first of these, the Proteome Analysis database (http://www.ebi.ac.uk/proteome/), contains 89 proteomes, including *M. tuberculosis*, and provides information on protein families, domains, and functions of the proteins from a specific proteome and allows comparisons between the individual proteomes (153). The second database, JVirGel (http://prodoric.tu-bs.de/proteomics.php), provides the ability to determine the expected 2-D position of the proteins and generation of virtual 2-D gels based on the calculated molecular mass and pI of deduced amino acid sequences (93). So far, six prokaryotic and six eukaryotic proteomes are accessible. The *M. tuberculosis* proteome is not yet included but is expected to be available in the near future (D. Jahn, personal communication).

Application of Proteomics to Strain Comparisons

Besides the standard 2-D mapping and identification of proteins, proteomic evaluations are ideally suited to assess phenotypic variations among strains. Although it is widely accepted that *M. tuberculosis* presents considerable phenotypic and genetic variation among strains, there are only a few proteomic studies comparing various *M. tuberculosis* strains. One such study compared the whole-cell lysates of the laboratory strain H37Rv and the clinical isolate CDC 1551 and demonstrated surprisingly similar protein profiles between the two strains (23). In total, only 17 protein spots differed between the two strains, and only 3 and 7 spots were unique to strain H37Rv and CDC 1551, respectively. The remaining spot differences were quantitative. Two of the unique protein spots in both strain H37Rv and CDC 1551 were identified as the transcriptional regulator MoxR (Rv1479). The differential mobility of this protein in the 2-D gel patterns of these strains was found to be associated with a single point mutation between the *moxR* gene of strains H37Rv and CDC 1551, but it remains unknown whether this point mutation affects protein function. Interestingly, a separate study observed a similar mobility shift between MoxR of *M. tuberculosis* strains H37Rv and Erdman (103). This latter study also showed that Rv2296, Ald/Rv2780, and SppA/Rv0724 were present in the proteome of strain H37Rv but absent from that of strain Erdman, while Rv3213c and CadI/Rv2641 were absent from the H37Rv proteome but present in that of strain Erdman. The number of protein differences observed between the 2-D gel patterns of strains H37Rv and CDC 1551 is relatively small in comparison to the differences predicted by the genome sequences (23), and it is possible that a larger number of differences might have been observed if subcellular fractions of these two strains were compared instead of whole-cell lysate.

Genomic comparisons between *M. tuberculosis* and *M. bovis* BCG revealed 13 regions (116 ORFs) of the *M. tuberculosis* H37Rv genome that are missing in BCG Copenhagen and BCG Chicago (15). In a series of studies, Mattow et al. (123, 124) compared the proteomes of *M. tuberculosis* and *M. bovis* BCG. Analysis of the cellular protein profiles of these two organisms characterized 32 protein spots unique to *M. tuberculosis* (123). Of these 32 proteins, 12 were encoded by genes known to be missing in *M. bovis* BCG. The remaining 20 *M. tuberculosis*-specific spots represented products of genes not deleted in *M. bovis* BCG. For 11 of the unique *M. tuberculosis* protein spots (representing eight gene products), corresponding proteins in *M. bovis* BCG were identified, but they had altered electrophoretic mobilities, most probably caused by strain-specific posttranslational modifications or amino acid substitutions. However, 10 proteins (FusA2/Rv0120c, NadC/Rv1596, LinB/Rv2579, Ald/Rv2780, PurE/Rv3275c, Rv0036c, Rv2449c, Rv2557, Rv3407, and Rv3881c) unique to *M. tuberculosis* did not have corresponding mobility variants in *M. bovis* BCG. A similar comparative analysis of the culture filtrate proteins led to the identification of 39 specific *M. tuberculosis* H37Rv protein spots, representing five ORFs known to be deleted in *M. bovis* BCG, and 22 not reported as deleted (124). Of this latter group of proteins, 16 had electrophoretic mobility variants in *M. bovis* BCG and 6 (AroF/Rv2540c, FadA2/Rv0243, Rv1684, Rv3046c, Rv3881c, and Rv1498A) were truly unique to the *M. tuberculosis* culture filtrate proteins.

Proteomic Studies for Definition of Stress Responses and Virulence Factors

A powerful application of 2-D protein maps is the characterization of global changes induced by different environmental stimuli. This method has proven very useful for elucidating metabolic pathways and identifying proteins associated with virulence. For *M. tuberculosis*, such analyses are important, not only to understand the basic physiology of the bacterium but also to provide key input for drug and vaccine target discovery programs. The first proteomic analyses of the *M. tuberculosis* response to environmental stress were performed well before the completion of the genome sequence and assessed heat shock and oxidative stress (70, 181, 219). Specifically, Young and Garbe (219) identified seven gene products (DnaK [Rv0350], GroEL [Rv0440], GroES [Rv3418c], and four novel proteins) of *M. tuberculosis* induced during heat shock. The *M. tuberculosis* response to oxidative stress was relatively limited, resulting in the increased production of KatG (Rv1908c) (181) and a small number of other proteins (70). This was in contrast to the oxidative stress response observed in other bacteria and was consistent with the observation that in *M. tuberculosis* a regulatory gene involved in the oxidative response (*oxyR*) contains multiple inactivating mutations (54, 181). This led to the hypothesis that *M. tuberculosis* may have developed a constitutive oxidative stress response and that the thioredoxin-like protein AhpD (Rv2429), together with the enzymes SucB (Rv2215), Lpd (Rv0462), and AhpC (Rv2428), serves as an antioxidant defense in *M. tuberculosis* (36). The response of *M. tuberculosis* to different nitric oxide donors was also studied by Garbe et al. (71) by using 2-D gels, and induction of α-crystallin (Acr/Nox16/Rv2031c) and bacterioferritin (Nox19/BfrB/Rv3841) was reported. The completed genome and the extensive proteome maps available today would make an updated version of these early studies a useful and very timely endeavor.

M. tuberculosis is able to persist in a latent state for long periods under conditions characterized by low oxygen levels, low pH, and nutrient deprivation. A detailed characterization of the *M. tuberculosis* proteome under conditions which mimic latent infection is important for the understanding of the mechanism and dynamics of surviving persistent bacilli. Oxygen limitation is the most frequently used model of "dormant" TB, and the major molecule that accumulates under hypoxic conditions and in the stationary phase of *M. tuberculosis* cultures is the Acr protein (224). In two different studies of hypoxic growth of *M. bovis* BCG, six proteins (Acr, Rv2623, Rv2626c, Rv3133c, CysA2/CysA3 [Rv0815c/Rv3117], and Gap

[Rv1436]) were found to be upregulated (28, 67). Recently, *M. tuberculosis* was found to upregulate three of the same proteins (Acr, Rv2623, and Rv2626c) during oxygen limitation, but Fba (Rv0363c), Rv0569, Ald (Rv2780), and BfrB were also found to be induced in hypoxic cultures (164). These proteome-based studies complement the whole-genome microarray study of the hypoxic response in *M. tuberculosis*, in which the two-component response regulator pair Rv3133c-Rv3132c was identified as a genetic system that regulates Acr in response to hypoxia (182). Similarly, proteome analysis of an *M. bovis* BCG mutant lacking the Rv3133c gene demonstrated loss of induction of three previously identified dormancy proteins (Acr, Rv2623, and Rv2626c) (27). Another model for persistent *M. tuberculosis* is nutrient starvation, and in a combined proteome and microarray study, the response to starvation in phosphate-buffered saline buffer was characterized and a number of differentially expressed genes were identified (24). Interestingly, Acr and Ald (L-alanine dehydrogenase) production was increased in both the hypoxia and nutrient starvation studies, whereas induction of other gene products was specific to a single condition (24, 164, 182). Also, the influence of iron depletion has been studied for *M. tuberculosis*. When bacteria were cultured with low and high concentrations of iron, proteomic analyses identified 10 iron-regulated proteins (213). Among these were Fur (FurA/Rv1909c), aconitase (Acn/Rv1475c), and Acr. Both Fur and aconitase are regulated by iron in other bacteria and may therefore also function as transcriptional regulators in *M. tuberculosis*.

Proteins of importance for intracellular growth are best studied by analyzing the composition of the *M. tuberculosis* proteome during in vivo growth. So far, two proteome studies have attempted a comparison between mycobacterial proteins expressed in broth and in human THP-1 cells (114, 131). Using *M. bovis* BCG, six macrophage-induced proteins were identified, including Acr, Rv2623, and InhA (Rv1484) (131). However, a limitation of these studies is the presence of contaminating host proteins that decrease the resolution and detection of bacterial gene products. Thus, until new methods or technologies are introduced to overcome the problem of interfering host proteins, the use of in vitro systems that mimic specific aspects of in vivo growth will continue to provide the most useful information on the *M. tuberculosis* response to intracellular growth.

PROTEIN LOCALIZATION

One of the most important properties related to the function of a specific protein is its subcellular localization. Many of the early studies with *M. tuberculosis* proteins focused on polypeptides actively secreted or released by the cell during replication (221). However, most of this work was focused on defining the antigenicity of these proteins. Studies by Andersen et al. (8) later revealed that the protein profiles of culture filtrate from early- and late-stage cultures differed significantly, leading to the idea that *M. tuberculosis* generates a subset of actively secreted proteins and another group that is released from the cell wall during the growth process. In support of this idea, Wiker et al. (210) developed a quantitative localization index to differentiate between truly secreted proteins and those that are cell associated. Unlike these two approaches, which are based on actual observations with *M. tuberculosis* cultures, there are several bioinformatics methods for differentiating between exported and nonexported proteins. The most noted of these is SignalP (135), which is based on the ability to identify signal sequences associated with proteins translocated by the Sec-dependent system (see below). A second program, LocateProtein, also predicts exported proteins, but this neural network is trained on the entire sequence of known exported and secreted proteins (179). Using LocateProtein and a third program (ExProt) (167), it has been determined that approximately one-quarter of the proteins produced by *M. tuberculosis* are targeted for export or secretion (167, 179). While these programs are of significant value, they are limited in their abilities and do not define the precise extracytoplasmic location of proteins. Proteomic techniques are ideal for addressing this question and should be capable of providing a quantitative measure of protein localization. The majority of proteomic studies of *M. tuberculosis*, to date, have focused on proteins of the culture filtrate, cytosol, or whole-cell lysate. At present there are few studies that applied directed proteomic approaches to the cell wall proteins (165) and membrane proteins (80). The study of the *M. tuberculosis* cell wall fraction identified 413 protein spots by 2-D PAGE, 23 of which were identified at a molecular level. Interestingly, several of the cell wall-associated proteins were also observed in the culture filtrate or cytosol, but a distinct quantitative difference in the amounts of these proteins in the various subcellular fractions could be observed (Fig. 1) (165). The analysis of the membrane proteins relied on sodium dodecyl sulfate (SDS)-PAGE and the identification of multiple proteins in a single SDS-PAGE band by microcapillary high-performance liquid chromatography tandem MS and not on conventional proteomic techniques (80). In all, 739 proteins were identified in the membrane fraction; 85 of these were predicted to be transmembrane proteins and approximately 120 proteins were

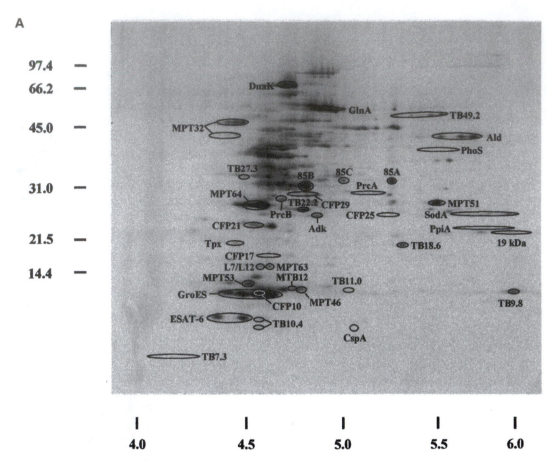

Figure 1. 2-D PAGE of the culture filtrate (A), cytosol (B), and cell wall (C) proteins of *M. tuberculosis* H37Rv. Reprinted from reference 165 with permission.

predicted to be membrane associated based on their predicted biochemical function. These two studies clearly demonstrate the power of proteomic techniques to define protein localization, but they also underscore the primary problem of subcellular-fraction mixing associated with the lysis of cells by mechanical means. Nevertheless, these types of approach, coupled with a quantitative index such as that implemented by Wiker et al. (210), should provide a wealth of information about protein localization in *M. tuberculosis*.

The continued definition of a specific protein's subcellular niche is important to defining protein function. This is particularly true for several of the cell wall and secreted proteins (such as glutamine synthetase [Rv2220], malate synthetase [Rv1837c], Ef-TU [Rv0685], and RplL [Rv0652] [85, 165, 185], which have known or predicted activities consistent with localization in the cytosol but do not contain canonical export motifs. For proteins such as these, there remains considerable debate about whether their unexpected identification in an extracytoplasmic location is an artifact of in vitro culture and sub-

cellular fractionation techniques or whether they play a dual role, such as was shown for the members of the Ag85 complex (17).

PROTEIN TRANSLOCATION AND SECRETION

In bacteria, proteins are localized to their extracytoplasmic compartments through active protein export systems that selectively translocate the appropriate proteins out of the cytoplasm. Because virulence factors and protective antigens are among the exported proteins of *M. tuberculosis*, the protein export systems of *M. tuberculosis* are important not only to the physiology of the bacillus but also to pathogenesis of disease. Given the unique structure of the mycobacterial cell envelope (discussed in chapters 17–19), novel protein export systems may be required to transport proteins into and across this "atypical" structure. Research into the protein export systems of mycobacteria has uncovered examples of both highly conserved export pathways and new systems.

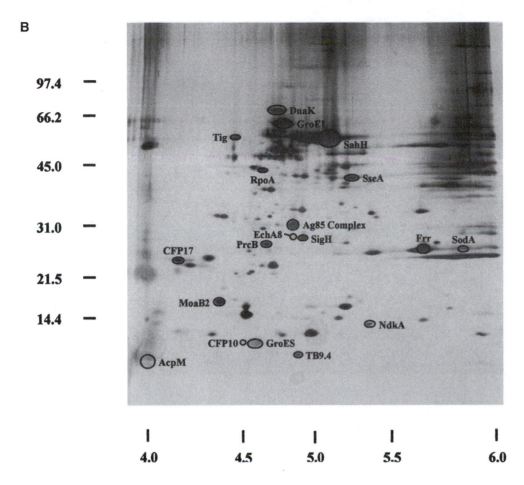

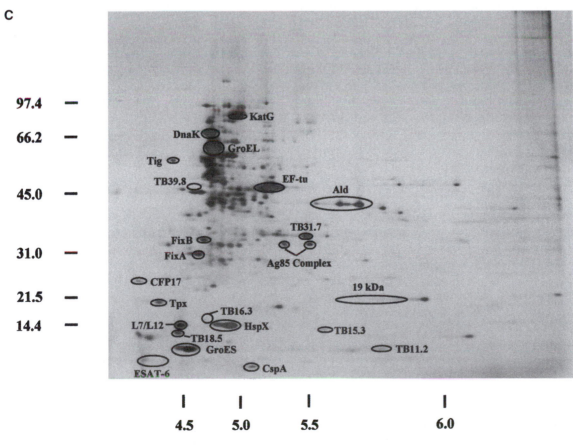

Figure 1. *Continued*

Sec Pathway

The Sec pathway is essential, highly conserved, and the primary pathway for protein transport across the cytoplasmic membrane of bacteria. Over two decades of study, primarily with *Escherichia coli*, has resulted in an advanced understanding of this pathway. Proteins transported by the Sec pathway are synthesized as precursors with a Sec signal sequence at their amino terminus. The Sec signal sequence is composed of a charged amino terminus, a hydrophobic core, and a polar region containing a site for cleavage by a signal peptidase (154). Sec precursor proteins are transported in an unfolded state through the core of the translocase, which is the membrane-embedded channel composed of SecY and SecE proteins (154). Shortly after or during translocation, the signal sequence is cleaved to generate the mature protein. The ultimate location of translocated Sec substrates is either the cell wall or complete release from the cell.

An essential component of the Sec pathway is the multifunctional SecA protein. SecA binds to precursor proteins, chaperones that deliver precursor to the translocase, acidic phospholipids in the membrane, and integral membrane components of the translocase (62). Furthermore, SecA is an ATPase that provides energy for protein translocation. Through cycles of ATP binding and hydrolysis, SecA delivers bound precursor proteins to the translocase and undergoes conformational changes that drive the stepwise export of the protein across the membrane (63). Energy from ATP hydrolysis is required to initiate translocation, and it alone is sufficient to carry out the process in vitro; however, the proton motive force can help drive protein export (176). SecG and the complex of SecD, SecF, and YajC are proteins that increase the efficiency of Sec-dependent export (61). The Sec pathway also participates in the delivery and insertion of integral membrane proteins. The bacterial signal recognition particle and the signal recognition particle receptor FtsY can target these proteins to the Sec translocase (200), and YidC appears to function in the stable integration of membrane proteins in the lipid bilayer (171).

M. tuberculosis has a functional Sec pathway. The genome sequence includes homologues of all the Sec pathway components, with the exception of SecB, a protein not found in all Sec systems (31, 43). In addition, there are examples of proven exported and secreted proteins of *M. tuberculosis* synthesized with consensus Sec signal sequences, and these signal sequences can promote the export of heterologous proteins in mycobacteria (34, 60, 117, 138, 211). Interestingly, Wiker et al. (211) noted that a high proportion of *M. tuberculosis* Sec translocated proteins possess a mature N terminus with an aspartic acid (D) in the +1 position and a proline (P) in the +2 position. The significance of this DP motif to mycobacterial protein export has yet to be tested.

So far, the only detailed analyses of Sec pathway components in mycobacteria have focused on the SecA proteins. The *M. tuberculosis* genome contains two *secA* homologues (*secA1* [Rv3240c] and *secA2* [Rv1821]), and this property seems to be shared by all *Mycobacterium* species, including the nonpathogenic *M. smegmatis*. This was surprising because studies of *secA* in diverse bacteria consistently identified a single and essential *secA* (178). More recently, additional examples of bacteria with multiple *secA* genes in their genome have been identified. All these new examples are gram-positive bacteria, and they include many pathogenic species (*Staphylococcus aureus*, *Streptococcus pneumoniae*, *Streptococcus gordonii*, *Listeria monocytogenes*, *Corynebacterium diphtheriae*, and *Bacillus anthracis*).

Both SecA1 and SecA2 of *M. tuberculosis* have significant amino acid similarity to other SecA homologues and contain the hallmark ATP-binding motifs. However, of the two proteins, SecA1 is more similar to SecA in other bacteria. The available data indicate that SecA1 is the primary housekeeping SecA and functions in a similar manner to the well-characterized SecA proteins of other bacteria. For example, *secA1* is essential in mycobacteria like *secA* in *E. coli*. This was directly shown for *M. smegmatis*, where the *secA1* gene cannot be deleted in a wild-type strain but can be deleted in a recombinant merodiploid strain (32). In *M. tuberculosis*, *secA1* also appears to be a gene that cannot be disrupted, as indicated by transposon site hybridization (174). Furthermore, it was shown that the N-terminal region of SecA1 can substitute for the corresponding region of *E. coli* SecA to complement an *E. coli secA51*(Ts) mutant (142).

SecA2

Unlike *secA1*, *secA2* of mycobacteria is nonessential, as revealed by the successful construction of *secA2* deletion mutants of *M. smegmatis* and *M. tuberculosis* (32, 33). Two different approaches demonstrated that the nonessential SecA2 functions in protein export in mycobacteria. First, it was shown that the Δ*secA2* mutant of *M. smegmatis* has a partial defect in exporting certain PhoA fusion proteins (32). Because the PhoA fusion proteins tested contained recognizable Sec signal sequences, these data suggest that SecA2 assists SecA1 in the translocation of proteins with consensus Sec signal sequences. However, not all exported PhoA fusion proteins were affected in the Δ*secA2* mutant, thus indicating a degree of substrate specificity that is not currently understood. In a second approach, the culture filtrate proteins secreted into media by wild-type and a Δ*secA2* mutant strain of *M. tuberculosis* were compared by proteomic methods (2-D PAGE and MS), and a small number of proteins whose release depends on *secA2* were identified (33). Because these proteins lack Sec signal sequences, it suggests a second role for SecA2 in the nonconventional export of a specific subset of proteins. The 2-D PAGE analysis also identified three proteins apparently upregulated in the *M. tuberculosis* Δ*secA2* mutant, the basis of which remains to be established. The comparative analysis was limited to the secreted protein fractions. It is likely that additional substrates localized to other extracytoplasmic fractions, such as the cell wall, also depend on SecA2 for export and will be identified as this system is fully elucidated.

One of the proteins released into the medium in a SecA2-dependent fashion was SodA (superoxide dismutase A [Rv3846] (33). Multiple laboratories had previously identified SodA in the culture media of growing *M. tuberculosis* (2, 8, 86, 158, 186, 198, 227). Because SodA lacks a recognizable Sec signal sequence, it was long debated whether release was attributable to a specific secretion mechanism or autolysis. Given that the release of endogenous SodA, expressed from its chromosomal locus, has now been demonstrated to depend on the accessory secretion factor SecA2, it appears that SodA is secreted by an unconventional protein export pathway.

Much work remains to characterize the mechanistic basis of SecA2-dependent secretion. Proteins that work with SecA2 in export are undefined, as is the mechanism for substrate recognition and targeting to SecA2. The virulence of the Δ*secA2* mutant of *M. tuberculosis* is attenuated in the mouse model of infection. This indicates that some SecA2-dependent proteins are exported virulence factors (33). The hypothesis promoting SecA2 as a newly identified strategy of some bacterial pathogens to localize virulence factors is further supported by findings that SecA2 of *L. monocytogenes* contributes to virulence and SecA2 of *S. gordonii* exports an adhesin (19, 115).

Twin-Arginine Translocation (Tat) Pathway

The twin-arginine translocation (Tat) pathway is a relatively recent discovery in bacteria, and our understanding of the mechanics of the process is limited. Like the Sec pathway, the Tat system transports proteins across the cytoplasmic membrane, and Tat substrates are synthesized as precursors with an N-terminal signal sequence that resembles a Sec signal sequence. However, the similarities between the Sec and Tat pathways end there. A Tat signal sequence is distinguished by the hallmark "twin-arginine" motif, which directs the precursor to the Tat pathway: (S/T)-R-R-X-#-# (# = hydrophobic residue). Site-directed mutagenesis experiments indicate that the twin arginines play an important role in export since simultaneous replacement of both with conservative lysine substitutions eliminates the export of numerous Tat substrates (52, 188, 214). Another distinctive feature of the Tat pathway is that the precursor protein can be exported in a fully folded state, with some substrates bound to cofactors and others being multimeric complexes (161, 172, 173, 206).

The Tat pathway operates independently of the Sec pathway (173) and requires a minimum of two structural components, both of which are predicted membrane proteins, TatA and TatC (55, 216). Some bacteria additionally contain TatB and TatE proteins, which are structurally similar to and share homology with TatA. The protein sequence of Tat factors is largely uninformative in deducing function. The energy source for Tat export also distinguishes it from the Sec pathway in being exclusively the proton motive force.

Based on genomic analysis, the Tat pathway appears to be present in mycobacteria. *M. tuberculosis* genes encoding homologues of TatA (Rv2094c), TatC (Rv2093c), and a less convincing TatB (Rv1224) are present in the genome (43, 55, 216). Consistent with these Tat homologues in *M. tuberculosis*, the TATFIND program, a Tat substrate recognition program based on published Tat signal sequences, identified potential Tat substrates in *M. tuberculosis* (31 substrates in the H37Rv strain, and 29 in CDC 1551) (55). Candidate Tat substrates include phospholipase C (Rv2439c), which is localized to the cell wall and contributes to the virulence of *M. tuberculosis* (159). A role for the Tat pathway in *M. tuberculosis* pathogenesis has not been tested, but a role in virulence was demonstrated in *Pseudomonas aeruginosa*, enterohemorrhagic *E. coli*, and *Agrobacterium tumefaciens* (57, 137, 152). Interestingly, recent experiments suggest that the Tat pathway in mycobacteria is essential, which is unlike the case in other bacteria studied so far. The *tatC* gene in *M. tuberculosis* appears to be essential for optimal growth, as shown by transposon site hybridization (174).

ESAT-6 Secretion

In 1995, a small highly immunogenic protein (ESAT-6 [Rv3875], secreted by *M. tuberculosis* was identified (7, 187), and it has since received much attention as a diagnostic and vaccine candidate (29, 157). The attenuated *M. bovis* BCG strains lack the

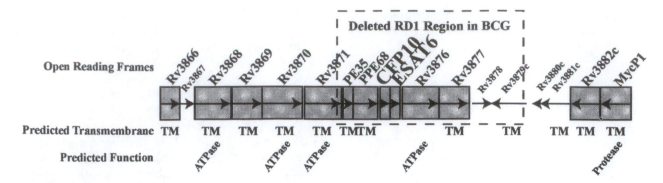

Figure 2. Schematic of the conserved ESAT-6 cluster region 1 of *M. tuberculosis* H37Rv. ORFs are depicted as black arrows showing the direction of transcription. The conserved genes in the cluster are boxed. The names of each ORF are listed above the diagram. Predicted transmembrane domains were identified with the Tmpred prediction software (94).

esat6 gene due to its location within RD1, a region of the *M. tuberculosis* and *M. bovis* chromosome that is deleted in BCG (spanning genes *rv3871* to *rv3879c*) (84, 121) (see Fig. 2). Furthermore, RD1 and ESAT-6 specifically were shown by multiple research groups to contribute to the virulence of *M. tuberculosis* and *M. bovis* (81, 96, 116, 155, 175, 189, 205).

The genome sequence revealed that *M. tuberculosis* contains a family of ESAT-6-like proteins (22 members in *M. tuberculosis*), and genomic analysis recently defined a superfamily of ESAT-6/WXG100 proteins in mycobacteria and some gram-positive bacteria (74, 143, 193). Although the overall sequence similarity can be low, ESAT-6/WXG100 superfamily members exhibit strong conservation around a WXG motif, small size (approximately 100 amino acids), and clustering with homologous genes. In *M. tuberculosis*, genes encoding ESAT-6 like proteins are generally found as pairs. This is true for *esat6* in RD1, which is located in an operon with a gene encoding another family member, *cfp10* (also referred to as *rv3874*, *esxB*, and *lhp*).

ESAT-6 is classified as a secreted protein on the basis of its being released by *M. tuberculosis* after short periods of growth and in the absence of obvious autolysis; however, it should be noted that it has also been reported to be associated with the cell wall (7, 8, 156, 165, 187). ESAT-6 lacks a recognizable Sec signal sequence; consequently, the responsible export mechanism was not immediately obvious. It is likely that most ESAT-6 family members are secreted since there are other examples of these proteins (CFP-10 and Rv0288) being secreted by *M. tuberculosis*, again in the absence of Sec signal sequences (21, 184).

Analysis of the genes adjacent to *esat6* was the first step toward understanding ESAT-6 secretion. In general, a secretion system requires a protein channel through which the substrate travels and energy to drive the process. Genes encoding components of a

specialized secretion system are often clustered in the genome with the genes encoding the secreted substrates. It was proposed early on that the genes adjacent to *esat6* participate in the secretion process (43). In *M. tuberculosis*, there are homologous genes clustered around *esat6* family members, and the largest clusters of conserved genes have been defined as ESAT-6 cluster regions 1 to 5 (74, 193). RD1 and *esat6* are located in cluster region 1, which spans genes *rv3866* to *rv3883c* (Fig. 2). Many of the conserved genes in the cluster encode membrane proteins, nucleotide-binding proteins, and ATPases. Of note is one conserved ORF which encodes a predicted membrane-bound ATPase that is homologous to YukA of *Bacillus subtilis*. In every bacterium with *esat6* family members, examples of clustering with *yukA* homologues is found (143). This strong conservation in genomic organization suggests that YukA provides energy for the secretion process. In some ESAT-6 cluster regions, this homologue is encoded by one large gene; however, in cluster region 1, the motifs of the homologue are split among two smaller adjacent genes (*rv3870* and *rv3871*).

Complementary approaches have begun to identify the genes in the conserved cluster required for ESAT-6 secretion. Starting with BCG, which, due to the RD1 deletion, does not express ESAT-6, Pym et al. (156) reintroduced missing genes to identify those required for secretion of ESAT-6 and CFP-10. The introduction of plasmids expressing only transcriptional fusions of *esat6* or *cfp10* into BCG leads to production of the respective proteins, but they remain cytoplasmic and are not secreted into the culture medium (13, 156). This indicates that BCG lacks not only ESAT-6 but also the system for secreting it. Testing different "knock-in" constructs that carry the *esat6* and *cfp10* genes, along with additional upstream or downstream genes, revealed that several genes upstream of *rv3872* (PE35) and at least one gene downstream of *esat6* are required for the secretion process (156) (Fig. 2). Strong candidates for the products of the ORFs involved are Rv3871 (YukA homologue), Rv3876, (putative membrane ATPase), and/or Rv3877 (predicted polytopic membrane protein). The opposite approach of disrupting or deleting genes in RD1 in *M. tuberculosis* has further defined the genes required. This analysis showed that Rv3870, Rv3871, and Rv3877 are specifically required for secretion of ESAT-6 and CFP-10 (81, 96, 189). A role for Rv3876 is also likely, but it may be less critical to the process than are the other proteins (81). *M. tuberculosis* mutants lacking these proteins are also attenuated for virulence. This implies that ESAT-6 must be secreted to function in pathogenesis. It remains a possibility that the contribution of this secretion system to pathogenesis extends beyond ESAT-6 and includes the secretion of additional virulence factors. Proteomic experiments to compare the culture filtrate proteins secreted by one of the above-described *M. tuberculosis* mutants defective in ESAT-6 export with wild-type *M. tuberculosis* will serve to address the issue of whether additional substrates are secreted by this new system.

Although there has been progress in identifying some of the genes required for ESAT-6 secretion, the mechanistic basis of the secretion machinery remains unknown. Protein interactions among system components are just starting to be identified. ESAT-6 and CFP-10 physically interact and form a stable 1:1 complex (160, 189). Whether this complex is important for secretion, stability and/or function remains to be resolved. Rv3870 and Rv3871 interact, as shown by the yeast two-hybrid system (160, 189), and this is consistent with each of these proteins representing a functional domain of YukA. Furthermore, the yeast two-hybrid system identified the C terminus of Rv3871 as being capable of binding to CFP-10 (160, 189). This latter interaction connects a component of the secretion apparatus with a secreted substrate and represents an important step toward understanding the secretion mechanism.

These recent experiments all help us to understand the ESAT-6 secretion system, but many basic questions remain unanswered. What is the minimal complement of the ESAT-6 secretion system? What are the functions of the conserved components? Is there cross talk between the multiple ESAT-6 clusters? How are proteins targeted to this system? Finally, what are the substrates of the system? If ESAT-6 is the primary secreted substrate, then it must perform a function common to many different bacteria. An alternative possibility is that ESAT-6 is a conserved component of the secretion apparatus and might be secreted during the assembly of the secretion machine,

or an extracellular location may be required for ESAT-6 function, perhaps as a regulator that triggers secretion in the appropriate environment. This alternative is consistent with other types of specialized secretion systems in bacteria, where there are examples of secreted components of the machinery and where the components of the secretion apparatus tend to be more highly conserved than the substrates themselves (150).

POSTTRANSLATIONAL MODIFICATIONS

Annotation of the genome and 2-D PAGE analyses provides a rough template of proteome function and composition. However, the full complexity of the proteome includes posttranslational modifications such as acylation, phosphorylation, glycosylation, methylation, and acetylation. In some cases, bioinformatic interrogation of protein sequences provides strong evidence for potential modifications, such as acylation or phosphorylation, but other modifications, such as O glycosylation, are more difficult to predict due to the lack of defined consensus sequences. Application of proteomic techniques to the global identification of posttranslational modifications in *M. tuberculosis* has yet to be undertaken and is warranted in the coming phase of *M. tuberculosis* proteome research.

Protein Phosphorylation

Phosphorylation and dephosphorylation of proteins is universally used as an intracellular signaling mechanism and for regulation of protein function. The most commonly recognized of the bacterial phosphoproteins are those of the two-component regulatory modules (190). At its most basic level, a two-component regulatory module is composed of a sensor kinase, which is generally a transmembrane protein, and a response regulator. The sensor kinase detects an environmental signal on the outside of the cytoplasmic membrane and transmits this signal through conformational change, allowing for autophosphorylation of a His residue in the N-terminal cytosolic domain of the sensor kinase. In turn, the phosphate is donated by the sensor kinase to an Asp residue of the response regulator. Phosphorylation of the response regulator activates this protein to bind with specific DNA sequences or other proteins to modulate gene expression or protein function. The N-terminal and C-terminal regions of sensor kinases and response regulators, respectively, are highly conserved. Thus, they are easily identified, and their sites of phosphorylation can be determined via homology comparisons.

Table 1. Known phosphorylated proteins of *M. tuberculosis*

Protein	Function	Reference(s)
DevR (Rv3133c)[a]	Response regulator	144
MprB (Rv0982)[b]	Sensor kinase	225
MprA (Rv0981)[a]	Response regulator	225
TrcS (Rv1032c)[b]	Sensor kinase	88
TrcR (Rv1033c)[a]	Response regulator	88
MtrA (Rv3246c)[b]	Response regulator	203
PknB (Rv0014c)[c, d]	Ser/Thr kinase	10, 223
PknA (Rv0015c)[c]	Ser/Thr kinase	38
PknD (Rv0931c)[c]	Ser/Thr kinase	145
PknE (Rv1743)[c]	Ser/Thr kinase	129
PknF (Rv1746)[c]	Ser/Thr kinase	109
PknG (Rv0410c)[c]	Ser/Thr kinase	109
Ndk (Rv2445c)	Secreted diphosphate nucleotide kinase	39

[a]Phosphorylation presumed to be on a conserved Asp residue.
[b]Phosphorylation presumed to be on a conserved His residue.
[c]Phosphorylation of Thr and Ser residues shown.
[d]Actual sites of phosphorylation defined.

In all, 15 sensor kinases and 15 response regulators are encoded by the *M. tuberculosis* genome (43). These form 11 histidine kinase-response regulator pairs and several unpaired sensor kinases and response regulators (Table 1). In comparison to *E. coli* and *B. subtilis*, *M. tuberculosis* encodes a relatively small number of two-component regulatory modules (43). It has been argued that the scarcity of these regulatory elements may be compensated for by the presence of several Ser/Thr kinases (see below). However, an alternative hypothesis is that the small number of two-component regulatory proteins is a reflection of the narrow biological niche of *M. tuberculosis*.

Studies associated with the two-component regulatory proteins of *M. tuberculosis* have been largely conducted at a genetic level and have identified putative regulatory functions for several of these modules (discussed in chapter 22). In contrast, there are a limited number of studies evaluating the actual proteins of these *M. tuberculosis* regulatory modules. The best studied of these is DevR (Rv3133c), a response regulator responsible for the phenotypic response of *M. tuberculosis* to hypoxia (144, 182). Recently, a DNA consensus sequence bound by DevR (note that in this study DevR is called DosR) and located upstream of a large number of hypoxia-induced genes was identified (144). Binding of DevR to this consensus sequence was inhibited by introducing a point mutation (Asp54-Glu) at the putative phosphorylation site of this response regulator protein. These data clearly demonstrate the involvement of DevR and protein phosphorylation in the regulatory response to hypoxia. However, the apparent nonparticipation by the corresponding sensor kinase (DevS [Rv3132c]) is unexpected (182). Thus, DevR may be interacting with multiple sensor kinases, potentially explaining why nearly identical gene expression patterns are produced by exposure of *M. tuberculosis* to hypoxia and nitric oxide (139, 204).

Other proteins of *M. tuberculosis* two-component regulatory modules have also been assessed for their ability to act as phosphate acceptors (Table 1). Using recombinant proteins, MprA and MprB were shown to be a true signal-transducing pair with autophosphorylation of MprB and subsequent transfer of the phosphate to MprA (225). Similarly, a truncated form of TrcS containing only the C-terminal domain was shown to undergo autophosphorylation and transfer of the phosphate to TrcR (Rv1033c) (88). The response regulator MtrA was shown to be phosphorylated in an in vitro system that used the *E. coli* CheA sensor kinase as the phosphate donor (203).

Proteomic analyses coupled with metabolic labeling would seem to be a likely method to assess the global production and phosphorylation of two-component regulatory systems. However, a phosphoramidate modification of a sensor kinase possesses a free energy of −14 kcal/mol (191). Therefore, dephosphorylation of the modified His residue rapidly occurs via hydrolysis in an aqueous solution. Although slightly more stable based on free-energy values, the acylphosphate modification of an Asp residue in a response regulator may also undergo hydrolysis or be dephosphorylated by a specific phosphatase (191). This instability of phosphate modifications on the sensor kinases and response regulators creates a major impediment to studying two-component regulatory modules on a proteomic scale. Nevertheless, proteomics is a valid means of assessing mutants of two-component regulatory proteins and identifying proteins that are regulated via these mechanisms.

A second group of phosphorylated regulatory molecules are Ser/Thr kinases, once thought to be specific for eukaryotes (104). However, prokaryotic genomics proves that Ser/Thr kinases and Tyr kinases are not restricted to eukaryotes (149). Eleven Ser/Thr protein kinases and no Tyr protein kinases are encoded by *M. tuberculosis* (43). *M. leprae*, with its minimal genome, encodes four orthologues and has pseudogenes of four others (44). Like the two-component regulatory proteins, several Ser/Thr kinases of *M. tuberculosis* are demonstrated to undergo phosphate modification (Table 1).

The most widely studied of the *M. tuberculosis* Ser/Thr protein kinases is PknB (Rv0014c). Initially, autophosphorylation on both Ser and Thr residues was demonstrated (10), but more detailed structural studies defined six sites of phosphorylation on PknB (223), four in the Ser/Thr kinase domain and two in the linker region between the Ser/Thr kinase domain and the transmembrane domain. PknB possesses a C-terminal extracytoplasmic domain, similar to the targeting domain of the *Streptococcus pneumoniae* penicillin-binding protein 2x (223), designated the penicillin-binding protein and Ser/Thr kinase attachment (PASTA) domain (215). This suggests a role for PknB in the regulation of *M. tuberculosis* cell wall biosynthesis. Further analyses of the potential mechanism of regulation employed by PknB demonstrate that the phosphate esters of Thr171 and Thr173 are targets of the protein phosphatase PstP (Rv0018c) and that site-directed mutagenesis of these two residues significantly decreases the kinase activity of PknB (26), thus indicating their critical role in the regulatory activity of PknB.

The other Ser/Thr protein kinases previously assessed include PknA (Rv0015c), PknD (Rv0931c), PknE (Rv1743), PknF (Rv1746), and PknG (Rv0410c) (38, 109, 129, 145, 146). Recombinant PknA autophosphorylates at Ser and Thr residues and catalyzes phosphotransfer to myelin basic protein and histones, and when overexpressed in *E. coli,* PknA induces the elongation of *E. coli* cells (38). However, in *M. tuberculosis,* an association of PknA with cell division has yet to be demonstrated. PknD was the first Ser/Thr protein kinase to be identified in *M. tuberculosis,* with its corresponding gene located within the *pst* gene cluster (145), and the recombinant enzyme has been characterized. PknD is localized in the cytoplasmic membrane of *M. tuberculosis,* and in several *M. bovis* strains the *pknD* gene has a point mutation resulting in a truncated cytoplasmic protein with the kinase domain (146). However, it is unknown whether this change in subcellular location alters the function of PknD. PknE, PknF, and PknG were also shown to autophosphorylate Ser and Thr residues (109, 129). PknF is a transmembrane protein, and PknG is located in the cytosol. The *M. tuberculosis* genome sequence does not encode putative Tyr protein kinases. This is in contrast to a pregenome sequence report of a 55-kDa *M. tuberculosis* protein that reacted to an antiphosphotyrosine antibody (41). Conformation of phosphotyrosine activity in *M. tuberculosis* or molecular identification of this 55-kDa protein has not been reported. However, the tubercle bacillus does encode two Tyr protein phosphatases (MptpA [Rv2234] and MptpB [Rv0153c]) that are reported to be secreted and directly involved in host-pathogen interactions (108, 183). This is in contrast to the single Ser/Thr phosphatase (PstP) that is membrane bound and proposed to function in the regulatory processes of the Ser/Thr kinases (26, 40).

Beyond the two-component regulatory modules and the Ser/Thr protein kinases, it is likely that *M. tuberculosis* contains many more phosphorylated pro-

teins. In fact, a secreted diphosphate nucleotide kinase (Ndk [Rv2445c]) that is proposed to act as a cytotoxic factor for host cells was found to autophosphorylate (39), and indirect evidence suggests the phosphorylation of an anti-anti-sigma factor (Rv3687c) similar to those observed in *B. subtilis* (14). There are multiple bacterial processes such as catabolite repression in both gram-negative and gram-positive bacteria that are modulated via protein phosphorylation (14). Moreover, recent proteomic studies with *Corynebacterium glutamicum* revealed 59 protein spots that were metabolically labeled with ^{33}P and approximately 90 protein spots that reacted to antiphosphoserine or antiphosphothreonine antibodies (18). Interestingly, the majority of these phosphorylated *C. glutamicum* proteins were identified as metabolic enzymes, not regulatory proteins. Thus, it is likely that protein phosphorylation plays a much broader role in bacterial physiology than was previously realized.

Protein Acylation

The association of bacterial proteins with membrane structures is achieved through hydrophobic domains or N-terminal acylation. The N-terminally acylated bacterial lipoproteins have a highly conserved structure, with an N-terminal Cys residue modified by a diacylglycerol moiety bound through a thioether linkage and a third acyl function attached to the α-amine via an amide bond (30) (Fig. 3). In other bacterial species, the phospholipid pool serves as the fatty acid donor for lipoprotein synthesis (16, 99). Thus, the composition of a lipoprotein's fatty acids mimics that of the organism's phospholipids. Although

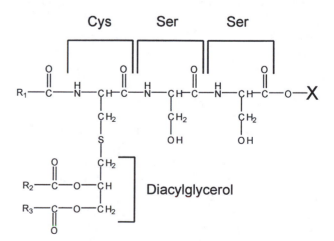

Figure 3. Triacylated Cys residue of the mature N terminus of the *M. tuberculosis* 19-kDa lipoprotein (LpqH [Rv3763]). R$_1$, R$_2$, and R$_3$ indicate palmitic acid, palmitoleic acid, oleic acid, or tuberculostearic acid; with the acylation at each site presumably being heterogeneous.

this is not proven for the lipoproteins of *M. tuberculosis*, it is presumed that the lipoprotein fatty acids are the same as those associated with the phospholipids: palmitic acid, palmitoleic acid, oleic acid, and tuberculostearic acid (77). Prolipoproteins are translocated across the cytoplasmic membrane via the Sec translocation machinery, and release of the signal peptide via signal peptidase II provides the N-terminal Cys residue of the mature protein (30). The conserved N-terminal signal peptide, with its signal peptidase recognition and cleavage site followed by a Cys residue, provides a motif for the easy identification of bacterial lipoproteins. Annotation of the *M. tuberculosis* genome identified 89 genes encoding proteins with a "prokaryotic membrane lipoprotein lipid attachment site" (Prosite entry PS00013) (43). Although mycobacterial lipoproteins are observed in several proteomic studies, to date there is only a single study that has directly targeted the *M. tuberculosis* lipoproteins on a proteomic scale. This work, conducted by Young and Garbe (220) well before the sequencing of the *M. tuberculosis* genome, utilized metabolic labeling with [^{3}H]palmitate, enrichment of membrane proteins by Triton X-114 biphase partitioning, and 2-D PAGE. This analysis allowed the visualization of five [^{3}H]palmitate-labeled protein spots. Two proteins reacted with antibodies that identified them as the 38-kDa antigen (PstS1 [Rv0934]) and the 19-kDa lipoprotein antigen (LpqH [Rv3763]). The remaining spots migrated with molecular masses of 26, 27, and 65 kDa and were not identified at a molecular level. The paucity of lipoproteins observed, in comparison to the number of putative lipoproteins encoded by the genome, is most probably a result of the difficulty associated with solubilization and isoelectric focusing of these proteins rather than a reflection of gene expression. Improved solubilization techniques for membrane proteins (90, 113) and the use of immobilized pH gradient strips for isoelectric focusing (78) or non-gel-based proteomic techniques (68) should help to uncover the true population of lipoproteins produced by *M. tuberculosis*.

The function of protein acylation in bacteria is thought to be largely structural and one of localization. In gram-negative bacteria, lipoproteins can be localized to the inner or outer membrane depending on the amino acids at positions 2 and 3 of the mature protein and the Lol system responsible for lipoprotein release from the inner membrane (194). In gram-positive bacteria, lipoproteins are found in the outer leaflet of the cytoplasmic membrane (30, 192). The role of acylation as a localization mechanism is underscored when comparing gram-negative and gram-positive organisms where homologues of nonlipidated periplasmic gram-negative proteins are acylated in gram-positive organisms to ensure localization to the outer surface of the cytoplasmic membrane in the absence of a periplasmic space (134). The exact localization of lipoproteins in *M. tuberculosis* is unknown, but some, such as Pst1 (a protein involved in phosphate transport), would be predicted to be associated with the cytoplasmic membrane based on their function. However, it is likely that other lipoproteins are associated with the outer lipid layer of the cell wall.

Bacterial lipoproteins are well known for their immunomodulatory activity (22, 53, 87, 128). The best-studied *M. tuberculosis* lipoproteins (PstS1, the 19-kDa lipoprotein, and P27 [Rv1411c]) are dominant immunogens, consistent with early studies demonstrating that recombinant acylation of proteins increases their immunogenicity (22, 53). More recently, the immunomodulatory activity of mycobacterial lipoproteins was discovered to be an outcome of their interaction with Toll-like receptor 2 (TLR 2) of host cells. Lipoprotein-TLR2 interaction induces interleukin-12 production and bactericidal activity (195, 196) or down-regulation of major histocompatibility complex expression and antigen processing (73, 136, 197). This later activity of immune down-regulation potentially explains why overexpression of the recombinant 19-kDa lipoprotein in *M. vaccae* or *M. smegmatis* and vaccination with these recombinants exacerbated subsequent infection with virulent *M. tuberculosis* (217). The dichotomy associated with the immunomodulatory activities of mycobacterial lipoproteins is probably a property of how the antigen is presented and the time of interaction with TLR2, not of the structural differences of the proteins evaluated.

Protein Glycosylation

The modification of proteins with glycosyl residues is well known to occur in eukaryotic organisms, where differential glycosylation has a significant impact on protein function (119). Glycoproteins, in particular the proteins comprising the outer crystalline coat (S-layer), are also well described in the archaea (20). Over the last decade, it has become apparent that a wide array of eubacteria also produce glycoproteins, but in comparison to eukaryotes, a bacterium glycosylates a relatively small percentage of its proteome (20). Early lectin-binding studies with the culture filtrate proteins of *M. tuberculosis* suggested that the 38-kDa antigen 5 (PstS1), the 19-kDa lipoprotein, and a 55- to 50-kDa complex (Apa [MPT32, Rv1860]) were glycosylated (49, 64–66). However, other analyses of these purified glycoproteins indicated that lectin binding was due to nonspecific contamination of the proteins by cell wall glycoconjugates such as lipoarabinomannan or lipoman-nan (48). The work of Dobos et al. (58, 59) provided definitive chemical proof by MS and N-terminal sequencing that the Apa (MPT32) secreted protein was indeed O glycosylated on Thr residues with mannose, mannobiose, and mannotriose. A similar study with the MPB83 antigen (Rv2873) of *M. bovis* also demonstrated O mannosylation of Thr residues (127). However, the linkage of the mannose units within the oligosaccharides was (1 → 3) and not (1 → 2) as observed with MPT32. For the 19-kDa lipoprotein, a combination of site-directed mutagenesis and lectin binding was used to demonstrate glycosylation, but the nature and precise location of the glycosylation modification remain to be identified (92). More recently, top-down proteomic approaches using electrospray ionization Fourier transform MS on culture filtrate proteins of *M. tuberculosis* separated by concanavalin A (ConA) affinity chromatography yielded a 9-kDa product with 7 hexose residues and two 20-kDa products with 20 hexose residues each, but the molecular identity of these three products was not determined (72).

Unlike sites of N glycosylation, there is no consensus sequence for O glycosylation; however, general structural features are proposed (76). An alignment of the known glycosylation sites of Apa and MPB83 indicates a significant degree of similarity (Fig. 4). Specifically, all the glycosylation sites are in Pro-, Ala-, Thr-, and Ser-rich domains, and the glycosylated Thr residues are 1 or 2 amino acids downstream of a Pro residue. Two Ala residues are located within 1 to 2 amino acids downstream of the first and second glycosylation sites of Apa as well as the glycosylation site of MPB83. Interestingly, the putative glycosylation sites of the 19-kDa lipoprotein are in an Ala- and Thr-rich region, but no Pro residues are present. Efforts to define an O glycosylation motif for eukaryotes led to the development of a neural network (NetOglyc) to predict potential sites of O glycosylation (83). Using this neural network, Herrmann et al. (91) identified 35 *M. tuberculosis* lipoproteins with at least two putative O glycosylation sites within the first 30 amino acids of the mature protein sequence. Several of these protein sequences were expressed in a *phoA* fusion cassette in *M. smegmatis*, and the resulting fusion proteins were tested for reactivity with ConA. Of the 11 sequences tested, 7 (19 kDa, PstS1, LppN [Rv2270], LppQ [Rv2341], MPT83 [Rv2873], SodC [Rv0432], and GlnH [Rv0411c]) yielded strong ConA reactivity. Although these studies did not confirm glycosylation of native proteins, the fact that three known glycosylated lipoproteins (19 kDa, PstS1, and MBT83) were identified argues that the use of predictive neural networks and recombinant fusion products is an effective method to screen for the glycoproteins of *M. tuberculosis*. These data also suggest that protein glycosylation in *M. tuberculosis* may be more prevalent than was originally thought and that high-throughput proteomic systems will aid in identifying proteins with this form of post-translational modification.

In eukaryotes, the glycosylation of proteins provides many functions including antigen recognition, receptor binding, regulation of protein activity, and protection from proteolysis (101, 119). While the importance of protein glycosylation in bacterial systems is not yet fully appreciated, there are specific examples of this type of modification affecting enzymatic activity, pathogen-host cell interactions, antigen recognition, and protein stability (177). During the analysis of putative glycosylation domains of the 19-kDa lipoprotein produced as a recombinant form in *M. smegmatis*, several point mutations were introduced at Thr residues suspected of being O glycosylated (92). These mutations not only decreased the ConA-binding activity of the recombinant 19-kDa lipoprotein but also resulted in the proteolytic cleavage of the protein. Thus, at least for this one mycobacterial protein, glycosylation may serve to prevent proteolytic digestion. Protein glycosylation in *M. tuberculosis* may also play an important role in antigen recognition, as was demonstrated using recombinant and native forms of the Apa (MPT32) glycoprotein to assess T-cell recognition and skin test reactivity (95, 162).

Protein	Glycopeptide	Position
Apa glycosylation site 1	P P V P [T] T A A S	6–14
Apa glycosylation site 2	S P P S [T] A A A P	14–22
Apa glycosylation site 3	P A P A [T] P V A P	22–31
Apa glycosylation site 4	P T P T [T] P T P Q	273–281
MPB83 glycosylation site	A A P V [T T] A A M A	20–29

Figure 4. Alignment of the glycosylation sites of Apa (Rv1860) and MBP83 (Rv2873). "Position" indicates the location of the peptide shown in the mature protein sequence.

Other Forms of Posttranslational Modifications

Beyond the posttranslational modifications discussed above, there remain a large number of modifications that are associated primarily with eukaryotic proteomes such as prenylation (166), acetylation (110), methylation (112), nitrosylation (98), and glycation (218). Although significant data for these modifications are lacking for prokaryotic systems, it is not safe to simply assume their absence in *M. tuberculosis*. For example, there is a recent report of protein methylation in *M. tuberculosis*. A comparison of recombinant and native forms of the heparin-binding hemagglutinin adhesin (HBHA) protein (Rv0475) by MS indicated a molecular mass difference originally thought to be due to the presence of two hexose residues covalently bound to the native HBHA (125). The difference in the molecular mass was localized to a 50-amino-acid Lys-rich C-terminal domain of HBHA and found to be a result not of glycosylation but of modification of 13 Lys residues with up to 26 methyl groups, with each Lys being mono- or dimethylated (148). Except for eukaryotic histone proteins, where methylation appears to regulate the interaction of this protein with nucleic acids (112), the role of protein methylation is relatively unknown. The C-terminal domain is responsible for the attachment of HBHA to host cells (126), and methylation of this protein appears to prevent proteolytic degradation by the proteases of bronchoalveolar lavage fluids (148). Thus, given the cell surface location of HBHA and its biological activity, protein methylation may prove to be an important function in regulating the interaction of *M. tuberculosis* with host cells.

PROTEOMIC IDENTIFICATION OF DIAGNOSTIC AND VACCINE CANDIDATES

T-Cell Antigens

The protective immune response to tuberculosis is mediated by T cells rather than B cells, and both the current vaccine (*M. bovis* BCG) and the diagnostic reagent PPD target the T-cell response (45, 69). This fundamental concept has had a profound influence on antigen discovery programs, since the identification of T-cell antigens relies on the in vitro stimulation of T cells with antigen preparations and the subsequent monitoring of cellular proliferation, activation, or cytokine release. Therefore, each protein to be investigated (native or recombinant) has to be purified, and after the last purification step, the protein needs to be in a buffer compatible with cellular assays. Early T-cell antigen discovery efforts were relatively random and focused on the more abundant and easily purified pro-

teins, such as Ag85 and MPT64 (Rv1980c) (133). The first attempts to systematically analyze the T-cell antigens in complex mixtures were performed by a T-cell Western blot method in which proteins separated by SDS-PAGE were transferred to nitrocellulose, which was subsequently cut into strips and added to cell cultures (1, 222). However, this method suffered from the uncontrolled influence of nitrocellulose particles on cell culture viability and the inability to quantify the protein content in each fraction. Realizing the limitations of earlier approaches, Andersen and Heron (9) developed a multielution method in which short-term culture filtrate (ST-CF) was separated into narrow-molecular-mass fractions by preparative SDS-PAGE and electroelution, leading to nontoxic protein fractions that did not contain SDS and were compatible with cellular assays. A 2-D application of this method was also attempted, although low yields made the subsequent identification of reactive fractions very difficult (82). The multielution method was used in several studies with mice, cattle, and humans (7, 9, 25, 151). The results of these studies all pointed to two highly reactive regions of the ST-CF filtrate, those at 5 to 12 kDa and 25 to 36 kDa. A detailed study of the low-molecular-mass region led to the identification of ESAT-6, already described earlier in this chapter (7, 187). Weldingh et al. (207) used more powerful methods of resolving proteins and succeeded in identifying six novel T-cell antigens by N-terminal sequence analysis (Table 2). In a similar but larger-scale approach, more than 600 fractions obtained from preparative 2-D liquid-phase electrophoresis were screened for a gamma interferon response in splenocytes of mice infected with *M. tuberculosis*. This resulted in the identification of nearly 40 cytosol and culture filtrate protein fractions with dominant T-cell immunoreactivity. When this technique was coupled with liquid chromatography-tandem MS, it was observed that there was considerable protein overlap among several of the immunodominant fractions, and 30 individual proteins from these fractions were identified, 17 of which were novel (46) (Table 2).

Although these approaches provided many useful data, the complete genome sequence allowed more efficient strategies for the identification of T-cell antigens and epitopes. In this regard, the strong interest in secreted proteins was pursued by computer-based analysis: all proteins predicted by the genome sequence were analyzed for the presence of a secretory signal peptide, and the 52 most likely secreted proteins were identified and selected for immunological characterization (75). Using an in silico T-cell epitope prediction program, De Groot et al. (51) predicted the peptides capable of binding to the class I or class II major histocompatibility complex alleles for

Table 2. T-cell antigens identified via proteomics

Protein	Subcellular location	Identification method	Reference(s)
Rv1984c	ST-CF	N-Term[c]	207
PpiA (Rv0009)	ST-CF	N-Term	207
Cut2 (Rv2301)	ST-CF	N-Term	207
CFP28[b]	ST-CF	N-Term	207
Apa (Rv1860)[a]	CF	Tandem MS	46
PstS1 (Rv0934)[a]	CF	Tandem MS	46
Rv0577	CF and cytosol	Tandem MS	46
Rv1827	ST-CF, CF and cytosol	Tandem MS and N-Term	46, 207
BfrB (Rv3841)	CF	Tandem MS	46
Tpx (Rv1932)	ST-CF, CF and cytosol	Tandem MS and N-Term	46, 207
Rv1352	CF	Tandem MS	46
GroES (Rv3148c)[a]	CF and cytosol	Tandem MS	46
ESAT-6 (Rv3875)[a]	CF	Tandem MS	46
Rv1810	CF	Tandem MS	46
Mpt64 (Rv1980c)[a]	CF	Tandem MS	46
FbpB (Rv1886c)[a]	CF	Tandem MS	46
FbpA (Rv3804c)[a]	CF	Tandem MS	46
FbpC (Rv0129c)[a]	CF	Tandem MS	46
DnaK (Rv0350)[a]	CF	Tandem MS	46
FecB (Rv3044)	CF	Tandem MS	46
Ssb (Rv0054)	Cytosol	Tandem MS	46
RplL (Rv0652)	Cytosol	Tandem MS	46
FixA (Rv3029c)	Cytosol	Tandem MS	46
FixB (Rv3028c)	Cytosol	Tandem MS	46
AhpC2 (Rv2428)	Cytosol	Tandem MS	46
GroEL2 (Rv0440)[a]	Cytosol	Tandem MS	46
HspX (Rv2031c)[a]	Cytosol	Tandem MS	46
Rv2626c	Cytosol	Tandem MS	46
Rv1211	Cytosol	Tandem MS	46
Mdh (Rv1240)	Cytosol	Tandem MS	46
Rv1626	Cytosol	Tandem MS	46
Adk (Rv0733)	Cytosol	Tandem MS	46
ClpP (Rv2461c)	Cytosol	Tandem MS	46
SucD (Rv0952)	Cytosol	Tandem MS	46

[a]Protein previously shown to be a T cell immunogen by other approaches.
[b]Identity to a gene product in the TubercuList database (http://genolist.pasteur.fr/TubercuList/) could not be found by BLAST or FASTA search.
[c]N-term, N-terminal amino acid sequencing by Edman degradation.

which matrices exist by the EpiMatrix algorithm. This resulted in a 99.8% reduction of the number of putative *M. tuberculosis* epitopes to be tested experimentally (51). Together with the large number of T-cell antigens identified in culture filtrate (recently reviewed by Okkels et al. [141]), inclusion of these molecules in the 2-D maps will allow a future generation of the "T-cell immunoproteome."

B-Cell Antigens

Although it is generally thought that the humoral immune response plays no major role in protection against *M. tuberculosis* infection, the field of tuberculosis research has always maintained a certain focus on the identification of antigens recognized by antibodies. One attraction of such antigens has been their potential use in a rapid serodiagnostic test for tuberculosis, but in many cases the antigens initially identified by antibodies were later demonstrated to be potent T-cell antigens as well, e.g., Ag85B (HYT27) (6) and CFP10 (56). Unlike the identification of T-cell antigens, antigens recognized by antibodies are easily identified by detection on 2-D Western blots. In an *M. tuberculosis* immunoproteome investigation, 2-D blots of culture filtrate proteins were probed with pools of sera from healthy controls and tuberculosis patients at different stages of disease. Sera from patients with early tuberculosis identified three potential serodiagnostic candidates, Ag85C, MPT32, and an 88-kDa protein, as well as eight proteins that were not identified (169). A similar proteome-based study also identified the 88-kDa protein as malate synthase (GlcB [Rv1837c]) (89). Testing of recombinant GlcB by enzyme-linked immunosorbent assay against human sera demonstrated greater sensitivity than the "gold standard" 38-kDa PstS1 and was able to recognize a significant number of patients coinfected with human immunodeficiency virus (HIV) (111, 170). 2-D Western blots were also used by Samanich et al. (168) for investigation of the serum response of individual tuberculosis patients (non-HIV-infected cavitary and noncavitary tuberculosis patients, and HIV-infected noncavitary tuberculosis patients). In contrast to an earlier study based on recombinant *M. tuberculosis* proteins that reported very heterogeneous human antibody responses (120), Samanich et al. demonstrated homogeneity in antibody responses, where MPT32 and the 38-kDa antigen were recognized primarily by patients with cavitary lesions and MPT51 (Rv3803c) and GlcB were recognized by sera from patients with noncavitary as well as cavitary tuberculosis (168). These activities have so far resulted in the identification of more than 10 human B-cell antigens, and the first attempts to combine these molecules into a practical test for serodiagnosis are under way.

FUTURE DIRECTIONS FOR PROTEOMICS AND THE STUDY OF TUBERCULOSIS

The completion of the determination of the *M. tuberculosis* genome sequence undoubtedly allowed logarithmic advances in knowledge concerning the overall composition and function of the proteome. However, for the majority of gene products assigned a putative enzymatic activity, experimental confirmation of these activities or the specific metabolic pathways involved is lacking. Functional predictions are not available for 48% of the putative gene products (37), and we have a poor understanding of large families of proteins such as the PE and PPE proteins. Moreover, the important issue of defining the composition of the *M. tuberculosis* proteome during in vivo growth in the host is unknown and demands attention. The answers to these issues will take many years to resolve, and some will not be addressed until new technologies are created that facilitate their investigation. Nevertheless, there are several issues that can be immediately addressed through current and emerging proteomic technologies.

The completion of proteomic maps and data sets with a focus on elucidating the subcellular location of proteins will provide a wealth of data pertinent to determining protein function. In particular, assessing the true localization of proteins that are observed extracytoplasmically but possess functions associated with the cytosol is very important. Rigorously defined subcellular fractions are needed for this work, and such fractions should allow the distinction of outer cell components from the subset of proteins with an extracellular function. Similarly, the localization of PE

and PPE proteins needs to be addressed. Limited studies of these two protein families suggest that they are localized to the cell wall (12, 35, 50, 140). If this is true, it is interesting that numerous genetic screens conducted on mycobacteria to identify exported *M. tuberculosis* proteins, including membrane proteins, never identified a member of these families (34, 60, 117, 211), raising the question of the localization process.

There remains a dearth of proteomic data with regard to clinical isolates. A large comparative proteomic approach that utilizes subcellular fractions of *M. tuberculosis* to achieve high resolution has the potential to provide molecular markers associated with pathogenesis or disease presentation, as well as to potentially identify new diagnostic or vaccine antigens. Such experimentation needs to go beyond the basic mapping of proteins by 2-D PAGE. The analysis of differential posttranslational modification of proteins among strains of *M. tuberculosis* could provide additional information about the importance and potential biological function of specific protein modifications. Similarly, assessment of protein profile changes in response to environmental stress among a large group of clinical isolates could further direct research efforts toward the most important of the regulatory pathways. Along with the continued development of proteome maps, reagents such as antibodies to individual proteins need to be generated for determining subcellular localization and protein production during in vivo growth of the bacillus.

The elucidation of enzymatic or signaling pathways by analysis of comparative proteome profiles is an approach that is currently underutilized for *M. tuberculosis*. This may be due to the success of DNA microarray technologies in helping to define a proposed pathway for mycolic acid biosynthesis (212) and the regulatory mechanism associated with a shift to hypoxic growth (182). Nevertheless, proteomic and microarray techniques are highly complementary (79). Further, as proteomics moves away from gel-based technologies (147, 228), comparative proteomic analyses will become more high throughput and reproducible. Proteome comparisons under different sets of environmental conditions and of *M. tuberculosis* mutants hold great potential for understanding protein function.

The introduction of new technologies such as protein microarray chips (228) will also facilitate the continued identification of serodiagnostic antigens, development of serodiagnostic profiles associated with different states of disease, and assessment of protein-protein interactions or drug-protein interactions. These applications could have a significant impact on elucidating metabolic pathways and regulatory networks of *M. tuberculosis,* on defining host-pathogen protein interactions, and on understanding posttranslational modifications.

REFERENCES

1. **Abou-Zeid, C., E. Filley, J. Steele, and G. A. Rook.** 1987. A simple new method for using antigens separated by polyacrylamide gel electrophoresis to stimulate lymphocytes in vitro after converting bands cut from Western blots into antigen-bearing particles. *J. Immunol. Methods* **98:**5–10.

2. **Abou-Zeid, C., I. Smith, J. M. Grange, T. L. Ratliff, J. Steele, and G. A. Rook.** 1988. The secreted antigens of *Mycobacterium tuberculosis* and their relationship to those recognized by the available antibodies. *J. Gen. Microbiol.* **134:**531–538.

3. **Affronti, L. F., and F. B. Seibert.** 1965. Some early investigations of *Mycobacterium tuberculosis. Am. Rev. Respir. Dis.* **92:**1–8.

4. **Andersen, A. B.** 1994. *Mycobacterium tuberculosis* proteins. Structure, function, and immunological relevance. *Dan. Med. Bull.* **41:**205–215.

5. **Andersen, Å. B., and E. B. Hansen.** 1989. Structure and mapping of antigenic domains of protein antigen b, a 38,000-molecular-weight protein of *Mycobacterium tuberculosis. Infec. Immun.* **57:**2481–2488.

6. **Andersen, Å. B., Z.-L. Yuan, K. Hasl¢v, B. Vergmann, and J. Bennedsen.** 1986. Interspecies reactivity of five monoclonal antibodies to *Mycobacterium tuberculosis* as examined by immunoblotting and enzyme-linked immunosorbent assay. *J. Clin. Microbiol.* **23:**446–451.

7. **Andersen, P., Å. B. Andersen, A. L. Sørensen, and S. Nagai.** 1995. Recall of long-lived immunity to *Mycobacterium tuberculosis* infection in mice. *J. Immunol.* **154:**3359–3372.

8. **Andersen, P., D. Askgaard, L. Ljungqvist, J. Bennedsen, and I. Heron.** 1991. Proteins released from *Mycobacterium tuberculosis* during growth. *Infect. Immun.* **59:**1905–1910.

9. **Andersen, P., and I. Heron.** 1993. Simultaneous electroelution of whole SDS-polyacrylamide gels for the direct cellular analysis of complex protein mixtures. *J. Immunol. Methods* **161:**29–39.

10. **Av-Gay, Y., S. Jamil, and S. J. Drews.** 1999. Expression and characterization of the *Mycobacterium tuberculosis* serine/threonine protein kinase PknB. *Infect. Immun.* **67:**5676–5682.

11. **Banerjee, A., E. Dubnau, A. Quemard, V. Balasubramanian, K. S. Um, T. Wilson, D. Collins, G. de Lisle, and W. R. Jacobs, Jr.** 1994. *inhA,* a gene encoding a target for isoniazid and ethionamide in *Mycobacterium tuberculosis. Science* **263:**227–230.

12. **Banu, S., N. Honore, B. Saint-Joanis, D. Philpott, M. C. Prevost, and S. T. Cole.** 2002. Are the PE-PGRS proteins of *Mycobacterium tuberculosis* variable surface antigens? *Mol. Microbiol.* **44:**9–19.

13. **Bao, L., W. Chen, H. Zhang, and X. Wang.** 2003. Virulence, immunogenicity, and protective efficacy of two recombinant *Mycobacterium bovis* bacillus Calmette-Guérin strains expressing the antigen ESAT-6 from *Mycobacterium tuberculosis. Infect. Immun.* **71:**1656–1661.

14. **Beaucher, J., S. Rodrigue, P. E. Jacques, I. Smith, R. Brzezinski, and L. Gaudreau.** 2002. Novel *Mycobacterium tuberculosis* anti-sigma factor antagonists control sigmaF activity by distinct mechanisms. *Mol. Microbiol.* **45:**1527–1540.

15. **Behr, M. A., M. A. Wilson, W. P. Gill, H. Salamon, G. K. Schoolnik, S. Rane, and P. M. Small.** 1999. Comparative genomics of BCG vaccines by whole-genome DNA microarray. *Science* **284:**1520–1523.

16. **Belisle, J. T., M. E. Brandt, J. D. Radolf, and M. V. Norgard.** 1994. Fatty acids of *Treponema pallidum* and *Borrelia burgdorferi* lipoproteins. *J. Bacteriol.* **176:**2151–2157.

17. **Belisle, J. T., V. D. Vissa, T. Sievert, K. Takayama, P. J. Brennan, and G. S. Besra.** 1997. Role of the major antigen of *Mycobacterium tuberculosis* in cell wall biogenesis. *Science* **276:**1420–1422.

18. **Bendt, A. K., A. Burkovski, S. Schaffer, M. Bott, M. Farwick, and T. Hermann.** 2003. Towards a phosphoproteome map of *Corynebacterium glutamicum. Proteomics* **3:**1637–1646.

19. **Bensing, B. A., and P. M. Sullam.** 2002. An accessory *sec* locus of *Streptococcus gordonii* is required for export of the surface protein GspB and for normal levels of binding to human platelets. *Mol. Microbiol.* **44:**1081–1094.

20. **Benz, I., and M. A. Schmidt.** 2002. Never say never again: protein glycosylation in pathogenic bacteria. *Mol. Microbiol.* **45:**267–276.

21. **Berthet, F. X., P. B. Rasmussen, I. Rosenkrands, P. Andersen, and B. Gicquel.** 1998. A *Mycobacterium tuberculosis* operon encoding ESAT-6 and a novel low-molecular-mass culture filtrate protein (CFP-10). *Microbiology* **144:**3195–3203.

22. **Bessler, W. G., W. Baier, U. vd Esche, P. Hoffmann, L. Heinevetter, K. H. Wiesmuller, and G. Jung.** 1997. Bacterial lipopeptides constitute efficient novel immunogens and adjuvants in parenteral and oral immunization. *Behring Inst. Mitt.* **98:**390–399.

23. **Betts, J. C., P. Dodson, S. Quan, A. P. Lewis, P. J. Thomas, K. Duncan, and R. A. McAdam.** 2000. Comparison of the proteome of *Mycobacterium tuberculosis* strain H37Rv with clinical isolate CDC 1551. *Microbiology* **146:**3205–3216.

24. **Betts, J. C., P. T. Lukey, L. C. Robb, R. A. McAdam, and K. Duncan.** 2002. Evaluation of a nutrient starvation model of *Mycobacterium tuberculosis* persistence by gene and protein expression profiling. *Mol. Microbiol.* **43:**717–731.

25. **Boesen, H., B. N. Jensen, T. Wilcke, and P. Andersen.** 1995. Human T-cell responses to secreted antigen fractions of *Mycobacterium tuberculosis. Infect. Immun.* **63:**1491–1497.

26. **Boitel, B., M. Ortiz-Lombardia, R. Duran, F. Pompeo, S. T. Cole, C. Cervenansky, and P. M. Alzari.** 2003. PknB kinase activity is regulated by phosphorylation in two Thr residues and dephosphorylation by PstP, the cognate phospho-Ser/Thr phosphatase, in *Mycobacterium tuberculosis. Mol. Microbiol.* **49:**1493–1508.

27. **Boon, C., and T. Dick.** 2002. *Mycobacterium bovis* BCG response regulator essential for hypoxic dormancy. *J. Bacteriol.* **184:**6760–6767.

28. **Boon, C., R. Li, R. Qi, and T. Dick.** 2001. Proteins of *Mycobacterium bovis* BCG induced in the Wayne dormancy model. *J. Bacteriol.* **183:**2672–2676.

29. **Brandt, L., M. Elhay, I. Rosenkrands, E. B. Lindblad, and P. Andersen.** 2000. ESAT-6 subunit vaccination against *Mycobacterium tuberculosis. Infect. Immun.* **68:**791–795.

30. **Braun, V., and H. C. Wu.** 1994. Lipoproteins, structure, function, biosynthesis and model for protein export. *New Compr. Biochem.* **27:**319–341.

31. **Braunstein, M., and J. T. Belisle.** 2000. Genetics of protein secretion, p. 203–220. *In* G. F. Hatfull and W. R. Jacobs (ed.), *Molecular Genetics of Mycobacteria.* ASM Press, Washington, D.C.

32. **Braunstein, M., A. M. Brown, S. Kurtz, and W. R. Jacobs, Jr.** 2001. Two nonredundant SecA homologues function in mycobacteria. *J. Bacteriol.* **183:**6979–6990.

33. **Braunstein, M., B. J. Espinosa, J. Chan, J. T. Belisle, and W. R. Jacobs, Jr.** 2003. SecA2 functions in the secretion of

superoxide dismutase A and in the virulence of *Mycobacterium tuberculosis*. *Mol. Microbiol.* **48**:453–464.

34. Braunstein, M., T. I. Griffin, J. I. Kriakov, S. T. Friedman, N. D. Grindley, and W. R. Jacobs, Jr. 2000. Identification of genes encoding exported *Mycobacterium tuberculosis* proteins using a Tn*552'phoA* in vitro transposition system. *J. Bacteriol.* **182**:2732–2740.

35. Brennan, M. J., G. Delogu, Y. Chen, S. Bardarov, J. Kriakov, M. Alavi, and W. R. Jacobs, Jr. 2001. Evidence that mycobacterial PE_PGRS proteins are cell surface constituents that influence interactions with other cells. *Infect. Immun.* **69**:7326–7333.

36. Bryk, R., C. D. Lima, H. Erdjument-Bromage, P. Tempst, and C. Nathan. 2002. Metabolic enzymes of mycobacteria linked to antioxidant defense by a thioredoxin-like protein. *Science* **295**:1073–1077.

37. Camus, J. C., M. J. Pryor, C. Medigue, and S. T. Cole. 2002. Re-annotation of the genome sequence of *Mycobacterium tuberculosis* H37Rv. *Microbiology* **148**:2967–2973.

38. Chaba, R., M. Raje, and P. K. Chakraborti. 2002. Evidence that a eukaryotic-type serine/threonine protein kinase from *Mycobacterium tuberculosis* regulates morphological changes associated with cell division. *Eur. J. Biochem.* **269**:1078–1085.

39. Chopra, P., A. Singh, A. Koul, S. Ramachandran, K. Drlica, A. K. Tyagi, and Y. Singh. 2003. Cytotoxic activity of nucleoside diphosphate kinase secreted from *Mycobacterium tuberculosis*. *Eur. J. Biochem.* **270**:625–634.

40. Chopra, P., B. Singh, R. Singh, R. Vohra, A. Koul, L. S. Meena, H. Koduri, M. Ghildiyal, P. Deol, T. K. Das, A. K. Tyagi, and Y. Singh. 2003. Phosphoprotein phosphatase of *Mycobacterium tuberculosis* dephosphorylates serine-threonine kinases PknA and PknB. *Biochem. Biophys. Res. Commun.* **311**:112–120.

41. Chow, K., D. Ng, R. Stokes, and P. Johnson. 1994. Protein tyrosine phosphorylation in *Mycobacterium tuberculosis*. *FEMS Microbiol. Lett.* **124**:203–207.

42. Closs, O., M. Harboe, N. H. Axelsen, K. Bunch-Christensen, and M. Magnusson. 1980. The antigens of *Mycobacterium bovis*, strain BCG, studied by crossed immunoelectrophoresis: a reference system. *Scand. J. Immunol.* **12**:249–263.

43. Cole, S. T., R. Brosch, J. Parkhill, T. Garnier, C. Churcher, D. Harris, S. V. Gordon, K. Eiglmeier, S. Gas, C. E. Barry III, F. Tekaia, K. Badcock, D. Basham, D. Brown, T. Chillingworth, R. Connor, R. Davies, K. Devlin, T. Feltwell, S. Gentles, N. Hamlin, S. Holroyd, T. Hornsby, K. Jagels, A. Krogh, J. McLean, S. Moule, L. Murphy, K. Oliver, J. Osborne, M. A. Quail, M.-A. Rajandream, J. Rogers, S. Rutter, K. Seeger, J. Skelton, R. Squares, S. Squares, J. E. Sulston, K. Taylor, S. Whitehead, and B. G. Barrell. 1998. Deciphering the biology of *Mycobacterium tuberculosis* from the complete genome sequence. *Nature* **393**:537–544.

44. Cole, S. T., K. Eiglmeier, J. Parkhill, K. D. James, N. R. Thomson, P. R. Wheeler, N. Honore, T. Garnier, C. Churcher, D. Harris, K. Mungall, D. Basham, D. Brown, T. Chillingworth, R. Connor, R. M. Davies, K. Devlin, S. Duthoy, T. Feltwell, A. Fraser, N. Hamlin, S. Holroyd, T. Hornsby, K. Jagels, C. Lacroix, J. Maclean, S. Moule, L. Murphy, K. Oliver, M. A. Quail, M.-A. Rajandream, K. M. Rutherford, S. Rutter, K. Seeger, S. Simon, M. Simmonds, J. Skelton, R. Squares, S. Squares, K. Stevens, K. Taylor, S. Whitehead, J. R. Woodward, and B. G. Barrell. 2001. Massive gene decay in the leprosy bacillus. *Nature* **409**:1007–1011.

45. Cooper, A. M., D. K. Dalton, T. A. Stewart, J. P. Griffin, D. G. Russell, and I. M. Orme. 1993. Disseminated tuberculo-

sis in interferon gamma gene-disrupted mice. *J. Exp. Med.* **178**:2243–2247.

46. Covert, B. A., J. S. Spencer, I. M. Orme, and J. T. Belisle. 2001. The application of proteomics in defining the T cell antigens of *Mycobacterium tuberculosis*. *Proteomics* **1**:574–586.

47. Damiani, G., A. Biano, A. Beltrame, D. Vismara, M. F. Mezzopreti, V. Colizzi, D. B. Young, and B. R. Bloom. 1988. Generation and characterization of monoclonal antibodies to 28-, 35-, and 65-kilodalton proteins of *Mycobacterium tuberculosis*. *Infec. Immun.* **56**:1281–1287.

48. Daniel, T. M. 1989. The chemical composition of immunoaffinity-purified *Mycobacterium tuberculosis* antigen 5. *Am. Rev. Respir. Dis.* **139**:1566–1567.

49. Daniel, T. M., N. J. Gonchoroff, J. A. Katzmann, and G. R. Olds. 1984. Specificity of *Mycobacterium tuberculosis* antigen 5 determined with mouse monoclonal antibodies. *Infect. Immun.* **45**:52–55.

50. Daugelat, S., J. Kowall, J. Mattow, D. Bumann, R. Winter, R. Hurwitz, and S. H. Kaufmann. 2003. The RD1 proteins of *Mycobacterium tuberculosis*: expression in *Mycobacterium smegmatis* and biochemical characterization. *Microbes Infect.* **5**:1082–1095.

51. De Groot, A. S., A. Bosma, N. Chinai, J. Frost, B. M. Jesdale, M. A. Gonzalez, W. Martin, and C. Saint-Aubin. 2001. From genome to vaccine: in silico predictions, ex vivo verification. *Vaccine* **19**:4385–4395.

52. DeLisa, M. P., P. Samuelson, T. Palmer, and G. Georgiou. 2002. Genetic analysis of the twin arginine translocator secretion pathway in bacteria. *J. Biol. Chem.* **277**:29825–29831.

53. Deres, K., H. Schild, K. H. Wiesmuller, G. Jung, and H. G. Rammensee. 1989. In vivo priming of virus-specific cytotoxic T lymphocytes with synthetic lipopeptide vaccine. *Nature* **342**:561–564.

54. Deretic, V., J. Song, and E. Pagan-Ramos. 1997. Loss of oxyR in *Mycobacterium tuberculosis*. *Trends Microbiol.* **5**:367–372.

55. Dilks, K., R. W. Rose, E. Hartmann, and M. Pohlschroder. 2003. Prokaryotic utilization of the twin-arginine translocation pathway: a genomic survey. *J. Bacteriol.* **185**:1478–1483.

56. Dillon, D. C., M. R. Alderson, C. H. Day, T. Bement, A. Campos-Neto, Y. A. Skeiky, T. Vedvick, R. Badaro, S. G. Reed, and R. Houghton. 2000. Molecular and immunological characterization of *Mycobacterium tuberculosis* CFP-10, an immunodiagnostic antigen missing in *Mycobacterium bovis* BCG. *J. Clin. Microbiol.* **38**:3285–3290.

57. Ding, Z., and P. J. Christie. 2003. *Agrobacterium tumefaciens* twin-arginine-dependent translocation is important for virulence, flagellation, and chemotaxis but not type IV secretion. *J. Bacteriol.* **185**:760–771.

58. Dobos, K. M., K. H. Khoo, K. M. Swiderek, P. J. Brennan, and J. T. Belisle. 1996. Definition of the full extent of glycosylation of the 45-kilodalton glycoprotein of *Mycobacterium tuberculosis*. *J. Bacteriol.* **178**:2498–2506.

59. Dobos, K. M., K. Swiderek, K. H. Khoo, P. J. Brennan, and J. T. Belisle. 1995. Evidence for glycosylation sites on the 45-kilodalton glycoprotein of *Mycobacterium tuberculosis*. *Infect. Immun.* **63**:2846–2853.

60. Downing, K. J., R. A. McAdam, and V. Mizrahi. 1999. Staphylococcus aureus nuclease is a useful secretion reporter for mycobacteria. *Gene* **239**:293–299.

61. Duong, F., and W. Wickner. 1997. Distinct catalytic roles of the SecYE, SecG and SecDFyajC subunits of preprotein translocase holoenzyme. *EMBO J.* **16**:2756–2768.

62. Economou, A. 1998. Bacterial preprotein translocase: mechanism and conformational dynamics of a processive enzyme. *Mol. Microbiol.* **27:**511–518.

63. Economou, A., and W. Wickner. 1994. SecA promotes preprotein translocation by undergoing ATP-driven cycles of membrane insertion and deinsertion. *Cell* **78:**835–843.

64. Espitia, C., R. Espinosa, R. Saavedra, R. Mancilla, F. Romain, A. Laqueyrerie, and C. Moreno. 1995. Antigenic and structural similarities between *Mycobacterium tuberculosis* 50- to 55-kilodalton and *Mycobacterium bovis* BCG 45- to 47-kilodalton antigens. *Infect. Immun.* **63:**580–584.

65. Espitia, C., and R. Mancilla. 1989. Identification, isolation and partial characterization of *Mycobacterium tuberculosis* glycoprotein antigens. *Clin. Exp. Immunol.* **77:**378–383.

66. Fifis, T., C. Costopoulos, A. J. Radford, A. Bacic, and P. R. Wood. 1991. Purification and characterization of major antigens from a *Mycobacterium bovis* culture filtrate. *Infect. Immun.* **59:**800–807.

67. Florczyk, M. A., L. A. McCue, R. F. Stack, C. R. Hauer, and K. A. McDonough. 2001. Identification and characterization of mycobacterial proteins differentially expressed under standing and shaking culture conditions, including Rv2623 from a novel class of putative ATP-binding proteins. *Infect. Immun.* **69:**5777–5785.

68. Flory, M. R., T. J. Griffin, D. Martin, and R. Aebersold. 2002. Advances in quantitative proteomics using stable isotope tags. *Trends Biotechnol.* **20:**S23–S29.

69. Flynn, J. L., J. Chan, K. J. Triebold, D. K. Dalton, T. A. Stewart, and B. R. Bloom. 1993. An essential role for interferon-gamma in resistance to *Mycobacterium tuberculosis* infection. *J. Exp. Med.* **178:**2249–2254.

70. Garbe, T. R., N. S. Hibler, and V. Deretic. 1996. Response of *Mycobacterium tuberculosis* to reactive oxygen and nitrogen intermediates. *Mol. Med.* **2:**134–142.

71. Garbe, T. R., N. S. Hibler, and V. Deretic. 1999. Response to reactive nitrogen intermediates in *Mycobacterium tuberculosis*: induction of the 16-kilodalton alpha-crystallin homolog by exposure to nitric oxide donors. *Infect. Immun.* **67:**460–465.

72. Ge, Y., M. El-Naggar, S. K. Sze, H. B. Oh, T. P. Begley, F. W. McLafferty, H. Boshoff, and C. E. Barry III. 2003. Top down characterization of secreted proteins from *Mycobacterium tuberculosis* by electron capture dissociation mass spectrometry. *J. Am. Soc. Mass. Spectrom.* **14:**253–261.

73. Gehring, A. J., R. E. Rojas, D. H. Canaday, D. L. Lakey, C. V. Harding, and W. H. Boom. 2003. The *Mycobacterium tuberculosis* 19-kilodalton lipoprotein inhibits gamma interferon-regulated HLA-DR and Fc gamma R1 on human macrophages through Toll-like receptor 2. *Infect. Immun.* **71:**4487–4497.

74. Gey Van Pittius, N. C., J. Gamieldien, W. Hide, G. D. Brown, R. J. Siezen, and A. D. Beyers. 2001. The ESAT-6 gene cluster of *Mycobacterium tuberculosis* and other high G+C Gram-positive bacteria. *Genome Biol.* **2:**RESEARCH0044. Epub 2001 Sep 19.

75. Gomez, M., S. Johnson, and M. L. Gennaro. 2000. Identification of secreted proteins of *Mycobacterium tuberculosis* by a bioinformatic approach. *Infec. Immun.* **68:**2323–2327.

76. Gooley, A. A., and K. L. Williams. 1994. Towards characterizing O-glycans: the relative merits of in vivo and in vitro approaches in seeking peptide motifs specifying O-glycosylation sites. *Glycobiology* **4:**413–417.

77. Goren, M. B., and P. J. Brennan. 1979. Mycobacterial lipids: chemistry and biological activities, p. 63–193. *In* G. P. Youmans (ed.), *Tuberculosis*. The W. B. Saunders Co., Philadelphia, Pa.

78. Gorg, A., C. Obermaier, G. Boguth, A. Harder, B. Scheibe, R. Wildgruber, and W. Weiss. 2000. The current state of two-dimensional electrophoresis with immobilized pH gradients. *Electrophoresis* **21:**1037–1053.

79. Griffin, T. J., S. P. Gygi, T. Ideker, B. Rist, J. Eng, L. Hood, and R. Aebersold. 2002. Complementary profiling of gene expression at the transcriptome and proteome levels in *Saccharomyces cerevisiae*. *Mol. Cell. Proteomics* **1:**323–333.

80. Gu, S., J. Chen, K. M. Dobos, E. M. Bradbury, J. T. Belisle, and X. Chen. 2003. Comprehensive proteomic profiling of the membrane constituents of a *Mycobacterium tuberculosis* strain. *Mol. Cell. Proteomics* **2:**1284–1296.

81. Guinn, K. M., M. J. Hickey, S. K. Mathur, K. L. Zakel, J. E. Grotzke, D. M. Lewinsohn, S. Smith, and D. R. Sherman. Individual RD1-region genes are required for export of ESAT-6/CFP-10 and for virulence of *Mycobacterium tuberculosis*. *Mol. Microbiol.* **51:**359–370.

82. Gulle, H., B. Schoel, and S. H. Kaufmann. 1990. Direct blotting with viable cells of protein mixtures separated by two-dimensional gel electrophoresis. *J. Immunol. Methods* **133:**253–261.

83. Hansen, J. E., O. Lund, N. Tolstrup, A. A. Gooley, K. L. Williams, and S. Brunak. 1998. NetOglyc: prediction of mucin type O-glycosylation sites based on sequence context and surface accessibility. *Glycoconj. J.* **15:**115–130.

84. Harboe, M., T. Oettinger, H. G. Wiker, I. Rosenkrands, and P. Andersen. 1996. Evidence for occurrence of the ESAT-6 protein in *Mycobacterium tuberculosis* and virulent *Mycobacterium bovis* and for its absence in *Mycobacterium bovis* BCG. *Infect. Immun.* **64:**16–22.

85. Harth, G., D. L. Clemens, and M. A. Horwitz. 1994. Glutamine synthetase of *Mycobacterium tuberculosis*: extracellular release and characterization of its enzymatic activity. *Proc. Natl. Acad. Sci. USA* **91:**9342–9346.

86. Harth, G., and M. A. Horwitz. 1999. Export of recombinant *Mycobacterium tuberculosis* superoxide dismutase is dependent upon both information in the protein and mycobacterial export machinery. A model for studying export of leaderless proteins by pathogenic mycobacteria. *J. Biol. Chem.* **274:**4281–4292.

87. Hauschildt, S., P. Hoffmann, H. U. Beuscher, G. Dufhues, P. Heinrich, K. H. Wiesmuller, G. Jung, and W. G. Bessler. 1990. Activation of bone marrow-derived mouse macrophages by bacterial lipopeptide: cytokine production, phagocytosis and Ia expression. *Eur. J. Immunol.* **20:**63–68.

88. Haydel, S. E., N. E. Dunlap, and W. H. Benjamin, Jr. 1999. In vitro evidence of two-component system phosphorylation between the *Mycobacterium tuberculosis* TrcR/TrcS proteins. *Microb. Pathog.* **26:**195–206.

89. Hendrickson, R. C., J. F. Douglass, L. D. Reynolds, P. D. McNeill, D. Carter, S. G. Reed, and R. L. Houghton. 2000. Mass spectrometric identification of mtb81, a novel serological marker for tuberculosis. *J. Clin. Microbiol.* **38:**2354–2361.

90. Henningsen, R., B. L. Gale, K. M. Straub, and D. C. DeNagel. 2002. Application of zwitterionic detergents to the solubilization of integral membrane proteins for two-dimensional gel electrophoresis and mass spectrometry. *Proteomics* **2:**1479–1488.

91. Herrmann, J. L., R. Delahay, A. Gallagher, B. Robertson, and D. Young. 2000. Analysis of post-translational modification of mycobacterial proteins using a cassette expression system. *FEBS Lett.* **473:**358–362.

92. Herrmann, J. L., P. O'Gaora, A. Gallagher, J. E. Thole, and D. B. Young. 1996. Bacterial glycoproteins: a link between

glycosylation and proteolytic cleavage of a 19 kDa antigen from *Mycobacterium tuberculosis*. *EMBO J.* **15**:3547–3554.

93. Hiller, K., M. Schobert, C. Hundertmark, D. Jahn, and R. Munch. 2003. JVirGel: calculation of virtual two-dimensional protein gels. *Nucleic Acids Res.* **31**:3862–3865.

94. Hofmann, K., and W. Stoffel. 1993. Tmbase—A database of membrane spanning protein segments. *Biol. Chem. Hoppe-Seyler* **374**:166–170.

95. Horn, C., A. Namane, P. Pescher, M. Riviere, F. Romain, G. Puzo, O. Barzu, and G. Marchal. 1999. Decreased capacity of recombinant 45/47-kDa molecules (Apa) of *Mycobacterium tuberculosis* to stimulate T lymphocyte responses related to changes in their mannosylation pattern. *J. Biol. Chem.* **274**:32023–32030.

96. Hsu, T., S. M. Hingley-Wilson, B. Chen, M. Chen, A. Z. Dai, P. M. Morin, C. B. Marks, J. Padiyar, C. Goulding, M. Gingery, D. Eisenberg, R. G. Russell, S. C. Derrick, F. M. Collins, S. L. Morris, C. H. King, and W. R. Jacobs, Jr. 2003. The primary mechanism of attenuation of bacillus Calmette-Guérin is a loss of secreted lytic function required for invasion of lung interstitial tissue. *Proc. Natl. Acad. Sci. USA* **100**:12420–12425.

97. Hunter, S. W., B. Rivoire, V. Mehra, B. R. Bloom, and P. J. Brennan. 1990. The major native proteins of the leprosy bacillus. *J. Biol. Chem.* **265**:14065–14068.

98. Ischiropoulos, H. 2003. Biological selectivity and functional aspects of protein tyrosine nitration. *Biochem. Biophys. Res. Commun.* **305**:776–783.

99. Jackowski, S., and C. O. Rock. 1986. Transfer of fatty acids from the 1 position of phosphatidylethanolamine to the major outer membrane lipoprotein of *Escherichia coli*. *J. Biol. Chem.* **261**:1328–1333.

100. Jacobs, W. R., Jr., G. V. Kalpana, J. D. Cirillo, L. Pascopella, S. B. Snapper, R. A. Udani, W. Jones, R. G. Barletta, and B. R. Bloom. 1991. Genetic systems for mycobacteria. *Methods Enzymol.* **204**:537–555.

101. Jentoft, N. 1990. Why are proteins O-glycosylated? *Trends Biochem. Sci.* **15**:291–294.

102. Jungblut, P. R., E. C. Muller, J. Mattow, and S. H. Kaufmann. 2001. Proteomics reveals open reading frames in *Mycobacterium tuberculosis* H37Rv not predicted by genomics. *Infect. Immun.* **69**:5905–5907.

103. Jungblut, P. R., U. E. Schaible, H. Mollenkopf, U. Zimny-Arndt, B. Raupach, J. Mattow, P. Halada, S. Lamer, K. Hagens, and S. H. Kaufmann. 1999. Comparative proteome analysis of *Mycobacterium tuberculosis* and *Mycobacterium bovis* BCG strains: towards functional genomics of microbial pathogens. *Mol. Microbiol.* **33**:1103–1117.

104. Kennelly, P. J., and M. Potts. 1996. Fancy meeting you here! A fresh look at "prokaryotic" protein phosphorylation. *J. Bacteriol.* **178**:4759–4764.

105. Khanolkar Young, S., A. H. Kolk, Å. B. Andersen, J. Bennedsen, P. J. Brennan, B. Rivoire, S. Kuijper, K. P. McAdam, C. Abe, H. V. Batra, S. D. Chaparas, G. Damiani, M. Singh, and H. D. Engers. 1992. Results of the third immunology of leprosy/immunology of tuberculosis antimycobacterial monoclonal antibody workshop. *Infect. Immun.* **60**:3925–3927.

106. Klatser, P. R., M. Y. De Wit, A. H. Kolk, and R. A. Hartskeerl. 1991. Characterization of murine B-cell epitopes on the *Mycobacterium leprae* proline-rich antigen by use of synthetic peptides. *Infect. Immun.* **59**:433–436.

107. Koch, R. 1891. Weitere Mitteilung uber das Tuberkulin. *Dtsche. Med. Wochnschr.* **43**:1189–1192.

108. Koul, A., A. Choidas, M. Treder, A. K. Tyagi, K. Drlica, Y. Singh, and A. Ullrich. 2000. Cloning and characterization of

secretory tyrosine phosphatases of *Mycobacterium tuberculosis*. *J. Bacteriol.* **182**:5425–5432.

109. Koul, A., A. Choidas, A. K. Tyagi, K. Drlica, Y. Singh, and A. Ullrich. 2001. Serine/threonine protein kinases PknF and PknG of *Mycobacterium tuberculosis*: characterization and localization. *Microbiology* **147**:2307–2314.

110. Kurdistani, S. K., and M. Grunstein. 2003. Histone acetylation and deacetylation in yeast. *Nat. Rev. Mol. Cell. Biol.* **4**:276–284.

111. Laal, S., K. M. Samanich, M. G. Sonnenberg, J. T. Belisle, J. O'Leary, M. S. Simberkoff, and S. Zolla-Pazner. 1997. Surrogate marker of preclinical tuberculosis in human immunodeficiency virus infection: antibodies to an 88-kDa secreted antigen of *Mycobacterium tuberculosis*. *J. Infect. Dis.* **176**:133–143.

112. Lachner, M., and T. Jenuwein. 2002. The many faces of histone lysine methylation. *Curr. Opin. Cell Biol.* **14**:286–298.

113. Lanne, B., F. Potthast, A. Hoglund, H. Brockenhuus von Lowenhielm, A. C. Nystrom, F. Nilsson, and B. Dahllof. 2001. Thiourea enhances mapping of the proteome from murine white adipose tissue. *Proteomics* **1**:819–828.

114. Lee, B.-Y., and M. A. Horwitz. 1995. Identification of macrophage and stress-induced proteins of *Mycobacterium tuberculosis*. *J. Clin. Investig.* **96**:245–249.

115. Lenz, L. L., and D. A. Portnoy. 2002. Identification of a second *Listeria secA* gene associated with protein secretion and the rough phenotype. *Mol. Microbiol.* **45**:1043–1056.

116. Lewis, K. N., R. Liao, K. M. Guinn, M. J. Hickey, S. Smith, M. A. Behr, and D. R. Sherman. 2003. Deletion of RD1 from *Mycobacterium tuberculosis* mimics bacille Calmette-Guérin attenuation. *J. Infect. Dis.* **187**:117–123.

117. Lim, E. M., J. Rauzier, J. Timm, G. Torrea, A. Murray, B. Gicquel, and D. Portnoi. 1995. Identification of *Mycobacterium tuberculosis* DNA sequences encoding exported proteins by using phoA gene fusions. *J. Bacteriol.* **177**:59–65.

118. Ljungqvist, L., A. Worsaae, and I. Heron. 1988. Antibody responses against *Mycobacterium tuberculosis* in 11 strains of inbred mice: novel monoclonal antibody specificities generated by fusions, using spleens from BALB.B10 and CBA/J mice. *Infect. Immun.* **56**:1994–1998.

119. Lowe, J. B., and J. D. Marth. 2003. A genetic approach to mammalian glycan function. *Annu. Rev. Biochem.* **72**:643–691.

120. Lyashchenko, K., R. Colangeli, M. Houde, H. Al Jahdali, D. Menzies, and M. L. Gennaro. 1998. Heterogeneous antibody responses in tuberculosis. *Infect. Immun.* **66**:3936–3940.

121. Mahairas, G. G., P. J. Sabo, M. J. Hickey, D. C. Singh, and C. K. Stover. 1996. Molecular analysis of genetic differences between *Mycobacterium bovis* BCG and virulent *M. bovis*. *J. Bacteriol.* **178**:1274–1282.

122. Mattow, J., P. R. Jungblut, E. C. Muller, and S. H. Kaufmann. 2001. Identification of acidic, low molecular mass proteins of *Mycobacterium tuberculosis* strain H37Rv by matrix-assisted laser desorption/ionization and electrospray ionization mass spectrometry. *Proteomics* **1**:494–507.

123. Mattow, J., P. R. Jungblut, U. E. Schaible, H. J. Mollenkopf, S. Lamer, U. Zimny-Arndt, K. Hagens, E. C. Muller, and S. H. Kaufmann. 2001. Identification of proteins from *Mycobacterium tuberculosis* missing in attenuated *Mycobacterium bovis* BCG strains. *Electrophoresis* **22**:2936–2946.

124. Mattow, J., U. E. Schaible, F. Schmidt, K. Hagens, F. Siejak, G. Brestrich, G. Haeselbarth, E. C. Muller, P. R. Jungblut, and S. H. Kaufmann. 2003. Comparative proteome analysis of culture supernatant proteins from virulent *Mycobacterium tuberculosis* H37Rv and attenuated *M. bovis* BCG Copenhagen. *Electrophoresis* **24**:3405–3420.

125. Menozzi, F. D., R. Bischoff, E. Fort, M. J. Brennan, and C. Locht. 1998. Molecular characterization of the mycobacterial heparin-binding hemagglutinin, a mycobacterial adhesin. *Proc. Natl. Acad. Sci. USA* 95:12625–12630.

126. Menozzi, F. D., J. H. Rouse, M. Alavi, M. Laude-Sharp, J. Muller, R. Bischoff, M. J. Brennan, and C. Locht. 1996. Identification of a heparin-binding hemagglutinin present in mycobacteria. *J. Exp. Med.* 184:993–1001.

127. Michell, S. L., A. O. Whelan, P. R. Wheeler, M. Panico, R. L. Easton, A. T. Etienne, S. M. Haslam, A. Dell, H. R. Morris, A. J. Reason, J. L. Herrmann, D. B. Young, and R. G. Hewinson. 2003. The MPB83 antigen from *Mycobacterium bovis* contains O-linked mannose and (1→3)-mannobiose moieties. *J. Biol. Chem.* 278:16423–16432.

128. Modlin, R. L. 2001. Activation of toll-like receptors by microbial lipoproteins: role in host defense. *J. Allergy Clin. Immunol.* 108:S104–S106.

129. Molle, V., C. Girard-Blanc, L. Kremer, P. Doublet, A. J. Cozzone, and J. F. Prost. 2003. Protein PknE, a novel transmembrane eukaryotic-like serine/threonine kinase from *Mycobacterium tuberculosis. Biochem. Biophys. Res. Commun.* 308:820–825.

130. Mollenkopf, H. J., P. R. Jungblut, B. Raupach, J. Mattow, S. Lamer, U. Zimny-Arndt, U. E. Schaible, and S. H. Kaufmann. 1999. A dynamic two-dimensional polyacrylamide gel electrophoresis database: the mycobacterial proteome via Internet. *Electrophoresis* 20:2172–2180.

131. Monahan, I. M., J. Betts, D. K. Banerjee, and P. D. Butcher. 2001. Differential expression of mycobacterial proteins following phagocytosis by macrophages. *Microbiology* 147:459–471.

132. Nagai, S., J. Matsumoto, and T. Nagasuga. 1981. Specific skin-reactive protein from culture filtrate of *Mycobacterium bovis* BCG. *Infect. Immun.* 31:1152–1160.

133. Nagai, S., H. G. Wiker, M. Harboe, and M. Kinomoto. 1991. Isolation and partial characterization of major protein antigens in the culture fluid of *Mycobacterium tuberculosis. Infec. Immun.* 59:372–382.

134. Navarre, W. W., and O. Schneewind. 1999. Surface proteins of gram-positive bacteria and mechanisms of their targeting to the cell wall envelope. *Microbiol. Mol. Biol. Rev.* 63:174–229.

135. Nielsen, H., J. Engelbrecht, S. Brunak, and G. von Heijne. 1997. A neural network method for identification of prokaryotic and eukaryotic signal peptides and prediction of their cleavage sites. *Int. J. Neural. Syst.* 8:581–599.

136. Noss, E. H., R. K. Pai, T. J. Sellati, J. D. Radolf, J. Belisle, D. T. Golenbock, W. H. Boom, and C. V. Harding. 2001. Toll-like receptor 2-dependent inhibition of macrophage class II MHC expression and antigen processing by 19-kDa lipoprotein of *Mycobacterium tuberculosis. J. Immunol.* 167:910–918.

137. Ochsner, U. A., A. Snyder, A. I. Vasil, and M. L. Vasil. 2002. Effects of the twin-arginine translocase on secretion of virulence factors, stress response, and pathogenesis. *Proc. Natl. Acad. Sci. USA* 99:8312–8317.

138. O'Donnell, M. A., A. Aldovini, R. B. Duda, H. Yang, A. Szilvasi, R. A. Young, and W. C. DeWolf. 1994. Recombinant *Mycobacterium bovis* BCG secreting functional interleukin-2 enhances gamma interferon production by splenocytes. *Infect. Immun.* 62:2508–2514.

139. Ohno, H., G. Zhu, V. P. Mohan, D. Chu, S. Kohno, W. R. Jacobs, Jr., and J. Chan. 2003. The effects of reactive nitrogen intermediates on gene expression in *Mycobacterium tuberculosis. Cell. Microbiol.* 5:637–648.

140. Okkels, L. M., I. Brock, F. Follmann, E. M. Agger, S. M. Arend, T. H. M. Ottenhoff, F. Oftung, I. Rosenkrands, and P. Andersen. 2003. PPE protein (Rv3873) from DNA segment RD1 of *Mycobacterium tuberculosis*: strong recognition of both specific T-cell epitopes and epitopes conserved within the PPE family. *Infect. Immun.* 71:6116–6123.

141. Okkels, L. M., T. M. Doherty, and P. Andersen. 2003. Selecting the components for a safe and efficient tuberculosis subunit vaccine—recent progress and post-genomic insights. *Curr. Pharm. Biotechnol.* 4:69–83.

142. Owens, M. U., W. E. Swords, M. G. Schmidt, C. H. King, and F. D. Quinn. 2002. Cloning, expression, and functional characterization of the *Mycobacterium tuberculosis secA* gene. *FEMS Microbiol. Lett.* 211:133–141.

143. Pallen, M. J. 2002. The ESAT-6/WXG100 superfamily—and a new Gram-positive secretion system? *Trends Microbiol.* 10:209–212.

144. Park, H. D., K. M. Guinn, M. I. Harrell, R. Liao, M. I. Voskuil, M. Tompa, G. K. Schoolnik, and D. R. Sherman. 2003. Rv3133c/dosR is a transcription factor that mediates the hypoxic response of *Mycobacterium tuberculosis. Mol. Microbiol.* 48:833–843.

145. Peirs, P., L. De Wit, M. Braibant, K. Huygen, and J. Content. 1997. A serine/threonine protein kinase from *Mycobacterium tuberculosis. Eur. J. Biochem.* 244:604–612.

146. Peirs, P., B. Parmentier, L. De Wit, and J. Content. 2000. The *Mycobacterium bovis* homologous protein of the *Mycobacterium tuberculosis* serine/threonine protein kinase Mbk (PknD) is truncated. *FEMS Microbiol. Lett.* 188:135–139.

147. Peng, J., J. E. Elias, C. C. Thoreen, L. J. Licklider, and S. P. Gygi. 2003. Evaluation of multidimensional chromatography coupled with tandem mass spectrometry (LC/LC-MS/MS) for large-scale protein analysis: the yeast proteome. *J. Proteome Res.* 2:43–50.

148. Pethe, K., P. Bifani, H. Drobecq, C. Sergheraert, A. S. Debrie, C. Locht, and F. D. Menozzi. 2002. Mycobacterial heparin-binding hemagglutinin and laminin-binding protein share antigenic methyllysines that confer resistance to proteolysis. *Proc. Natl. Acad. Sci. USA* 99:10759–10764.

149. Petrickova, K., and M. Petricek. 2003. Eukaryotic-type protein kinases in *Streptomyces coelicolor*: variations on a common theme. *Microbiology* 149:1609–1621.

150. Plano, G. V., J. B. Day, and F. Ferracci. 2001. Type III export: new uses for an old pathway. *Mol. Microbiol.* 40:284–293.

151. Pollock, J. M., and P. Andersen. 1997. Predominant recognition of the ESAT-6 protein in the first phase of infection with *Mycobacterium bovis* in cattle. *Infec. Immun.* 65:2587–2592.

152. Pradel, N., C. Ye, V. Livrelli, J. Xu, B. Joly, and L. F. Wu. 2003. Contribution of the twin arginine translocation system to the virulence of enterohemorrhagic *Escherichia coli* O157:H7. *Infect. Immun.* 71:4908–4916.

153. Pruess, M., W. Fleischmann, A. Kanapin, Y. Karavidopoulou, P. Kersey, E. Kriventseva, V. Mittard, N. Mulder, I. Phan, F. Servant, and R. Apweiler. 2003. The Proteome Analysis database: a tool for the in silico analysis of whole proteomes. *Nucleic Acids Res.* 31:414–417.

154. Pugsley, A. P. 1993. The complete general secretory pathway in gram-negative bacteria. *Microbiol. Rev.* 57:50–108.

155. Pym, A. S., P. Brodin, R. Brosch, M. Huerre, and S. T. Cole. 2002. Loss of RD1 contributed to the attenuation of the live tuberculosis vaccines *Mycobacterium bovis* BCG and *Mycobacterium microti. Mol. Microbiol.* 46:709–717.

156. Pym, A. S., P. Brodin, L. Majlessi, R. Brosch, C. Demangel, A. Williams, K. E. Griffiths, G. Marchal, C. Leclerc, and S. T. Cole. 2003. Recombinant BCG exporting ESAT-6 confers enhanced protection against tuberculosis. *Nat. Med.* 9:533–539.

157. Ravn, P., A. Demissie, T. Eguale, H. Wondwosson, D. Lein, H. A. Amoudy, A. S. Mustafa, A. K. Jensen, A. Holm, I. Rosenkrands, F. Oftung, J. Olobo, F. von Reyn, and P. Andersen. 1999. Human T cell responses to the ESAT-6 antigen from *Mycobacterium tuberculosis*. *J. Infect. Dis.* **179:**637–645.

158. Raynaud, C., G. Etienne, P. Peyron, M. A. Laneelle, and M. Daffe. 1998. Extracellular enzyme activities potentially involved in the pathogenicity of *Mycobacterium tuberculosis*. *Microbiology* **144:**577–587.

159. Raynaud, C., C. Guilhot, J. Rauzier, Y. Bordat, V. Pelicic, R. Manganelli, I. Smith, B. Gicquel, and M. Jackson. 2002. Phospholipases C are involved in the virulence of *Mycobacterium tuberculosis*. *Mol. Microbiol.* **45:**203–217.

160. Renshaw, P. S., P. Panagiotidou, A. Whelan, S. V. Gordon, R. G. Hewinson, R. A. Williamson, and M. D. Carr. 2002. Conclusive evidence that the major T-cell antigens of the *Mycobacterium tuberculosis* complex ESAT-6 and CFP-10 form a tight, 1:1 complex and characterization of the structural properties of ESAT-6, CFP-10, and the ESAT-6*CFP-10 complex. Implications for pathogenesis and virulence. *J. Biol. Chem.* **277:**21598–21603.

161. Rodrigue, A., A. Chanal, K. Beck, M. Muller, and L. F. Wu. 1999. Co-translocation of a periplasmic enzyme complex by a hitchhiker mechanism through the bacterial *tat* pathway. *J. Biol. Chem.* **274:**13223–13228.

162. Romain, F., C. Horn, P. Pescher, A. Namane, M. Riviere, G. Puzo, O. Barzu, and G. Marchal. 1999. Deglycosylation of the 45/47-kilodalton antigen complex of *Mycobacterium tuberculosis* decreases its capacity to elicit in vivo or in vitro cellular immune responses. *Infect. Immun.* **67:**5567–5572.

163. Rosenkrands, I., A. King, K. Weldingh, M. Moniatte, E. Moertz, and P. Andersen. 2000. Towards the proteome of *Mycobacterium tuberculosis*. *Electrophoresis* **21:**3740–3756.

164. Rosenkrands, I., R. A. Slayden, J. Crawford, C. Aagaard, C. E. Barry III, and P. Andersen. 2002. Hypoxic response of *Mycobacterium tuberculosis* studied by metabolic labeling and proteome analysis of cellular and extracellular proteins. *J. Bacteriol.* **184:**3485–3491.

165. Rosenkrands, I., K. Weldingh, S. Jacobsen, C. V. Hansen, W. Florio, I. Gianetri, and P. Andersen. 2000. Mapping and identification of *Mycobacterium tuberculosis* proteins by two-dimensional gel electrophoresis, microsequencing and immunodetection. *Electrophoresis* **21:**935–948.

166. Roskoski, R., Jr. 2003. Protein prenylation: a pivotal post-translational process. *Biochem. Biophys. Res. Commun.* **303:**1–7.

167. Saleh, M. T., M. Fillon, P. J. Brennan, and J. T. Belisle. 2001. Identification of putative exported/secreted proteins in prokaryotic proteomes. *Gene* **269:**195–204.

168. Samanich, K., J. T. Belisle, and S. Laal. 2001. Homogeneity of antibody responses in tuberculosis patients. *Infect. Immun.* **69:**4600–4609.

169. Samanich, K. M., J. T. Belisle, M. G. Sonnenberg, M. A. Keen, S. Zolla-Pazner, and S. Laal. 1998. Delineation of human antibody responses to culture filtrate antigens of *Mycobacterium tuberculosis*. *J. Infect. Dis.* **178:**1534–1538.

170. Samanich, K. M., M. A. Keen, V. D. Vissa, J. D. Harder, J. S. Spencer, J. T. Belisle, S. Zolla-Pazner, and S. Laal. 2000. Serodiagnostic potential of culture filtrate antigens of *Mycobacterium tuberculosis*. *Clin. Diagn. Lab. Immunol.* **7:**662–668.

171. Samuelson, J. C., M. Chen, F. Jiang, I. Moller, M. Wiedmann, A. Kuhn, G. J. Phillips, and R. E. Dalbey. 2000. YidC mediates membrane protein insertion in bacteria. *Nature* **406:**637–641.

172. Santini, C. L., B. Ize, A. Chanal, M. Muller, G. Giordano, and L. F. Wu. 1998. A novel *sec*-independent periplasmic protein translocation pathway in *Escherichia coli*. *EMBO J.* **17:**101–112.

173. Sargent, F., E. G. Bogsch, N. R. Stanley, M. Wexler, C. Robinson, B. C. Berks, and T. Palmer. 1998. Overlapping functions of components of a bacterial Sec-independent protein export pathway. *EMBO J.* **17:**3640–3650.

174. Sassetti, C. M., D. H. Boyd, and E. J. Rubin. 2003. Genes required for mycobacterial growth defined by high density mutagenesis. *Mol. Microbiol.* **48:**77–84.

175. Sassetti, C. M., and E. J. Rubin. 2003. Genetic requirements for mycobacterial survival during infection. *Proc. Natl. Acad. Sci. USA* **100:**12989–12994.

176. Schiebel, E., A. J. Driessen, F. U. Hartl, and W. Wickner. 1991. Delta mu H$^+$ and ATP function at different steps of the catalytic cycle of preprotein translocase. *Cell* **64:**927–939.

177. Schmidt, M. A., L. W. Riley, and I. Benz. 2003. Sweet new world: glycoproteins in bacterial pathogens. *Trends Microbiol.* **11:**554–561.

178. Schmidt, M. G., and K. B. Kiser. 1999. SecA: the ubiquitous component of preprotein translocase in prokaryotes. *Microbes Infect.* **1:**993–1004.

179. Schneider, G. 1999. How many potentially secreted proteins are contained in a bacterial genome? *Gene* **237:**113–121.

180. Seibert, F. B., and J. T. Glenn. 1941. Tuberculin purified protein derivative: preparation and analyses of a large quantity for standard. *Am. Rev. Tuberc.* **44:**9–25.

181. Sherman, D. R., P. J. Sabo, M. J. Hickey, T. M. Arain, G. G. Mahairas, Y. Yuan, C. E. Barry III, and C. K. Stover. 1995. Disparate responses to oxidative stress in saprophytic and pathogenic mycobacteria. *Proc. Natl. Acad. Sci. USA* **92:**6625–6629.

182. Sherman, D. R., M. Voskuil, D. Schnappinger, R. Liao, M. I. Harrell, and G. K. Schoolnik. 2001. Regulation of the *Mycobacterium tuberculosis* hypoxic response gene encoding alpha-crystallin. *Proc. Natl. Acad. Sci. USA* **98:**7534–7539.

183. Singh, R., V. Rao, H. Shakila, R. Gupta, A. Khera, N. Dhar, A. Singh, A. Koul, Y. Singh, M. Naseema, P. R. Narayanan, C. N. Paramasivan, V. D. Ramanathan, and A. K. Tyagi. 2003. Disruption of mptpB impairs the ability of *Mycobacterium tuberculosis* to survive in guinea pigs. *Mol. Microbiol.* **50:**751–762.

184. Skjot, R. L., T. Oettinger, I. Rosenkrands, P. Ravn, I. Brock, S. Jacobsen, and P. Andersen. 2000. Comparative evaluation of low-molecular-mass proteins from *Mycobacterium tuberculosis* identifies members of the ESAT-6 family as immunodominant T-cell antigens. *Infect. Immun.* **68:**214–220.

185. Smith, C. V., C. C. Huang, A. Miczak, D. G. Russell, J. C. Sacchettini, and K. Honer zu Bentrup. 2003. Biochemical and structural studies of malate synthase from *Mycobacterium tuberculosis*. *J. Biol. Chem.* **278:**1735–1743.

186. Sonnenberg, M. G., and J. T. Belisle. 1997. Definition of *Mycobacterium tuberculosis* culture filtrate proteins by two-dimensional polyacrylamide gel electrophoresis, N-terminal amino acid sequencing, and electrospray mass spectrometry. *Infect. Immun.* **65:**4515–4524.

187. Sørensen, A. L., S. Nagai, G. Houen, P. Andersen, and Å. B. Andersen. 1995. Purification and characterization of a low-molecular-mass T-cell antigen secreted by *Mycobacterium tuberculosis*. *Infect. Immun.* **63:**1710–1717.

188. Stanley, N. R., T. Palmer, and B. C. Berks. 2000. The twin arginine consensus motif of Tat signal peptides is involved in Sec-independent protein targeting in Escherichia coli. *J. Biol. Chem.* **275:**11591–11596.

189. Stanley, S. A., S. Raghavan, W. W. Hwang, and J. S. Cox. 2003. Acute infection and macrophage subversion by *Mycobacterium tuberculosis* require a specialized secretion system. *Proc. Natl. Acad. Sci. USA* 100:13001–13006.

190. Stock, A. M., V. L. Robinson, and P. N. Goudreau. 2000. Two-component signal transduction. *Annu. Rev. Biochem.* 69:183–215.

191. Stock, J. B., A. M. Stock, and J. M. Mottonen. 1990. Signal transduction in bacteria. *Nature* 344:395–400.

192. Sutcliffe, I. C., and R. R. Russell. 1995. Lipoproteins of gram-positive bacteria. *J. Bacteriol.* 177:1123–1128.

193. Tekaia, F., S. V. Gordon, T. Garnier, R. Brosch, B. G. Barrell, and S. T. Cole. 1999. Analysis of the proteome of *Mycobacterium tuberculosis* in silico. *Tubercle Lung Dis.* 79:329–342.

194. Terada, M., T. Kuroda, S. I. Matsuyama, and H. Tokuda. 2001. Lipoprotein sorting signals evaluated as the LolA-dependent release of lipoproteins from the cytoplasmic membrane of *Escherichia coli. J. Biol. Chem.* 276:47690–47694.

195. Thoma-Uszynski, S., S. M. Kiertscher, M. T. Ochoa, D. A. Bouis, M. V. Norgard, K. Miyake, P. J. Godowski, M. D. Roth, and R. L. Modlin. 2000. Activation of toll-like receptor 2 on human dendritic cells triggers induction of IL-12, but not IL-10. *J. Immunol.* 165:3804–3810.

196. Thoma-Uszynski, S., S. Stenger, O. Takeuchi, M. T. Ochoa, M. Engele, P. A. Sieling, P. F. Barnes, M. Rollinghoff, P. L. Bolcskei, M. Wagner, S. Akira, M. V. Norgard, J. T. Belisle, P. J. Godowski, B. R. Bloom, and R. L. Modlin. 2001. Induction of direct antimicrobial activity through mammalian toll-like receptors. *Science* 291:1544–1547.

197. Tobian, A. A., N. S. Potter, L. Ramachandra, R. K. Pai, M. Convery, W. H. Boom, and C. V. Harding. 2003. Alternate class I MHC antigen processing is inhibited by Toll-like receptor signaling pathogen-associated molecular patterns: *Mycobacterium tuberculosis* 19-kDa lipoprotein, CpG DNA, and lipopolysaccharide. *J. Immunol.* 171:1413–1422.

198. Tullius, M. V., G. Harth, and M. A. Horwitz. 2001. High extracellular levels of *Mycobacterium tuberculosis* glutamine synthetase and superoxide dismutase in actively growing cultures are due to high expression and extracellular stability rather than to a protein-specific export mechanism. *Infect. Immun.* 69:6348–6363.

199. Urquhart, B. L., S. J. Cordwell, and I. Humphery-Smith. 1998. Comparison of predicted and observed properties of proteins encoded in the genome of *Mycobacterium tuberculosis* H37Rv. *Biochem. Biophys. Res. Commun.* 253:70–79.

200. Valent, Q. A., P. A. Scotti, S. High, J. W. de Gier, G. von Heijne, G. Lentzen, W. Wintermeyer, B. Oudega, and J. Luirink. 1998. The *Escherichia coli* SRP and SecB targeting pathways converge at the translocon. *EMBO J.* 17:2504–2512.

201. Verbon, A., S. Kuijper, H. M. Jansen, P. Speelman, and A. H. Kolk. 1990. Antigens in culture supernatant of *Mycobacterium tuberculosis*: epitopes defined by monoclonal and human antibodies. *J. Gen. Microbiol.* 136:955–964.

202. Verstijnen, C. P., R. Schoningh, S. Kuijper, J. Bruins, R. J. von Ketel, D. G. Groothuis, and A. H. Kolk. 1989. Rapid identification of cultured *Mycobacterium tuberculosis* with a panel of monoclonal antibodies in western blot and immunofluorescence. *Res. Microbiol.* 140:653–666.

203. Via, L. E., R. Curcic, M. H. Mudd, S. Dhandayuthapani, R. J. Ulmer, and V. Deretic. 1996. Elements of signal transduction in *Mycobacterium tuberculosis*: in vitro phosphorylation and in vivo expression of the response regulator MtrA. *J. Bacteriol.* 178:3314–3321.

204. Voskuil, M. I., D. Schnappinger, K. C. Visconti, M. I. Harrell, G. M. Dolganov, D. R. Sherman, and G. K. Schoolnik. 2003. Inhibition of respiration by nitric oxide induces a *Mycobacterium tuberculosis* dormancy program. *J. Exp. Med.* 198:705–713.

205. Wards, B. J., G. W. de Lisle, and D. M. Collins. 2000. An esat6 knockout mutant of *Mycobacterium bovis* produced by homologous recombination will contribute to the development of a live tuberculosis vaccine. *Tubercle Lung Dis.* 80:185–189.

206. Weiner, J. H., P. T. Bilous, G. M. Shaw, S. P. Lubitz, L. Frost, G. H. Thomas, J. A. Cole, and R. J. Turner. 1998. A novel and ubiquitous system for membrane targeting and secretion of cofactor-containing proteins. *Cell* 93:93–101.

207. Weldingh, K., I. Rosenkrands, S. Jacobsen, P. B. Rasmussen, M. J. Elhay, and P. Andersen. 1998. Two-dimensional electrophoresis for analysis of *Mycobacterium tuberculosis* culture filtrate and purification and characterization of six novel proteins. *Infect. Immun.* 66:3492–3500.

208. Wiker, H. G., M. Harboe, J. Bennedsen, and O. Closs. 1988. The antigens of *Mycobacterium tuberculosis*, H37Rv, studied by crossed immunoelectrophoresis. Comparison with a reference system for *Mycobacterium bovis* BCG. *Scand. J. Immunol.* 27:223–239.

209. Wiker, H. G., M. Harboe, and T. E. Lea. 1986. Purification and characterization of two protein antigens from the heterogeneous BCG85 complex in *Mycobacterium bovis* BCG. *Int. Arch. Allergy Appl. Immunol.* 81:298–306.

210. Wiker, H. G., M. Harboe, and S. Nagai. 1991. A localization index for distinction between extracellular and intracellular antigens of *Mycobacterium tuberculosis. J. Gen. Microbiol.* 137:875–884.

211. Wiker, H. G., M. A. Wilson, and G. K. Schoolnik. 2000. Extracytoplasmic proteins of *Mycobacterium tuberculosis*—mature secreted proteins often start with aspartic acid and proline. *Microbiology* 146:1525–1533.

212. Wilson, M., J. DeRisi, H. H. Kristensen, P. Imboden, S. Rane, P. O. Brown, and G. K. Schoolnik. 1999. Exploring drug-induced alterations in gene expression in *Mycobacterium tuberculosis* by microarray hybridization. *Proc. Natl. Acad. Sci. USA* 96:12833–12838.

213. Wong, D. K., B. Y. Lee, M. A. Horwitz, and B. W. Gibson. 1999. Identification of Fur, aconitase, and other proteins expressed by *Mycobacterium tuberculosis* under conditions of low and high concentrations of iron by combined two-dimensional gel electrophoresis and mass spectrometry. *Infect. Immun.* 67:327–336.

214. Yahr, T. L., and W. T. Wickner. 2001. Functional reconstitution of bacterial Tat translocation in vitro. *EMBO J.* 20:2472–2479.

215. Yeats, C., R. D. Finn, and A. Bateman. 2002. The PASTA domain: a beta-lactam-binding domain. *Trends Biochem. Sci.* 27:438.

216. Yen, M. R., Y. H. Tseng, E. H. Nguyen, L. F. Wu, and M. H. Saier, Jr. 2002. Sequence and phylogenetic analyses of the twin-arginine targeting (Tat) protein export system. *Arch. Microbiol.* 177:441–450.

217. Yeremeev, V. V., I. V. Lyadova, B. V. Nikonenko, A. S. Apt, C. Abou-Zeid, J. Inwald, and D. B. Young. 2000. The 19-kD antigen and protective immunity in a murine model of tuberculosis. *Clin. Exp. Immunol.* 120:274–279.

218. Yim, M. B., H. S. Yim, C. Lee, S. O. Kang, and P. B. Chock. 2001. Protein glycation: creation of catalytic sites for free radical generation. *Ann. N.Y. Acad. Sci.* 928:48–53.

219. Young, D., and T. R. Garbe. 1991. Heat shock proteins and antigens of *Mycobacterium tuberculosis. Infec. Immun.* 59:3086–3093.

220. Young, D. B., and T. R. Garbe. 1991. Lipoprotein antigens of *Mycobacterium tuberculosis. Res. Microbiol.* 142:55–65.

221. Young, D. B., S. H. Kaufmann, P. W. Hermans, and J. E. Thole. 1992. Mycobacterial protein antigens: a compilation. *Mol. Microbiol.* **6:**133–145.

222. Young, D. B., and J. R. Lamb. 1986. T lymphocytes respond to solid-phase antigen: a novel approach to the molecular analysis of cellular immunity. *Immunology* **59:**167–171.

223. Young, T. A., B. Delagoutte, J. A. Endrizzi, A. M. Falick, and T. Alber. 2003. Structure of *Mycobacterium tuberculosis* PknB supports a universal activation mechanism for Ser/Thr protein kinases. *Nat. Struct. Biol.* **10:**168–174.

224. Yuan, Y., D. D. Crane, R. M. Simpson, Y. Q. Zhu, M. J. Hickey, D. R. Sherman, and C. E. Barry III. 1998. The 16-kDa alpha-crystallin (Acr) protein of *Mycobacterium tuberculosis* is required for growth in macrophages. *Proc. Natl. Acad. Sci. USA* **95:**9578–9583.

225. Zahrt, T. C., C. Wozniak, D. Jones, and A. Trevett. 2003. Functional analysis of the *Mycobacterium tuberculosis* MprAB two-component signal transduction system. *Infect. Immun.* **71:**6962–6970.

226. Zhang, Y., B. Heym, B. Allen, D. Young, and S. Cole. 1992. The catalase-peroxidase gene and isoniazid resistance of *Mycobacterium tuberculosis. Nature* **358:**591–593.

227. Zhang, Y., R. Lathigra, T. Garbe, D. Catty, and D. Young. 1991. Genetic analysis of superoxide dismutase, the 23 kilodalton antigen of *Mycobacterium tuberculosis. Mol. Microbiol.* **5:**381–391.

228. Zhu, H., M. Bilgin, R. Bangham, D. Hall, A. Casamayor, P. Bertone, N. Lan, R. Jansen, S. Bidlingmaier, T. Houfek, T. Mitchell, P. Miller, R. A. Dean, M. Gerstein, and M. Snyder. 2001. Global analysis of protein activities using proteome chips. *Science* **293:**2101–2105.

Tuberculosis and the Tubercle Bacillus
Edited by Stewart T. Cole et al.
© 2005 ASM Press, Washington, D.C.

Chapter 17

The Cell Envelope of *Mycobacterium tuberculosis* with Special Reference to the Capsule and Outer Permeability Barrier[†]

PHILIP DRAPER AND MAMADOU DAFFÉ

The major purposes of the study of mycobacterial envelopes may be considered as follows:

- determination of the structures of the components of the envelope
- determination of the arrangement of the various components in the intact envelope
- determination of the functions of the components in protecting the bacterium from, and interacting with, its environment
- determination of biological activities of the components or combinations of them
- identification of the enzymes responsible for synthesizing the structures
- development of drugs able to interfere with biosynthesis of the components or with their biological actions.

Mycobacterial envelopes have been objects of chemical and biochemical study for many decades. Apart from their intrinsic interest as unusual natural products, their immunological adjuvant properties were clearly important, and the possibility existed that the chemical requirements for adjuvant action could be defined. It was also likely that other components of the envelope had biological activities and that these activities were involved in the pathogenesis of tuberculosis. Success in achieving the practical aims of these investigations was partial: a minimal adjuvant active structure was defined, although its activity was much lower than that of whole mycobacterial cells, while several compounds with impressive biological activities were identified, although it was not clear how these activities related to the pathogenesis of the disease. On the other hand, an impressive body of chemical and structural information was accumulated.

More recently, there has been an urgent need for new antituberculosis drugs to combat the rising incidence of drug-resistant disease. Bacterial envelopes are, in general, essential for survival under normal conditions; for a pathogen, they provide the vital interface between bacterium and host, resisting destructive mechanisms and probably modifying host-cell behavior in favor of the parasite. Since mycobacterial envelopes contain many unique chemical structures, they are obvious targets for novel drugs, and this has led to renewed interest in structures and biosynthetic pathways. Although it is very unlikely that every component of the envelope is essential for survival in a host, some are already known to be so (for example, the mycolic acids). Now that the molecular biology of *Mycobacterium tuberculosis* is beginning to be understood, the production of knockout mutants offers a convenient way of checking whether there is a requirement for a given component and also of determining biological activities in the context of whole organisms, which avoids objections that can be raised against experiments with isolated components.

Probably the most important recent development affecting this aspect of tuberculosis research, as well as most other aspects, has been the completion of the sequencing of the genome of *M. tuberculosis* H37Rv (14). Additionally, sequences of a clinical strain of *M. tuberculosis* and of the related mammalian pathogen *Mycobacterium bovis* are becoming available. Once open reading frames (ORFs) in the sequences have been correctly identified, one has, in principle, knowledge about all the enzymes and regulatory and structural proteins present in the organism. In practice, matters are not quite so simple. Although ORFs may be discovered with fair certainty,

Philip Draper • Philip@borehamh.demon.co.uk (Retired). **Mamadou Daffé** • Department of Molecular Mechanisms of Mycobacterial Infections, Institute of Pharmacology and Structural Biology, Mixed Research Unit (UMR 5089), Centre National de la Recherche Scientifique and Université Paul Sabatier, 205 route de Narbonne, 31077 Toulouse Cedex 04, France.

[†]This chapter is dedicated to the memory of Jo Colston, who died in 2003, in recognition of his outstanding contribution to the understanding of mycobacterial diseases.

identification of the proteins whose structures they encode depends on sequence homologies to already identified proteins in other organisms. For enzymes responsible for biochemical reactions unique to *M. tuberculosis*, this method of identification is ineffective. Furthermore, not all genes are expressed under all conditions, and expression must be confirmed. In spite of these problems, though, the sequencing has had a major effect on envelope research.

This review concentrates on a few topics of current interest in the field of envelope studies, particularly the permeability of the cell envelope of *M. tuberculosis*. There are a number of recent reviews where a more complete general coverage may be found (10, 15, 23). The biosynthesis of envelope components, where recent progress has been striking, is dealt with by other authors in this volume (see chapters 18 and 19).

OVERVIEW OF THE *M. TUBERCULOSIS* ENVELOPE

Figure 1 shows the assumed arrangement of the components of the envelope, based on ultrastructural, physical, and chemical evidence. The basis of the envelope is peptidoglycan, a structure common, with minor variants, to most eubacteria. Because this is a cross-linked macromolecule entirely surrounding the bacterial cell, it is mainly responsible for the size and shape of the cell. Covalently linked to the peptidoglycan are two types of molecule characteristic of mycobacteria: arabinogalactan and mycolic acids. Arabinogalactan has unusual component monosaccharides and linkages, while the mycolic acids, which esterify the distal ends of the arabinogalactan units, are unique to mycobacteria. Mycolic acids form a large family of related lipids, and particular mycobacterial species often contain unique selections from the family. The structures of all these components are known in considerable, though not complete, detail, and there is extensive knowledge of the biochemical pathways involved in their biosynthesis. Their arrangement in the envelope is partially understood. The covalently linked components may be isolated essentially free from any of the other substances normally associated with the envelope; the name "cell wall skeleton" has usefully been applied to the material.

Inside the call wall skeleton is the plasma membrane. A good deal of research was done on the plasma membranes of rapidly growing mycobacteria, but rather little is known specifically about the membrane of *M. tuberculosis*. There is every reason to suppose that mycobacterial membranes are struc-

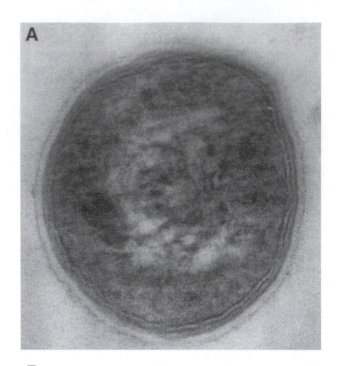

A

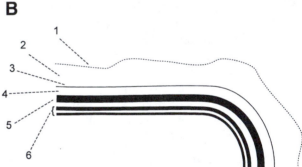

B

Figure 1. Envelope of *M. tuberculosis*. (A) Electron micrograph of ultrathin section of a strain of the *M. tuberculosis* complex. Photograph courtesy of J. L. Koeck, Laboratory of Electron Microscopy, HIA Val-de-Grace, France. (B) Diagram of the construction of the envelope (the layers are only roughly to scale). 1, position of superficial lipids of the capsule. 2, capsule mainly of polysaccharide and protein (the outer margin is ill defined unless the bacterium is within a phagocytic cell); 3, position of "buried" lipids in the capsule; 4, mycolate layer, probably including other lipids; 5, peptidoglycan plus arabinogalactan (arrangement not established); 6, triple-layer plasma membrane, with the outer layer being somewhat thicker (in electron micrographs) than the inner layer.

turally and functionally very similar to other bacterial plasma membranes. Since there has been little recent development of our knowledge of the plasma membrane of *M. tuberculosis*, it is not considered further in this chapter.

There is good evidence that undisturbed *M. tuberculosis* accumulates a capsule around itself. This consists of proteins and polysaccharides with minor amounts of lipid, and it forms the interface between the bacterium and its environment. The arrangement of the components and their functions are not really known, although they are presumably protective and may be bioactive as well. In addition, there are a very large number of "envelope-associated" substances, mostly lipids and glycolipids. Some of these are known to have powerful biological activities in experimental systems, but their situation in the envelope and contribution to disease process are incompletely known and in some cases controversial.

Porins are recently discovered components of the envelope. Quantitatively, their amount is trivial, but they are apparently important. One major and largely understood function of the envelope is to form a passive barrier, impermeable to potentially harmful water-soluble substances in the environment. This barrier is based on the mycolic acids and is physically and functionally quite separate from the plasma membrane of the bacterium. It is a highly successful barrier, as discussed below, but carries a potential penalty in that access by essential hydrophilic nutrients is impeded. The solution to this problem as developed by gram-negative bacteria, which also have highly impermeable outer membranes as part of their envelopes, is to embed pore-forming proteins in the impermeable layer. The pores are of controlled size, and their number and type are regulated according to the environment in which the bacterium finds itself. Mycobacterial porins are different from gram-negative bacterial porins, and there is much less information about most aspects of them, but the topic is being actively studied.

Cell Wall Skeleton

Numerous reviews have been written about the cell wall skeleton, so the present section restricts the discussion to some details of special interest. Mycobacterial peptidoglycan belongs to a family of structures possessed by almost all eubacteria but by no other type of living organism (22). It consists of chains of a glycan formed from alternating units of N-acetylglucosamine linked 1→4 to muramic acid (1) (see chapter 18). Tetrapeptide chains attached to the muramic acid residues cross-link the glycan chains. In the mycobacterial species examined, except *Mycobacterium leprae*, the peptide consists of L-alanyl-D-isoglutaminyl-*meso*-diaminopimelyl-D-alanine and the diaminopimelic acid is amidated (76). The structure of mycobacterial peptidoglycan (59, 76) differs slightly from that of the common type, e.g., peptidoglycan of *Escherichia coli*. First, the muramic acid is N acylated with a glycolyl residue rather than the usual acetyl residue (1). Second, a substantial number of unusual cross-links between two chains of peptidoglycan occur in mycobacterial peptidoglycan;

a proportion of bonds involving two residues of diaminopimelic acid, in addition to the usual D-alanyl-diaminopimelate linkages, have been characterized in mycobacteria (75). In the purified peptidoglycan of *M. leprae*, however, L-alanine is specifically replaced by glycine (24). Because conventional peptidoglycan tetrapeptide constituents occur in walls of *Mycobacterium lepraemurium* prepared from bacteria grown in mice (21), the formation of an unusual peptidoglycan structure in *M. leprae* is apparently not a general consequence of growth in vivo. It has been shown that the enzyme involved in forming this structure in *M. leprae* has some sequence differences from that of *M. tuberculosis* but that the kinetics of the two enzymes are similar (41), so that there is no obvious explanation for this variation in *M. leprae*. Biosynthesis of the peptidoglycan of mycobacteria has been assumed to be similar to that of the homologous structure in other bacteria and has not been much studied, although genes for many of the required enzymes have been identified in the genome of *M. tuberculosis*. The arabinogalactan and mycolic acid moieties are unique to mycobacteria and their close relatives, and their biosynthesis has received considerable attention recently. Some of this progress is reviewed in chapter 18.

The arabinogalactan is composed of D-arabinofuranosyl and D-galactofuranosyl residues. Structural analyses of the arabinogalactans from *M. tuberculosis* (18), many rapidly and slowly growing mycobacterial species, and *M. leprae* (19) showed that all possess the same structural features: two or three arabinan chains attached to the homogalactan core of linear alternating 5- and 6-linked β-D-galactofuranosyl residues. The homoarabinan chains are composed of linear α-D-arabinofuranosyl residues with branching produced by 3,5-linked α-D-arabinofuranosyl units substituted at both positions by α-D-arabinofuranosyl residues (see chapter 18). The nonreducing termini of the arabinan chains consist of penta-arabinosyl units. Some problems remain in understanding the function of the curious structure of the arabinogalactan. Its use of the furanose forms of the component monosaccharides may make the structure stiff and so help the formation of the mycolic acid monolayer (see below). The function of the long galactan "tail" of the molecule, which seems unnecessary for the structure of the cell wall skeleton as it is currently understood, is mysterious. Arabinogalactan of slow-growing mycobacteria (only) also contains a single residue of unacylated galactosamine per arabinogalactan unit (25).

Mycolic acids are long chain α-branched-β-hydroxy fatty acids elaborated by all mycobacteria and contain up to 90 carbon atoms (6). *M. tuberculosis* elaborates dicyclopropanated α-mycolates and monocyclopropanated keto- and methoxymycolates. The same types of mycolates are produced by some slow-growing mycobacterial species, such as *Mycobacterium gordonae*, *Mycobacterium kansasii*, and *Mycobacterium gastri*. The absence of oxygenated mycolates reduces the permeability of the cell wall of *M. tuberculosis* to small molecules (26), whereas a decrease in the number of mycolates linked to arabinogalactan enhances the permeability of the outer barrier of the tubercle bacillus (30).

Residues of *M. leprae* and (to a lesser extent) *M. tuberculosis* persist in formerly infected tissues long after all the organisms are dead, and all the pathogenic mycobacteria thrive in an environment—a phagocytic cell—normally able to kill and disintegrate microorganisms. At least some of this resistance to destruction may be analyzed in terms of the chemical structure of the cell wall skeleton, where the layer of mycolate protects the arabinogalactan and peptidoglycan from the effects of lytic enzymes. The arabinogalactan itself, with its unusual D-arabino configuration and galactofuranosyl units, is in any case likely to be a poor substrate for animal glycosidases. A major problem with this analysis is the difference in persistence between walls from rapidly growing, nonpathogenic species (which are destroyed quite rapidly) and the slowly growing pathogens (which are not). This difference is reflected by an in vitro model, the susceptibility of the walls to lysozyme and other wall-lytic enzymes, where the slowly growing species are less affected than the rapidly growing ones (32). However, according to present knowledge, there is no chemical difference between the cell wall

skeleton of different mycobacterial species (with the minor exception of *M. leprae*, as noted above).

The cell wall skeleton is primarily responsible for the formation of the outer permeability barrier of the mycobacterial envelope. The mycolic acids, which are attached in groups of four to the terminal arabinose moieties of a penta-arabinoside unit that terminates the arabinogalactan, are known to form a close-packed monolayer. In *M. tuberculosis*, the amount of mycolic acids present is calculated to be sufficient to form a monolayer covering the whole bacterial cell (30). The probable arrangement is shown in Fig. 2. It is likely that other lipids are associated with the mycolic acids to form the barrier, but the nature of these lipids and the exact arrangement of the whole structure is uncertain. However, it is certain that the structure exists and that it is an efficient barrier, giving *M. tuberculosis* a permeability to small hydrophilic molecules similar to that of *Pseudomonas aeruginosa* and lower than that of *E. coli* (see below).

Capsule

The recent discovery of the mixture of proteins and polysaccharides that accumulates around unstirred *M. tuberculosis* in vitro (36, 37, 53, 54), and presumably around the bacterium as it grows within a vacuole in a cell of its human host, is unexpected. Early microscopic and ultrastructural studies had led to the conclusion that pathogenic mycobacteria possessed a capsule, and more recently Rastogi et al. (60) identified such a structure on all mycobacterial species, although in a morphologically altered form.

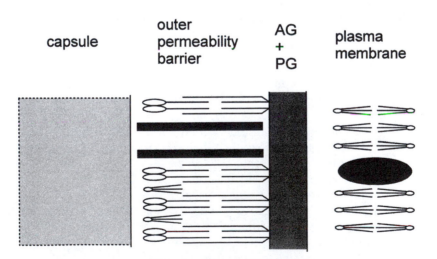

Figure 2. Permeability barriers of mycobacteria. The diagram shows the capsule, the outer permeability barrier comprising mycolates and other lipids, arabinogalactan (AG) plus peptidoglycan (PG), and the plasma membrane. The capsule and AG+PG are hydrophilic but are likely to impede the diffusion of large molecules. The outer permeability barrier and the plasma membrane allow the diffusion of lipophilic molecules. A porin is represented in the outer permeability barrier, and a transport protein is shown in the plasma membrane; these proteins allow the passage of hydrophilic molecules.

However, it was supposed that the layer was composed of lipid or glycolipid. The conventional view has been that the outer part of *M. tuberculosis* cells consists of lipid, which explains the hydrophobic properties of the cells and their tendency to stick together in aqueous media. It now seems that the lipid-bounded cells are an artifact of agitated cultures in bacteriological media, usually in the presence of low concentrations of nonionic detergents. Under these conditions, the capsule (strictly a pseudocapsule, because it is not covalently bound to the rest of the envelope) falls away, leaving the lipophilic surface of the envelope exposed. It may be noted that the carbohydrate components of the capsule were well known as occurring in culture filtrates of *M. tuberculosis* (64). Images of the capsule obtained by ultrastructural techniques intended to reduce distortion of the structure have been obtained by Beveridge and his group (56, 57). Unfortunately, the technical problem of handling a dangerous pathogen in the freeze-substitution procedure has prevented *M. tuberculosis* itself from being examined in this way.

Chemical nature of the capsule

The main polysaccharide components of the capsule are a glucan, an arabinomannan, and a mannan. The glucan, the major capsular polysaccharide of *M. tuberculosis* and other slow-growing mycobacteria, has an apparent molecular mass of 100 kDa by gel permeation chromatography (36, 37, 53), 1,000-fold lower than that of the cytosolic glycogen (4). However, the mass estimated by analytical centrifugation was twice that of mycobacterial cytosolic glycogen (P. Dinadayala, A. Lemassu, and M. Daffé, unpublished data). Glycosyl-linkage composition analysis, as well as chemical and enzymatic degradation techniques, showed that the glucan is composed of repeating units of five or six 4-linked α-D-glucosyl residues substituted at position 6 with an oligoglucosyl (mono- to pentaglucosyl) residue. Thus, the mycobacterial glucan probably corresponds to the "highly branched glycogen-type glucan" found associated with cell wall preparations of *M. tuberculosis* (3) and *M. bovis* bacille Calmette-Guérin (BCG) (43). Although the chains described for mammalian glycogen are longer (4), data from comparative analyses of the mycobacterial glycogen and glucan showed that the two polysaccharides have common structural features. However, mycobacterial glucan and glycogen differ in parameters deduced from both polarimetry and dynamic light scattering (Dinadayala et al., unpublished). Further, the inactivation of genes encoding enzymes putatively involved in the biosynthesis of capsular glucan reduced the amount of glucan and, in

some cases, altered the polysaccharide structurally, but did not affect the cytosolic glycogen (P. Dinadayala, M. Jackson, A. Lemassu, and M. Daffé, unpublished data). Based on its presence in the culture medium of several mycobacterial species (20) and its similar apparent molecular mass (34), polysaccharide II of Seibert et al. (64) probably corresponds to the capsular glucan of Daffé and colleagues despite the different structure proposed earlier (34). It is also worth noting that the glucan identified in cultures of BCG, whose structure has been described as a 6-linked-D-glucan (74), is in fact structurally similar to the glycogen-like glucan found in all other mycobacterial species examined so far (20a).

The heteropolysaccharide, D-arabino-D-mannan, has an apparent molecular mass of 13 kDa and possesses a mannan chain composed of a -6-linked α-D-mannosyl-1 core substituted at some positions 2 with an α-D-mannosyl unit. The D-arabinan segment of the arabinomannan has a structure related to that of the cell wall arabinogalactan (see above); in slow-growing species, this segment of arabinomannan is capped on the nonreducing termini by oligomannosides (36, 37, 49, 53, 54), a feature that had been noted by Ohashi as early as in 1970 (52) and that is not found in the wall AG (18, 19). The capsular mannan is a 4-kDa polysaccharide composed of a -6-linked α-D-mannosyl-1 core substituted at some positions 2 with an α-D-mannosyl unit. In *M. tuberculosis*, the structure is identical to that of the mannan moiety of the lipomannan isolated from the species.

The capsule also contains several proteins (15, 16). Some of these seem to be secreted proteins being transported to the exterior, but others may be "resident" capsular proteins. Although the putative resident proteins are present in culture filtrates, they also exist in substantial amounts in the material extracted by mild mechanical treatment of cells, suggesting that they are true capsular components shed from the surface of the cells into the medium along with the rest of the capsule (53). The potential role of the capsular proteins has been discussed in an earlier review (16).

The mycobacterial capsule contains only a tiny amount of lipid (2 to 3%), and most of this is not on the capsular surface. Progressive removal of the capsular material shows that most of the lipid is in the inner rather than the outer part of the capsule (55).

Envelope-associated compounds and the capsule

Extraction of the envelope of *M. tuberculosis* with solvents releases a bewildering variety of substances, especially lipids and glycolipids. The chemical structures of many of these are known, but in most cases their function is more or less mysterious. The identified substances have been catalogued and discussed on numerous occasions and are not reviewed exhaustively here. It is evident, however, that some of them are mainly or exclusively capsular components, which is important when their biological availability is being considered. In agreement with serological and ultrastructural findings (15) is the observation that some of the species- and type-specific glycolipids (phenolic glycolipids and glycopeptidolipids) are found in the outer layer of the capsule (55). Several other lipids traditionally considered to be wall-associated components, notably trehalose dimycolates, which in the isolated state have striking biological activity (15), evidently occur also in the capsule, a situation in which they are presumably much better able to exert any biological effects they may have. The structures, known biological activities, and biosynthetic pathways leading to the capsular lipids have been extensively reviewed recently (15–17).

The capsule as a dynamic structure

Components now known to belong to the capsule have long been recognized in culture filtrates of mycobacteria grown in laboratory media. It appears, though, that capsular substances are in a constant state of turnover even in mycobacteria growing inside host cells. A special instance of this occurs in the case of the "obligate" intracellular bacterium *M. leprae*, where the serologically active glycolipid PGL-I can be detected in the blood of patients with lepromatous leprosy (78). Similarly the morphologically and chemically distinctive glycopeptidolipid of *M. lepraemurium* can be observed within vacuoles, not containing bacteria, in phagocytic cells of infected animals (12). Both these types of lipid occur in the superficial layers of the mycobacterial capsule (55).

A more general and detailed demonstration of this shedding of putative capsular components has been made recently, using radiolabeling and fluorescence techniques to increase sensitivity. The experiments have not been done with *M. tuberculosis* itself, but the use of the fairly attenuated BCG seems an excellent model. The substances include mycobacterial polar lipids, particularly glycolipids (7), proteins (8), and carbohydrates (9). Most of these materials might be interpreted as capsular components. The substances were released into vacuoles within the infected cells; for glycolipids, at least, they could also be found in (normal) extracellular vacuoles which could be taken up by bystander cells. Although it has not yet been directly demonstrated, it seems highly likely that some of these mycobacterial products,

continuously released in vivo, affect the host in ways significant to the disease process.

Outer Permeability Barrier and the Problems It Poses to the Mycobacterium

The current view of the nature of the outer permeability layer is based on a hypothesis by Minnikin (42) that the mycolate residues of the cell wall skeleton are arranged as a close-packed monolayer all around the periphery of the structure, as shown in Fig. 2. Excellent evidence for this close packing of mycolates, obtained by a variety of physicochemical techniques by Nikaido and collaborators (39, 40, 51), has been reviewed by one of us quite recently (23). It is highly probable that other envelope-associated lipids are involved with the mycolate layer, but there is no clear evidence of their exact nature or of their arrangement. The presence of such a monolayer is, no doubt, an efficient protection for the mycobacterial cell, and direct measurements of the permeabilities of mycobacteria shows that they are, indeed, extremely impermeable (see below). However, the impermeability presents the mycobacterium with a problem: how can hydrophilic nutrients be acquired? The solution is apparently the presence of pore-forming proteins called porins in the envelope.

Porins

It is worthwhile to summarize the general properties of porins, so that the resemblances and differences found in the mycobacterial porins may be appreciated. Porins were discovered in gram-negative bacteria, where they mediate the controlled transfer of small hydrophilic molecules across the outer membrane (50). This structure is remote from sources of cellular energy, so that transfer is a passive (diffusive) process driven by concentration gradients and regulated largely by molecular size. Typically, molecules with masses up to 600 Da can pass through the pores. The process is often quite nonspecific as regards chemical structure, but there may be selection by charge or by chemical nature in the case of particular porins. Expression of porin genes is regulated by a sensor-regulator pair responding to environmental conditions (2, 44). The crystal structures of several porins and related proteins are known. They typically fold to form cylindrical structures composed of β-sheets; the internal cavity is hydrophilic and filled with water, and the diffusing molecules pass through this in solution, while the outer surface of the cylinder bears many hydrophobic residues which interact with the lipids of the outer membrane (35). Many common gram-negative porins form trimers, with each monomer supplying one pore.

Mycobacterial porins

Convincing evidence for the exceptionally low permeability of the mycobacterial envelope to aqueous solutes and for the presence of water-filled channels which allow controlled diffusion across the barrier (analogues of gram-negative porins) was obtained with *Mycobacterium chelonae*, a (relatively) nonpathogenic species noted for its generalized resistance to antimycobacterial drugs (31). Extracts of *M. chelonae*, made with detergents commonly used to extract porins from the envelopes of gram-negative bacteria, contained proteins that were able to form pores in liposomes and artificial lipid bilayers, but no progress has been made in identifying these proteins (73). Progress is restricted by general ignorance of the properties of this species, and especially of its genome, and its slight clinical significance. It shares with the significant pathogens *Mycobacterium avium* and *Mycobacterium intracellulare* a rather general resistance to antibacterial drugs and disinfectants, thought to be related to its extremely low permeability. Thus, its physiological need for some sort of porin analogue is clear, and it was a good subject for preliminary investigations.

Porin-like proteins have been identified in the envelope of the rapidly growing nonpathogen *Mycobacterium smegmatis*, and one of these has been sequenced (46, 48). It turns out that *M. smegmatis* possesses a family of genes for four related proteins, of which MspA seems to be the most important (68). The proteins differ only in minor details of their amino acid sequences. Experiments with knockout mutants have shown that MspA is responsible for the diffusion of small hydrophilic molecules across the envelope: diffusion of glucose is reduced fourfold in the mutants. In spite of this, mutant *M. smegmatis* strains show no growth defect in media containing glucose as the carbon source. This is unlikely to be because the outer permeability barrier of the rapidly growing mycobacteria is less effective than that of the slowly growing species, since the measured permeability of *M. smegmatis* is about 10 times that of *M. chelonae* (72) and therefore very similar to that of *M. tuberculosis* (13). It may be that other porins of this family are sufficiently expressed in the mutant for glucose to be transported at a rate adequate for growth. Most probably, however, this nutritionally versatile and successful species has considerable redundancy built into its mechanisms for getting nutrients, so that the loss of a single porin species is not a serious disability.

MspA has several remarkable and unique properties. Its active form is a tetramer, which has great stability against denaturation even at elevated temperatures (27). In contrast to the trimer porins of gram-negative bacteria, which have a triple pore, MspA forms only a single pore. Moreover, the pore is nearly three times longer than that typically found in gram-negative porins, which is consistent with the considerably greater thickness of the outer permeability barrier of mycobacteria. X-ray analysis of MspA revealed a homooctameric goblet-like conformation with a single central channel. MspA contains two consecutive β barrels with nonpolar outer surfaces that form a ribbon around the porin, which is too narrow to fit the thickness of the mycobacterial outer membrane model (27a). The properties of MspA are extensively discussed in a recent review (47).

Comparison of nucleotide and amino acid sequences shows that this porin of *M. smegmatis* has no homologue in *M. tuberculosis*. Therefore, one cannot extrapolate information about it directly to *M. tuberculosis*. However, knowledge of MspA illustrates some important principles. One is the use of a multimer of relatively small individual proteins to form a pore of sufficient length to cross the thick outer permeability barrier of mycobacteria. Another is that although MspA, like the gram-negative bacterial porins and proteins of the OmpA family, makes use of a β-barrel structure to form a pore, it does this in a novel way.

Porins of *M. tuberculosis*

The permeability of *M. tuberculosis* has been measured (13); while it is some 10 times greater than that of *M. chelonae*, it is comparable to that of *P. aeruginosa* and still 100 times lower than that of *E. coli*. Therefore, this species would also be expected to need some type of pore-forming molecule in its outer permeability barrier to allow access by nutrients. Within the *M. tuberculosis* complex, both BCG and *M. tuberculosis* itself have been studied, and several porin-like proteins have been discovered. Two approaches have been used: first, bacteria or isolated envelopes may be extracted under various conditions and the extracts may be examined for the presence of proteins with the distinctive properties of porins. Alternatively, the genome may be searched for genes having some sequence resemblance to known porin molecules. The identified ORFs may be cloned and expressed in some convenient system, and the properties of the recombinant proteins may be studied.

The first approach has the advantage that one is seeking proteins with appropriate properties directly and that methods of extracting, purifying, and studying porins from bacteria are well worked out. In the case of *M. tuberculosis* and its relatives, it has yielded evidence for at least two different proteins (33, 38). One of these is remarkable for its very small molecular size and its ability to be extracted, with retention of biological function, by mixtures of chloroform and methanol, a property it shares with MspA of *M. smegmatis* (48). Its active form appears to be a highly stable oligomer. The other is a larger protein which is extracted in a more conventional fashion by porin detergents and forms a larger pore. Unfortunately, the amounts of these proteins present in the mycobacterial envelope seem to be very small, so that although a good deal is now known about their physicochemical behavior, it has not yet been possible to obtain enough material for sequencing or to identify their genes in the genome.

The second approach, i.e., screening the genome, offers the potential for obtaining relatively unlimited quantities of the proteins but is limited by the known low sequence homologies between porins from various species. In fact, it turns out that *M. tuberculosis* and its close relatives possess one such similar ORF, identified as *ompA* in the published sequence. The gene is referred to as *ompA*$_{Tb}$ in this chapter to avoid confusion with the gene of *E. coli*. It has been cloned and expressed (with some difficulty, since it appears to be toxic) in *E. coli*, and the purified recombinant protein can form pores with porin-like properties in liposomes and in artificial lipid bilayers (45, 66). Material with similar apparent molecular size in SDS-PAGE gels, cross-reacting with antibodies to the recombinant protein, can be extracted from intact bacteria or from purified envelopes, although the amounts obtained are very small—too small, so far, to allow the sequencing of bands on SDS-PAGE. These extracts can also form pores, but the interpretation of this fact is uncertain, because although the extracts contain proteins reacting with antiserum to recombinant OmpA$_{Tb}$, they would also be expected to contain at least one of the proteins discovered by direct extraction. The pores formed by the extracts appeared to have roughly the same properties as those formed by recombinant OmpA$_{Tb}$ (65), but the amount of activity obtained did not allow the properties of the pores to be measured in great detail.

The original OmpA is a major outer membrane protein of *E. coli*, but its function is a matter of some controversy, since its activity in pore formation in experimental systems, though clear, is low. Pores are formed, but relatively large amounts of purified protein are needed, compared with the amounts of other porins, to obtain a specified number of pores (63, 70). The protein is one of a quite extensive family of bacterial proteins whose common feature is a particular carboxy-terminal se-

quence. This sequence probably does not form part of the β-cylinder; in gram-negative species it projects into the periplasm and may have a binding function (62, 71). Unlike those porins of gram-negative bacteria, whose biological activity is well characterized, proteins of the OmpA family occur as monomers rather than trimers. A modified, recombinant version of OmpA has been crystallized (58), and the crystal structure seems to rule out a role as a pore-forming molecule. The configuration in the crystals includes a β-cylinder (formed from the monomer protein), and water molecules are present in the cavity, but they do not form a continuous pore because the diameter is too small. It was originally reported that the form of the protein that can be persuaded to crystallize had no activity in pore formation in experimental systems, but this has subsequently been shown to be untrue. The engineered protein forms small pores in planar lipid bilayers; complete OmpA forms both small and large pores in such systems (5). A similar ability to form two types of channel is noted with OprF, a major outer membrane protein of *P. aeruginosa* which also belongs to the OmpA family (11). OprF is, in fact, more homologous to OmpA$_{Tb}$ than is OmpA.

OmpA$_{Tb}$ is clearly a member of the OmpA family, with a good sequence homology in the characteristic carboxy-terminal region. There is only weak, probably not significant, similarity elsewhere in the molecule. Like OmpA, it appears to contain a signal sequence at its amino-terminal end, but the precise site at which proteolytic cleavage normally occurs after the protein has been transferred across the plasma membrane differs from the consensus (65). It is not clear whether the signal sequence of OmpA$_{Tb}$ is present in the final native protein. The recombinant molecule contains the signal sequence of necessity, since its purification from detergent extracts of recombinant *E. coli* envelopes depends on the presence of an amino-terminal His$_6$ tag, which is joined to the rest of the protein through the signal sequence. Mouse antiserum raised to the amino-terminal sequence of OmpA$_{Tb}$ reacts with recombinant OmpA$_{Tb}$, showing that this sequence is still present (P. Jenner, R. Butler, and P. Draper, unpublished data). A recombinant molecule with the signal sequence removed was also expressed (66); this lacked the toxicity to *E. coli* of the parent polypeptide, was soluble in aqueous media without the need for detergents, and appeared to have no capacity for forming pores. Detergent extracts of broken *M. tuberculosis* contained a protein band reacting with antiserum to recombinant OmpA$_{Tb}$. This band appeared to have about the same size as the recombinant protein, and so no light is thrown on the problem of whether the putative signal sequence is removed in the native protein. The mouse antiserum mentioned above had insufficient affinity for OmpA$_{Tb}$ to detect the very small amounts of material that could be extracted from mycobacteria.

It may be noted that OmpA$_{Tb}$ is quite a small protein (with a molecular mass of about 38 kDa as estimated by SDS-PAGE), with somewhat fewer amino acid residues than OmpA, and so it is highly unlikely that it could form a pore in the outer permeability barrier of *M. tuberculosis* (see the discussion of MspA [above]). In SDS-PAGE gels there is a minor but very sharp band corresponding in size to a dimer (P. Draper, unpublished data); the system used would probably not have resolved higher oligomers, but the overwhelming majority of the recombinant protein is present as a monomer. The need to assemble the protein into its active, oligomeric form is a possible explanation of the low efficiency of pore formation in experimental systems.

It seems from its size and pore-forming properties that OmpA$_{Tb}$ is different from either of the proteins independently discovered by direct extraction. It therefore seems that there may be at least three envelope proteins of *M. tuberculosis* capable of forming pores in the outer permeability barrier. There has to be some skepticism about whether this is a primary function in the case of OmpA$_{Tb}$, because of the controversy surrounding OmpA proper, but apart from the properties of the protein in experimental membrane systems, there is more direct evidence of a physiological pore-forming function. Mutants of *M. tuberculosis* without *ompA* show reduced permeability to a number of small water-soluble substances (serine, glucose, and glycerol) (61). The reduction was only a partial one, but the effect was clear even at the earliest time at which measurements could be made (a few minutes after addition of the labeled substrate). This reduction is not reflected in any reduction in growth rate in laboratory media, but that is also the case with MpsA knockout mutants of *M. smegmatis*. It was noted that uptake of glycine was increased in the knockout mutant, in contrast to the other substances tried. This puzzling fact may be explained by supposing that OmpA$_{Tb}$ is not normally involved in the uptake of glycine. Interpretation of the results obtained with knockout mutants of this sort is not quite straightforward, since it is necessary to cultivate the mutant before any experiments can be done. The cells are therefore preadapted to any changes in growth conditions caused by the presence of the mutation. In this case, it may well be that increased expression of alternative porin-like molecules capable of transporting glycine produces this apparently paradoxical result.

In contrast to its behavior in laboratory media, the OmpA$_{Tb}$ knockout mutant is impaired in its ability to grow in macrophages and severely defective in its ability to grow in normal mice compared with wild-type *M. tuberculosis* (61). The defect in growth in animals becomes increasingly evident with time, consistent with the suggestion that it is especially severe after cell-mediated immunity begins to control the growth of the pathogen in these animals. That cell-mediated immunity is indeed involved is supported by the fact that the knockout mutant shows no defect in growth in immunologically deficient (nu^-/nu^-) animals, which are as highly susceptible to the mutant as to the wild type. Among the important early events in the response of host cells to invasion by *M. tuberculosis* is an acidification of the parasite-containing vacuole. This acidification is partially restricted by virulent bacteria; this restriction is thought to be one of the mechanisms by which the pathogen counters the antibacterial responses of the host. The OmpA$_{Tb}$ knockout mutant proves to be extremely susceptible to mild acidification of laboratory media, with a dramatic initial reduction in growth rate from which recovery occurs only after several days. The conclusion is that OmpA$_{Tb}$ is involved in the response of *M. tuberculosis* to mildly acidic conditions (such as might be found in a host phagosome, especially when cell-mediated immune processes begin to function). It is not yet clear whether this property is distinct from any general porin function.

Some data on the regulation of the expression of OmpA$_{Tb}$ have been obtained (67). The structural gene is associated in the genome with an identified sensor-regulator pair, and it is known that the regulator protein can bind to two sites, one within and one adjacent to *ompA$_{Tb}$*. Further, the binding of the putative regulator protein is much enhanced by phosphorylation, which is a distinctive feature of this type of regulatory system. Extensive attempts to produce knockout mutants of the regulator protein were unsuccessful, and so the protein may be essential. Studies by real-time PCR provided some evidence that growth in medium with high osmotic strength upregulated the expression of *ompA$_{Tb}$*, although the effect was not great. More dramatic changes were noted during growth after mild acidification of the growth medium and also in macrophages (61). This is consistent with the poor performance of the *ompA$_{Tb}$* knockout mutant under these circumstances, since it is unable to produce any OmpA$_{Tb}$ in response to the lowered pH.

Some consideration may be given to the site of mycobacterial porins. This is assumed to be the mycolate monolayer of the cell wall skeleton, which is where such pores are needed. Several publications illustrate the porins in this position, as does Fig. 2, but this has not yet been unequivocally demonstrated. Mycobacterial porins may be extracted from intact mycobacteria by mild treatment, which implies a peripheral site. OmpA$_{Tb}$ can be extracted from purified walls of *Mycobacterium microti*, a member of the *M. tuberculosis* group (Draper, unpublished), and so it must be located in the envelope and not, for example, in the plasma membrane. Recently, there has been a preliminary observation of localization using the anti-OmpA$_{Tb}$ serum (C. Raynaud, personal communication). Raynaud used confocal microscopy and the antiserum to demonstrate the presence of OmpA$_{Tb}$ on the surface of intact *M. tuberculosis*; no fluorescence was observed on the OmpA$_{Tb}$ knockout mutant. Curiously, the fluorescence was not uniformly distributed but occurred as clumps on the bacteria. Whether this is an artifact of preparation or represents a real situation remains to be demonstrated.

The investigation of mycobacterial porins, including those from *M. tuberculosis*, has already produced some exciting data, but our understanding is far from complete. Their site within the envelope needs to be determined. It would be useful to identify the genes for the two porin-like proteins discovered by detergent extraction. This would allow the production of recombinant protein in quantity and the production of knockout mutants. The status of OmpA$_{Tb}$ as a conventional porin needs to be confirmed, and a more complete understanding of its role in response to lowered pH would be valuable. A better understanding is needed of the regulation of the levels of all these proteins and of the changes produced by changing environmental conditions, especially by growth inside cells.

THE ENVELOPE AND THE DISEASE

M. tuberculosis, with its complex structure and metabolic capabilities and its ability to grow in several contrasting environments, is a fascinating subject for research. However, it also causes a fatal infectious disease. Consideration must be given to the relevance of research on the envelope to control or cure of the disease, which must include an understanding of how the pathogen can thrive in the host despite the host's normally efficient mechanisms for eliminating pathogens.

First, the envelope is protective in a passive manner. Passive resistance is the ability to be unaffected by, or to recover from, any attempts by the animal host to damage the pathogen. This is obviously a real phenomenon: pathogenic mycobacteria multiply in macrophages, which are capable of destroying many types of microorganism. It is also fairly clear how such resistance is achieved by *M. tuberculosis*: the envelope contains structures which are inherently resistant to degradation by host enzymes or which, because of their impermeability, limit access by host agents to structures which might be susceptible. The old (and correct) idea of a "thick waxy coat" has been broadened by a knowledge of the actual arrangement of the lipids involved and the truly low permeability that they allow. The realization that there is probably an even thicker layer of carbohydrate and protein outside the lipid offers the possibility that this layer impedes the diffusion of large molecules—for example, enzymes that might destroy the lipid layer—toward the bacterial surface. Evidence from Russell's group shows that material from the capsule, both lipid and carbohydrate, is shed into and escapes from the cell; clearly, the capsule is being continuously replaced during intracellular infection.

Second, components of the envelope are likely to be partly responsible for the active effect of the bacteria on the host cell, particularly in the observed modification of the properties and development of the bacterium-containing vacuole so that it becomes quite different from a vacuole containing an indifferent particle. A critical feature of this alteration is failure of proton-ATPase to be transferred to the vacuolar membrane, which prevents the acidification of phagocytic vacuoles (69) and inhibits their normal development. The shed components of the capsule might be particularly important in this activity; it has been suggested that lipoarabinomannan is involved in this process (28, 77), but the situation of lipoarabinomannan in the construction of the mycobacterial envelope is obscure, and it is not clear that it is a capsular component. It is noteworthy that these experiments involving lipoarabinomannan were done with *M. tuberculosis* itself, helping to support the validity of model systems involving BCG.

Third, components of the envelope are likely to play a substantial role in the generation of immunity to (and control of and eventual recovery from) the infection. It is important to realize that the envelope is a dynamic structure and that continuously produced labile components may be involved; this may explain why killed *M. tuberculosis* gives only poor protection against the disease.

Fourth, antibacterial drugs must pass through the envelope. They must either diffuse through the outer permeability barrier, a process likely to be slow and to require that the molecule be rather lipophilic, or pass through the pores provided by porins, which demands that the molecules be highly water soluble and relatively small. In either case, knowledge of mechanisms of transfer across the envelope is required.

Finally, the unusual nature of the mycobacterial envelope, and its evident importance to success as a pathogen, is an Achilles' heel, because interference with the formation or functioning of the envelope is likely to be harmful to the bacterium. In an interesting inversion of this principle, discovery of the mode of action of the efficacious antituberculosis drug isoniazid has enhanced our knowledge of how its target, biosynthesis of mycolic acids essential for the outer permeability barrier, proceeds.

It should be clear from this review, and from earlier ones concerning the envelope, that information about all these topics has accumulated slowly and that recently the rate of acquisition has increased, particularly because of the availability of molecular biological methods. We hope that the present chapter will draw attention to some aspects of envelope research relevant to control of tuberculosis.

REFERENCES

1. **Adam, A., J. F. Petit, J. Wietzerbin-Falszpan, P. Sinay, D. W. Thomas, and E. Lederer.** 1969. L'acide N-glycolyl-muramique, constituant des parois de *Mycobacterium smegmatis*: identification par spectrométrie de masse. *FEBS Lett.* 4:87–92.

2. **Aiba, H., F. Nakasai, S. Mizushima, and T. Mizuno.** 1989. Evidence for the physiological importance of the phosphotransfer between the two regulatory components, EnvZ and OmpR, in osmoregulation in *Escherichia coli*. *J. Biol. Chem.* 264:14090–14094.

3. **Amar-Nacasch, C., and E. Vilkas.** 1970. Étude des parois de *Mycobacterium tuberculosis*. II. Mise en évidence d'un mycolate d'arabinobiose et d'un glucane dans les parois de *M. tuberculosis* H37Ra. *Bull. Soc. Chim. Biol.* 52:145–151.

4. **Antoine, A. D., and B. S. Tepper.** 1969. Characterization of glycogen from mycobacteria. *Arch. Biochem. Biophys.* 134:207–213.

5. **Arora, A., D. Rinehart, G. Szabo, and L. K. Tamm.** 2000. Refolded outer membrane protein A of *Escherichia coli* forms ion channels with two conductive states in planar lipid bilayers. *J. Biol. Chem.* 275:1594–1600.

6. **Asselineau, C., J. Asselineau, G. Lanéelle, and M. A. Lanéelle.** 2002. The biosynthesis of mycolic acids by mycobacteria: current and alternative hypotheses. *Prog. Lipid Res.* 41:501–523.

7. **Beatty, W. L., E. R. Rhoades, H. J. Ullrich, D. Chatterjee, J. E. Heuser, and D. G. Russell.** 2000. Trafficking and release of mycobacterial lipids from infected macrophages. *Traffic* 1:235–247.

8. **Beatty, W. L., and D. G. Russell.** 2000. Identification of mycobacterial surface proteins released into subcellular compartments of infected macrophages. *Infect. Immun.* 68:6997–7002.

9. **Beatty, W. L., H. J. Ullrich, and D. G. Russell.** 2001. Mycobacterial surface moieties are released from infected macrophages by a constitutive exocytic event. *Eur. J. Cell Biol.* 80:31–40.

10. **Brennan, P. J., and H. Nikaido.** 1995. The envelope of mycobacteria. *Annu. Rev. Biochem.* 64:29–63.

11. **Brinkman, F. S. L., M. Bains, and R. E. W. Hancock.** 2000. The amino terminus of *Pseudomonas aeruginosa* outer membrane protein OprF forms channels in lipid bilayers membranes: correlation with a three-dimensional model. *J. Bacteriol.* 182:5251–5255.

12. **Brown, I. N., and P. Draper.** 1976. Growth of *Mycobacterium lepraemurium* in the mouse bone marrow: an ultrastructural study. *Infect. Immun.* 13:1199–1204.

13. **Chambers, H. F., D. Moreau, D. Yaijko, C. Miick, C. Wagner, C. Hackbarth, S. Kocagöz, and H. Nikaido.** 1995. Can penicillins and other beta-lactam antibiotics be used to treat tuberculosis? *Antimicrob. Agents Chemother.* 39:2620–2624.

14. **Cole, S. T., R. Brosch, J. Parkhill, T. Garnier, C. Churcher, D. Harris, S. V. Gordon, K. Eiglmeier, S. Gas, C. E. Barry III, F. Tekaia, K. Badcock, D. Basham, D. Brown, T. Chillingworth, R. Connor, R. Davies, K. Devlin, T. Feltwell, S. Gentles, N. Hamlin, S. Holroyd, T. Hornsby, K. Jagels, A. Krogh, J. McLean, S. Moule, L. Murphy, K. Oliver, J. Osborne, M. A. Quail, M.-A. Rajandream, J. Rogers, S. Rutter, K. Seeger, J. Skelton, R. Squares, S. Squares, J. E. Sulston, K. Taylor, S. Whitehead, and B. G. Barrell.** 1998. Deciphering the biology of *Mycobacterium tuberculosis* from the complete genome sequence. *Nature* 393:537–544.

15. **Daffé, M., and P. Draper.** 1998. The envelope layers of mycobacteria with reference to their pathogenicity. *Adv. Microb. Physiol.* 39:131–203.

16. **Daffé, M., and G. Etienne.** 1999. The capsule of *Mycobacterium tuberculosis* and its implications for pathogenicity. *Tubercle Lung Dis.* 79:153–169.

17. **Daffé, M., and A. Lemassu.** 2000. Glycomicrobiology of the mycobacterial cell surface: structure and biological activities of the cell envelope glycoconjugates, p. 225–273. In R.J. Doyle (ed.), *Glycomicrobiology*. Kluwer Academic/Plenum Press, New York, N.Y.

18. **Daffé, M., P. J. Brennan, and M. McNeil.** 1990. Predominant structural features of the cell wall arabinogalactan of *Mycobacterium tuberculosis* as revealed through characterization of oligoglycosyl alditol fragments by gas chromatography/mass spectrometry and by ^{1}H- and ^{13}C-NMR analyses. *J. Biol. Chem.* 265:6734–6743.

19. **Daffé, M., P. J. Brennan, and M. McNeil.** 1993. Major structural features of the cell wall arabinogalactans of *Mycobacterium*, *Rhodococcus*, and *Nocardia* spp. *Carbohydr. Res.* 249:383–398.

20. **Daniel, T. M.** 1984. Soluble mycobacterial antigens, p. 417–465. In G. P. Kubica and L. G. Wayne (ed.), *The Mycobacteria: a Sourcebook*, part A. Marcel Dekker, Inc., New York, N.Y.

20a. **Dinadayala, P., A. Lemassu, P. Granovski, S. Cerantola, N. Winter, and M. Daffé.** 2004. Revisiting the structure of the anti-neoplastic glucans of *Mycobacterium bovis* Bacille Calmette-Guerin. Structural analysis of the extracellular and boiling water extract-derived glucans of the vaccine substrains. *J. Biol. Chem.* 279:12369–12378.

21. **Draper, P.** 1971. The walls of *Mycobacterium lepraemurium*: chemistry and ultrastructure. *J. Gen. Microbiol.* 69:313–324.

22. **Draper, P.** 1982. The anatomy of mycobacteria, p. 9–52. In C. Ratledge and J. Stanford (ed.), *The Biology of the Mycobacteria*, vol. 1. *Physiology, Identification and Classification*. Academic Press, Ltd., London, United Kingdom.

23. **Draper, P.** 1998. The outer parts of the mycobacterial envelope as permeability barriers. *Front. Biosci.* 3:1253–1261.

24. **Draper, P., O. Kandler, and A. Darbre.** 1987. Peptidoglyacn and arabinogalactan of *Mycobacterium leprae*. *J. Gen Microbiol.* 133:1187–1194.

25. **Draper, P., K. H. Khoo, D. Chatterjee, A. Dell, and H. R. Morris.** 1997. Galactosamine in walls of slow-growing mycobacteria. *Biochem. J.* 327:519–525.

26. Dubnau, E., J. Chan, C. Raynaud, V. P. Mohan, M. A. Lanéelle, K. Yu, A. Quémard, I. Smith, and M. Daffé. 2000. Oxygenated mycolic acids are necessary for virulence of *M. tuberculosis* in mice. *Mol. Microbiol.* **36**:630–637.

27. Engelhardt, H., C. Heinz, and M. Niederweis. 2002. A tetrameric porin limits the cell wall permeability of *Mycobacterium smegmatis*. *J. Biol. Chem.* **277**:37567–37572.

27a. Faller, M., M. Niederweis, and G. E. Schulz. 2004. The structure of a mycobacterial outer-membrane channel. *Science* **303**:1189–1192.

28. Fratti, R. A., J. Chua, I. Vergne, and V. Deretic. 2003. *Mycobacterium tuberculosis* glycosylated phosphatidylinositol causes phagosome maturation arrest. *Proc. Natl. Acad. Sci. USA* **100**:5437–5442.

29. Heinz, C., H. Engelhardt, and M. Niederweis. 2003. The core of the tetrameric mycobacterial porin MspP is an extremely stable β-sheet domain. *J. Biol. Chem.* **278**:8678–8685.

30. Jackson, M., C. Raynaud, M. A. Lanéelle, C. Guilhot, C. Laurent-Winter, D. Ensergueix, B. Gicquel, and M. Daffé. 1999. Inactivation of the antigen 85C gene profoundly affects the mycolate content and alters the permeability of the *Mycobacterium tuberculosis* cell envelope. *Mol. Microbiol.* **31**:1573–1587.

31. Jarlier, V., and H. Nikaido. 1990. Permeability barrier to hydrophilic solutes in *Mycobacterium chelonei*. *J. Bacteriol.* **172**:1418–1423.

32. Kanetsuna, F. 1968. Chemical analyses of mycobacterial cell walls. *Biochim. Biophys. Acta* **158**:130–143.

33. Kartmann, B., S. Stenger, and M. Niederweis. 1999. Porins in the cell wall of *Mycobacterium tuberculosis*. *J. Bacteriol.* **181**:6543–6546.

34. Kent, P. W. 1951. Structure of an antigenic polysaccharide isolated from tuberculin *J. Chem. Soc.* **1**:364–368.

35. Koebnik, R., K. P. Locher, and P. van Gelder. 2000. Structure and function of bacterial outer membrane proteins: barrels in a nutshell. *Mol. Microbiol.* **37**:239–253.

36. Lemassu, A., and M. Daffé. 1994. Structural features of the exocellular polysaccharides of *Mycobacterium tuberculosis*. *Biochem. J.* **297**:351–357.

37. Lemassu, A., A. Ortalo-Magné, F. Bardou, G. Silve, M. A. Lanéelle, and M. Daffé. 1996. Extracellular and surface-exposed polysaccharides of non-tuberculous mycobacteria. *Microbiology* **142**:1513–1520.

38. Lichtinger, T., B. Heym, E. Maier, H. Eichner, and S. T. Cole. 1999. Evidence for a small anion-selective channel in the cell wall of *Mycobacterium bovis* BCG besides a wide cation-selective pore. *FEBS Lett.* **454**:349–355.

39. Liu, J., C. E. Barry III, G. S. Besra, and H. Nikaido. 1996. Mycolic acid structure determines the fluidity of the mycobacterial cell wall. *J. Biol. Chem.* **271**:29545–29551.

40. Liu, J., E. Y. Rosenberg, and H. Nikaido. 1995. Fluidity of the lipid domain of cell wall from *Mycobacterium chelonae*. *Proc. Natl. Acad. Sci. USA* **92**:11254–11258.

41. Mahapatra, S., D. C. Crick, and P. J. Brennan. 2000. Comparison of the UDP-N-acetylmuramate:L-alanine ligase enzymes from *Mycobacterium tuberculosis* and *Mycobacterium leprae*. *J. Bacteriol.* **182**:6827–6830.

42. Minnikin, D. E. 1982. Lipids: complex lipids, their chemistry, biosynthesis and roles, p. 95–184. *In* C. Ratledge and J. Stanford, (ed.), *The Biology of the Mycobacteria*, vol. 1. *Physiology, Identification and Classification*. Academic Press Ltd., London, United Kingdom.

43. Misaki, A., and S. Yukawa. 1966. Studies on cell walls of mycobacteria. II. Constitution of polysaccharides from BCG cell walls. *J. Biochem.* **59**:511–520.

44. Mizuno, T., and S. Mizushima. 1990. Signal transduction and gene regulation through the phosphorylation of two regulatory components: the molecular basis for the osmotic regulation of the porin genes. *Mol. Microbiol.* **4**:1077–1082.

45. Mobasheri, H., R. H. Senaratne, P. Draper, and E. J. A. Lea. 1998. Single channel properties of a porin-like protein from *Mycobacterium tuberculosis* H37Rv in planar lipid bilayers. *Biophys. J.* **74**:A320.

46. Mukhopadhyay, S., D. Basu, and P. Chakrabarti. 1997. Characterization of a porin from *Mycobacterium smegmatis*. *J. Bacteriol.* **179**:6205–6207.

47. Niederweis, M. 2003. Mycobacterial porins—new channel proteins in unique outer membranes. *Mol. Microbiol.* **49**:1167–1177.

48. Niederweis, M., S. Ehrt, C. Heinz, U. Klocker, S. Karosi, K. M. Swiderek, L. W. Riley, and R. Benz. 1999. Cloning of the *mspA* gene encoding a porin from *Mycobacterium smegmatis*. *Mol. Microbiol.* **33**:933–945.

49. Nigou, G., M. Gilleron, T. Brando, A. Vercellone, and G. Puzo. 1999. Structural definition of arabinomannans from *Mycobacterium bovis* BCG. *Glycoconj. J.* **16**:257–264.

50. Nikaido, H. 1994. Porins and specific diffusion channels in bacterial outer membranes. *J. Biol. Chem.* **269**:3905–3908.

51. Nikaido, H., S. H. Kim, and E. Y. Rosenberg. 1993. Physical organization of lipids in the cell wall of *Mycobacterium chelonae*. *Mol. Microbiol.* **8**:1025–1030.

52. Ohashi, M. 1970. Studies on the chemical structure of serologically active arabinomannan from mycobacteria. *Jpn. J. Exp. Med.* **40**:1–14.

53. Ortalo-Magné, A., M. A. Dupont, A. Lemassu, Å. B. Andersen, P. Gounon, and M. Daffé. 1995. Molecular composition of the outermost capsular material of the tubercle bacillus. *Microbiology* **141**:1609–1620.

54. Ortalo-Magné, A., Å. B. Andersen, and M. Daffé. 1996. The outermost capsular arabinomannans and other mannoconjugates of virulent and avirulent tubercle bacilli. *Microbiology* **142**:927–935.

55. Ortalo-Magné, A., A. Lemassu, M. A. Lanéelle, F. Bardou, G. Silve, P. Gounon, G. Marchal, and M. Daffé. 1996. Identification of the surface-exposed lipids on the cell envelope of *Mycobacterium tuberculosis* and other mycobacterial species. *J. Bacteriol.* **178**:456–461.

56. Paul, T. R., and T. J. Beveridge. 1992. Reevaluation of envelope profiles and cytoplasmic ultrastructure of mycobacteria processed by conventional embedding and freeze-substitution protocols. *J. Bacteriol.* **174**:6508–6517.

57. Paul, T. R., and T. J. Beveridge. 1994. Preservation of surface lipids and determination of ultrastructure of *Mycobacterium kansasii* by freeze-substitution. *Infect. Immun.* **62**:1542–1550.

58. Pautsch, A., and G. E. Schulz. 1998. Structure of the outer membrane protein A transmembrane domain. *Nat. Struct. Biol.* **5**:1013–1017.

59. Petit, J. F., A. Adam, J. Wietzerbin-Falszpan, E. Lederer, and J. M. Ghuysen. 1969. Chemical structure of the cell wall of *Mycobacterium smegmatis*. I. Isolation and partial characterization of the peptidoglycan. *Biochem. Biophys. Res. Commun.* **35**:478–485.

60. Rastogi, N., C. Fréhel, and H. L. David. 1986. Triple-layered structure of mycobacterial cell wall: evidence for the existence of a polysaccharide-rich outer layer in 18 mycobacterial species. *Curr. Microbiol.* **13**:237–242.

61. Raynaud, C., K. G. Papavinasasundaram, R. A. Speight, B. Springer, P. Sander, E. Böttger, M. J. Colston, and P. Draper. 2002. The functions of OmpATb, a pore-forming protein of *Mycobacterium tuberculosis*. *Mol. Microbiol.* **46**:191–201.

62. Ried, G., R. Koebnik, I. Hindennach, B. Mutschler, and U. Henning. 1994. Membrane topology and assembly of outer membrane protein OmpA of *Escherichia coli*. *Mol. Gen. Genet.* **243:**127–135.

63. Saint, N., E. De, N. Julien, N. Orange, and G. Molle. 1992. Ionophore properties of OmpA of *Escherichia coli*. *Biochim. Biophys. Acta* **1145:**119–123.

64. Seibert, F. B. 1949. The isolation of three different proteins and two polysaccharides from tuberculin by alcohol fractionation. Their chemical and biological properties. *Am. Rev. Tuberc.* **59:**86–101.

65. Senaratne, R. H. 1999. *Porin-Like Proteins from* Mycobacterium tuberculosis. Ph.D. thesis. Open University, Milton Keynes, United Kingdom.

66. Senaratne, R. H., H. Mobasheri, K. G. Papavinasasundaram, P. Jenner, E. J. A. Lea, and P. Draper. 1998. Expression of a gene for a porin-like protein of the OmpA family from *Mycobacterium tuberculosis* H37Rv. *J. Bacteriol.* **180:**3541–3547.

67. Speight, R. A. 2000. *The Structure, Function and Regulation of Mycobacterial Porin-Encoding Genes*. Ph.D. thesis. University College, London, United Kingdom.

68. Stahl, C., S. Kubetzko, I. Kaps, S. Seeber, H. Engelhardt, and M. Niederweis. 2001. MspA provides the main hydrophobic pathway through the cell wall of *Mycobacterium smegmatis*. *Mol. Microbiol.* **40:**451–464.

69. Sturgill-Koszycki, S., P. H. Schlesinger, P. Chakraborty, P. L. Hadix, H. L. Collins, A. K. Fok, R. D. Allen, S. D. Gluck, J. Heuser, and D. G. Russell. 1994. Lack of acidification in *Mycobacterium* phagosomes produced by exclusion of the vesicular proton-ATPase. *Science* **263:**678–681.

70. Sugawara, E., and H. Nikaido. 1992. Pore-forming activity of OmpA porin of *Escherichia coli*. *J. Biol. Chem.* **267:**2507–2511.

71. Sugawara, E., M. Steiert, S. Rouhani, and H. Nikaido. 1996. Secondary structure of the outer membrane proteins OmpA of *Escherichia coli* and OprF of *Pseudomonas aeruginosa*. *J. Bacteriol.* **178:**6067–6069.

72. Trias, J., and R. Benz. 1994. Permeability of the cell wall of *Mycobacterium smegmatis*. *Mol. Microbiol.* **14:**283–290.

73. Trias, J., V. Jarlier, and R. Benz. 1992. Porins in the cell wall of mycobacteria. *Science* **258:**1479–1481.

74. Wang, R., M. E. Klegerman, I. Marsden, M. Sinnott, and M. J. Groves. 1995. An anti-neoplastic glycan isolated from *Mycobacterium bovis* (BCG vaccine). *Biochem. J.* **311:**867–872.

75. Wietzerbin, J., B. C. Das, J.-F. Petit, E. Lederer, M. Leyh-Bouille, and J.-M. Ghuysen. 1974. Occurrence of D-alanyl-(D)-*meso*-diaminopimelic acid and *meso*-diaminopimelyl-*meso*-diaminopimelic acid interpeptide linkages in the peptidoglycan of *Mycobacteria* (sic). *Biochemistry* **13:**3471–3476.

76. Wietzerbin-Falszpan, J., B. C. Das, I. Azuma, A. Adam, J. F. Petit, and E. Lederer. 1970. Isolation and mass spectrometric identification of the peptide subunits of mycobacterial cell walls. *Biochem. Biophys. Res. Commun.* **40:**57–63.

77. Xu, S., A. Cooper, S. Sturgill-Koszycki, T. van Heyningen, D. Chatterjee, I. Orme, P. Allen, and D. G. Russell. 1994. Intracellular trafficking in *Mycobacterium tuberculosis* and *Mycobacterium avium*-infected macrophages. *J. Immunol.* **153:**2568–2578.

78. Young, D. B., J. P. Harnish, J. Knight, and T. M. Buchanan. 1985. Detection of phenolic glycolipid I in sera from patients with lepromatous leprosy. *J. Infect. Dis.* **152:**1078–1081.

Tuberculosis and the Tubercle Bacillus
Edited by Stewart T. Cole et al.
© 2005 ASM Press, Washington, D.C.

Chapter 18

Structure, Biosynthesis, and Genetics of the Mycolic Acid-Arabinogalactan-Peptidoglycan Complex

SEBABRATA MAHAPATRA, JOYOTI BASU, PATRICK J. BRENNAN, AND DEAN C. CRICK

The cell envelope of *Mycobacterium tuberculosis* is made up of three major components: a plasma membrane; a covalently linked complex of mycolic acid, arabinogalactan, and peptidoglycan (MAPc); and a polysaccharide-rich capsule-like layer. The plasma membrane of *Mycobacterium* is comparable to that of other gram-positive organisms except that it is rich in the phosphatidylinositol mannosides found in all members of the *Actinomycetales* (8). The MAPc is made up of a highly cross-linked peptidoglycan (PG), which is covalently linked to arabinogalactan (AG). The AG is in turn esterified to a variety of 60- to 90-carbon long, branched α-alkyl, β-hydroxy mycolic acids. This complex is associated with a variety of noncovalently linked lipids, glycans, proteins, and peptides as decribed in chapter 17.

The PG of *M. tuberculosis* has been classified as A1γ, as has that of *Escherichia coli* and a number of other organisms (59). However, mycobacterial PG does have some distinguishing features (Fig. 1). The glycan chains are composed of alternating units of (β 1→4)-linked *N*-acetylglucosamine (GlcNAc) and *N*-glycolylmuramic acid (MurNGlyc), whereas most other bacteria contain N-acetylmuramic acid, suggesting that the N-acetyl group has been oxidized to N-glycolyl at some stage of biosynthesis. A tetrapeptide (L-alanyl-D-isoglutamyl-*meso*-diaminopimelyl-D-alanine) side chain substitutes the carboxylic acid function of each muramic acid residue (35). In *Mycobacterium leprae* PG, the L-alanine residues are completely replaced with glycine (21).

The peptide chains of *Mycobacterium* spp. are heavily cross-linked, providing added structural integrity for the bacterium. The overall degree of cross-linking is 70 to 80% in *Mycobacterium* spp., compared to 20 to 30% in *E. coli* (42). About two-thirds of the cross-links are between the carboxyl group of a terminal D-Ala and the amino groups of the D-center of a *meso*-diaminopimelic acid (DAP) of another peptide, the typical cross-linking found in A1γ PG. Approximately one-third of the peptide cross-bridges occur between the carboxyl group of the L-center of one DAP residue and the amino group of the D-center of another DAP residue, forming an L,D-cross-link (66). Only recently have L,D-cross-links been found in the PG of stationary-phase *E. coli* (61). The free carboxylic acid groups of the DAP or D-isoglutamic acid residues of mycobacterial PG may be amidated, and some of the free carboxylic groups of the D-isoglutamic acid residues may also be modified by the addition of a glycine residue in peptide linkage (33). The C-6 of some of the muramic acid residues form phosphodiester bonds to C-1 of α-D-GlcNAc, which, in turn, is (1→3) linked to a α-L-rhamno-pyranose (Rha*p*) residue, providing the "linker unit" between the galactan of AG and PG (44).

AG is a unique polymer of arabinofuranose (ara*f*) and galactofuranose (gal*f*) (46) (Fig. 2). The galactan of AG consists of a linear chain of about 30 units of alternating 5- and 6-linked β-D-Gal*f* residues (14). The arabinan chains, of which there may be two or three, are attached to the C-5 of some of the 6-linked Gal*f* residues close to the reducing end of the molecule and are composed of 5-linked α-D-Ara*f* with branching introduced at the 2 and 3 positions, forming a [β-D-Ara*f*-(1→2)-α-D-Ara*f*]₂-3,5-α-D-Ara*f*-(1→5)-α-D-Ara*f* motif at the nonreducing termini (14). Mycolic acids are esterified, in clusters of four, to two-thirds of the terminal arabinofuranosides (45). Thus, the primary structure of the MAPc is quite well understood.

However, the secondary structure of the MAPc is still open to conjecture. Two models have been proposed to describe the physical organization of the

Sebabrata Mahapatra, Patrick J. Brennan, and Dean C. Crick   •   Department of Microbiology, Immunology and Pathology, Colorado State University, Fort Collins, CO 80523-1682.   **Joyoti Basu**   •   Department of Chemistry, Bose Institute, Kolkata 700 009, India.

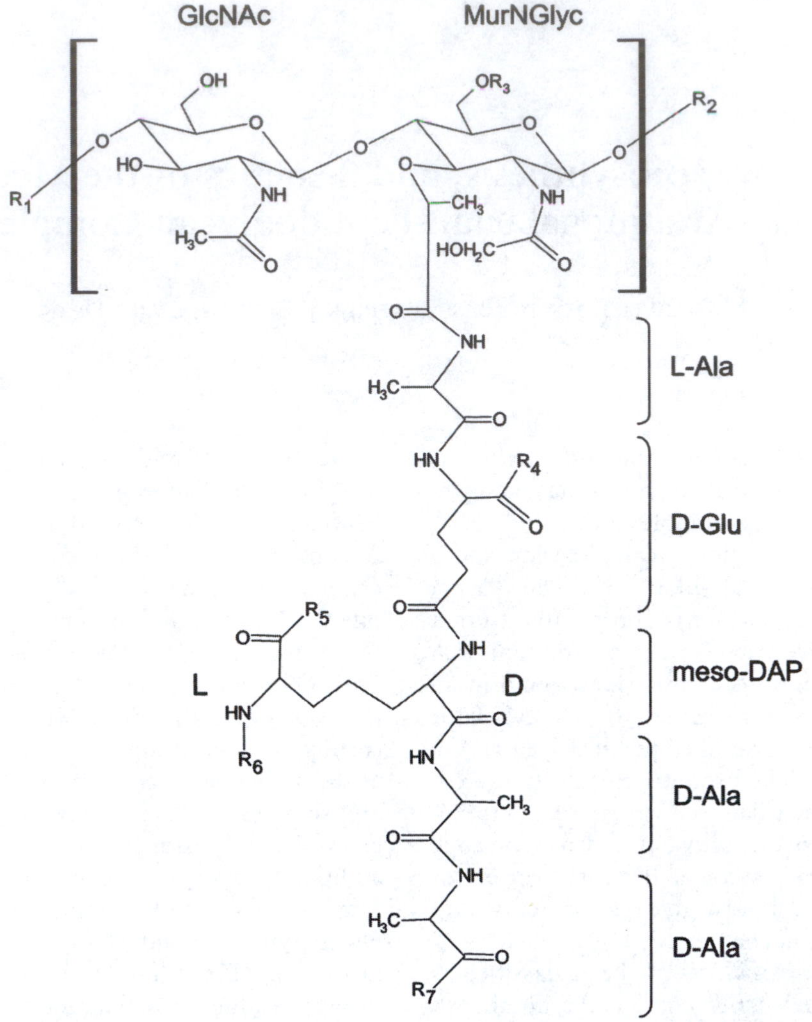

Figure 1. Structure of a representative monomer of mycobacterial PG prior to peptide trimming. R1, *N*-glycolylmuramic acid residue of another monomer; R2, *N*-acetylglucosamine residue of another monomer; R3, H or the linker unit of AG; R4, OH, NH₂ or glycine; R5, OH or NH₂; R6, H, or cross-linked to penultimate D-Ala or to the D-center of another *meso*-DAP residue; R7, OH or NH₂.

MAPc. One model predicts that the PG and galactan are parallel to the plasma membrane. This orientation is consistent with traditional models of PG structure (25, 47). However, recent application of molecular mechanics modeling indicates that it is possible that the PG and AG strands are coiled and perpendicular to the plane of the plasma membrane (19, 20).

Although the structural definition of the mycobacterial MAPc remains an area of interest, the current impetus for studying *M. tuberculosis* and other pathogenic mycobacteria is the need to identify targets for the development of new drugs. It is also felt that knowledge of the biosynthesis and genetics of this aspect of the cell wall biogenesis may provide insight into overall cell wall architecture, particularly the relationship between its soluble components and the insoluble MAPc. Therefore, emphasis has been

shifting to the study of cell envelope biosynthesis and the identification of enzymes that are essential to the viability of *M. tuberculosis*. The publication of the sequence of the complete *M. tuberculosis* genome in 1998 and a list of essential genes in 2003 (56) has greatly aided these studies.

BIOSYNTHESIS OF PEPTIDOGLYCAN PRECURSORS

PG biosynthesis in mycobacteria has not been investigated in detail but is generally assumed to be similar to that seen in *E. coli*. This notion is supported by genetic analysis. Most of the genes involved in the basic PG biosynthesis in *E. coli* are known (63, 64). Cole et al. have identified the homo-

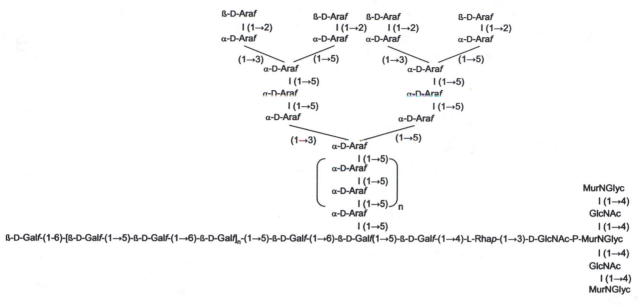

Figure 2. Schematic illustration of the cell wall AG and the Rha*p*-GlcNAc linker.

logues of most of those in the *M. tuberculosis* and *M. leprae* genomes (12); however, the genes involved in the biosynthesis of the distinguishing features of the PG of *Mycobacterium* spp., discussed above, have yet to be identified.

PG biosynthesis in *E. coli* can be divided into three stages based on subcellular localization (63, 64). The first stage, which occurs in the cytoplasm, is the formation of UDP-*N*-acetylmuramyl-L-alanyl-D-isoglutamyl-*meso*-diaminopimelyl-D-alanyl-D-alanine, or Park's nucleotide. In the second, membrane-associated stage, lipid-linked disaccharide–pentapeptide molecules are synthesized. Once synthesized, the disaccharide-pentapeptide unit is flipped to the outer surface of the membrane, which is the site for the final, periplasmic steps of PG biosynthesis. These periplasmic steps involve polymerization of the glycan chains by transglycosylation and cross-linking of the peptide side chains by transpeptidation, forming nascent PG, which is then incorporated into the existing cell wall. The current understanding of this process is summarized in Fig. 3.

The first committed step in the PG biosynthesis pathway is the transfer of an enolpyruvate residue to the 3 position of the GlcNAc residue of UDP-GlcNAc by MurA. *M. tuberculosis* MurA has been overexpressed and partially characterized by De Smet et al. (17). Their results indicate that wild-type *M. tuberculosis* is resistant to the antibiotic fosfomycin due to the presence of an aspartate residue instead of a cysteine residue at position 117. Replacement of aspartate-117 by a cysteine residue resulted in a mutant strain of *M. tuberculosis* that was not resistant to

fosfomycin (17), thus highlighting the need to use the proteins from the target organism when screening for new antibiotics.

The subsequent NADPH-dependent reaction, catalyzed by MurB, reduces the enolpyruvate moiety to D-lactate, yielding UDP-*N*-acetylmuramic acid (UDP-MurNAc). It has been reported that in *Nocardia asteroides* the oxidation of the *N*-acetyl group to the *N*-glycolyl function of muramic acid occurs at this stage (24), but data are not available for *Mycobacterium* spp. UDP-MurNAc-pentapeptide is then formed by the sequential addition of L-alanine, D-isoglutamic acid, DAP, and D-alanyl-D-alanine to the UDP-MurNAc in four reactions catalyzed by the MurC, MurD, MurE, and MurF ligases, respectively. The first reaction of this sequence is the addition of the L-alanine to the lactyl moiety of UDP-MurNAc, catalyzed by MurC, a UDP-MurNAc:L-alanine ligase. MurC from *M. tuberculosis* (Rv2152c) and *M. leprae* has been overexpressed and partially characterized (39). MurC cloned from *M. tuberculosis* and *M. leprae* has similar catalytic activities to those of other known alanine ligases, except for having much lower apparent K_m values for glycine. It is not clear from the kinetic data why *M. tuberculosis* should have L-alanine in its PG while *M. leprae* has glycine.

The addition of a D-isoglutamic acid to the carboxy terminus of the L-alanine residue of the UDP-MurNAc-L-alanine is catalyzed by MurD, a UDP-MurNAc-L-Ala:D-Glu ligase. The MurD (Rv2155c) of *M. tuberculosis* has also been overexpressed in active form (unpublished data) and is enzymatically similar to the MurD from *E. coli*. MurE and MurF,

A

B

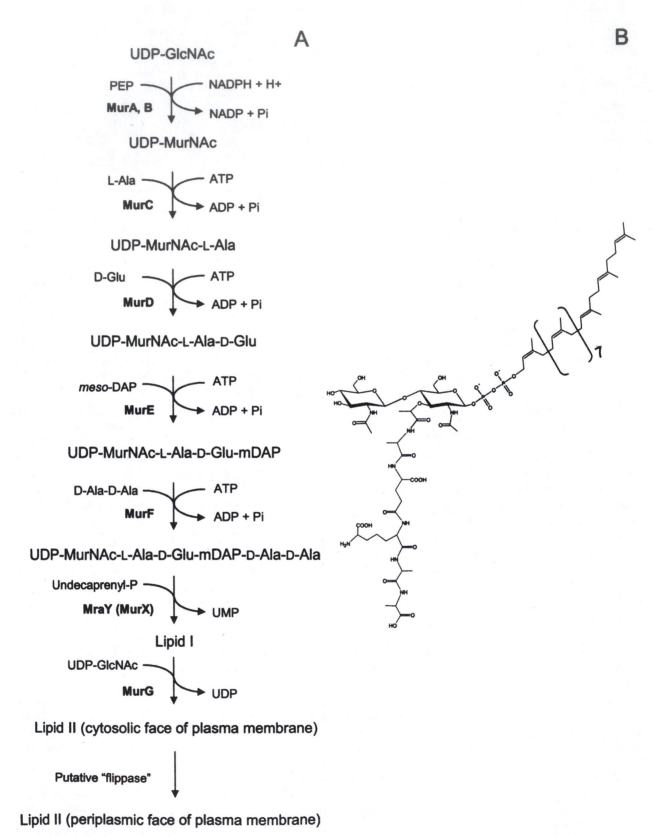

UDP-GlcNAc

PEP ⟶   ⟶ NADPH + H+
MurA, B ↓ ⟶ NADP + Pi

UDP-MurNAc

L-Ala ⟶   ⟶ ATP
MurC ↓   ⟶ ADP + Pi

UDP-MurNAc-L-Ala

D-Glu ⟶   ⟶ ATP
MurD ↓   ⟶ ADP + Pi

UDP-MurNAc-L-Ala-D-Glu

meso-DAP ⟶ ⟶ ATP
MurE ↓   ⟶ ADP + Pi

UDP-MurNAc-L-Ala-D-Glu-mDAP

D-Ala-D-Ala ⟶ ⟶ ATP
MurF ↓   ⟶ ADP + Pi

UDP-MurNAc-L-Ala-D-Glu-mDAP-D-Ala-D-Ala

Undecaprenyl-P ⟶
MraY (MurX) ↓ ⟶ UMP

Lipid I

UDP-GlcNAc ⟶
MurG ↓ ⟶ UDP

Lipid II (cytosolic face of plasma membrane)

Putative "flippase" ↓

Lipid II (periplasmic face of plasma membrane)

Figure 3. (A) Biosynthetic pathway leading to the formation of lipid II in *E. coli*. (B) Structure of lipid II from *E. coli*.

the remaining two ligases of this pathway, have yet to be studied.

Of the other enzymes related to UDP-MurNAc-pentapeptide synthesis in mycobacteria, the D-alanine racemase and D-alanine:D-alanine ligase from *Mycobacterium smegmatis* have been studied. *M. smegmatis* was found not to be dependent on the D-alanine racemase activity for growth (10), suggesting that there may be an alternative pathway for the biosynthesis of D-alanine in this organism. The D-alanine:D-alanine ligase activity of the *M. smegmatis* *ddl* gene product has been confirmed (23).

In *E. coli*, MraY (sometimes designated MurX) catalyzes the synthesis of lipid I by transferring phosphoryl-MurNAc-pentapeptide to a molecule of undecaprenyl phosphate. In a subsequent reaction catalyzed by MurG (48, 62), a GlcNAc residue is transferred from UDP-GlcNAc to form GlcNAc-MurNAc(pentapeptide)-prenol (lipid II, Fig. 3) (62). The lipid II of *M. smegmatis* has been synthesized in a cell-free assay system in our laboratory (unpublished data), and the lipid moiety has been identified as decaprenyl phosphate (unpublished data) instead of undecaprenyl phosphate as seen in *E. coli*, *Staphylococcus aureus*, and *Micrococcus luteus* (28, 29). The carboxylic acid functions of the peptide moiety of the mycobacterial lipid II are extensively modified by amidation, methylation, and addition of glycine residues in different combinations (unpublished data). The enzymes involved in these modifications are the subjects of continuing study. The disaccharide-pentapeptide of lipid II is thought to be translocated from the cytoplasmic face of the plasma membrane to the periplasmic face, where it is used directly in the assembly of PG. It is not clear how this translocation is mediated, but it is likely that a "flippase" similar in function, although not in sequence, to the protein encoded by the *wzxE* gene in *E. coli* (55) is responsible.

TRANSPEPTIDATION AND TRANSGLYCOSYLATION

Analysis of the genome of *M. tuberculosis* reveals the presence of a repertoire of putative penicillin binding proteins (PBPs), of which only a few have been characterized (Table 1). Four major PBPs, migrating at 94, 82, 52, and 37 kDa, have been detected in the membranes of exponentially growing cultures of *M. tuberculosis* H37Ra (11). Inactivation of the 94-, 82-, and 52-kDa PBPs in exponentially growing cells is associated with antibacterial activity of β-lactams. A β-lactam/β-lactamase inhibitor combination is bactericidal in the exponential phase of the *M. tuberculosis* cultures. In spite of this, β-lactam

Table 1. The putative penicillin binding proteins of *M. tuberculosis*

Gene	Annotation	Length (aa)
Rv0016c	Probable PBP	491
Rv0050	PBP	678
Rv0907	Probable PBP	532
Rv1367c	Probable PBP	377
Rv1730c	Probable PBP	517
Rv1922	Probable PBP	371
Rv2163c	PBP2	679
Rv2864c	Probable PBP	603
Rv2911	PBP	191
Rv3330	Probable PBP	405
Rv3627c	Probable PBP	461
Rv3682	PBP	810

antibiotics are ineffective as therapeutic agents of tuberculosis. The ineffectiveness of the β-lactams most probably lies largely in the production of β-lactamase (54) and failure to access the appropriate PBP targets (11, 31, 52).

The bimodular class A PBPs consist of a carboxy-terminal acyltransferase module fused at its N-terminal end to a glycosyltransferase module. *M. tuberculosis* and *M. leprae* each have a single β-lactam-sensitive class A high-molecular-mass, bimodular PBP encoded by *Rv0050* and *ML2688*, respectively. When expressed in *E. coli*, these PBPs, referred to as PBP1*, adopt the expected membrane topologies and are sensitive to a range of β-lactams, with k_{+2}/K (the second-order rate constant for enzyme acylation) ranging from 100,000 to 10,000 $M^{-1}s^{-1}$ (4, 6). Disruption of the gene encoding the ortholog of these proteins in *M. smegmatis* results in a strain that grows more slowly in the exponential phase (7), suggesting a role for this PBP in the exponential phase of growth. The β-lactam sensitivity of this PBP is in accord with the effectiveness of β-lactam/β-lactamase inhibitor combinations in exponentially growing cultures of *M. tuberculosis* (11). The genomes of both *M. tuberculosis* and *M. leprae* have the information for another pair of bimodular class A PBPs encoded by *Rv3682* and *ML2308*, with closely related acyltransferase modules. While the protein encoded by *Rv3682* has not been characterized, its ortholog in *M. leprae*, designated PBP1, when expressed in *E. coli* has low k_{+2}/K values of 1 to 10 $M^{-1} s^{-1}$ for β-lactams. The acyltransferase module expressed alone in *E. coli* has the same low affinity for β-lactams as the full-size protein fusion (38). The ortholog of PBP1 in *M. smegmatis*, when disrupted by transposition, results in a strain impaired in long-term survival (32). cDNA obtained from macrophage-grown bacilli indicates that the gene for a class A PBP is up-regulated during in vivo growth of *M. tuberculosis* (26), suggesting that cell wall remodeling is one of the features of in vivo growth of *M. tuberculosis*, a characteristic also observed in *Salmonella enterica* serovar Typhimurium grown in vivo (53).

Inferring from existing knowledge that the D,D-cross-linked PG predominates in exponentially growing cultures and that the L,D-cross-linked PG predominates in stationary-phase cultures in *E. coli* (61), and taking into account the fact that disruption of the *M. smegmatis* orthologs of PBP1* and PBP1 result in impaired exponential-phase growth and stationary-phase survival, respectively, it appears possible that PBP1* and PBP1 play distinct roles in synthesis of the D,D-cross-linked PG and the L,D-cross-linked PG, respectively.

Recently it was shown that the gram-positive bacterium *Enterococcus faecium* shifts its muropeptide composition from the usual D,D-cross-links to L,D-cross-links as a mechanism of acquiring β-lactam resistance (40). In *M. smegmatis* grown for 9 days at 37°C D,D-cross-linked and L,D-cross-linked peptides occur in a proportion of 2:1, raising the possibility that mycobacterial β-lactam resistance relates, at least in part, to the presence of the L,D-cross-links. It is of immediate interest to test the hypothesis that the penicillin-resistant acyltransferase module of PBP1 of *M. tuberculosis* and *M. leprae*, fused to a glycosyltransferase module, carries out L,D-cross-linked PG assembly from lipid II precursor molecules in a penicillin-resistant manner. It is also possible that a β-lactam-insensitive D,D-cross-link-specific carboxypeptidase operates to cleave the C-terminal D-Ala residue of the pentapeptide, causing accumulation of substrate for the L,D-transpeptidase, a situation that exists in β-lactam-resistant *E. faecium* (40).

Class B PBPs are characterized by a C-terminal acyltransferase module fused to an N-terminal module that, for PBP3 of *E. coli*, is involved in protein-protein interactions with components of the divisome (41). In *M. tuberculosis*, *Rv2163* encodes a putative PBP that appears to be closely related to PBP3 of *E. coli*. It is clustered on the chromosome with genes predicted to encode cell division proteins FtsQ (*Rv2151c*), FtsZ (*Rv2150c*), and FtsW (*Rv2154c*), as well as the genes encoding protein homologs of *E. coli* MurC, MurG, MurD, MurX (MraY), MurF, and MurE (*Rv2152c*, *Rv2153c*, *Rv2155c*, *Rv2156c*, *Rv2157c*, and *Rv2158c*, respectively). Together, these form the *M. tuberculosis* dcw cluster. Of the putative components of the *M. tuberculosis* divisome, FtsZ and FtsW have been expressed in *E. coli* and have been shown to interact directly through a cluster of oppositely charged residues present at the C termini of the two proteins (16). The interaction between

FtsZ and FtsW may serve to link cell division to septal PG biosynthesis (Fig. 4). Rv2163c has also been expressed in *E. coli*, binds penicillin, and interacts with FtsW (unpublished observations).

Monofunctional or low-molecular-mass PBPs have been implicated in cell morphogenesis in *E. coli*. The *M. tuberculosis* genome appears to contain the information for three such PBPs encoded by *Rv3627c*, *Rv3330*, and *Rv2911*, which contain the signature sequences SXXK, SXN, and KTG. None of these PBPs have yet been biochemically characterized. However, a 49.5-kDa PBP has been isolated and characterized from *M. smegmatis* (3). This PBP has a high affinity for benzylpencillin, ampicillin, and cefoxitin and has both carboxypeptidase and transpeptidase activities, marking it as a true low-molecular-mass PBP (51). Antibodies raised against this protein cross-react with a 52-kDa protein from *M. tuberculosis*, perhaps Rv3627c. Thus far, bioinformatics have not identified a one-to-one correspondence of open reading frames encoding the mycobacterial divisome and its *E. coli* counterpart, suggesting that mycobacteria lack some of the divisome components. Perhaps protein-protein interactions unique to mycobacteria, such as those between FtsZ and FtsW, are responsible for maintaining the functionality of the divisome and linking septal PG synthesis to cell division in the absence of some of the components found in *E. coli*.

A number of eukaryotic-type serine/threonine kinase-encoding genes have been found in the genome of *M. tuberculosis* (2). Of these, the genes *pknA* and *pknB*, encoding eukaryotic-type serine/threonine ki-

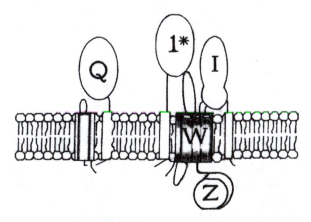

Figure 4. Hypothetical organization of the cell division apparatus of *M. tuberculosis*. FtsZ (Z) interacts with FtsW (W) through the C-tails of both proteins, thereby anchoring FtsZ to the membrane. FtsW is predicted to play a central role by linking cell division to PG biosynthesis through interactions with PBP1* (1*) and PBP3 (I). A putative FtsQ (Q) has also been identified. Its function is not yet known.

nases, are located adjacent to an open reading frame (*Rv0016c*) encoding a putative PBP. Heterologous expression of *pknA* of *M. tuberculosis* in *E. coli* shows elongation of the rods from 1–2 μm to 60–70 μm (9), implicating PknA in regulation of morphological changes associated with cell division.

A previously uncharacterized domain, the PASTA domain (for "penicillin-binding protein and serine/threonine kinase-associated domain") has been identified at the C-terminal ends of PknB and PBP1 (Rv3682) of *M. tuberculosis* (69), among several other proteins of gram-positive bacteria. Structural analyses have characterized the PASTA repeat as a small globular fold consisting of three β-strands and an α-helix with a loop of variable length between the first and second β-strands. This domain shows strong structural conservation but low sequence identity. By inference from the structure of PBP2x of *Streptococcus pneumoniae* (18), showing that the β-lactam ring of cefuroxime associates with a PASTA domain, it has been predicted that the PASTA domain acts as a sensor of presumably unlinked PG to regulate cell wall biosynthesis. The presence of an N-terminal cytosolic kinase domain linked to a C-terminal sensor-like domain is strongly suggestive of a role of PknB in cell wall modeling. PknB phosphorylates PBP3 and Rv0016c of *M. tuberculosis* (unpublished data), an observation whose implications are yet to be understood. It also remains to be seen whether the PASTA domain could be a viable antibiotic target.

ARABINOGALACTAN BIOSYNTHESIS AND LIGATION TO PEPTIDOGLYCAN

The AG biosynthetic pathway has been investigated mainly in *M. smegmatis* and *M. tuberculosis*. The first reaction of the pathway is the transfer of a GlcNAc-1-phosphate residue from UDP-GlcNAc to polyprenyl phosphate, giving rise to polyprenyl-P-P-GlcNAc, or GL-1 (49) (Fig. 5). In *E. coli* and other organisms, WecA (previously Rfe) catalyzes this reaction (1). A homologue of *wecA* has been identified in

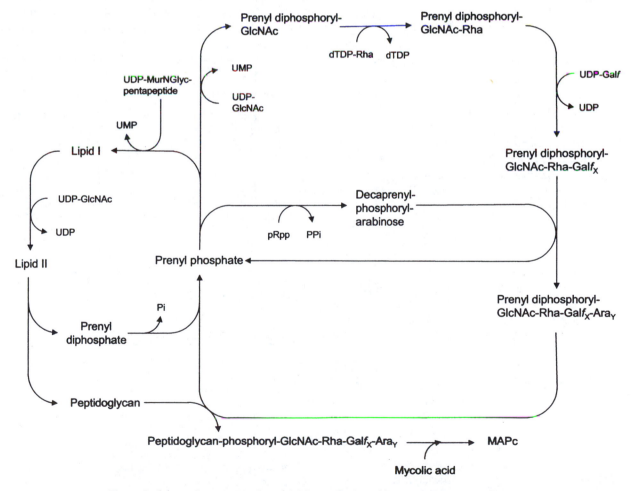

Figure 5. Schematic representation of AG biosynthesis and ligation to PG in mycobacteria.

the *M. tuberculosis* genome (12, 15); however, the enzyme catalyzing this reaction in mycobacteria has yet to be biochemically characterized. In the subsequent reaction, catalyzed by WbbL1 (Rv3265c), a rhamnose residue is transferred to the 3 position of the GlcNAc residue of GL-1, forming GL-2 or the "linker unit" (43). dTDP-rhamnose, the nucleotide donor of the above reaction, is synthesized from glucose-1-phosphate via a four-step reaction cascade (37, 43). RmlA (Rv0334) initiates the reaction dTTP + α-D-glucose 1-phosphate → dTDP-glucose + PP$_i$ (36). The dTDP-glucose is then converted to dTDP-rhamnose in three sequential reactions catalyzed by dTDP-D-glucose-4,6-dehydratase (Rv3464, RmlB), dTDP-4-keto-6-deoxy-D-glucose-3,5-epimerase (Rv 3465, RmlC), and dTDP-rhamnose synthase (Rv3266, RmlD) (30, 37, 60).

UDP-Gal*f* is the activated donor of the Gal*f* residues of the galactan (65). This molecule is synthesized from UDP-glucose. The first step of this synthesis is the conversion of UDP-glucose to UDP-galactopyranose (UDP-Gal*p*), catalyzed by UDP-Gal*p* epimerase. In *M. tuberculosis*, *Rv3634* possibly encodes the enzyme (65). Once UDP-Gal*p* is formed, the *glf* gene product, Rv3809c, converts UDP-Gal*p* to UDP-Gal*f* (65).

The Gal*f* residues are then added to the linker unit, and polymerization begins. Based on the structure of the galactan unit of AG, it is quite likely that there are at least two (and perhaps several) galactosyltransferases involved in the biosynthesis (13). One enzyme could transfer the first Gal*f* residue to the linker unit (GL-2); formation of the alternating (1→5) and (1→6) links could be catalyzed either by a bifunctional enzyme or by two linkage-specific enzymes. A Gal*f* transferase gene (*Rv3808c*, encoding GalT) of *M. tuberculosis* has been cloned, overexpressed, and partially characterized (34, 50). This enzyme is reported to catalyze the formation of both (1→5) and (1→6) linkages in cell-free assay systems using natural (50) or synthetic (34) substrate analogs. The arabinofuranose (Ara*f*) residues of arabinan are added to the linker unit-galactan polymer from a decaprenylphosphoryl-Ara*f* (DPA) precursor (50, 67). The Ara*f* moiety of DPA originates from the pentose phosphate pathway (57, 58). The structural complexity of arabinofuran present in AG indicates the possibility of multiple arabinosyltransferases in *Mycobacterium* spp. As yet, no arabinosyltransferase has been characterized from *M. tuberculosis*. The *embA* and *embB* gene products in *Mycobacterium avium* have been reported to be Ara*f* transferases (5), and the *embA* and *embB* gene products in *M. smegmatis* are involved in the biosynthesis of the terminal hexaarabinofuranosyl motif of AG (22). Current evi-

dence indicates that AG is sequentially built up on the prenyl diphosphate carrier lipid until it reaches mature or near mature size (49, 50, 68). It is not yet clear whether this polymerization takes place inside or outside of the plasma membrane.

Once the prenyl diphosphate-linked mature AG is synthesized, the GlcNAc of the linker unit of AG forms a 1-*O*-phosphoryl linkage with the 6 position of a MurNAc residue of PG, releasing the prenyl phosphate. This reaction is catalyzed by an unidentified ligase. The ligation of AG to PG has been demonstrated in experiments with cell-free preparations of *M. smegmatis*, and the nature of in vitro-synthesized material was confirmed by the observation that the newly ligated AG can be released from PG by muramidase treatment (68). It is likely that the ligation reaction occurs at the outer surface of the plasma membrane. In vivo radiolabeling experiments of the *M. smegmatis* cell wall demonstrated that the incorporation of AG into the cell wall requires newly synthesized PG and that the PG must be undergoing concomitant cross-linking (27). However, the subcellular location of the enzymes involved in the polymerization of the AG and the ligation of AG to PG remain unclear. The schematic pathway of the biosynthesis of AG and ligation to PG is summarized in Fig. 5. The mycosylation of the terminal Ara motifs of the nascent PG-AG complex probably occurs after ligation to PG. The synthesis of the mycolic acid portion of MAPc is dealt with in chapter 19.

Acknowledgments. Work conducted by the U.S.-based scientists was supported by grants AI18357, AI46393, and AI49151 from the National Institute of Allergy and Infectious Diseases.

REFERENCES

1. **Amer, A. O., and M. A. Valvano.** 2002. Conserved aspartic acids are essential for the enzymic activity of the WecA protein initiating the biosynthesis of O-specific lipopolysaccharide and enterobacterial common antigen in *Escherichia coli*. *Microbiology* **148:**571–582.

2. **Av-Gay, Y., and M. Everett.** 2000. The eukaryotic-like Ser/Thr protein kinases of *Mycobacterium tuberculosis*. *Trends Microbiol.* **8:**238–244.

3. **Basu, J., R. Chattopadhyay, M. Kundu, and P. Chakrabarti.** 1992. Purification and partial characterization of a penicillin-binding protein from *Mycobacterium smegmatis. J. Bacteriol.* **174:**4829–4832.

4. **Basu, J., S. Mahapatra, M. Kundu, S. Mukhopadhyay, M. Nguyen-Disteche, P. Dubois, B. Joris, J. Van Beeumen, S. T. Cole, P. Chakrabarti, and J. M. Ghuysen.** 1996. Identification and overexpression in *Escherichia coli* of a *Mycobacterium leprae* gene, *pon1*, encoding a high-molecular-mass class A penicillin-binding protein, PBP1. *J. Bacteriol.* **178:**1707–1711.

5. **Belanger, A. E., G. S. Besra, M. E. Ford, K. Mikusova, J. T. Belisle, P. J. Brennan, and J. M. Inamine.** 1996. The *embAB* genes of *Mycobacterium avium* encode an arabinosyl transferase involved in cell wall arabinan biosynthesis that is the

target for the antimycobacterial drug ethambutol. *Proc. Natl. Acad. Sci. USA* **93**:11919–11924.

6. Bhakta, S., and J. Basu. 2002. Overexpression, purification and biochemical characterization of a class A high-molecular-mass penicillin-binding protein (PBP), PBP1,* and its soluble derivative from *Mycobacterium tuberculosis. Biochem. J.* **361**:635–639.

7. Billman-Jacobe, H., R. E. Haites, and R. L. Coppel. 1999. Characterization of a *Mycobacterium smegmatis* mutant lacking penicillin binding protein 1. *Antimicrob. Agents Chemother.* **43**:3011–3013.

8. Brennan, P. J. 1988. *Mycobacterium* and other *Actinomycetes*, p. 203–298. *In* C. Ratledge and S. G. Wilkinson (ed.), *Microbial Lipids.* Academic Press, Ltd., London, United Kingdom.

9. Chaba, R., M. Raje, and P. K. Chakraborti. 2002. Evidence that a eukaryotic-type serine/threonine protein kinase from *Mycobacterium tuberculosis* regulates morphological changes associated with cell division. *Eur. J. Biochem.* **269**:1078–1085.

10. Chacon, O., Z. Y. Feng, N. B. Harris, N. E. Caceres, L. G. Adams, and R. G. Barletta. 2002. *Mycobacterium smegmatis* D-alanine racemase mutants are not dependent on D-alanine for growth. *Antimicrob. Agents Chemother.* **46**:47–54.

11. Chambers, H. F., D. Moreau, D. Yajko, C. Miick, C. Wagner, C. Hackbarth, S. Kocagoz, E. Rosenberg, W. K. Hadley, and H. Nikaido. 1995. Can penicillins and other beta-lactam antibiotics be used to treat tuberculosis. *Antimicrob. Agents Chemother.* **39**:2620–2624.

12. Cole, S. T., R. Brosch, J. Parkhill, T. Garnier, C. Churcher, D. Harris, S. V. Gordon, K. Eiglmeier, S. Gas, C. E. Barry III, F. Tekaia, K. Badcock, D. Basham, D. Brown, T. Chillingworth, R. Conner, R. Davies, K. Devlin, T. Feltwell, S. Gentles, N. Hamlin, S. Holroyd, T. Hornsby, K. Jagels, A. Krogh, J. McLean, S. Moule, L. Murphy, K. Oliver, J. Osborne, M. A. Quail, M.-A. Rajandream, J. Rogers, S. Rutter, K. Seeger, J. Skelton, R. Squares, S. Squares, J. E. Sulston, K. Taylor, S. Whitehead, and B. G. Barrell. 1998. Deciphering the biology of *Mycobacterium tuberculosis* from the complete genome sequence. *Nature* **396**:190–198.

13. Crick, D. C., S. Mahapatra, and P. J. Brennan. 2001. Biosynthesis of the arabinogalactan-peptidoglycan complex of *Mycobacterium tuberculosis. Glycobiology* **11**:107R–118R.

14. Daffé, M., P. J. Brennan, and M. McNeil. 1990. Predominant structural features of the cell wall arabinogalactan of *Mycobacterium tuberculosis* as revealed through characterization of oligoglycosyl alditol fragments by gas chromatography/mass spectrometry and by ¹H and ¹³C NMR analyses. *J. Biol. Chem.* **265**:6734–6743.

15. Dal Nogare, A. R., N. Dan, and M. A. Lehrman. 1998. Conserved sequences in enzymes of the UDP-GlcNAc/MurNAc family are essential in hamster UDP-GlcNAc:dolichol-P GlcNAc-1-P transferase. *Glycobiology* **8**:625–632.

16. Datta, P., A. Dasgupta, S. Bhakta, and J. Basu. 2002. Interaction between FtsZ and FtsW of *Mycobacterium tuberculosis. J. Biol. Chem.* **277**:24983–24987.

17. De Smet, K. A. L., K. E. Kempsell, A. Gallagher, K. Duncan, and D. B. Young. 1999. Alteration of a single amino acid residue reverses fosfomycin resistance of recombinant MurA from *Mycobacterium tuberculosis. Microbiology* **145**:3177–3184.

18. Dessen, A., N. Mouz, E. Gordon, J. Hopkins, and O. Dideberg. 2001. Crystal structure of PBP2x from a highly penicillin-resistant *Streptococcus pneumoniae* clinical isolate—a mosaic framework containing 83 mutations. *J. Biol. Chem.* **276**:45106–45112.

19. Dmitriev, B. A., S. Ehlers, and E. T. Rietschel. 1999. Layered murein revisited: a fundamentally new concept of bacterial cell wall structure, biogenesis and function. *Med. Microbiol. Immunol.* **187**:173–181.

20. Dmitriev, B. A., S. Ehlers, E. T. Rietschel, and P. J. Brennan. 2000. Molecular mechanics of the mycobacterial cell wall: from horizontal layers to vertical scaffolds. *Int. J. Med. Microbiol.* **290**:251–258.

21. Draper, P., O. Kandler, and A. Darbre. 1987. Peptidoglycan and arabinogalactan of *Mycobacterium leprae. J. Gen. Microbiol.* **133**:1187–1194.

22. Escuyer, V. E., M. A. Lety, J. B. Torrelles, K. H. Khoo, J. B. Tang, C. D. Rithner, C. Frehel, M. R. McNeil, P. J. Brennan, and D. Chatterjee. 2001. The role of the *embA* and *embB* gene products in the biosynthesis of the terminal hexaarabinofuranosyl motif of *Mycobacterium smegmatis* arabinogalactan. *J. Biol. Chem.* **276**:48854–48862.

23. Feng, Z. Y., and R. G. Barletta. 2003. Roles of *Mycobacterium smegmatis* D-alanine:D-alanine ligase and D-alanine racemase in the mechanisms of action of and resistance to the peptidoglycan inhibitor D-cycloserine. *Antimicrob. Agents Chemother.* **47**:283–291.

24. Gateau, O., C. Bordet, and G. Michel. 1976. Study of formation of N-glycolylmuramic acid from *Nocardia asteroides. Biochim. Biophys. Acta* **421**:395–405.

25. Ghuysen, J. M. 1968. Use of bacteriolytic enzymes in determination of wall structure and their role in cell metabolism. *Bacteriol. Rev.* **32**:425–464.

26. Graham, J. E., and J. E. Clark-Curtiss. 1999. Identification of *Mycobacterium tuberculosis* RNAs synthesized in response to phagocytosis by human macrophages by selective capture of transcribed sequences (SCOTS). *Proc. Natl. Acad. Sci. USA* **96**:11554–11559.

27. Hancock, I. C., S. Carman, G. S. Besra, P. J. Brennan, and E. Waite. 2002. Ligation of arabinogalactan to peptidoglycan in the cell wall of *Mycobacterium smegmatis* requires concomitant synthesis of the two wall polymers. *Microbiology* **148**:3059–3067.

28. Higashi, Y., J. L. Strominger, and C. C. Sweeley. 1967. Structure of a lipid intermediate in cell wall peptidoglycan synthesis: a derivative of a C55 isoprenoid alcohol. *Proc. Natl. Acad. Sci. USA* **57**:1878–1884.

29. Higashi, Y., J. L. Strominger, and C. C. Sweeley. 1970. Biosynthesis of the peptidoglycan of bacterial cell walls. XXI. Isolation of free C_{55}-isoprenoid alcohol and of lipid intermediates in peptidoglycan synthesis from *Staphylococcus aureus. J. Biol. Chem.* **245**:3697–3702.

30. Hoang, T. T., Y. Ma, R. J. Stern, M. R. McNeil, and H. P. Schweizer. 1999. Construction and use of low-copy number T7 expression vectors for purification of problem proteins: purification of *Mycobacterium tuberculosis* RmlD and *Pseudomonas aeruginosa* LasI and RhlI proteins, and functional analysis of purified RhlI. *Gene* **237**:361–371.

31. Jarlier, V., and H. Nikaido. 1994. Mycobacterial cell-wall structure and role in natural resistance to antibiotics. *FEMS Microbiol. Lett.* **123**:11–18.

32. Keer, J., M. J. Smeulders, K. M. Gray, and H. D. Williams. 2000. Mutants of *Mycobacterium smegmatis* impaired in stationary-phase survival. *Microbiology* **146**:2209–2217.

33. Kotani, S., I. Yanagida, K. Kato, and T. Matsuda. 1970. Studies on peptides, glycopetides and antigenic polysaccharide-glycopeptide complexes isolated from an L-11 enzyme lysate of cell walls of *Mycobacterium tuberculosis* strain H37Rv. *Biken J.* **13**:249–275.

34. Kremer, L., L. G. Dover, C. Morehouse, P. Hitchin, M. Everett, H. R. Morris, A. Dell, P. J. Brennan, M. R. McNeil, C. Flaherty, K. Duncan, and G. S. Besra. 2001. Galactan biosynthesis in *Mycobacterium tuberculosis*—identification of

a bifunctional UDP-galactofuranosyltransferase. *J. Biol. Chem.* **276**:26430–26440.

35. Lederer, E., A. Adam, R. Ciorbaru, J. F. Petit, and J. Wietzerbin. 1975. Cell walls of mycobacteria and related organisms; chemistry and immunostimulant properties. *Mol. Cell. Biochem.* **7**:87–104.

36. Ma, Y., J. A. Mills, J. T. Belisle, V. Vissa, M. Howell, K. Bowlin, M. S. Scherman, and M. McNeil. 1997. Determination of the pathway for rhamnose biosynthesis in mycobacteria: cloning, sequencing and expression of the *Mycobacterium tuberculosis* gene encoding alpha-D-glucose-1-phosphate thymidylyltransferase. *Microbiology* **143**:937–945.

37. Ma, Y., R. J. Stern, M. S. Scherman, V. D. Vissa, W. Yan, V. C. Jones, F. Zhang, S. G. Franzblau, W. H. Lewis, and M. R. McNeil. 2001. Drug targeting *Mycobacterium tuberculosis* cell wall synthesis: genetics of dTDP-rhamnose synthetic enzymes and development of a microtiter plate-based screen for inhibitors of conversion of dTDP-glucose to dTDP-rhamnose. *Antimicrob. Agents Chemother.* **45**:1407–1416.

38. Mahapatra, S., S. Bhakta, J. Ahamed, and J. Basu. 2000. Characterization of derivatives of the high-molecular-mass penicillin-binding protein (PBP) 1 of *Mycobacterium leprae*. *Biochem. J.* **350**:75–80.

39. Mahapatra, S., D. C. Crick, and P. J. Brennan. 2000. Comparison of the UDP-N-acetylmuramate:L-alanine ligase enzymes from *Mycobacterium tuberculosis* and *Mycobacterium leprae*. *J. Bacteriol.* **182**:6827–6830.

40. Mainardi, J. L., R. Legrand, M. Arthur, B. Schoot, J. van Heijenoort, and L. Gutmann. 2000. Novel mechanism of beta-lactam resistance due to bypass of DD-transpeptidation in *Enterococcus faecium*. *J. Biol. Chem.* **275**:16490–16496.

41. Marrec-Fairley, M., A. Piette, X. Gallet, R. Brasseur, H. Hara, C. Fraipont, J. M. Ghuysen, and M. Nguyen-Disteche. 2000. Differential functionalities of amphiphilic peptide segments of the cell-septation penicillin-binding protein 3 of *Escherichia coli*. *Mol. Microbiol.* **37**:1019–1031.

42. Matsuhashi, M. 1966. Biosynthesis in the bacterial cell wall. *Tanpakushitsu Kakusan Koso* **11**:875–886. (In Japanese.)

43. McNeil, M. 1999. Arabinogalactan in mycobacteria: structure, biosynthesis, and genetics, p. 207–223. *In* J. B. Goldberg (ed.), *Genetics of Bacterial Polysaccharides*. CRC Press, Washington, D.C.

44. McNeil, M., M. Daffe, and P. J. Brennan. 1990. Evidence for the nature of the link between the arabinogalactan and peptidoglycan of mycobacterial cell walls. *J. Biol. Chem.* **265**:18200–18206.

45. McNeil, M., M. Daffe, and P. J. Brennan. 1991. Location of the mycolyl ester substituents in the cell walls of mycobacteria. *J. Biol. Chem.* **266**:13217–13223.

46. McNeil, M., S. J. Wallner, S. W. Hunter, and P. J. Brennan. 1987. Demonstration that the galactosyl and arabinosyl residues in the cell wall arabinogalactan of *Mycobacterium leprae* and *Mycobacterium tuberculosis* are furanoid. *Carbohydr. Res.* **166**:299–308.

47. McNeil, M. R., and P. J. Brennan. 1991. Structure, function and biogenesis of the cell envelope of mycobacteria in relation to bacterial physiology, pathogenesis and drug resistance—some thoughts and possibilities arising from recent structural information. *Res. Microbiol.* **142**:451–463.

48. Mengin-Lecreulx, D., L. Texier, M. Rousseau, and J. van Heijenoort. 1991. The *murG* gene of *Escherichia coli* codes for the UDP-N-acetylglucosamine:N-acetylmuramyl-(pentapeptide) pyrophosphoryl-undecaprenol N-acetylglucosamine transferase involved in the membrane steps of peptidoglycan synthesis. *J. Bacteriol.* **173**:4625–4636.

49. Mikusova, K., M. Mikus, G. S. Besra, I. Hancock, and P. J. Brennan. 1996. Biosynthesis of the linkage region of the mycobacterial cell wall. *J. Biol. Chem.* **271**:7820–7828.

50. Mikusova, K., T. Yagi, R. Stern, M. R. McNeil, G. S. Besra, D. C. Crick, and P. J. Brennan. 2000. Biosynthesis of the galactan component of the mycobacterial cell wall. *J. Biol. Chem.* **275**:33890–33897.

51. Mukherjee, T., O. Basu, S. Mahapatra, C. Goffin, J. van Beeumen, and J. Basu. 1996. Biochemical characterization of the 49 kDa penicillin-binding protein of *Mycobacterium smegmatis*. *Biochem. J.* **320**:197–200.

52. Mukhopadhyay, S. and P. Chakrabarti. 1997. Altered permeability and beta-lactam resistance in a mutant of *Mycobacterium smegmatis*. *Antimicrob. Agents Chemother.* **41**:1721–1724.

53. Quintela, J. C., M. A. de Pedro, P. Zollner, G. Allmaier, and F. Garcia del Portillo. 1997. Peptidoglycan structure of *Salmonella typhimurium* growing within cultured mammalian cells. *Mol. Microbiol.* **23**:693–704.

54. Quinting, B., J. M. Reyrat, D. Monnaie, G. Amicosante, V. Pelicic, B. Gicquel, J. M. Frere, and M. Galleni. 1997. Contribution of beta-lactamase production to the resistance of mycobacteria to beta-lactam antibiotics. *FEBS Lett.* **406**:275–278.

55. Rick, P. D., K. Barr, K. Sankaran, J. Kajimura, J. S. Rush, and C. J. Waechter. 2003. Evidence that the *wzxE* gene of *Escherichia coli* K-12 encodes a protein involved in the transbilayer movement of a trisaccharide-lipid intermediate in the assembly of enterobacterial common antigen. *J. Biol. Chem.* **278**:16534–16542.

56. Sassetti, C. M., D. H. Boyd, and E. J. Rubin. 2003. Genes required for mycobacterial growth defined by high density mutagenesis. *Mol. Microbiol.* **48**:77–84.

57. Scherman, M., A. Weston, K. Duncan, A. Whittington, R. Upton, L. Deng, R. Comber, J. D. Friedrich, and M. McNeil. 1995. Biosynthetic origin of mycobacterial cell wall arabinosyl residues. *J. Bacteriol.* **177**:7125–7130.

58. Scherman, M. S., L. Kalbe-Bournonville, D. Bush, Y. Xin, L. Deng, and M. McNeil. 1996. Polyprenylphosphate-pentoses in mycobacteria are synthesized from 5-phosphoribose pyrophosphate. *J. Biol. Chem.* **271**:29652–29658.

59. Schleifer, K. H., and O. Kandler. 1972. Peptidoglycan types of bacterial cell walls and their taxonomic implications. *Bacteriol. Rev.* **36**:407–477.

60. Stern, R. J., T. Y. Lee, T. J. Lee, W. Yan, M. S. Scherman, V. D. Vissa, S. K. Kim, B. L. Wanner, and M. R. McNeil. 1999. Conversion of dTDP-4-keto-6-deoxyglucose to free dTDP-4-keto-rhamnose by the *rmlC* gene products of *Escherichia coli* and *Mycobacterium tuberculosis*. *Microbiology* **145**:663–671.

61. Templin, M. F., A. Ursinus, and J. V. Holtje. 1999. A defect in cell wall recycling triggers autolysis during the stationary growth phase of *Escherichia coli*. *EMBO J.* **18**:4108–4117.

62. van Heijenoort, J. 1994. Biosynthesis of bacterial peptidoglycan unit, p. 39–54. *In* J. M. Ghuysen and R. Hakenbeck (ed.), *Bacterial Cell Wall*. Elsevier Biomedical Press, Amsterdam, The Netherlands.

63. van Heijenoort, J. 2001. Formation of the glycan chains in the synthesis of bacterial peptidoglycan. *Glycobiology* **11**:25R–36R.

64. van Heijenoort, J. 2001. Recent advances in the formation of the bacterial peptidoglycan monomer unit. *Nat. Prod. Rep.* **18**:503–519.

65. Weston, A., R. J. Stern, R. E. Lee, P. M. Nassau, D. Monsey, S. L. Martin, M. S. Scherman, G. S. Besra, K. Duncan, and M. R. McNeil. 1997. Biosynthetic origin of mycobacterial cell wall galactofuranosyl residues. *Tubercle Lung Dis.* **78**:123–131.

66. Wietzerbin, J., B. C. Das, J. F. Petit, E. Lederer, M. Leyh-Bouille, and J. M. Ghuysen. 1974. Occurrence of D-alanyl-(D)-*meso*-diaminopimelic acid and *meso*-diaminopimelyl-

meso-diaminopimelic acid interpeptide linkages in the peptidoglycan of mycobacteria. *Biochemistry* **13:**3471–3476.

67. **Wolucka, B. A., M. R. McNeil, E. de Hoffmann, T. Chojnacki, and P. J. Brennan.** 1994. Recognition of the lipid intermediate for arabinogalactan/arabinomannan biosynthesis and its relation to the mode of action of ethambutol on mycobacteria. *J. Biol. Chem.* **269:**23328–23335.

68. **Yagi, T., S. Mahapatra, K. Mikuova, D. C. Crick, and P. J. Brennan.** 2003. Polymerization of mycobacterial arabinogalactan and ligation to peptidoglycan. *J. Biol. Chem.* **278:**26497–26504.

69. **Yeats, C., R. D. Finn, and A. Bateman.** 2002. The PASTA domain: a beta-lactam-binding domain. *Trends Biochem. Sci.* **27:**438–440.

Tuberculosis and the Tubercle Bacillus
Edited by Stewart T. Cole et al.
© 2005 ASM Press, Washington, D.C.

Chapter 19

A Waxy Tale, by *Mycobacterium tuberculosis*

LAURENT KREMER AND GURDYAL S. BESRA

The *Mycobacterium tuberculosis* cell envelope differs substantially from the canonical cell wall structures of both gram-negative and gram-positive bacteria. This unique cell wall structure accounts for its unusual low permeability and hence contributes to its resistance to common antibiotics and chemotherapeutic agents. The architecture of the mycobacterial cell wall has been thoroughly investigated over the past 50 years. Investigations, using chemical models (75) and electron microscopy (18, 39) conclude that the bacterium is protected by a highly lipophilic barrier. A key feature of the mycobacterial envelope is its high lipid content, up to 60% of the dry weight of the bacteria.

An updated model of the *M. tuberculosis* cell wall is shown in Fig. 1 (41, 76). The inner membrane barrier is composed of mycolic acids anchored to arabinogalactan (AG), which is linked to peptidoglycan. This complete structure is referred to as the mycolyl-arabinogalactan-peptidoglycan complex (19). The outer membrane barrier comprises an assortment of covalently bound mycolic acids and a vast array of "free" lipids, such as phthiocerol dimycocerosates (PDIMs), phenolic glycolipids (PGLs), trehalose-containing glycolipids, and sulfolipids (SL) (75). Interspersed somehow are the cell wall proteins, the phosphatidyl-*myo*-inositol mannosides (PIMs), lipomannan (LM), and lipoarabinomannan (LAM). PIMs, LM, and LAM are major glycolipids that are anchored to the plasma membrane through their phosphatidyl-*myo*-inositol anchor and extend to the exterior of the cell wall (12, 15).

Many of these cell wall waxes display potent biological activities when tested in vitro on eukaryotic cells and can be considered virulence factors. In that regard, these components represent central effectors in *M. tuberculosis* pathogenicity (39, 50). Emphasis has also shifted to the study of mycobacterial lipid biosynthesis in order to identify enzymes that are essential to the viability of *M. tuberculosis* and hence represent targets for future drug development. The publication of the complete *M. tuberculosis* genome sequence has greatly aided these studies (32). This article reviews the current understanding of the major cell wall waxes found in *M. tuberculosis*, along with their functions and biosynthesis.

MYCOLIC ACIDS

Mycolic acids from *M. tuberculosis* differ from those from other related genera, such as *Corynebacterium*, *Nocardia*, and *Rhodococcus*, in that they are the largest (C_{70} to C_{90}). Mycolic acids are long-chain high-molecular-weight α-alkyl β-hydroxy fatty acids consisting of a meromycolate moiety, with carbon chain lengths of up to C_{56} and a long saturated α-branch, C_{20} to C_{24}. They possess at least two chiral centers at positions α and β to the carboxylic acid. The stereochemistry at these two centers is *R, R* (38) (Fig. 2).

The mycobacterial mycolic acids contain *cis* and *trans* cyclopropane rings, *cis* and *trans* double bonds, and keto, methoxy, epoxy, and wax-ester functionalities in addition to the β-hydroxy acid unit (Fig. 3). α-Mycolic acids contain no oxygen functionality other than the β-hydroxy acid group and can therefore be distinguished from oxygenated mycolic acids, such as keto- and methoxymycolates. Keto- and methoxymycolates have also been shown to contain *trans*-cyclopropane and *cis*-cyclopropane rings (74, 75). Polar modifications containing oxygen functions are found in the distal portion of the meromycolate chain, whereas nonpolar modifications, i.e., cyclopropane rings and unsaturations, are found in both the proximal (closest to the β-hydroxy group) and distal positions of the chain. Cyclopropane rings and double bonds occurring in a *trans* conformation

Laurent Kremer • Laboratoire des Mécanismes Moléculaires de la Pathogénie Microbienne, INSERM U447, Institut Pasteur de Lille/IBL, 1 rue du Pr. Calmette, 59 000 Lille, France.   **Gurdyal S. Besra** • School of Biosciences, The University of Birmingham, Edgbaston, Birmingham, B15 2TT, United Kingdom.

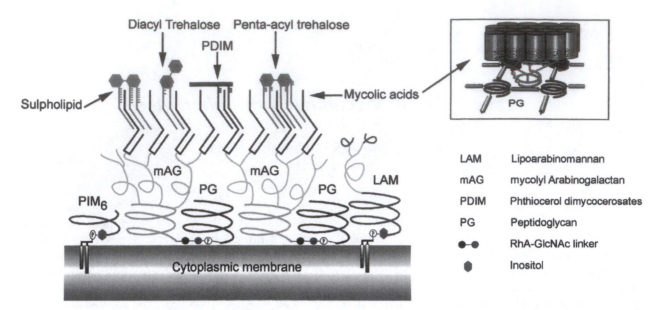

Figure 1. Simplified representation of the mycobacterial cell wall from *M. tuberculosis*. Adapted from references 41 and 76. © 2002 with permission from Elsevier.

also have an adjacent methyl group (75, 108, 109). The structure of mycolic acids lends itself to very efficient packing within the mycobacterial cell envelope, resulting in a highly impermeable barrier. With the exception of the β-hydroxy group, all other functionality leading to disruption of the highly ordered "linear" packing is found toward the distal end of the meromycolate chain. Thus, mycolic acids fall into species-specific subclasses according to the type and extent of functionality contained in them.

The α-mycolates have been found in all mycobacterial species examined and represent the most widely distributed class of mycolates. Ketomycolates are also abundant among mycobacterial species. ω-1-Methoxymycolates are the most restricted, occurring in a very few fast-growing strains. The α′-mycolic acids are shorter than α-mycolates, containing 60 carbons instead of 80, and are widely distributed within mycobacteria although absent from *M. tuberculosis*. The mycolic acids specific to *M. tuberculosis* are α-, keto-, and methoxymycolates. Studies of the carbon content of each class of mycolates within *M. tuberculosis* by Yuan et al. (116) and Watanabe et al. (108,

109) revealed that α-mycolates contain 76 to 82 carbons whereas keto- and methoxymycolates contain 84 to 89 and 83 to 90 carbons, respectively.

The mycolic acids give rise to important characteristics including resistance to chemical injury, resistance to dehydration, low permeability to hydrophobic antibiotics, and the ability to persist within the host (116). Mycolic acids have unique characteristics essential for maintaining the cell wall structure, and their physiological role may possibly be correlated to individual mycolates (48, 116). Generally, *cis* or *trans* olefin or cyclopropane functionalities at the proximal position are thought to play an important role in maintaining the viscosity of the cell wall at an appropriate level, through manipulation of the ratio of *cis* and *trans* geometries. The role of the oxygenated mycolates is less clear, although they allow possible hydrogen bond formation within the lipid-rich environment and are essential in maintaining cell wall function (75).

Mycolic acids are found primarily as esters of the nonreducing arabinan terminus of AG (19). The AG polysaccharide, which is unique to mycobacteria

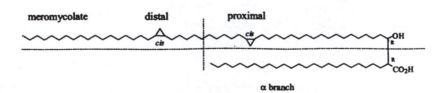

Figure 2. α-Mycolate from *M. tuberculosis*.

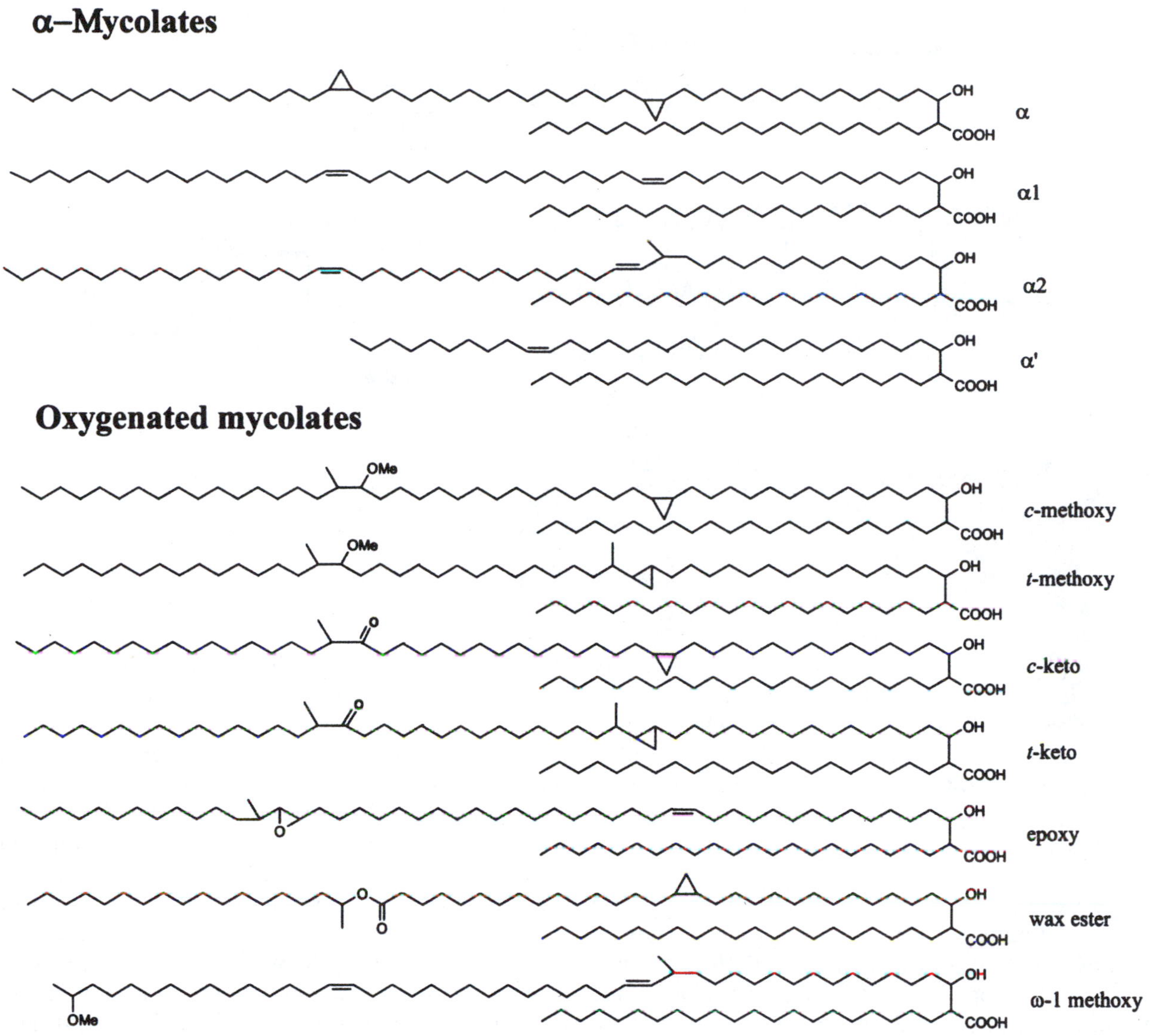

α–Mycolates

Oxygenated mycolates

Figure 3. Mycobacterial α-mycolates and oxygenated mycolates. *t*, trans; *c*, cis.

and other actinomycetes, is composed of D-arabino-furanose and D-galactofuranose residues. The arabinan chains are linked to the galactan chain toward the reducing end and are composed of linear α(1→5)-D-arabinofuranosyl (Ara*f*) residues with 3,5-branching. The nonreducing terminals of the arabinan are capped with a characteristic hexaarabinose motif [t-β-D-Ara*f*-(1→2)-α-D-Ara*f*]₂-3,5-α-D-Ara*f*-(1→5)-α-D-Ara*f*. The hexaarabinose motifs are esterified at the C-5 positions, in clusters of four, with mycolic acids, although only two-thirds of these motifs are mycolated in AG (Fig. 4).

Besides being esterified to AG, mycolic acids can be found as extractable "free" lipids within the cell wall, associated mainly with glucose, trehalose, or polyprenylphosphomannose (Man-P-C₃₅) to form glucose monomycolates (GMM), trehalose monomy-

colates (TMM), trehalose dimycolates (TDM), or 6-O-mycolyl-β-D-mannopyranosyl monophosphooc-tahydroheptaprenol (MycPL) (14) (Fig. 5).

The major biological functions associated with mycolic acid either bound to AG or associated with trehalose are summarized in Fig. 6.

COMPLEX LIPIDS

Mycolic acids are thought to make an ordered monolayer in the envelope and are probably associated with other free lipids, thus forming a bilayer representing an efficient permeability barrier against hydrophilic molecules. This barrier is likely to account for the high resistance of mycobacteria to toxic substances (19). These lipids have intrigued researchers for over

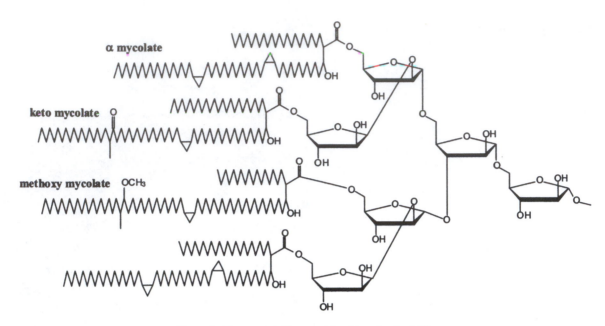

Figure 4. Tetramycolyl hexaarabinoside unit of mAGP.

five decades and encompass a extraordinary variety of exotic structures, TDM, multiacylated trehalose derivatives, SL, PDIM, and PGL. Knowledge of their functions in signalling events, in pathogenesis and in modulating the host immune system is now emerging.

Trehalose-6,6′-Dimycolate (Cord Factor)

A variety of glycosylated forms of mycolic acids exist in the outer layer of the mycobacterial cell wall, the most extensively studied being TDM, commonly called cord factor (Fig. 5). The long acyl chains of the mycolic acid residues differ in structure and chain length within TDM. Although TDM represents a relatively small percentage of the total amount of myco-

lic acid residues in the cell wall, it is suggested that it undergoes important interactions with the mammalian immune system. Its toxic properties may play a role in multiplication of the tubercle bacilli and their distribution in host cells (2). Woodbury and Barrow (112) demonstrated that TDM diffuses into the host cell membranes and damages their function. According to Kato (59), cord factor intoxication is attributable to a direct physical effect on mitochondrial membranes, resulting in disruption of electron flow along the mitochondrial respiratory chain and of oxidative phosphorylation. TDM also induces apoptosis when injected into mice (82) and displays immunostimulatory properties, presumably responsible for its antitumoral activity (10). One significant

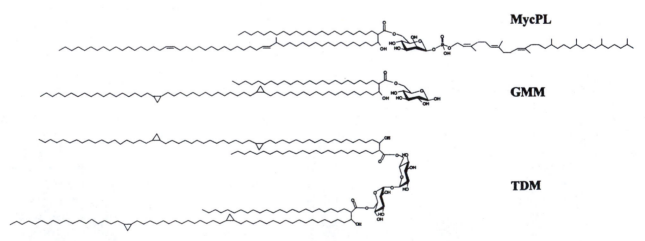

Figure 5. Representative structures of glucose monomycolate (GMM), trehalose dimycolate (TDM), and 6-O-mycolyl-β-D-mannopyranosyl monophosphooctahydroheptaprenol (MycPL).

Protection against environmental stress

Low cell wall permeability

Natural resistance against drugs

Persistence of the disease in mice

Participates in mycobacterial pathogenesis

Protection against oxydative radicals

Loss of body weight and induction of granulomas in rabbits

Thymic and splenic atrophy in mice and rabbtis

Immunostimulatory and adjuvant properties

Antitumoral activity

Pro-inflammatory and Th1 cytokine-inducing activities: TNF-α, IL-1, IL-12

Depletion of NKT cells

Upregulation of MHC-II and CD1d1 on macrophages

Induction of corneal angiogenesis in rats

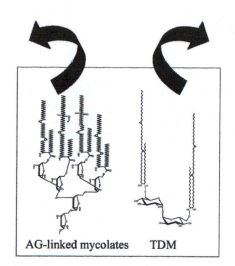

AG-linked mycolates   TDM

Figure 6. Major functions assigned to mycolic acids bound to AG or to TDM.

property established for TDM is its ability to induce lung granulomas (8, 9). Recent insights originated from the observation that TDM induces a loss of body weight and prominent granulomas in the liver and the lungs when injected into rabbits, which are the only animals that readily produce tuberculous cavities (54). Both nonimmune and immune mechanisms take part in granulomatous inflammation induced by mycobacterial infection (113). Although the mechanisms and receptors involved remain unknown, it is accepted that macrophages represent a major target of the immune-stimulating activity of TDM (83). The adjuvant and granulomatogenic activities of TDM can be further potentiated by costimulation with other cellular components, such as the cell wall skeleton derived from the tubercle bacilli (90). Recent studies also demonstrated that injection of TDM into mice was accompanied by a depletion of natural killer (NK) cells, an upregulation of major histocompatibility complex class II, and CD1d1 molecules on macrophages, and an increased proportion of Th1 cells (93).

Other Trehalose-Containing Lipids

Trehalose-containing glycolipids associated with the cell wall, other than TDM, include (i) SL, which are acylated by two to four very long, highly branched fatty acids, and (ii) di-, tri-, and pentaacyl trehalose (DAT, TAT, and PAT, respectively), which are acylated by multimethyl-branched fatty acids (76) (Fig. 7).

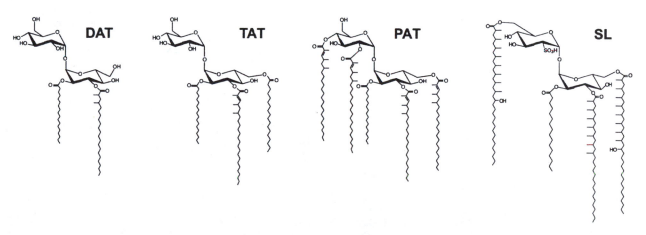

Figure 7. Representation of some complex lipids in *M. tuberculosis*. Adapted from reference 76. © 2002 with permission from Elsevier.

SLs are trehalose derivatives containing a sulfate group at the 2 position of trehalose and multimethyl-branched fatty acids, called the phthioceranic or hydroxy-phthioceranic acids (Fig. 7). A clear correlation exists between the presence of SLs in *M. tuberculosis* isolates and virulence for guinea pigs. SLs of *M. tuberculosis* have been implicated in the virulence of this organism by effectively antagonizing the phagosome-lysosome fusion in macrophages, thus probably promoting the intracellular survival of this pathogen (51), but this role was questioned in later work. In light of the controversial role of SLs in *M. tuberculosis* pathogenesis, new insights came from the generation of *M. tuberculosis* mutants devoid of SLs (34, 101). Indeed, a mycocerosic acid synthase (*mas*)-like *pks2* gene responsible for SL biosynthesis was identified and successfully disrupted by homologous recombination (101). However, the *pks2* mutant, defective in an early step in SL biosynthesis, had no obvious growth defect in infected mice. In contrast, a strain with a disruption of MmpL8, a transporter of SL in *M. tuberculosis*, was highly attenuated for growth in a mouse model of tuberculosis (34). It was therefore concluded that although SL is dispensable during the acute stage of infection, *mmpL8* is absolutely required for normal *M. tuberculosis* growth in vivo.

The di- and trimethyl-branched fatty acids, mycolipenates and mycosanoates, are found in some forms of DAT, TAT, and PAT and are present in the pathogenic species *M. tuberculosis*, *M. bovis* and *M. africanum* but not in the avirulent *M. tuberculosis* H37Ra or in the attenuated vaccine strain *M. bovis*

BCG (37). DAT inhibits the proliferation of murine T cells (94) and is a candidate antigen for the serodiagnosis of tuberculosis due to its antigenicity (13). An *M. tuberculosis*-derived mutant in which the polyketide synthase gene *msl3* was inactivated could no longer produce mycolipenates and mycosanoates (42). Therefore, this mutant defective in DAT and PAT was used to assess the in vivo contribution of these complex lipids to pathogenesis. Unexpectedly, it was observed that the *msl3* mutant was capable of binding and entering more efficiently into phagocytic and nonphagocytic host cells than the wild-type strain (91). Moreover, the absence of DAT and PAT did not affect the overall replication and persistence of the tubercle bacillus in the lungs, spleen, and liver of infected mice.

Phthiocerol Dimycocerosates and Phenolic Glycolipids

The PDIMs are major waxes of the tubercle bacillus (Fig. 8). PDIMs are also found in other related mycobacterial species. These unusual lipids are nonpolar waxes comprising two mycocerosic acids (long-chain polymethyl-branched fatty acids) attached to a phthiocerol diol backbone. The role of PDIMs in pathogenesis of *M. tuberculosis* has been addressed (22, 35). Using signature-tagged transposon mutagenesis, *M. tuberculosis* mutants with insertions in various genes involved in the biosynthsis of PDIMs were isolated. Inactivation of genes abolishing either biosynthesis or transport of PDIMs in *M. tuberculosis* led to mutants with replication defects in the

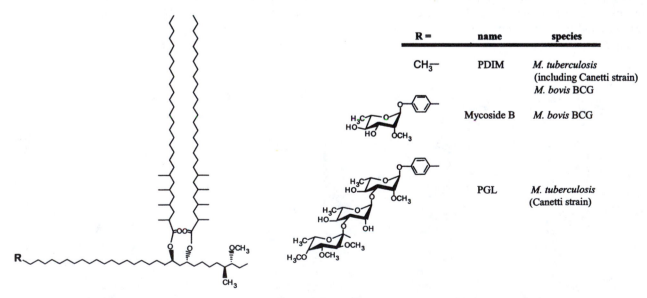

Figure 8. Representation of PDIM as well as PGLs from *M. bovis* BCG (also called mycoside B) and from the Canetti strain of *M. tuberculosis*.

lungs, demonstrating that synthesis and proper transport of PDIMs is necessary for organ-specific replication of *M. tuberculosis* (35). In addition, the PDIM mutants exhibited a more permeable cell wall, which was more sensitive to detergent, indicating that these complex lipids may play an important role in maintaining the integrity of the cell envelope.

Several members of the *M. tuberculosis* complex have alternative characteristic glycolipid antigens that are related to PDIMs, termed PGLs, in which the lipid core is ω-terminated by an aromatic nucleus, probably derived from *p*-hydroxybenzoic acid. *M. bovis* and the attenuated strain *M. bovis* BCG produce PGLs (Fig. 8), also designated mycoside B (75). The unusual *M. tuberculosis* "Canetti" strain, with smooth colony morphology, is characterized by the presence of a unique PGL (36), in contrast to most *M. tuberculosis* strains, which are devoid of PGLs. It was recently proposed that *M. tuberculosis* strains are natural mutants deficient in PGLs due to a frameshift in *pks15/1* whereas a single open reading frame for *pks15/1* is found in *M. bovis* BCG (33). PGLs were also found in *M. leprae* and shown to suppress lymphocyte responses (84, 105). Recently, they were shown to bind to peripheral nerve laminin and facilitate Schwann cell invasion by *M. leprae* (78). PGLs are immunogenic, with their carbohydrate at the nonreducing end as recognized epitopes. Leprosy patients have antibodies against PGLs, which make PGLs attractive candidates for serodiagnosis of leprosy (29).

The long-chain components of both PDIMs and PGLs are considered to interact with the mycolate chains to provide a type of outer membrane (Fig. 1). This arrangement may provide an effective barrier to the penetration of antibacterial agents (19, 75).

LIPOARABINOMANNAN AND LIPOMANNAN

PIMs, LM, and LAM constitute another group of free lipids playing crucial biological roles with regard to *M. tuberculosis* pathogenicity. LAM is a high-molecular-weight lipoglycan composed of two polysaccharides consisting of D-mannan and D-arabinan attached to a phosphatidyl-*myo*-inositol (PI) unit, anchoring the LAM structure to the plasma membrane (56). The biosynthesis of LAM involves the addition of mannopyranosyl (Man*p*) residues to PI to produce both the short PIMs (two to five Man*p* residues) and LM, which is further glycosylated with arabinan to form LAM. In all species, D-mannan has a highly branched structure with an α(1→6)-linked Man*p* backbone. This mannan core is substituted at C-2 by single Man*p* units in numerous species, including *M. tuberculosis*, *M. leprae*, and *M. smegmatis*,

and at C-3 by single Man*p* units in *Mycobacterium chelonae* (52). The mannan size and the degree of branching can vary depending on the species. The size and extent of branching of the mannan core of LAM is species specific. Studies of LAM from *M. tuberculosis* Erdman strain (27) estimated that the mannan core consists of 20 mannose residues, in comparison to 26 found in *M. smegmatis* (61). The arabinan domain consists of a linear α(1→5)-linked arabinofuranosyl backbone punctuated with branched hexaarabinofuranosides (Ara$_6$); [β-D-Ara*f*-(1→2)-α-D-Ara*f*-(1-]$_2$→3 and →5)-α-D-Ara*f*-(1→5)-α-D-Ara*f*→, and linear tetraarabinofuranosides (Ara$_4$), β-D-Ara*f*-(1→2)-α-D-Ara*f*-(1→5)-α-D-Ara*f*-(1→5)-α-D-Ara*f*→ (26, 27).

Comparative analysis of LAMs from different mycobacterial species has shown that the nonreducing termini of the arabinosyl side chains are differentially modified. *M. tuberculosis*, *M. leprae*, and *M. avium* modify the termini with caps consisting of a single Man*p*, a dimannoside [α-D-Man*p*(1→2)-α-D-Man*p*] or a trimannoside [α-D-Man*p*-(1→2)-α-D-Man*p*-(1→2)-α-D-Man*p*], with dimannosides predominating (79, 106), resulting in LAM being termed ManLAM. In the fast-growing species *M. smegmatis*, mannose caps are absent and branches of the terminal arabinan are terminated by inositol phosphate caps (61), resulting in LAM being termed PILAM. Is is thought that these modifications are responsible for the marked differences in the biological activities of ManLAM and PILAM. A third LAM family has recently been described on the basis of the finding that LAM from *M. chelonae* is devoid of both the mannooligosaccharide and the inositol phosphate cap (52); it is therefore designated AraLAM. A representation of PIM$_2$, LM, and ManLAM from *M. tuberculosis* is depicted in Fig. 9.

ManLAM is an important modulator of the immune response during the course of tuberculosis pathogenesis and exhibits a vast array of biological functions (28). One of the major activities associated with ManLAM is its capacity to inhibit the activation of macrophages, to inhibit the production of proinflammatory cytokines including interleukin-12 and tumor necrosis factor alpha, and to participate in *M. tuberculosis*-induced macrophage apoptosis (81). Among its main biological activities, ManLAM was shown to inhibit gamma interferon-mediated macrophage activation (24, 100), to suppress macrophage-dependent T-cell proliferation (77), and to induce the nitric oxide synthase (25). Thus, through its immunosuppressive effect, ManLAM appears as a virulence factor that enables the persistence of pathogenic mycobacteria within the infected host. In contrast, PILAM is a potent tumor necrosis factor alpha- and interleukin-8-inducing factor, and this release of

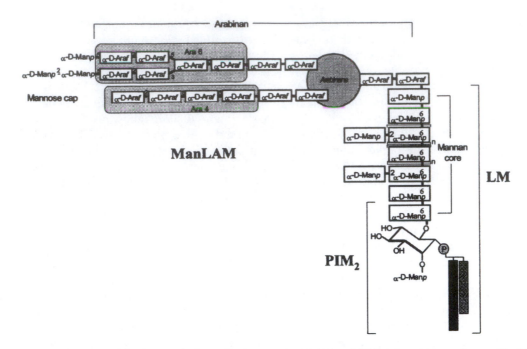

Figure 9. Representation of the structural relationship between LM, LAM, and PIM. Adapted from reference 62 with permission from the publisher.

proinflammatory cytokines is mediated by Toll-like receptor 2 activation. Therefore, by activating macrophages, PILAM can be considered to favor the killing of the nonpathogenic species *M. smegmatis*.

ManLAM has also been shown to mediate the phagocytosis of mycobacteria within phagocytic cells (98). It interacts with phagocytic cells in different ways, by binding to cell surface C-type lectin receptors, the mannose receptor (98), and the dendritic cell-specific intercellular cell adhesion molecule 3 (ICAM-3)-grabbing nonintegrin (DC-SIGN) (71). Recent studies have also reported that *M. tuberculosis* ManLAM causes phagosome maturation arrest by blocking the delivery of lysosomal constituents from the *trans*-Golgi network to the mycobacterial phagosome (47). ManLAM was shown to specifically inhibit the pathway dependent on phosphatidylinositol 3-kinase activity. Based on these observations, it was suggested that ManLAM biosynthesis might represent a prime target for the development of new antituberculosis drugs, with intracellular localization-altering properties.

LM is also an abundant cell wall component and is considered to be the direct precursor of LAM. However, the biological relevance of LM in host defense has not been thoroughly investigated yet. A recent study provided evidence that, in contrast to their respective LAMs, LM from *M. chelonae* and *M. kansasii* stimulated a strong proinflammatory response in human macrophages (107). This LM-mediated activation process was both CD14 and

Toll-like receptor 2 dependent. Progressive degradation of the arabinan domain of LAM restored the cytokine-inducing activity at a level similar to those of LMs, thus supporting the hypothesis that the arabinan domain hinders the capacity of LAMs to stimulate proinflammatory cytokine secretion. Thus, LM may also participate in the immunomodulation of the infected host, and the D-mannan core of this glycolipid is essential for this function (107). As a consequence, since ManLAM and LM display some antagonistic properties with respect to macrophage activation and since both molecules coexist within the mycobacterial cell wall, the LM/LAM ratio may be particularly important to a determination of the global effect of macrophage activation.

Interestingly, PIMs, which are known precursors of LM and LAM, have recently been proposed to recruit NK T cells, which play a primary role in the granulomatous response (1, 49). Moreover, a role for surface-exposed PIMs as *M. tuberculosis* adhesins that mediate attachment to nonphagocytic cells has also been established (44, 55).

Beatty et al. (7) demonstrated that intracellular mycobacteria release cell wall lipids and glycolipids into the endosomal network of infected macrophages. Relased BCG lipids have recently been identified as PIM$_2$, mono- and diphosphatidylglycerol, phosphatidylethanolamine, TMM, TDM, as well as mycoside B (89). In addition, some of these lipids, mainly PIM$_2$, were found to elicit the production of proinflammatory cytokines from macrophages that may participate in the granulomatous response. In a persistent infection, such as in tuberculosis, the continued presence of the bacillus provides an enduring source of these inflammatory lipids, thus contributing to the chronic response to the disease.

BIOSYNTHESIS OF *M. TUBERCULOSIS* CELL WALL LIPIDS

Understanding the pathways that are used for the synthesis of each separate component of the mycobacterial cell wall can facilitate the development of new antibacterial agents through the identification

of potential enzymatic targets. The elucidation of these pathways also allows the biosynthetic targets of established drugs, such as ethambutol and isoniazid (INH), to be confirmed.

Biosynthesis of Mycolic Acids

The biosynthesis of mycolic acids proposed by Takayama and Qureshi (103) involved five distinct stages, as presented in Fig. 10: (i) synthesis of C_{24} to C_{26} saturated straight-chain fatty acids to provide the α-alkyl branch of the mycolic acids; (ii) synthesis of C_{50} to C_{56} fatty acids providing the meromycolate backbone; (iii) introduction of functional groups to

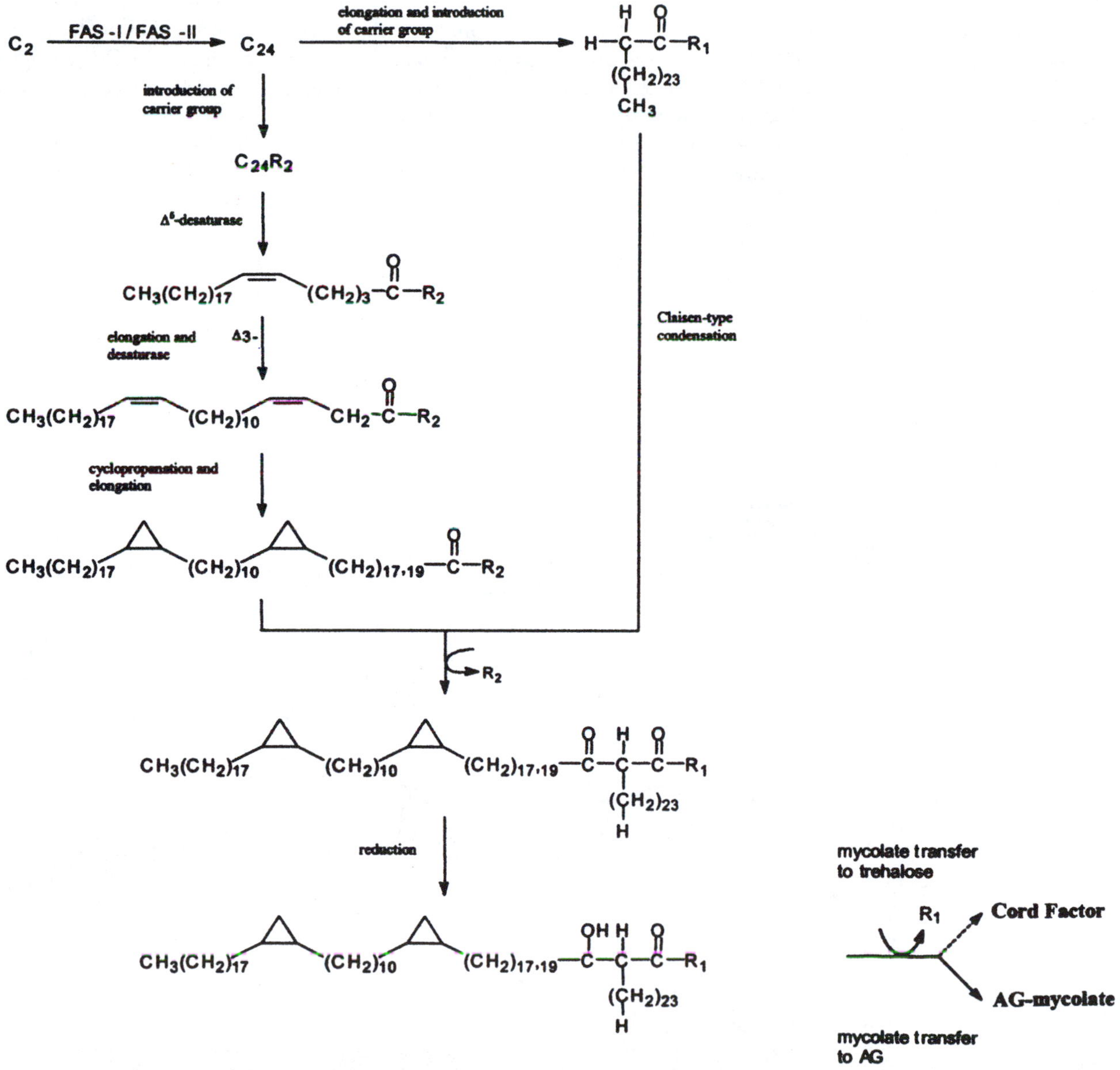

Figure 10. Biosynthesis of α-mycolic acids in *M. tuberculosis.*

the meromycolate chain; (iv) Claisen-type condensation between the two chains before a final reduction to give the mycolic acid; and (v) transfer of the mycolic acid to AG and other acceptors (103).

The biosynthesis of mycolic acids in *M. tuberculosis* is achieved through repetitive cycles of condensation, keto reduction, dehydration, and enoyl reduction catalyzed by a β-ketoacyl synthase, a β-ketoacyl-reductase, a β-hydroxyacyl dehydratase, and an enoyl reductase, respectively. Two types of fatty acid-synthesizing systems, fatty acid synthase I (FAS-I) and fatty acid synthase II (FAS-II), achieve these enzymatic cycles (Fig. 11). FAS-I is usually found only in eukaryotes and catalyzes the de novo synthesis of C_{12} to C_{16} fatty acids from acetyl coenzyme A (acetyl-CoA). In contrast, FAS-II is found in bacteria and plants and is composed of four dissociable enzymes, acting repetitively and successively to elongate the growing acyl chain. Mycobacteria are unusual in that they possess both FAS-I and FAS-II systems (Fig. 11). Acyl primers are continually activated via a thioester linkage to the prosthetic group of CoA for FAS-I or an acyl carrier protein (ACP) for FAS-II. The function of ACP in FAS-II is to shuttle acyl intermediates between enzymes. The *M. tuberculosis* ACP, termed AcpM, contains residues conserved with respect to the *E. coli* ACP (111). The difference between these two ACPs is the ability of AcpM to handle long-acyl-chain intermediates ($>C_{16}$), with the aid of an extended carboxyl terminus (111). In mycobacteria, the FAS-I system catalyzes the de novo synthesis of short-chain fatty acids from acetyl-CoA, which are further elongated by the FAS-II system, leading to fatty acids ranging from C_{26} to C_{56}.

FAS-I and short-chain fatty acid biosynthesis

In *M. tuberculosis*, as in other actinomycetes, FAS-I is capable of de novo synthesis, and the first step in fatty acid synthesis is always conserved (17). Acetyl-CoA and malonyl-CoA are condensed to a β-keto thioester before repetition of keto-reduction, dehydration, and enoyl reduction affords the elongated saturated product with retention of the thioester function (Fig. 11). FAS-I is a homodimer of a multifunctional protein in which each subunit protein contains seven catalytic activities plus an ACP (21). All intermediates generated remain bound to the enzyme throughout the process of elongation and undergo transacylation to other catalytic sites within the enzyme. The specificity of the condensing enzyme and transacylase determines the chain length of the product. The specificity is not absolute; therefore, products with different chain lengths are produced. It is thought that FAS-I produces both the α-branch and the meromycolate primers.

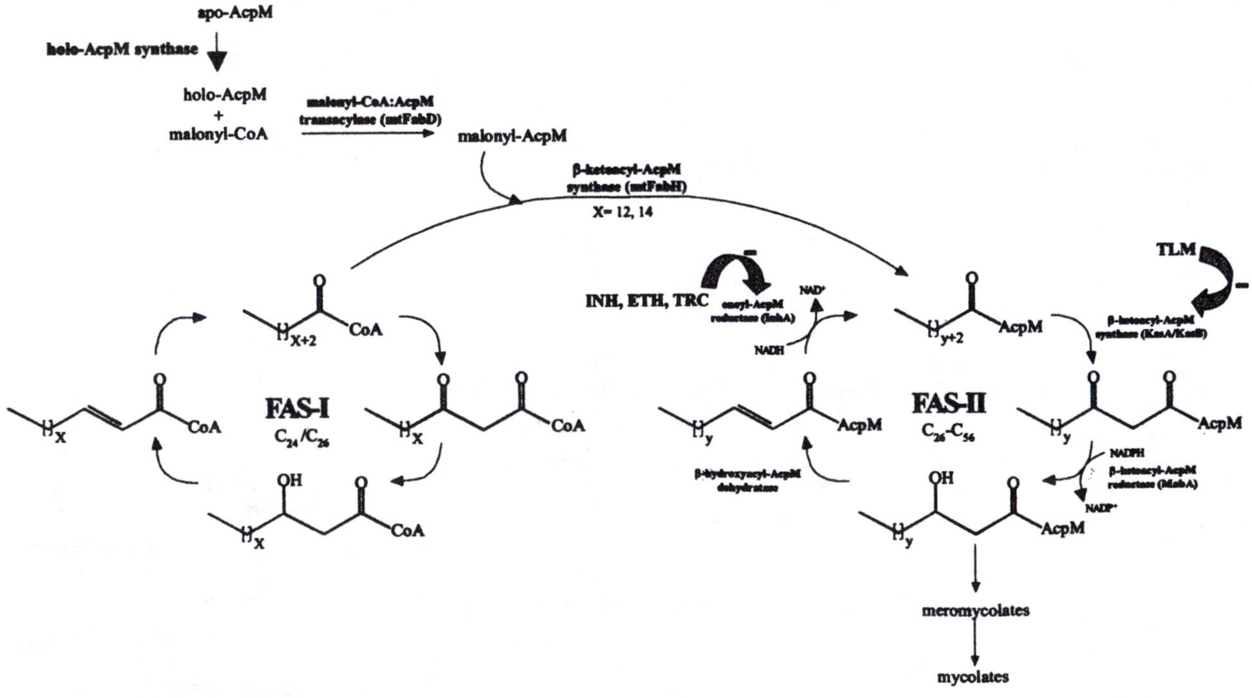

Figure 11. FAS-I and FAS-II systems in *M. tuberculosis*. Inhibition of the FAS-II enzymes InhA and KasA by various antitubercular agents is shown by an arrow. TLM, thiolactomycin; ETH, ethionamide; TRC, triclosan.

FAS-II and long-chain fatty acid biosynthesis

The *M. tuberculosis* FAS-II system is analogous to other bacterial FAS-II systems, except that it is not capable of de novo synthesis but, instead, elongates acyl CoA primers generated by FAS-I to a mixture of homologous fatty acids with longer chains (20). Malonyl-CoA:AcpM transacylase (mtFabD) is essential to the biosynthesis of mycolic acids (Fig. 11). This enzyme catalyzes the transacylation of malonyl-CoA with holo-AcpM to generate malonyl-AcpM, an elongation substrate essential to FAS-II in mycolic acid biosynthesis (66). Holo-AcpM consists of the activated form of AcpM, due to the addition of a phosphopantotheine group to the inactive apo-AcpM. First, acyl-CoA primers undergo a condensation reaction with malonyl-AcpM catalyzed by mtFabH. The acyl-AcpM precursors then undergo a cycle of keto reduction, dehydration, and enoyl reduction catalyzed by the β-ketoacyl-AcpM reductase, the β-hydroxyacyl-AcpM dehydratase, and the enoyl-AcpM reductase, respectively (Fig. 11). Two genes encoding enoyl- and keto-reductases are *inhA* and *mabA*, respectively. InhA has been identified through studies involving isoniazid-resistant mutants of *M. smegmatis* (6). The MabA protein from *M. tuberculosis* has been expressed in *E. coli* and shown to catalyze the NADPH-specific reduction of β-ketoacyl derivatives (72). Crystal structure studies of MabA (31) and InhA (92) demonstrate conservation in the location of binding of the acyl chain. Further elongation lengthens the acyl-AcpM, by an additional two carbon units, by condensation with malonyl-AcpM, catalyzed by KasA/KasB, and a complete cycle of FAS II (Fig. 11).

Mechanistically, elongation by the FAS-II system in *M. tuberculosis* is achieved by a Claisen-type condensation reaction which takes place in three distinct stages: (i) transfer of the pantotheine-bound acyl primer to a cysteine residue within the active site of mtFabH, KasA, and KasB; (ii) decarboxylation of the donor malonyl-AcpM substrate to yield an acetyl-AcpM carbanion; and (iii) nucleophilic attack of the carbanion with the carbonyl group on the enzyme-bound primer to yield the elongated β-ketoacyl-AcpM product (Fig. 12).

M. tuberculosis FabH

The role of mtFabH is to catalyze the condensation of long-chain acyl-CoA primers, formed by FAS-I, and malonyl-AcpM and to funnel the generated precursors into the FAS-II system (Fig. 11). In doing so, it plays a pivotal role in linking the two FAS cycles and initiating mycolic acid biosynthesis (30).

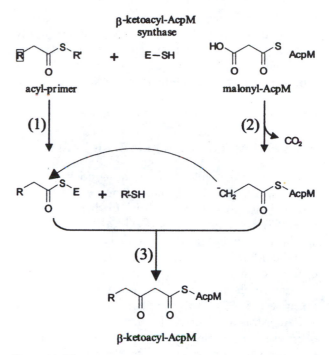

Figure 12. Three-step mechanism of the Claisen-type condensation reaction. *R′*, CoA, specific for mtFabH; *R′*, AcpM, specific for KasA/KasB.

Inhibition of mycolic acid biosynthesis is known to be effective in combating mycobacterial infection; given the importance of mtFabH in mycolic acid biosynthesis, it represents an attractive target. However, no existing drugs or new compounds have been shown to be a specific target of mtFabH. A key feature in developing novel antimycobacterial agents is the understanding of distinct features that separate mtFabH from other condensing enzymes. Investigations carried out by Choi et al. (30) determined the substrate specificity of mtFabH, with optimum activity being obtained with lauroyl-CoA. These observations are consistent with structural studies conducted by Scarsdale et al. (95). The structure of mtFabH has led to the identification of key active-site residues Cys112, His244, and Asn274. *E. coli* FabH and mtFabH both contain a CoA/malonyl-ACP binding channel that originates from the enzyme surface to the cysteine residue within the active site. They also contain a second hydrophobic pocket leading from the active site, which is blocked by Phe87 in *E. coli* and Thr87 in *M. tuberculosis*. The difference in these amino acid residues is postulated to account for the difference in substrate specificities between the two enzymes; Phe87 constrains specificity to acetyl-CoA in *E. coli*, whereas Thr87 allows the binding of long-chain acyl CoAs in mtFabH. This second hydrophobic pocket in mtFabH is capped by an α-helix, which restricts the bound acyl chain length to 16 carbons, thus limiting the length of the acyl chain to 16 carbons and excluding long-chain acyl-CoA products (C_{24} to C_{26}) from chain elongation. These observations are consistent with the proposed role of mtFabH as the initiator of fatty acid elongation and clearly distinguish it from the chain extension steps involved in mycolic biosynthesis catalyzed by KasA/KasB.

β-Ketoacyl-ACP synthases KasA/KasB

KasA and KasB catalyze the condensation of acyl-AcpM and malonyl-AcpM, hence elongating the growing meromycolate chain by a further two carbon units (67, 97) (Fig. 11). KasA and KasB contain many similarities, including the specificity for long chain acyl-AcpM primers (97). There are also significant differences in sensitivity to antimycobacterial agents, such as thiolactomycin, with KasA being the most sensitive (65, 97). However, both are able to utilize C_{16}-AcpM as a substrate, leading to some ambiguity over whether inhibition of one enzyme would lead to overcompensation of activity by the other. The Kas enzymes, ecFabB/ecFabF and KasA/KasB, have been compared, and a high degree of sequence homology has been observed (65). A three-dimensional model of KasA, based on the crystallographic coordinates of the *E. coli* FabF protein, revealed the putative residues of the catalytic triad in the active site (65). Participation of Cys171, His311, Lys340, and His345 in catalysis was subsequently confirmed by replacing these residues with alanine, which abolished the overall elongation activity of KasA (67).

Through genetic and biochemical approaches, two genes of the FAS-II system, *inhA* and *kasA*, have been postulated to encode the primary target of INH (6, 73). Therefore, due to conflicting reports, the mode of action of INH has recently been reexamined. First, studies performed in vivo demonstrated that overexpression of InhA, but not KasA, in *M. smegmatis*, *M. bovis* BCG, and *M. tuberculosis* conferred increased resistance to INH (70). Second, in vitro assays using purified KasA or InhA demonstrated that KatG-activated INH inhibited InhA activity but not KasA activity (69). Taken together, these findings clearly establish the role of InhA as the primary target of INH in *M. tuberculosis*.

Modification of the meromycolate chain

The meromycolate chain is functionalized prior to condensation with the α-branch to afford the complete mycolic acid (87). Biosynthesis of oxygenated meromycolates is less well developed than that of α-mycolates, although Watanabe et al. (109) have demonstrated the possibility that their synthesis involves different enzyme systems than that of the α-mycolates. Desaturation of the alkyl chain during elongation of the meromycolate chain constitutes the first modification step. The hypothesis that desaturation is coupled to elongation is further clarified through identification of cyclopropanated and unsaturated fatty acids that are shorter than the full-length mero-chains (86, 102). It is thought that they are precursors of full-length meromycolates, suggesting that modification occurs while the acyl group is attached to the AcpM. The *M. tuberculosis* genome has identified three potential desaturates, namely, DesA1, DesA2, and DesA3, which use ACP esters (32, 57). The double bonds can then be further modified to yield a wide range of mycolic acids. Yuan et al. (114) identified that the *cma1* gene, encoding CMAS-1, leads to the production of *cis*-cyclopropane-containing mycolates at the distal position. The *cma2* gene was subsequently found to introduce a *cis*-cyclopropane ring at the proximal position in the meromycolate (48). Since it is possible to identify both *cis*- and *trans*-cyclopropane rings, there must be additional genes encoding proteins which are able to produce *trans*-cyclopropane-containing mycolates. Glickman et al. (50) demonstrated that the *cma2* gene, previously designated as encoding the *cis*-synthase, is required for the synthesis of *trans*-cyclopropane rings of both keto and methoxy mycolates, thus defining *cma2* as a *trans*-cyclopropane synthetase-encoding gene.

A cluster of genes highly similar to *cma1* and *cma2* have been identified by Yuan and Barry (115) as *mma1* to *mma4*, encoding MMAS1 to MMAS-4. They have been shown to modify double bonds in the meromycolate chain through action of *S*-adenosyl-L-methionine-dependent methyltransferases. MMAS-4 catalyzes the *S*-adenosyl-L-methionine-dependent transformation of the distal *cis*-olefin into a secondary alcohol with an adjacent methyl branch. MMAS-3 methylates this secondary alcohol to form the corresponding methyl ether, and MMAS-2 introduces a *cis*-cyclopropane in the proximal position of the methoxy series (115). MMAS-1 is responsible for the conversion of a *cis*-olefin into a *trans*-olefin, with concomitant introduction of an allylic methyl branch in a precursor to both methoxy- and ketone-containing mycolic acids (116). Quémard et al. (85) postulated that very small amounts of hydroxymycolic acids exist in the *M. tuberculosis* complex compared to other types of mycolic acids. It also may represent the biosynthetic precursor of both keto- and methoxymycolic acids before transfer of a methyl group from SAM in the latter case.

With the aim of unraveling the mechanism of mycolic acid biosynthesis, it was found that a mutant *M. tuberculosis* strain inactivated in *mma4* (also termed *hma*) no longer synthesizes oxygenated mycolic acids (43). It was subsequently demonstrated that the *hma*-disrupted strain produces new types of mycolic acids that are absent from the parent strain (40). These new molecules consisted of a mixture of monoethylenic monocyclopropanated α-mycolates and a tiny amount of *cis*-epoxy-containing monocyclopropanated mycolates. Since the accumulation of large amounts of ethylenic α-mycolates in the *hma*-disrupted mutant was comparable to the accumulation of oxygenated mycolates of the parent strain, it reinforces the hypothesis that ethylenic long-chain fatty acid derivatives may be used for the synthesis of oxygenated mycolates in *M. tuberculosis* (40). In addition, this mutant displayed profound cell wall permeability alterations and was highly attenuated in a mouse model of infection (43). It has also been suggested that cyclopropanation of mycolic acids may play an important role in the survival and pathogenesis of *M. tuberculosis* in macrophages. Accordingly, disruption of the *pcaA* gene, encoding a *cis*-cyclopropane synthase, is essential for persistence in mice (50).

A recent review of mycolic acid biosynthesis (3) discusses the possibility that mycobacteria may use more than one pathway for the biosynthesis of mycolates. A model proposing the building of the meromycolate chain through condensation of four molecules of fatty acids, two of them being ω-oxidized before or after condensation, was proposed by Asselineau et al. (3). An alternative hypothesis to the addition of functional groups to unsaturated precursors yielding a range of mycolates, methylations following the initial condensation of two fatty acids may facilitate the building of very long aliphatic chains and determine the location of double bonds (3, 99, 114–116). Structural modifications can take place on methylation sites to yield a range of mycolates (116).

Claisen-type condensation of the meromycolate chain and the α-chain

A biological equivalent of the Claisen condensation reaction, with the carbonyl carbon of the meromycolate acting as an electrophile and the α-carbon of the α-branch acting as the nucleophile, yields the 3-ketoester intermediate. Reduction of the intermediate yields the mature mycolic acid, which contains two chiral centers, at positions α and β to the carboxylic acid. The gene(s) encoding the Claisen condensation step has yet to be identified but represents an attractive drug target that merits exploration in the future. This condensation step generates mature mycolic acids, which are *trans* esterified to AG or associated with other cell wall components, for instance glucose, trehalose, or polyprenylphosphomannose.

Biosynthesis of Phthiocerol Dimycoserosates

There has been much recent progress on the biosynthesis of PDIMs. Recently, a DNA segment comprising at least 15 genes was identified in *M. tuberculosis* and shown to encode various activities participating in the biosynthesis of either mycocerosic acids or phthiocerol. The *mas* gene, encoding the mycocerosic acid synthase, is located in the middle of this operon. This enzyme is an iterative polyketide synthase that acts like FAS-I but produces C_{29} to C_{32} mycocerosic acids after several rounds of extension on a C_{18} fatty acid precursor, using methylmalonyl-CoA instead of malonyl-CoA, which is the source of the methyl branches of mycocerosic acids (5, 46, 88). Targeted disruption of *mas* from *M. bovis* BCG generated a mutant lacking mycocerosic acids and phenolic glycolipids but still producing PDIMs with shorter mycocerosic acids (C_{23} and C_{26}) (4). One study has implicated a second enzyme, termed short-chain mycocerosic acid synthase, in catalyzing the synthesis of such acids (46).

Upstream of *mas* and transcribed in the opposite direction is the *ppsA* to *ppsE* cluster (5). Disruption of this gene cluster and subsequent analysis of the *pps* mutant demonstrated that these genes are involved in both phthiocerol and phenolphthiocerol biosynthesis due to the absence of PDIMs and PGLs (5). Pps proteins are acting though a modular polyketide synthase mechanism. Modules 1 and 2 (PpsA and PpsB) contain an acyltransferase domain, a ketoacyl synthase domain, and a keto reductase domain, allowing the introduction of the hydroxyl group. PpsD and PpsE use methylmalonyl-CoA, allowing the introduction of the characteristic methyl branches of phthiocerol. Following reduction and decarboxylation steps to produce phthiocerol, the acyl-CoA synthase (FadD28) attaches the mycocerosic acids, synthesized by MAS, to the phthiocerol synthesised by the Pps modules (23, 35).

Biosynthesis of Phosphatidyl-*myo*-Inositol Mannosides, Lipomannan, and Lipoarabinomannan

Although the structures of PIMs, LM and LAM have been extensively studied during the last decade, biosynthesis of these glycoconjugates has recently been investigated by genetic approaches in the light of the *M. tuberculosis* genome sequence (80).

Only a few mannosyltransferases involved in the different mannosylation steps have been reported so far. These enzymes can be discriminated according to the mannose donor they are using, either GDP-Man, which is incorporated early in PIM biosynthesis, or C_{35}/C_{50}-P-Man*p*, which is involved later in the process.

LAM biosynthesis is initiated by α-mannosyltransferases, which utilize the mannose donor GDP-Man and the PI acceptor precursor, yielding PIM$_2$ (Fig. 13). PIM biosynthesis is initiated by two distinct mannosyltransferases, which use GDP-mannose as the sugar donor. Initially, Man$p$ is transferred to the 2 position of the *myo*-inositol ring of PI to form PIM$_1$, in a reaction catalyzed by PimA (63), whose gene has been shown to be essential, demonstrating that PIM$_1$ and presumably more highly mannosylated PIMs are required for cell growth. Interestingly, *pimA* belongs to an operon of five genes that are likely to be involved in the synthesis of PIMs (63). In addition to *pimA*, this gene cluster contains the *pgsA* gene encoding the PI synthase, which allows the condensation of inositol and the diglyceride of the CDP-diacylglycerol derivative (58), as well as a gene encoding a protein (Rv2611c) with high similarity to bacterial acyltransferases. The presence of a putative acyltransferase is consistent with the occurrence of acylation and deacylation processes in the biosynthesis of PIMs. Rv2611c catalyzes the acylation of the 6 position of the mannose residue linked to the 2 position of *myo*-inositol in PI mono- and dimannosides (64). A second Man$p$ residue is then transferred to the 6 position of the *myo*-inositol ring of PIM$_1$ to form PIM$_2$, in a reaction catalyzed by PimB, as previously shown by Schaeffer et al. (96). Finally, a third Man$p$ unit is introduced onto the growing molecule to form PIM$_3$, in a reaction encoded by the *pimC* gene identified in *M. tuberculosis* CDC 1551 (68) (Fig. 13). However, inactivation of *pimC* in *M. bovis* BCG did not affect cell growth and did not alter the PIM-LM-LAM composition of the mutant, suggestive of an alternative pathway occurring in *M. bovis* BCG and *M. tuberculosis* CDC 1551. This hypothesis was supported by

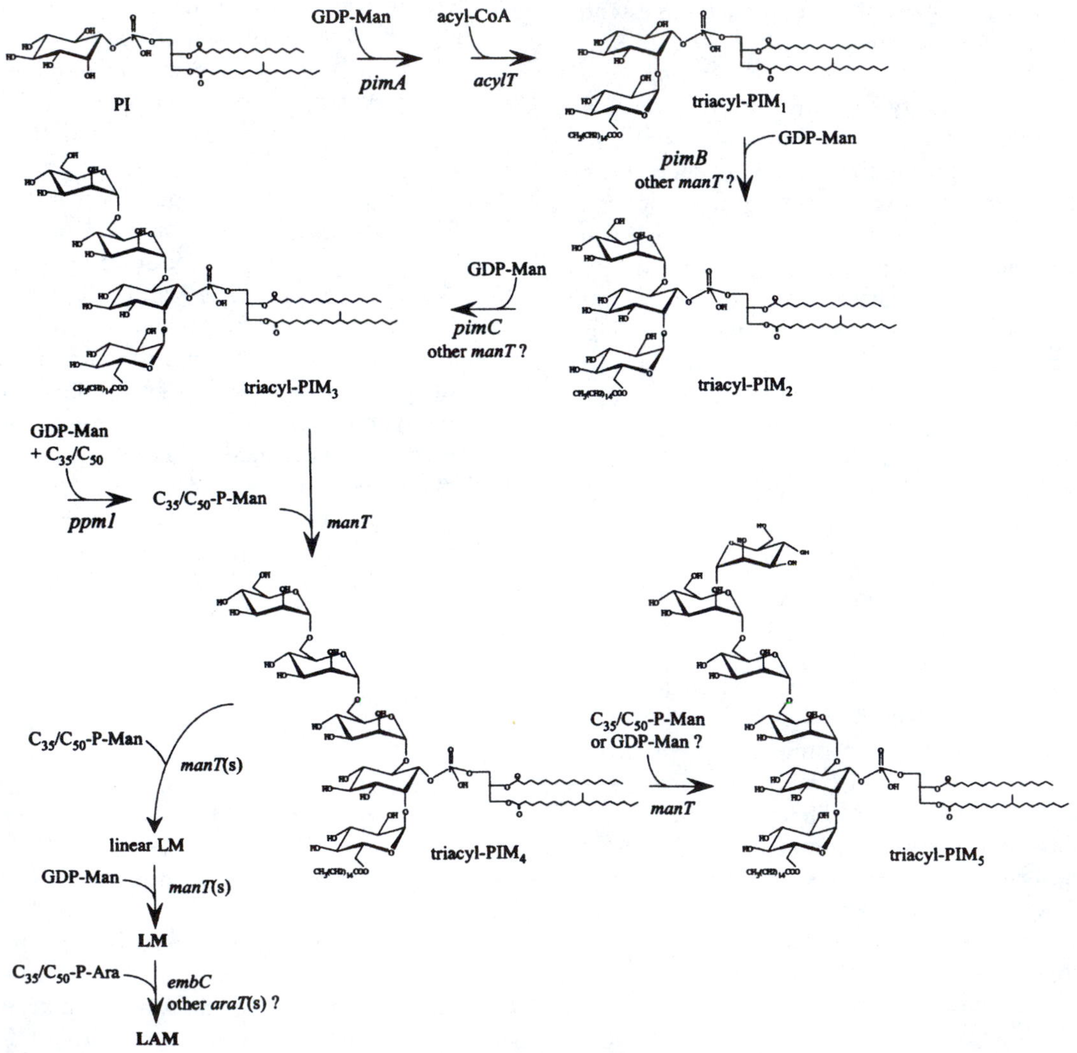

Figure 13. Proposed pathway for the biosynthesis of the PIMs, linear LM, native LM, and LAM of mycobacteria. Adapted from references 65 and 80 with permission from the publishers.

the fact that *pimC* was absent from *M. tuberculosis* H37Rv, a strain that produces PIMs, LM, and LAM (68). The mannose unit at the 6 position of PIM_3 is further elongated with mannose residues to generate PIM_{4-6}. Investigations conducted by Besra et al. (16) established that PIMs are extended with additional Man*p* residues from the alkali-stable C_{35}/C_{50}-P-Man*p* donor to form linear LM, containing only $\alpha(1\rightarrow6)$ Man*p* residues. C_{35}/C_{50}-P-Man*p* is synthesized from GDP-Man and polyprenols by the polyprenol monophosphomannose synthase, encoded by the *ppm1* gene (53). Linear LM is then further mannosylated to produce $\alpha(1\rightarrow2)$-linked Man*p*, representing "mature" LM, which is subsequently glycosylated with arabinan to form LAM (16). Regarding the mannosyltransferases participating in the mannose capping of Man-LAM, no gene candidate has been reported yet.

Very little is known regarding arabinan synthesis. C_{35}/C_{50}-P-Ara*f* is the only Ara*f* sugar donor yet identified (110). The EmbB protein, initially found to be the major target of ethambutol (11, 104), and its homologue EmbA have been reported to participate in the formation of the proper Ara_6 motif in AG (45). These two proteins have been proposed to catalyze $\alpha(1\rightarrow3)$-arabinosyltranferase activity in AG arabinan biosynthesis. *M. smegmatis* mutants that have been inactivated in either *embA* or *embB* display normal LAM arabinan biosynthesis. Interestingly, preliminary results suggested that an *embC*-deficient mutant strain is affected in arabinosylation of LAM (45, 60). Thus, EmbC, a protein that is highly homologuous to EmbA and EmbB, appears to catalyze arabinosyltransferase activity in LAM arabinan biosynthesis, although this merits further investigation.

Although the early genes in the PIM biosynthetic pathway appear to be essential for mycobacterial growth, it should now be possible to generate LM- or LAM-deficient mutants in order to explore the biological functions of these two glycolipids during in vivo growth.

Acknowledgments. G.S.B. acknowledges support as a Lister Institute-Jenner Research Fellow. This work was supported by the Medical Research Council, the Wellcome Trust, and INSERM.

REFERENCES

1. **Apostolou, I., Y. Takahama, C. Belmant, T. Kawano, M. Huerre, G. Marchal, J. Cui, M. Taniguchi, H. Nakauchi, J. J. Fournié, P. Kourilsky, and G. Gachelin.** 1999. Murine natural killer T (NKT) cells contribute to the granulomatous reaction caused by mycobacterial cell walls. *Proc. Natl. Acad. Sci. USA* 96:5141–5146.

2. **Asselineau, C., and J. Asselineau.** 1978. Trehalose-containing glycolipids. *Prog. Chem. Fats Other Lipids* 16:59–99.

3. **Asselineau, C., J. Asselineau, G. Lanéelle, and M. Lanéelle.** 2002. The biosynthesis of mycolic acids by mycobacteria: current and alternative hypotheses. *Prog. Lipid Res.* 41:501–523.

4. **Azad, A. K., T. D. Sirakova, L. M. Rogers, and P. E. Kolattukudy.** 1996. Targeted replacement of the mycocerosic acid synthase gene in *Mycobacterium bovis* BCG produces a mutant that lacks mycosides. *Proc. Natl. Acad. Sci. USA* 93:4787–4792.

5. **Azad, A. K., T. D. Sirakova, N. D. Fernandes, and P. E. Kolattukudy.** 1997. Gene knockout reveals a novel gene cluster for the synthesis of a class of cell wall lipids unique to pathogenic mycobacteria. *J. Biol. Chem.* 272:16741–16745.

6. **Banerjee, A., E. Dubnau, A. Quémard, V. Balasubramanian, K. S. Um, T. Wilson, D. Collins, G. de Lisle, and W. R. Jacobs, Jr.** 1994. *inhA*, a gene encoding a target for isoniazid and ethionamide in *Mycobacterium tuberculosis*. *Science* 263:227–230.

7. **Beatty, W. L., E. R. Rhoades, H. J. Ullrich, D. Chatterjee, J. E. Heuser, and D. G. Russell.** 2000. Trafficking and release of mycobacterial lipids from infected macrophages. *Traffic* 1:235–247.

8. **Bekierkunst, A.** 1968. Acute granulomatous response produced in mice by trehalose-6,6'-dimycolate. *J. Bacteriol.* 96:958–961.

9. **Bekierkunst, A., I. S. Levij, E. Yarkoni, E. Vilkas, A. Adam, and E. Lederer.** 1969. Granuloma formation induced in mice by chemically defined mycobacterial fractions. *J. Bacteriol.* 100:95–102.

10. **Bekierkunst, A., I. S. Levij, E. Yarkoni, E. Vilkas, and E. Lederer.** 1971. Suppression of urethane-induced lung adenome in mice treated with trehalose-6,6'-dimycolate (cord factor) and living bacillus Calmette-Guérin. *Science* 174:1240–1242.

11. **Belanger, A. E., G. S. Besra, M. E. Ford, K. Mikusová, J. T. Belisle, P. J. Brennan, and J. M. Inamine.** 1996. The *embAB* genes of *Mycobacterium avium* encode an arabinosyl transferase involved in cell wall arabinan biosynthesis that is the target for the antimycobacterial drug ethambutol. *Proc. Natl. Acad. Sci. USA* 93:11919–11924.

12. **Belanger, A. E., and J. M. Inamine.** 2000. Genetics of cell wall biosynthesis, p. 191–202. *In* G. F. Hatfull and W. R. Jacobs, Jr. (ed.), *Molecular Genetics of Mycobacteria*. ASM Press, Washington, D.C.

13. **Besra, G. S., R. Bolton, M. R. McNeil, M. Ridell, K. E. Simpson, J. Glushka, H. Halbeek, P. J. Brennan, and D. E. Minnikin.** 1992. Structure elucidation and antigenicity of a novel family of glycolipid antigens from *Mycobacterium tuberculosis* H37Rv. *Biochemistry* 31:9832–9837.

14. **Besra, G. S., T. Sievert, R. E. Lee, R. A. Slayden, P. J. Brennan, and K. Takayama.** 1994. Identification of the apparent carrier in mycolic acid synthesis. *Proc. Natl. Acad. Sci. USA* 91:12735–12739.

15. **Besra, G. S., and P. J. Brennan.** 1997. The mycobacterial cell wall: biosynthesis of arabinogalactan and lipoarabinomannan. *Biochem. Soc. Trans.* 25:845–850.

16. **Besra, G. S., C. B. Moorhouse, C. M. Rittner, C. J. Waechter, and P. J. Brennan.** 1997. Biosynthesis of mycobacterial lipoarabinomannan. *J. Biol. Chem.* 272:18460–18466.

17. **Bloch, K.** 1975. Fatty acid synthases from *Mycobacterium phlei*. *Methods Enzymol.* 35:84–90.

18. **Brennan, P. J., and P. Draper.** 1994. Ultrastructure of *Mycobacterium tuberculosis*, p. 271–306. *In* B. R. Bloom (ed.), *Tuberculosis: Pathogenesis, Protection and Control*. ASM Press, Washington, D.C.

19. **Brennan, P. J., and H. Nikaido.** 1995. The envelope of mycobacteria. *Annu. Rev. Biochem.* 65:215–239.

20. **Brindley, D. N., S. Matsumura, and K. Bloch.** 1969. *Mycobacterium phlei* fatty acid synthase—a bacterial multienzyme complex. *Nature* 224:666–669.

21. Brink, J., S. J. Ludtke, C. Y. Yang, Z. W. Gu, S. J. Wakil, and W. Chiu. 2002. Quaternary structure of human fatty acid synthase by electron cryomicroscopy. *Proc. Natl. Acad. Sci USA* 99:138–143.

22. Camacho, L. R., D. Ensergueix, E. Perez, B. Gicquel, and C. Guilhot. 1999. Identification of a virulence gene cluster of *Mycobacterium tuberculosis* by signature-tagged transposon mutagenesis. *Mol. Microbiol.* 34:257–267.

23. Camacho, L. R., P. Constant, C. Raynaud, M. A. Lanéelle, J. A. Triccas, B. Gicquel, M. Daffé, and C. Guilhot. 2001. Analysis of the phthiocerol dimycocerosate locus of *Mycobacterium tuberculosis*. Evidence that this lipid is involved in the cell wall permeability barrier. *J. Biol. Chem.* 276:19845–19854.

24. Chan, J., X. D. Fan, S. W. Hunster, P. J. Brennan, and B. R. Bloom. 1991. Lipoarabinomannan, a possible virulence factor involved in persistence of *Mycobacterium tuberculosis* within macrophages. *Infect. Immun.* 59:1755–1761.

25. Chan, E. D., K. R. Morris, J. T. Belisle, P. Hill, L. K. Remigio, P. J. Brennan, and D. W. Riches. 2001. Induction of inducible nitric oxide synthase-NO* by lipoarabinomannan of *Mycobacterium tuberculosis* is mediated by MEK1-ERK, MKK7-JNK, and NF-κB signaling pathways. *Infect. Immun.* 69:2001–2010.

26. Chatterjee, D., C. M. Bozic, M. McNeil, and P. J. Brennan. 1991. Structural features of the arabinan component of the lipoarabinomannan of *Mycobacterium tuberculosis*. *J. Biol. Chem.* 266:9652–9660.

27. Chatterjee, D., K. H. Khoo, M. R. McNeil, A. Dell, H. R. Morris, and P. J. Brennan. 1993. Structural definition of the nonreducing termini of mannose-capped LAM from *Mycobacterium tuberculosis* through selective enzymatic degradation and fast-atom-bombardment mass-spectrometry. *Glycobiology* 3:497–506.

28. Chatterjee, D., and K. H. Khoo. 1998. Mycobacterial lipoarabinomannan: an extraordinary lipoheteroglycan with profound physiological effects. *Glycobiology* 8:113–120.

29. Cho, S. N., D. L. Yanagihara, S. W. Hunter, R. H. Gelber, and P. J. Brennan. 1983. Serological specificity of phenolic glycolipid I from *Mycobacterium leprae* and use in serodiagnosis of leprosy. *Infect. Immun.* 41:1077–1083.

30. Choi, K. H., L. Kremer, G. S. Besra, and C. O. Rock. 2000. Identification and substrate specificity of β-ketoacyl (acyl carrier protein) synthase III (mtFabH) from *Mycobacterium tuberculosis*. *J. Biol. Chem.* 275:28201–28207.

31. Cohen-Gonsaud, M., S. Ducasse, F. Hoh, D. Zerbib, G. Labesse, and A. Quémard. 2002. Crystal structure of MabA from *Mycobacterium tuberculosis*, a reductase involved in long-chain fatty acid biosynthesis. *J. Mol. Biol.* 320:249–261.

32. Cole, S. T., R. Brosch, J. Parkhill, T. Garnier, C. Churcher, D. Harris, S. V. Gordon, K. Eiglmeier, S. Gas, C. E. Barry III, F. Tekaia, K. Badcock, D. Basham, D. Brown, T. Chillingworth, R. Connor, R. Davies, K. Devlin, T. Feltwell, S. Gentles, N. Hamlin, S. Holroyd, T. Hornsby, K. Jagels, A. Krogh, J. McLean, S. Moule, L. Murphy, K. Oliver, J. Osborne, M. A. Quail, M.-A. Rajandream, J. Rogers, S. Rutter, K. Saeger, J. Skelton, R. Squares, S. Squares, J. E. Sulston, K. Taylor, S. Whitehead, and B. G. Barrell. 1998. Deciphering the biology of *Mycobacterium tuberculosis* from the complete genome sequence. *Nature* 393:537–544.

33. Constant, P., E. Perez, W. Malaga, M. A. Lanéelle, O. Saurel, M. Daffé, and C. Guilhot. 2002. Role of the *pks15/1* gene in the biosynthesis of phenolglycolipids in the *Mycobacterium tuberculosis* complex. Evidence that all strains synthesize glycosylated *p*-hydroxybenzoic methyl esters and that strains devoid of phenolglycolipids harbor a frameshift mutation in the *pks15/1* gene. *J. Biol. Chem.* 277:38148–38158.

34. Converse, S. E., J. D. Mougous, M. D. Leavell, J. A. Leary, C. R. Bertozzi, and J. S. Cox. 2003. MmpL8 is required for sulfolipid-1 biosynthesis and *Mycobacterium tuberculosis* virulence. *Proc. Natl. Acad. Sci. USA* 100:6121–6126.

35. Cox, J. S., B. Chen, M. McNeil, and W. R. Jacobs, Jr. 1999. Complex lipid determines tissue-specific replication of *Mycobacterium tuberculosis* in mice. *Nature* 402:79–83.

36. Daffé, M., C. Lacave, M. A. Lanéelle, and G. Lanéelle. 1987. Structure of the major triglycosyl phenol-phthiocerol of *Mycobacterium tuberculosis* (strain Canetti). *Eur. J. Biochem.* 167:155–160.

37. Daffé, M., C. Lacave, M. A. Lanéelle, M. Gillois, and G. Lanéelle. 1988. Polyphthienoyl trehalose, glycolipids specific for virulent strains of the tubercle bacillus. *Eur. J. Biochem.* 172:579–584.

38. Daffé, M., M. A. Lanéelle, and C. Lacave. 1991. Structure and stereochemistry of mycolic acids of *Mycobacterium marinum* and *Mycobacterium ulcerans*. *Res. Microbiol.* 142:397–403.

39. Daffé, M., and P. Draper. 1998. The envelope layers of mycobacteria with reference to their pathogenicity. *Adv. Microb. Physiol.* 39:131–203.

40. Dinadayala, P., F. Laval, C. Raynaud, A. Lemassu, M. A. Lanéelle, G. Lanéelle, and M. Daffé. 2003. Tracking the putative biosynthetic precursors of oxygenated mycolates of *Mycobacterium tuberculosis*. Structural analysis of fatty acids of a mutant strain devoid of methoxy- and ketomycolates. *J. Biol. Chem.* 278:7310–7319.

41. Dmitriev, B. A., S. Ehlers, E. T. Rietschel, and P. J. Brennan. 2000. Molecular mechanics of the mycobacterial cell wall: from horizontal layers to vertical scaffolds. *Int. J. Med. Microbiol.* 290:251–258.

42. Dubey, V. S., T. D. Sirakova, and P. E. Kolattukudy. 2002. Disruption of *msl3* abolishes the synthesis of mycolipanoic and mycolipenic acids required for polyacyltrehalose synthesis in *Mycobacterium tuberculosis* H37Rv and causes cell aggregation. *Mol. Microbiol.* 45:1451–1459.

43. Dubnau, E., J. Chan, C. Raynaud, V. P. Mohan, M. A. Lanéelle, K. Yu, A. Quémard, I. Smith, and M. Daffé. 2000. Oxygenated mycolic acids are necessary for virulence of *Mycobacterium tuberculosis* in mice. *Mol. Microbiol.* 36:630–637.

44. Ehlers, M. R., and M. Daffé. 1998. Interactions between *Mycobacterium tuberculosis* and host cells: are mycobacterial sugars the key? *Trends Microbiol.* 6:328–335.

45. Escuyer, V. E., M. A. Lety, J. B. Torrelles, K. H. Khoo, J. B. Tang, C. D. Rithner, C. Frehel, M. R. McNeil, P. J. Brennan, and D. Chatterjee. 2001. The role of the *embA* and *embB* gene products in the biosynthesis of the terminal hexaarabinofuranosyl motif of *Mycobacterium smegmatis* arabinogalactan. *J. Biol. Chem.* 276:48854–48862.

46. Fernandes, N. D., and P. E. Kolattukudy. 1998. A newly identified methyl-branched chain fatty acid synthesizing enzyme from *Mycobacterium tuberculosis* var. *bovis* BCG. *J. Biol. Chem.* 273:2823–2828.

47. Fratti, R. A., J. Chua, I. Vergne, and V. Deretic. 2003. *Mycobacterium tuberculosis* glycosylated phosphatidylinositol causes phagosome maturation arrest. *Proc. Natl. Acad. Sci. USA* 100:5437–5442.

48. George, K. M., Y. Yuan, D. R. Sherman, and C. E. Barry III. 1995. The biosynthesis of cyclopropanated mycolic acids in *Mycobacterium tuberculosis*. Identification and functional analysis of CMAS-2. *J. Biol. Chem.* 270:27292–27298.

49. Gilleron, M., C. Ronet, M. Mempel, B. Monsarrat, G. Gachelin, and G. Puzo. 2001. Acylation state of the phosphatidylinositol mannosides from *Mycobacterium bovis* bacillus Calmette Guérin and ability to induce granuloma and recruit natural killer T cells. *J. Biol. Chem.* **276:**34896–34904.

50. Glickman, M. S., J. S. Cox, and W. R. Jacobs, Jr. 2000. A novel mycolic acid cyclopropane synthetase is required for cording, persistence, and virulence of *Mycobacterium tuberculosis*. *Mol. Cell* **5:**717–727.

51. Goren, M. B., P. D. Hart, M. R. Young, and J. A. Armstrong. 1976. Prevention of phagosome-lysosome fusion in cultured macrophages by sulfatides of *Mycobacterium tuberculosis*. *Proc. Natl. Acad Sci USA* **73:**2510–2514.

52. Guérardel, Y., E. Maes, E. Elass, Y. Leroy, P. Timmerman, G. S. Besra, C. Locht, G. Strecker, and L. Kremer. 2002. Structural study of lipomannan and lipoarabinomannan from *Mycobacterium chelonae*: presence of unusual components with alpha-1,3-mannopyranose side chains. *J. Biol. Chem.* **277:**30635–30648.

53. Gurcha, S. S., A. R. Baulard, L. Kremer, C. Locht, D. B. Moody, W. Muhlecker, C. E. Costello, D. C. Crick, P. J. Brennan, and G. S. Besra. 2002. Ppm1, a novel polyprenol monophosphomannose synthase from *Mycobacterium tuberculosis*. *Biochem. J.* **365:**441–450.

54. Hamasaki, N., K. I. Isowa, K. Kamada, Y. Terano, T. Matsumoto, T. Arakawa, K. Kobayashi, and I. Yano. 2000. In vivo admnistration of mycobacterial cord factor (trehalose 6,6'-dimycolate) can induce lung and liver granulomas and thymic atrophy in rabbits. *Infect. Immun.* **68:**3704–3709.

55. Hoppe, H. C., B. J. M. De Wet, C. Cywes, M. Daffé, and M. R. W. Ehlers. 1997. Identification of phosphatidylinositol mannoside as a mycobacterial adhesin mediating both direct and opsonic binding to nonphagocytic mammalian cells. *Infect. Immun.* **65:**3896–3905.

56. Hunter, S. W., and P. J. Brennan. 1990. Evidence for the presence of a phosphatidylinositol anchor on the lipoarabinomannan of *Mycobacterium tuberculosis*. *J. Biol. Chem.* **265:**9272–9279.

57. Jackson, M., D. Portnoi, D. Catheline, L. Dumail, J. Rauzier, P. Legrand, and B. Gicquel. 1997. *Mycobacterium tuberculosis* Des protein: an immunodominant target for the humoral response of tuberculosis patients. *Infect. Immun.* **65:**2883–2889.

58. Jackson, M., D. C. Crick, and P. J. Brennan. 2000. Phosphatidylinositol is an essential phospholipid of mycobacteria. *J. Biol. Chem.* **275:**30092–30099.

59. Kato, M. 1970. Site II-specific inhibition of mitochondria oxidative phosphorylation by trehalose-6,6'-dimycolate (cord factor) of *Mycobacterium tuberculosis*. *Arch. Biochem. Biophys.* **140:**379–390.

60. Kaur, D., T. L. Lowary, V. D. Vissa, D. C. Crick, and P. J. Brennan. 2002. Characterization of the epitope of antilipoarabinomannan antibodies as the terminal hexaarabinofuranosyl motif of mycobacterial arabinans. *Microbiology* **148:**3049–3057.

61. Khoo, K. H., A. Dell, H. R. Morris, P. J. Brennan, and D. Chatterjee. 1995. Inositol phosphate capping of the nonreducing termini of lipoarabinomannan from rapidly growing strains of *Mycobacterium*. *J. Biol. Chem.* **270:**12380–12389.

62. Khoo, K. H., E. Douglas, P. Parastoo, J. M. Inamine, G. S. Besra, K. Mikusová, P. J. Brennan, and D. Chatterjee. 1996. Truncated structural variants of lipoarabinomannan in ethambutol drug-resistant strains of *Mycobacterium smegmatis*. *J. Biol. Chem.* **271:**28682–28690.

63. Kordulakova, J., M. Gilleron, K. Mikusová, G. Puzo, P. J. Brennan, B. Gicquel, and M. Jackson. 2002. Definition of the first mannosylation step in phosphatidylinositol mannoside synthesis. PimA is essential for growth of myocbacteria. *J. Biol. Chem.* **277:**31335–31344.

64. Kordulakova, J., M. Gilleron, G. Puzo, P. J. Brennan, B. Gicquel, K. Mikusova, and M. Jackson. 2003. Identification of the required acyltransferase step in the biosynthesis of the phosphatidylinositol mannosides of *Mycobacterium* species. *J. Biol. Chem.* **278:**36285–36295.

65. Kremer, L., J. D. Douglas, A. R. Baulard, C. Morehouse, M. R. Guy, D. Alland, L. G. Dover, J. H. Lakey, W. R. Jacobs, Jr., P. J., Brennan, D. E. Minnikin, and G. S. Besra. 2000. Thiolactomycin and related analogues as novel antimycobacterial agents targeting KasA and KasB condensing enzymes in *Mycobacterium tuberculosis*. *J. Biol. Chem.* **275:**16857–16864.

66. Kremer, L., K. M. Nampoothiri, S. Lesjean, L. G. Dover, S. Graham, J. Betts, P. J. Brennan, D. E. Minnikin, C. Locht, and G. S. Besra. 2001. Biochemical characterization of acyl carrier protein (AcpM) and malonyl-CoA:AcpM transacylase (mtFabD), two major components of *Mycobacterium tuberculosis* fatty acid synthase II. *J. Biol. Chem.* **276:**27967–27974.

67. Kremer, L., L. G. Dover, S. Carrère, K. M. Nampoothiri, S. Lesjean, A. K. Brown, P. J. Brennan, D. E. Minnikin, C. Locht, and G. S. Besra. 2002. Mycolic acid biosynthesis and enzymic characterization of the β-ketoacyl-ACP synthase A-condensing enzyme from *Mycobacterium tuberculosis*. *Biochem. J.* **364:**423–430.

68. Kremer, L., S. S. Gurcha, P. Bifani, P. G. Hitchen, A. Baulard, H. R. Morris, A. Dell, P. J. Brennan, and G. S. Besra. 2002. Characterization of a putative α-mannosyltransferase involved in phosphatidylinositol trimannoside biosynthesis in *Mycobacterium tuberculosis*. *Biochem. J.* **363:**437–447.

69. Kremer, L., L. G. Dover, H. R. Morbidoni, C. Vilchèze, W. N. Maughan, A. Baulard, S. C. Tu, N. Honoré, V. Deretic, J. C. Sacchettini, C. Locht, W. R. Jacobs, Jr., and G. S. Besra. 2003. Inhibition of InhA activity, but not KasA activity, induces formation of a KasA-containing complex in mycobacteria. *J. Biol. Chem.* **278:**20547–20554.

70. Larsen, M. H., C. Vilchèze, L. Kremer, G. S. Besra, L. Parsons, M. Salfinger, L. Heifets, M. H. Hazbon, D. Alland, J. C. Sacchettini, and W. R. Jacobs, Jr. 2002. Overexpression of *inhA*, but not *kasA*, confers resistance to isoniazid and ethionamide in *Mycobacterium smegmatis*, *M. bovis* BCG, and *M. tuberculosis*. *Mol. Microbiol.* **46:**453–466.

71. Maeda, N., J. Nigou, J. L. Herrmann, M. Jackson, A. Amara, P. H. Lagrange, G. Puzo, B. Gicquel, and O. Neyrolles. 2003. The cell surface receptor DC-SIGN discriminates between *Mycobacterium* species through selective recognition of the mannose caps on lipoarabinomannan. *J. Biol. Chem.* **278:**5513–5516.

72. Marrakchi, H., S. Ducasse, G. Labesse, H. Montrozier, E. Margeat, L. Emorine, X. Charpentier, M. Daffé, and A. Quémard. 2002. MabA (FabG1), a *Mycobacterium tuberculosis* protein involved in the long-chain fatty acid elongation system FAS-II. *Microbiology* **148:**951–960.

73. Mdluli, K., R. A. Slayden, Y. Zhu, S. Ramaswamy, X. Pan, D. Mead, D. D. Crane, J. M. Musser, and C. E. Barry III. 1998. Inhibition of a *Mycobacterium tuberculosis* β-ketoacyl ACP synthase by isoniazid. *Science* **280:**1607–1610.

74. Minnikin, D. E., and M. Goodfellow. 1980. Lipid composition in the classification and Identification of acid fast bacteria, p. 189–256. *In* M. Goodfellow and R. G. Board (ed.),

Microbiological Classification and Identification. Academic Press, Ltd., London, United Kingdom.

75. **Minnikin, D. E.** 1982. Lipids: complex lipids, their chemistry, biosynthesis and roles, p. 95–184. *In* C. Ratledge and J. Stanford (ed.), *The Biology of Mycobacteria.* Academic Press, Ltd., London, United Kingdom.

76. **Minnikin, D. E., L. Kremer, L. G. Dover, and G. S. Besra.** 2002. The methyl-branched fortifications of *Mycobacterium tuberculosis. Chem. Biol.* 9:545–553.

77. **Molloy, A., G. Gaudernack, W. R. Levis, Z. A. Cohn, and G. Kaplan.** 1990. Suppression of T-cell proliferation by *Mycobacterium leprae* and its products: the role of lipopolysaccharide. *Proc. Natl. Acad Sci. USA* 8:973–977.

78. **Ng, V., G. Zanazzi, R. Timpl, J. F. Talts, J. L. Salzer, P. J. Brennan, and A. Rambukkana.** 2000. Role of the cell wall phenolic glycolipid-1 in the peripheral nerve predilection of *Mycobacterium leprae. Cell* 103:511–524.

79. **Nigou, J., M. Gilleron, B. Cahuzac, J. D. Bounéri, M. Herold, M. Thurnher, and G. Puzo.** 1997. The phosphatidyl-*myo*-inositol anchor of the lipoarabinomannans from *Mycobacterium bovis* bacillus Calmette Guérin. Heterogeneity, structure, and role in the regulation of cytokine secretion. *J. Biol. Chem.* 272:23094–23103.

80. **Nigou, J., M. Gilleron, and G. Puzo.** 2003. Lipoarabinomannans: from structure to biosynthesis. *Biochimie* 85:153–166.

81. **Nigou, J., M. Gilleron, M. Rojas, L. F. Garcia, M. Thurnher, and G. Puzo.** 2002. Mycobacterial lipoarabinomannans: modulators of dendritic cell function and the apoptotic response. *Microbes Infect.* 4:945–953.

82. **Ozeki, Y., K. Kaneda, N. Fujiwara, M. Morimoto, S. Oka, and I. Yano.** 1997. In vivo induction of apoptosis in the thymus by administration of mycobacterial cord factor (trehalose 6,6'-dimycolate). *Infect. Immun.* 65:1793–1799.

83. **Porcelli, S. A., and G. S. Besra.** 2002. Immune recognition of the mycobacterial cell wall, p. 230–249. *In* J. P. Gorvel (ed.), *Intracellular Pathogens in Membrane Interactions and Vacuole Biogenesis.* ASM Press, Washington, D.C.

84. **Prasad, H. K., R. S. Misrah, and I. Nath.** 1987. Phenolic glycolipid-I of *Mycobacterium leprae* induces general suppression of *in vitro* concanavalin A responses unrelated to leprosy type. *J. Exp. Med.* 165:239–244.

85. **Quémard, A., M. A. Lanéelle, H. Marrakchi, D. Prome, E. Dubnau, and M. Daffé.** 1997. Structure of a hydroxymycolic acid potentially involved in the synthesis of oxygenated mycolic acids of the *Mycobacterium tuberculosis* complex. *Eur. J. Biochem.* 250:758–763.

86. **Qureshi, N., K. Takayama, and H. K. Schnoes.** 1980. Purification of C_{30-56} fatty acids from *Mycobacterium tuberculosis* H37Ra. *J. Biol. Chem.* 255:182–189.

87. **Qureshi, N., N. Sathyamoorthy, and K. Takayama.** 1984. Biosynthesis of C-30 to C-56 fatty-acids by an extract of *Mycobacterium tuberculosis* H37Ra. *J. Bacteriol.* 157:46–52.

88. **Rainwater, D. L., and P. E. Kolattukudy.** 1985. Fatty acid biosynthesis in *Mycobacterium tuberculosis* var. *bovis* bacillus Calmette-Guérin. Purification and characterization of a novel fatty acid synthase, mycocerosic acid synthase, which elongates n-fatty acyl-CoA with methylmalonyl-CoA. *J. Biol. Chem.* 260:616–623.

89. **Rhoades, E., F. F. Hsu, J. B. Torrelles, J. Turk, D. Chatterjee, and D. G. Russell.** 2003. Indentification and macrophage-activating activity of glycolipids released from intracellular *Mycobacterium bovis* BCG. *Mol. Microbiol.* 48:875–888.

90. **Ribi, E., D. L. Granger, K. C. Milner, K. Yamamoto, S. M. Strain, R. Parker, R. W. Smith, W. Brehmer, and I. Azuma.** 1982. Induction of resistance to tuberculosis in mice with defined components of mycobacteria and with some unrelated materials. *Immunology* 46:297–305.

91. **Rousseau, C., O. Neyrolles, Y. Bordat, S. Giroux, T. D. Sirakova, M. C. Prevost, P. E. Kolattukudy, B. Gicquel, and M. Jackson.** 2003. Deficiency in mycolipenate- and mycosanoate-derived acyltrehaloses enhances early interactions of *Mycobacterium tuberculosis* with host cells. *Cell. Microbiol.* 5:405–415.

92. **Rozwarski, D. A., C. Vilchèze, M. Sugantino, R. Bittman, and J. C. Sacchettini.** 1999. Crystal structure of the *Mycobacterium tuberculosis* enoyl-ACP reductase, InhA, in complex with NAD$^+$ and a C_{16} fatty acyl substrate. *J. Biol. Chem.* 274:15582–15589.

93. **Ryll, R., K. Watanabe, N. Fujiwara, H. Takimoto, R. Hasunuma, Y. Kumazawa, M. Okada, and I. Yano.** 2001. Mycobacterial cord factor, but not sulfolipid, causes depletion of NKT cells and upregulation of CD1d1 on murine macrophages. *Microbes Infect.* 3:611–619.

94. **Saavedra, R., E. Segura, R. Leyva, L. A. Esparza, and L. M. López-Marin.** 2001. Mycobacterial di-O-acyl-trehalose inhibits mitogen- and antigen-induced proliferation of murine T cells in vitro. *Clin. Diagn. Lab. Immunol.* 8:1081–1088.

95. **Scarsdale, N., G. Kazanina, X. He, K. A. Reynolds, and H. T. Wright.** 2001. Crystal structure of the *Mycobacterium tuberculosis* β-keto-acyl carrier protein synthase III. *J. Biol. Chem.* 276:20516–20522.

96. **Schaeffer, M., K. H. Khoo, G. S. Besra, D. Chatterjee, P. J. Brennan, J. T. Belisle, and J. Inamine.** 1999. The *pimB* gene of *Mycobacterium tuberculosis* encodes a mannosyltransferase involved in lipoarabinomannan biosynthesis. *J. Biol. Chem.* 274:31625–31631.

97. **Schaeffer, M. L., G. Agnihotri, C. Volker, H. Kallender, P. J. Brennan, and J. T. Lonsdale.** 2001. Purification and biochemical characterization of the *Mycobacterium tuberculosis* beta-ketoacyl-acyl carrier protein synthases KasA and KasB. *J. Biol. Chem.* 276:47029–47037.

98. **Schlesinger, L. S., S. R. Hull, and T. M. Kaufman.** 1994. Binding of the terminal mannosyl units of lipoarabinomannan from a virulent strain of *Mycobacterium tuberculosis* to human macrophages. *J. Immunol.* 152:4070–4079.

99. **Schroeder, B. G., and C. E. Barry III.** 2001. The specificity of methyl transferases involved in trans mycolic acid biosynthesis in *Mycobacterium tuberculosis* and *Mycobacterium smegmatis. Bioorg. Chem.* 29:164–177.

100. **Sibley, L. D., S. W. Hunter, P. J. Brennan, and J. L. Krahenbuhl.** 1988. Mycobacterial lipoarabinomannan inhibits gamma interferon-mediated activation of macrophages. *Infect. Immun.* 56:1232–1236.

101. **Sirakova, T. D., A. K. Thirumala, V. S. Dubey, H. Sprecher, and P. E. Kolattukudy.** 2001. The *Mycobacterium tuberculosis pks2* gene encodes the synthase for the hepta- and octamethyl-branched fatty acids required for sulfolipid synthesis. *J. Biol. Chem.* 276:16833–16839.

102. **Takayama, K., N. Qureshi, and H. K. Schnoes.** 1978. Isolation and characterization of monounsaturated long-chain fatty acids in *Mycobacterium tuberculosis. Lipids* 13:575–579.

103. **Takayama, K., and N. Qureshi.** 1984. Structure and synthesis of lipids, p. 315–344. *In* G. B. Kubica and L. G. Wayne (ed.), *The Mycobacteria. A Sourcebook.* Marcel Dekker, Inc., New York, N.Y.

104. **Telenti, A., W. J. Philipp, S. Sreevatsan, C. Bernasconi, K. E. Stockbauer, B. Wieles, J. M. Musser, and W. R. Jacobs, Jr.** 1997. The *emb* operon, a gene cluster of *Mycobacterium*

tuberculosis involved in resistance to ethambutol. *Nat. Med.* **3:**567–570.

105. **Vachula, M., T. J. Holzer, and B. R. Andersen.** 1989. Suppression of monocyte oxidative response by phenolic glycolipid I of *Mycobacterium leprae. J. Immunol.* **142:**1696–1701.

106. **Vercellone, A., J. Nigou, and G. Puzo.** 1998. Relationships between the structure and the roles of lipoarabinomannans and related glycoconjugates in tuberculosis pathogenesis. *Front. Biosci.* **3:**e149–e163.

107. **Vignal, C., Y. Guérardel, L. Kremer, M. Masson, D. Legrand, J. Mazurier, and E. Elass.** 2003. Lipomannans, but not lipoarabinomannans, purified from *Mycobacterium chelonae* and *Mycobacterium kansasii* induce TNF-α and IL-8 secretion by a CD14-TLR2 dependent mechanism. *J. Immunol.* **171:**2014–2023.

108. **Watanabe, M., Y. Aoyagi, M. Ridell, and D. E. Minnikin.** 2001. Separation and characterization of individual mycolic acids in representative mycobacteria. *Microbiology* **147:** 1825–1837.

109. **Watanabe, M., Y. Aoyagi, H. Mitome, T. Fujita, H. Naoki, M. Ridell, and D. E. Minnikin.** 2002. Location of functional groups in mycobacteria meromycolate chain: the recognition of new structural principles in mycolic acids. *Microbiology* **148:**1881–1902.

110. **Wolucka, P. J., M. McNeil, E. de Hoffmann, T. Chojnacki, and P. J. Brennan.** 1994. Recognition of the lipid intermediate for arabinogalactan/arabinomannan biosynthesis and its relation to the mode of action of ethambutol on mycobacteria. *J. Biol. Chem.* **269:**23328–23335.

111. **Wong, H. C., G. Liu, Y. M. Zhang, C. O. Rock, and J. Zheng.** 2002. The solution structure of acyl carrier protein from *Mycobacterium tuberculosis. J. Biol. Chem.* **277:** 15874–15880.

112. **Woodbury, J. L., and W. W. Barrow.** 1989. Radiolabelling of *Mycobacterium avium* oligosaccharide determinant and use in macrophage studies. *J. Gen. Microbiol.* **135:**1875–1884.

113. **Yamagami, H., T. Matsumoto, N. Fujiwara, T. Arakawa, K. Kaneda, I. Yano, and K. Kobayashi.** 2001. Trehalose 6,6′-dimycolate (cord factor) of *Mycobacterium tuberculosis* induces foreign-body and hypersensitivity-type granulomas in mice. *Infect. Immun.* **69:**810–815.

114. **Yuan, Y., R. E. Lee, G. S. Besra, J. T. Belisle, and C. E. Barry III.** 1995. Identification of a gene involved in the biosynthesis of cyclopropanated mycolic acids in *Mycobacterium tuberculosis. Proc. Natl. Acad. Sci. USA* **92:**6630–6634.

115. **Yuan, Y., and C. E. Barry III.** 1996. A common mechanism for the biosynthesis of methoxy and cyclopropyl mycolic acids in *Mycobacterium tuberculosis. Proc. Natl. Acad. Sci. USA* **93:**12828–12833.

116. **Yuan, Y., D. C. Crane, J. M. Musser, S. Streevatsan, and C. E. Barry III.** 1997. MMAS-1, the branch point between *cis-* and *trans-*cyclopropane containing oxygenated mycolates in *Mycobacterium tuberculosis. J. Biol. Chem.* **272:** 10041–10049.

VIII. METABOLISM

Chapter 20

General Metabolism and Biochemical Pathways of Tubercle Bacilli

PAUL R. WHEELER AND JOHN S. BLANCHARD

There has been a great shift in the way we are able to think about metabolism in the *Mycobacterium tuberculosis* complex since the subject was reviewed in the last edition of this book (165). Since then, the complete, annotated genome sequences of *M. tuberculosis* (34) (http://genolist.pasteur.fr/TubercuList/) and *M. bovis* (48) have become available. Before that, one had to hypothesize about the key areas to investigate based on what was known about the chemistry and biology of the tubercle bacilli. Now, consideration of their genomes itself generates hypotheses. Some of these hypotheses are consistent with established ideas, for example, that lipid metabolism is especially important and that genus- and even species-specific pathways of lipid biosynthesis may represent good targets for selective antimicrobials. Another example is the determination of the genes required for iron acquisition and storage that are necessary activities for most pathogenic microbes (125).

However, new hypotheses are generated too. For example, does the so-called "redundancy" in many genes for intermediary metabolism, along with the surprising number of alternate, anaerobic electron transport chains, provide the organism with the metabolic versatility to allow it to survive in a wide range of niches? Within the host, the aerobic alveolar macrophage, the granuloma, and the liquefied centre of the caseous lesion represent very different environments. Furthermore, genes that are likely to encode products never seen in *M. tuberculosis* were discovered: there appear to be far more genes encoding polyketide synthases than the number of polyketide-like lipids that have been discovered in years of systematic lipid analysis (90). Novel multigene families of glycine-rich PE and PPE proteins, hitherto unknown and unsuspected, were revealed. Could these be essential for pathogenicity during so far unexplored periods of the life of *M. tuberculosis* in the host?

Having the complete genome sequences means that all the genes that can be expressed under all conditions are now catalogued (28). In the past, most of the work on metabolism in *M. tuberculosis* was done with bulk, aerobically grown liquid cultures. Alternatively, adaptation to anaerobic conditions was explored in a model developed from studying metabolic and antigenic changes in tubercle bacilli allowed to settle to the bottom of flasks (156, 158). This appears to have been an incredibly far-sighted piece of work since the inside of the granuloma is an oxygen-limited environment, so that the Wayne model is a working model for persisting tubercle bacilli during infection—a theme that is revisited and explored throughout this chapter. In vivo, a few studies were performed with macrophage cultures and host-grown bacteria from an advanced stages of disease when sufficient bacteria could be obtained (13, 24, 91, 162).

In the future, it should be possible to investigate *M. tuberculosis* metabolism and gene expression in a much wider range of environments, such as those outlined above, by extracting its mRNAs or proteins and identifying them by referring back to the genome. Since both technology and our knowledge of gene expression under carefully defined conditions improves, that future work will itself generate new hypotheses about which genes are key to pathogenicity in the different environments encountered in the host.

Currently, the role of regulatory genes in pathogenicity is a major area of investigation, since these genes, by definition, are involved in the response to changing environments during infection. This work is important since these genes may encode regulatory proteins that control virulence. Since there are a discrete number of regulatory functions, it should be possible to understand the response to a wide range of conditions by investigating a relatively small number of genes. Functionally investigating genes involved in

Paul R Wheeler • Tuberculosis Research Unit, Veterinary Laboratories Agency (Weybridge), New Haw, Addlestone, Surrey KT15 3NB, United Kingdom. **John S. Blanchard** • Department of Biochemistry, Albert Einstein College of Medicine, 1300 Morris Park Ave., Bronx, NY 10461.

sulfur metabolism is also productive, since their activities are key to a wide range of fundamental biological activities. Indeed, we argue that sulfur metabolism is a major area of current research that has arisen in a piecemeal way. These two areas—regulomics and thiomics—are highlighted in this chapter. Since regulation in general is being dealt with in chapters 15 and 22, we deal with the regulation of each pathway and area of metabolism we discuss. More generally, we focus on the postgenomic advances, where a functional understanding of the genes and pathways predicted for intermediary metabolism in the *M. tuberculosis* complex has been obtained, as the framework for this chapter.

AMINO ACID BIOSYNTHESIS

Historically, the functions of key genes in amino acid biosynthesis were tested relatively early in molecular biology research in *M. tuberculosis*. Starting in the mid-1990s, transposon libraries were made and screened (85, 120, 169) for amino acid auxotrophs at a time before site-directed mutagenesis and targeted knocking out of genes had been developed for the tubercle bacilli. The driving force behind this work was the need to obtain attenuated strains suitable for vaccine development. An interesting spectrum of attenuation was obtained, from very slight in mutants with mutations in sulfur amino acid biosynthesis through strongly attenuated for proline, tryptophan, and leucine auxotrophs to lethal deletions that could not be rescued by the addition of amino acids to culture media for aspartokinase and for the *aroK* gene in the shared part of aromatic amino biosynthesis. The details of the metabolic pathways, illustrated with figures to show the metabolic function of the genes disrupted in these experiments, are dealt with in turn.

L-Lysine

L-Lysine is one of four amino acids derived from L-aspartate and shares the first two steps in its biosynthetic pathway in common with L-methionine and L-threonine (Fig. 1; Table 1). Genetic knockouts of genes in this pathway have demonstrated its essentiality in *Mycobacterium smegmatis* (120). These first two steps, catalyzed by aspartokinase and aspartate semialdehyde dehydrogenase, are catalyzed by the adjacent *ask* and *asd* genes (Rv3709c and Rv3708c, respectively [33]). There do not appear to be multiple aspartokinases that are differentially feedback regulated by the end products of these amino acid pathways, as has been observed in other bacteria. Together, the two enzymes catalyze the conversion of the γ-carboxyl group of L-aspartate to the corresponding aldehyde. The first committed step in the lysine pathway is the aldol condensation of pyruvate to aspartate semialdehyde to generate the cyclic hydroxytetrahydropicolinate, which undergoes nonenzymatic dehydration to yield dihydropicolinate. This reaction is likely to be catalyzed by the Rv2753c gene product, although this gene product has not been expressed and functionally characterized (Table 1). Dihydrodipicolinate is subsequently reduced in an NAD(H)-dependent reaction catalyzed by the Rv2773c gene product (121), which has been expressed, purified, and crystallized (M. Cirilli, personal communication). The next step involves enzyme-assisted cyclic imine hydrolysis to generate 2-amino-6-oxopimelate, followed by acylation to generate the stable acyclic α-*N*-acyl-2-amino-6-oxopimelate. While it is likely that the acyl group is the succinyl moiety, no firm biochemical evidence for this exists, nor is there an obvious open reading frame with similarity to the only biochemically and structurally characterized *dapD*-encoded *N*-succinylase (16). Following acylation, a pyridoxal-5′ phosphate-dependent transamination yields *N*-succinyl-L,L-diaminopimelate. The *Escherichia coli* enzyme that catalyzes this reaction was shown to be identical to the *argD*-encoded *N*-acetylornithine aminotransferase, and an *M. tuberculosis* homologue of *argD* exists (Rv1165) and has been demonstrated to catalyze this reaction (R. Ledwidge and J. S. Blanchard, unpublished data). Deacylation, to generate L,L-diamin-opimelic acid (L,L-DAP), is catalyzed by the *dapE*-encoded desuccinylase, for which there is a homologue in the *M. tuberculosis* genome (Rv1202). The conversion of L,L-DAP to D,L-DAP is catalyzed by the *dapF*-encoded diaminopimelate epimerase, one of the very few examples of a PLP-independent amino acid racemase. The *Haemophilus influenzae* enzyme has been thoroughly characterized, both mechanistically and structurally (32, 73), and the Rv2726c gene product is likely to catalyze this reaction since it can be modeled on the *H. influenzae* DapF. In the final step, the *lysA*-encoded diaminopimelate decarboxylase cata-lyzes the PLP-dependent decarboxylation of the D-amino acid stereocenter. The Rv1293-encoded gene was cloned from *M. tuberculosis* and shown to complement an *E. coli lysA* strain (5); the three-dimensional structure of this enzyme appears to confirm the unique reaction mechanism shown for LysA enzymes (53).

The biosynthesis of both L-threonine and L-methionine proceeds via the NADH-dependent reduction of L-aspartate semialdehyde catalyzed by the *thrA*-encoded homoserine dehydrogenase. None of the annotated genes have had their enzymatic functions confirmed, but the Rv1294 gene product is the likely mycobacterial homoserine dehydrogenase.

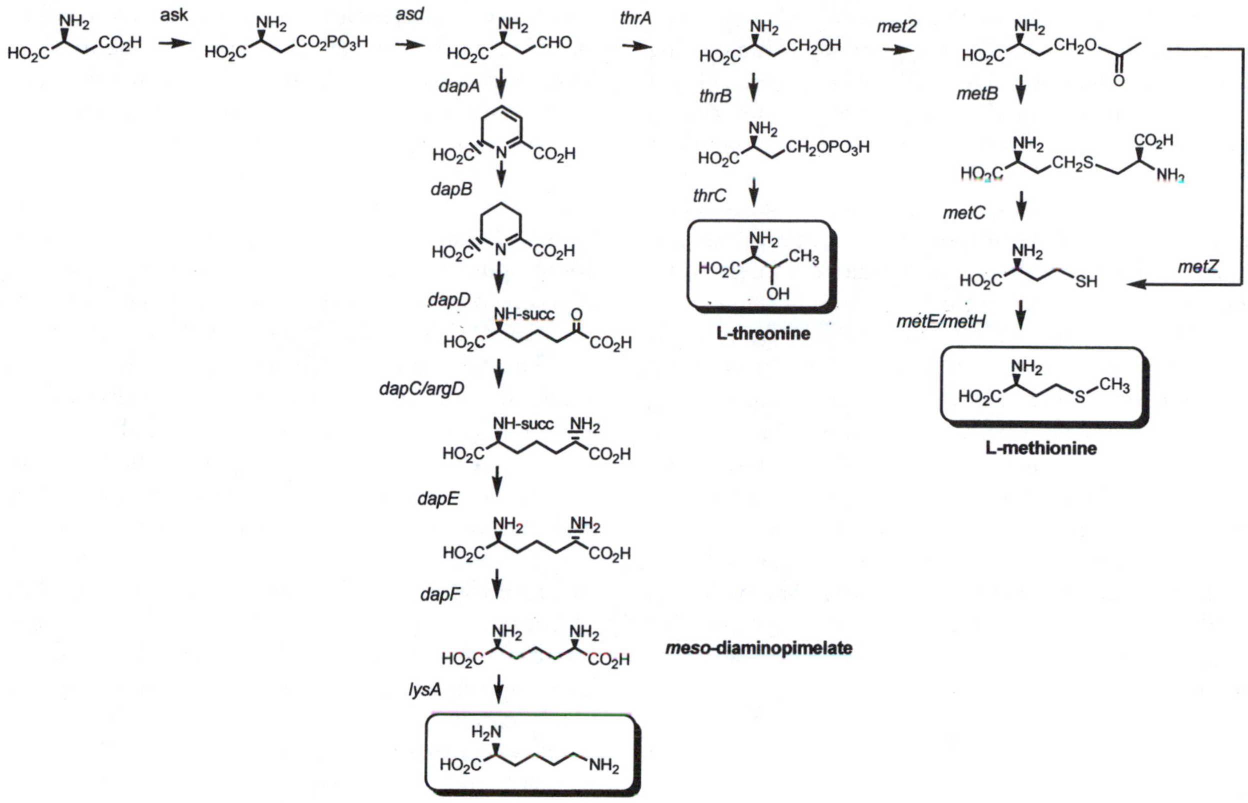

Figure 1. Biosynthesis of the aspartate family of amino acids. Unbroken arrows show chemical transformations, and broken arrows show pathways of several transformations.

Table 1. Genes in biosynthesis of the aspartate family of amino acids

Gene	Rv no.[a]	Size (aa)	EC	Enzyme name	Comment
ask	**Rv3709c**	421	2.7.2.4	Aspartokinase	
asd	Rv3708c	345	1.2.1.11	Aspartate semialdehyde dehydrogenase	
dapA	Rv2753c	300	4.2.1.52	Dihydrodipicolinate synthase	
dapB	**Rv2773c**	400	1.3.1.26	Dihydrodipicolinate reductase	
dapD			2.3.1.117	2-Amino-6-oxo-pimelate succinylase	
dapC	Rv1655	400	2.6.1.17	N-Succinyl-2-amino-6-oxo-pimelate transaminase	See also argD
dapE	Rv1202	354	3.5.1.18	N-Succinyl-L,L-DAP desuccinylase	
dapF	Rv2726c	289	5.1.1.7	L,L-DAP epimerase	
lysA	**Rv1293**	447	4.1.1.20	D,L-DAP decarboxylase	
thrA	Rv1294	441	1.1.1.3	Homoserine dehydrogenase	
thrB	Rv1296	316	2.7.1.39	Homoserine kinase	
thrC	Rv1295	360	4.2.99.2	Threonine synthase	
met2	Rv3341	379	2.3.1.31	Homoserine O-acetyltransferase	metA in tuberculist
metB	Rv1079	388	4.2.99.9	Cystathionine γ-synthase	
metC	Rv3340	449	4.4.1.8	Cystathionine β-lyase	
metE	Rv1133c	759	2.1.1.14	Methionine synthase	
metH	Rv2124c	1192	2.1.1.13	Methionine synthase	
metZ	Rv0391	406	4.2.99.-	O-succinylhomoserine sulfhydrylase	

[a]Boldface Rv numbers indicate that the enzyme activity corresponding to the CDS has been confirmed by isolation or cloning of the enzyme, complementation, or the loss of activity when the gene is inactive for at least one of the M. tuberculosis complex. Similar evidence obtained with orthologous genes in mycobacteria if their counterpart in the M. tuberculosis complex is essentially unambiguous. For all others, the enzyme name is derived from the gene annotation.

The alcohol product of the dehydrogenase reaction is phosphorylated by the *thrB*-encoded homoserine kinase, for which Rv1296 is the likely gene in *M. tuberculosis*. In the final step, phosphohomoserine is converted into L-threonine by the PLP-dependent threonine synthase. The *thrC*-encoded synthase is likely to be encoded by Rv1295. The mechanism involves an unusual β-elimination of inorganic phosphate, to generate the PLP-linked iminobutenoate, followed by the addition of water to the β position.

The first unique step in the biosynthesis of L-methionine is the activation of the γ-hydroxy group of homoserine (Fig. 1). This is accomplished using succinyl coenzyme A (succinyl-CoA) in some bacteria, including *E. coli* (*metA* and homologs) (19) or acetyl-CoA in *Haemophilus influenzae* and mycobacteria (*met2* and homologues, including Rv3341) (20). In either case, the product of the reaction is the ester that is activated for the next step (Fig. 1). The pathways for the addition of the thiol group to give L-methionine are discussed in the section on sulfur metabolism (see below).

Branched-Chain Amino Acids

The biosynthetic pathways leading to L-valine and L-leucine are shown in Fig. 2. Several of the activities discussed below were identified before the genes to encode them were predicted (2–4). Two molecules of pyruvate are condensed to generate acetolactate by the acetolactate synthase complex. A number of homologues are predicted to encode both the large and small subunits of the enzyme present in the *M. tuberculosis* genome, including homologues of the *ilvG* (Rv1820)-, *ilvB* (Rv3003c)-, *ilvB2* (Rv3407c)-, and *ilvX* (Rv3509c)-encoded large subunit (Table 2). There is a single homologue to the *ilvN*-encoded small subunit (Rv3002c). The gene products have not been expressed or purified. The second step converts acetolactate into 1,2-dihydroxyisovalerate. This reaction is catalyzed by the *ilvC*-encoded isomeroreductase in *E. coli*, and a homologue has been identified in *M. tuberculosis* (Rv3001c). The isomeroreductase is one of only two enzymes that have been demonstrated to catalyze vitamin B_{12}-independent alkyl migration chemistry (the other is involved in the biosynthesis of isoprenoids via the nonmevalonate pathway that is present in *M. tuberculosis*). The reaction involves an initial 1,2-methyl migration followed by the pyridine nucleotide-dependent reduction of the α-keto acid. It is unclear whether both reactions are catalyzed by the same enzyme in mycobacteria, since the two activities have been reported to be separable (4). The conversion of 1,2-dihydroxyisovalerate to α-ketoisovalerate is catalyzed by the *ilvD*-encoded

dihydroxy acid dehydratase, and Rv0189c has been identified as the gene encoding the enzyme in *M. tuberculosis*. α-Ketoisovalerate is the precursor of both L-valine and L-leucine, as well as pantothenate (vitamin B_5) and CoA. The direct transamination of α-ketoisovalerate, using L-glutamate as the amino donor, to generate L-valine is catalyzed by the *ilvE*-encoded branched-chain aminotransferase. The mycobacterial homologue, Rv2210c, has not been biochemically characterized. It shows relatively broad substrate specificity for α-ketoacids with alkyl substituents.

The first unique step in L-leucine biosynthesis is the addition of the acetyl group of acetyl-CoA to α-ketoisovalerate to generate isopropylmalate (Fig. 2). This reaction is catalyzed by the *leuA*-encoded 2-isopropylmalate synthase. This reaction is analogous to the addition reaction catalyzed by citrate synthase, where two carbon units from glycolysis enter the tricarboxylic acid cycle. The homologous protein in *M. tuberculosis* is Rv3710. 2-Isopropylmalate is converted to 3-isopropylmalate by the *leuC/leuD*-encoded isopropylmalate dehydratase in a reaction analogous to that catalyzed by aconitase. The mycobacterial homologues of these two subunits are the Rv2988c and Rv2987c (60), respectively. An attenuated strain of *M. tuberculosis* has been generated by allelic exchange of the wild-type *leuD* gene by a truncated variant and shown to be auxotrophic for leucine (60). In the penultimate step, the oxidative decarboxylation of 3-isopropylmalate generates α-ketoisocaproate. This reaction is catalyzed by the *leuB*-encoded isopropylmalate dehydrogenase, for which the *M. tuberculosis* homologue is Rv2995c. In the final step, the *ilvE*-encoded branched-chain aminotransferase that also catalyzes the final step in L-valine and L-isoleucine biosynthesis converts α-ketoisocaproate into L-leucine.

Other Biosynthetic Pathways Required for Virulence (Aromatic Amino Acids, Proline, and Histidine) and Their Control

Very few genes for other biosynthetic pathways have been confirmed by showing the enzyme activity of their products or by complementation of mutants with defined effects. Therefore, we have not included figures for these pathways, but pathways showing the annotated genes can be viewed at http://www.genome.ad.jp/kegg/. However, the information that currently exists is very interesting. Mutations in genes predicted to function in both aromatic amino acid and proline biosynthesis have been shown to be attenuating. When the genes for *trpD* or *proC* were knocked out, the effect was strongly attenuating. These two knockouts were auxotrophs, verifying the pathways in which the genes were predicted to function (146).

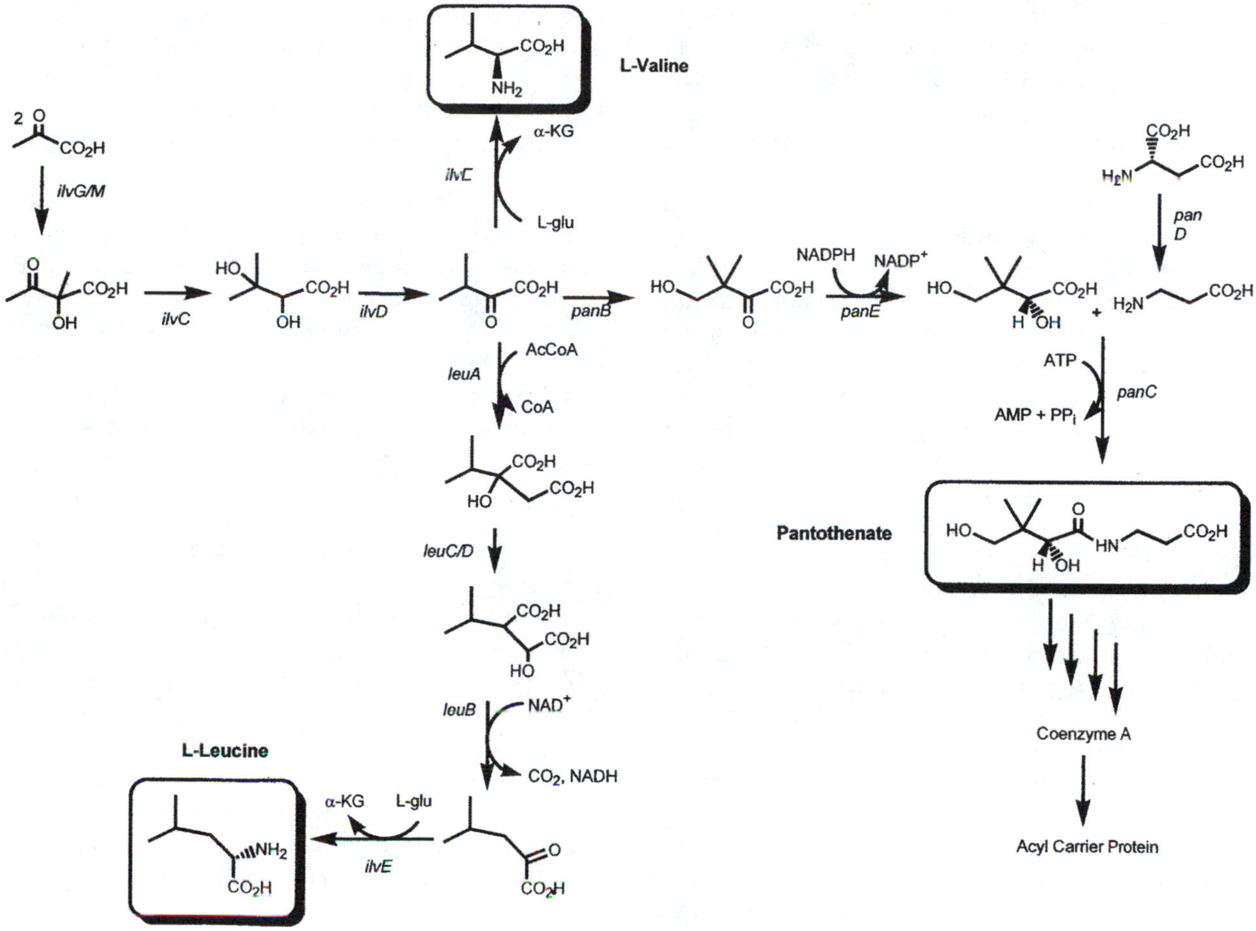

Figure 2. Branched chain amino acid biosynthesis. Unbroken arrows show chemical transformations, and broken arrows show pathways of several transformations.

Table 2. Genes in branched chain amino acid biosynthesis

Gene	Rv no.[a]	Size (aa)	EC	Enzyme name
ilvG	Rv1820	547	4.1.3.8	Acetolactate synthase (large subunit)
ilvB	Rv3003c	618	4.1.3.8	Acetolactate synthase (large subunit)
ilvB2	Rv3407c	552	4.1.3.8	Acetolactate synthase (large subunit)
ilvX	Rv3509c	515	4.1.3.8	Acetolactate synthase (large subunit)
ilvN	Rv3002c	168	4.1.3.8	Acetolactate synthase (small subunit)
ilvC	Rv3001c	333	1.1.1.86	Ketol acid reductoisomerase
ilvD	Rv0189c	575	4.2.1.9	Dihydroxy acid dehydratase
ilvE	Rv2210c	368	2.6.1.42	Branched chain aminotransferase
leuA	Rv3710	644	4.1.3.12	2-Isopropylmalate synthase
leuC	**Rv2988c**	473	4.2.1.33	Isopropylmalate dehydratase (large subunit)
leuD	**Rv2987c**	198	4.2.1.33	Isopropylmalate dehydratase (small subunit)
leuB	Rv2995c	336	1.1.1.85	Isopropylmalate dehydrogenase
panB	**Rv2225**	281	2.1.2.11	3-Methyl-2-oxobutanoate hydroxymethyltransferase
panE	Rv2573	246	1.1.1.169	Ketopantoate reductase
panD	**Rv3601c**	139	4.1.1.11	Asparate 1-decarboxylase
panC	**Rv3602c**	309	6.3.2.1	Pantothenate synthase

[a]Boldface Rv numbers indicate that the enzyme activity corresponding to the CDS has been confirmed by isolation or cloning of the enzyme, complementation, or the loss of activity when the gene is inactive for at least one of the *M. tuberculosis* complex. Similar evidence obtained with orthologous genes in mycobacteria if their counterpart in the *M. tuberculosis* complex is essentially unambiguous. For all others, the enzyme name is derived from the gene annotation.

A knockout of *aroK* was lethal. Since it could not be rescued by adding the end products of the biosynthetic pathway to the medium but could be rescued only by introducing an active copy of the gene into the bacteria, *aroK* is termed an essential gene. Only a single copy of *aroK*, predicted to encode shikimate kinase, occurs in the *M. tuberculosis* genome, as opposed to two copies in *E. coli*, offering one possible explanation for its essentiality (115). Both *aroK* and the gene for the subsequent step in the pathway, *aroA*, have been cloned and overexpressed, and their enzyme activities have been demonstrated (110). As predicted, *aroK* was found to encode shikimate kinase and *aroA* was found to encode 5-enolpyruvylshikimate-3-phosphate synthase (110) using phosphenolpyruvate as its co-substrate.

The first step of the shikimate pathway, like the AroK and AroA steps, is common to all the aromatic amino acids. It involves the condensation of phosphoenolpyruvate with D-erythrose-4-phosphate. These are products of glycolysis and the pentose cycle, and some significant findings on their generation are discussed in the section on carbon and energy metabolism (below).

Mutations in *proC*, *trpD*, and *hisD* had similar effects on intracellular survival in a human macrophage-like cell line and under starvation for the single amino acid for which they were auxotrophic (114). The tryptophan and histidine auxotrophs lost viability, but the proline auxotroph survived as well as its parent strain, H37Rv, even though it was attenuated in mice. Since a complete-starvation model gave a different pattern of survival, the findings suggested that the intracellular environment was deficient in some but not all amino acids. The results could not be explained as a result of conflict between the regulatory effects of the stringent response and unavailability of a single amino acid, since neither tryptophan nor histidine repressed the activity of their respective promoter loci (114). The promoter activity findings add to a growing body of evidence suggesting that most amino acid biosynthetic genes are constitutively expressed (114). Even for cysteine biosynthesis, for which there is evidence of transcriptional control (reviewed below in the section on sulfur metabolism), sulfate transport is barely affected by growing tubercle bacilli in the presence of a sulfur-containing amino acid (169). Instead, control at the posttranslational level is highlighted by the recent solving of the structure of N-1-(5′-phosphoribosyl)-ATP transferase from *M. tuberculosis*, the first enzyme in the pathway for histidine biosynthesis. This *hisG*-encoded enzyme exhibits allosteric inhibition by AMP and the end point of the pathway, histidine (30).

Finally, it has been discovered that the Rv1603 gene encodes an enzyme that is shared by the pathways for both tryptophan and histidine biosynthesis.

Like its orthologue from *Streptomyces coelicolor*, it can complement both *trpF* and *hisA* auxotrophic mutants of *E. coli*, indicating that it has both N-(5-phospho-β-D-ribosyl)anthranilate ketol-isomerase and 1-(5-phosphoribosyl)-5-[(5- phosphoribosylamino)methylideneamino]imidazole-4-carboxamide ketol-isomerase activities and is an ancient, broad-specificity enzyme (14). There are several other examples in amino acid biosynthesis of enzymes in different pathways having analogous catalytic mechanisms, and it will be intriguing to find if any more of them are encoded by a single gene in *M. tuberculosis*. This would have implications for the evolution of amino acid biosynthesis and its control in actinomycetes in general and *M. tuberculosis* in particular.

SULFUR METABOLISM

Sulfate is readily available in tissues, body fluids, and culture media. With a sulfate transport system encoded by the *cysTWA subI* genes and shown to be the sole sulfate transport system in the *M. tuberculosis* complex (169), the bacteria are equipped to take up this mineral. There are then two routes for assimilation of its sulfur: a nonreductive route into sulfatides, including trehalose sulfate, and a reductive pathway to give thiols (Fig. 3 and Table 3).

Sulfated Compounds

Sulfolipids, essentially acylated trehalose 2′-sulfate, have long been known to occur in *M. tuberculosis*. They were found only in strains virulent in guinea pigs. The attenuated strains elaborated lipids that were similar but lacked the sulfate group (see references 17 and 89 for reviews). Since variation among the sulfolipids is due solely to differences in their acyl moieties, a single sulfotransferase should be sufficient for sulfation of all the sulfolipids. The gene (*Rv1373*; new suggested name, *stf2*) that encodes the sulfotransferase has been cloned and expressed, and its enzymatic activity has been demonstrated (130). In *M. bovis*, *Rv1373* is a pseudogene, explaining why sulfolipids have never been observed in this organism (48, 130). It has been suggested that sulfolipids inhibit phagosome activation and thus promote intracellular survival of virulent strains of *M. tuberculosis* (174), perhaps by disrupting cell signaling (21, 94). However, *M. bovis* lacks sulfolipids and its virulence is not compromised. The sulfotransferase probably uses trehalose as its substrate, since trehalose 2′-sulfate was observed in addition to sulfolipids in an analysis of all the sulfated metabolites (95) that could be produced by a *cysH* mutant unable to reduce sulfate (Fig. 3).

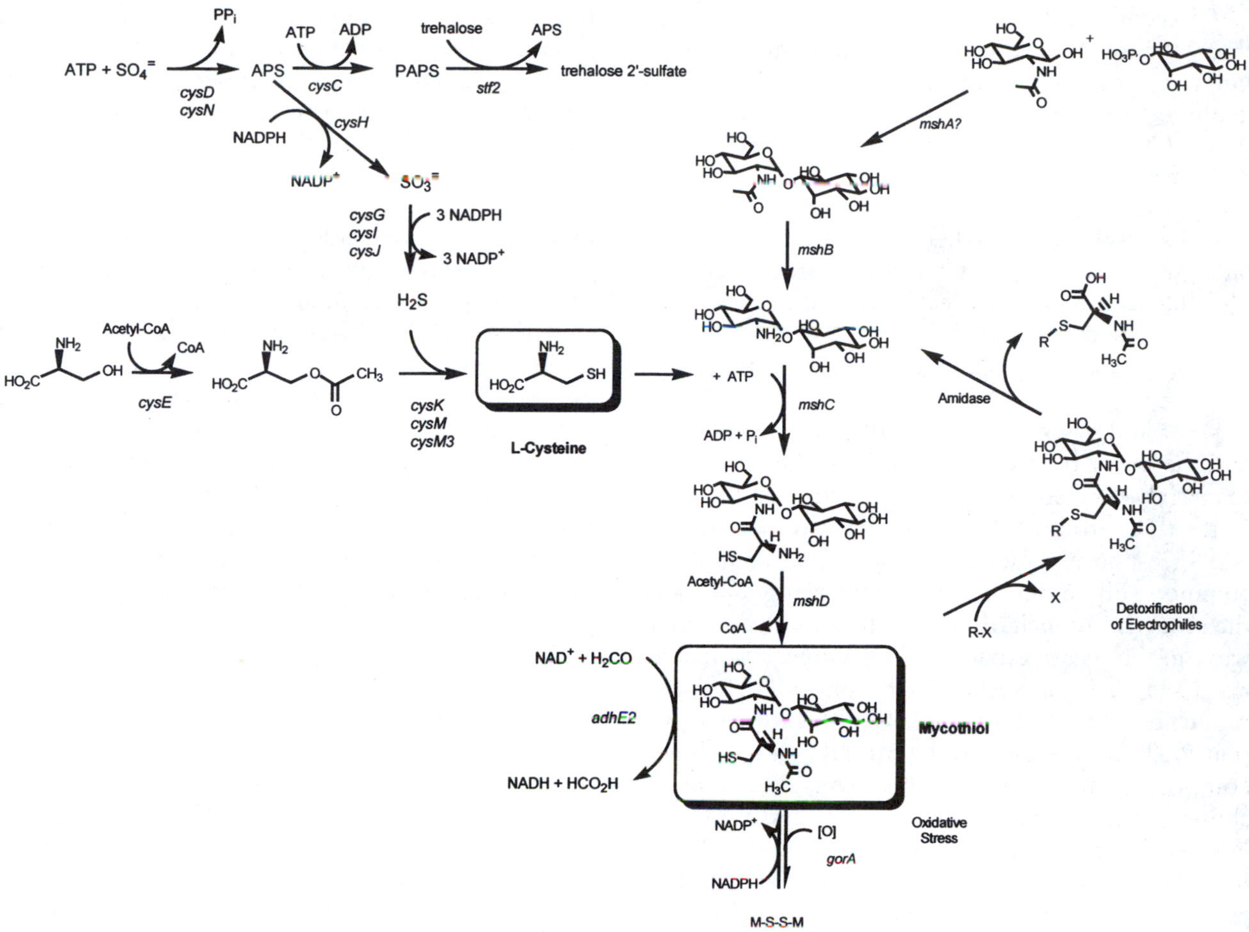

Figure 3. Sulfur metabolism—cysteine. Unbroken arrows show chemical transformations, and broken arrows show pathways of several transformations.

Table 3. Genes in sulfur metabolism—cysteine

Gene	Rv no.[a]	Size (aa)	EC	Enzyme name	Comments
cysN	**Rv1286***	614	2.7.7.4	ATP sulfurylase	
cysD	Rv1285	332	2.7.7.4	ATP sulfurylase	
cysC	**Rv1286***		2.7.1.25	APS kinase	*Fused to cysN
cysH	**Rv2392**	254	1.8.-.-	APS reductase	
cysG	Rv0511	565	1.8.1.2	Sulfite reductase	
cysE	Rv2335	229	2.3.1.30	Serine O-acetyltransferase	
cysM	Rv1336	323	4.2.99.8	O-Acetylserine sulfhydrylase	
cysK	Rv2334	310	4.2.99.8	O-Acetylserine sulfhydrylase	
cysM3	Rv0848	372	4.2.99.8	O-Acetylserine sulfhydrylase	
mshA	**Rv0486**	480		Glycosyltransferase	
mshB	**Rv1170**	303		Deacetylase	
mshC	**Rv2130c**	414		Ligase	
mshD	**Rv0819**	315		Acetyltransferase	
gorA	**Rv2855**	459		Mycothiol disulfide reductase	
adhE2	**Rv2259**	361		Mycothiol-dependent formaldehyde dehydrogenase	
mca	**Rv1082**	288		S-Alkylmycothiol amidase	

[a] Boldface Rv numbers indicate that the enzyme activity corresponding to the CDS has been confirmed by isolation or cloning of the enzyme, complementation, or the loss of activity when the gene is inactive for at least one of the *M. tuberculosis* complex. Similar evidence obtained with orthologousf genes in mycobacteria if their counterpart in the *M. tuberculosis* complex is essentially unambiguous. For all others, the enzyme name is derived from the gene annotation.

Recently, a bioinformatic approach identified three *stf* (for "sulfotransferase") paralogues and six putative *ats* (sulfatase) genes in the *M. tuberculosis* genome (94), suggesting that other sulfated compounds exist and that sulfate can be recycled by the Ats enzymes. Intriguingly, one of the sulfatase genes, *atsA*, is missing in *M. bovis*, along with *stf2* (mentioned above) (48). Whether they are functionally related, with *atsA* being lost when there are no trehalose 2′-sulfate compounds to desulfate, is unclear.

Reductive Pathway of Sulfur Metabolism

Far and away the majority of sulfur compounds, and the many biochemical reactions that depend on them, rely on a supply of reduced sulfur in the form of the thiol group. While gram-negative bacteria use PAPS (3′-phosphoadenosine 5′-phosphosulfate) as a common sulfate donor for sulfated compounds and the reductive branch of the sulfate assimilation pathway, gram-negative bacteria, including mycobacteria, have APS (adenosine 5′-phosphosulfate) at this branch point of the pathways (Fig. 3). Clear evidence that PAPS is used only in the production of sulfated compounds in *M. tuberculosis* was obtained by showing that its *cysH* complements *cysC* (APS kinase) mutants of *E. coli*, suggesting that *cysH M. tuberculosis* must encode an APS reductase (166) (the genes that have been identified are listed in Table 3). The ability of the *M. tuberculosis* complex to grow on sulfate as the sole sulfur source indicates the operation of the complete pathway predicted from sulfate transport to sulfide production (Fig. 3).

Sulfur Transfer Steps for the Biosynthesis of L-Cysteine and L-Methionine

The transfer of the thiol of L-cysteine to the γ-carbon of *O*-acylhomoserine generates cystathionine. This reaction is catalyzed by *metB*-encoded cystathionine γ-synthase. In *M. tuberculosis*, the Rv1079 gene product has been ascribed this function. Cystathionine is subsequently cleaved into homocysteine, pyruvate, and ammonia by the PLP-dependent cystathionine β-lyase. The *metC*-encoded lyase has been identified in mycobacteria as Rv3340 and is directly adjacent to the homoserine *O*-acetyltransferase. There is a second, direct route that may be present in mycobacteria to produce homocysteine from *O*-acetylhomoserine, since a homologue of the *metZ*-encoded *O*-succinylhomoserine sulfhydrylase has been identified (Rv0391). This uses sulfide to displace the acetyl group from *O*-succinylhomoserine. This second route for assimilating sulfur into homocysteine (Fig. 1) probably explains why a Rv1079 mutant was not auxo-

trophic (146). Functionally analogous genes exist in *Corynebacterium glutamicum*. In that actinomycete, *metY* encodes an *O*-acetylhomoserine sulf-hydrylase, and neither *metB* nor *metY* gene disruption alone confers auxotrophy. Finally, there are two possible homologues that can catalyze the S-methyltransfer reaction in mycobacteria, either the *metE*- or *metH*-encoded methionine synthases. Neither of these genes (Rv1133c or Rv2124c, respectively) have been expressed and shown to catalyze the methylation reaction.

Although the source of the sulfur atom of methionine is cysteine in this biosynthetic sequence known as transsulfuration, as we will see, the sulfur atom of cysteine can also be derived from methionine in a pathway referred to as reverse transsulfuration (Fig. 4 and Table 4). That pathway is reviewed, along with methionine metabolism in general, after a discussion of anabolic pathways in which cysteine is used—mycothiol and CoA biosynthesis.

Mycothiol

Mycothiol [MSH; 1-D-*myo*-inosityl 2-deoxy-2-(*N*-acetamido-L-cystein-amido-α-D-glucopyranoside)] was first isolated in 1994 from both *Streptomyces* sp. strain AJ94663 and *M. bovis* (42). It is the major low-molecular-weight thiol in actinomycetes, where it is uniquely produced (43, 103, 105). It has been proposed to function analogously to glutathione, and all of the appropriate enzymatic machinery to assist in these functions have been very recently identified. Mutants of *M. smegmatis* in which mycothiol biosynthesis has been abrogated exhibit high-level resistance to isoniazid and are more susceptible than wild-type strains to oxidative stress and antibiotics (107, 126). However, mycothiol is essential for growth of the Erdman strain of *M. tuberculosis*, since disruption of the *mshC* gene (Fig. 3) is lethal (135).

Mycothiol is capable of reacting with electrophiles to generate the MSH S conjugates, and in fact, it was the bimane derivative whose structure was solved by nuclear magnetic resonance spectroscopy. These S conjugates are cleaved at the amide bond between the N-acetylcysteine and the glucosamine ring to generate the N-acetylcysteine S conjugate (mercapturic acid) and the pseudodisaccharide (104). The mercapturic acid is efficiently excreted from the cell, while the pseudodisaccharide is recycled, as discussed below. The Rv1082-encoded amidase that catalyzes this reaction was one of the first of the mycothiol-specific enzymes to be identified (Fig. 3 and Table 3).

Also like glutathione, the oxidized form of the compound, mycothiol disulfide, is enzymatically reduced by a flavoenzyme, disulfide reductase. This enzyme, encoded by Rv2855 (*gor*), was identified as a

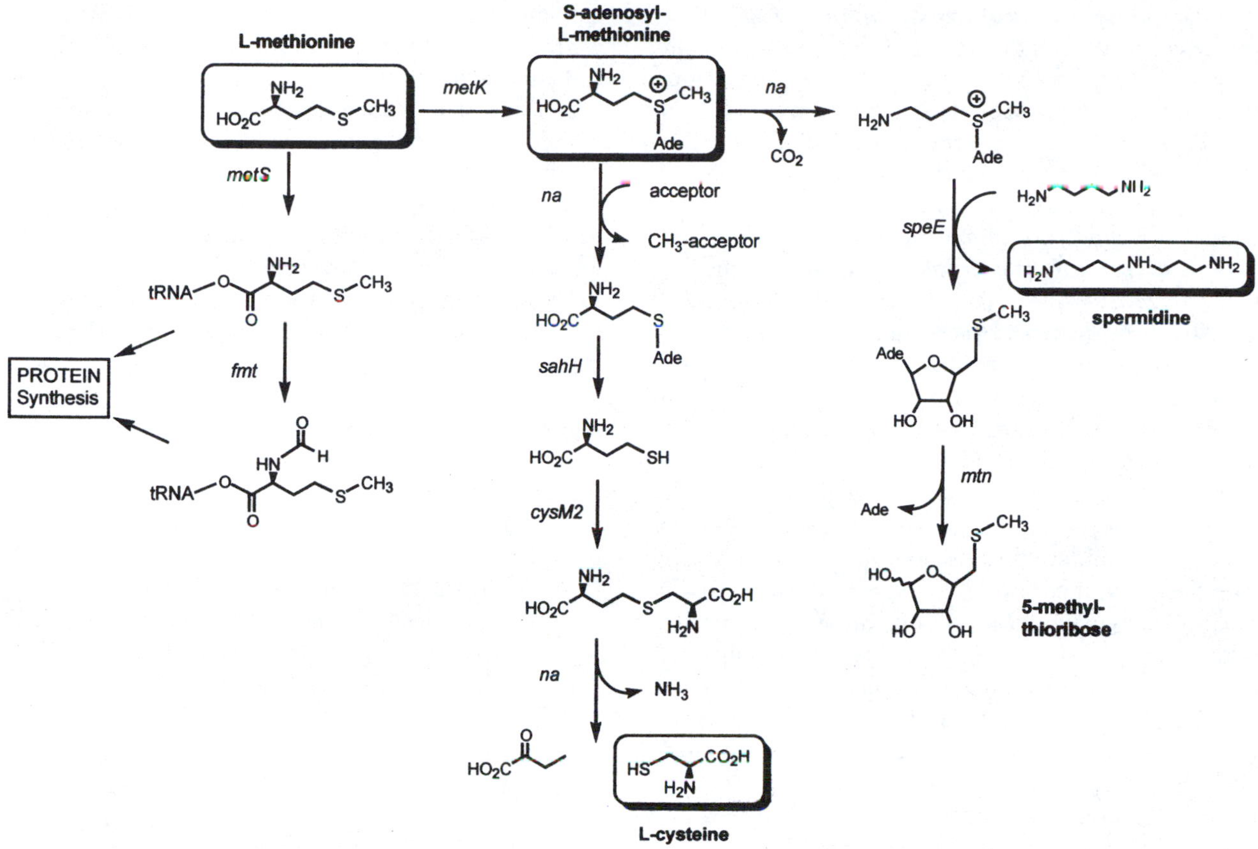

Figure 4. Sulfur metabolism—methionine. Unbroken arrows show chemical transformations, and broken arrows show pathways of several transformations.

homologue of glutathione reductase that contained both the flavin and pyridine nucleotide-binding motifs, the N-terminal catalytic redox cysteines that function in reversible disulfide-dithiol redox chemistry, and the C-terminal His-Glu dyad responsible for thiolate product protonation (116). The substrate specificity of this enzyme has been explored, and the enzyme reacts only with mycothiol disulfide or a truncated synthetic disulfide lacking the inositol ring, but not with glutathione or trypanothione. A mycothiol-dependent formaldehyde dehydrogenase activity has also been identified and purified from *M. smegmatis* (42, 109).

Table 4. Genes in sulfur metabolism—methionine

Gene	Rv no.[a]	Size (aa)	EC	Enzyme name	Comment
metS	Rv1007c		6.1.1.10		
fmt	Rv1406		2.1.2.9		
metK	Rv1392	403	2.5.1.6	SAM synthetase	
Many?			2.1.1.37	Methyltransferases	Includes *mma*, *cma*, *pca* genes
sahH	Rv3248c		3.3.1.1.	SAH hydrolase	
cysM2	Rv1077		4.2.1.22		
?	NA		4.4.1.1.	Cystathionine γ-lyase	
?	NA		4.1.1.50	SAM decarboxylase	
speE	Rv2601		2.5.1.16	Spermidine synthase	
mtn	Rv0091		3.2.2.16	5-Methylthioadenosine hydrolase	

[a]Boldface Rv numbers indicate that the enzyme activity corresponding to the CDS has been confirmed by isolation or cloning of the enzyme, complementation, or the loss of activity when the gene is inactive for at least one of the *M. tuberculosis* complex. Similar evidence obtained with orthologous genes in mycobacteria if their counterpart in the *M. tuberculosis* complex is essentially unambiguous. For all others, the enzyme name is derived from the gene annotation. NA, not available.

The biosynthesis of mycothiol has been very recently characterized due to the efforts of R. C. Fahey, G. L. Newton, and Y. Av-Gay (Fig. 3). Using a combination of genetics, in which mutants unable to make mycothiol were generated, and classic biochemistry, the major steps in this restricted biosynthetic pathway have been identified. The first step, where N-acetylglucosamine and *myo*-inositol are condensed to generate the α-linked psuedodisaccharide, is catalyzed by the Rv0846-encoded enzyme. The gene from *M. tuberculosis* complements a mutant of its orthologue in *M. smegmatis*, enabling the pseudodisaccharide and mycothiol to be synthesized, although the precise nature of the substrates has yet to be determined (106). The next step is the deacetylation of the 2-N-acetyl group, catalyzed by the Rv1170-encoded deacetylase (104). This enzyme is homologous to the amidase discussed above, involved in electrophile detoxification. The expressed and partially purified enzyme exhibits significantly higher activity with GlcNAc-Ins than with S-alkylmycothiol. Once deacetylated, the 2-amine is coupled to L-cysteine via an ATP-dependent synthase reaction that generates the amide linkage between the pseudodisaccharide and the thiol-containing amino acid (136). This Rv2130c-encoded synthase has been expressed and biochemically characterized. Finally, in 2002, the final enzyme in the pathway was identified (72). This Rv0819-encoded α-N-acetyltransferase catalyzes the acetyl-CoA-dependent acetylation of Cys-Gln-Ins to generate mycothiol, and the *M. tuberculosis* enzyme has been heterologously expressed and shown to catalyze the reaction with a specific activity of 0.5 U/mg.

Pantothenate and Coenzyme A Biosynthesis

The cysteine molecule is also incorporated into CoA in a reaction in which pantothenate must first be synthesized (Fig. 2). The first unique step in the biosynthesis of pantothenate (vitamin B_5) is the hydroxymethylation of α-ketoisovalerate to generate ketopantoate. This reaction is catalyzed by the *panB*-encoded methylenetetrahydrofolate-dependent 3-methyl-2-oxobutanoate hydroxymethyltransferase. The *M. tuberculosis* Rv2225 gene product has been purified and demonstrated to catalyze the reaction (149). The next reaction in the sequence is catalyzed by the *panE*-encoded ketopantoate reductase. This enzyme catalyzes the reduced pyridine nucleotide-dependent reduction of ketopantoate to form D-(−)-hydroxypantoate. There is no annotated gene corresponding to *panE*; however, the Rv2573 gene has some similarity to the *E. coli* gene encoding reductase. Hydroxypantoate is then condensed with β-alanine by the Rv3602c-encoded pantothenate synthase. This

enzyme has been kinetically and mechansitically characterized (175). The β-alanine substrate for pantothenate synthase is generated by the *panD*-encoded L-aspartate-1-decarboxylase. This is a small enzyme, which uses a posttranslationally generated pyruvyl group as the site of L-aspartate binding and catalysis. The *M. tuberculosis* homologue is the Rv3601c gene product, which has recently been expressed (31). These four enzymatic steps are found only in bacteria, fungi and plants and are not present in higher eukaryotes, which are pantothenate auxotrophs. Recently, strains of *M. tuberculosis* in which the adjacent *panC* and *panD* genes were deleted have been shown to be highly attentuated (133). Many of the *M. tuberculosis* homologues of the enzymes that convert pantothenate to CoA have been annotated, as has the enzyme that transfers the pantotheinyl arm to apo-ACP to generate the active holo-ACP molecule (Table 2). Considering the large number of enzymes that catalyze fatty acid synthesis and metabolism in *M. tuberculosis*, the early steps leading to pantothenate seem logical targets for inhibitor assessment.

METHIONINE METABOLISM

Methionine as the Sole Sulfur Source

Methionine auxotrophs of the *M. tuberculosis* complex have been isolated by several groups. Disruption of sulfate transport at either the *cysA* (169) or *subI* (86) locus resulted in complete abolition of sulfate transport (169) and methionine auxotrophy. A *cysH* mutant, disrupted in the sulfate reduction pathway, also resulted in methionine auxotrophy (95). None of these auxotrophs could be rescued by cysteine, and no cysteine auxotrophs were ever isolated, suggesting that methionine could be used as the sole source of sulfur. Indeed, on solid media, cysteine toxicity has been observed (169). However, in standard liquid culture media containing an excess of sulfur as 4 mM sulfate, L-cysteine could be used as the sole nitrogen source (29). This differential toxic effect of cysteine might be a result of its oxidation to more toxic products on the surface of the solid medium or its greater accumulation in intracellular metabolic pools. Some evidence about the small metabolic pool size of cysteine in tubercle bacilli grown in liquid culture, supporting the latter view, is presented below.

Since methionine, but not cysteine, can be used as the sole source of sulfur, the operation of the reverse transsulfuration pathway is required (Fig. 4 and Table 4). This pathway has been demonstrated in the actinomycete, *Streptomyces phaeochromogenes* (101). However, the only evidence for its existence in mycobacteria was, until recently, the demonstration of the key enzyme activity of the pathway, cystathionine γ-lyase, in crude extracts of *M. phlei* (101). The problem with relying on this assay is that enzymes of the γ-family of pyridoxal-5'-phosphate-dependent enzymes that include cystathionine γ-lyase (1) have notoriously broad substrate specificity. That problem was overcome recently when the enzyme activity was demonstrated in *M. tuberculosis* H37Rv and *M. bovis* BCG strains that incorporated the sulfur atom from [^{35}S]methionine into mycothiol (P. R. Wheeler, N. G. Coldham, E. E. Wooff, and R. G. Hewinson. *Abstr. 5th Int. Conf. Pathog. Mycobact. Infect.*, abstr. P136, 2002), which, as already explained (Fig. 3), contains the cysteine moiety. The identity of the gene that encodes this cystathionine γ-lyase activity is as yet unknown: three homologues of the protein family have been identified (Rv0391, Rv1079, and Rv3340 [see Table 4]), although all have been assigned alternative predicted functions (Table 1). During the investigation of reverse transsulfuration in the *M. tuberculosis* complex, cysteine was never detected in the pool metabolites, although N-acetylcysteine and mycothiol were detected. This failure to detect cysteine indicates that, as in many other organisms (127), the pool concentration of cysteine is kept very low to avoid its intracellular toxicity.

Metabolism of Methionine into Activated Metabolites

All cells have to assimilate the methionine molecule into two key metabolites required for metabolic reactions that are not confined to amino acid or sulfur metabolism. These metabolites are N-formylmethioninyl-transfer RNA (N-fMet-tRNA) and S-adenosylmethionine (S-AdoMet).

N-fMet-tRNA is required for the initiation of polypeptide biosynthesis on the ribosome in bacteria. Its production occurs in *M. tuberculosis* by charging the tRNA with methionine followed by formylation (Fig. 4). Both genes have been annotated (34), and the first one, the methionyl-tRNA synthetase, has been cloned and characterized (69).

S-AdoMet is involved in methyl transfer reactions. The gene, *metK*, encoding the enzyme for the biosynthesis of S-AdoMet has been annotated in the *M. tuberculosis* genome, although the corresponding enzyme activity has not been demonstrated. In contrast, there is a wealth of information on reactions involving transfer of the methyl group of S-AdoMet. Many methyltransferases (Table 4) are involved in lipid biosynthesis (89), notably in the conversion of double bonds to cyclopropane rings, and the introduction of methoxy groups into mycolic acids (172) and phthiocerol (89). Crystal structures of three of

the cyclopropane synthases have been solved, and the conserved nature of their interaction with S-AdoMet has been revealed (63). The functional activity of most of the genes predicted to be lipid:methyltransferases was shown by making mutants and demonstrating that their mycolates retained double bonds in place of the cyclopropane groups in the corresponding parental strain (50, 51). Additionally, when certain methyltransferase genes from *M. tuberculosis* were cloned into *M. smegmatis*, which naturally makes unsaturated α-mycolates, cyclopropanated α-mycolates could be isolated (173). Direct demonstration of transfer of the methyl group from S-AdoMet has been shown by using strains overexpressing a methyltransferase (*mma1*) (141). Further, in an earlier study using cell extracts of H37Ra, the transfer of labeled methyl groups from S-AdoMet occurred into intermediates with 48- to 56-carbon acids, showing that they were used as substrates rather than complete, unsaturated mycolic acids (122). Several mutants lacking methyltransferases involved in mycolic acid biosynthesis are attenuated (50–52), even though they still produce mycolic acids, albeit unsaturated ones. A *metK* mutant is likely to be lethal, since it would abolish almost all methylation reactions in all classes of metabolites (Fig. 4). An example of a methyltransferase acting outside of lipid metabolism is that encoded by Rv2118c. Its crystal structure has been determined, and domains for binding S-AdoMet and the transfer of the methyl group have been identified. Sequence alignments and structural analysis suggest that Rv2118c could be an RNA methyltransferase (56).

An unusual end product of the predicted pathway of S-AdoMet metabolism is 5-methythioribose (Fig. 4). The product has actually been identified as a 5-methylthiopentose and is linked to lipoarabinomannan (LAM), a lipopolysaccharide including 60 to 100 sugar residues (152). One residue of this sugar is linked to one LAM molecule via the nonreducing terminus of a mannosyl cap. Its role is unknown, although 5'-methylthioadenosine, which has the same functional group, is known to inhibit a tyrosine kinase (83). Thus, it is possible that this thiosugar might contribute to the immunomodulatory properties associated only with mannose-capped LAM (152). The pathway that may be used for its biosynthesis has been shown to be used for recycling methionine in several bacteria, including *Klebsiella pneumoniae* (100) and *Bacillus subtilis* (142). The second and third, but not the first, genes have been annotated in the *M. tuberculosis* genome (Table 4), even though the genome annotation was done before the discovery of the 5-methylthiopentose and thus the need for the pathway. SpeE was demonstrated in *M. bovis* by the formation of its product, methylthioadenosine

(119), long before it could be determined whether it is encoded by Rv2601, the gene predicted to encode this enzyme.

SULFUR METABOLISM OF *M. TUBERCULOSIS* IN THE HOST AND ITS REGULATION

Disruption of the genes for methionine and cysteine biosynthesis in the *M. tuberculosis* complex had a weak effect, if any, in attenuating the bacteria, contrasting with the strongly attenuating or even lethal effect of knocking out genes in the biosynthetic pathways for other amino acids. Transposon mutants of *M. bovis* BCG with mutations in the *cysA* (169) and *subI* (86) genes persisted in BALB/c mice as well as their parental strains did, although the *subI* mutant was attenuated when it was tested in SCID mice (55). A *metB* mutant of *M. tuberculosis* H37Rv, obtained by homologous recombination, was only weakly attenuated in DBA or SCID mice (146), although this mutant was not an auxotroph and disruption of *metB* is predicted to be bypassed by the operation of the *metZ* gene (Fig. 1). Together with the prediction, based on its genome annotation, that *M. leprae* is a natural methionine auxotroph (35, 161), this suggests that methionine is available to pathogenic mycobacteria, perhaps as the principal source of sulfur, in the host.

Several biosynthetic genes discussed in the preceding section, including *subI*, *cysD*, and *cysH*, are all essential for growth on minimal medium including sulfate (137). However, sulfate transport and cysteine biosynthesis may also be induced by a SigH-dependent mechanism, which has been linked to virulence (84). The *cysTWA* and *cysM* genes are part of the *sigH* regulon, as shown by their upregulation in H37Rv but not in a *sigH* mutant after exposure to an environmental stress (diamide) that induces *sigH*. The link with virulence is supported by the demonstration that an *M. tuberculosis* CDC 1551 mutant lacking *sigH* exhibits reduced immunopathology and mortality despite showing tissue persistence in C57BL/6 and C3H mice (67). However, other genes induced under the control of *sigH* are known to be virulence factors, including those for the microbe's thiol-based antioxidant defense. Thus, the expression of the *cys* genes mentioned above may not be related to virulence but, rather, may be related to their coregulation with virulence-associated genes in the *sigH* regulon.

CARBON AND ENERGY METABOLISM

The principal carbon sources that are supplied to *M. tuberculosis* in culture are glucose, glycerol, lipids, and the carbon skeletons of amino acids. Regardless of which are used, they must be both dissimilated, via acetyl-CoA, to provide energy, and assimilated, notably into the copious glycans and lipids that characterize the mycobacteria (Fig. 5 and Table 5).

Lipids as a Carbon Source

Before the genome of *M. tuberculosis* had been sequenced, it was argued that *M. tuberculosis* and other pathogenic mycobacteria might be lipolytic rather than lipogenic. Thus, although they would have to synthesize their own characteristic lipids, lipids might be the major available carbon source in the host (165). The detection of lipolytic enzymes, including phospholipases, and the ability of host-grown tubercle bacilli (*M. microti* in these experiments) simultaneously to catabolize and anabolize fatty acids provides powerful circumstantial evidence to support that view (164).

Analysis of the genome sequence has strengthened the view of *M. tuberculosis* as using lipids as a principal carbon source. Arguably, the most immediately apparent feature of the genome was a remarkable commitment to lipid catabolism. An astonishing 36 homologous *fadE* genes, encoding the first step in the catabolic β-oxidation cycle, were annotated (34). Similarly, a high degree of *fadE* paralogy (22, 39) (http://ca.expasy.org/cgi-bin/prosite-search-ac?PDOC00070) is known to exist in another microbe known to have a lipolytic metabolism, *Aspergillus fumigatus* (79). In contrast, *E. coli* and *Salmonella enterica* serovar Typhimurium each have a single *fadE* gene (27). A similar situation exists with *fadD* genes, predicted to encode acyl-CoA ligases (EC 6.2.1.3) in *M. tuberculosis*, where 36 paralogues were annotated (34). Generally, the evolution of homologues of this gene is a mechanism by which an organism can build up a repertoire of being able to use a diverse range of fatty acids (59), although the degree of parology in *M. tuberculosis* seems exceptional (http://ca.expasy.org/cgi-bin/prosite-search-ac?PDOC00427).

FadD-encoded enzyme activity is needed to convert fatty acids to fatty acyl-CoAs. In turn, fatty acyl-CoAs are the substrates for FadE, fatty acyl-CoA dehydrogenase (Fig. 5). Together with the rest of the β-oxidation complex (see Fig. 4 in reference 34), they are needed to account for the observed oxidation of exogenous fatty acids to CO_2 (26, 164). However, *fadD* genes are involved in anabolic as well as catabolic activities. Recently, it was shown, using a cloning approach followed by purification, enzyme assay, and analysis by thin-layer chromatography and electrospray ionization mass spectrometry, that these

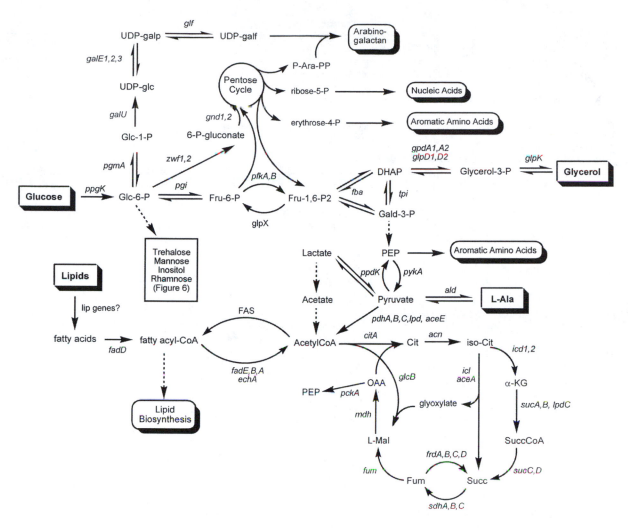

Figure 5. Carbon metabolism and its links to metabolism in general, including lipid metabolism. Unbroken arrows show chemical transformations, and broken arrows show pathways of several transformations. OAA, oxaloacetate; PEP, phospho-*enol*pyruvate.

Table 5. Genes in pathways of carbon metabolism

Gene	Rv no.[a]	Size (aa)	EC	Enzyme name	Comment

Gene	Rv no.[a]	Size (aa)	EC	Enzyme name	Comment
Glycolosis, gluconeogenesis and related activities[b]					
	Rv0650	302	2.7.1.2	Glucokinase	Annotated as sugar kinase. Could be a hexokinase
ppgK	**Rv2702**	265	2.7.1.63	Polyphosphate glucokinase	Also uses ATP (62)
pgi	Rv0946c	553	5.3.1.9	Glucose-6-phosphate isomerase	
pfkA	Rv3010c	343	2.7.1.11	6-Phosphofructokinase	Exclusive to glycolysis
pfkB	Rv2029c	339	2.7.1.11	6-Phosphofructokinase	Exclusive to glycolysis
glpX	**Rv1099c**	328	3.1.3.11	Fructose-biphosphatase	Not annotated but needed for growth. Exclusive to gluconeogenesis
fba	Rv0363c	344	4.1.2.13	Bisphosphate aldolase	This is a class II aldolase; enzymatic data suggest a second, class I aldolase, but that was not annotated
tpi	Rv1438	261	5.3.1.1	Triosephosphate isomerase	
glpK	**Rv3696c**	517	2.7.1.30	Glycerol kinase	Inactive in *M. bovis* field strain, 2122/97 (48)
gpdA1	Rv0564c	341	1.1.1.94	Glycerol-3-phosphate dehydrogenase (NAD(P)+)	

Continued on following page

Table 5. *Continued*

Gene	Rv no.[a]	Size (aa)	EC	Enzyme name	Comment
gpdA2	Rv2982c	334	1.1.1.94	Glycerol-3-phosphate dehydrogenase (NAD(P)+)	
glpD1	Rv2249c	516	1.1.99.5	Glycerol-3-phosphate dehydrogenase (acceptor)	Predicted acceptor *not* NAD(P) for GlpD enzymes—possibly quinone
glpD2	Rv3302c	585	1.1.99.5	Glycerol-3-phosphate dehydrogenase (acceptor)	

Glyceraldehyde-3-phosphate to phosphoenolpyruvate[b]

Gene	Rv no.[a]	Size (aa)	EC	Enzyme name	Comment
pykA	**Rv1617**	472	2.7.1.40	Pyruvate kinase	Cannot be used for gluconeogenesis. Inactive gene in *M. bovis* field strain, 2122/97 (48)
ppdK	Rv1127c	490	2.7.9.1	Pyruvate, phosphate dikinase precursor	Conversion of pyruvate to phospho*enol*pyruvate
ald	**Rv2780**	371	1.4.1.1	L-Alanine dehydrogenase	Inactive gene in *M. bovis* field strain, 2122/97 (48)
pca	**Rv2967c**	1127	6.4.1.1	Pyruvate carboxylase	These two enzymes are likely to be used to convert pyruvate to phospho*enol*pyruvate
pckA	**Rv0211**	606	4.1.1.32	Phospho*enol*pyruvate carboxykinase (GTP)	

Catabolism of pyruvate to acetyl-CoA and lactate[c]

Gene	Rv no.[a]	Size (aa)	EC	Enzyme name	Comment
	Rv0843	334	1.2.4.1	Pyruvate dehydrogenase E1 component alpha subunit	
aceE	Rv2241	901	1.2.4.1	Pyruvate dehydrogenase E1 component	
pdhA	Rv2497c	367	1.2.4.1	Pyruvate dehydrogenase E1 component, alpha subunit	
pdhB	Rv2496c	348	1.2.4.1	Pyruvate dehydrogenase E1 component, beta subunit	
pdhC	Rv2495c	393	2.3.1.12	Dihydrolipoamide acetyltransferase	A pyruvate dehydrogenase E2 component
lpd	**Rv0462**	464	1.8.1.4	Dihydrolipoamide dehydrogenase	Also required for 2-oxoglutarate dehydrogenase activity
lldD1	Rv0694	396	1.1.2.3	L-Lactate dehydrogenase (cytochrome)	Quinone is likely to be the electron acceptor (Fig. 6)
lldD2	Rv1872c	414	1.1.2.3	L-Lactate dehydrogenase (cytochrome)	See below
?	?	NA[d]	1.13.12.4	Lactate 2-monooxygenase	Rv1872c product is very similar to the *M. smegmatis* enzyme (see Swiss-Prot P21795).

Krebs cycle[e]

Gene	Rv no.[a]	Size (aa)	EC	Enzyme name	Comment
citA	Rv0889c	373	2.3.3.1	Citrate synthase	
gltA1	Rv1131	393	2.3.3.1	Citrate synthase	
gltA2	Rv0896	431	2.3.3.1	Citrate synthase	
acn	Rv1475c	943	4.2.1.3	Aconitate hydratase	
icd1	Rv3339c	409	1.1.1.42	Isocitrate dehydrogenase	
icd2	Rv0066c	745	1.1.1.42	Isocitrate dehydrogenase	
sucA	Rv1248c	1,214	1.2.4.2	2-Oxoglutarate dehydrogenase	Also referred to as alpha-ketoglutarate dehydrogenase
sucB	Rv2215	553	2.3.1.61	Dihydrolipoamide succinyltransferase	2-Oxoglutarate dehydrogenase E2 component. Lipoate content of SucB shown.
	Rv2455c	653	1.2.7.3	2-Oxoglutarate ferredoxin oxidoreductase, alpha subunit	
	Rv2454c	373	1.2.7.3	2-Oxoglutarate ferredoxin oxidoreductase, beta subunit	
sucC	Rv0951	387	6.2.1.5	Succinyl-CoA synthetase beta chain	
sucD	Rv0952	303	6.2.1.5	Succinyl-CoA synthetase alpha chain	
sdhA	Rv3318	590	1.3.99.1	Succinate dehydrogenase flavoprotein subunit	
sdhB	Rv3319	263	1.3.99.1	Succinate dehydrogenase iron-sulfur protein	

Continued on following page

Table 5. *Continued*

Gene	Rv no.[a]	Size (aa)	EC	Enzyme name	Comment
sdhC	Rv3316	112	1.3.99.1	Succinate dehydrogenase cytochrome b-556 subunit	
sdhD	Rv3317	114	1.3.99.1	Succinate dehydrogenase hydrophobic membrane anchor protein	
	Rv0247c	248	1.3.99.1	Similar to succinate dehydrogenase iron-sulfur protein	
	Rv0248c	646	1.3.99.1	Similar to succinate dehydrogenase flavoprotein subunit	
fum	Rv1098c	474	4.2.1.2	Fumarate hydratase	
mdh	Rv1240	329	1.1.1.37	Malate dehydrogenase	
mez	Rv2332	652	1.1.1.38	Malate oxidoreductase (decarboxylating)	
Glyoxylate cycle					
icl	**Rv0467**	428	4.1.3.1	Isocitrate lyase	MT0483 in CDC 1551
aceA	See comment	611	4.1.3.1	Isocitrate lyase	MT1966 in CDC 1551-Rv1915/6; 367/398 aa-aceA pseudogenes in H37Rv
glcB	**Rv1837c**	741	2.3.3.9	Malate synthase	
Hexose monophosphate pathway[f]					
zwf1	Rv1121	466	1.1.1.49	Glucose-6-phosphate 1-dehydrogenase	
zwf2	Rv1447c	514	1.1.1.49	Glucose-6-phosphate 1-dehydrogenase	
gnd1	Rv1844c	485	1.1.1.44	6-Phosphogluconate dehydrogenase	
gnd2	Rv1122	340	1.1.1.44	6-Phosphogluconate dehydrogenase	
Genes in lipid metabolism, linked to general carbon metabolism, reviewed in this article					
fadD28	**Rv2941**	580	6.2.1.3	This fadD is absolutely required, at least in *M. tuberculosis*, to make phthioceroldimycocerosate	
fadD19	**Rv3515c**	548	6.2.1.3	Ortholog of the *M. avium mig* gene	
fas	**Rv2524c**	3069	2.3.1.-	Fused fatty acid synthase	

Classes of genes involved in general lipid metabolism referred to in this chapter

	Paralogues	EC	Enzyme name/comments
fadD	36*	6.2.1.-	Fatty acyl-CoA synthetase. *One of the 36 in H37Rv, fadD11, may be a psuedogene
fadE	36	1.3.99.-	Acyl-CoA dehydrogenase—the first dedicated step in beta-oxidation
echA	21	4.2.1.17	Enoyl-CoA hydratase/isomerase, participates in the beta, oxidation complex
fadB	5	1.1.1.157	3-Hydroxybutyryl-CoA dehydrogenase
fadA	6	2.3.1.9	Acetyl-CoA acetyltransferase
lip	22	3.1.-.-	Excluding lipA and lipB, lip genes are predicted to be esterases involved in releasing fatty acids

[a]Boldface Rv numbers indicate that the enzyme activity corresponding to the CDS has been confirmed by isolation or cloning of the enzyme, complementation, or the loss of activity when the gene is inactive for at least one of the *M. tuberculosis* complex. Similar evidence obtained with orthologous genes in mycobacteria if their counterpart in the *M. tuberculosis* complex is essentially unambiguous. For all others, the enzyme name is derived from the gene annotation.
[b]Individual steps are not reviewed for glyceraldehyde-3-phosphate to phospho*enol*pyruvate.
[c]Recycling acetate to acetyl-CoA is not reviewed in this chapter. See reference 161.
[d]NA, Not applicable.
[e]For fumararate reductase (*frdI* genes), see Table 7.
[f]Pentose cycle enzymes are all annotated, but they are not reviewed individually here.

genes encode two classes of enzymes (153). One class, including *fadD15*, *fadD17*, and *fadD19*, encode fatty acyl-CoA ligases. A previously undescribed new class, including *fadD26*, *fadD28*, *fadD30*, and *fadD32*, encode fatty acyl-AMP ligases. Both classes synthesize acyl-AMP in the presence of ATP alone, but only the CoA ligases synthesize acyl-CoA in the presence of ATP and CoA (reduced) (the classic assay constituents for this enzyme): the acyl-AMP ligases still synthesize acyl-AMP. However, all of the new class of FadD proteins are associated with a polyketide synthase (Pks). When incubated with ATP and their cognate Pks protein, the acyl moiety is transferred to the protein. This indicates that each is dedicated to the synthesis of a single polyketide. FadD28 is required for the biosynthesis of the wax phthiocerol dimycocerosate (25, 38, 46), with the *fadD28* gene clustered with the other genes for making that complex lipid. These results are consistent with previous work suggesting that FadD28 is an acyl-CoA ligase, since in the older work the assay used could not distinguish CoA and AMP esters (47).

Several FadD proteins are required for pathogenicity, including FadD19, FadD28, and FadD33. A gene designated *mig* (for "macrophage-induced gene") in *M. avium*, associated with virulence, has been shown enzymatically to encode a medium-chain acyl-CoA synthetase. The *mig* gene is similar to *M. tuberculosis fadD* genes and most closely similar to *fadD19* (93). In *M. tuberculosis*, both *fadD28* (25, 38) and *fadD33* (128) are required for the full virulence of the organism in mice. The *fadD28* gene, together with other genes in the same gene cluster, such as *mas*, is in one of the five predominant functional groups of genes that are upregulated during growth in macrophages (77). In *M. smegmatis*, the close homologue of *fadD33* is required for the accurate acylation of mycobactin, since mutants with mutations in this gene have a mycobactin with an altered fatty acyl moiety (75).

Compelling evidence for the utilization of lipids as a carbon source when *M. tuberculosis* is in the host (or inside host cells in vitro) comes from the expression of isocitrate lyase (Icl) during growth under those conditions and the attenuation of the bacilli by knocking out the *icl* gene. Isocitrate lyase is one of the two enzymes in the glyoxylate cycle (Fig. 5). Operation of this cycle when organisms are metabolizing lipids enables the acetyl-CoA produced by β-oxidation to be recycled (Fig. 5). In the year after the publication of the *M. tuberculosis* genome, a spot on two-dimensional protein gels that was strongly upregulated when *M. avium* was grown in macrophages was sequenced and identified as isocitrate lyase (61). This isocitrate lyase was shown to be the *icl* gene product and had 80% similarity to the *M. tuberculosis* Icl. Icl was shown to be functionally homologous in the two organisms. In both *M. tuberculosis* and *M. avium*, Icl was expressed in macrophages, was upregulated when palmitate or acetate was the limiting carbon source, had isocitrate lyase activity, and bound to the same polyclonal antibody (61). Using an *icl-gfp* construct that maintained enzymatic activity, it was shown that in *M. tuberculosis*, *icl* is continuously expressed in activated macrophages and transiently expressed in resting macrophages over 24 h (87). An *icl* knockout mutant of *M. tuberculosis* was attenuated in mice, although they grew until adaptive immunity started to operate. However, the strain with a disrupted *icl* was as virulent as its parent strain, Erdman, in gamma interferon knockout mice. Thus, *icl* is required for persistence in mice (87). More recently, transcript data indicate that *icl* is strongly upregulated when *M. tuberculosis* is in macrophages (140), and its transcript persists to some extent in chronic infections (151). There is a second gene, *aceA*, which encodes isocitrate lyase in some mycobacteria, including *M. tuberculosis* Erdman and CDC 1551, but not H37Rv (34). In contrast to *icl*, *aceA* was not upregulated by growth of *M. avium* on palmitate (61) and could not rescue an isocitrate lyase-deficient mutant of *M. smegmatis* (87). Thus, it appears that *icl* plays the major role in enabling mycobacteria to use lipids as a carbon source.

Both *icl* and the *glcB* gene, which encodes malate synthase—the other glyoxylate cycle enzyme—have been cloned and expressed, and crystal structures of the *M. tuberculosis* enzymes have been resolved. The catalytic mechanism of isocitrate lyase (Icl protein) was elucidated with its covalent modification of an active-site residue, Cys191, by the inhibitor 3-bromopyruvate (143). Analogues or metabolites of the products (succinate and glyoxylate) inhibited Icl activity, but the products themselves had no effect. Furthermore, glycolytic intermediates had no effect on Icl activity. In contrast, phosphoenolpyruvate (Fig. 5) was a highly potent inhibitor of malate synthase (145). The *icl* and *glcB* genes are on separate parts of the *M. tuberculosis* chromosome and are clearly differentially regulated (145). With the role of the glyoxylate cycle in persistence and lipolysis established, it will be fascinating to determine the carbon fluxes through the cycle and the role of *aceA* (Table 5), where it is active. Moreover, the role of glycine dehydrogenase in the flux of glyoxylate out of the cycle needs to be elucidated. This enzyme activity was more markedly upregulated than that of the glyoxylate cycle enzymes (Fig. 5) when *M. tuberculosis* was adapted to anoxic conditions in early studies (157), yet the gene that encodes glycine dehydrogenase has not been revealed. A proposal that this enzyme might be encoded by *ald*, the alanine dehydrogenase gene, seems unlikely since the *M. smegmatis ald* gene encodes the alanine, but not the glycine, dehydrogenase (44). The *M. smegmatis* Ald has 80% identity and similar regulation to *M. tuberculosis* Ald (44), suggesting functional similarity. The *gcvB* gene is predicted to encode glycine decarboxylase, not the dehydrogenase. The physiological role suggested for glycine dehydrogenase, consistent with its K_{eq} (4 × 10^{10}), was to recycle NAD under anoxic conditions. Subsequently, both *ndh* and *mdh* were shown to share this key role (88) (reviewed below). Intriguingly, the glyoxylate cycle is also required for the virulence of the pathogenic yeast *Candida albicans*, although, in contrast to *M. tuberculosis*, both the yeast genes for the cycle—*ICL1* and *MLS1*—are coordinately upregulated when the yeast cells are grown in macrophages (78).

Fatty Acid Biosynthesis De Novo and Elongation Are Catalyzed by the Same Synthase

The *fas* gene encodes a multifunctional fatty acid synthase that has been expressed and sequenced (45) and shown to correspond to the native synthase purified and characterized from *M. bovis* BCG (68). This synthase has two copies of all the functional domains of a fatty acid synthase, and its organization appears to be a head-to-tail fusion of two yeast-like synthases. Its products are fatty acyl-CoAs up to 26 carbons, but, uniquely, it can perform both the de novo synthesis starting with acetyl-CoA and the elongation reaction, adding successive C_2 units to preformed fatty acyl-CoA primers. C_{16}-CoA was readily elongated, suggesting that it may be a product of one of the two Fas subunits and that the mycobacterial Fas may play a role in anabolic scavenging of fatty acids. In turn, the C_{26} products are used for complex lipid biosynthesis (Fig. 5).

Glycan Biosynthesis: Role of Gluconeogenesis

The monosaccharides required for biosynthesis of arabinogalactan and arabinomannan, as well as trehalose for glycolipids, can all be synthesized readily from glucose (Fig. 5 and 6). First, though, we consider how the acetyl-CoA, generated by β-oxidation of fatty acids, can be used to generate the sugar molecules (Fig. 5). The glyoxylate cycle generates oxaloacetate, which must then be converted to phosphoenolpyruvate, the first step in the gluconeogenesis pathway. The gene for this step, *pckA*, encoding the enzyme phosphoenolpyruvate carboxykinase, has been annotated in the *M. tuberculosis* genome (34). Its extremely close orthologue (88% identity) in *M. smegmatis* encodes a GTP-dependent enzyme with a clear gluconeogenic function (98). When *pckA* was disrupted by illegitimate recombination in *M. bovis*, strains were attenuated in mice (36). The *pckA* gene was also shown by TraSH mutation to be required for survival during infection (138) and to be expressed in *M. tuberculosis* in macrophages (140), and in the lungs of both chronically infected mice and human patients (151).

All but one of the subsequent enzymes for gluconeogenesis is shared with glycolysis (the reverse pathway). The one that is dedicated to gluconeogenesis is fructose-1,6-bisphosphate phosphatase (Fbpase), where the interconversion of fructose-6-phosphate and fructose-1,6-bisphosphate is catalyzed by two enzymes working in opposite directions; this step is the control point for both pathways in nature (Fig. 5). Fbpase has only recently been found in any of the actinomycetes (http://www.genome.ad.jp/kegg/). The Rv1099c gene both complements an *E. coli* mutant lacking Fbpase, allowing it to grow on glycerol as the sole carbon source. The gene, a homologue of *glpX* and not *fbp*, also conferred enzyme activity (95a). Its very close orthologue from *Corynebacterium glutamicum* has been cloned, expressed, and characterized (129). These recent findings explain why Rv1099c was the most seriously attenuating TraSH mutation (138): the Fbpase it encodes is an activity essential for converting the lipids used by *M. tuberculosis* as its carbon source in the host to cell wall glycans (Fig. 5).

Glycan Biosynthesis: Transformations from Glycolytic Intermediates

Many of the genes used in making the sugar monomers needed for glycan and glycolipid biosynthesis are essential. This has been a rewarding discovery, given that the pathways (Fig. 6 and Table 6) were investigated in the first place because they appeared to be attractive potential targets for drug development. Enzymes for the final step in making galactofuran (112), for the final step in the formation of dTDP-rhamnose needed to make a linker between peptidoglycan and arabinogalactan (81), and for both the synthesis of phosphatidylinositol (65) and its first mannosylation in the pathway for making lipomannans (74) are all encoded by essential genes.

All four essential genes mentioned above have been functionally characterized. The *glf*-encoded UDP-galactopyranose mutase gene has been cloned, its enzyme activity has been shown (160), and its unique catalytic mechanism has been deduced from its structure (134).

All of the genes in the pathway from glucose-1-phosphate to dTDP-rhamnose, including *rmlD*, are essential (81) and have been cloned, and their enzyme activities have been shown (80, 82). Although the process of genome annotation initially suggested the existence of isoenzymes for RmlA and RmlB, only one gene for each step expressed enzyme activity (82) (Fig. 6) suggesting that *rmlA*, *rmlB*, and *rmlC* could also possibly be essential.

In the inositol pathway (Fig. 6), the *pgsA* gene of *M. tuberculosis* restores both the phosphatidylinositol content and the ability of a mutant of *M. smegmatis* with its *pgsA* orthologue deleted to grow. In the mutant, viability was lost as its phosphatidylinositol content fell below 30 to 50% of that in the parental strain (65). Although one might expect phosphatidylinositol to restore membrane bilayer integrity, that is not enough for viability. The ability to mannosylate this lipid is also required, with the *pimA* gene product, catalyzing the first mannosylation step (Fig. 6), being essential too. A similar strategy to that used with *pgsA*, of rescuing a lethal mutant of *M. smegmatis* with the

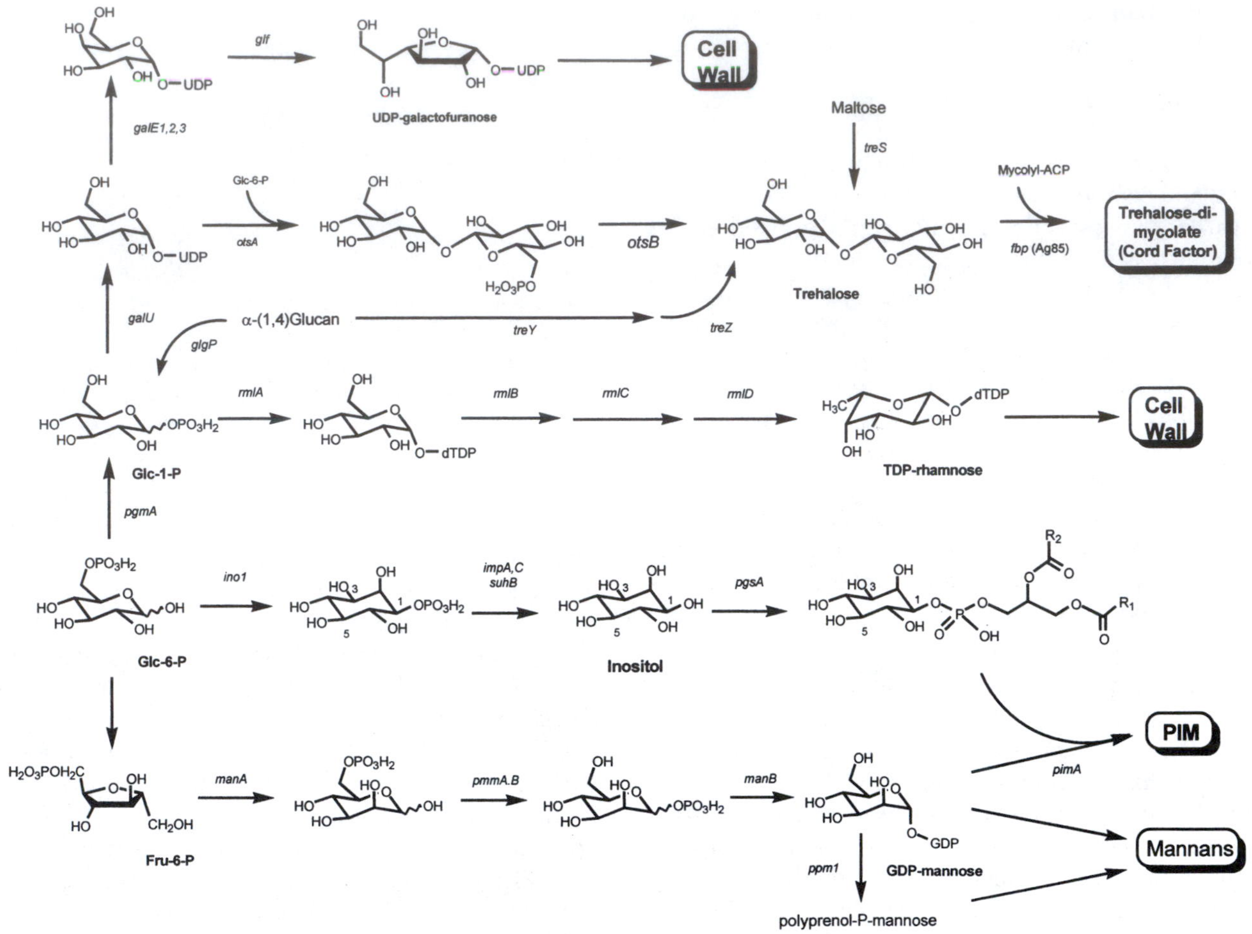

Figure 6. Carbon metabolism and its relation to cell wall biosynthesis. Unbroken arrows show chemical transformations, and broken arrows show pathways of several transformations.

M. tuberculosis pimA gene, showed its essentiality and biochemical function of mannosylation of phosphatidylinositol (74). The early steps in the inositol pathway are being defined too. First, glucose-6-phosphate is converted to inositol-1-phosphate by the *ino1* gene product. The *ino1* gene of *M. tuberculosis* was able to complement a yeast lacking any functional *INO1* gene, with its participation in the pathway being confirmed by giving (in the yeast) an inositol-secreting phenotype (8). Further evidence for this gene encoding the inositol-1-phosphate synthase comes from inactivation of the *ino1* gene, which results in a phenotype that is attenuated and can be rescued by inositol (96). The product of the Ino1-catalyzed transformation is inositol-1-phosphate. For the inositol to be used, it must be liberated by a phosphatase. There are several candidates (Fig. 6; Table 6) for the gene to encode such an enzyme, but so far only the *suhB* gene has been shown functionally to encode an enzyme with inositol-1-phosphatase activity (108). When the SuhB enzyme

was purified, it was shown to have a range of phosphatase activities, with inositol-1-phosphatase activity as the principal one (108), but other genes that encode sugar phosphatases still need to be investigated.

The other glycosidic building block for phosphatidylinositol mannoside and, ultimately, lipomannan biosynthesis is mannose (Fig. 6). This must be available as the GDP-mannose intermediate. The enzyme activity responsible for the transfer of GDP to the mannose was revealed when assaying the activity encoded by the cloned Rv3264 gene, then annotated *rmlA2*. Like *rmlA*, Rv3264 encodes a sugar-1-phosphate:nucleotide transferase, but it was clearly shown to encode ManB (80). Mannosyltransferases in lipomannan biosynthesis use both GDP-mannose and a lipid-linked mannose substrate (18). The *ppm1* (Rv2051c) gene, required for production of the lipid intermediate, encodes polyprenol-phosphomannose synthase (57). The catalytic domains and membrane-spanning domains of the Ppm1 protein of *M. tuberculosis*

Table 6. Biosynthesis of monomers for cell envelope glycans and glycolipids

Gene	Rv no.[a]	Size (aa)	EC	Enzyme name	Comment
pgmA	Rv3068c	547	5.4.2.2	Phosphoglucomutase	
Galactose					
galU	Rv0993	306	2.7.7.9	UTP:glucose-1-phosphate uridylyltransferase	
galE1	Rv3634c	314	5.1.3.2	UDP-glucose 4-epimerase	*rmlB3* (Rv3468c) is also now
galE2	Rv0501	376	5.1.3.2	UDP-glucose 4-epimerase	considered to encode for this
galE3	Rv0536	346	5.1.3.2	UDP-glucose 4-epimerase	enzyme
glf	**Rv3809c**	399	5.4.99.9	UDP-galactopyranose mutase	
Rhamnose					
rmlA	**Rv0334**	288	2.7.7.24	α-D-Glucose-1-phosphate thymidilyl-transferase	
rmlB	**Rv3464**	331	4.2.1.46	dTDP-glucose-4,6-dehydratase	
rmlC	**Rv3465**	202	5.1.3.13	dTDP-4-dehydrorhamnose 3,5-epimerase	
rmlD	**Rv3266c**	304	1.1.1.133	dTDP-4-dehydrorhamnose reductase	
Inositol					
ino1	**Rv0046c**	367	5.5.1.4	*myo*-inositol-1-phosphate synthase	
impA	Rv1604	270	3.1.3.25	Inositol monophosphatase	*Rv3137* and *cysQ* also have inositol
suhB	**Rv2701c**	290	3.1.3.25	Inositol monophosphatase	monophosphatase signatures (108)
First steps in phosphatidylinositolmannoside biosynthesis					
pgsA	**Rv2612c**	217	2.7.8.5	CDPdiacylglycerol:glycerol-3-phosphate 3-phosphatidyltransferase	Essential gene. However, DGBET predicts two other possible *pgsA* genes (http://www.genome.ad.jp/dbget-bin)
pimA	**Rv2610c**	378	2.4.1.57	Phosphatidylinositol:GPD-mannose alpha-mannosyltransferase	
Mannose					
pmmA	Rv3257c	465	5.4.2.8	Phosphomannomutase	
pmmB	Rv3308	534	5.4.2.8	Phosphomannomutase	
mrsA	Rv3441c	448	5.4.2.8	Phosphomannomutase	
manB	**Rv3264c**	359	2.7.7.13	Mannose-1-phosphate guanyltransferase	Annotated as *rmlA2*, but this activity has been shown
ppm1	**Rv2051c**	874	2.4.1.83	Polyprenolphosphate-mannose synthase	
Arabinose[b]					
Trehalose and other glucans					
glgP	Rv1328	863	2.4.1.1	Glycogen phosphorylase	
treY	**Rv1563c**	765	5.4.99.15	Maltooligosyl trehalose synthase	A pseudogene in many *M. bovis* strains (48)
treZ	**Rv1562c**	580	5.4.99.15	Maltooligosyltrehalose trehalohydrolase	Inactive in *M. leprae*
treS	**Rv0126**	601	5.4.99.-	Trehalose synthase	
otsA	**Rv3490**	500	2.4.1.15	Alpha, alpha-trehalose-phosphate synthase	
otsB1	Rv2006	1327	3.1.3.12	Trehalose-6-phosphate phosphatase	
otsB2	Rv3372	391	3.1.3.12	Trehalose-6-phosphate phosphatase	

[a]Boldface Rv numbers indicate that the enzyme activity corresponding to the CDS has been confirmed by isolation or cloning of the enzyme, complementation, or the loss of activity when the gene has been inactivated for at least one of the *M. tuberculosis* complex. Similar evidence obtained with orthologous genes in mycobacteria if their counterpart in the *M. tuberculosis* complex is essentially unambiguous. For all others, the enzyme name is derived from the gene annotation.

[b]The individual genes for incorporating the carbon of ribose, from the pentose cycle, to the monomer polyprenol phosphoarabinose, have not yet been identified.

were characterized and shown to be in a fused protein, in contrast to *M. smegmatis*, where the homologous domains are encoded by two separate *ppm* genes (15).

In the cell envelope of mycobacteria, mannose and galactofuranose residues exist in complex glycans that also include arabinose. The arabinose monomer for the necessary biosynthetic reactions is polyprenol-phosphoarabinose (76, 168). However, the route for formation of the monomer is proving hard to elucidate, given that epimerase activities to convert ribosyl compounds to arabinosyl compounds cannot be detected in mycobacteria and that the genes encoding the enzymes are unknown. On the basis of labeling experiments with *M. smegmatis*, the pentose cycle, substantially bypassing the decarboxylation step in the hexose monophosphate pathway (Fig. 5), via 6-phosphogluconate, leads to polyprenolphosphoribose (70, 139), followed by epimerization to polyprenolphosphoarabinose (167, 170).

There are three routes for trehalose biosynthesis in *M. tuberculosis* (Fig. 6), with one, the TreYZ pathway, being apparently lost in *M. leprae* (40) and some strains of *M. bovis* (48). When the *treZ* or both the *treYZ* genes of *M. tuberculosis* were cloned into *M. smegmatis*, they accelerated the rate of trehalose biosynthesis, confirming their predicted role and suggesting that TreZ is the rate-limiting step (40). Recently, the *otsA* gene was cloned and enzymatically characterized as acting on all the common nucleotide-glucosides in the reaction with glucose-6-phosphate to generate trehalose phosphate (113). However, the *otsB*-encoded phosphatase has been characterized only from *M. smegmatis*, in which it is highly specific for trehalose-6-phosphate (71). Although OtsB activity has been detected in extracts of *M. bovis* BCG (40), the predicted *otsB* genes in *M. tuberculosis* have reasonable similarity to the *M. smegmatis otsB* gene. It will be interesting to elucidate the role of the *M. tuberculosis otsB1* since it is upregulated over fourfold under anoxic conditions (144). Production of trehalose from glucan has been shown to be catalyzed by TreS by demonstrating enzymatic activity in a purified, recombinant, histidine-tagged form (40). An alternative metabolic fate for glucan is predicted to be glucose-1-phosphate (Fig. 6) since a glucan phosphorylase (encoded by *glgP*) has been annotated and expression of the corresponding protein has been observed by proteomic analysis (132).

Glucose and Glycerol Dissimilation

So far, this section has focussed on how lipids can be used as carbon sources. However, carbohydrates are possible sources of carbon, and glucose and glycerol are the major carbon sources available

in many standard culture media. The seminal work on the pathway for their dissimilation was done in India in the 1960s (12, 123, 155) and exhaustively reviewed in the context of mycobacterial culture (124). Essentially, in that work, key enzymes for glycolysis and the pentose cycle (Fig. 5) were detected and the operation of the complete pathways was established. One gene, *ppgK*, has been expressed and characterized from *M. tuberculosis*. This gene encodes a polyphosphate glucokinase that uses both polyphosphate and ATP as phosphate donors (62). Subsequently, all the genes for these pathways were annotated in the genome of *M. tuberculosis* H37Rv and CDC 1551. An interesting new finding of that analysis was that more than one gene was predicted for several of the steps (34). For example, there were two *pfk* genes for phosphofructokinase and two for each of the hexose monophosphate pathway enzymes, *zwf* and *gnd* (Table 5), that channel carbon from glucose into the pentose cycle (Fig. 5). Four genes for the oxidation of glycerol-3-phosphate to dihydroxyacetone phosphate (Fig. 5) have been annotated: the enzyme activity corresponding to GpdA1 and GpdA2 [NAD(P) reducing] was detected in the 1960s (see reference 124 for a review), but evidence for glycerol-3-phosphate: quinol oxidoreductase enzyme activity, corresponding to GlpD1 and GlpD2 (see Fig. 7) was never sought. This gene parology may allow differential expression of each paralogue. Preliminary evidence for this view comes from upregulation of *pfkB* gene expression (a 12-fold increase in transcript) during a shift to anoxic conditions in batch cultures (144). Further evidence comes from the increase in the amount of a protein corresponding to Fba as a spot in two-dimensional gels during oxygen limitation (131). Fba is a "type II," metal ion-dependent, fructose-1,6-bisphosphate aldolase associated with low oxygen tension. This proteomic approach was consistent with an earlier, enzymatic approach in which type II aldolase was found in *M. tuberculosis* grown in oxygen-limited cultures while a distinct, type I, aldolase was found predominantly in well-oxygenated, fermentor-grown cultures (9–11). Unfortunately, no gene corresponding to the type I aldolase could be found (28). In general, it should be noted that gene annotation and enzymatic analyses were separate events, and confirmation of the enzymes encoded by genes in these pathways may be needed before drawing conclusions about their differential regulation.

The End Product of Glycolysis Is Different in *M. tuberculosis* and *M. bovis*

The final product of glycolysis in *M. tuberculosis* is pyruvate. However, in *M. bovis* it is phosphoenolpyruvate, as indicated by a point mutation in the $Mg2^+$-binding site of the *pykA* gene, which encodes pyruvate kinase in the sequenced strain (strain 2122/97) (48). This mutation explains the lack of pyruvate kinase activity in *M. bovis* 2122/97. In contrast, pyruvate kinase activity has been demonstrated in *M. bovis* BCG, where the mutation has corrected during serial subculture. This explains why pyruvate must be included in routine media to isolate *M. bovis* (48). It also suggests a very limited role for glycolysis in *M. bovis* (Fig. 5). Furthermore, analysis of the genome revealed further lesions in the carbon metabolism of *M. bovis* 2122/97. Substrates containing the glycerol moiety cannot be used by *M. bovis* 2122/97, since genes for both glycerol kinase (*glpK*) and glycerol-3-phosphate transport (*ugpA*) are pseudogenes.

Substrates That Provide the Carbon for the Krebs Cycle

Pyruvate is converted to acetyl-CoA to provide carbon for the Krebs cycle. The genes predicted to encode two pyruvate dehydrogenase complexes for this step (Fig. 5) have been annotated (34). Previously, the enzyme activity was detected (154), but a review of the old work cannot elucidate whether both systems were operating. However, the single functional *lpd* gene that encodes the lipoamide dehydrogenase component of the complex has been identified, and its enzyme kinetics and properties have been elucidated (6). Lpd is a component of both the pyruvate dehydrogenase complex and the α-ketoglutarate dehydrogenase enzyme complexes in the Krebs cycle (Fig. 5). An alternative source of acetyl-CoA is from the β-oxidation of fatty acids (reviewed earlier in this chapter).

Amino acids including alanine, glutamate, and aspartate can be converted to keto acid intermediates by deamination reactions. Alanine dehydrogenase (Ald) converts alanine to pyruvate since BCG strains, naturally deficient in this enzyme, can have their inability to grow on alanine rescued by transformation with the *M. tuberculosis ald* gene (29). Although the equilibrium constant ($K_{eq} = 5 \times 10^{11}$) strongly favors the reaction in the direction of reductive amination of pyruvate, the sufficiency of Ald to allow growth on alanine shows that it can be used metabolically to provide pyruvate. Expression of the *ald* gene is downregulated by growth in the presence of ammonium ions (29) but upregulated during a shift to anoxic growth (131). The reason that *M. bovis* cannot grow on alanine as the sole nitrogen source (29) is that it has a nonfunctional *ald* gene. In contrast to the *M. tuberculosis ald* gene, the *M. bovis ald* gene contains a frameshift mutation (29). An important impli-

cation of this is that *M. bovis* can metabolize neither alanine nor glycolytic substrates to pyruvate.

An alternative source of pyruvate is from lactate oxidation. Genes have been annotated only for lactate:quinone oxidoreductase (*lldD1, lldD2*), but the corresponding enzyme activity was never investigated. The NAD-dependent lactate dehydrogenase (7) (reviewed in reference 13) and an unusual, *Mycobacterium*-specific lactate oxidase (decarboxylating), with acetate as a product, have both been characterized enzymatically (99), but their genes have not been identified (34). For lactate oxidase, the mechanism of action of the enzyme from *M. smegmatis* has been extensively studied (97, 150) and its amino acid sequence has been determined (49). Lld2 of *M. tuberculosis* has a strikingly high similarity (31% identity) to the *M. smegmatis* lactate oxidase, and thus *lld2* is a good candidate to investigate functionally. Alternatively, lactate oxidase could be encoded by one of the many oxidoreductase genes of unknown function in the *M. tuberculosis* genome. Pyruvate could theoretically be converted to acetyl-CoA via the lactate oxidase route (Fig. 5), but the part of this pathway where CoA is ligated to acetate could be a way of recycling acetate used in intermediary metabolism.

The Krebs Cycle

Our knowledge of the Krebs cycle enzymes and activity is similar to that of glycolysis: the enzyme activities (54, 99, 124, 155) and genes (34) were demonstrated independently, but none of the genes have been cloned or knocked out to confirm the functions ascribed to them. Gene redundancy or parology is apparent for citrate synthase, isocitrate dehydrogenase, pyruvate dehydrogenase, and probably lactate dehydrogenase (34). At the time of writing, no data had been obtained to suggest differential regulation of any of the redundant genes in the Krebs cycle, in contrast to the findings (reviewed above) on parologous genes in glycolysis. Gene "redundancy" in *M. tuberculosis* may reflect an ability to survive and grow in very different environments (compare, for example the center of a caseous lesion with an active, alveolar macrophage) within the host. In contrast, it has been suggested that the loss of "redundancy" in the *M. leprae* genome reflects a specialized life-style (35).

Aerobic and Anaerobic Respiration

NADH and reduced flavin adenine dinucleotide produced in the Krebs cycle and β-oxidation of fatty acids are fed into the respiratory chains (Fig. 5), enabling ATP to be generated via oxidative phosphorylation (Fig. 7 and Table 7). Electron transport is emphazised in Fig. 7, but, concomitant with electron transport, proton translocation occurs at various sites in the electron transport chain. These sites are suggested, with NADH dehydrogenase (NDH) I and the heme-containing oxidoreductases being highlighted, in other reviews (23, 124, 161). Acting in concert with ATP synthases (AtpA to AtpH), the sum of electron transport and proton translocation generates ATP through oxidative phosphorylation, together with recycling of NAD and flavin adenine dinucleotide. The complete annotation of all the genes for these functions is consistent with the functional demonstration of the sum of all the predicted reactions long ago.

Mycobacteria were regarded as the epitome of aerobes to the extent that they were chosen as the paradigm for demonstrating cytochromes and aero-bic respiration in bacteria (23). That fundamental biochemical research was done on *M. phlei*, while *M. avium* and *M. lepraemurium* (a member of the avium clade) were used to study cytochromes in host-grown mycobacteria (13, 64, 92). It was therefore of considerable interest when the *M. tuberculosis* genome annotation (34) revealed respiratory systems for aerobic, microaerophilic, and anoxic electron transport (Fig. 7, Table 7).

Although there are still few functional data, the data we have are interesting. The oxidative electron transport system that should operate in low oxygen tension, the cytochrome *bd*-quinol oxidase, has been shown functionally by complementation of an *M. smegmatis* mutant (66). In that work, inactivation of the *cydA* or *cydB* genes conferred a growth disadvantage at 0.5 to 1% O_2 saturation while there was no phenotype under fully aerobic conditions. A

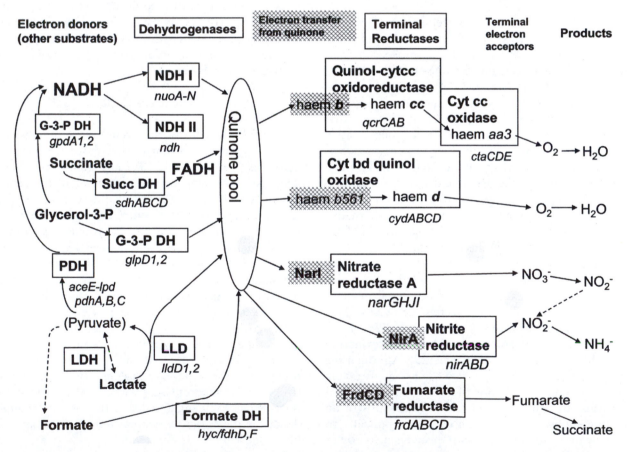

Figure 7. Respiration of *Mycobacterium tuberculosis*. Electron flow is shown by unbroken arrows; broken arrows are used to show three other metabolic steps linking involved substrates. Some functional data are required for respiratory pathways to be shown in this figure for at least some of the steps in any electron transport chain. Where genes or their close orthologues have been shown to encode heme proteins, the hemes are shown in bold. See Table 5 and Table 7 for evidence that genes encode individual proteins. Quinone components are not distinguished here, but are discussed in reviews by Minnikin (89), Ratledge (124) and Brodie & Gutnick (23). Translocatioon of protons is omitted from this figure to avoid overcomplication, but translocation has been reviewed by Ratledge (124) and Wheeler (161) with the annotation of intact ATP synthases (AtpA-H) so that the protons translocated can be used by *M. tuberculosis* to generate ATP.

Table 7. Energy generation: genes for electron transport components[a]

Gene	Rv no.[b]	Size (aa)	EC	Enzyme name	Comment
nuoA	Rv3145	Cluster: 15.70 kb	1.6.5.3	NADH dehydrogenase I	See tuberculist for details of individual genes
-N	Rv3158				
ndh	**Rv1854c**	463	1.6.99.3	NADH dehydrogenase II	
ndhA	Rv0392c	470	1.6.99.3	NADH dehydrogenase II	
qcrC	**Rv2194**	280	1.10.2.-	Ubiquinol-cytochrome C reductase	
qcrA	**Rv2195**	429	1.10.2.-	Ubiquinol-cytochrome C reductase iron-sulfur subunit	
qcrB	**Rv2196**	549	1.10.2.-	Ubiquinol-cytochrome C reductase cytochrome B subunit	
ctaC	Rv2200c	363	1.9.3.1	Cytochrome C oxidase (subunit II)	
ctaD	Rv3043c	573	1.9.3.1	Cytochrome C oxidase polypeptide I	
ctaE	Rv2193	203	1.9.3.1	Probable cytochrome C oxidase polypeptide III (cox3)	
cydA	**Rv1623c**	485	1.10.3.-	Cytochrome D ubiquinol oxidase subunit I	Previously known as appC, but renamed to conform with *M. smegmatis* nomenclature
cydB	**Rv1622c**	346	1.10.3.-	Cytochrome D ubiquinol oxidase subunit II	
cydC	**Rv1620c**	576	1.10.3.-	Transmembrane ATP-binding protein ABC	
cydD	**Rv1621c**	577	1.10.3.-	Transmembrane ATP-binding protein ABC	
narG	**Rv1161**	1,232	1.7.99.4	Nitrate reductase alpha chain	
narH	**Rv1162**	558	1.7.99.4	Nitrate reductase beta chain	
narJ	**Rv1163**	201	1.7.99.4	Nitrate reductase delta chain	
narI	**Rv1164**	246	1.7.99.4	Nitrate reductase gamma chain	
nirA	Rv2391	563	1.7.7.1	Ferredoxin-dependant nitrite reductase	
nirB	Rv0252	853	1.6.6.4	Nitrite reductase [NAD(P)H] large subunit	
nirD	Rv0253	118	1.6.6.4	Nitrite reductase [NAD(P)H] small subunit	
frdA	Rv1552	583	1.3.99.1	Fumarate reductase flavoprotein subunit	
frdB	Rv1553	247	1.3.99.1	Fumarate reductase iron-sulfur protein	
frdC	Rv1554	126	1.3.99.1	Fumarate reductase subunit C	
frdD	Rv1555	125	1.3.99.1	Fumarate reductase subunit D	
hycD	Rv0084	316	1.-.-.-	Formate hydrogenlyase	
hycE	Rv0087	492	1.-.-.-	Formate hydrogenlyase	
fdhD	Rv2899c	276		Protein required for formate dehydrogenase activity	
fdhF	Rv2900c	779	1.2.1.2	Formate hydrogenlyase	

[a] Genes shown in Fig. 7 not listed in this table are in Table 5.

[b] Boldface Rv numbers indicate that the enzyme activity corresponding to the CDS has been confirmed by isolation or cloning of the enzyme, complementation, or the loss of activity when the gene is inactive for at least one of the *M. tuberculosis* complex. Similar evidence obtained with orthologous genes in mycobacteria if their counterpart in the *M. tuberculosis* complex is essentially unambiguous. For all others, the enzyme name is derived from the gene annotation.

characteristic peak for reduced heme in cytochrome *d* was present in the parental strain, absent in the mutants, and restored in the mutant by transformation with the *M. tuberculosis cydABCD* gene cluster (66). Although upregulation of *M. smegmatis cyd* gene expression was evident below 1% O_2 in batch cultures in a fermentor, no data on the regulation of these genes have been obtained (66) in experiments with anoxic cultures of *M. tuberculosis*.

A second *M. tuberculosis* gene associated with

respiration that complements an *M. smegmatis* mutant with its orthologous gene disrupted is *ndh*. The effect of *ndh* disruption in *M. smegmatis* was pleiotropic: unable to grow at 42°C, a multiple amino acid auxotroph, 25-fold loss of NADH oxidase activity, and isoniazid resistance. All those effects are compatible with a failure to recycle NAD from NADH (88) and thus are consistent with the predicted function of *ndh*. The Ndh enzyme is annotated as a type II NADH oxidase (34), which is not coupled to electron transport (Fig. 7) or energy generation. Although there are no data showing differential regulation of *ndh* under axenic conditions, *ndh* is downregulated when *M. tuberculosis* is in macrophages (140). In contrast, the entire *nuo* regulon for the coupled, type I NADH oxidase shows lower gene expression both in macrophages and under axenic conditions at 0.2% O_2 saturation. Compared with 20% O_2, the transcript for individual genes was repressed by 1.5- to 3.4-fold (144) (see http://schoolniklab.stanford. edu/projects/tb.html). Although repression of less than twofold for individual genes is not very striking, the repression of all the genes in this operon provides compelling evidence for downregulation under anoxic conditions. Thus, as the oxygen tension falls, NAD recycling by Ndh must become increasingly important. Given the data for *M. tuberculosis*, it is extremely interesting that *M. leprae* has an intact *ndh* gene but that deletions and mutations have accumulated in all its *nuo* genes. This might have happened as leprosy bacilli became confined to a microaerophilic niche in which the *nuo* genes were always repressed, so that their loss had little or no deleterious effect (161).

Another gene predicted to encode a respiratory function, as a cytochrome *c*, is *qcrC*. Gels specifically stained for the heme *c* of this cytochrome from *M. tuberculosis* revealed a single band of 28 kDa that had the same mobility as its *Corynebacterium glutamicum* counterpart (147). The *C. glutamicum qcrC* orthologue has 54% identity to the *M. tuberculosis qcrC* (147). These are both atypically large genes for this cytochrome and probably arise from a tandem repeat. Consistent with that view, when the *C. glutamicum* gene was expressed and purified, it revealed a product with two heme *c* moieties, and so this product is referred to as cytochrome *cc*. The complete *qcr* operon encodes a cytochrome *c* reductase system containing cytochromes *b* and *cc*, suggesting that it functions in an aerobic respiratory pathway in *M. tuberculosis* (Fig. 7). As with *ndh*, there are no data to elucidate the regulation of either the *qcr* or the *cta* (Fig. 7) genes for cytochrome oxidoreductases under axenic conditions, but all five genes are downregulated when *M. tuberculosis* is in macrophages (140).

Diffusion of oxygen into bacterial cells would not normally be considered rate limiting, although the dual lipophilic membranes of mycobacteria are formidable barriers to polar molecules. Therefore, the discovery of two small hemoglobins in the genome (34) was interesting. The trHbO (truncated hemoglobin O), encoded by the *glbO* gene, has high affinity for molecular oxygen and stimulates the cytochrome oxidase system (118). When membrane vesicles containing cytochrome *o* prepared from *E. coli* were mixed with trHbO, O_2 uptake was stimulated, but not in vesicles prepared

from *cyo* mutants lacking, suggesting a possible function in oxygen delivery. Since *M. tuberculosis* lacks a cytochrome *o* (Fig. 7), trHbO would need to associate with the cytochrome *bd* oxidase in native membranes.

The second hemoglobin, hemoglobin N (trHbN), is encoded by the *glbN* gene. It has only 15% similarity to trHbO (111, 118) and binds oxygen at a level about 50-fold higher than trHbO. trHbN neither transfers bound oxygen to cytochrome oxidase (171), nor stimulates oxygen uptake in membrane vesicles containing cytochrome *o* (118). The high affinity of trHbN for oxygen has been proposed to be due to the presence of its Tyr33, a claim supported by the results of site-directed mutagenesis (171). An enzymatic activity has recently been demonstrated for trHbN, involving its ability to bind nitric oxide (NO) and catalyze its oxygen-dependent decomposition to nitrate (111, 117). *glbN* knockout strains of *M. bovis* BCG are unable to consume NO, and oxygen consumption by the mutant is strongly inhibited by NO compared to that of the parent strain. Finally, the different patterns of expression of trHbO and trHbN are consistent with the very different roles proposed for them, with trHbO being produced throughout agitated, aerobic culture (117) and trHbN being produced only in the stationary phase (37). The role of trHbN in protecting against the toxic effects of NO produced by the macrophage nitric oxide synthase is still unclear, since other mechanisms appear to be capable of NO detoxification (102).

Genes proposed to encode formate dehydrogenase were annotated in the *M. tuberculosis* genome (34). Although the corresponding enzyme activity has not been shown in *M. tuberculosis*, the genes are included in the respiration diagram (Fig. 7) based on the demonstration of a NAD-independent formate dehydrogenase activity that reduced thiazolyl dyes and cytochrome *c* in the particulate fraction of in *M. phlei* (41). The production of formate probably depends on a pyruvate-formate lyase, but only the activating enzyme, PflA, and not the lyase itself, has been annotated (34).

One of the anaerobic respiration systems predicted for *M. tuberculosis* that has now been shown to be functional is the *narGHJI* operon. When *M. smegmatis* mc²155 (naturally lacking nitrate reductase) was transformed with this gene cluster from *M. tuberculosis* H37Rv, the cluster was seen to confer anaerobic nitrate reductase activity. Furthermore, the ability of *M. bovis* BCG to produce nitrite when induced in anaerobic culture including nitrate was abrogated in a *narG* mutant (159). Independently, 1.6-fold induction of the transcript for *narG* and *narH*, together with stronger upregulation of Rv2454/5c, *narXZ*, encoding a putative fused nitrate reductase-nitrate transporter, was demonstrated on exposure of H37Rv to anoxic (0.2% O_2) conditions (144). However, *narXZ* did not compensate for the *narG* mutation (159). Further, in intracellular *M. tuberculosis*, *narX* was upregulated only in activated, and not naive, macrophages, suggesting that its function may be related to defense against toxic NO radicals. Interestingly, differential regulation of the *sdh* and *frd* gene clusters (Fig. 5) was not observed because of changes in oxygen tension axenically, and only weak upregulation of *frd* occurred in *M. tuberculosis* in macrophages (140), although in *E. coli* they are coordinately regulated with nitrate reductase (148). The *narG* mutant had reduced virulence in SCID mice, adding support to the view that genes that are expressed under anaerobic or low-oxygen conditions are important for pathogenicity and persistence (159).

CONCLUSIONS AND SUMMARY

The publication of the *M. tuberculosis* annotated genome sequence has provided the basis for renewed interest in its metabolism. All the annotated genes have been modeled into biochemical pathways (http://www.genome.ad.jp/kegg/), and functional genomics has already provided new insights into its physiology, its regulation, and its relation to virulence. Patterns are already emerging, with genes involved in stress response, lipid catabolism, and anaerobiosis being linked to the persistence of tubercle bacilli. Some of the predicted genes have had their functions confirmed, and it appears that a single isocitrate lyase and a single nitrate reductase are required for virulence. As in facultative pathogens (58, 163), the loss of biosynthetic genes is often highly attenuating. In amino acid biosynthesis, this loss has been linked to auxotrophy, providing a confirmation of the function of the gene lost. With tuberculosis still being a huge global burden in terms of mortality and morbidity, new interventions are needed. Thus, it is exciting that, already, essential genes in the pathways linking general carbohydrate metabolism to the biosynthesis of characteristic cell envelope components have been revealed: these genes may represent good targets for novel antimycobacterial agents. With the worldwide tuberculosis structural-genomics initiative, the expression and functional characterization of hundreds of genes continues apace.

Insights into evolution of the pathogenic mycobacteria are becoming possible by comparing the mycobacterial genomes as they are sequenced. We have emphasized the biochemical changes underlying the evolution of *M. bovis* as a member of the tubercle bacillus clade exhibiting marked host tropism. The ability to make deductions with such closely related bacilli enables the continuing epidemic of bovine tuberculosis, resulting in worldwide losses to agriculture of 3 billion dollars annually, to be addressed (48).

However transcript, gene, or proteomic data are generated—from differential growth conditions, comparative genomics, gaps in metabolic pathways generated from annotated genes, or even host tissue-derived bacteria—the functions of the genes identified is sensu stricto a set of predictions. The hypotheses thus generated about the functions of the bacteria that are expressed or that are important in pathogenicity must eventually be tested formally. Together with biochemical demonstrations to verify suggested metabolic pathways or confirmation that individual genes encode key enzymes, these approaches provide a powerful weapon against the tubercle bacilli. This is an exciting time to be involved in mycobacterial biochemistry.

Acknowledgments. We thank Lisa Keating, Huma Mansoor, and Stephen Gordon for their intellectually stimulating and helpful advice. P.R.W. acknowledges DEFRA (U.K.) for financial support.

REFERENCES

1. **Alexander, F. W., E. Sandmeier, P. K. Mehta, and P. Christen.** 1994. Evolutionary relationships among pyridoxal-5′-phosphate-dependent enzymes. Regio-specific alpha, beta and gamma families. *Eur. J. Biochem.* **219:**953–960.
2. **Allaudeen, H. S., and T. Ramakrishnan.** 1971. Biosynthesis of isoleucine and valine in *Mycobacterium tuberculosis* H 37 Rv. 3. Purification and properties of acetohydroxy acid isomeroreductase. *Indian J. Biochem.* **8:**23–27.
3. **Allaudeen, H. S., and T. Ramakrishnan.** 1968. Biosynthesis of isoleucine and valine in *Mycobacterium tuberculosis* H37 Rv. *Arch. Biochem. Biophys.* **125:**199–209.
4. **Allaudeen, H. S., and T. Ramakrishnan.** 1970. Biosynthesis of isoleucine and valine in *Mycobacterium tuberculosis* H37Rv. II. Purification and properties of acetohydroxy acid isomerase. *Arch. Biochem. Biophys.* **140:**245–256.
5. **Andersen, A. B., and E. B. Hansen.** 1993. Cloning of the *lysA* gene from *Mycobacterium tuberculosis*. *Gene* **124:**105–109.
6. **Argyrou, A., and J. S. Blanchard.** 2001. *Mycobacterium tuberculosis* lipoamide dehydrogenase is encoded by Rv0462 and not by the *lpdA* or *lpdB* genes. *Biochemistry* **40:**11353–11363.
7. **Artman, M., and A. Bekierkunst.** 1961. Studies on *Mycobacterium tuberculosis* H37Rv grown *in vivo*. *Am. Rev. Respir. Dis.* **83:**100–106.
8. **Bachhawat, N., and S. C. Mande.** 1999. Identification of the *INO1* gene of *Mycobacterium tuberculosis* H37Rv reveals a novel class of inositol-1-phosphate synthase enzyme. *J. Mol. Biol.* **291:**531–536.
9. **Bai, N. J., M. R. Pai, P. S. Murthy, and T. A. Venkitasubramanian.** 1974. Effect of oxygen tension on the aldolases of *Mycobacterium tuberculosis* H37Rv. *FEBS Lett.* **45:**68–70.
10. **Bai, N. J., M. R. Pai, P. S. Murthy, and T. A. Venkitasubramanian.** 1975. Fructose-1,6-diphosphate aldolase of *Mycobacterium tuberculosis* H37Rv. *Indian J. Biochem. Biophys.* **12:**181–183.

11. Bai, N. J., M. R. Pai, P. S. Murthy, and T. A. Venkitasubramanian. 1982. Fructose-bisphosphate aldolases from mycobacteria. *Methods Enzymol. Ser. E* **90:**241–250.

12. Bai, N. J., M. R. Pai, P. S. Murthy, and T. A. Venkitasubramanian. 1975. Pathways of carbohydrate metabolism in *Mycobacterium tuberculosis* H37Rv. *Can. J. Microbiol.* **21:**1688–1691.

13. Barclay, R., and P. R. Wheeler. 1989. Metabolism of mycobacteria in tissues, p. 37–106. *In* C. Ratledge, J. Stanford, and G. Grange (ed.), *The Biology of the Mycobacteria*, vol. 3. Academic Press, Ltd., London, United Kingdom.

14. Barona-Gomez, F., and D. A. Hodgson. 2003. Occurrence of a putative ancient-like isomerase involved in histidine and tryptophan biosynthesis. *EMBO Rep.* **4:**296–300.

15. Baulard, A. R., S. S. Gurcha, C. Gouffi, C. Locht, and G. S. Besra. 2003. In vivo interaction between the polyprenol phosphate mannose synthase Ppm1 and the integral membrane protein ppm2 from *Mycobacterium smegmatis* revealed by a bacterial two-hybrid system. *J. Biol. Chem.* **278:**2242–2248.

16. Beaman, T. W., J. S. Blanchard, and S. L. Roderick. 1998. The conformational change and active site structure of tetrahydrodipicolinate N-succinyltransferase. *Biochemistry* **37:**10363–10369.

17. Besra, G. S., and D. Chatterjee. 1994. Lipids and carbohydrates of *Mycobacterium tuberculosis*, p. 285–306. *In* B. R. Bloom (ed.), *Tuberculosis: Pathogenesis, Protection, and Control*. ASM Press, Washington, D.C.

18. Besra, G. S., C. B. Morehouse, C. M. Rittner, C. J. Waechter, and P. J. Brennan. 1997. Biosynthesis of mycobacterial lipoarabinomannan. *J. Biol. Chem.* **272:**18460–18466.

19. Born, T. L., and J. S. Blanchard. 1999. Enzyme-catalyzed acylation of homoserine: mechanistic characterization of the *Escherichia coli metA*-encoded homoserine transsuccinylase. *Biochemistry* **38:**14416–14423.

20. Born, T. L., M. Franklin, and J. S. Blanchard. 2000. Enzyme-catalyzed acylation of homoserine: mechanistic characterization of the *Haemophilus influenzae met2*-encoded homoserine transacetylase. *Biochemistry* **39:**8556–8564.

21. Bowman, K. G., and C. R. Bertozzi. 1999. Carbohydrate sulfotransferases: mediators of extracellular communication. *Chem. Biol.* **6:**R9–R22.

22. Brakhage, A. A., and K. Langfelder. 2002. Menacing mold: the molecular biology of *Aspergillus fumigatus*. *Annu. Rev. Microbiol.* **56:**433–455.

23. Brodie, A. F., and D. L. Gutnick. 1972. Electron transport and oxidative phosphorylation in microbial systems, p. 599–681. *In* T. E. King and M. Klingenberg (ed.), *Electron and Coupled Energy Transfer Systems*, vol. 1B. Marcel Dekker Inc., New York, N.Y.

24. Butcher, P. D., J. A. Mangan, and I. M. Monahan. 1998. Intracellular gene expression. Analysis of RNA from mycobacteria in macrophages using RT-PCR. *Methods Mol. Biol.* **101:**285–306.

25. Camacho, L. R., D. Ensergueix, E. Perez, B. Gicquel, and C. Guilhot. 1999. Identification of a virulence gene cluster of *Mycobacterium tuberculosis* by signature-tagged transposon mutagenesis. *Mol. Microbiol.* **34:**257–267.

26. Camargo, E. E., J. A. Kertcher, S. M. Larson, B. S. Tepper, and H. N. Wagner, Jr. 1982. Radiometric measurement of differential metabolism of fatty acid by mycobacteria. *Int. J. Lepr. Other Mycobact. Dis.* **50:**200–204.

27. Campbell, J. W., and J. E. Cronan, Jr. 2002. The enigmatic *Escherichia coli fadE* gene is *yafH*. *J. Bacteriol.* **184:**3759–3764.

28. Camus, J. C., M. J. Pryor, C. Medigue, and S. T. Cole. 2002. Re-annotation of the genome sequence of *Mycobacterium tuberculosis* H37Rv. *Microbiology* **148:**2967–2973.

29. Chen, J. M., D. C. Alexander, M. A. Behr, and J. Liu. 2003. *Mycobacterium bovis* BCG vaccines exhibit defects in alanine and serine catabolism. *Infect. Immun.* **71:**708–716.

30. Cho, Y., V. Sharma, and J. C. Sacchettini. 2003. Crystal structure of ATP phosphoribosyltransferase from *Mycobacterium tuberculosis*. *J. Biol. Chem.* **278:**8333–8339.

31. Chopra, S., H. Pai, and A. Ranganathan. 2002. Expression, purification, and biochemical characterization of *Mycobacterium tuberculosis* aspartate decarboxylase, PanD. *Protein Expression Purif.* **25:**533–540.

32. Cirilli, M., R. Zheng, G. Scapin, and J. S. Blanchard. 1998. Structural symmetry: the three-dimensional structure of *Haemophilus influenzae* diaminopimelate epimerase. *Biochemistry* **37:**16452–16458.

33. Cirillo, J. D., T. R. Weisbrod, L. Pascopella, B. R. Bloom, and W. R. Jacobs, Jr. 1994. Isolation and characterization of the aspartokinase and aspartate semialdehyde dehydrogenase operon from mycobacteria. *Mol. Microbiol.* **11:**629–639.

34. Cole, S. T., R. Brosch, J. Parkhill, T. Garnier, C. Churcher, D. Harris, S. V. Gordon, K. Eiglmeier, S. Gas, C. E. Barry III, F. Tekaia, K. Badcock, D. Basham, D. Brown, T. Chillingworth, R. Connor, R. Davies, K. Devlin, T. Feltwell, S. Gentles, N. Hamlin, S. Holroyd, T. Hornsby, K. Jagels, A. Krogh, J. Mclean, S. Moule, L. Murphy, K. Oliver, J. Osborne, M. A. Quail, M.-A. Rajandream, J. Rogers, S. Rutter, K. Seeger, J. Skelton, R. Squares, S. Squares, J. E. Sulstron, K. Taylor, S. Whitehead, and B. G. Barrell. 1998. Deciphering the biology of *Mycobacterium tuberculosis* from the complete genome sequence. *Nature* **393:**537–544. (Erratum, **396:**190, 1998).

35. Cole, S. T., K. Eiglmeier, J. Parkhill, K. D. James, N. R. Thomson, P. R. Wheeler, N. Honore, T. Garnier, C. Churcher, D. Harris, K. Mungall, D. Basham, D. Brown, T. Chillingworth, R. Connor, R. M. Davies, K. Devlin, S. Duthoy, T. Feltwell, A. Fraser, N. Hamlin, S. Holroyd, T. Hornsby, K. Jagels, C. Lacroix, J. Maclean, S. Moule, L. Murphy, K. Oliver, M. A. Quail, M.-A. Rajandream, K. M. Rutherford, S. Rutter, K. Seeger, S. Simon, M. Simmonds, J. Skelton, R. Squares, S. Squares, K. Stevens, K. Taylor, S. Whitehead, J. R. Woodward, and B. G. Barrell. 2001. Massive gene decay in the leprosy bacillus. *Nature* **409:**1007–1011.

36. Collins, D. M., T. Wilson, S. Campbell, B. M. Buddle, B. J. Wards, G. Hotter, and G. W. De Lisle. 2002. Production of avirulent mutants of *Mycobacterium bovis* with vaccine properties by the use of illegitimate recombination and screening of stationary-phase cultures. *Microbiology* **148:**3019–3027.

37. Couture, M., S. R. Yeh, B. A. Wittenberg, J. B. Wittenberg, Y. Ouellet, D. L. Rousseau, and M. Guertin. 1999. A cooperative oxygen-binding hemoglobin from *Mycobacterium tuberculosis*. *Proc. Natl. Acad. Sci. USA* **96:**11223–11228.

38. Cox, J. S., B. Chen, M. McNeil, and W. R. Jacobs, Jr. 1999. Complex lipid determines tissue-specific replication of *Mycobacterium tuberculosis* in mice. *Nature* **402:**79–83.

39. Denning, D. W., M. J. Anderson, G. Turner, J. P. Latge, and J. W. Bennett. 2002. Sequencing the *Aspergillus fumigatus* genome. *Lancet Infect. Dis.* **2:**251–253.

40. De Smet, K. A., A. Weston, I. N. Brown, D. B. Young, and B. D. Robertson. 2000. Three pathways for trehalose biosynthesis in mycobacteria. *Microbiology* **146:**199–208.

41. Deyhle, R. R., and L. L. Barton. 1977. Nicotinamide adenine dinucleotide-independent formate dehydrogenase in *Mycobacterium phlei*. *Can. J. Microbiol.* **23:**125–130.

42. Duine, J. A. 1999. Thiols in formaldehyde dissimilation and detoxification. *Biofactors* **10:**201–206.

43. Fahey, R. C. 2001. Novel thiols of prokaryotes. *Annu. Rev. Microbiol.* **55:**333–356.

44. Feng, Z., N. E. Caceres, G. Sarath, and R. G. Barletta. 2002. *Mycobacterium smegmatis* L-alanine dehydrogenase (Ald) is required for proficient utilization of alanine as a sole nitrogen source and sustained anaerobic growth. *J. Bacteriol.* **184:**5001–5010.

45. Fernandes, N. D., and P. E. Kolattukudy. 1996. Cloning, sequencing and characterization of a fatty acid synthase-encoding gene from *Mycobacterium tuberculosis* var. *bovis* BCG. *Gene* **170:**95–99.

46. Fitzmaurice, A. M., and P. E. Kolattukudy. 1998. An acyl-CoA synthase (*acoas*) gene adjacent to the mycocerosic acid synthase (*mas*) locus is necessary for mycocerosyl lipid synthesis in *Mycobacterium tuberculosis* var. *bovis* BCG. *J. Biol. Chem.* **273:**8033–8039.

47. Fitzmaurice, A. M., and P. E. Kolattukudy. 1997. Open reading frame 3, which is adjacent to the mycocerosic acid synthase gene, is expressed as an acyl coenzyme A synthase in *Mycobacterium bovis* BCG. *J. Bacteriol.* **179:**2608–2615.

48. Garnier, T., K. Eiglmeier, J. C. Camus, N. Medina, H. Mansoor, M. Pryor, S. Duthoy, S. Grondin, C. Lacroix, C. Monsempe, S. Simon, B. Harris, R. Atkin, J. Doggett, R. Mayes, L. Keating, P. R. Wheeler, J. Parkhill, B. G. Barrell, S. T. Cole, S. V. Gordon, and R. G. Hewinson. 2003. The complete genome sequence of *Mycobacterium bovis*. *Proc. Natl. Acad. Sci. USA* **100:**7877–7882.

49. Giegel, D. A., V. Massey, and C. H. Williams. 1990. L-Lactate 2-monooxygenase from *Mycobacterium smegmatis*. Cloning, nucleotide sequence and primary structure homology within an enzyme family. *J. Biol. Chem.* **265:**6626–6632.

50. Glickman, M. S., S. M. Cahill, and W. R. Jacobs, Jr. 2001. The *Mycobacterium tuberculosis cmaA2* gene encodes a mycolic acid *trans*-cyclopropane synthetase. *J. Biol. Chem.* **276:**2228–2233.

51. Glickman, M. S., J. S. Cox, and W. R. Jacobs, Jr. 2000. A novel mycolic acid cyclopropane synthetase is required for cording, persistence, and virulence of *Mycobacterium tuberculosis*. *Mol. Cell* **5:**717–727.

52. Glickman, M. S., and W. R. Jacobs, Jr. 2001. Microbial pathogenesis of *Mycobacterium tuberculosis*: dawn of a discipline. *Cell* **104:**477–485.

53. Gokulan, K., B. Rupp, M. S. Pavelka, Jr., W. R. Jacobs, Jr., and J. C. Sacchettini. 2003. Crystal structure of *Mycobacterium tuberculosis* diaminopimelate decarboxylase, an essential enzyme in bacterial lysine biosynthesis. *J. Biol. Chem.* **278:**18588–18596.

54. Goldman, D. S. 1961. Enzyme systems in mycobacteria. *Adv. Tuberc. Res.* **11:**1–44.

55. Guleria, I., R. Teitelbaum, R. A. McAdam, G. Kalpana, W. R. Jacobs, Jr., and B. R. Bloom. 1996. Auxotrophic vaccines for tuberculosis. *Nat. Med.* **2:**334–337.

56. Gupta, A., P. H. Kumar, T. K. Dineshkumar, U. Varshney, and H. S. Subramanya. 2001. Crystal structure of Rv2118c: an AdoMet-dependent methyltransferase from *Mycobacterium tuberculosis* H37Rv. *J. Mol. Biol.* **312:**381–391.

57. Gurcha, S. S., A. R. Baulard, L. Kremer, C. Locht, D. B. Moody, W. Muhlecker, C. E. Costello, D. C. Crick, P. J. Brennan, and G. S. Besra. 2002. Ppm1, a novel polyprenol monophosphomannose synthase from *Mycobacterium tuberculosis*. *Biochem. J.* **365:**441–450.

58. Hensel, M., J. E. Shea, C. Gleeson, M. D. Jones, E. Dalton, and D. W. Holden. 1995. Simultaneous identification of bacterial virulence genes by negative selection. *Science* **269:**400–403.

59. Hiltunen, J. K., and Y. Qin. 2000. Beta-oxidation—strategies for the metabolism of a wide variety of acyl-CoA esters. *Biochim. Biophys. Acta* **1484:**117–128.

60. Hondalus, M. K., S. Bardarov, R. Russell, J. Chan, W. R. Jacobs, Jr., and B. R. Bloom. 2000. Attenuation of and protection induced by a leucine auxotroph of *Mycobacterium tuberculosis*. *Infect. Immun.* **68:**2888–2898.

61. Honer Zu Bentrup, K., A. Miczak, D. L. Swenson, and D. G. Russell. 1999. Characterization of activity and expression of isocitrate lyase in *Mycobacterium avium* and *Mycobacterium tuberculosis*. *J. Bacteriol.* **181:**7161–7167.

62. Hsieh, P. C., B. C. Shenoy, D. Samols, and N. F. Phillips. 1996. Cloning, expression, and characterization of polyphosphate glucokinase from *Mycobacterium tuberculosis*. *J. Biol. Chem.* **271:**4909–4915.

63. Huang, C. C., C. V. Smith, M. S. Glickman, W. R. Jacobs, Jr., and J. C. Sacchettini. 2002. Crystal structures of mycolic acid cyclopropane synthases from *Mycobacterium tuberculosis*. *J. Biol. Chem.* **277:**11559–11569.

64. Ishaque, M. 1992. Energy generation mechanisms in the in vitro-grown *Mycobacterium lepraemurium*. *Int. J. Lepr. Other Mycobact. Dis.* **60:**61–70.

65. Jackson, M., D. C. Crick, and P. J. Brennan. 2000. Phosphatidylinositol is an essential phospholipid of mycobacteria. *J. Biol. Chem.* **275:**30092–30099.

66. Kana, B. D., E. A. Weinstein, D. Avarbock, S. S. Dawes, H. Rubin, and V. Mizrahi. 2001. Characterization of the *cydAB*-encoded cytochrome *bd* oxidase from *Mycobacterium smegmatis*. *J. Bacteriol.* **183:**7076–7086.

67. Kaushal, D., B. G. Schroeder, S. Tyagi, T. Yoshimatsu, C. Scott, C. Ko, L. Carpenter, J. Mehrotra, Y. C. Manabe, R. D. Fleischmann, and W. R. Bishai. 2002. Reduced immunopathology and mortality despite tissue persistence in a *Mycobacterium tuberculosis* mutant lacking alternative sigma factor, SigH. *Proc. Natl. Acad. Sci. USA* **99:**8330–8335.

68. Kikuchi, S., D. L. Rainwater, and P. E. Kolattukudy. 1992. Purification and characterization of an unusually large fatty acid synthase from *Mycobacterium tuberculosis* var. *bovis* BCG. *Arch. Biochem. Biophys.* **295:**318–326.

69. Kim, S., Y. J. Jo, S. H. Lee, H. Motegi, K. Shiba, M. Sassanfar, and S. A. Martinis. 1998. Biochemical and phylogenetic analyses of methionyl-tRNA synthetase isolated from a pathogenic microorganism, *Mycobacterium tuberculosis*. *FEBS Lett.* **427:**259–262.

70. Klutts, J. S., K. Hatanaka, Y. T. Pan, and A. D. Elbein. 2002. Biosynthesis of D-arabinose in *Mycobacterium smegmatis*: specific labeling from D-glucose. *Arch. Biochem. Biophys.* **398:**229–239.

71. Klutts, S., I. Pastuszak, V. K. Edavana, P. Thampi, Y. T. Pan, E. C. Abraham, J. D. Carroll, and A. D. Elbein. 2003. Purification, cloning, expression, and properties of mycobacterial trehalose-phosphate phosphatase. *J. Biol. Chem.* **278:**2093–2100.

72. Koledin, T., G. L. Newton, and R. C. Fahey. 2002. Identification of the mycothiol synthase gene (*mshD*) encoding the acetyltransferase producing mycothiol in actinomycetes. *Arch. Microbiol.* **178:**331–337.

73. Koo, C. W., and J. S. Blanchard. 1999. Chemical mechanism of *Haemophilus influenzae* diaminopimelate epimerase. *Biochemistry* **38:**4416–4422.

74. Kordulakova, J., M. Gilleron, K. Mikusova, G. Puzo, P. J. Brennan, B. Gicquel, and M. Jackson. 2002. Definition of the first mannosylation step in phosphatidylinositol mannoside synthesis. PimA is essential for growth of mycobacteria. *J. Biol. Chem.* **277:**31335–31344.

75. LaMarca, B. B. D., W. Zhu, J. E. L. Arcenaux, B. R. Byers, and M. D. Lundrigan. 2004. Participation of *fad* and *mbt* genes in synthesis of mycobactin in *Mycobacterium smegmatis*. *J. Bacteriol.* **186**:374–382.

76. Lee, R. E., P. J. Brennan, and G. S. Besra. 1998. Synthesis of beta-D-arabinofuranosyl-1-monophosphoryl polyprenols: examination of their function as mycobacterial arabinosyl transferase donors. *Bioorg. Med. Chem. Lett.* **8**:951–954.

77. Li, M. S., I. M. Monahan, S. J. Waddell, J. A. Mangan, S. L. Martin, M. J. Everett, and P. D. Butcher. 2001. cDNA-RNA subtractive hybridization reveals increased expression of mycocerosic acid synthase in intracellular *Mycobacterium bovis* BCG. *Microbiology* **147**:2293–2305.

78. Lorenz, M. C., and G. R. Fink. 2001. The glyoxylate cycle is required for fungal virulence. *Nature* **412**:83–86.

79. Losel, D. M. 1988. Fungal lipids, p. 699–806. *In* C. Ratledge and S. G. Wilkinson (ed.), *Microbial Lipids*, vol. 1. Academic Press, Ltd., London, United Kingdom.

80. Ma, Y., J. A. Mills, J. T. Belisle, V. Vissa, M. Howell, K. Bowlin, M. S. Scherman, and M. McNeil. 1997. Determination of the pathway for rhamnose biosynthesis in mycobacteria: cloning, sequencing and expression of the *Mycobacterium tuberculosis* gene encoding alpha-D-glucose-1-phosphate thymidylyltransferase. *Microbiology* **143**:937–945.

81. Ma, Y., F. Pan, and M. McNeil. 2002. Formation of dTDP-rhamnose is essential for growth of mycobacteria. *J. Bacteriol.* **184**:3392–3395.

82. Ma, Y., R. J. Stern, M. S. Scherman, V. D. Vissa, W. Yan, V. C. Jones, F. Zhang, S. G. Franzblau, W. H. Lewis, and M. R. McNeil. 2001. Drug targeting *Mycobacterium tuberculosis* cell wall synthesis: genetics of dTDP-rhamnose synthetic enzymes and development of a microtiter plate-based screen for inhibitors of conversion of dTDP-glucose to dTDP-rhamnose. *Antimicrob. Agents Chemother.* **45**:1407–1416.

83. Maher, P. A. 1993. Inhibition of the tyrosine kinase activity of the fibroblast growth factor receptor by the methyltransferase inhibitor 5′-methylthioadenosine. *J. Biol. Chem.* **268**:4244–4249.

84. Manganelli, R., M. I. Voskuil, G. K. Schoolnik, E. Dubnau, M. Gomez, and I. Smith. 2002. Role of the extracytoplasmic-function sigma factor sigma(H) in *Mycobacterium tuberculosis* global gene expression. *Mol. Microbiol.* **45**:365–374.

85. McAdam, R. A., S. Quan, D. A. Smith, S. Bardarov, J. C. Betts, F. C. Cook, E. U. Hooker, A. P. Lewis, P. Woollard, M. J. Everett, P. T. Lukey, G. J. Bancroft, W. R. Jacobs, Jr., and K. Duncan. 2002. Characterization of a *Mycobacterium tuberculosis* H37Rv transposon library reveals insertions in 351 ORFs and mutants with altered virulence. *Microbiology* **148**:2975–2986.

86. McAdam, R. A., T. R. Weisbrod, J. Martin, J. D. Scuderi, A. M. Brown, J. D. Cirillo, B. R. Bloom, and W. R. Jacobs, Jr. 1995. In vivo growth characteristics of leucine and methionine auxotrophic mutants of *Mycobacterium bovis* BCG generated by transposon mutagenesis. *Infect. Immun.* **63**:1004–1012.

87. McKinney, J. D., K. Honer zu Bentrup, E. J. Munoz-Elias, A. Miczak, B. Chen, W. T. Chan, D. Swenson, J. C. Sacchettini, W. R. Jacobs, Jr., and D. G. Russell. 2000. Persistence of *Mycobacterium tuberculosis* in macrophages and mice requires the glyoxylate shunt enzyme isocitrate lyase. *Nature* **406**:735–738.

88. Miesel, L., T. R. Weisbrod, J. A. Marcinkeviciene, R. Bittman, and W. R. Jacobs, Jr. 1998. NADH dehydrogenase defects confer isoniazid resistance and conditional lethality in *Mycobacterium smegmatis*. *J. Bacteriol.* **180**:2459–2467.

89. Minnikin, D. E. 1982. Lipids: complex lipids, their chemistry, biosynthesis and roles, p. 95–184. *In* C. Ratledge and J. Stanford (ed.), *The Biology of the Mycobacteria*, vol. 1. Academic Press Ltd., London, United Kingdom.

90. Minnikin, D. E., L. Kremer, L. G. Dover, and G. S. Besra. 2002. The methyl-branched fortifications of *Mycobacterium tuberculosis*. *Chem. Biol.* **9**:545–553.

91. Monahan, I., J. Betts, D. Banerjee, and P. Butcher. 2001. Differential expression of mycobacterial proteins following phagocytosis by macrophages. *Microbiology* **147**:459–471.

92. Mori, T. 1975. Biochemical properties of cultivated *Mycobacterium lepraemurium*. *Int. J. Lepr. Other Mycobact. Dis.* **43**:210–217.

93. Morscreck, C., S. Berger, and G. Plum. 2001. The macrophage-induced gene (*mig*) of *Mycobacterium avium* encodes a medium-chain acyl-coenzyme A synthetase. *Biochim. Biophys. Acta.* **1521**:59–65.

94. Mougous, J. D., R. E. Green, S. J. Williams, S. E. Brenner, and C. R. Bertozzi. 2002. Sulfotransferases and sulfatases in mycobacteria. *Chem. Biol.* **9**:767–776.

95. Mougous, J. D., M. D. Leavell, R. H. Senaratne, C. D. Leigh, S. J. Williams, L. W. Riley, J. A. Leary, and C. R. Bertozzi. 2002. Discovery of sulfated metabolites in mycobacteria with a genetic and mass spectrometric approach. *Proc. Natl. Acad. Sci. USA* **99**:17037–17042.

95a. Movahedzadeh, F., S. C. G. Rison, P. R. Wheeler, S. L. Kendall, T. J. Larson, and N. G. Stoker. The *Mycobacterium tuberculosis* Rv1099c gene encodes a GlpX-like class II fructose 1,6 bisphosphatase. *Microbiology*, in press.

96. Movahedzadeh, F., D. A. Smith, R. A. Norman, P. Dindayala, J. Murray-Rust, D. G. Russell, S. L. Kendall, S. C. G. Rison, M. S. McAlister, G. J. Bancroft, N. Q. McDonald, M. Daffe, Y. Av-Gay, and N. G. Stoker. 2004. The *Mycobacterium tuberculosis ino1* gene is essential for growth and virulence. *Mol. Microbiol.* **51**:1003–1014.

97. Muh, U., V. Massey, and C. H. Williams, Jr. 1994. Lactate monooxygenase. I. Expression of the mycobacterial gene in *Escherichia coli* and site-directed mutagenesis of lysine 266. *J. Biol. Chem.* **269**:7982–7988.

98. Mukhopadhyay, B., E. M. Concar, and R. S. Wolfe. 2001. A GTP-dependent vertebrate-type phosphoenolpyruvate carboxykinase from *Mycobacterium smegmatis*. *J. Biol. Chem.* **276**:16137–16145.

99. Murthy, P. S., M. M. Sisri, and T. Ramakrishnan. 1962. Tricarboxylic acid cycle and related enzymes in cell-free extracts of *Mycobacterium tuberculosis* H37Rv. *Biochem. J.* **84**:263–269.

100. Myers, R. W., J. W. Wray, S. Fish, and R. H. Abeles. 1993. Purification and characterization of an enzyme involved in oxidative carbon-carbon bond cleavage reactions in the methionine salvage pathway of *Klebsiella pneumoniae*. *J. Biol. Chem.* **268**:24785–24791.

101. Nagasawa, T., H. Kanzaki, and H. Yamada. 1984. Cystathionine gamma-lyase of *Streptomyces phaeochromogenes*. The occurrence of cystathionine gamma-lyase in filamentous bacteria and its purification and characterization. *J. Biol. Chem.* **259**:10393–10403.

102. Nathan, C., and M. U. Shiloh. 2000. Reactive oxygen and nitrogen intermediates in the relationship between mammalian hosts and microbial pathogens. *Proc. Natl. Acad. Sci. USA* **97**:8841–8848.

103. Newton, G. L., K. Arnold, M. S. Price, C. Sherrill, S. B. Delcardayre, Y. Aharonowitz, G. Cohen, J. Davies, R. C. Fahey, and C. Davis. 1996. Distribution of thiols in microorganisms: mycothiol is a major thiol in most actinomycetes. *J. Bacteriol.* **178**:1990–1995.

104. Newton, G. L., Y. Av-Gay, and R. C. Fahey. 2000. *N*-Acetyl-1-D-*myo*-inosityl-2-amino-2-deoxy-alpha-D-glucopyranoside deacetylase (MshB) is a key enzyme in mycothiol biosynthesis. *J. Bacteriol.* 182:6958–6963.

105. Newton, G. L., C. A. Bewley, T. J. Dwyer, R. Horn, Y. Aharonowitz, G. Cohen, J. Davies, D. J. Faulkner, and R. C. Fahey. 1995. The structure of U17 isolated from *Streptomyces clavuligerus* and its properties as an antioxidant thiol. *Eur. J. Biochem.* 230:821–825.

106. Newton, G. L., T. Koledin, B. Gorovitz, M. Rawat, R. C. Fahey, and Y. Av-Gay. 2003. The glycosyltransferase gene encoding the enzyme catalyzing the first step of mycothiol biosynthesis (*mshA*). *J. Bacteriol.* 185:3476–3479.

107. Newton, G. L., M. D. Unson, S. J. Anderberg, J. A. Aguilera, N. N. Oh, S. B. delCardayre, Y. Av-Gay, and R. C. Fahey. 1999. Characterization of *Mycobacterium smegmatis* mutants defective in 1-D-*myo*-inosityl-2-amino-2-deoxy-alpha-D-glucopyranoside and mycothiol biosynthesis. *Biochem. Biophys. Res. Commun.* 255:239–244.

108. Nigou, J., L. G. Dover, and G. S. Besra. 2002. Purification and biochemical characterization of *Mycobacterium tuberculosis* SuhB, an inositol monophosphatase involved in inositol biosynthesis. *Biochemistry* 41:4392–4398.

109. Norin, A., P. W. Van Ophem, S. R. Piersma, B. Persson, J. A. Duine, and H. Jornvall. 1997. Mycothiol-dependent formaldehyde dehydrogenase, a prokaryotic medium-chain dehydrogenase/reductase, phylogenetically links different eukaroytic alcohol dehydrogenases—primary structure, conformational modelling and functional correlations. *Eur. J. Biochem.* 248:282–289.

110. Oliveira, J. S., C. A. Pinto, L. A. Basso, and D. S. Santos. 2001. Cloning and overexpression in soluble form of functional shikimate kinase and 5-enolpyruvylshikimate 3-phosphate synthase enzymes from *Mycobacterium tuberculosis*. *Protein Expression Purif.* 22:430–435.

111. Ouellet, H., Y. Ouellet, C. Richard, M. Labarre, B. Wittenberg, J. Wittenberg, and M. Guertin. 2002. Truncated hemoglobin HbN protects *Mycobacterium bovis* from nitric oxide. *Proc. Natl. Acad. Sci. USA* 99:5902–5907.

112. Pan, F., M. Jackson, Y. Ma, and M. McNeil. 2001. Cell wall core galactofuran synthesis is essential for growth of mycobacteria. *J. Bacteriol.* 183:3991–3998.

113. Pan, Y. T., J. D. Carroll, and A. D. Elbein. 2002. Trehalosephosphate synthase of *Mycobacterium tuberculosis*. Cloning, expression and properties of the recombinant enzyme. *Eur. J. Biochem.* 269:6091–6100.

114. Parish, T. 2003. Starvation survival response of *Mycobacterium tuberculosis*. *J. Bacteriol.* 185:6702–6706.

115. Parish, T., and N. G. Stoker. 2002. The common aromatic amino acid biosynthesis pathway is essential in *Mycobacterium tuberculosis*. *Microbiology* 148:3069–3077.

116. Patel, M. P., and J. S. Blanchard. 1999. Expression, purification, and characterization of *Mycobacterium tuberculosis* mycothione reductase. *Biochemistry* 38:11827–11833.

117. Pathania, R., N. K. Navani, A. M. Gardner, P. R. Gardner, and K. L. Dikshit. 2002. Nitric oxide scavenging and detoxification by the *Mycobacterium tuberculosis* haemoglobin, HbN in *Escherichia coli*. *Mol. Microbiol.* 45:1303–1314.

118. Pathania, R., N. K. Navani, G. Rajamohan, and K. L. Dikshit. 2002. *Mycobacterium tuberculosis* hemoglobin HbO associates with membranes and stimulates cellular respiration of recombinant *Escherichia coli*. *J. Biol. Chem.* 277:15293–15302.

119. Paulin, L. G., E. E. Brander, and H. J. Poso. 1985. Specific inhibition of spermidine synthesis in *Mycobacterium* spp. by the dextro isomer of ethambutol. *Antimicrob. Agents Chemother.* 28:157–159.

120. Pavelka, M. S., Jr., and W. R. Jacobs, Jr. 1996. Biosynthesis of diaminopimelate, the precursor of lysine and a component of peptidoglycan, is an essential function of *Mycobacterium smegmatis*. *J. Bacteriol.* 178:6496–6507.

121. Pavelka, M. S., Jr., T. R. Weisbrod, and W. R. Jacobs, Jr. 1997. Cloning of the *dapB* gene, encoding dihydrodipicolinate reductase, from *Mycobacterium tuberculosis*. *J. Bacteriol.* 179:2777–2782.

122. Qureshi, N., N. Sathyamoorthy, and K. Takayama. 1984. Biosynthesis of C_{30} to C_{56} fatty acids by an extract of *Mycobacterium tuberculosis* H37Ra. *J. Bacteriol.* 157:46–52.

123. Ramakrishnan, T., P. S. Murthy, and K. P. Gopinathan. 1972. Intermediary metabolism of mycobacteria. *Bacteriol. Rev.* 36:65–108.

124. Ratledge, C. 1982. Nutrition, growth and metabolism, p. 186–272. *In* C. Ratledge and J. Stanford (ed.), *The Biology of the Mycobacteria*, vol. 1. Academic Press, Ltd., London, United Kingdom.

125. Ratledge, C., and L. G. Dover. 2000. Iron metbolism in pathogenic bacteria. *Annu. Rev. Microbiol.* 54:881–941.

126. Rawat, M., G. L. Newton, M. Ko, G. J. Martinez, R. C. Fahey, and Y. Av-Gay. 2002. Mycothiol-deficient *Mycobacterium smegmatis* mutants are hypersensitive to alkylating agents, free radicals, and antibiotics. *Antimicrob. Agents Chemother.* 46:3348–3355.

127. Reed, D. J. 1995. Cystathionine. *Methods Enzymol.* 252:92–102.

128. Rindi, L., L. Fattorini, D. Bonanni, E. Iona, G. Freer, D. Tan, G. Deho, G. Orefici, and C. Garzelli. 2002. Involvement of the *fadD33* gene in the growth of *Mycobacterium tuberculosis* in the liver of BALB/c mice. *Microbiology* 148:3873–3880.

129. Rittmann, D., S. Schaffer, V. F. Wendisch, and H. Sahm. 2003. Fructose 1,6-bisphosphatase from *Corynebacterium glutamicum*: expression and deletion of the fbp gene and biochemical characterization of the enzyme. *Arch. Microbiol.* 180:285–292.

130. Rivera-Marrero, C. A., J. D. Ritzenthaler, S. A. Newburn, J. Roman, and R. D. Cummings. 2002. Molecular cloning and expression of a novel glycolipid sulfotransferase in *Mycobacterium tuberculosis*. *Microbiology* 148:783–792.

131. Rosenkrands, I., R. A. Slayden, J. Crawford, C. Aagaard, C. E. Barry III, and P. Andersen. 2002. Hypoxic response of *Mycobacterium tuberculosis* studied by metabolic labeling and proteome analysis of cellular and extracellular proteins. *J. Bacteriol.* 184:3485–3491.

132. Rosenkrands, I., K. Weldingh, S. Jacobsen, C. V. Hansen, W. Florio, I. Gianetri, and P. Andersen. 2000. Mapping and identification of *Mycobacterium tuberculosis* proteins by two-dimensional gel electrophoresis, microsequencing and immunodetection. *Electrophoresis* 21:935–948.

133. Sambandamurthy, V. K., X. Wang, B. Chen, R. G. Russell, S. Derrick, F. M. Collins, S. L. Morris, and W. R. Jacobs, Jr. 2002. A pantothenate auxotroph of *Mycobacterium tuberculosis* is highly attenuated and protects mice against tuberculosis. *Nat. Med.* 8:1171–1174.

134. Sanders, D. A., A. G. Staines, S. A. McMahon, M. R. McNeil, C. Whitfield, and J. H. Naismith. 2001. UDP-galactopyranose mutase has a novel structure and mechanism. *Nat. Struct. Biol.* 8:858–863.

135. Sareen, D., G. L. Newton, R. C. Fahey, and N. A. Buchmeier. 2003. Mycothiol is essential for growth of *Mycobacterium tuberculosis* Erdman. *J. Bacteriol.* 185:6736–6740.

136. Sareen, D., M. Steffek, G. L. Newton, and R. C. Fahey. 2002. ATP-dependent L-cysteine:1D-*myo*-inosityl 2-amino-2-deoxy-alpha-D-glucopyranoside ligase, mycothiol biosynthesis enzyme MshC, is related to class I cysteinyl-tRNA synthetases. *Biochemistry* 41:6885–6890.

137. Sassetti, C. M., D. H. Boyd, and E. J. Rubin. 2001. Comprehensive identification of conditionally essential genes in mycobacteria. *Proc. Natl. Acad. Sci. USA* 98:12712–12717.

138. Sassetti, C. M., and E. J. Rubin. 2003. Genetic requirements for mycobacterial survival during infection. *Proc. Natl. Acad. Sci. USA* 100:12989–12984.

139. Scherman, M. S., L. Kalbe-Bournonville, D. Bush, Y. Xin, L. Deng, and M. McNeil. 1996. Polyprenylphosphate-pentoses in mycobacteria are synthesized from 5-phosphoribose pyrophosphate. *J. Biol. Chem.* 271:29652–29658.

140. Schnappinger, D., S. Ehrt, M. I. Voskuil, Y. Liu, J. A. Mangan, I. Monahan, G. Dolganov, B. Efron, P. D. Butcher, C. Nathan, and S. G.K. 2003. Transcriptional adaptation of *Mycobacterium tuberculosis* within macrophages: insights into the phagosomal environment. *J. Exp. Med.* 198:693–704.

141. Schroeder, B. G., and C. E. Barry III. 2001. The specificity of methyl transferases involved in trans mycolic acid biosynthesis in *Mycobacterium tuberculosis* and *Mycobacterium smegmatis*. *Bioorg. Chem.* 29:164–177.

142. Sekowska, A., and A. Danchin. 2002. The methionine salvage pathway in *Bacillus subtilis*. *BMC Microbiol.* 2:8–12.

143. Sharma, V., S. Sharma, K. Hoener zu Bentrup, J. D. McKinney, D. G. Russell, W. R. Jacobs, Jr., and J. C. Sacchettini. 2000. Structure of isocitrate lyase, a persistence factor of *Mycobacterium tuberculosis*. *Nat. Struct. Biol.* 7:663–668.

144. Sherman, D. R., M. Voskuil, D. Schnappinger, R. Liao, M. I. Harrell, and G. K. Schoolnik. 2001. Regulation of the *Mycobacterium tuberculosis* hypoxic response gene encoding alpha-crystallin. *Proc. Natl. Acad. Sci. USA* 98:7534–7539.

145. Smith, C. V., C. C. Huang, A. Miczak, D. G. Russell, J. C. Sacchettini, and K. Honer zu Bentrup. 2003. Biochemical and structural studies of malate synthase from *Mycobacterium tuberculosis*. *J. Biol. Chem.* 278:1735–1743.

146. Smith, D. A., T. Parish, N. G. Stoker, and G. J. Bancroft. 2001. Characterization of auxotrophic mutants of *Mycobacterium tuberculosis* and their potential as vaccine candidates. *Infect. Immun.* 69:1142–1150.

147. Sone, N., K. Nagata, H. Kojima, J. Tajima, Y. Kodera, T. Kanamaru, S. Noguchi, and J. Sakamoto. 2001. A novel hydrophobic diheme c-type cytochrome. Purification from *Corynebacterium glutamicum* and analysis of the QcrCBA operon encoding three subunit proteins of a putative cytochrome reductase complex. *Biochim. Biophys. Acta* 1503:279–290.

148. Spiro, S., and J. R. Guest. 1991. Adaptive responses to oxygen limitation in *Eschericia coli*. *Trends Biochem. Sci.* 16:310–314.

149. Sugantino, M., R. Zheng, M. Yu, and J. S. Blanchard. 2003. *Mycobacterium tuberculosis* ketopantoate hydroxymethyltransferase: tetrahydrofolate-independent hydroxymethyltransferase and enolization reactions with alpha-keto acids. *Biochemistry* 42:191–199.

150. Sun, W., C. H. Williams, Jr., and V. Massey. 1997. The role of glycine 99 in L-lactate monooxygenase from *Mycobacterium smegmatis*. *J. Biol. Chem.* 272:27065–27076.

151. Timm, J., F. A. Post, L. G. Bekker, G. B. Walther, R. Manganelli, W. T. Chan, L. Tsenova, B. Gold, I. Smith, G. Kaplan, and J. D. McKinney. 2003. Differential expression of iron-, carbon-, and oxygen-responsive mycobacterial genes in the lungs of chronically infected mice and tuberculosis patients. *Proc. Natl. Acad. Sci. USA* 100:14321–14326.

152. Treumann, A., F. Xidong, L. McDonnell, P. J. Derrick, A. E. Ashcroft, D. Chatterjee, and S. W. Homans. 2002. 5-Methylthiopentose: a new substituent on lipoarabinomannan in *Mycobacterium tuberculosis*. *J. Mol. Biol.* 316:89–100.

153. Trivedi, O. A., P. Arora, V. Sridharan, R. Tickoo, D. Mohanty, and R. S. Gokhale. 2004. Enzyme activation and transfer of fatty acids as acyl-adenylates in mycobacteria. *Nature* 428:441–445.

154. Tyagi, A. K., T. L. Reddy, and T. A. Venkitasubramanian. 1976. Effect of oxygen tension on oxidative phosphorylation in *Mycobacterium phlei*. *Indian J. Biochem. Biophys.* 13:93–95.

155. Tyagi, A. K., T. L. Reddy, and T. A. Venkitasubramanian. 1976. Oxidative phosphorylation in *Mycobacterium tuberculosis* BCG. *Indian J. Biochem. Biophys.* 13:43–45.

156. Wayne, L. G., and G. A. Diaz. 1967. Autolysis and secondary growth of *Mycobacterium tuberculosis* in submerged culture. *J. Bacteriol.* 93:1374–1381.

157. Wayne, L. G., and K. Y. Lin. 1982. Glyoxylate metabolism and adaptation of *Mycobacterium tuberculosis* to survival under anaerobic conditions. *Infect. Immun.* 37:1042–1049.

158. Wayne, L. G., and C. D. Sohaskey. 2001. Nonreplicating persistence of *Mycobacterium tuberculosis*. *Annu. Rev. Microbiol.* 55:139–163.

159. Weber, I., C. Fritz, S. Ruttkowski, A. Kreft, and F. C. Bange. 2000. Anaerobic nitrate reductase (*narGHJI*) activity of *Mycobacterium bovis* BCG in vitro and its contribution to virulence in immunodeficient mice. *Mol. Microbiol.* 35:1017–1025.

160. Weston, A., R. J. Stern, R. E. Lee, P. M. Nassau, D. Monsey, S. L. Martin, M. S. Scherman, G. S. Besra, K. Duncan, and M. R. McNeil. 1997. Biosynthetic origin of mycobacterial cell wall galactofuranosyl residues. *Tubercle Lung Dis.* 78:123–131.

161. Wheeler, P. R. 2003. Leprosy—clues about the biochemistry of *Mycobacterium leprae* and its host-dependency from the genome. *World J. Microbiol. Biotechnol.* 19:1–16.

162. Wheeler, P. R. 1990. Recent research into the physiology of *Mycobacterium leprae*. *Adv. Microb. Physiol.* 31:71–124.

163. Wheeler, P. R. 2001. Understanding the physiology of difficult, pathogenic bacteria from analysis of their genome sequences. *J. Med. Microbiol.* 51:1–4.

164. Wheeler, P. R., K. Bulmer, and C. Ratledge. 1991. Fatty acid oxidation and the beta-oxidation complex in *Mycobacterium leprae* and two axenically cultivable mycobacteria that are pathogens. *J. Gen. Microbiol.* 137:885–893.

165. Wheeler, P. R., and C. Ratledge. 1994. Metabolism of *Mycobacterium tuberculosis*, p. 353–388. *In* B. R. Bloom (ed.), *Tuberculosis. Pathogenesis, Protection, and Control*. ASM Press, Washington, D.C.

166. Williams, S. J., R. H. Senaratne, J. D. Mougous, L. W. Riley, and C. R. Bertozzi. 2002. 5′-Adenosinephosphosulfate lies at a metabolic branch point in mycobacteria. *J. Biol. Chem.* 277:32606–32615.

167. Wolucka, B. A., and E. De Hoffmann. 1995. The presence of beta-D-ribosyl-1-monophosphodecaprenol in mycobacteria. *J. Biol. Chem.* 270:20151–20155.

168. Wolucka, B. A., M. R. McNeil, E. de Hoffmann, T. Chojnacki, and P. J. Brennan. 1994. Recognition of the lipid intermediate for arabinogalactan/arabinomannan biosynthesis and its relation to the mode of action of ethambutol on mycobacteria. *J. Biol. Chem.* 269:23328–23335.

169. Wooff, E., S. L. Michell, S. V. Gordon, M. A. Chambers, S. Bardarov, W. R. Jacobs, Jr., R. G. Hewinson, and P. R.

Wheeler. 2002. Functional genomics reveals the sole sulfate transporter of the *Mycobacterium tuberculosis* complex and its relevance to the acquisition of sulfur *in vivo*. *Mol. Microbiol.* **43:**653–663.

170. Xin, Y., R. E. Lee, M. S. Scherman, K. H. Khoo, G. S. Besra, P. J. Brennan, and M. McNeil. 1997. Characterization of in vitro synthesized arabinan of mycobacterial cell walls. *Biochim. Biophys. Acta* **1335:**231–234.

171. Yeh, S. R., M. Couture, Y. Ouellet, M. Guertin, and D. L. Rousseau. 2000. A cooperative oxygen binding hemoglobin from *Mycobacterium tuberculosis*. Stabilization of heme ligands by a distal tyrosine residue. *J. Biol. Chem.* **275:**1679–1684.

172. Yuan, Y., and C. E. Barry III. 1996. A common mechanism for the biosynthesis of methoxy and cyclopropyl mycolic acids in *Mycobacterium tuberculosis*. *Proc. Natl. Acad. Sci. USA* **93:**12828–12833.

173. Yuan, Y., R. E. Lee, G. S. Besra, J. T. Belisle, and C. E. Barry III. 1995. Identification of a gene involved in the biosynthesis of cyclopropanated mycolic acids in *Mycobacterium tuberculosis*. *Proc. Natl. Acad. Sci. USA* **92:**6630–6634.

174. Zhang, L., M. B. Goren, T. J. Holzer, and B. R. Andersen. 1988. Effect of *Mycobacterium tuberculosis*-derived sulfolipid I on human phagocytic cells. *Infect. Immun.* **56:**2876–2883.

175. Zheng, R., and J. S. Blanchard. 2001. Steady-state and pre-steady-state kinetic analysis of *Mycobacterium tuberculosis* pantothenate synthetase. *Biochemistry* **40:**12904–12912.

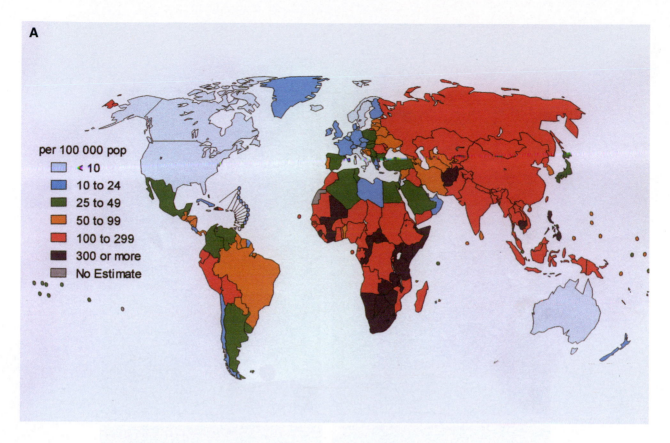

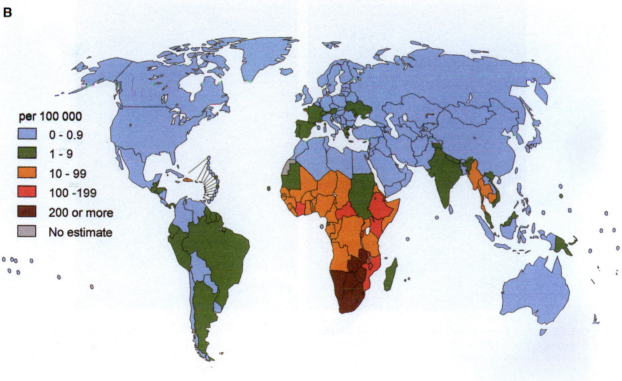

Color Plate 1. (Chapter 1) Global TB incidence rates (per 100,000 population per year) at the start of 2000 (13). (A) All forms of TB. (B) HIV-related TB. The boundaries and names shown and the designations used on this map do not imply the expression of any opinion whatsoever on the part of the World Health Organization concerning the legal status of any country, territory, city or area or of its authorities, or concerning the delimitation of its frontiers or boundaries. Dotted lines on maps represent approximate border lines for which there may not yet be full agreement. Panel A is reprinted from reference 68a in chapter 1. Panel B is reprinted from reference 13 in chapter 1. Copyrighted © 2003, American Medical Association. All rights reserved.

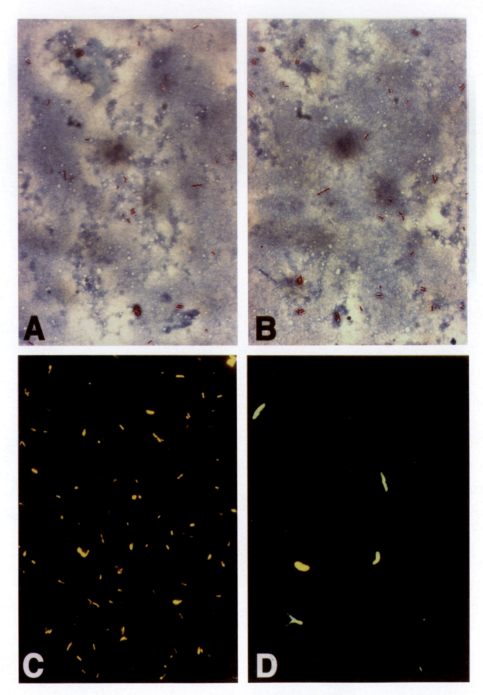

Color Plate 2. (Chapter 4) *M. tuberculosis* in smears from concentrated sputum specimens. (A and B) Ziehl-Neelsen stain (total magnification, x1,125); (C) auramine stain, fluorescent microscopy (total magnification x1,440); (D) auramine stain, fluorescent microscopy (total magnification, x2,000).

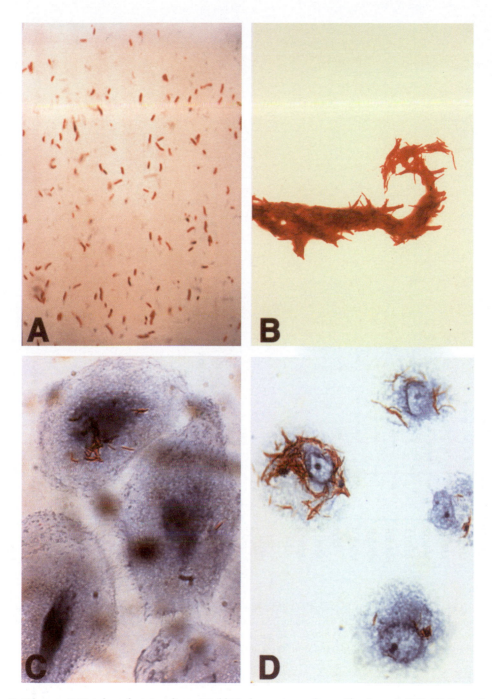

Color Plate 3. (Chapter 4) *M. tuberculosis* in cultures (Ziehl-Neelsen stain, total magnification, x1,125). (A) Smear from a culture grown on 7H11 agar; (B) smear from 7H12 broth culture showing "cord formation"; (C and D) intracellular growth in human monocyte-derived macrophages.

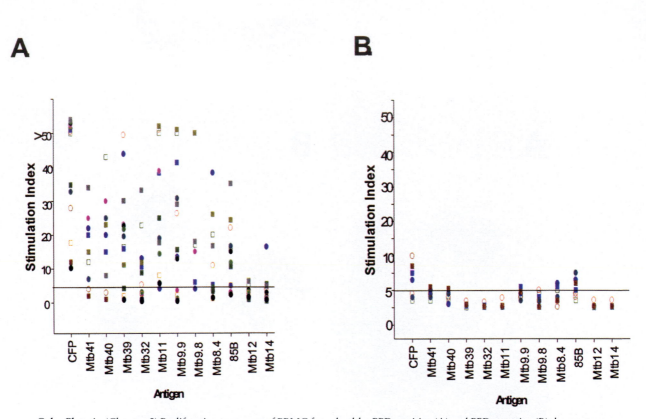

Color Plate 4. (Chapter 5) Proliferative responses of PBMC from healthy PPD-positive (A) and PPD-negative (B) donors to selected recombinant antigens. Donor PBMC were stimulated in vitro with CFP or the indicated recombinant antigens. Mtb12 and Mtb14 are two poorly immunogenic *M. tuberculosis* antigens included in this assay to serve as controls. Identical symbols indicate responses of the same donor PBMC to the different antigens.

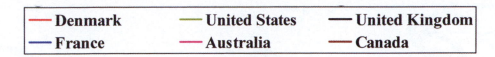

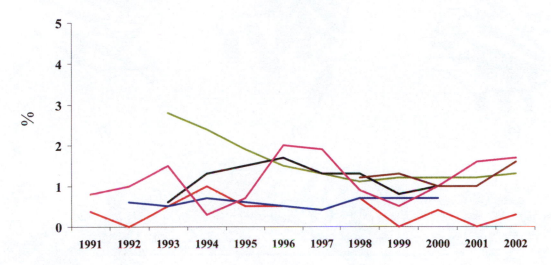

Color Plate 5. (Chapter 7) Trends of MDR-TB in selected high-income countries. MDR-TB in high-income countries has remained at very low levels after the sound implementation of measures to prevent, contain, and monitor this form of tuberculosis in the early 1990s. The majority of MDR-TB cases in these countries are reported in foreign-born individuals. Data from references 13a, 29, 30, 81a, 97, and 109 in chapter 7; Staten Serum Institute, National Surveillance of Communicable Diseases, *Epi-News* (http://www.ssi.dk); and CDC, Reported tuberculosis in the United States, 2002 (http://www.cdc.gov/nchstp/bb/surv).

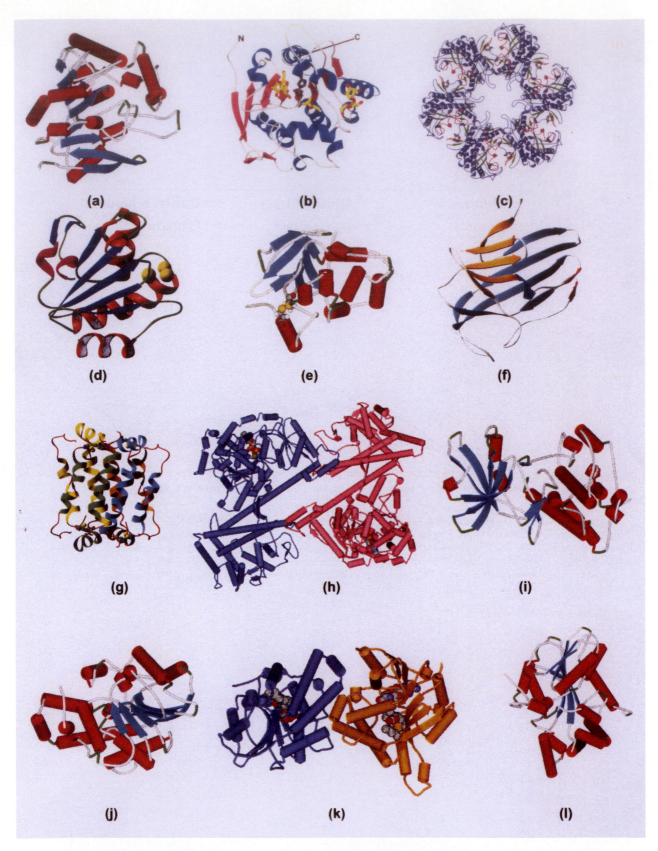

Color Plate 6. (Chapter 11) Ribbon diagrams of representative protein structures determined by the TB Structural Genomics Consortium. In general. α-helices and β-strands are colored red and cyan, respectively; if the PDB file contains more than one monomer, each subunit is colored differently. For each structure, the PDB code and the Rv number are given and, where known, the anotated function. These figures were prepared with the program WebLabViewerPro and RIBBONS. (a) 1dgy, Rv0129c—Ag85C; (b) 1f0p, Rv1886c—Ag85B; (c) 1hto, Rv2220—GlnA; (d) 1lu4, Rv2878c—MPT53; (e) 1nyo, Rv2875—MPB70; (f) 1lmi, Rv1926c—MPT63; (g) no pdb code, Rv0203; (h) 1nkt, Rv3240c—SecA1; (i) 1mru, Rv0014c—PknB; (j) 1lle, Rv0470c—PcaA; (k) 1kpg, Rv3392c—CcmA1; (l) 1kpi, Rv0503c—CcmA2. Reprinted from reference 41 in chapter 11. © 2003 with permission from Elsevier.

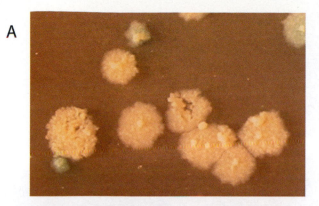

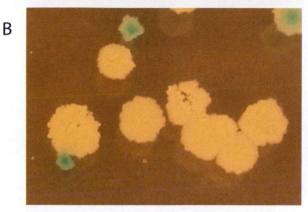

Color Plate 7. (Chapter 12) Section of colonies in whch a second crossover has taken place by using counter-selection and color screening. Bacteria carrying a single crossover of a plasmid carrying *sacB* and *IacZ* (i.e., sucrose-sensitive, *IacZ*⁺) are plated onto medium containing sucrose and 5-bromo-4-chloro-3-indolyl-β-D-galactoside. Most bacteria are killed through sucrose sensitivity. Colonies that grow are resistant through loss of the vector by a double crossover (*lacZ*, white) or through a spontaneous mutation and still contain the vector (*lacZ*⁺, blue). The same colonies are shown from the top (A) and bottom (B); the photograph in panel B has been reversed to make the comparison clearer. Plate courtesy of F. Mova-hedzadeh.

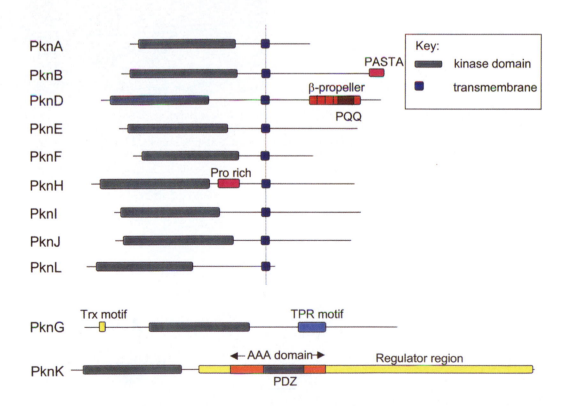

Color Plate 8. (Chapter 22) Structural analyses of *M. tuberculosis* STPKs. The motifs were drawn on a schematic representation of the linear peptide sequence. Reprinted from Y. Av-Gay and M. Everett, *Trends Microbiol.* 8:238–244, 2000. © 2000 with permission from Elsevier.

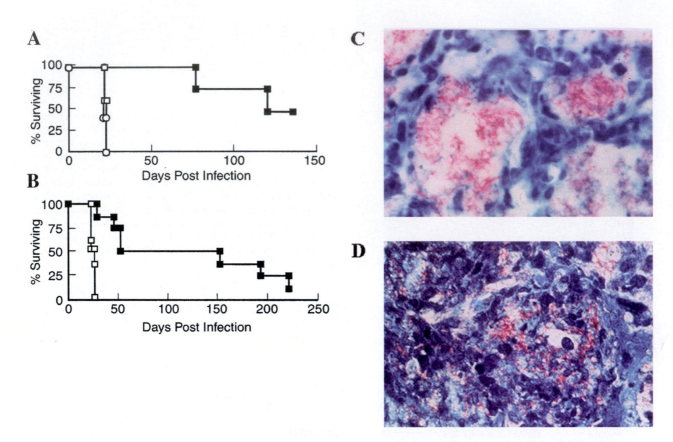

Color Plate 9. (Chapter 32) (A and B) Survival of mice infected inratracheally with *M. tuberculosis* Erdman which has been incubated with MAb 9d8 (Mtb-9d8) (black squares) or conrols (open symbols). (A) Experiment performed with C57BL/6 mice, using ascites. (B) Experiment performed with BALB/c mice, using purified MAb preparations (MAb 9d8 or an isotype-matched anti-cryptococcal MAb). Survival was significantly longer in the presence of MAb 9d8 (P < 0.01). (C and D) Lung histology of mice infected with *M. tuberculosis* preincubated with MAb 9d8 or control. (C) In the lungs of mice receiving Mtb-9d8, acid-fast bacilli are contained inside well-delineated granulomatous structures. (D) In the lungs of control mice, acid-fast bacilli are dispersed throughout the tissue, without well-defined granulomatous formation (B). Adapted from R. Teitelbaum et al., *Proc. Natl. Acad. Sci.* USA **95**:15688-15693, 1998.

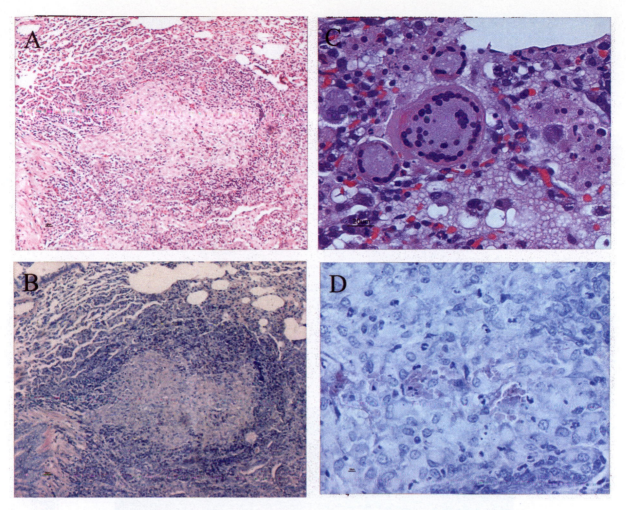

Color Plate 10. (Chapter 36) Histopathology of caseous necrosis in rabbit pulmonary tubercles 5 weeks following infection with *M. bovis.* (A) A caseous center (hematoxylin and eosin stain), revealing disintegrating epithelioid macrophages at the center and a rim of basophilic mononuclear cells and early capillary formation on the periphery. (B) Same caseous center as in panel A (acid-fast stain), showing the relative paucity of acid-fast bacilli in rabbit tubercles at 5 weeks. (C) Multinucleated (Langhans') giant cell in rabbit lung tissues at 5 weeks (hematoxylin and eosin stain). (D) Acid-fast stain and high-power (magnification, ×400) view of a peripheral region of a 5-week old-caseous rabbit tubercle showing several acid-fast bacilli and some weakly acid-fast debris from destroyed bacilli. Courtesy of M. Yoder, Johns Hopkins University.

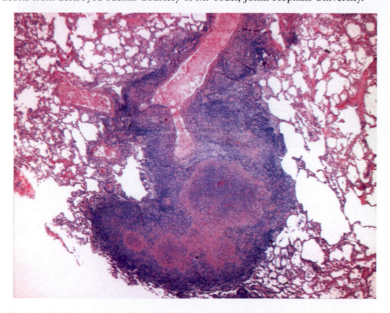

Color Plate 11. (Chapter 36) Caseous granuloma in the lung of a cynomolgus macaque infected for 6 weeks with *M. tuberculosis.* In monkeys, solid as well as caseous granulomas can be observed.

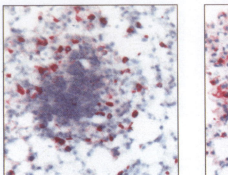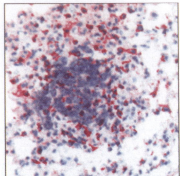

Color Plate 12. (Chapter 37) Immunohistochemical staining of infected mouse lung lesions for the presence of CD4 cells (left) or CD8 cells (right).

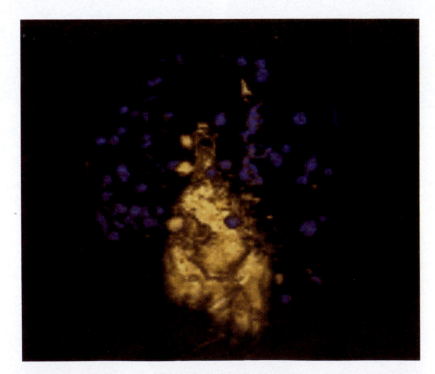

Color Plate 13. (Chapter 37) Magnetic resonance image of a guinea pig lung section 30 days after aerosol infection. Each individual granulomatous lesion has been colorized blue. The streak on the right corresponds to inflammation in the pleural space. The large object in the center is the mediastinal lymph node, which becomes extremely large (and heavily necrotic) in unprotected animals. Computer analysis of such images can provide data on both lesion number and distribution, as well as lesion volumes.

Chapter 21

Iron Metabolism in the Tubercle Bacillus and Other Mycobacteria

LUIS E. N. QUADRI AND COLIN RATLEDGE

Iron is an essential nutrient for the well-being of humans. Without an adequate supply of it in our diet, anemia and its various complications quickly result. Equally, iron is essential for the growth of bacteria, except perhaps for the lactic acid bacteria; in order for bacteria to be successful pathogens within an animal host, it is essential that they acquire iron and, of course, all their other nutrients from the host tissues and fluids. A priority for a bacterium being able to grow in vivo is therefore considered to be the acquisition of iron, since iron, alone among the nutrients, is effectively insoluble at neutral pH values. [The solubility of ferric iron, Fe(III), at pH 7 has been recently recalculated at approximately 10^{-10} M (4, 10), which, although much higher than the previously used, and often quoted, figure of 10^{-18} M, is still 4 orders of magnitude lower than that needed to support microbial growth without the intervention of some solubilizing agent.] While pathogenicity is clearly a multifactorial process and the defenses of the host against the invading bacteria can be many and varied, if the would-be pathogen cannot gain its essential iron from the animal it has chosen to invade, then it cannot grow and will be eliminated from the body. Iron is essential because it is required for the functioning of numerous enzymes and other proteins; these include synthesis of the heme nucleus of various cytochromes (these are involved with energy production and in the metabolism of a number of compounds including desaturase reactions in the formation of mycobacterial lipids), in the functioning of oxygenases and oxidases, and by acting as an essential cofactor with many enzymes, including aconitase as part of the essential tricarboxylic acid cycle.

The mechanism of iron acquisition by mycobacteria, and by the tubercle bacillus in particular, is therefore one of the central issues concerning the pathogenicity of this group of bacteria. In this chapter we describe the key components of the iron acquisition system, how they interlink in the sequestration of iron from the host sources of iron, and how the iron is then made available to the bacterial cell for its own purposes. The biochemistry of this process has been established for some years now, but it is only over the past decade that the key genes involved in the regulation of iron uptake and metabolism have been identified. The major impetus for this genetic understanding has, of course, come about as a result of the sequencing of the tubercle bacillus genome, which has revealed much about how, and when, the key components are synthesized to meet the changing demands of the bacterial cell for iron. How the whole biochemistry of the cell then responds to the availability—or lack of availability—of iron is now being understood through the use of proteomics and transcriptomics. There is, however, still some considerable way to go before the intricate details of the process are finally unraveled. Perhaps as a means of encouraging further research in this area, the fact that iron metabolism is central to the pathogenicity of the mycobacteria could well form one of the key areas for the design of future antimycobacterial agents. Knock out iron acquisition or metabolism within the bacteria, and you have effectively stopped them from growing.

A number of reviews have been written on iron metabolism in pathogenic bacteria in general (6, 8, 13, 34, 56) and in mycobacteria in particular (15, 55, 59, 68) over the past few years. Other recent general reviews of mycobacteria have also included details of iron metabolism, and these may also be useful (28, 49, 73).

COMPONENTS OF THE MYCOBACTERIAL IRON ACQUISITION SYSTEM

The sources of iron within a host that are accessed by pathogenic bacteria are primarily (i) hemo-

Luis E. N. Quadri • Department of Microbiology and Immunology, Medical College of Cornell University, New York, NY 10021. Colin Ratledge • Department of Biological Sciences, University of Hull, Hull HU6 7RX, United Kingdom.

globin, which is utilized by hemolytic bacteria, thereby causing jaundice and various septicemias; (ii) various iron-transporting molecules present in the blood or various fluids of the body and known as the transferrins and lactoferrins, which are two structurally related proteins; and (iii) ferritin, which is the ubiquitous iron storage protein found in all cell types in the body.

It is only the last two sources that are usable by the mycobacteria. Hemoglobin is not usually used by mycobacteria, although the species known as *Mycobacterium haemophilum* is able to use the iron within the heme nucleus. Removal of iron from transferrin, lactoferrin, and ferritin is considered to require the presence of iron-binding compounds specifically produced by the bacteria for this purpose. These compounds are collectively known as siderophores. The production of siderophores by pathogenic and nonpathogenic bacteria has been widely reviewed (29, 66, 78). The synthesis of all siderophores is greatly increased when there is a lack of iron for microbial growth; synthesis of siderophores is therefore an early, if not the earliest, response of a pathogen when it encounters iron deprivation in vivo. Conversely, the infected host attempts to withhold the availability of free iron from the invading bacteria in order to check their multiplication (56, 75). However, the strength of iron binding by the siderophores is considerably greater than that of transferrin, lactoferrin, and ferritin; consequently, bacteria are able to acquire iron and commence their infective process.

In the pathogenic mycobacteria, the extracellular siderophore is carboxymycobactin, which is structurally related to mycobactin (Fig. 1), a molecule that was first isolated and characterized in the 1950s and 1960s by Snow and colleagues (67). Mycobactin has been found in all mycobacteria, pathogens and nonpathogens alike, except for some strains of *M. vaccae*, *M. avium*, *M. paratuberculosis* (55), and possibly *M. chelonae*, *M. parafortuitum*, and *M. thermoresistible* (67). Its presence in *M. leprae* has been ruled out in view of the absence of key genes for its biosynthesis (12, 76). Mycobactin itself, though, does not occur extracellularly and thus cannot be the means of sequestering iron from the host. Instead, mycobactin is considered to be involved in the short-term storage of iron within the cell envelope of the mycobacterium, serving to hold the iron, which was brought to the cell via carboxymycobactin, in a form that can be used by the cell as needed (55, 56). This is shown diagrammatically in Fig. 2. The mechanism by which the iron is removed from mycobactin, so that it can be transported across the cell membrane into the cytoplasm, involves reduction of Fe(III) to Fe(II) by a ferrimycobactin reductase. It has been suggested that, following reduction, salicylic acid (2-hydroxybenzoic acid) would be involved in the process as a possible acceptor and transporter of ferrous ions into the cell (55) (Fig. 2).

Salicylic acid is a precursor of both mycobactin and carboxymycobactin (Fig. 1), and, although it is not involved in the biosynthesis of any other cell component, neither mycobactin nor carboxymy-

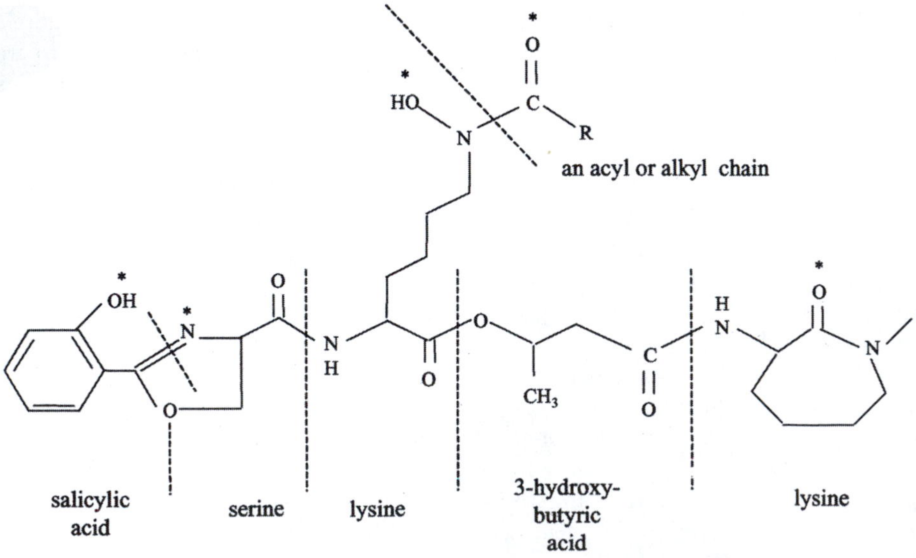

Figure 1. Structures of mycobactin and carboxymycobactin T from *M. tuberculosis*. The siderophores differ only in the nature of the R side chain. The side chain usually has a *cis* double bond at C-2 and a length of 17 to 20 carbons in mycobactin T (67) or 2 to 9 carbons followed by a carboxylic group (or its methyl ester form) in carboxymycobactin T (26, 42). The atoms involved in iron binding are indicated by asterisks.

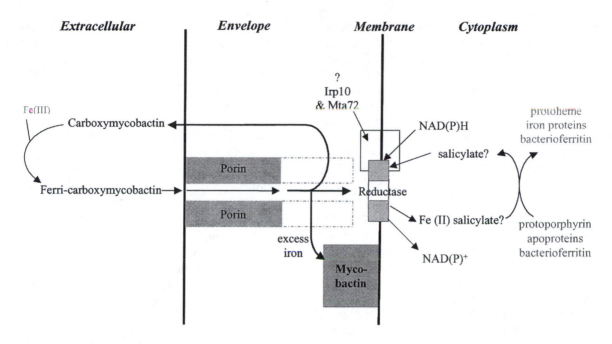

Figure 2. Diagram showing the suggested route of uptake of iron into *M. tuberculosis* via the carboxymycobactin route.

cobactin (or both together) can satisfy the growth requirement of salicylate auxotrophs (1), thus implying a secondary function(s) for this molecule. One such function is, as suggested above, to be the means of transferring Fe(II) from the reduced ferromycobactin across the membrane for subsequent insertion into protoporphyrins, apoproteins, or, for long-term storage within the cytoplasm, bacterioferritin.

Bacterioferritins occur in many bacteria, including *M. tuberculosis*, *M. leprae*, and a number of other mycobacteria, where their presence has been determined either directly or by recognition of one of the two genes, *brf1* or *brf2*, involved in their synthesis (7, 39, 46, 50). Bacterioferritins differ from animal ferritins in that they contain, for some unknown purpose, between 8 and 12 heme groups bound between two polypeptides that make up a 24-subunit complex. Each subunit has a molecular size of about 18 kDa. Within the hollow sphere created by this structure may reside up to 4,000 atoms of iron as a crystalline ferric oxide. Since bacterioferritin occurs within the cytoplasm of the bacterial cell, it serves to provide an iron store that can then be used by the cell machinery as required for metabolic activities: it is therefore the cytoplasmic iron store as opposed to mycobactin which acts as an intraenvelope iron store. The reason why both iron storage systems are needed has been discussed in some detail elsewhere (55). Essentially, two separate iron storage mechanisms are needed because, during iron deprivation, which is probably experienced by the pathogens during their growth in the

macrophages of the host, the biosynthesis of heme and other iron-containing molecules, including bacterioferritin, is repressed. Unlike *Escherichia coli* and other bacteria which have only one iron storage system, mycobacteria are able to repress porphyrin biosynthesis when deprived of iron so that, when iron is restored to them, there are no acceptor molecules available within the cell to take up the available iron. A transition period is therefore required during which porphyrins, and other precursors of the iron-containing compounds, need to be synthesized. Since iron would be cytotoxic if left uncomplexed within the cytoplasm, it is then withheld from entry into the cytoplasm until acceptor molecules for it are synthesized. Since it would be disadvantageous for mycobacteria to be unable to acquire iron should it suddenly become available to them when they are in an iron-deprived state, they use mycobactin as a means of holding the iron temporarily within the envelope and then pass this into the cytoplasm as the demand for iron dictates. The ferrimycobactin reductase, as depicted in Fig. 2, is therefore a crucial system for controlling the influx of iron into the cytoplasm.

In nonpathogenic mycobacteria, the principal extracellular siderophores are known as exochelins. This term was originally applied collectively to all mycobacterial siderophores before their structures were determined; subsequently, it became clear that the pathogenic species and the nonpathogens produced structurally different molecules and that two different names were needed. Some confusion has arisen because one or two research groups continue to use the term "exochelin" for the extracellular siderophores from *M. tuberculosis* and related species; this is incorrect, and the term "carboxymycobactin" should be used instead. The structures of the exochelins from *M. smegmatis* and *M. neoaurum,* designated, respectively, exochelin MS and exochelin MN, have been described previously (63, 64). Exochelins have also been found to occur in *M. vaccae* (48), an "armadillo-derived" *Mycobacterium* species (30), and several other saprophytic mycobacteria (C. Ratledge and M. Ewing, unpublished work). They are linear penta- and hexapeptides in which hydroxamate groups form the main iron-binding centers, although exochelin MN contains a unique β-hydroxyhistidine moiety in the iron chelation center (Fig. 3).

One of the key differences between the mode of iron uptake via exochelin MS and the carboxymycobactins is that the former occurs by an active transport system, thus involving the use of ATP, whereas the latter occurs by a facilitated-diffusion system which is insensitive to energy poisons and uncouplers of oxidative phosphorylation (70, 71). This is shown diagrammatically in Fig. 4, which should then be contrasted with the uptake system shown in Fig. 2. However, the uptake of iron from exochelin MN also appears to occur by a facilitated diffusion process (30, 32), indicating that each exochelin probably has its own mechanism of uptake. In spite of the uptake of ferri-exochelin MN being by a facilitated diffusion process, this compound cannot be assimilated by

M. smegmatis (30), indicating that there is some inherent specificity in the process, possibly being due to the ferri-exochelin MN being in a highly charged state at physiological pH values (17). This property could well facilitate proton-assisted Fe(III) exchange between exochelin MN and the lipophilic mycobactin in the cell envelope but does not entirely explain why it cannot be taken up by *M. smegmatis*. It is, however, taken up by *M. leprae* (see below).

One further complication should be mentioned. In the nonpathogenic species, as typified by *M. smegmatis* and *M. neoaurum*, small amounts of carboxymycobactin are also synthesized. Although the amounts produced are normally less than 5% of the amount of exochelin (57), it does mean that mutants designed to show auxotrophy for exochelin cannot be produced since the cells then switch to using the carboxymycobactin route of iron acquisition.

GENETICS OF IRON ACQUISITION, IRON STORAGE, AND IRON-DEPENDENT REGULATION OF GENE EXPRESSION IN MYCOBACTERIA

The work of several groups has allowed significant advances in the identification of genes with demonstrated or predicted functions in iron acquisition, iron storage, and iron-dependent regulation of gene expression in *Mycobacterium* species. In particular, considerable progress has been made toward the

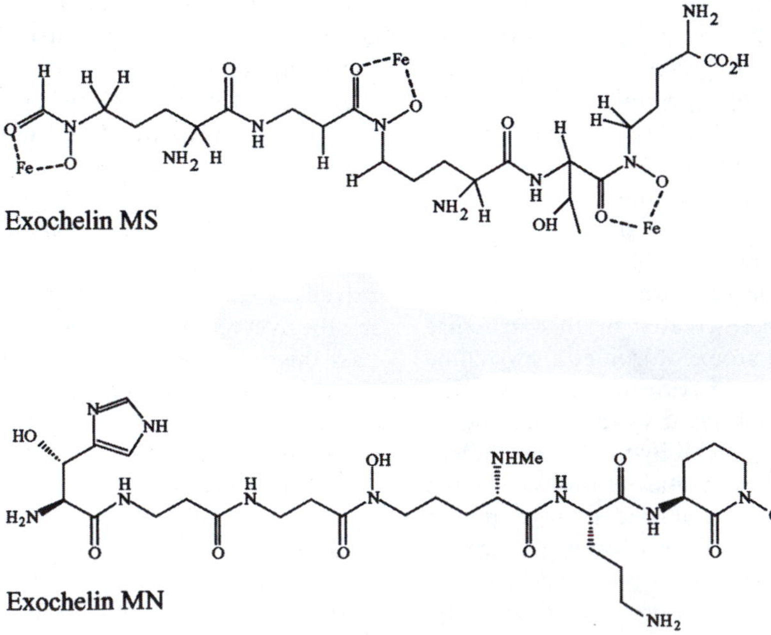

Figure 3. (Top) Structure of exochelin MS from *M. smegmatis.* Reproduced with permission from reference 64. © The Biochemical Society. (Bottom) Structure of exochelin MN from *M. neoaurum.* Reprinted from reference 63. © 1995, with permission from Elsevier.

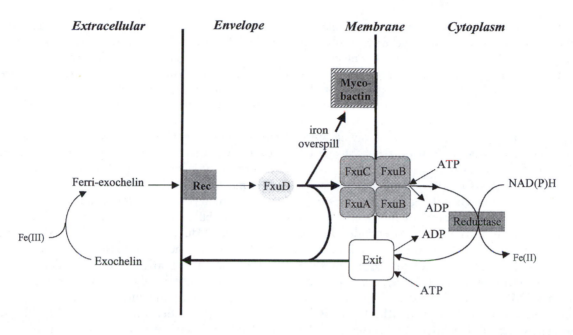

Figure 4. Diagram showing the suggested route of uptake of iron into *M. smegmatis* via the exochelin-mediated route.

identification of the biosynthesis pathways for the peptidosiderophores (i.e., exochelins) and peptide-polyketide hybrid siderophores (i.e., mycobactins and carboxymycobactins) produced by *Mycobacterium* species. The sequence analysis of the enzymes encoded in the gene clusters involved in siderophore biosynthesis has led to several models being proposed for the biosynthesis of these iron chelators within the frame of the multiple-carrier thiotemplate mechanism for the assembly of nonribosomally synthesized peptide and polyketide products. By this mechanism, the structural cores of the siderophores are synthesized from simple building blocks by the concerted action of peptide arylation enzymes, nonribosomal peptide synthetases, and polyketide synthases. Tremendous progress has also been made toward understanding how mycobacteria regulate gene expression in response to iron. Recent studies of this subject have uncovered a mechanism for iron-dependent regulation of gene expression that controls the transcription of many mycobacterial genes, including those required for siderophore production and iron storage. These studies have also illustrated that adequate iron homeostasis could be a matter of life or death for some mycobacteria and suggested the activation of an iron-starvation adaptive response in mycobacteria growing in the host environment.

Mycobactin/Carboxymycobactin Gene Cluster of *M. tuberculosis*

In 1998, more than 30 years after the first mycobactin structure was reported (67), the first gene cluster encoding the core of the biosynthetic machinery needed for the production of mycobactin and carboxymycobactin was identified in the genome of *M. tuberculosis* H37Rv (11, 53). Notably, neither possible siderophore transport genes (which may not be necessary since the uptake of ferri-carboxymycobactin occurs by facilitated diffusion and not active transport [Fig. 2]) nor ferri-mycobactin reductase [which might be a general NAD(P)$^+$-linked enzyme rather than a specific siderophore reductase] is present in the cluster. The cluster is referred to as the *mbt* cluster, spans 24 kb, and is the only locus in the genome with the potential to encode an enzymatic machinery that, based on the model for nonribosomal peptide and polyketide biosynthesis, could be capable of assembling peptide-polyketide hybrid compounds with the structural characteristics of mycobactin and carboxymycobactin of *M. tuberculosis* (53). This observation reinforced the early hypothesis that both families of siderophores were derived from a structural core synthesized by the same enzymes. More recently, De Voss and coworkers (16) reported that deletion of the peptide synthetase gene *mbtB* of the *mbt* cluster of *M. tuberculosis* resulted in a mutant unable to produce either mycobactin or carboxymycobactin. Furthermore, the mutant showed a dramatic decrease in growth both in iron-deficient medium and inside macrophages (16). The phenotype of the mutant conclusively linked the production of mycobactin and carboxymycobactin to the *mbt* gene cluster and clearly illustrated the relevance of one or both of these siderophores for bacterial multiplication in iron-limiting medium and intracellularly. However, the relative importance of mycobactin and carboxymycobactin could not be assessed since the mutant was blocked in the pathway common to both siderophores. Interestingly, the decreased yet significant growth of the *mbtB* mutant in iron-deficient environments might suggest the existence of additional iron acquisition systems in *M. tuberculosis*, perhaps involving citric acid or some other cationic transporter, as suggested by Calder and Horwitz (9).

Sequence analysis of the *mbt* gene cluster revealed that it encompasses 10 genes, named *mbtA* through *mbtJ* (Fig. 5). The catalytic functions and domain organization of the enzymes encoded in the cluster have been assigned based on analysis of their amino acid sequences (53). Among these enzymes are a peptide arylation enzyme (MbtA), three peptide synthetases (MbtB, MbtE, and MbtF), and two polyketide synthases (MbtC and MbtD). A model for the MbtABCDEF-dependent biosynthesis of the mycobactin/carboxymycobactin peptide-polyketide hybrid core via a multiple-carrier thiotemplate mechanism has been proposed within the framework of the current model for nonribosomal peptide and polyketide biosynthesis (15, 52, 53). In line with this model, MbtABCDEF are thought to synthesize the peptide-polyketide core of the siderophores from salicylate, serine, lysine, and acyl coenzyme A thioesters as donors for the biosynthesis of the polyketide moiety of the siderophores. Consistent with this model, MbtA has been shown to utilize ATP to activate sali-

cylate, as an enzyme-bound salicyloyl-adenylate (salicyloyl-AMP), and to selectively recognize the posttranslationally phosphopantetheinylated N-terminal aryl carrier protein domain of MbtB as a target for transfer of the salicyloyl moiety of salicyloyl-AMP (53). The transfer produces the salicyloyl-MbtB intermediate, which represents an initial and committed covalent acyl enzyme intermediate in the acyl chain assembly of mycobactin and carboxymycobactin. Recent results indicate that the MbtA homolog found in *M. smegmatis* (see below) is also able to add salicylate to the aryl carrier protein domain of *M. tuberculosis* MbtB and that the *M. tuberculosis* peptide synthetase, MbtF, activates Lys (L. E. N. Quadri, unpublished results). Two possible tailoring enzymes, MbtG and MbtJ/LipK, are also encoded in the cluster. MbtG is a predicted lysine-N-oxygenase, presumably involved in the hydroxylation of the lysine residues of the siderophores, while MbtJ/LipK is a probable esterase/acetyl hydrolase that might be involved in the transfer of alkyl substituents to the side chain of the internal lysine residue of the peptide-polyketide backbone. Also encoded in the cluster is the enzyme MbtI/TrpE2, which could be involved in salicylate biosynthesis. Finally, the hypothetical protein MbtH, which is encoded by a small gene at the 3' end of the cluster, has no predictable function based on its amino acid sequence. Interestingly, MbtH homologs have been noted in several gene clusters involved in the biosynthesis of nonribosomally synthesized peptides, including several siderophores (53).

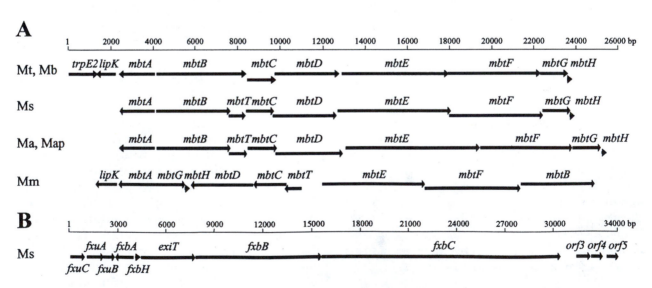

Figure 5. Organization of *Mycobacterium* gene clusters encoding the core of the biosynthetic machinery involved in the production of siderophores. (A) Gene clusters involved in the production of the aryl-capped peptide-polyketide mycobactin and carboxymycobactin siderophores in various *Mycobacterium* species. (B) Gene clusters involved in the production of the peptide siderophore exochelin MS. Mt, *M. tuberculosis*; Mb, *M. bovis*; Ms, *M. smegmatis*; Ma, *M. avium*; Map, *M. avium* subsp. *paratuberculosis*; Mm, *M. marinum*. See the text for details of gene functions.

Two phosphopantetheinyl transferases (PptT and AcpS) encoded by two unlinked genes (*pptT* and *acpS*) apart from the *mbt* cluster are thought to be required for siderophore synthesis as well. PptT has been shown to cause posttranslational phosphopantetheinylation of carrier protein domains in the peptide synthetases encoded in the *mbt* cluster, while AcpS is the predicted enzyme for phosphopantetheinylation of the carrier protein domains in the polyketide synthase MbtD (53).

Mycobactin/Carboxymycobactin Gene Clusters of Mycobacteria Other than *M. tuberculosis*

Mycobactins have been isolated from *M. tuberculosis* and most other mycobacteria, both pathogens and nonpathogens alike. The only exceptions would appear to be some (but not necessarily all) strains of *M. paratuberculosis*, *M. vaccae*, *M. chelonae*, *M. parafortuium*, and *M. thermoresistible* (3, 55, 67).

As detailed in the section on components of the mycobacterial iron acquisition system (above), the extracellular siderophores of mycobacteria fall into two types. Although initially both types were termed exochelins, this was before their structures were established. Those from the pathogenic species are now known to be structurally related to mycobactin itself and are termed carboxymycobactins (Fig. 1), whereas those from the nonpathogenic species are peptido-derivatives for which the collective name of "exochelins" is retained (Fig. 3). Although no exochelins have been found in any pathogenic species, carboxymycobactins have been recognized in both *M. smegmatis* and *M. neoaurum*, but only at about 5 to 10% of the total amount of siderophores (41, 57), and thus not only the genes for production of their corresponding exochelins but also those for production of carboxymycobactin and mycobactin will occur in these species.

BLAST searches for homologs of the *M. tuberculosis* proteins encoded in the *mbt* cluster in the partially sequenced genomes of other *Mycobacterium* species revealed that similar gene clusters are present in *M. smegmatis*, *M. bovis*, *M. avium*, *M. avium* subsp. *Paratuberculosis*, and *M. marinum* (Fig. 5) (Quadri, unpublished). No *mbt* cluster was found in the finished genome of *M. leprae* (12), a *Mycobacterium* species considered to lack mycobactin and presumably also carboxymycobactin production (40). Nevertheless, the possibility that some of the peptide/polyketide synthetase genes in *M. leprae* are involved in the synthesis some type of peptidosiderophore cannot be ruled out (76). In connection with this possibility, the ability of *M. leprae* to acquire iron attached to *M. neoaurum* exochelin MN has been established

(30). The effect, however, appears to be fairly specific, since ferri-exochelins and ferri-carboxymycobactins from other mycobacteria were not assimilated. Thus, even though exochelin MN was taken up by *M. leprae* by a facilitated-diffusion type of process, it is a process with some inherent specificity.

The comparison of the *mbt* clusters of *M. tuberculosis*, *M. smegmatis*, *M. bovis*, *M. avium*, *M. avium* subsp. *paratuberculosis,* and *M. marinum* indicates that there are significant differences in the organization of the genes present in the clusters of the different species (Fig. 5) (Quadri, unpublished). The clusters of *M. tuberculosis* and *M. bovis* appear to be identical in their *mbtA-mbtH* gene organization. The gene clusters of *M. smegmatis*, *M. avium*, and *M. avium* subsp. *paratuberculosis* appear to lack the *mbtJ/lipK* and *mbtI/irpE2* genes, which were not found at the 5' ends or in close proximity to the clusters. A significant change in gene organization can be seen in the cluster of *M. marinum*. This cluster also appears to lack the *mbtI/irpE2* gene. As with the *M. tuberculosis mbt* cluster, no siderophore transport genes or ferric reductase genes appear to be present in the *mbt* clusters of the other mycobacteria.

One additional noticeable difference among the *mbt* clusters mentioned above is that the possible thioesterase domain predicted at the C terminus of the synthetase MbtB of *M. tuberculosis* and *M. bovis* is replaced by a nonintegrated stand-alone predicted thioesterase, MbtT, encoded downstream of MbtB in the clusters of *M. avium*, *M. avium* subsp. *paratuberculosis*, and *M. smegmatis* or upstream of MbtE in *M. marinum* (Fig. 6). A second difference can be found in the domain organization of the MbtE homologs; *M. avium* MbtE has an additional adenylylation domain upstream of the peptidyl carrier protein domain (Fig. 6). MbtE of *M. avium* subsp. *paratuberculosis* has an additional domain as well, although it is interrupted by a frameshift (perhaps arising from a sequencing error). The *mbt* clusters of *M. tuberculosis*, *M. bovis*, *M. smegmatis*, and *M. marinum* have a total of four adenylylation domains each, which are predicted to be required for the adenylylation of a salicylate molecule, a serine residue, and two lysine residues and their subsequent loading onto their target carrier domains (52). The presence of a fifth adenylylation domain in the *mbt* clusters of *M. avium* and *M. avium* subsp. *paratuberculosis* is unexpected, since it would appear to be unnecessary based on the logic of nonribosomal peptide assembly. The role of these additional domains remains obscure. Interestingly, sequence analysis indicates that the gene cluster required for synthesis of the non-salicyloyl-containing exochelin MS of *M. smegmatis* has a total of six adenylylation domains (81), one more than would be

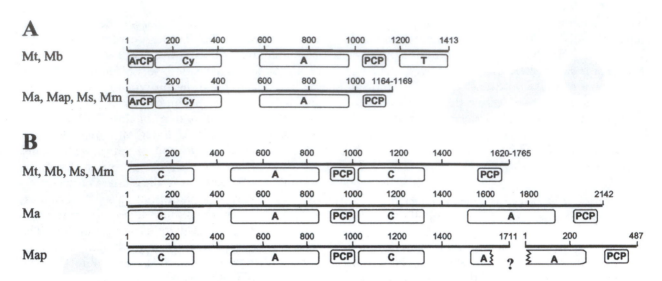

Figure 6. Differences in organization of predicted functional domains in the nonribosomal peptide synthetases MbtB and MbtE of various *Mycobacterium* species. Species abbreviations are the same as in Fig. 5. (A) Domain organization of MbtB homologs. The thioesterase domain in Mt and Mb is replaced by a separate thioesterase subunit in Ma, Map, Ms, and Mm. (B) Domain organization of MbtE homologs. The Ma and Map homologs appear to have an additional adenylation domain. The Map genome sequence corresponding to the MbtE coding region is frameshifted. Since the final annotation of the genome is not finished, it remains to be determined whether the frameshift is a sequencing error. Domain abbreviations: ArCP, aryl carrier protein domain; PCP, peptidyl carrier domain; Cy, cyclization domain; C, condensation domain; A, adenylation domain; T, thioesterase domain. The scale indicates the number of amino acids.

needed for synthesis of the major exochelin MS pentapeptide siderophore (64). However, other hexapeptidesiderophores have since been recognized in this species, providing a biosynthetic correlate to the presence of the additional domain (see below).

Exochelin MS Cluster of *M. smegmatis*

The first genes shown to be involved in the production of exochelin MS (Fig. 3) were identified by Fiss et al. (23) (Fig. 5). The genes were identified by genetic analysis of a DNA fragment able to complement an exochelin MS-deficient strain generated by UV mutagenesis. The gene responsible for the complementation was *fxbA*, which encoded a protein with homology to formyltransferases. The complementing fragment contained three additional open reading frames (ORFs), which are now known as *fxuA*, *fxuB*, and *fxuC* and encoded proteins with homology to the ferri-enterobactin permeases FepG, FepC, and FepD of *E. coli*, respectively. Based on these observations, Fiss et al. (23) suggested that FxbA would be involved in formylation of the exochelin MS molecule and that the Fxu proteins were likely to constitute an exochelin MS permease.

Additional genetic characterization of the exochelin MS locus was reported by Yu et al. in 1998 (81). These investigators noted that a single *M. smegmatis* cosmid complemented 13 chemically

mutagenized clones of *M. smegmatis* deficient in the production (or secretion) of exochelin MS. The sequence of the ~30-kb complementing fragment revealed a total of nine ORFs. The previously reported *fxbA* gene (23) was located at the 5' end of the sequenced region. The locus also encompassed, from the 5' to the 3' end, (i) *orf1* and *orf2*, encoding proteins with homology to ABC transporters; (ii) *fxbB* and *fxbC*, encoding proteins with homology to nonribosomal peptide synthetases; (iii) *fxuD*, encoding a protein with homology to periplasmic siderophore receptors; (iv) *orf3*, encoding a protein with an ATP-binding domain; and (v) *orf4* and *orf5*, encoding proteins with multiple transmembrane-spanning segments and no homology to proteins of known functions. Based on sequence homology analysis, the investigators proposed that *orf1*, *orf2*, and *fxuD* were good candidates to be involved in exochelin MS transport whereas *fxbB* and *fxbC* would be likely to have functions in exochelin MS biosynthesis. The investigators confirmed the essential role of *fxbB* and *fxbC* for exochelin MS production by performing further complementation and Tn*10* mutagenesis analysis of the two genes. Based on the available structural information of exochelin MS and the requirement of nonribosomal peptide synthetases for its production, the investigators proposed that the siderophore was synthesized nonribosomally via the multiple-carrier thiotemplate mechanism. Interestingly, they noted that while five adenylylation domains would be predicted to be required for the synthesis of the exochelin MS pentapeptide, the FxbB and FxbC proteins contained a total of six such domains. Although this was initially confusing, the reason for this extra domain arrangement is now clear: *M. smegmatis* produces at least six distinct exochelins (64), of which only the structure of the major component as a pentapeptide derivative has been determined (Fig. 3). However, the structures of four of the minor exochelins have recently been examined (G. Sharman and C. Ratledge, unpublished results), and three of these turn out to be hexapeptide derivatives. The metabolic relationship between the major exochelin and minor ones is not yet understood.

Zhu et al. also reported the results of complementation studies of exochelin MS-deficient mutants (generated by UV light or transposon mutagenesis) and the genetic characterization of the exochelin MS locus of *M. smegmatis* (82). These investigators mapped and sequenced a ~15-kb region involved in exochelin MS production. The sequence analysis revealed a total of four ORFs. One of them, located at the 5′ end of the sequenced region, was the previously reported *fxbA* gene (23). The remaining ORFs were named *exiT*, *fxbB*, and *fxbC* (Fig. 5). ExiT was noted to have sequence similarity to ABC transporters, and, because the genetic analysis demonstrated that *exiT* was required for exochelin MS production, the protein was proposed to be involved in siderophore secretion. Interestingly, the fact that the *exiT* mutant did not accumulate exochelin MS led the investigators to hypothesize that synthesis might be tightly coupled to export. It should be noted that the sequence of ExiT (from *M. smegmatis* strain LR222) corresponds to a fusion between the sequences of Orf1 and Orf2 reported by Yu et al. for *M. smegmatis* strain mc²155 (81) and deduced from the unfinished genome sequence of this strain (National Center for Biotechnology Information, microbial genome database). The predicted nonribosomal peptide synthetases FxbB and FxbC were shown by mutagenesis and complementation analysis to be required for exochelin MS production.

GENES INVOLVED IN IRON STORAGE

Two different types of ferritins involved in iron storage have been identified, the heme-containing bacterioferritins and the heme-free ferritins (2, 35). In contrast to the genes of bacterial iron acquisition systems, which are upregulated under low-iron conditions, the genes encoding iron storage proteins ap-

pear to be upregulated under high-iron conditions. This increased production of iron storage proteins is thought to protect against oxidative stress by sequestering ferrous iron and consequently limiting toxic hydroxy radical (OH·) formation by Fenton chemistry (2, 33).

Interestingly, the first mycobacterial bacterioferritins were identified during the characterization of immunodominant and highly expressed mycobacterial proteins in the early 1990s. In 1991, Brooks et al. purified and characterized *M. paratuberculosis* (referred to in this chapter as *M. avium* subsp. *paratuberculosis*) antigen D as a bacterioferritin (7). Similarly, Deshpande et al. found that one of the immunodominant proteins of *M. leprae* was a bacterioferritin (14). The first mycobacterial bacterioferritin genes were detected in 1994 (39, 50). Pessolani et al. sequenced the *M. leprae* bacterioferritin gene (*bfr*) and showed that the bacterioferritin was the major membrane protein (MMP-II) of in vivo-grown *M. leprae* (50). They also detected homologous *bfr* sequences in *M. avium* subsp. *paratuberculosis*, *M. avium*, *M. tuberculosis*, *M. intracellulare*, and *M. scrofulaceum* by Southern hybridization analysis. In the same year, Inglis et al. reported the sequence of the gene encoding the bacterioferritin of *M. avium* subsp. *silvaticum* (39). In 1998, the released sequence of the *M. tuberculosis* genome revealed the presence of two bacterioferritins in this bacterium: the 18-kDa BfrA and the 20-kDa BfrB (a ferritin-like protein), which are encoded by Rv1876 and Rv3841, respectively (11). More recently, the complete annotation of the *M. leprae* genome included two bacterioferritin genes as well (12). One of these genes (ML2038) encodes the 18-kDa BfrA, which corresponds to the previously identified *M. leprae* bacterioferritin (50). The second gene is a pseudogene (ML0075) which encodes the ferritin-like protein BfrB.

Protein similarity searches to identify homologs of *M. tuberculosis* BfrA and BfrB in the unfinished genome sequence of *M. bovis* revealed the presence of the two respective homologs, both with 100% identity to the *M. tuberculosis* proteins. Similarly, a search for *M. tuberculosis* BfrA and BfrB homologs in the unfinished genome sequences of *M. marinum* and *M. smegmatis* permitted the identification of the corresponding bacterioferritin homologs in these species (with ≥73% identity to the *M. tuberculosis* proteins). However, only BfrA homologs could be found in the unfinished genome sequences of *M. avium* subsp. *paratuberculosis* and *M. avium* (both with 88% identity to *M. tuberculosis* BfrA) (Quadri, unpublished).

Several recent lines of evidence suggest that *M. tuberculosis bfrB* is regulated in response to oxygen levels and reactive nitrogen intermediates and that both *bfrB* and *bfrA* are regulated by iron in *M. tuberculosis*. In 1998, during studies of differential gene expression in *M. tuberculosis* grown at different oxygen tensions, Imboden and Schoolnik prepared and characterized a library of cDNA clones corresponding to genes expressed during in vitro growth under low-oxygen conditions (38). One of the cDNAs that was overrepresented in the library was that of the gene known today to encode BfrB. RNA-slot blot hybridization and reverse transcription-PCR (RT-PCR) analysis was used to demonstrate that *bfrB* mRNA levels were indeed differentially decreased in culture sediments (considered to be under nearly anaerobic conditions) compared with shaken cultures under high- or low-oxygen conditions. Since iron storage proteins are thought to reduce iron-dependent reactive oxygen intermediate generation under aerobic conditions by sequestering ferrous iron, the investigators suggested that repression of bacterioferritin production might be expected under the low-iron and hypoxic conditions present in the culture sediments. Sherman et al. also determined that *bfrB* was among the *M. tuberculosis* genes whose mRNA levels increased under hypoxia, as judged by the results of a DNA microarray-based transcriptome analysis of the hypoxic response of the bacterium (65). Further evidence suggesting *bfrB* regulation by oxygen levels was provided by the proteome analysis of the hypoxic response of *M. tuberculosis*, reported by Rosenkrands et al. (61). The analysis involved two-dimensional gel electrophoresis of bacterial proteins followed by identification of several individual protein spots by mass spectrometry techniques. BfrB was identified in this study as one of the main upregulated proteins in bacteria grown under low-oxygen conditions.

The effect of nitric oxide donors on bacterioferritin levels was studied by Garbe et al. (25). These investigators showed that *M. tuberculosis* BfrB was one of the proteins highly induced by nitroprusside and to a lesser extent by SNAP (*S*-nitroso-*N*-acetyl-DL-penicillamine), as determined in a two-dimensional gel electrophoresis-based proteome analysis of the bacterium response to the nitric oxide donors. Finally, a more recent study by Rodriguez et al. reported a DNA microarray-based transcriptional profiling aimed at studying iron- and IdeR-regulated gene expression (see below) in *M. tuberculosis* (60). In this study, the investigators determined that both *bfrA* and *bfrB* mRNA levels increased in bacteria grown under high-iron conditions. Furthermore, the study showed that the decrease of *bfrA* and *bfrB* mRNA levels under the low-iron condition required the regulator IdeR (see below).

IRON-DEPENDENT REGULATION OF GENE EXPRESSION IN MYCOBACTERIA

Early Studies of Iron-Regulated Mycobacterial Proteins

Starting in the late 1980s, several groups began reporting studies centered on the use of one- and two-dimensional gel electrophoresis analysis to detect iron-regulated proteins (IRPs) in mycobacteria. The first direct evidence of mycobacterial IRPs was provided by the work of Hall et al. in 1987 (31). The investigators compared the protein profiles of preparations of walls and membranes of *M. smegmatis* grown under low- or high-iron conditions and demonstrated the existence of many iron-regulated envelope proteins (IREPs). The analysis clearly showed the synthesis of four additional proteins (180, 84, 29, and 25 kDa) under the low-iron conditions. Interestingly, antibodies against the 29-kDa IREP prevented exochelin MS-mediated iron uptake into iron-starved cells but not into iron-replete cells. The authors proposed that this IREP was involved in ferri-exochelin MS uptake. More recently, Dover and Ratledge (18) presented evidence of direct binding between ferri-exochelin MS and the 29- and 25-kDa envelope proteins of *M. smegmatis*. They suggested that the 29-kDa protein was a ferri-exochelin MS-binding protein and that the 25-kDa protein played a role in complex assembly or stability. Additional studies with *M. smegmatis* were reported more recently by Lundrigan et al., who showed the induction of at least five IRPs (180, 84, 62, 48, and 38 kDa) in *M. smegmatis* grown under low-iron conditions, with only one of them (84 kDa) being associated with the cell envelope (44).

In 1989, soon after the report by Hall et al. (31), Sritharan and Ratledge described the induction of four IREPs (120, 29, 21, and 14 kDa) and the repression of two IREPs (240 and 250 kDa) in *M. neoaurum* grown under low-iron conditions (69). Additional work by Sritharan and Ratledge investigated the IREPs in *M. smegmatis*, *M. avium*, and *M. vaccae* grown in vitro under low- and high-iron conditions (69). This work also covered the analysis of cell envelope proteins in *M. avium* grown in mice and *M. leprae* grown in an armadillo. Overall, several IREPs (ranging from 11 to 180 kDa) induced under the low-iron conditions were identified in the study. Most notably, two IREPs of 240 and 250 kDa were identified as iron repressed in *M. smegmatis* and *M. avium* but shown to be produced irrespective of the iron level in both *M. leprae* and *M. vaccae*. Three of the four IREPs (14, 21, and 29 kDa) identified in *M. avium* grown in vitro were also visualized in bacteria grown in mice. The latter cells also contained the 240- and 250-kDa proteins shown to be repressed under high-iron conditions in *M. smegmatis* and *M. avium*. Finally, *M. leprae* grown in armadillos also had cell envelope proteins of 29, 240, and 250 kDa.

The first studies of IREPs in *M. tuberculosis* were reported by Raghu and Sarma in 1993 (54). These investigators studied IREPs in *M. tuberculosis* virulent strain H37Rv, in a low-virulence strain from South India, and in the avirulent strain H37Ra. They also extended the previous studies of *M. smegmatis* IREPs. Overall, Raghu and Sarma detected (i) eight IREPs (25, 29, 45, 85, 90, 110, 120, and 180 kDa) induced under low-iron conditions in *M. smegmatis*, (ii) three IREPs (60, 80, and 90 kDa) induced under low-iron conditions in the virulent *M. tuberculosis* strain, (iii) three IREPs (29, 60, and 90 kDa) induced under low-iron conditions in the low-virulence *M. tuberculosis* strain, (iv) one IREP (90 kDa) induced under low-iron conditions in the avirulent *M. tuberculosis* strain, and (v) three high-molecular-weight IREPs (~250 kDa) induced under high-iron conditions in the low-virulence *M. tuberculosis* strain.

The work on IREPs of *M. tuberculosis* continued with the contributions of Calder and Horwitz (9), who reported two IRPs (15 and 24 kDa) induced under high-iron conditions and three IRPs (10, 13, and 23 kDa) induced under low iron conditions on analysis of whole-cell protein extracts. Furthermore, amino acid sequencing was used to identify the 13-kDa IRP as the major membrane protein of *M. tuberculosis* (43) and to deduce probes that were utilized for cloning of the gene (*irpA*) of the 10-kDa IRP and its adjacent gene (*mtaA*, encoding a metal transporting P-type ATPase homolog). Calder and Horwitz also performed Northern blot analysis and showed that *irpA* and *mtaA* were induced at the transcriptional level under low-iron conditions (9). The investigators suggested that the *irpA* and *mtaA* pair encoded a metal transport system in *M. tuberculosis*. The reported induction of *irpA* and *mtaA* provided the first example of iron-regulated transcription in pathogenic mycobacteria.

In 1999, Wong et al. presented a more extensive analysis of IRPs of *M. tuberculosis* grown under conditions of high and low iron (79). The two-dimensional gel electrophoresis analysis permitted high-resolution separation and visualization of hundreds of proteins from whole-cell extracts. The investigators reported that at least 27 IRPs were visualized in the gels, with the production of 15 and 12 proteins being increased and decreased, respectively, under the low-iron conditions. Several of the IRPs were identified.

The proteins upregulated under high-iron conditions were an iron-responsive ferric uptake regulator (Fur) protein homolog, an aconitase, a homolog of the LSR2 protein antigen of *M. leprae*, a heat shock protein of the α-crystallin family (an NADP-dependent dehydrogenase), a peptidyl-prolyl *cis-trans*-isomerase, and EF-Tu. Only one protein, a GTP-dependent phosphoenolpyruvate carboxykinase homolog, was identified among those upregulated under low-iron conditions. Based on their results, the investigators suggested that Fur and aconitase, which can affect the translation and stability of mammalian mRNAs involved in iron storage (47), might play a role in the iron-dependent regulation of protein levels in *M. tuberculosis*.

Studies of Iron-Regulated Transcription of Mycobacterial Genes

While the studies of iron-regulated proteins in mycobacteria addressed above started in the late 1980s, most of the studies of iron-regulated transcription of mycobacterial genes have been reported since the mid-1990s. (For a recent review of the subject, see reference 59.) These studies have revealed the magnitude of the iron-dependent regulation of gene expression in mycobacteria and established the relevance of the iron-dependent regulatory protein called IdeR as a key player at the center of the mechanism of iron-dependent regulation of gene expression. Overall, only the sequences of the *M. tuberculosis*, *M. smegmatis*, and *M. leprae ideR* genes have been reported, and the function of the regulators have been investigated in *M. tuberculosis* and *M. smegmatis*. As could be expected, highly similar IdeR homologs can be found in the unfinished genome sequences of *M. bovis*, *M. avium*, *M. avium* subsp. *paratuberculosis*, and *M. marinum* (National Center for Biotechnology Information microbial genome database; http://www. ncbi.nlm.nih.gov). Although it is likely that the IdeR homologs are involved in the control of iron homeostasis in these mycobacteria, the function of these proteins remains to be established experimentally.

The first mycobacterial IdeR was described by Schmitt et al. in 1995 (62). The investigators identified the regulatory gene *ideR* in the genome of *M. tuberculosis* based on the homology of its products to the diphtheria toxin repressor (DtxR) of *Corynebacterium diphtheriae*. DtxR, the first iron-dependent regulator discovered (5), acts as a repressor only in complex with Fe(II) and represses the transcription of iron-regulated genes by binding to a target sequence in the operators of the promoter regions (72). Schmitt et al. demonstrated that the *M. tuberculosis ideR* allele repressed transcription from the *C. diphtheriae tox*, IRP1, and IRP2 promoters in an *E. coli* background only under high-iron conditions and that the allele restored the wild-type iron-dependent expression of the corynebacterial siderophore in a *C. diphtheriae dtxR* mutant (62). Gel mobility shift and DNase I footprint analysis revealed that recombinantly produced IdeR could bind to a DNA fragment that included the *tox* promoter/operator sequence of *C. diphtheriae* and that the binding was activated by Fe(II) and other divalent metals (62). The similarity of IdeR and DtxR has been recently extended from the functional level to the structural one. The comparison of the crystal structures of the repressors revealed that the overall architectures of the two structures are very similar (22).

It was not until 1999 that the first gene expression studies demonstrating IdeR-dependent regulated transcription in *M. tuberculosis* were reported (58). The work by Rodriguez et al. identified a potential IdeR binding site in the *M. tuberculosis* genome. The site was flanked by two divergently oriented genes, Rv2122c (possibly involved in histidine biosynthesis and referred to by the authors as *irg1/hisE*) and Rv2123 (encoding a protein member of the PPE family and referred to by the authors as *irg2*). The analysis of transcriptional fusions of *irg1* and *irg2* to β-galactosidase (*lacZ*) revealed that the expression of *irg1* and *irg2* decreased in *M. tuberculosis* and in the surrogate *M. smegmatis* host grown under high-iron conditions. The analysis also showed that iron-dependent repression was lost in an *M. smegmatis ideR* mutant. The investigators also used footprinting and gel shift analysis to demonstrate IdeR binding to the predicted binding site.

Additional studies by Gold et al. (27) demonstrated the relevance of IdeR in iron-regulated gene expression. The authors identified ~50 potential IdeR-regulated genes by searching the entire *M. tuberculosis* genome for promoter regions containing the consensus IdeR/DtxR-binding sequence by using a computer algorithm. As expected, several of the identified genes encoded proteins annotated to be involved in iron acquisition (i.e., *mbtA*, *mbtB*, *mbtI*, Rv1348, and Rv1347c) or storage (i.e., *bfrA* and *bfrB*). However, many other genes encoded proteins whose annotation indicated their involvement in various metabolic pathways and cellular functions (e.g., *hisB*, *pheA*, lysyl-tRNA, *murB*, *hemL*, and *rpmB*) with no immediately apparent relationship to iron metabolism. Many genes with no predicted functional assignment were also present among those identified as potentially regulated by IdeR. The investigators analyzed the functionality of four predicted IdeR boxes (those located between *mbtA* and *mbtB* and between *bfrA* and *bfd* or upstream of *mbtI* and Rv3402c). While gel retardation and footprinting analysis was used to demonstrate that IdeR bound these boxes, primer extension analysis was used to

map the binding sequence to a region close to the −10 position of each promoter. The latter observation led the investigators to suggest that, like DtxR, IdeR repressed by blocking RNA polymerase binding.

Gold et al. also performed transcription analysis to demonstrate that *mbtA*, *mbtB*, *mbtI*, Rv3402c, and *bfd* were iron regulated and significantly repressed in iron-replete *M. tuberculosis* cells compared with iron-starved cells (27). Notably, expression of *bfrA* (a gene with not one but two IdeR boxes) was shown to be significantly upregulated in the iron-replete cells. Further expression analysis using an *M. tuberculosis bfrA-lacZ* fusion with or without deletion of the IdeR boxes in *M. smegmatis* and the *M. smegmatis ideR* mutant as surrogate hosts showed that IdeR could indeed act as an activator of *bfrA* transcription. Finally, the investigators also studied the expression of *mbtB*, *mbtI*, Rv3402, and *bfrA* in *M. tuberculosis* recovered from infected human THP-1 macrophages by using real-time RT-PCR. The analysis demonstrated that, except for *bfrA*, the IdeR-regulated genes were induced during infection, suggesting that the intracellular environment presented an iron-limiting condition to the bacterium. Interestingly, *mbtB* is strongly upregulated in mouse lungs (J. D. McKinney, unpublished results), suggesting that the bacterium experiences iron starvation in the human host and that siderophore production might be needed to overcome this condition.

In 2002, Rodriguez et al. reported the first genome-wide DNA microarray-based transcriptional profiling aimed at studying IdeR- and iron-regulated gene expression in *M. tuberculosis* (60). The investigators identified 153 genes whose expression was modulated by iron by comparing the transcriptomes of wild-type *M. tuberculosis* grown under low- and high-iron conditions. Genes belonging to many different functional categories and several genes encoding conserved hypothetical proteins with no functional assignment were represented among the iron-responsive genes. As expected, the mRNA levels of several genes involved in iron homeostasis were affected by iron. Among them, the genes required for mycobactin and carboxymycobactin biosynthesis and the iron storage protein genes *bfrA* and *bfrB* were upregulated and downregulated under low-iron conditions, respectively.

As part of the same study, Rodriguez et al. extended their transcriptome analysis to identify genes regulated by IdeR (60). This was done by comparing the transcriptomes of the wild-type strain, an *ideR* mutant (strain ST22) with an undefined second-site suppressor mutation that permitted deletion of the essential *ideR*, and the *ideR*-complemented mutant (strain ST52). Only the gene expression of cultures grown under high-iron conditions was analyzed, since only under these conditions did the three strains have similar growth characteristics. The analysis revealed that regulation of one-third of the 153 identified iron-regulated genes required the presence of IdeR. Among the genes that were shown to be both iron and IdeR regulated were, for example, the *mbt* genes involved in mycobactin and carboxymycobactin production (which were not downregulated in the presence of high iron levels in the absence of IdeR) and the *bfrA* gene involved in iron storage (which was not upregulated in the presence of high iron levels in the absence of IdeR). Consistent with the loss of repression of *mbt* genes under high-iron conditions in the absence of IdeR, the *ideR* mutant was shown to have increased production of siderophores; the mutant produced the same quantity of mycobactin under low- and high-iron conditions. This quantity was comparable to that produced by the wild-type strain under low-iron conditions. Finally, the group of genes that were identified as being iron regulated but IdeR independent was composed of genes with unknown functions and genes with functions in several metabolic pathways and cellular functions. Interestingly, no genes with clear links to iron metabolism were found in this group.

In addition to providing a wealth of information regarding iron- and IdeR-dependent regulation of gene expression in *M. tuberculosis*, the work of Rodriguez et al. demonstrated the crucial need to maintain proper iron homeostasis and the essential nature of *ideR* in this bacterium (60). The investigators reported that *ideR* could be disrupted only in the presence of a second copy of *ideR* or a second-site suppressor mutation which restricted iron acquisition ability and thus alleviated the lethal effects of *ideR* inactivation. The essential nature of *M. tuberculosis ideR* contrasted with the dispensability of *ideR* reported for *M. smegmatis* (19) (see below). Additionally, the work of Rodriguez et al. showed that although no obvious genes involved in oxidative stress protection were identified among the IdeR-regulated genes, the repressor was required for wild-type levels of resistance to oxidative stress; the *ideR* mutant displayed higher sensitivity to hydrogen peroxide treatment (60). This result was similar to that obtained earlier with an *ideR* mutant of *M. smegmatis* (19).

The relevance of proper IdeR-dependent regulation for the virulence of *M. tuberculosis* was established by Manabe et al. in 1999 (45). These investigators constructed an *M. tuberculosis* strain expressing an iron-independent, positive dominant, corynebacterial *dtxR* hyperrepressor, DtxR(E175K). The in vitro growth rates of wild-type and DtxR(E175K)-expressing strains were comparable; however, an

altered colony morphology was noted for the strain expressing DtxR(E175K). More importantly, the DtxR(E175K)-expressing strain was shown to be attenuated compared with the wild-type strain in a mouse infection model with tail vein injection. The DtxR(E175K)-expressing strain was reported to display a 1.2-log-unit reduction in bacterial CFU in both the spleen and the lungs at 16 weeks postinfection. Supporting the viable bacterial counts, histopathologic analysis of the spleen and the lungs revealed fewer acid-fast bacilli. The investigators also performed a computerized search for the IdeR/DtxR consensus binding sequence in the *M. tuberculosis* genome and identified six potential binding sites (referred to as IB1 to IB6) within 200 bp upstream of predicted genes. Only five of the potential binding sites (IB1 to IB5) were shown to bind DtxR in gel shift assays. The genes downstream of the binding sites encoded a homolog of the sensor PhoP, a homolog of the HtrA serine protease, the 16S rRNA, an alcohol dehydrogenase (AdhB), and a homolog of the *M. tuberculosis* 19-kDa antigen. Based on their observations, the investigators postulated that IdeR might control genes essential for virulence in *M. tuberculosis*. Interestingly, Hobson et al. utilized quantitative real-time RT-PCR analysis and analysis of an *ideR* promoter-*lacZ* fusion to demonstrate upregulation of *M. tuberculosis ideR* in bacteria growing in human THP-1 macrophages (36). This report presented the first evidence that the expression of the regulator is regulated in the host.

The function of IdeR in *M. smegmatis* has also been investigated. In 1996, soon after the first reported studies with *M. tuberculosis ideR* (62), Dussurget et al. reported the results of the first study with *M. smegmatis ideR* (19): they constructed two *ideR* mutants of *M. smegmatis* mc^{2}155 by allelic replacement and characterized the phenotype of the mutants (strains SM1 and SM3) and an *ideR*-complemented control strain (SM4, with an ectopic single *ideR* copy). The *ideR* mutants, but not the complemented strain, displayed constitutive siderophore production.

Furthermore, IdeR was shown to be required for the iron-dependent repression of mycobactin and exochelin MS production under high-iron conditions. Interestingly, quantitative analysis of the amounts of mycobactin and exochelin MS showed that the derepression observed in the *M. smegmatis ideR* mutant was not complete; the production of both siderophores under high-iron conditions was lower than that observed under low-iron conditions. These observations led the authors to postulate the existence of a second repressor of siderophore production. Unexpectedly, the production of both siderophores under low-iron conditions, measured for the *ideR* mutant and the complemented strain, was significantly lower than in the wild-type *M. smegmatis* strain. Adilakshmi et al. (1) have recently extended the work to show that the biosynthesis of carboxymycobactin (the second type of secreted siderophores of *M. smegmatis*) and salicylate (the precursor of mycobactin and carboxymycobactin [Fig. 1]) was also derepressed under high-iron conditions in the absence of IdeR.

More recently, Dussurget et al. showed that *M. smegmatis* IdeR regulates the expression of *fxbA* (21), encoding the predicted formyltransferase essential for exochelin MS biosynthesis (23). In this study, the investigators interpreted the results of mobility shift, primer extension, and DNase I footprinting analyses to demonstrate that IdeR could bind to the *fxbA* promoter region and protect a 28-bp palindromic sequence (IdeR box) in the presence of Fe(II) and other divalent metals. The investigators also analyzed *fxbA* promoter-*lacZ* transcriptional fusions in wild-type *M. smegmatis* and in an *ideR* mutant strain to corroborate the notion that *fxbA* expression was negatively regulated by iron in an IdeR-dependent manner. Interestingly, the levels of *fxbA* derepression in the *ideR* mutant were ~50% lower than in the wild-type strain grown under iron limitation. Based on this observation, the authors suggested that IdeR may exert, in some way, a positive regulation on *fxbA*.

The initial work of Dussurget et al. also demonstrated that IdeR played a role beyond iron metabolism by showing that the regulator was required for a wild-type oxidative stress response (19). The *ideR* mutant (but not the complemented strain tested) had an increased sensitivity to hydrogen peroxide killing and decreased activities of the oxidative stress protective enzymes SodA (manganese-cofactored superoxide dismutase) and KatG (catalase/peroxidase). However, the activity of the catalase KatE remained unchanged in the mutant. In a subsequent study, Dussurget et al. established that the decrease in SodA and KatG activities paralleled a decrease in the amounts of the corresponding proteins and mRNAs in the *ideR* mutant (20). Interestingly, the *ideR* mutant was reported to also have increased sensitivity to the antituberculosis drug, isoniazid (whose activation in the cell generates reactive oxygen species), the oxidizing transition metal cadmium, and the superoxide radical generator plumbagin, but not to rifampin or sodium dodecyl sulfate. Based on the phenotype of the *ideR* mutant, it has been proposed that *M. smegmatis* IdeR acts as a pleiotropic regulator that not only regulates iron uptake genes but also affects the synthesis of selective oxidative stress protective enzymes by a mechanism that is not yet clear (19, 20).

CONCLUSIONS: IRON AND TUBERCULOSIS

Iron is essential for the growth of mycobacteria and the development of mycobacterial virulence in animals. Several key papers have now established that the acquisition of iron from host tissues is essential for the virulence and growth of mycobacteria in vivo (16, 27, 36; see also reviews in references 56 and 59). These recent results then indirectly confirm what has long been suspected, i.e., that administration of iron to a person with tuberculosis is to be avoided at all costs. When a person becomes infected with the tubercle bacillus or, indeed, other bacteria, one of the earliest defense mechanisms put into operation by the infected host is the withholding of iron from the invading bacteria by the transfer of all free iron into transferrin or lactoferrin, both of which deliberately have spare iron-binding capacity for this very purpose (55, 56). In practice, this means that partial anemia of a patient with tuberculosis is not a bad thing, since iron is then automatically in limiting supply not only to the host but also to the bacteria. Trousseau in 1872, in his lectures in Paris (74), was already alerting medical students to the dangers of administering iron to patients with quiescent tuberculosis. Since then, there have been a number of regrettable examples of well-meaning medical practitioners giving iron to anemic patients being admitted to hospital in the early stages of tuberculosis or other diseases, with the result that the pathogenic bacteria get the iron before the host and then overwhelm the host defense systems. Death of the patient then quickly follows. Even the diet of tuberculosis patients can be crucial for their survival: a recent survey in Zimbabwe of 98 patients with pulmonary tuberculosis showed that those who were exposed to high levels of dietary iron (from the local beer) had a 17-fold increase in the estimated odds of developing active tuberculosis (24). Thus, iron plays a major role in the development of tuberculosis, especially in the earliest stages of infection, when the bacilli stand the greatest chance of being successfully dealt with by the host defense system. Medical practitioners interfere with this "nutritional defense" state of the host at their peril.

Does, then, this vital role of iron in the growth of mycobacteria in vivo represent a possible target for the development of potential antitubercular agents? The short answer to this is probably "yes," in that we already have one such compound: the old drug *para*-aminosalicylic acid (PAS). PAS functions not as an antifolate compound, as the textbooks would have us believe, but as an antisalicylic acid compound, thereby inhibiting the synthesis of the key siderophore components, carboxymycobactin and mycobactin, of the mycobacterial iron uptake system (1). Thus, it is entirely feasible to inhibit the growth of mycobacteria in vivo and thus to prevent the development of tuberculosis by using a drug that inhibits some aspect of iron acquisition. The work by Miller and his group (37, 80) has indicated that mycobactin analogs might be potential inhibitors of *M. tuberculosis* grown in laboratory cultures, presumably by interfering with the transfer of iron into the bacteria, although more recent work by Poreddy et al., using analogs of carboxymycobactin, has not confirmed this concept (51). However, the number of such analogues that have been tested is rather limited, and so the opportunity for synthesizing a greater range of siderophore analogs could still represent a useful route for tuberculosis chemotherapy. However, opportunities to develop further analogs of salicylate, based on the structure of PAS itself, would seem to be unlikely in view of the previous attempts at this and the realization that even small changes to the structure of PAS result in loss of its activity (77).

As we begin to appreciate more of the mycobacterial iron acquisition pathway at the molecular level (53), the design of specific inhibitors for any of the enzymes of the salicylate-mycobactin pathway (Fig. 5 and 6) becomes an attractive proposition for chemotherapy of tuberculosis. The next steps toward this goal must therefore lie in the structural determination of the old proteins and then in the design of appropriate inhibitors. Hopefully, the work reviewed in this chapter will encourage the pursuit of this goal.

REFERENCES

1. **Adilakshmi, T., P. D. Ayling, and C. Ratledge.** 2000. Mutational analysis of a role for salicylic acid in iron metabolism of *Mycobacterium smegmatis. J. Bacteriol.* **182:**264–271.
2. **Andrews, S. C.** 1998. Iron storage in bacteria. *Adv. Microb. Physiol.* **40:**281–351.
3. **Barclay, R., D. F. Ewing, and C. Ratledge.** 1985. Isolation, identification, and structural analysis of the mycobactins of *Mycobacterium avium, Mycobacterium intracellulare, Mycobacterium scrofulaceum,* and *Mycobacterium paratuberculosis. J. Bacteriol.* **164:**896–903.
4. **Boukhalfa, H., and A. L. Crumbliss.** 2002. Chemical aspects of siderophore mediated iron transport. *Biometals* **15:**325–339.
5. **Boyd, J., M. N. Oza, and J. R. Murphy.** 1990. Molecular cloning and DNA sequence analysis of a diphtheria tox iron-dependent regulatory element (*dtxR*) from *Corynebacterium diphtheriae. Proc. Natl. Acad. Sci. USA* **87:**5968–5972.
6. **Braun, V.** 2001. Iron uptake mechanisms and their regulation in pathogenic bacteria. *Int. J. Med. Microbiol.* **291:**67–79.
7. **Brooks, B. W., N. M. Young, D. C. Watson, R. H. Robertson, E. A. Sugden, K. H. Nielsen, and S. A. Becker.** 1991. *Mycobacterium paratuberculosis* antigen D: characterization and evidence that it is a bacterioferritin. *J. Clin. Microbiol.* **29:**1652–1658.
8. **Bullen, J. J., and E. Griffiths (ed.).** 1999. *Iron and Infection: Molecular, Physiological and Clinical Aspects,* 2nd ed. John Wiley & Sons, Ltd., Chichester, United Kingdom.

9. **Calder, K. M., and M. A. Horwitz.** 1998. Identification of iron-regulated proteins of *Mycobacterium tuberculosis* and cloning of tandem genes encoding a low iron-induced protein and a metal transporting ATPase with similarities to two-component metal transport systems. *Microb. Pathog.* **24:**133–143.
10. **Chipperfield, J. R., and C. Ratledge.** 2000. Salicylic acid is not a bacterial siderophore: a theoretical study. *Biometals* **13:**165–168.
11. **Cole, S. T., R. Brosch, J. Parkhill, T. Garnier, C. Churcher, D. Harris, S. V. Gordon, K. Eiglmeier, S. Gas, C. E. Barry III, F. Tekaia, K. Badcock, D. Basham, D. Brown, T. Chillingworth, R. Connor, R. Davies, K. Devlin, T. Feltwell, S. Gentles, N. Hamlin, S. Holroyd, T. Hornsby, K. Jagels, A. Krogh, J. McLean, S. Moule, L. Murphy, K. Oliver, J. Osborne, M. A. Quail, M.-A. Rajandream, J. Rogers, S. Rutter, K. Seeger, J. Skelton, S. Squares, R. Squares, J. E. Sulston, K. Taylor, S. Whitehead, and B. G. Barrett.** 1998. Deciphering the biology of *Mycobacterium tuberculosis* from the complete genome sequence. *Nature* **393:**537–544.
12. **Cole, S. T., K. Eiglmeier, J. Parkhill, K. D. James, N. R. Thomson, P. R. Wheeler, N. Honore, T. Garnier, C. Churcher, D. Harris, K. Mungall, D. Basham, D. Brown, T. Chillingworth, R. Connor, R. M. Davies, K. Devlin, S. Duthoy, T. Feltwell, A. Fraser, N. Hamlin, S. Holroyd, T. Hornsby, K. Jagels, C. Lacroix, J. Maclean, S. Moule, L. Murphy, K. Oliver, M. A. Quail, M.-A. Rajandream, K. M. Rutherford, S. Rutter, K. Saeger, S. Simon, M. Simmonds, J. Skelton, R. Squares, S. Squares, K. Stevens, K. Taylor, S. Whitehead, J. R. Woodward, and B. G. Barrell.** 2001. Massive gene decay in the leprosy bacillus. *Nature* **409:**1007–1011.
13. **Collins, H. L.** 2003. The role of iron in infections with intracellular bacteria. *Immunol. Lett.* **85:**193–195.
14. **Deshpande, R. G., M. B. Khan, D. A. Bhat, and R. G. Navalkar.** 1995. Immunoaffinity chromatographic isolation of a high molecular weight seroreactive protein from *Mycobacterium leprae* cell sonicate. *FEMS Immunol. Med. Microbiol.* **11:**163–169.
15. **De Voss, J. J., K. Rutter, B. G. Schroeder, and C. E. Barry III.** 1999. Iron acquisition and metabolism by mycobacteria. *J. Bacteriol.* **181:**4443–4451.
16. **De Voss, J. J., K. Rutter, B. G. Schroeder, H. Su, Y. Zhu, and C. E. Barry III.** 2000. The salicylate-derived mycobactin siderophores of *Mycobacterium tuberculosis* are essential for growth in macrophages. *Proc. Natl. Acad. Sci. USA* **97:**1252–1257.
17. **Dhungana, S., M. J. Miller, L. Dong, C. Ratledge, and A. L. Crumbliss.** 2003. Iron chelation properties of an extracellular siderophore exochelin MN. *J. Am. Chem. Soc.* **125:**7654–7663.
18. **Dover, L. G., and C. Ratledge.** 1996. Identification of a 29-kDa protein in the envelope of *Mycobacterium smegmatis* as a putative ferri-exochelin receptor. *Microbiology* **142:**1521–1530.
19. **Dussurget, O., M. Rodriguez, and I. Smith.** 1996. An *ideR* mutant of *Mycobacterium smegmatis* has derepressed siderophore production and an altered oxidative-stress response. *Mol. Microbiol.* **22:**535–544.
20. **Dussurget, O., M. Rodriguez, and I. Smith.** 1998. Protective role of the *Mycobacterium smegmatis* IdeR against reactive oxygen species and isoniazid toxicity. *Tubercle Lung Dis.* **79:**99–106.
21. **Dussurget, O., J. Timm, M. Gomez, B. Gold, S. Yu, S. Z. Sabol, R. K. Holmes, W. R. Jacobs, Jr., and I. Smith.** 1999. Transcriptional control of the iron-responsive *fxbA* gene by the mycobacterial regulator IdeR. *J. Bacteriol.* **181:**3402–3408.

22. Feese, M. D., B. P. Ingason, J. Goranson-Siekierke, R. K. Holmes, and W. G. Hol. 2001. Crystal structure of the iron-dependent regulator from *Mycobacterium tuberculosis* at 2.0-Å resolution reveals the Src homology domain 3-like fold and metal binding function of the third domain. *J. Biol. Chem.* 276:5959–5966.

23. Fiss, E. H., S. Yu, and W. R. Jacobs, Jr. 1994. Identification of genes involved in the sequestration of iron in mycobacteria: the ferric exochelin biosynthetic and uptake pathways. *Mol. Microbiol.* 14:557–569.

24. Gangaidzo, I. T., V. M. Moyo, E. Mvundura, G. Aggrey, N. L. Murphree, H. Khumalo, T. Saungweme, I. Kasvosve, Z. A. Gomo, T. Rouault, J. R. Boelaert, and V. R. Gordeuk. 2001. Association of pulmonary tuberculosis with increased dietary iron. *J. Infect. Dis.* 184:936–939.

25. Garbe, T. R., N. S. Hibler, and V. Deretic. 1999. Response to reactive nitrogen intermediates in *Mycobacterium tuberculosis*: induction of the 16-kilodalton alpha-crystallin homolog by exposure to nitric oxide donors. *Infect. Immun.* 67:460–465.

26. Gobin, J., C. H. Moore, J. R. Reeve, Jr., D. K. Wong, B. W. Gibson, and M. A. Horwitz. 1995. Iron acquisition by *Mycobacterium tuberculosis*: isolation and characterization of a family of iron-binding exochelins. *Proc. Natl. Acad. Sci. USA* 92:5189–5193.

27. Gold, B., G. M. Rodriguez, S. A. Marras, M. Pentecost, and I. Smith. 2001. The *Mycobacterium tuberculosis* IdeR is a dual functional regulator that controls transcription of genes involved in iron acquisition, iron storage and survival in macrophages. *Mol. Microbiol.* 42:851–865.

28. Gomez, M., and I. Smith. 2000. Determinants of mycobacterial gene expression, p. 111–129. *In* G. F. Hatfull and W. R. Jacobs, Jr. (ed.), *Molecular Genetics of Mycobacteria*. ASM Press, Washington, D.C.

29. Griffiths, E., and P. Williams. 1999. The iron-uptake systems of pathogenic bacteria, fungi and protozoa, p. 87–212. *In* J. J. Bullen and E. Griffiths (ed.), *Iron and Infection: Molecular, Physiological and Clinical Aspects*, 2nd ed. John Wiley & Sons, Ltd., Chichester, United Kingdom.

30. Hall, R. M., and C. Ratledge. 1987. Exochelin-mediated iron acquisition by the leprosy bacillus, *Mycobacterium leprae*. *J. Gen. Microbiol.* 133:193–199.

31. Hall, R. M., M. Sritharan, A. J. Messenger, and C. Ratledge. 1987. Iron transport in *Mycobacterium smegmatis*: occurrence of iron-regulated envelope proteins as potential receptors for iron uptake. *J. Gen. Microbiol.* 133:2107–2114.

32. Hall, R. M., P. R. Wheeler, and C. Ratledge. 1983. Exochelin-mediated iron uptake into *Mycobacterium leprae*. *Int. J. Lepr. Other Mycobact. Dis.* 51:490–494.

33. Halliwell, B., and J. M. Gutteridge. 1984. Oxygen toxicity, oxygen radicals, transition metals and disease. *Biochem. J.* 219:1–14.

34. Hantke, K. 2001. Iron and metal regulation in bacteria. *Curr. Opin. Microbiol.* 4:172–177.

35. Harrison, P. M., P. D. Hempstead, P. J. Artymiuk, and S. C. Andrews. 1998. Structure-function relationships in the ferritins. *Metal Ions Biol. Syst.* 35:435–477.

36. Hobson, R. J., A. J. McBride, K. E. Kempsell, and J. W. Dale. 2002. Use of an arrayed promoter-probe library for the identification of macrophage-regulated genes in *Mycobacterium tuberculosis*. *Microbiology* 148:1571–1579.

37. Hu, J., and M. J. Miller. 1997. Total synthesis of a mycobactin S, a siderophore and growth promoter of *Mycobacterium Smegmatis*, and determination of its growth inhibitory activity against *Mycobacterium tuberculosis*. *J. Am. Chem. Soc.* 119:3462–3468.

38. Imboden, P., and G. K. Schoolnik. 1998. Construction and characterization of a partial *Mycobacterium tuberculosis* cDNA library of genes expressed at reduced oxygen tension. *Gene* 213:107–117.

39. Inglis, N. F., K. Stevenson, A. H. Hosie, and J. M. Sharp. 1994. Complete sequence of the gene encoding the bacterioferritin subunit of *Mycobacterium avium* subspecies *silvaticum*. *Gene* 150:205–206.

40. Kato, L. 1985. Absence of mycobactin in *Mycobacterium leprae*: probably a microbe dependent microorganism implications. *Indian. J. Lepr.* 57:58–70.

41. Lane, S. J., P. S. Marshall, R. J. Upton, and C. Ratledge. 1998. Isolation and characterization of carboxymycobactins as the second extracellular siderophores in *Mycobacterium smegmatis*. *Biometals* 11:13–20.

42. Lane, S. J., P. S. Marshall, R. J. Upton, C. Ratledge, and M. Ewing. 1995. Novel extracellular mycobactins, the carboxymycobactins from *Mycobacterium avium*. *Tetrahedron Lett.* 36:4129–4132.

43. Lee, B. Y., S. A. Hefta, and P. J. Brennan. 1992. Characterization of the major membrane protein of virulent *Mycobacterium tuberculosis*. *Infect. Immun.* 60:2066–2074.

44. Lundrigan, M. D., J. E. Arceneaux, W. Zhu, and B. R. Byers. 1997. Enhanced hydrogen peroxide sensitivity and altered stress protein expression in iron-starved *Mycobacterium smegmatis*. *Biometals* 10:215–225.

45. Manabe, Y. C., B. J. Saviola, L. Sun, J. R. Murphy, and W. R. Bishai. 1999. Attenuation of virulence in *Mycobacterium tuberculosis* expressing a constitutively active iron repressor. *Proc. Natl. Acad. Sci. USA* 96:12844–12848.

46. Matzanke, B. F., R. Bohnke, U. Mollmann, R. Reissbrodt, V. Schunemann, and A. X. Trautwein. 1997. Iron uptake and intracellular metal transfer in mycobacteria mediated by xenosiderophores. *Biometals* 10:193–203.

47. Melefors, O., and M. W. Hentze. 1993. Translational regulation by mRNA/protein interactions in eukaryotic cells: ferritin and beyond. *Bioessays* 15:85–90.

48. Messenger, A. J., R. M. Hall, and C. Ratledge. 1986. Iron uptake processes in *Mycobacterium vaccae* R877R, a mycobacterium lacking mycobactin. *J. Gen. Microbiol.* 132:845–852.

49. Pavelka, M. S. J. 2000. Genetics of mycobacterial metabolism, p. 221–234. *In* G. F. Hatfull and W. R. Jacobs, Jr. (ed.), *Molecular Genetics of Mycobacteria*. ASM Press, Washington, D.C.

50. Pessolani, M. C., D. R. Smith, B. Rivoire, J. McCormick, S. A. Hefta, S. T. Cole, and P. J. Brennan. 1994. Purification, characterization, gene sequence, and significance of a bacterioferritin from *Mycobacterium leprae*. *J. Exp. Med.* 180:319–327.

51. Poreddy, A. R., O. F. Schall, G. D. Marshall, C. Ratledge, and U. Slomczynska. 2003. Solid-phase synthesis of methyl carboxymycobactin T7 and analogs as potential antimycobacterial agents. *Bioorg. Med. Chem. Lett.* 13:2553–2556.

52. Quadri, L. E. N. 2000. Assembly of aryl-capped siderophores by modular peptide synthetases and polyketide synthases. *Mol. Microbiol.* 37:1–12.

53. Quadri, L. E. N., J. Sello, T. A. Keating, P. H. Weinreb, and C. T. Walsh. 1998. Identification of a *Mycobacterium tuberculosis* gene cluster encoding the biosynthetic enzymes for assembly of the virulence-conferring siderophore mycobactin. *Chem. Biol.* 5:631–645.

54. Raghu, B., and G. R. Sarma. 1993. Isolation and characterization of siderophores and envelope proteins from mycobacteria. *Biochem. Mol. Biol. Int.* 31:333–339.

55. Ratledge, C. 1999. Iron metabolism, p. 260–286. *In* C.

Ratledge and J. Dale (ed.), *Mycobacteria: Molecular Biology and Virulence*. Blackwell Science, Oxford, United Kingdom.

56. **Ratledge, C., and L. G. Dover.** 2000. Iron metabolism in pathogenic bacteria. *Annu. Rev. Microbiol.* **54:**881–941.

57. **Ratledge, C., and M. Ewing.** 1996. The occurrence of carboxymycobactin, the siderophore of pathogenic mycobacteria, as a second extracellular siderophore in *Mycobacterium smegmatis. Microbiology* **142:**2207–2212.

58. **Rodriguez, G. M., B. Gold, M. Gomez, O. Dussurget, and I. Smith.** 1999. Identification and characterization of two divergently transcribed iron regulated genes in *Mycobacterium tuberculosis. Tubercle Lung Dis.* **79:**287–298.

59. **Rodriguez, G. M., and I. Smith.** 2003. Mechanisms of iron regulation in mycobacteria: role in physiology and virulence. *Mol. Microbiol.* **47:**1485–1494.

60. **Rodriguez, G. M., M. I. Voskuil, B. Gold, G. K. Schoolnik, and I. Smith.** 2002. *ideR*, an essential gene in *Mycobacterium tuberculosis*: role of IdeR in iron-dependent gene expression, iron metabolism, and oxidative stress response. *Infect. Immun.* **70:**3371–3381.

61. **Rosenkrands, I., R. A. Slayden, J. Crawford, C. Aagaard, C. E. Barry III, and P. Andersen.** 2002. Hypoxic response of *Mycobacterium tuberculosis* studied by metabolic labeling and proteome analysis of cellular and extracellular proteins. *J. Bacteriol.* **184:**3485–3491.

62. **Schmitt, M. P., M. Predich, L. Doukhan, I. Smith, and R. K. Holmes.** 1995. Characterization of an iron-dependent regulatory protein (IdeR) of *Mycobacterium tuberculosis* as a functional homolog of the diphtheria toxin repressor (DtxR) from *Corynebacterium diphtheriae. Infect. Immun.* **63:**4284–4289.

63. **Sharman, G. J., D. H. Williams, D. F. Ewing, and C. Ratledge.** 1995. Determination of the structure of exochelin MN, the extracellular siderophore from *Mycobacterium neoaurum. Chem. Biol.* **2:**553–561.

64. **Sharman, G. J., D. H. Williams, D. F. Ewing, and C. Ratledge.** 1995. Isolation, purification and structure of exochelin MS, the extracellular siderophore from *Mycobacterium smegmatis. Biochem. J.* **305:**187–196.

65. **Sherman, D. R., M. Voskuil, D. Schnappinger, R. Liao, M. I. Harrell, and G. K. Schoolnik.** 2001. Regulation of the *Mycobacterium tuberculosis* hypoxic response gene encoding alpha-crystallin. *Proc. Natl. Acad. Sci. USA* **98:**7534–7539.

66. **Sigel, A., and H. Sigel (ed.).** 1999. Iron transport and storage in microorganisms, plants and animals. *Metal Ions Biol. Syst.* **35:**37–66.

67. **Snow, G. A.** 1970. Mycobactins: iron-chelating growth factors from mycobacteria. *Bacteriol. Rev.* **34:**99–125.

68. **Sritharan, M.** 2000. Iron as a candidate in virulence and pathogenesis in mycobacteria and other microorganisms. *World J. Microbiol. Biotechnol.* **16:**769–780.

69. **Sritharan, M., and C. Ratledge.** 1990. Iron-regulated envelope proteins of mycobacteria grown in vitro and their occurrence in *Mycobacterium avium* and *Mycobacterium leprae* grown *in vivo. Biol. Metals* **2:**203–208.

70. **Stephenson, M. C., and C. Ratledge.** 1979. Iron transport in *Mycobacterium smegmatis*: uptake of iron from ferriexochelin. *J. Gen. Microbiol.* **110:**193–202.

71. **Stephenson, M. C., and C. Ratledge.** 1980. Specificity of exochelins for iron transport in three species of mycobacteria. *J. Gen. Microbiol.* **116:**521–523.

72. **Tao, X., N. Schiering, H. Y. Zeng, D. Ringe, and J. R. Murphy.** 1994. Iron, DtxR, and the regulation of diphtheria toxin expression. *Mol. Microbiol.* **14:**191–197.

73. **Timm, J., M. Gomez, and I. Smith.** 1999. Gene expression and regulation, p. 59–92. *In* C. Ratledge and J. Dale (ed.), *Mycobacteria: Molecular Biology and Virulence*. Blackwell Science, Oxford, United Kingdom.

74. **Trousseau, A.** 1872. True and false chlorosis. *Lect. Clin. Med.* **5:**95–117.

75. **Weinberg, E. D.** 1993. The development of awareness of iron-withholding defense. *Perspect. Biol. Med.* **36:**215–221.

76. **Wheeler, P. R.** 2003. Leprosy—clues about the biochemistry of *Mycobacterium leprae* and its host-dependency from the genome. *World J. Microbiol. Biotechnol.* **19:**1–16.

77. **Winder, F. G.** 1982. Mode of action of antimycobacterial agents and associated aspects of the molecular biology of the mycobacteria, p. 353–438. *In* C. Ratledge and J. Standford (ed.), *The Biology of the Mycobacteria*, vol. 1. Academic Press, Ltd., London, United Kingdom.

78. **Winkelmann, G., and H. Drechsel.** 1997. Microbial siderophores, p. 199–246. *In* H. J. Rehm and R. Reed (ed.), *Biotechnology*, 2nd ed, vol. 7. Wiley-VCH, Weinheim, Germany.

79. **Wong, D. K., B. Y. Lee, M. A. Horwitz, and B. W. Gibson.** 1999. Identification of fur, aconitase, and other proteins expressed by *Mycobacterium tuberculosis* under conditions of low and high concentrations of iron by combined two-dimensional gel electrophoresis and mass spectrometry. *Infect. Immun.* **67:**327–336.

80. **Xu, Y., and M. J. Miller.** 1998. Total syntheses of mycobactin analogues as potent antimycobacterial agents using a minimal protecting group strategy. *J. Org. Chem.* **63:**4314–4322.

81. **Yu, S., E. Fiss, and W. R. Jacobs, Jr.** 1998. Analysis of the exochelin locus in *Mycobacterium smegmatis*: biosynthesis genes have homology with genes of the peptide synthetase family. *J. Bacteriol.* **180:**4676–4685.

82. **Zhu, W., J. E. Arceneaux, M. L. Beggs, B. R. Byers, K. D. Eisenach, and M. D. Lundrigan.** 1998. Exochelin genes in *Mycobacterium smegmatis*: identification of an ABC transporter and two non-ribosomal peptide synthetase genes. *Mol. Microbiol.* **29:**629–639.

Tuberculosis and the Tubercle Bacillus
Edited by Stewart T. Cole et al.
© 2005 ASM Press, Washington, D.C.

Chapter 22

Two-Component Systems, Protein Kinases, and Signal Transduction in *Mycobacterium tuberculosis*

YOSSEF AV-GAY AND VOJO DERETIC

This chapter covers two types of regulatory signal transduction elements in *Mycobacterium tuberculosis*: (i) histidine protein kinase response regulators, referred to as two-component systems, and (ii) eucaryotic-type Ser/Thr protein kinases (STPKs.). Based on the data available so far and on analogies to systems studied in other bacteria, these factors play a role in physiology and virulence of *M. tuberculosis*. The chapter is divided into two parts, covering the two types of phosphotransfer signaling systems individually.

BACTERIAL TWO-COMPONENT SIGNAL TRANSDUCTION SYSTEMS

The existence of a large superfamily of two-component signal transduction systems in bacteria (47) was first recognized nearly three decades ago (39, 48). The prototypical two-component systems consist of a histidine protein kinase (often functioning as an environmental sensor), which, as a manifestation of signal transduction, phosphorylates an aspartate residue on its cognate response regulator (a transcriptional regulator or a regulator of other proteins). The genes encoding histidine protein kinase-response regulator pairs are often genetically linked, hence the term "two-component systems," reflecting the telltale tandem chromosomal arrangement of the cognate kinase-response regulator pairs. There are variations on this theme, ranging from isolated, orphan components without an obvious cognate sensor kinase or response regulator to complex phosphorelay systems. Kinases sometimes incorporate response regulator domains within their sequence. Depending on the type of signaling involved, kinases are either membrane or cytosolic proteins. In general, the chemistry of the phosphotransfer reaction between

phosphohistidines in kinases and recipient aspartate residues in response regulators (corresponding to the prototypical active site composed of Asp-12, Asp-13, Asp-57, and Lys-109 in CheY) is nearly unique to bacterial systems. Although it has been found in eucaryotic organisms, it is not present in the animal kingdom (54). The two-component signaling elements can control gene expression or nontranscriptional responses, resulting in adaptations to environmental stimuli or internal metabolic changes. The regulated processes include gene activation, direct effects on bacterial physiology such as chemotaxis, programmed developmental events in sporulation, and bacterial virulence in pathogenic organisms (47).

Pregenomic Studies, Genomic Information, and Postgenomic Analyses of *M. tuberculosis* Two-Component Systems

A number of pregenomic studies using conventional approaches have identified the presence in *M. tuberculosis* of elements corresponding to bacterial two-component systems (12, 51). The existence of phosphotransfer reactions with purified *M. tuberculosis* proteins has been biochemically demonstrated (24, 26, 51). According to the *M. tuberculosis* H37Rv genome sequence (7), there are 11 complete, genetically linked two-component systems (Table 1). One of these systems represents a more complex cluster of three linked genes: a response regulator and two histidine kinases. There are also seven additional solitary genes annotated as sensor kinases or response regulator genes that are scattered around the chromosome. They are termed orphan genes (Table 1) since their interacting partners are not obvious.

The studies of two-component systems have intensified since the cataloging of the 30 genes in this category by genomic and boinformatics approaches

Yossef Av-Gay • Division of Infectious Diseases, University of British Columbia, Vancouver, BC, Canada V5Z-3J5. **Vojo Deretic** • University of New Mexico Medical School, Albuquerque, NM 87131.

Table 1. *M. tuberculosis* two-component signal transduction systems[a]

Gene name	Rv no. (H37Rv genome)	Gene type and arrangement	Functional information or bioinformatic predictions	Macrophage phenotype	Animal model phenotype	References
devR-devS	*Rv3133c-Rv3132c*	RR-S/K	Identified by subtractive hybridization (H37Rv vs. H37Ra); induced by hypoxic conditions; affects α-crystallin expression and stationary-phase survival in vitro	*devR* mutant—paradoxical enhancement of early (24-h) survival in activated macrophages; expression (by GFP) in macrophages gradually increases with time	*devR* mutant—hypervirulent in SCID mice; also early (<60 days) hypervirulence in DBA mice	13, 31, 34, 42
kdpD-kdpE	*Rv1028c-Rv1027c*	S/K-RR	*kdpD-kdpE* designation based on bioinformatics including linkage to *kdpABC*, homologs of a high-affinity potassium uptake system	—	*kdpDE* mutant hypervirulent in SCID mice	7, 34
mprA-mprB	*Rv0981-Rv0982*	RR-S/K	Required for persistence	*mprA* mutant—enhanced growth in resting macrophages	*mprA* mutant attenuated for long-term persistence in the lungs	58
mtrA-mtrB	*Rv3246c-Rv3245c*	RR-S/K	Essential gene(s); seroconversion predictor of future active disease	NA (essential genes)	NA (essential genes)	12, 45, 51, 57
narL-narS	*Rv0844c-Rv0345*	RR divergent from S/K	*narL* designation based on bioinformatics	No phenotype in activated macrophages	*narL* mutant no phenotype in SCID mice	7, 34
orrA	*Rv0260c*	RR orphan	—	—	—	7
orrB	*Rv0818*	RR orphan	—	Constitutively expressed (by GFP)	—	7, 58
orrC	*Rv1626*	RR orphan	—	Expression studied by GFP	—	7, 58
orrD	*Rv2884*	RR orphan	—	Expression studied by GFP	—	7, 58
orrE	*Rv3143*	RR orphan	—	Induced intracellular expression (by GFP) in BCG but not detected in H37Rv	—	7, 58
oskA	*Rv2027c*	S/K orphan	High similarity to *devS*	—	—	7, 13, 42
oskB	*Rv3220c*	S/K orphan	—	—	*Rv3220c* mutant—no phenotype in SCID mice	7, 34
phoP-phoR	*Rv0757-Rv0758*	RR-S/K	*phoP-phoR* designation based on bioinformatics; affects LAM acylation and cording	*PhoP* mutant—reduced growth in macrophages; constitutively expressed (by GFP)	*phoP* mutant attenuated in mice	29, 37, 58
prrA-prrB	*Rv0903c-Rv0902c*	RR-S/K	Differentially expressed in macrophages	*prrA* mutant—transient (early) defect in intracellular growth	*prrA*—no phenotype in BALB/c mice (short term)	16, 19
senX3- regX3	*Rv0490-Rv0491*	S/K-RR	—	*regX3* not affected for growth in macrophages	*regX3* mutant—no phenotype in BALB/c mice (short term)	16
tcrX-tcrY	*Rv3765c-Rv3764c*	RR-S/K	—	—	*tcrXY* mutant—hypervirulent in SCID mice	34
trcR-trcS	*Rv1033c-Rv1032c*	RR-S/K	Expressed during log-phase growth in broth; gradually shuts down during intracellular growth	*trcS* mutant not affected in macrophages	*trcS* mutant—hypervirulent in SCID mice; no phenotype in BALB/c mice (short term)	16, 23, 34
tcrA-Rv601c-Rv600c	*Rv602c-Rv601c-Rv600c*	RR-S/K-S/K	—	—	—	7

[a]RR, response regulator; S/K, sensor kinase. Gene designations for orphan genes (with no linked or identified cognate second component): *orrA* to *orrE*, orphan response regulators A through E; *oskA* and *oskB*, orphan sensor-kinases A and B; —, information not available; NA, not applicable.

(7). To date, functional or expression studies of some type have been carried out with all but three of the systems. Knockout mutations have been generated in 9 of 11 complete two-component systems and in 1 out of the 7 orphan genes. The only two complete systems that have not been inactivated to date are *tcrA-Rv601c-Rv600c* and *mtrA-mtrB*. The former system has three linked genes, complicating interpretations with mutants once they are generated, but there are no other a priori reasons for it not to be studied. Attempts to inactivate the latter have been unsuccessful (34, 57). Since inactivation could be accomplished in an artificially constructed *mtrA* merodiploid, with a second copy of *mtrA* present on a plasmid, it was concluded that the *mtrA-mtrB* system must be essential in *M. tuberculosis* (57).

The bioinformatics approach (7) used in predicting/assigning functions to some of the two-component systems in *M. tuberculosis* has yielded only one likely ortholog (*kdpDE*) of a previously characterized two-component system. The *kdpDE* gene products show convincing similarity to the *Escherichia coli* regulators of a high-affinity potassium transport system (KdpABC), which imports potassium when it is scarce (52). The *M. tuberculosis kdpDE* genes are located immediately upstream of the putative *kdpABC* genes.

Global Genomic Analyses of *M. tuberculosis* Two-Component Systems

There have been a number of global approaches focused exclusively on *M. tuberculosis* two-component systems or including them within a broader search for genes of interest. The studies to date include (i) subtractive hybridization comparing H37Rv and H37Ra (*devRS*) (13), (ii) selective capture of transcribed sequences (*pprA*) (19), (iii) global expression analyses by using microarrays (*devRS*) (42), (iv) identification of mutants (*trcS*, *regX3*, and *prrA*) in an ordered transposon mutagenesis library of *M. tuberculosis* (16), (v) conventional generation of mutants in two-component systems (*devR*, *kdpDE*, *narL*, *tcrXY*, *trcS*, and *Rv3220c*) for simultaneous comparative analysis (34), and (vi) global expression analyses during intracellular growth (58).

Functional Studies of *M. tuberculosis* Two-Component Systems

At this point, the available information regarding the exact function of individual two-component systems in *M. tuberculosis* is limited. The majority of the reported studies have focused on expression profiles of these systems, biochemistry of the phospho-

transfer reaction, and DNA binding. Purified mycobacterial response regulators (MtrA, RegX3, and TrcR) have been shown to serve as typical substrates for the phosphotransfer reaction using heterologous (CheA) (51) or cognate (TrcS, SenX3) (23, 26) histidine protein kinases. Another sensor, DevS, has been purified and shown to undergo autophosphorylation typical of bacterial histidine protein kinases (41). DNA binding and autoregulation have been shown for RegX3 and TrcR (23). To date, no subordinate genes controlled by the response regulators in *M. tuberculosis* have been positively identified. One exception is a correlation in hypoxic expression between *devSR* and *acr* (encoding α-crystallin) detected by microarrays and a follow-up mutational analysis indicating that the disruption of a gene (*Rv3134c*) upstream of *devR* abrogates hypoxia-induced expression of *acr* (42). Since many mutants are now available, the door is open to apply microarray and other approaches to identify individual two-component regulons in *M. tuberculosis*.

M. tuberculosis Virulence and Two-Component Systems

Bacterial two-component systems often directly regulate bacterial virulence factors or control physiological functions affecting the fitness of a pathogen during infection. *M. tuberculosis* mutants with mutations in 9 of the 11 complete two-component systems and in one orphan sensor kinase gene have been tested for their phenotype during infection in mice and growth in resting or activated macrophages ex vivo. Different routes of infection (aerosol and intravenous) and murine models, including inbred strains of normal mice (BALB/c and DBA) or mice with severe combined immunodeficiency (SCID mice), have been used, complicating direct comparisons. A compilation of the available data is given in Table 1.

Two response regulators, *mprA* and *devR*, have been implicated in persistence and latency (42, 58). The *mprA* mutant has been tested in a murine model of tuberculosis and shown to be attenuated for long-term persistence in the lungs. The *devR* gene is induced under microaerobic conditions (42), considered by some investigators to approximate dormancy or latency. According to in vivo green fluorescent protein (GFP) analyses, the *devR* gene seems to be induced specifically in H37Rv infecting human monocyte-derived macrophages, and its expression levels increase later during infection, consistent with its proposed role in persistence (58). A *phoP* mutant was found to be attenuated in mice but not essential for persistence, as stated by the authors of the report (58). Studies of animal models with a number of other two-component mutants have yielded observations that may appear paradoxical. It has been reported (34) that in SCID mice (lacking T-cell responses but nevertheless having innate defense components), inactivation of a number of two-component systems (devR, tcrXY, trcS, and kdpDE) increased virulence (determined by time to death in SCID mice infected i.v. with 10^6 bacteria). A follow-up analysis with one of the mutants (the devR mutant) also showed enhanced survival in normal (DBA) mice and in activated macrophages. An independent study with another response regulator, mprA, showed enhanced growth of the knockout mutant in resting macrophages (58). The observations that inactivation of five different two-component systems increases the ability of M. tuberculosis to kill the murine host or enhances the growth of the mutant strains in mice or macrophages may reflect evolutionary adaptations of M. tuberculosis important for propagation and infectious cycle of the pathogen.

In a global approach to the examinination of intracellular expression of response regulators using transcriptional GFP fusions (58), the majority of response regulators (mtrA, narL, phoP, prrA, mprA, trcR, devR, tcrX, orrB, orrC, and orrD) have been tested for expression in murine and human macrophages infected with either the vaccine strain M. tuberculosis. subsp. bovis bacillus Calmette-Guérin (BCG) or virulent M. tuberculosis H37Rv. The response regulators showed patterns falling into one of the following four categories. (i) Class I includes response regulators (phoP and orrB) constitutively expressed in vivo and in vitro and in both BCG and H37Rv. (ii) Class II includes response regulators (mtrA) expressed in BCG and in H37Rv during infection of macrophages, with signs of induction during intracellular growth. (iii) Class III includes response regulators (mprA and orrB) expressed in BCG but repressed in H37Rv grown in murine or human macrophages. (iv) Class IV includes response regulators (devR) not expressed in BCG but induced in H37Rv. These patterns indicate that, in vivo, at least some two-component systems may be expressed at higher levels in the avirulent strain BCG relative to the virulent M. tuberculosis H37Rv. This theme parallels, at least in its first approximation, some of the surprising results with two-component knockout mutants enhancing virulence in mice (34) and increasing their growth in macrophages (34, 58).

Intracellular survival is a time-honored virulence property of M. tuberculosis and is linked to its ability to inhibit phagosome-lysosome fusion (40). A number of genes (narL, regX3, and trcS) have been tested for effects on growth in macrophages ex vivo, and no growth defect was detected (16, 34). The prrA mutant tested for survival in macrophages showed only transient (early) defects in intracellular growth. As mentioned above, devR and mprA mutants showed a paradoxical increase in survival or outright growth enhancement, respectively, although the intracellular growth-enhancing effect of mprA inactivation was abrogated in gamma interferon- and lipopolysaccharide-activated macrophages (34, 58). A phoP mutant displayed reduced growth in macrophages (37), and this property has been linked to lipoarabinomannan structure (mostly its extent of acylation) (29). Since lipoarabinomannan contributes significantly to the phagosome maturation arrest (i.e., inhibition of phagosome-lysosome fusion) (17, 18), this is a potentially relevant finding that may link the role of at least one of the two-component systems in M. tuberculosis with the intraphagosomal survival of this pathogen in the host macrophage.

SERINE/THREONINE PROTEIN KINASES OF MYCOBACTERIUM TUBERCULOSIS

Protein phosphorylation is a principal mechanism by which extracellular signals are translated into cellular responses. Protein phosphorylation is carried out by specific protein kinases and is coupled to dephosphorylation reactions carried out by protein phosphatases. As discussed above, the molecular system that is primarily responsible for stimulus response coupling in bacteria involves the so-called two-component systems, consisting of histidine kinase sensors and their associated response regulators (47), which are also present in mycobacteria (7, 51). In contrast, protein phosphorylation in eukaryotes occurs mainly on phosphoester (serine, threonine, or tyrosine) residues. The eukaryotic protein kinases and phosphatases form the backbone of this signal transduction pathway. Phosphoester protein kinases and their coupled phosphatases were previously thought to be unique to eukaryotes. As a result of accumulation of bacterial genome-sequencing data and the use of antiphosphoprotein antibodies, it has been shown that some prokaryotes, including M. tuberculosis, also contain phosphoester kinases and phosphatases (1, 2, 27, 59).

Thus far, STPKs have been shown to be involved in three different processes in prokaryotes, namely, development regulation, stress responses, and pathogenicity. Bacteria capable of differentiating into a new developmental state, including Streptomyces (30, 33, 50), Anabaena (60, 61), and Myxococcus xanthus (22, 49), contain a large number of STPK-encoding genes. In these bacteria, kinases are involved in the control of late stages of development, sporulation, or secondary-metabolite production. Interestingly, the dormant state of *M. tuberculosis*, associated with prolonged latent infection, has been proposed to involve the development of an extreme stationary phase that may be analogous to a spore-like state (14). Additionally, STPKs are involved in the survival of human pathogens within the host, as typified by the *Yersinia pseudotuberculosis* plasmid-encoded protein kinase YopO (20) and the *Pseudomonas aeruginosa* STPK (53). Both of these kinases are required for full virulence of these pathogens in mouse models.

In addition to their proposed roles in pathogenesis, several of the bacterial eukaryotic-like protein kinases are involved in the regulation of different developmental states of the bacterium. For example, the Ser/Thr kinase Pkn1 of *Myxococcus xanthus* is expressed exclusively during sporulation, and inactivation of this gene inhibits spore formation in this bacterium (59). *M. tuberculosis* encodes and expresses at least eight eukaryotic-like protein kinases, and six proteins can be phosphorylated in vitro, suggesting the presence of functional kinases in *M. tuberculosis* (1). The completion of the *M. tuberculosis* genome-sequencing project provided a list of 11 putative eukaryotic-like protein kinases (STPKs) and four protein phosphatases (7). An earlier review (2) provided the bioinformatic background about this newly discovered family of kinases, while in this chapter we summarize the current experimental, structural, and genomics information.

M. tuberculosis Serine/Threonine Protein Kinase Structure and Homology Analysis

The protein kinase signature, including all 11 domains that are conserved, as described by Hanks and Quinn (21), is present in all *M. tuberculosis* STPKs and was used as the criterion for their annotation during the sequencing project. An additional gene, *pknM*, which has previously been annotated as encoding a putative STPK, does not possess any recognizable kinase signatures. Not surprisingly, the homologues with highest sequence similarity were identified in the accumulating sequence data of *Mycobacterium leprae* and other actinomycetes such as *Streptomyces coelicolor*. Phylogenetic analysis comparing the kinase domains from all of the *M. tuberculosis* STPKs with other prokaryotic and eukaryotic kinases show that all but two of the *M. tuberculosis* STPKs, PknG and PknK, are present in a large cluster with most other prokaryotic sequences (2). PknG and PknK do not cluster with the rest of the *M. tuberculosis* STPKs and appear to be most similar to the eukaryotic STPKs. Four of the *M. tuberculosis* STPKs, PknA, PknB, PknG, and PknL, are present in *M. leprae*,

which has undergone a process of genetic drift and massive gene decay (8). None of the members of the *M. tuberculosis* STPK family are present in the missing chromosomal regions in bacillus Calmette-Guérin (BCG) (4). Transposon mutant libraries of *M. tuberculosis* H37Rv have also failed to disrupt except PknD (32), suggesting that these STPKs may play important roles in mycobacterial growth.

Functional Predictions

Since their discovery, five of the STPKs, PknA (6), PknB (3), PknD (36), PknF (28), and PknG (28), have been expressed as recombinant proteins in *E. coli* and shown to be active kinases. Table 2 summarizes our present knowledge of the *M. tuberculosis* STPKs, obtained from both experimental and bioinformatic analyses. Bioinformatic analysis has provided the majority of clues to possible STPK functions, which, together with location information from the genome, have allowed us to assign putative roles to certain STPKs (2). Of the 11 STPKs, 8 contain a single transmembrane helix (Color Plate 8). With the exception of PknL, the transmembrane region is located proximal to the amino-terminal kinase domain and is followed by a carboxy-terminal region of variable length. Topology prediction revealed that the N-terminal regions are on the inside and the C-terminal regions are on the outside (2), consistent with these proteins acting as signaling molecules between the cell exterior and interior. Recent crystal structure data for PknB support this prediction (56).

PknA is a 46-kDa protein that phosphorylates itself and artificial substrates (6). PknA modifies the morphology of *E. coli* when ectopically expressed in an overexpression system (6). *pknA* and *pknB* reside within an operon with a penicillin-binding protein and are probably used to control the switch between peptidoglycan elongation and septum formation in other bacteria (25, 43). The most extensively studied Ser/Thr kinase thus far is PknB. The *pknB* gene was cloned and expressed in *E.coli* and shown to encode an active protein capable of phosphorylating the artificial substrate myelin basic protein (3). Inhibition of PknB in BCG was shown to be associated with bacterial killing, suggesting that the STPKs can be used as drug targets in mycobacteria (15). The crystal structure of PknB revealed that it is a transmembrane signaling kinase (56). The predicted fold of the PknB extracellular domain, which was named the PASTA domain, matches the proposed targeting domain of penicillin-binding protein 2x (55).

The third member of the *M. tuberculosis* STPK family, PknD, was also shown to be an active kinase in an in vitro assay (36) and was found to be trun-

Table 2. Summary of *M. tuberculosis* STpK properties

Name	ORF[a]	Mol wt	TM[b]	Unique features	*M. leprae* homolog	Auto-P[c]	Proposed regulatory role	Response to:	Reference(s)
PknA	*Rv0015c*	45,598	+		+	+	Cell elongation and division		6
PknB	*Rv0014c*	66,511	+	PastA domain	+	+	Cell elongation and division	Starvation/ hypoxia	3, 15, 56
PknD	*Rv0931c*	69,514	+	β-propeller, PQQ domain		+	Phosphate transport	Starvation	35
PknE	*Rv1743*	60,513	+				Membrane transport		
PknF	*Rv1746*	50,669	+			+	Membrane transport		28
PknG	*Rv0410c*	81,579	−	Trx motif, TPR motif	+	+	Aminoacid uptake, stationary-phase metabolism	Hypoxia	28
PknH	*Rv1266c*	66,755	+	AFSK-like		+	Arabinan metabolism		
PknI	*Rv2914c*	61,806	+	Asn in active site		+	Cell division		
PknJ	*Rv2088*	61,564	+			+	?		
PknK	*Rv3080c*	119,420	−	PDZ and AAA domains			Transcription, secondary metabolites		
PknL	*Rv2176*	42,803	+		+		Transcription?		

[a]H37Rv open reading frame (ORF) designation.
[b]Predicted transmembrane-spanning region.
[c]Experimental evidence of autophosphorylation.

cated in *Mycobacterium bovis* (36). PknD contains a β-propeller structure in its carboxy terminus similar to the ones present in lipoprotein and scavenger receptors, extracellular matrix components, and tyrosine kinases (46). The funnel-shaped β-propeller structure is thought to act as the receptor module in these proteins. Interestingly, this structure also encompasses a pyrroloquinoline quinone (PQQ) binding site. PQQ is a redox coenzyme that serves as a cofactor for a number of enzymes, including some bacterial dehydrogenases (11).

The *pknE* and *pknF* genes are located in an operon with ABC transporter genes, indicating a possible role in regulation of transport systems. PknF was shown to be an active transmembrane kinase protein (28), while knowledge about PknE is still limited. The *pknH* gene is also located downstream of genes encoding ABC transporter components but is also proximal to the gene encoding the transcriptional regulator EmbR, which controls cell wall arabinosyltransferases, the target of the antimycobacterial drug ethambutol (5). EmbR is homologous to *S. coelicolor* AfsR, which is phosphorylated by the Ser/Thr kinase AfsK (30). Transcriptional analysis revealed that the *pknH* promoter is constitutively expressed in in vitro *Mycobacterium smegmatis* culture (10) and is down regulated on exposure to heat, acid, and microaerophylic conditions (9).

Few functional clues are available for PknI, PknJ, or PknL. It has been suggested that PknI is in-

volved in the regulation of cell division (2). The gene for PknJ is situated directly downstream of several transposon genes, whereas the gene for PknL, which is unique among the *M. tuberculosis* STPKs in having a carboxy-terminal transmembrane region, is in the same operon as a putative transcriptional regulator gene.

The last two members of the family, PknG and PknK, have no apparent transmembrane regions and are thus predicted to be soluble proteins. Immunoblot analysis of various cellular fractions of *M. tuberculosis* H37Rv revealed that PknG is predominantly a cytosolic enzyme, and in vitro activity assays revealed that it is an active kinase (28). PknG is the only STPK that has an N-terminal region preceeding the kinase domain; in this respect, it is similar to the secreted YopO kinase of *Yersinia*. PknG contains a short thioredoxin motif in its N terminus and a single TPR signaling domain (44) in its C terminus. The *pknG* gene is located in an operon with *glnH* (RV 1411c), which in other bacteria is part of a glutamine uptake system that is induced under nitrogen-limiting conditions. Thus, it seems likely that PknG plays a role in glutamine uptake and may be cotranscribed with *glnH* under nitrogen-limiting conditions. Indeed, GFP transcriptional fusion studies have demonstrated that PknG expression is up regulated on entry into stationary phase (9a).

PknK shows homology to the regulatory regions of transcriptional regulators of the LuxR family, such as *Klebsiella pneumoniae* AcoK and *Escherichia coli* MalT, and contains an ATP-binding motif (AAA) characteristic of molecules with ATPase activity. This AAA domain also encompasses a PDZ domain, which is involved in targeting signaling molecules to sub-membranous sites (38) and was proposed to regulate the production of a secondary metabolite(s) in *M. tuberculosis* (2).

Control of cell development, stress response, and pathogenesis are some of the functions that have been putatively assigned to the *M. tuberculosis* STPKs (Table 2). From the available evidence, at least three STPKs could be involved in cell growth and development, namely, PknA, PknB, and PknI, all of which appear to regulate aspects of cell division and elongation. Regulation of this crucial step in the cell cycle by STPKs has not been previously described, and this mode of regulation could be important with respect to the characteristically slow growth of *M. tuberculosis* and its ability to enter an extreme stationary phase or dormant state, associated with prolonged latent infection. The role of *M. tuberculosis* STPKs in pathogenicity is difficult to predict prior to thorough analysis of available mutants; however, the involvement of intra- and/or extracellular phosphorylation mechanisms in *M. tuberculosis* infection is likely. Interference with the normal immune response of the host during mycobacterial infection could be mediated by disabling host signaling pathways. Indeed, it has been recently shown that the signaling pattern of the host response is modified upon infection (26a).

ADDENDUM IN PROOF

Since the writing of this chapter, the following findings regarding two-component systems have been reported. (i) Autoregulation has been demonstrated for *prrA* (F. Ewann, C. Locht, and P. Supply, *Microbiology* 150:241–246, 2004). SenX3 has been found to contain a PAS-like domain involved in sensing oxygen or redox status in other systems (L. Rickman, J. W. Saldanha, D. M. Hunt, D. N. Hoar, M. J. Colston, J. B. Millar, and R. S. Buxton, *Biochem. Biophys. Res. Commun.* 314:259–267, 2004). DevS-DevR (also known as DosS-DosR or Rv 3133c-Rv3132c; see Table 1) have been found to engage in a phosphotransfer reaction, and one of the orphan kinases, OskA (Rv2027c, also named DosT) can cross-talk with DosR (D. M. Roberts, R. P. Liao, G. Wisedchaisri, W. G. Hol, and D. R. Sherman, *J. Biol. Chem.* 279: 23082–23087, 2004; D. K. Saini, V. Malhotra, and J. S. Tyagi, *FEBS Lett.* 565:75–80, 2004). A phosphotransfer reaction has also been shown for the MprA-MprB pair (T. C. Zahrt, C. Wozniak, D. Jones, and A. Trevett, *Infect. Immun.* 71:6962–6970, 2003). (ii) A new global analysis using selective capture of transcribed sequences has been reported (S. E. Haydel and J. E. Clark-Curtiss, *FEMS Microbiol. Lett.* 236:341–347, 2004). (iii) Effects on virulence have been reinvestigated for DevR, and a 3-log-lower bacterial burden in spleens of guinea pigs has been reported (V. Malhotra, D. Sharma, V. D. Ramanathan, H. Shakila, D. K. Saini, S. Chakravorty, T. K. Das, Q. Li, R. F. Silver, P. R. Narayanan, and J. S. Tyagi, *FEMS Microbiol. Lett.* 231:237–245, 2004). Two

studies on *senX-regX3* now show that they affect virulence (T. Parish, D. A. Smith, G. Roberts, J. Betts, and N. G. Stoker, *Microbiology* 149:1423–1435, 2003; Rickman et al., *Biochem. Biophys. Res. Commun.* 314:259–267, 2004). (iv) Candidate subordinate genes have been identified for *senX3-regX3* (Parish et al., *Microbiology* 149:1423–1435, 2003).

For SPTKs, an FHA phosphoprotein recognition domain has been found to mediate EmbR phosphorylation by PknH (V. Molle, D. Soulat, J. M. Jault, C. Grangeasse, A. J. Cozzone, and J. F. Prost, *FEMS Microbiol. Lett.* 234:215–223, 2004). A deletion mutant of *M. tuberculosis* PknG has been reported to control glutamine-glutamate metabolism. This mutant shows severe in vitro and in vivo growth attenuation (S. Cowley, M. Ko, N. Pick, R. Chow, K. J. Downing, B. G. Gordhan, J. C. Betts, V. Mizrahi, D. A. Smith, R. W. Stokes, and Y. Av-Gay, *Mol. Microbiol.* 52:1691–1702, 2004). Another study, using *M. bovis* BCG mutant and chemical intervention, suggests that PknG promotes survival within the macrophage by inhibiting phagosome-lysosome fusion, although no mechanistic studies have been provided (A. Walburger, A. Koul, G. Ferrari, L. Nguyen, C. Prescianotto-Baschong, K. Huygen, B. Klebl, C. Thompson, G. Bacher, and J. Pieters, *Science* 304:1800–1804, 2004). Walburger et al. (*Science* 304:1800–1804, 2004) indicate that PknG is unique to pathogenic mycobacteria, but the TIGR database suggests otherwise. The attenuated in vitro growth of the *pknG* mutant observed in *M. tuberculosis* (Cowley et al., *Mol. Microbiol.* 52:1691–1702, 2004) indicates that PknG may be of significance for mycobacterial metabolism and growth in general.

REFERENCES

1. **Av-Gay, Y., and J. E. Davies.** 1997. Components of eukaryotic-like signaling pathways in *Mycobacterium tuberculosis*. *Microb. and Comp. Genomics* 2:63–73.
2. **Av-Gay, Y., and M. Everett.** 2000. The eukaryotic-like Ser/Thr protein kinases of *Mycobacterium tuberculosis*. *Trends Microbiol.* 8:238–244.
3. **Av-Gay, Y., S. Jamil, and S. J. Drews.** 1999. Expression and characterization of the *Mycobacterium tuberculosis* serine/threonine protein kinase PknB. *Infect. Immun.* 67:5676–5682.
4. **Behr, M. A., M. A. Wilson, W. P. Gill, H. Salamon, G. K. Schoolnik, S. Rane, and P. M. Small.** 1999. Comparative genomics of BCG vaccines by whole-genome DNA microarray. *Science* 284:1520–1523.
5. **Belanger, A. E., G. S. Besra, M. E. Ford, K. Mikusova, J. T. Belisle, P. J. Brennan, and J. M. Inamine.** 1996. The *embAB* genes of *Mycobacterium avium* encode an arabinosyl transferase involved in the cell wall arabinan biosynthesis that is the target for the antimycobacterial drug ethambutol. *Proc. Natl. Acad. Sci. USA* 93:11919–11924.
6. **Chaba, R., M. Raje, and P. K. Chakraborti.** 2002. Evidence that a eukaryotic-type serine/threonine protein kinase from *Mycobacterium tuberculosis* regulates morphological changes associated with cell division. *Eur. J. Biochem.* 269:1078–1085.
7. **Cole, S. T., R. Brosch, J. Parkhill, T. Garnier, C. Churcher, D. Harris, S. V. Gordon, K. Eiglmeier, S. Gas, C. E. Barry III, F. Tekaia, K. Badcock, D. Basham, D. Brown, T. Chillingworth, R. Connor, R. Davies, K. Devlin, T. Feltwell, S. Gentles, N. Hamlin, S. Holroyd, T. Hornsby, K. Jagels, A. Krogh, J. McLean, S. Moule, L. Murphy, K. Oliver, J. Osborne, M. A. Quail, M.-A. Rajandream, J. Rogers, S. Rutter, K. Seeger, J. Skelton, R. Squares, S. Squares, J. E. Sulston, K. Taylor, S. Whitehead, and B. G. Barrell.** 1998. Deciphering the biol-

ogy of *Mycobacterium tuberculosis* from the complete genome sequence. *Nature* 393:537–544.

8. Cole, S. T., K. Eiglmeier, J. Parkhill, K. D. James, N. R. Thomson, P. R. Wheeler, N. Honore, T. Garnier, C. Churcher, D. Harris, K. Mungall, D. Basham, D. Brown, T. Chillingworth, R. Connor, R. M. Davies, K. Devlin, S. Duthoy, T. Feltwell, A. Fraser, N. Hamlin, S. Holroyd, T. Hornsby, K. Jagels, C. Lacroix, J. Maclean, S. Moule, L. Murphy, K. Oliver, M. A. Quail, M.-A. Rajandream, K. M. Rutherford, S. Rutter, K. Seeger, S. Simon, M. Simmonds, M. Skelton, R. Squares, S. Squares, K. Stevens, K. Taylor, S. Whitehead, J. R. Woodward, and B. G. Barrell. 2001. Massive gene decay in the leprosy bacillus. *Nature* 409:1007–1011.

9. Cowley, S., and Y. Av-Gay. 2001. Monitoring promoter activity and protein localization in *Mycobacterium* spp. using green fluorescent protein. *Gene* 264:225–231.

9a. Cowley, S., S. J. Drews, O. Tang, S. Jamil, M. Ko, and Y. Av-Gay. 2000. Investigations of the eukaryotic serine/threonine kinases of *M. tuberculosis. Tubercle Lung Dis.* 80:96.

10. Cowley, S. C., R. Babakaiff, and Y. Av-Gay. 2002. Expression and localization of the *Mycobacterium tuberculosis* protein tyrosine phosphatase PtpA. *Res. Microbiol.* 153:233–241.

11. Cozier, G. E., I. G. Giles, and C. Anthony. 1995. The structure of the quinoprotein alcohol dehydrogenase of *Acetobacter aceti* modelled on that of methanol dehydrogenase from *Methylobacterium extorquens. Biochem. J.* 308:375–379.

12. Curcic, R., S. Dhandayuthapani, and V. Deretic. 1994. Gene expression in mycobacteria: transcriptional fusions based on xylE and analysis of the promoter region of the response regulator *mtrA* from *Mycobacterium tuberculosis. Mol. Microbiol.* 13:1057–1064.

13. Dasgupta, N., V. Kapur, K. K. Singh, T. K. Das, S. Sachdeva, K. Jyothisri, and J. S. Tyagi. 2000. Characterization of a two-component system, *devR-devS*, of *Mycobacterium tuberculosis. Tubercle Lung Dis.* 80:141–159.

14. DeMaio, J., Y. Zhang, C. Ko, D. B. Young, and W. R. Bishai. 1996. A stationary-phase stress-response sigma factor from *Mycobacterium tuberculosis. Proc. Natl. Acad. Sci. USA* 93:2790–2794.

15. Drews, S. J., F. Hung, and Y. Av-Gay. 2001. A protein kinase inhibitor as an antimycobacterial agent. *FEMS Microbiol. Lett.* 205:369–374.

16. Ewann, F., M. Jackson, K. Pethe, A. Cooper, N. Mielcarek, D. Ensergueix, B. Gicquel, C. Locht, and P. Supply. 2002. Transient requirement of the PrrA-PrrB two-component system for early intracellular multiplication of *Mycobacterium tuberculosis Infect. Immun.* 70:2256–2263.

17. Fratti, R. A., J. M. Backer, J. Gruenberg, S. Corvera, and V. Deretic. 2001. Role of phosphatidylinositol 3-kinase and Rab5 effectors in phagosomal biogenesis and mycobacterial phagosome maturation arrest. *J. Cell Biol.* 154:631–644.

18. Fratti, R. A., J. Chua, I. Vergne, and V. Deretic. 2003. *Mycobacterium tuberculosis* glycosylated phosphatidylinositol causes phagosome maturation arrest. *Proc. Natl. Acad. Sci USA* 100:5437–5442.

19. Graham, J. E., and J. E. Clark-Curtiss. 1999. Identification of *Mycobacterium tuberculosis* RNAs synthesized in response to phagocytosis by human macrophages by selective capture of transcribed sequences (SCOTS). *Proc. Natl. Acad. Sci. USA* 96:11554–11559.

20. Hakansson, S., E. E. Galyov, R. Rosqvist, and H. Wolf-Watz. 1996. The *Yersinia* YpkA Ser/Thr kinase is translocated and subsequently targetted to the inner surface of the HeLa cell plasma membrane. *Mol. Microbiol.* 20:593–603.

21. Hanks, S. K., and A. M. Quinn. 1991. Protein kinase catalytic domain sequence database: identification of conserved fea-

tures of primary structure and classification of family members. *Methods Enzymol.* 200:38–62.

22. Hanlon, W. A., M. Inouye, and S. Inouye. 1997. Pkn9, a Ser/Thr protein kinase involved in the development of *Myxococcus xanthus. Mol. Microbiol.* 23:459–471.

23. Haydel, S. E., W. H. Benjamin, Jr., N. E. Dunlap, and J. E. Clark-Curtiss. 2002. Expression, autoregulation, and DNA binding properties of the *Mycobacterium tuberculosis* TrcR response regulator. *J. Bacteriol.* 184:2192–2203.

24. Haydel, S. E., N. E. Dunlap, and W. H. Benjamin, Jr. 1999. In vitro evidence of two-component system phosphorylation between the *Mycobacterium tuberculosis* TrcR/TrcS proteins. *Microb. Pathog.* 26:195–206.

25. Henriques, A. O., P. Glaser, P. J. Piggot, and C. P. Moran, Jr. 1998. Control of cell shape and elongation by the *rodA* gene in *Bacillus subtilis. Mol. Microbiol.* 28:235–247.

26. Himpens, S., C. Locht, and P. Supply. 2000. Molecular characterization of the mycobacterial SenX3–RegX3 two-component system: evidence for autoregulation. *Microbiology* 146:3091–3098.

26a. Karlsgot Hestrik, A. L., Z. Hmama, and Y. Av-Gay. 2003. Kinome analysis of host response to mycobacterial infection. *Infect. Immun.* 71:5514–5522.

27. Kennelly, P. J., and M. Potts. 1996. Fancy meeting you here! A fresh look at "prokaryotic" protein phosphorylation. *J. Bacteriol.* 178:4759–4764.

28. Koul, A., A. Choidas, A. K. Tyagi, K. Drlica, Y. Singh, and A. Ullrich. 2001. Serine/Threonine protein kinases PknF and PknG of *Mycobacterium tuberculosis*: characterization and localization. *Microbiology* 147:2307–2314.

29. Ludwiczak, P., M. Gilleron, Y. Bordat, C. Martin, B. Gicquel, and G. Puzo. 2002. *Mycobacterium tuberculosis phoP* mutant: lipoarabinomannan molecular structure. *Microbiology* 148:3029–3037.

30. Matsumoto, A., S. K. Hong, H. Ishizuka, S. Horinouchi, and T. Beppu. 1994. Phosphorylation of the AfsR protein involved in secondary metabolism in *Streptomyces* species by a eukaryotic-type protein kinase. *Gene* 146:47–56.

31. Mayuri, G. Bagchi, T. K. Das, and J. S. Tyagi. 2002. Molecular analysis of the dormancy response in *Mycobacterium smegmatis*: expression analysis of genes encoding the DevR-DevS two-component system, Rv3134c and chaperone alpha-crystallin homologues. *FEMS Microbiol. Lett.* 211:231–237.

32. McAdam, R. A., S. Quan, D. A. Smith, S. Bardarov, J. C. Betts, F. C. Cook, E. U. Hooker, A. P. Lewis, P. Woollard, M. J. Everett, P. T. Lukey, G. J. Bancroft, W. R. J. Jacobs, and K. Duncan. 2002. Characterization of a *Mycobacterium tuberculosis* H37Rv transposon library reveals insertions in 351 ORFs and mutants with altered virulence. *Microbiology* 148:2975–2986.

33. Nadvornik, R., T. Vomastek, J. Janecek, Z. Technikova, and P. Branny. 1999. Pkg2, a novel transmembrane protein Ser/Thr kinase of *Streptomyces granaticolor. J. Bacteriol.* 181:15–23.

34. Parish, T., D. A. Smith, S. Kendall, N. Casali, G. J. Bancroft, and N. G. Stoker. 2003. Deletion of two-component regulatory systems increases the virulence of *Mycobacterium tuberculosis. Infect. Immun.* 71:1134–1140.

35. Peirs, P., L. De Wit, M. Braibant, K. Huygen, and J. Content. 1997. A serine/threonine protein kinase from *Mycobacterium tuberculosis. Eur. J. Biochem.* 244:604–612.

36. Peirs, P., B. Parmentier, L. De Wit, and J. Content. 2000. The *Mycobacterium bovis* homologous protein of the *Mycobacterium tuberculosis* serine/threonine protein kinase Mbk (PknD) is truncated. *FEMS Microbiol. Lett.* 188:135–139.

37. Perez, E., S. Samper, Y. Bordas, C. Guilhot, B. Gicquel, and

C. Martin. 2001. An essential role for *phoP* in *Mycobacterium tuberculosis* virulence. *Mol. Microbiol.* **41:**179–187.

38. Ponting, C. P., C. Phillips, K. E. Davies, and D. J. Blake. 1997. PDZ domains: targeting signalling molecules to sub-membranous sites. *Bioessays* **19:**469–479.

39. Ronson, C. W., B. T. Nixon, and F. M. Ausubel. 1987. Conserved domains in bacterial regulatory proteins that respond to environmental stimuli. *Cell* **49:**579–581.

40. Russell, D. G., H. C. Mwandumba, and E. E. Rhoades. 2002. *Mycobacterium* and the coat of many lipids. *J. Cell Biol.* **158:**421–426.

41. Saini, D. K., N. Pant, T. K. Das, and J. S. Tyagi. 2002. Cloning, overexpression, purification, and matrix-assisted refolding of DevS (Rv 3132c) histidine protein kinase of *Mycobacterium tuberculosis. Protein Expression Purif.* **25:**203–208.

42. Sherman, D. R., M. Voskuil, D. Schnappinger, R. Liao, M. I. Harrell, and G. K. Schoolnik. 2001. Regulation of the *Mycobacterium tuberculosis* hypoxic response gene encoding alpha-crystallin. *Proc. Natl. Acad. Sci. USA* **98:**7534–7539.

43. Signoretto, C., F. Di Stefano, and P. Canapari. 1996. Modified peptidoglycan chemical composition in shape-altered *Escherichia coli. Microbiology* **142:**1919–1926.

44. Sikorski, R. S., M. S. Boguski, M. Goebl, and P. Hieter. 1990. A repeating amino acid motif in CDC23 defines a family of proteins and a new relationship among genes required for mitosis and RNA sythesis. *Cell* **60:**307–317.

45. Singh, K. K., X. Zhang, A. S. Patibandla, P. Chien, Jr., and S. Laal. 2001. Antigens of *Mycobacterium tuberculosis* expressed during preclinical tuberculosis: serological immunodominance of proteins with repetitive amino acid sequences. *Infect. Immun.* **69:**4185–4191.

46. Springer, T. A. 1998. An extracellular beta-propeller module predicted in lipprotein and scavenger receptors, tyrosine kinases, epidermal growth factor precursor, and extracellular matrix components. *J. Mol. Biol.* **283:**837–862.

47. Stock, J. B., A. J. Ninfa, and A. M. Stock. 1989. Protein phosphorylation and regulation of adaptive responses in bacteria. *Microbiol. Rev.* **53:**450–490.

48. Trach, K. A., J. W. Chapman, P. J. Piggot, and J. A. Hoch. 1985. Deduced product of the stage 0 sporulation gene *spo0F* shares homology with the Spo0A, OmpR, and SfrA proteins. *Proc. Natl. Acad. Sci. USA* **82:**7260–7264.

49. Udo, H., M. Inouye, and S. Inouye. 1997. Biochemical characterization of Pkn2, a protein Ser/Thr kinase from *Myxococcus xanthus*, a Gram-negative developmental bacterium. *FEBS Lett.* **400:**188–192.

50. Urabe, H., and H. Ogawara. 1995. Cloning, sequencing, and expression of serine/threonine kinase-encoding genes from *Streptomyces coelicolor* A3(2). *Gene* **153:**99–104.

51. Via, L. E., R. Curcic, M. H. Mudd, S. Dhandayuthapani, R. J. Ulmer, and V. Deretic. 1996. Elements of signal transduction and *Mycobacterium tuberculosis*: in vitro phosphorylation and in vivo expression of the response regulator MtrA. *J. Bacteriol.* **178:**3314–3321.

52. Walderhaug, M. O., J. W. Polarek, P. Voelkner, J. M. Daniel, J. E. Hesse, K. Altendorf, and W. Epstein. 1992. KdpD and KdpE, proteins that control expression of the kdpABC operon, are members of the two-component sensor-effector class of regulators. *J. Bacteriol.* **174:**2152–2159.

53. Wang, J., C. Li, H. Yang, A. Mushegian, and S. Jin. 1998. A novel serine/threonine protein kinase homologue of *Pseudomonas aeruginosa* is specifically inducible within the host infection site and is required for full virulence in neutropenic mice. *J. Bacteriol.* **180:**6764–6768.

54. Wolanin, P. M., P. A. Thomason, and J. B. Stock. 2002. Histidine protein kinases: key signal transducers outside the animal kingdom. *Genome Biol.* **3:**REVIEWS3013.

55. Yates, C., R. D. Finn, and A. Bateman. 2002. The PASTA domain: a beta-lactam-binding domain. *Trends Biochem. Sci.* **27:**438.

56. Young, T. A., B. Delagoutte, J. A. Endrizzi, A. M. Falick, and T. Alber. 2003. Structure of *Mycobacterium tuberculosis* PknB supports a universal activation mechanism for Ser/Thr protein kinases. *Nat. Struct. Biol.* **10:**168–174.

57. Zahrt, T. C., and V. Deretic. 2000. An essential two-component signal transduction system in *Mycobacterium tuberculosis. J Bacteriol.* **182:**3832–3838.

58. Zahrt, T. C., and V. Deretic. 2001. *Mycobacterium tuberculosis* signal transduction system required for persistent infections. *Proc. Natl. Acad. Sci. USA* **98:**12706–12711.

59. Zhang, C. C. 1996. Bacterial signalling involving eukaryotic-type protein kinases. *Mol. Microbiol.* **20:**9–15

60. Zhang, C. C., A. Friry, and L. Peng. 1998. Molecular and genetic analysis of two closely linked genes that encode, respectively, a protein phosphatase 1/2A/2B homolog and a protein kinases homolog in the cyanobacterium *Anabaena* sp. strain PCC 7120. *J. Bacteriol.* **180:**2616–2622.

61. Zhang, C. C., and L. Libs. 1998. Cloning and characterisation of the *pknD* gene encoding an eukaryotic-type protein kinase in the cyanobacterium *Anabaena* sp. PCC7120. *Mol. Gen. Genet.* **258:**26–33.

Tuberculosis and the Tubercle Bacillus
Edited by Stewart T. Cole et al.
© 2005 ASM Press, Washington, D.C.

Chapter 23

Nucleic Acid Metabolism

Valerie Mizrahi, Michael Buckstein, and Harvey Rubin

In recent years, our understanding of nucleic acid metabolism in *Mycobacterium tuberculosis* has been informed by major advances on three fronts: (i) the availability of the genome sequences of *M. tuberculosis* and other mycobacteria, (ii) the development of robust methods for creating mutant strains, and (iii) the wide-scale application of postgenomic tools for analyzing global gene expression patterns and for comparing the genomes of strains of *M. tuberculosis* and closely related species. In addition, a significant number of mycobacterial proteins involved in nucleic acid metabolism have been the subject of in-depth structural and biochemical investigation (see, e.g., references 1 and 2), and the structures of many more are expected to become available soon through the efforts of the TB Structural Genomics Consortium. In the first part of this chapter, we review the biosynthesis, salvage, and interconversion of purine and pyrimidine ribonucleotides; the biosynthesis of deoxyribonucleotides; and the biosynthesis and function of (p)ppGpp in *M. tuberculosis*. In the second part, we review the processes of DNA replication, repair, and mutagenesis in the context of the mechanisms of genome evolution, pathogenesis, and the development of drug resistance in *M. tuberculosis*. The reader is referred to reference 54 for detailed background information on the genes and pathways reviewed herein.

BIOSYNTHESIS, SALVAGE, AND INTERCONVERSION OF RIBONUCLEOTIDES

Purine Ribonucleotide Synthesis

The genome sequence of *M. tuberculosis* confirmed that the de novo synthesis of purines is mediated by the same highly conserved pathways seen in other bacteria. The synthetic machinery and pathways that convert the starting product of IMP to AMP and GMP are essentially intact in *M. tuberculosis*, with the exception being the absence of *purR*, the purine repressor seen in other microorganisms. A possible candidate for *purR*, Rv3575c, does, however, exist but remains untested. Although few rate constants are known, it is hypothesized that the slow growth rate of *M. tuberculosis* and other mycobacteria might be a function of reduced rates at critical steps in the pathway of making nucleotides. Purine repression thus might never be necessary for *M. tuberculosis*.

Interesting work has been done targeting various enzymes in the purine synthesis pathway and has revealed novel functions for some of these enzymes. For instance, *M. smegmatis* mutants with mutations in amidophosphoribosyl transferase (*purF*), which replaces the pyrophosphate group of phosphororibosyl-α-phosphate with the amide nitrogen of glutamine, show a precipitous reduction in viability for the first 5 to 10 days in an O_2-starved stationary-phase culture, even in medium supplemented with purines (39). After 10 to 20 days, near-wild-type culturability is regained. Sequence analysis shows very close homology between *M. smegmatis*, *M. leprae*, and *M. tuberculosis*, suggesting similar functions. Whether this phenotype represents utilization of a novel synthesis pathway reflecting other needs for purine synthesis intermediates or is simply a function of the fact that the cells are entering a dormant state remains to be determined.

While detailed kinetic analyses of most of the intermediate enzymes have yet to be performed, the enzymes involved in the final steps of purine nucleotide synthesis that convert GMP and AMP to triphosphate species in mycobacteria have been well studied. Adenylate kinase from *M. tuberculosis* is a member of the "short"-isoform adenylate kinases, where the

Valerie Mizrahi • Molecular Mycobacteriology Research Unit, School of Pathology, National Health Laboratory Service and University of the Witwatersrand, Johannesburg, South Africa. **Michael Buckstein and Harvey Rubin** • Division of Infectious Diseases, Department of Medicine, University of Pennsylvania Medical Center, Philadelphia, PA 19104-6073.

solvent-exposed LID domain is reduced in amino acid number to an irregular loop (56). As predicted, the specific activity of *M. tuberculosis* adenylate kinase is approximately threefold lower than that of *Escherichia coli*. The lower kinetic rate might reflect an overall decreased rate of nucleotide synthesis that could contribute to the slow growth of *M. tuberculosis*. Nucleoside disphosphate kinase (Ndk), which nonspecifically transfers phosphate groups from ATP or GTP to nucleotide or deoxynucleotide diphosphates for DNA, RNA, and polysaccharide synthesis, has been crystallized in *M. tuberculosis* (12). Functional studies demonstrated an elegant mechanism by which one set of *M. smegmatis* proteins can complex nucleoside disphosphate kinase to channel nucleoside triphosphate synthesis toward the GTP product while two other proteins channel the Ndk toward either CTP or UTP synthesis (72). These studies suggest that the Ndk and its binding proteins form a network that controls the synthesis of nucleotide-linked sugars necessary for nucleic acid and cell wall polysaccharide production. Interestingly, Ndk is also secreted by *M. bovis* BCG (94) and *M. tuberculosis* (13) and serves to enhance ATP-induced macrophage cell death (13).

Pyrimidine Ribonucleotide Synthesis

Like purine synthesis, the six enzymes involved in pyrimidine biosynthesis have been identified in the *M. tuberculosis* genome and appear to be highly conserved. Although this pathway is superficially similar to that of *E. coli* and even mammalian cells, it is expected that *M. tuberculosis* will exhibit unique regulatory properties in correlation with its slow growth. For instance, aspartate carbomoyltransferase (*pyrB*) in *E. coli* has a well-characterized allosteric activation by ATP and inactivation by CTP, presumably balancing purine and pyrimidine synthesis. Exactly how *M. tuberculosis* achieves such regulation in the context of its GC-rich genome remains a mystery. Evolutionary analyses of *pyrB* show *M. tuberculosis* clustering closest with *P. aeuroginosa* and *P. putida* (11). The large phylogenetic distance from *E. coli* certainly leaves potential for alternative regulation in the context of a GC-rich genome. In terms of regulatory elements, *M. tuberculosis* also possesses *pyrR*, the first gene in the *pyr* operon and one which encodes a putative regulatory protein. In *B. subtilis*, PyrR is bifunctional: it attenuates transcription by binding specifically to the *pyr* operon mRNA and is also a uracil phosphoribosyltransferase (79). Site-directed mutagenesis with *B. subtilis* has identified several amino acids essential for RNA binding that are concentrated in two segments (71). Many of these residues

are conserved in *M. tuberculosis*. Whether *M. tuberculosis* has the same regulatory and catalytic properties as PyrR in *B. subtilis* remains to be determined experimentally, although some critical residues involved in regulation are strongly implicated by sequence homology.

Salvage and Interconversion Pathways

Although the formation of AMP and GMP from IMP is irreversible, purine and pyrimidine nucleotides can be interconverted based on metabolic need through the activities of several enzymes in mycobacteria, including purine nucleotide phosphorylase (DeoD), adenosine deaminase (Add), and hypoxanthine-guanine phosphoribosyltransferase (Hgprt). Purine nucleotide phosphorylase catalyzes the phosphorolysis of the N-ribosidic bonds of purine nucleosides and deoxynucleosides. *M. tuberculosis* PNP is a trimeric protein, unlike its hexameric counterpart in *E. coli*. It has recently been cocrystallized with a transition state analogue, immucillin-H, revealing three distinct catalytic sites (74). The crystal structure, as well as its slow-onset inhibition and picomolar dissociation constants with immucillin-H, supports a catalytic mechanism of reactant destabilization by electrostatic interactions, transition-state stabilization, and leaving-group activation. This information should facilitate specific drug development. A *Listeria hgprt* mutant shows a deficiency in survival under nutritionally limited conditions. This phenotype is very similar to that of a *rel* mutant (see below) and indicates that this gene might also play an important role in linking purine synthesis and the stringent response (77). Such a link has yet to be shown experimentally in mycobacteria but would be expected to play a role in regulating nucleotide concentrations under stringent conditions.

Wheeler measured the activity of the purine and pyrimidine salvage systems in *M. leprae*, *M. microti*, and *M. avium* and found phosphoribosyltransferases specific for certain metabolites in each of the species (87–90). Under various growth conditions, different activities were observed. Of the pathways found, only the gene encoding a uracil phosphoribosyltransferase (*upp*) was identified in the *M. tuberculosis* genome. The genome of *M. tuberculosis* does not contain a specific thymidine kinase, making it one of few organisms that lack this enzyme (58). However, *M. tuberculosis* does contain the genes encoding deoxycytidine triphosphate deaminase (*dcd*), which converts dCTP to dUTP; deoxyuridine triphosphatase (*dut*), which converts dUTP to duMP; and thymidylate synthase (both *thyA* and *thyX* [Rv2754c] [58]), which converts dUMP to dTMP. Interestingly, *dcd* was found to be activated in granulomas in frogs chronically infected with *M. marinum* (63), suggesting a possible role for nucleotide salvage in persistence.

The thymidine generated by both the salvage and de novo pathways is converted by thymidylate kinase to TTP. Thymidylate kinase catalyzes phosphate group transfer, preferentially from ATP, to convert thymidine diphosphate to thymidine triphosphate. Some recent work has focused on thymidylate kinase in *M. tuberculosis* and has raised hopes for its exploitation as a novel drug target. Crystal structures, with and without substrate, have been solved (42, 43). Some features such as the dimerization mode and binding domains are unique to *M. tuberculosis*, in contrast to yeast, human, and *E. coli* thymidylate kinase, and thus provide candidates for specific drug targeting (33).

Formation of Deoxyribonucleotides from Ribonucleotides

Ribonucleotide reductase (RNR), the two-subunit enzyme that catalyzes the reduction of nucleoside diphosphates to deoxynucleoside diphosphates, is responsible for the first committed step in DNA synthesis. This step is the rate-limiting step for replicating the genome and thus is an ideal candidate for drug targeting. Previous biochemical studies had suggested that the active RNR in *M. tuberculosis* is of the class Ib type encoded by *nrdE* and *nrdF2* (91, 92). While a second small-subunit (NrdF1) does exist and contains all of the necessary residues to constitute an active subunit, it does not appear to function with the NrdE large subunit (91). Genetic evidence in support of this conclusion is that targeted knockout of *nrdF2* could be achieved only in the presence of a complementing allele, confirming that *nrdF2* is essential and cannot be functionally substituted by *nrdF1* (22), which is non-essential (48). *M. tuberculosis* RNR has been studied extensively at the biochemical and biophysical levels, revealing many unique features in the *nrdEF* system. For example, the tyrosyl free radical on the small subunit is located in a rigid hydrophobic pocket, as determined by electron paramagnetic resonance spectrum analysis (44). The consequent inaccessibility of the radical makes the *M. tuberculosis* enzyme particularly resistant to drugs that act as radical scavengers, such as phenols, thiols, and hydroxyurea (24).

In addition to the class Ib RNR, *M. tuberculosis* encodes a putative class II RNR encoded by *nrdZ*. The class II RNRs contain a single subunit, are also active under anaerobic conditions, utilize cobalt instead of iron, and reduce nucleoside di- and triphosphates. *nrdZ* is part of the hypoxia-induced DosR

regulon (73, 83) and, as such, is an obvious candidate for ensuring bacterial survival in the limiting environment of the granuloma. However, survival of an *nrdZ* null mutant was not impaired under hypoxic conditions in vitro, and the lungs of B6D2/F$_1$ mice infected with the *nrdZ* mutant showed equal bacterial loads to those infected with the parental wild-type strain up to 1 year postinfection. Combined with the inability of *nrdZ* alone to compensate for loss of *nrdF2*, these observations argue against a significant role for *nrdZ* in growth and survival of *M. tuberculosis*, at least in a murine infection model (22).

The Stringent Response

The ability to withstand limiting nutrient availability and low O$_2$ tension is evident in *M. tuberculosis*, which can remain dormant in granulomatous lesions in a host for decades. The biochemistry of nucleotides, most notably through the conversion of GTP to hyperphosphorylated moieties, ppGpp and pppGpp [(p)ppGpp], is a central process in the response of other microorganisms to the environmental stress of amino acid or carbon source depletion. It is now known from both in vitro and in vivo studies that production and hydrolysis of (p)ppGpp are carried out in *M. tuberculosis* by *relA*, originally identified in the *M. tuberculosis* genome based on its homology to the gene that encodes the enzyme that catalyzes the synthesis and degradation of (p)ppGpp in *E. coli* (3). In *M. tuberculosis*, *relA* encodes a bifunctional enzyme that carries out a synthetic activity, 3'-pyrophosphoryltransferase, to form (p)ppGpp and a degradative activity, (p)ppGpp-specific 3'-pyrophosphohydrolase. It appears that gram-positive organisms contain both the RelA and SpoT functions encoded on a single gene (reference 46 and references cited therein). The separate catalytic domains of these bifunctional enzymes have been experimentally documented by using truncated proteins in *Streptomyces equisimilis* (49) and *M. tuberculosis* (A. Avarbock, D. Avarbock, J. S. Teh, M. Buckstein, Z. Wang, and H. Rubin, unpublished data).

The biochemistry of Rel$_{Mtb}$ has been studied (3). Mn^{2+} can replace the requirement for Mg^{2+} in the synthesis reaction, but excess Mg^{2+} results in a dramatic reduction of enzymatic function in vitro (3). In contrast, hydrolysis of the 3'-pyrophosphoryl group of (p)ppGpp by Rel$_{Mtb}$ is an exclusively manganese-dependent reaction, similar to the action of SpoT from other organisms (3, 50). The catalytic activity of Rel$_{Mtb}$ is increased manyfold when it is mixed with uncharged tRNA and ribosomes (4), consistent with the current Rel model in other bacteria that amino acid starvation activates the (p)ppGpp synthesis pathway. Although truncated forms of Rel can exhibit single catalytic kinetics at baseline levels, they lose the ability to be activated by uncharged tRNA and ribosomes. These data suggest that the regulatory domain(s) of the protein is located along the C terminal.

Protein synthesis is thought to be decreased in dormant *M. tuberculosis*, but the dormant bacteria remain poised to initiate protein synthesis once environmental conditions become favorable (36). Given the ability of (p)ppGpp to decrease protein synthesis by inhibiting rRNA and tRNA transcription, we suggest that (p)ppGpp levels may play an important role in entry into and emergence from dormancy. Additionally, (p)ppGpp may lower *M. tuberculosis* protein synthesis by increasing the levels of RpoS-like sigma factors (28). A *rel*$_{\text{Mtb}}$ knockout strain shows a significant reduction in aerobic growth rate in both minimal and rich media, suggesting that Rel might play a functional role in unstarved bacteria as well; also, as predicted, long-term survival during in vitro starvation or nutrient run-out is dramatically impaired in the mutant strain (61). In subsequent studies, loss of Rel$_{\text{Mtb}}$ accordingly was found to severely compromise the ability of *M. tuberculosis* to establish a persistent infection in mice (16).

DNA REPLICATION, REPAIR, AND MUTAGENESIS

Genome Plasticity in *M. tuberculosis*

Currently, there is considerable interest in understanding the forces driving genome evolution in mycobacteria, particularly with respect to the development of pathogenicity and phylogenetic diversity (9, 55). Microbial evolution is driven by a variety of genetic mechanisms, including lateral gene transfer, genetic rearrangements, and point mutations. However, the sterility of the ecological niche occupied by *M. tuberculosis* implies that its microevolution within

the human host is driven by mechanisms other than lateral gene transfer. Since the apparent scarcity of single-nucleotide polymorphisms (SNPs) in structural genes in the *M. tuberculosis* complex was first documented (76), the picture that has emerged is one in which insertion and deletion events (InDels) provide the major source of genome plasticity in the *M. tuberculosis* complex (8). The IS6110 element, which demonstrates variability in copy number and site of insertion (84) and promotes deletions by homologous recombination (26, 35), is an undisputedly important mediator of genome plasticity. Genome-wide comparisons using higher-resolution microarray techniques have also revealed a significant extent of genomic deletions among clinical isolates of *M. tuberculosis* (38, 78). Moreover, the high concentration of InDels in PE and PPE genes, coupled with the highly polymorphic character of these genes, suggests that repeat expansions and contractions at these loci provide another major source of genetic variability in *M. tuberculosis* (5, 8). However, the extent of sequence variation between isolates of *M. tuberculosis* attributable to SNPs is greater than previously thought (27, 37), thus implicating base substitution mutations as an additional and potentially important source of variation. The mechanisms leading to the various types of genetic alterations are summarized in Table 1 and discussed below.

Genetic Recombination

In addition to providing a mechanism for generating genetic diversity by creating novel combinations of elements that could confer selective advantages on the organism, genetic recombination plays a second important function in vivo, namely, the recombinational repair of DNA as a mechanism for maintaining genome integrity. Extensive studies over the past decade, which were predicated on the assumption that the ability of *M. tuberculosis* to survive in the harsh intracellular environment of its phagocytic host cell would depend on its ability to re-

Table 1. Mechanisms underlying genome plasticity in *M. tuberculosis*

Mechanism	Type of polymorphism	Responsible and/or affected loci	Genes and/or proteins involved
Recombination	Insertion, deletion	Repeats, e.g., IS6110	*recA* and other recombination genes
Transposition	Insertion	Various IS elements	Tranposases, resolvases
Replication errors	Insertions/deletions at tandem repeats	PE and PPE genes, MIRU elements, and simple repeats	DNA polymerase III, other?
Error-prone replication (conditional)	SNPs	Sites of DNA damage	*dnaE2*, other?
	Frameshifts		*dnaE2*?, others (*dinP*, *dinX*)?
DNA repair and/or detoxification defects (heritable)	SNPs	Global	*mutT* and *mutT2* or *ogt*?, others?

pair DNA damage, have provided a wealth of information on the RecA protein from this and other mycobacteria. X-ray crystal structures have revealed a weakening in the higher-order aggregation of filaments into bundles and explained its weakened interaction with ATP, which may have functional implications (18). Significant advances have also been made in defining the enzymatic activity of RecA (80) and the regulatory mechanisms governing its expression and function. *recA* is positively regulated at the transcriptional level in response to DNA damage via dual, *recA/lexA*-dependent and -independent pathways (21). Negative regulation of RecA has also been shown to occur posttranscriptionally by direct interaction of RecA with RecX, which suppresses ATPase and strand exchange activities (81). RecA also interacts specifically with the single-stranded DNA binding protein in vivo, suggesting a joint function for these two proteins in DNA repair and/or recombination processes (66). Finally, the RecA intein possesses both Mn^{2+}-ATP- and Mg^{2+}-dependent endonuclease activity for cleaving cognate and ectopic sites, respectively, and as such is a novel homing endonuclease, which may utilize its ectopic cleavage site ability to spread through natural populations (31, 32). However, the physiological role (if any) of this intein in recombination mediated by its cognate RecA is unclear.

Although some insights into the recombination process have been gained from its exploitation as a tool for genome manipulation (34, 60), the molecular details remain obscure (57). For instance, the efficiency of homologous recombination is dependent on the length of homology (59), but the minimal efficient processing segment below which recombination is inefficient has not yet been reported for any mycobacterial species. Similarly, insights into the constraints on recombination between similar but not identical (homeologous) sequences of DNA would be of significant interest since homeologous recombination not only plays an important role in the evolution of DNA sequences and genomes by lateral gene transfer but also raises a barrier to genetic exchange between related genera (65).

Dispersion of Mobile Genetic Elements and Replication Errors at Repeat Loci

The biology of mycobacterial transposons was recently reviewed by McAdam et al. (47). A total of 56 loci showing homology to insertion sequences (ISs) were identified in *M. tuberculosis* H37Rv (30). Of these, only the commonly used epidemiological marker IS*6110* has been shown to be capable of transposing from one site to another. However, DNA damage leads to widespread induction of transposases, resolvases, and IS elements in *M. tuberculosis*, including members of the 13E12 repeat family (6, 20, 64). Although their mobility remains to be ascertained, these observations suggest that such elements might be activated by genotoxic stress.

The formation of InDels at repeat loci has been proposed to occur as a result of replication errors mediated by repeat sequences (8). This hypothesis has been tested by using a reporter assay modeled on a deletion polymorphism observed in the Rv0746 gene of *M. bovis* BCG Pasteur (14). Preliminary results suggest that deletions of this type indeed occur primarily by slipped-strand mispairing events between neighboring (proximal and distal) PGRS elements (S. Durbach et al., unpublished data). However, the applicability of this type of slippage mechanism to other repeat loci remains to be investigated.

Heritable and Environment-Dependent Mutators

All drug resistance in *M. tuberculosis* is mediated by the introduction of mutations in chromosomal genes, a significant proportion of which correspond to base substitution and frameshift mutations (95). One of the factors determining the rate at which antibiotic resistance emerges in a bacterial population is the rate of formation of the resistant mutants, which, in turn, is dependent on the mutation rate of the organism and the population size. The rate of emergence of multidrug-resistant strains of *M. tuberculosis* (25) is higher than would be expected from the product of individual mutation frequencies, suggesting that the in vitro mutation frequencies determined for laboratory strains of *M. tuberculosis* (19) might not reflect the situation occurring during parasitism of the human host. For this reason, significant attention has focused recently on investigating mutational dynamics in *M. tuberculosis*.

Important new insights into the modulation of mutational dynamics in *M. tuberculosis* are emerging from studies of heritable and environment-dependent (conditional) mutator genes, respectively. The potential importance of heritable mutators with a constitutive mutator phenotype in the adaptation of bacterial populations is evidenced by their presence in pathogenic isolates of *E. coli*, *Salmonella* (41), and *Neisseria* (67), with most, but not all, of the pathogen mutator strains identified to date owing their increased mutation rate to defects in methyl-directed mismatch repair. Interestingly, a high percentage of *M. tuberculosis* strains of the W-Beijing genotype carry a missense mutation in *mutT4* (Rv3908) and a second mutation in either *mutT2* or *ogt* (62). Since the W-Beijing genotype is common among isolates responsible for multidrug-resistant *M. tuberculosis* outbreaks, it is tempting to speculate that defects in the elimination of damaged nucleotide pools (*mutT*) and/or in the reversal of alkylation damage (*ogt*) may facilitate the acquisition of a multidrug-resistant genotype by increasing the supply of mutants better equipped for survival during immune surveillance and/or drug selective pressure. However, the data available to date argue against an elevated rate of mutation to rifampin resistance in strains of the W-Beijing genotype (86).

Homogeneous populations of constitutive mutators can, however, be maladapted to survival (51). Environment-dependent mutators offer an alternate mechanism for enhancing survival in response to stressful conditions (52). The best-known examples of such mutators are the genes encoding SOS-inducible, error-prone repair polymerases (29). These enzymes participate in translesion synthesis under conditions that promote DNA damage, and they thereby enhance survival after DNA damage and generate mutations that may be beneficial for survival. *M. tuberculosis* possesses two Y-family polymerase-encoding genes, *dinP* and *dinX*, but neither was damage inducible by mitomycin C (7). However, another DNA polymerase-encoding gene, *dnaE2*, is SOS inducible in *M. tuberculosis* (6, 20) and is solely responsible for damage-induced point mutagenesis to rifampin and streptomycin resistance in *M. tuberculosis* and *M. smegmatis* and for protecting these organisms against the lethal effects of DNA damage in vitro (6). This alternate, catalytic (α) subunit of DNA polymerase III is therefore superficially analogous to the *E. coli* SOS polymerases IV and V and is the first example of a family C DNA polymerase displaying error-prone DNA repair. Loss of *dnaE2* resulted in a marked attenuation of *M. tuberculosis* in mice, in accordance with the observed induction of *dnaE2* during stationary infection. Moreover, rifampin-resistant mutants were found to arise less frequently in mice infected with the mutant strain than in the parental wild type, suggesting that ongoing *dnaE2*-dependent DNA repair is required for full virulence and contributes to the emergence of drug resistance in vivo (6). In contrast, the physiological roles of DinP, DinX, and the putative DNA polymerase Rv2328c (45) in DNA repair, genetic diversification, and long-term survival (93) remain to be elucidated.

DNA Repair Systems

In addition to their potential utility as vaccine candidates, mutants of *M. tuberculosis* and *M. bovis* BCG that are defective in various DNA repair pathways are being applied in delineating regulatory pathways of gene expression (21) and in probing the nature and extent of the genotoxic stresses imposed on these pathogens during an in vivo infection. A *recA* deletion mutant of *M. tuberculosis* has been used to distinguish damage-inducible genes that are regulated in a *recA*-dependent manner from those induced via *recA*-independent mechanisms (64). This has led to the discovery of a novel induction mechanism for the *recA* gene, which is independent of *recA* and *lexA* (21). A corresponding *recA* deletion mutant of *M. bovis* BCG was constructed as a genetically more stable BCG vaccine candidate (68). This strain was predictably hypersensitive to DNA damage in vitro but displayed no further attenuation in a mouse model of infection and showed the same protective efficacy as the wild type (69). The lack of an in vivo phenotype of this mutant contrasts with the profound attenuation of other intracellular pathogens with impaired recombinational repair function (10) and is particularly surprising in light of the critical role of recombinational repair in the survival of *E. coli* exposed to ˙NO (75). Interestingly, functional impairment of the specialized alkylation damage repair and reversal system of *M. tuberculosis* yielded similar results: deletion of the *adl-ogt* operon rendered *M. tuberculosis* hypersensitive to DNA damage but had no discernible effect on growth or persistence in mice. Since alkylation damage of DNA is a downstream consequence of nitrosative stress, these observations led to the conclusion that in the murine infection model, the permeation of nitrosative stress to the level of cytotoxic, alkyative damage to the DNA is restricted in *M. tuberculosis* (23). However, in stark contrast to these findings, other components of the base excision repair and nucleotide excision repair pathways, specifically UvrB and Ung (uracil DNA glycosylase), were subsequently shown to be crucial for resistance to nitrosative stress (17, 82). Screening of a saturation transposon mutant library of *M. tuberculosis* at various stages of growth in vivo underscored the importance of base excision repair by Ung and by exonuclease III (*xthA*) and endonuclease IV (*end*) for growth of this organism in mice (70). Therefore, the overall picture that has emerged from studies of DNA repair-defective mutants is that although the in vivo environment of *M. tuberculosis* is indeed DNA damaging (6), the nature of the predominant lesions, such as deaminated cytosine and other possible products of oxidative and/or nitrosative damage (70), necessitates repair by excision-based mechanisms rather than by recombination.

The repair of double-stranded breaks (DSBs) may also be of particular importance in *M. tuberculosis* on the grounds that lesions of this type might accumulate as a result of prolonged periods of replicative inactivity and, if unrepaired, would present a major threat to the reactivation of the organism in a viable form (53, 54). The recent identification of a functional Ku ligase system in *M. tuberculosis* for DSB repair by nonhomologous end joining (85) comprising the Ku-like protein, Rv0937c, and the ATP-dependent DNA ligase, Rv0938, offers a potentially important alternative pathway for DSB repair to that provided by homologous recombination.

Response of *M. tuberculosis* to DNA Damage

Whole-genome expression profiling has provided exciting insights into the global response of *M. tuberculosis* to DNA damage (6, 20, 64). On the one hand, comparisons with *E. coli* have revealed both striking similarities and differences in the damage-induced gene expression profiles between these two organisms (15, 40). On the other hand, comparison of the profiles of genes induced in wild-type *M. tuberculosis* and isogenic *recA* mutants have allowed the induced-genes to be classified according to whether they are *recA*/*lexA*- dependent, independent, or both. Other than the large number of genes associated with mobile genetic elements detected in the transcriptome of DNA-damaged *M. tuberculosis*, a notable feature is the fact that most induced genes are of unknown function. Included among these are genes which lack counterparts in *E. coli* but which have domains linking their functions to DNA repair.

PROSPECTS

The development of increasingly powerful technologies for exploring protein function, structure, and expression in *M. tuberculosis* has led to a quantum leap in understanding nucleic acid metabolism in this organism. However, as we have attempted to emphasize throughout this chapter, many compelling and fundamental questions have yet to be addressed. For example, the regulation of DNA metabolic pathways during persistence has not been investigated to any significant extent. In addition to questions of this type, discovery-based, postgenomic research has raised a host of new questions that warrant further investigation. Collectively, these questions are set to fuel this field of research for the foreseeable future.

Acknowledgments. V.M. was supported by an International Scholars grant from the Howard Hughes Medical Institute. We thank Elaine Davis and K. Muniyappa for providing data prior to publication and Helena Boshoff, Stephanie Dawes, and Digby Warner for helpful comments.

REFERENCES

1. Acharya, N., and U. Varshney. 2002. Biochemical properties of single-stranded DNA-binding protein from *Mycobacterium smegmatis*, a fast-growing mycobacterium and its physical interaction with uracil DNA glycosylases. *J. Mol. Biol.* **318**:1251–1264.

2. Arrigo, C. J., K. Singh, and M. J. Modak. 2002. DNA polymerase I of *Mycobacterium tuberculosis*: functional role of a conserved aspartate in the hinge joining the M and N helices. *J. Biol. Chem.* **277**:1653–1661.

3. Avarbock, D., J. Salem, L. S. Li, Z. M. Wang, and H. Rubin. 1999. Cloning and characterization of a bifunctional *relA*/*spoT* homologue from *Mycobacterium tuberculosis*. *Gene* **233**:261–269.

4. Avarbock, A., D. Avarbock, and H. Rubin. 2000. Differential regulation of opposing Rel_{Mtb} activities by the aminoacylation state of a tRNA ribosome·mRNA·Rel_{Mtb} complex. *Biochemistry* **39**:11640–11648.

5. Banu, S., N. Honore, B. Saint-Joanis, D. Philpott, M. C. Prevost, and S. T. Cole. 2002. Are the PE-PGRS proteins of *Mycobacterium tuberculosis* variable surface antigens? *Mol. Microbiol.* **44**:9–19.

6. Boshoff, H. I. M., M. B. Reed, C. E. Barry III, and V. Mizrahi. 2003. dnaE2 contributes to *in vivo* survival and the emergence of drug resistance in *Mycobacterium tuberculosis*. *Cell* **113**:183–193.

7. Brooks, P. C., F. Movahedzadeh, and E. O. Davis. 2001. Identification of some DNA damage-inducible genes of *Mycobacterium tuberculosis*: apparent lack of correlation with LexA binding. *J. Bacteriol.* **183**:4459–4467.

8. Brosch, R., A. S. Pym, S. V. Gordon, and S. T. Cole. 2001. The evolution of mycobacterial pathogenicity: clues from comparative genomics. *Trends Microbiol.* **9**:452–458.

9. Brosch, R., S. V. Gordon, M. Marmiesse, P. Brodin, C. Buchrieser, K. Eiglmeier, T. Garnier, C. Gutierrez, G. Hewinson, K. Kremer, L. M. Parsons, A. S. Pym, S. Samper, D. van Soolingen, and S. T. Cole. 2002. A new evolutionary scenario for the *Mycobacterium tuberculosis* complex. *Proc. Natl. Acad. Sci. USA* **99**:3684–3689.

10. Buchmeier, N. A., C. J. Lipps, M. Y. So, and F. Heffron. 1993. Recombination-deficient mutants of *Salmonella typhimurium* are avirulent and sensitive to the oxidative burst of macrophages. *Mol. Microbiol.* **7**:933–936.

11. Burns, B. P, S. L. Hazell, G. L. Mendz, T. Kolesnikow, D. Tillet, and B. A. Neilan. 2000. The *Heliobacter pylori pyrB* gene encoding aspartate carbamoyltransferase is essential for bacterial survival. *Arch. Biochem. Biophys.* **380**:78–84.

12. Chen, Y., S. Morera, J. Mocan, I. Lascu, and J. Janin. 2002. X-ray structure of *Mycobacterium tuberculosis* nucleoside diphosphate kinase. *Proteins* **47**:556–557.

13. Chopra, P., A. Singh, A. Koul, S. Ramachandran, K. Drlica, A.K. Tyagi and Y. Singh. 2003. Cytotoxic activity of nucleoside diphosphate kinase secreted from *Mycobacterium tuberculosis*. *Eur. J. Biochem.* **270**:625–634.

14. Cole, S. T., R. Brosch, J. Parkhill, T. Garnier, C. Churcher, D. Harris, S. V. Gordon, K. Eiglmeier, S. Gas, C. E. Barry III, F. Tekaia, K. Badcock, D. Basham, D. Brown, T. Chillingworth, R. Connor, R. Davies, K. Devlin, T. Feltwell, S. Gentles, N. Hamlin, S. Holroyd, T. Hornsby, K. Jagels, A. Krogh, J. McLean, S. Moule, L. Murphy, K. Oliver, J. Osborne, M. A. Quail, M.-A. Rajandream, J. Rogers, S. Rutter, K. Seeger, J. Skelton, R. Squares, S. Squares, J.E. Sulston, K. Taylor, S. Whitehead, and B.G. Barrell. 1998. Deciphering the biology of *Mycobacterium tuberculosis* from the complete genome sequence. *Nature* **393**:537–544.

15. Courcelle, J., A. Khodursky, B. Peter, P. O. Brown, and P. C. Hanawalt. 2001. Comparative gene expression profiles following UV exposure in wild-type and SOS-deficient *Escherichia coli. Genetics* **158**:41–64.

16. Dahl, J. L., C. N. Kraus, H. I. Boshoff, B. Doan, K. Foley, D. Avarbock, G. Kaplan, V. Mizrahi, H. Rubin, and C. E. Barry III. 2003. The role of Rel$_{MTb}$-mediated adaptation to stationary phase in long-term persistence of *Mycobacterium tuberculosis* in mice. *Proc. Natl. Acad. Sci. USA* **100**:10026–10031.

17. Darwin, K. H., S. Ehrt, J. C. Gutierrez-Ramos, N. Weich, and C. F. Nathan. 2003. The proteasome of *Mycobacterium tuberculosis* is required for resistance to nitric oxide. *Science* **302**:1963–1966.

18. Datta, S., M. M. Prabu, M. B. Vaze, N. Ganesh, N. R. Chandra, K. Muniyappa, and M. Vijayan. 2000. Crystal structures of *Mycobacterium tuberculosis* RecA and its complex with ADP-AIF4: implications for decreased ATPase activity and molecular aggregation. *Nucleic Acids Res.* **28**:4964–4973.

19. David, H. L. 1970. Probability distribution of drug-resistant mutants in unselected populations of *Mycobacterium tuberculosis. Appl. Microbiol.* **20**:810–814.

20. Davis, E. O., E. M. Dullaghan, and L. Rand. 2002. Definition of the mycobacterial SOS box and use to identify LexA-regulated genes in *Mycobacterium tuberculosis. J. Bacteriol.* **184**:3287–3295.

21. Davis, E. O., B. Springer, K. K. Gopaul, K. G. Papavinasasundaram, P. Sander, and E. C. Böttger. 2002. DNA damage induction of *recA* in *Mycobacterium tuberculosis* independently of LexA. *Mol. Microbiol.* **46**:791–800.

22. Dawes, S. S., D. F. Warner, L. Tsenova, J. Timm, J. D. McKinney, G. Kaplan, H. Rubin, and V. Mizrahi. 2003. Ribonucleotide reduction in *Mycobacterium tuberculosis*: function and expression of genes encoding class Ib and class II ribonucleotide reductases. *Infect. Immun.* **71**:6124–6131.

23. Durbach, S. I., B. Springer, E. E. Machowski, R. J. North, K. G. Papavinasasundaram, M. J. Colston, E. C. Böttger, and V. Mizrahi. 2003. DNA alkylation damage as a sensor of nitrosative stress in *Mycobacterium tuberculosis. Infect. Immun.* **71**:997–1000.

24. Elleingand, E., C. Gerez, S. Un, M. Knupling, G. Lu, J. Salem, H. Rubin, S. Sauge-Merle, J. P. Laulhere, and M. Fontecave. 1998. Reactivity studies of the tyrosyl radical in ribonucleotide reductase from *Mycobacterium tuberculosis* and *Arabidopsis thaliana*—comparison with *Escherichia coli* and mouse. *Eur. J. Biochem.* **258**:485–490.

25. Espinal, M. A., S. J. Kim, P. G. Suarez, K. M. Kam, A. G. Khomenko, G. B. Migliori, J. Baez, A. Kochi, C. Dye, and M. C. Raviglione. 2000. Standard short-course chemotherapy for drug-resistant tuberculosis: treatment outcomes in 6 countries. *JAMA* **283**:2537–2545.

26. Fang, Z., C. Doig, D. T. Kenna, N. Smittipat, P. Palittapongarnpim, B. Watt, and K. J. Forbes. 1999. IS*6110*–mediated deletions of wild-type chromosomes of *Mycobacterium tuberculosis. J. Bacteriol.* **181**:1014–1020.

27. Fleischmann, R. D., D. Alland, J. A. Eisen, L. Carpenter, O. White, J. Peterson, R. DeBoy, R. Dodson, M. Gwinn, D. Haft, E. Hickey, J. F. Kolonay, W. C. Nelson, L. A. Umayam, M. Ermolaeva, S. L. Salzberg, A. Delcher, T. Utterback, J. Weidman, H. Khouri, J. Gill, A. Mikula, W. Bishai, W. R. Jacobs, Jr., J. C. Venter, and C. M. Fraser. 2002. Whole-genome comparison of *Mycobacterium tuberculosis* clinical and laboratory strains. *J. Bacteriol.* **184**:5479–5490.

28. Gentry, D. R., V. J. Hernandez, L. H. Nguyen, D. B. Jensen, and M. Cashel. 1993. Synthesis of the stationary-phase sigma factor sigma s is positively regulated by ppGpp. *J. Bacteriol.* **175**:7982–7989.

29. Goodman, M. F. 2002. Error-prone repair DNA polymerases in prokaryotes and eukaryotes. *Annu. Rev. Biochem.* **71**:17–50.

30. Gordon, S. V., B. Heym, J. Parkhill, B. Barrell, and S. Cole. 1999. New insertion sequences and a novel repeated sequence in the genome of *Mycobacterium tuberculosis* H37Rv. *Microbiology* **145**:881–892.

31. Guhan, N., and K. Muniyappa. 2002. The RecA intein of *Mycobacterium tuberculosis* promotes cleavage of ectopic DNA sites. Implications for the dispersal of inteins in natural populations. *J. Biol. Chem.* **277**:40352–40361.

32. Guhan, N., and K. Muniyappa. 2002. *Mycobacterium tuberculosis* RecA intein possesses a novel ATP-dependent site-specific double-stranded DNA endonuclease activity. *J. Biol. Chem.* **277**:16257–16264.

33. Haouz, A., V. Vanheusden, H. Munier-Lehmann, M. Froeyen, P. Herdewijn, S. Van Calenbergh, and M. Delarue. 2003. Enzymatic and structural analysis of inhibitors designed against *M. tuberculosis* thymidylate kinase. New insights into the phosphoryl transfer mechanism. *J. Biol. Chem.* **278**:4963–4971.

34. Hinds, J., E. Mahenthiralingam, K. E. Kempsell, K. Duncan, R. W. Stokes, T. Parish, and N. G. Stoker. 1999. Enhanced gene replacement in mycobacteria. *Microbiology* **145**:519–527.

35. Ho, T. B., B. D. Robertson, G. M. Taylor, R. J. Shaw, and D. B. Young. 2000. Comparison of *Mycobacterium tuberculosis* genomes reveals frequent deletions in a 20 kb variable region in clinical isolates. *Yeast* **17**:272–282.

36. Hu, Y. M., P. D. Butcher, K. Sole, D. A. Mitchison, and A. R. Coates. 1998. Protein synthesis is shutdown in dormant *Mycobacterium tuberculosis* and is reversed by oxygen or heat shock. *FEMS Microbiol. Lett.* **158**:139–145.

37. Hughes, A. L., R. Friedman, and M. Murray. 2002. Genome-wide pattern of synonymous nucleotide substitution in two complete genomes of *Mycobacterium tuberculosis. Emerg. Infect. Dis.* **8**:1342–1346.

38. Kato-Maeda, M., J. T. Rhee, T. R. Gingeras, H. Salamon, J. Drenkow, N. Smittipat, and P. M. Small. 2001. Comparing genomes within the species *Mycobacterium tuberculosis. Genome Res.* **11**:547–554.

39. Keer, J., M. J. Smeulders, and H. D. Williams. 2001. A *purF* mutant of *Mycobacterium smegmatis* has impaired survival during oxygen-starved stationary phase. *Microbiology* **147**:473–481.

40. Khil, P. P., and R. D. Camerini-Otero. 2002. Over 1000 genes are involved in the DNA damage response of *Escherichia coli. Mol. Microbiol.* **44**:89–105.

41. LeClerc, J. E., B. Li, W. L. Payne, and T. A. Cebula. 1996. High mutation frequencies among *Escherichia coli* and *Salmonella* pathogens. *Science* **274**:1208–1211.

42. Li de la Sierra, I., H. Munier-Lehmann, A. M. Gilles, O. Barzu, and M. Delarue. 2000. Crystallization and preliminary X-ray analysis of the thymidylate kinase from *Mycobacterium tuberculosis. Acta Crystallogr. Ser. D.* **56**:226–228.

43. Li de la Sierra, I., H. Munier-Lehmann, A. M. Gilles, O. Barzu, and M. Delarue. 2001. X-ray structure of TMP kinase from *Mycobacterium tuberculosis* complexed with TMP at 1.95A resolution. *J. Mol. Biol.* **311**:87–100.

44. Liu, A., S. Potsch, A. Davydov, A. L. Barra, H. Rubin, and A. Graslund. 1998. The tyrosyl free radical of recombinant ribonucleotide reductase from *Mycobacterium tuberculosis* is located in a rigid hydrophobic pocket. *Biochemistry* **37**:16369–16477.

45. Makarova, K. S., L. Aravind, N. V. Grishin, I. B. Rogozin, and E. V. Koonin. 2002. A DNA repair system specific for theromophilic Archaea and bacteria predicted by genomic context analysis. *Nucleic Acids Res.* **30**:482–496.

46. Martinez-Costa, O. H., M. A. Fernandez-Moreno, and F. Malpartida. 1998. The *relA/spoT*-homologous gene in *Streptomyces coelicolor* encodes both ribosome-dependent (p)ppGpp-synthesizing and -degrading activities. *J. Bacteriol.* **180**:4123–4132.

47. McAdam, R. A., S. Quan, and C. Guilhot. 2000. Mycobacterial transposons and their applications, p. 69–84. *In* G. F. Hatfull and W. R. Jacobs, Jr. (ed.), *Molecular Genetics of Mycobacteria*. ASM Press, Washington, D.C.

48. McAdam, R. A., S. Quan, D. A. Smith, S. Bardarov, J. C. Betts, F. C. Cook, E. U. Hooker, A. P. Lewis, P. Woollard, M. J. Everett, P. T. Lukey, G. J. Bancroft, W. R. Jacobs, Jr., and K. Duncan. 2002. Characterization of a *Mycobacterium tuberculosis* H37Rv transposon library reveals insertions in 351 ORFs and mutants with altered virulence. *Microbiology* **148**:2975–2986.

49. Mechold, U., H. Murphy, L. Brown, and M. Cashel. 2002. Intramolecular regulation of the opposing (p)ppGpp catalytic activities of Rel(Seq), the Rel/Spo enzyme from *Streptococcus equisimilis*. *J. Bacteriol.* **184**:2878–2888.

50. Mechold, U., and H. Malke. 1997. Characterization of the stringent and relaxed responses of *Streptococcus equisimilis*. *J. Bacteriol.* **17**:2658–2667.

51. Merino, D., H. Reglier-Poupet, P. Berche, A. Charbit, and The European Listeria Genome Consortium. 2002. A hypermutator phenotype attenuates the virulence of *Listeria monocytogenes* in a mouse model. *Mol. Microbiol.* **44**:877–887.

52. Metzgar, D., and C. Wills. 2000. Evidence for the adaptive evolution of mutation rates. *Cell* **101**:581–584.

53. Mizrahi, V., and S. J. Andersen. 1998. DNA repair in *Mycobacterium tuberculosis*. What have we learnt from the genome sequence? *Mol. Microbiol.* **29**:1331–1339.

54. Mizrahi, V., S. S. Dawes, and H. Rubin. 2000. DNA replication, p. 159–172. *In* G. F. Hatfull and W. R. Jacobs, Jr. (ed.), *Molecular Genetics of Mycobacteria*. ASM Press, Washington, D.C.

55. Mostowy, S., D. Cousins, J. Brinkman, A. Aranaz, and M. A. Behr. 2002. Genomic deletions suggest a phyogeny for the *Mycobacterium tuberculosis* complex. *J. Infect. Dis.* **186**:74–80.

56. Munier-Lehmann, H., S. Burlacu-Miron, C. T. Craescu, H. H. Mantsch, and C. P. Schultz. 1999. A new subfamily of short bacterial adenylate kinases with the *Mycobacterium tuberculosis* enzyme as a model: a predictive and experimental study. *Proteins* **36**:238–248.

57. Muniyappa, K., M. B. Vaze, N. Ganesh, M. S. Reddy, N. Guhan, and R. Venkatesh. 2000. Comparative genomics of *Mycobacterium tuberculosis* and *Escherichia coli* for recombination (*rec*) genes. *Microbiology* **146**:2093–2095.

58. Myllykallio, H., G. Lipowski, D. Leduc, J. Filee, P. Forterre, and U. Liebl. 2002. An alternative flavin-dependent mechanism for thymidylate synthesis. *Science* **297**:105–107.

59. Parish, T., B. G. Gordhan, R. A. McAdam, K. Duncan, V. Mizrahi, and N. G. Stoker. 1999. Production of mutants in amino acid biosynthesis genes of *Mycobacterium tuberculosis* by homologous recombination. *Microbiology* **145**:3497–3503.

60. Pavelka, M. S., Jr., and W. R. Jacobs, Jr. 1999. Comparison of the construction of unmarked deletion mutations in *Mycobacterium smegmatis*, *Mycobacterium bovis* bacillus Calmette-Guérin, and *Mycobacterium tuberculosis* H37Rv by allelic exchange. *J. Bacteriol.* **181**:4780–4789.

61. Primm, T., S. Andersen, V. Mizrahi, D. Avarbock, H. Rubin, and C. E. Barry III. 2000. The stringent response of *Mycobacterium tuberculosis* is required for long-term survival. *J. Bacteriol.* **182**:4889–4898.

62. Rad, M. E., P. Bifani, C. Martin, K. Kremer, S. Samper, J. Rauzier, B. Kreiswirth, J. Blazquez, J. Jouan, D. van Soolingen, and B. Gicquel. 2003. Mutations in putative mutator genes of *Mycobacterium tuberculosis* strains of the W-Beijing family. *Emerg. Infect. Dis.* **9**:838–845.

63. Ramakrishnan, L., N. A. Federspiel, and S. Falkow. 2000. Granuloma-specific expression of *Mycobacterium* virulence proteins from the glycine-rich PE-PGRS family. *Science* **288**:1436–1439.

64. Rand, L., J. Hinds, B. Springer, P. Sander, R. S. Buxton, and E. O. Davis. 2003. The majority of inducible DNA repair genes in *Mycobacterium tuberculosis* are induced independently of RecA. *Mol. Microbiol.* **50**:1031–1042.

65. Rayssiguier, C., D. S. Thaler, and M. Radman. 1989. The barrier to recombination between *Escherichia coli* and *Salmonella typhimurium* is disrupted in mismatch-repair mutants. *Nature* **342**:396–401.

66. Reddy, M. S., N. Guhan, and K. Muniyappa. 2001. Characterization of single-stranded DNA-binding proteins from mycobacteria. The carboxy-terminal domain of SSB is essential for stable association with its cognate RecA protein. *J. Biol. Chem.* **276**:45959–45968.

67. Richardson, A. R., Z. Yu, T. Popovic, and I. Stojiljkovic. 2002. Mutator clones of *Neisseria meningitidis* in epidemic serogroup A disease. *Proc. Natl. Acad. Sci. USA* **99**:6103–6107.

68. Sander, P., K. G. Papavinasasundaram, T. Dick, E. Stavropolous, K. Ellrott, B. Springer, M. J. Colston, and E. C. Böttger. 2001. *Mycobacterium bovis* BCG *recA* deletion mutant shows increased susceptibility to DNA-damaging agents but wild-type survival in a mouse infection model. *Infect. Immun.* **69**:3562–3568.

69. Sander, P., E. C. Böttger, B. Springer, B. Steinmann, M. Rezwan, E. Stavropoulos, and M. J. Colston. 2003. A *recA* deletion mutant of *Mycobacterium bovis* BCG confers protection equivalent to that of wild type BCG but shows increased genetic stability. *Vaccine* **21**:4124–4127.

70. Sassetti, C. M., and E. J. Rubin. 2003. Genetic requirements for mycobacterial survival during infection. *Proc. Natl. Acad. Sci. USA* **100**:12989–12994.

71. Savacool, H. K., and R. L. Switzer. 2002. Characterization of the interaction of *Bacillus subtilis* PyrR with *pyr* mRNA by site-directed mutagenesis of the protein. *J. Bacteriol.* **184**:2521–2528.

72. Shankar, S., C. D. Hershberger, and A. M. Chakrabarty. 1997. The nucleoside diphosphate kinase of *Mycobacterium smegmatis*: identification of proteins that modulate specificity of nucleoside triphosphate synthesis by the enzyme. *Mol. Microbiol.* **24**:477–487.

73. Sherman, D. R., M. Voskuil, D. Schnappinger, R. Liao, M.I. Harrell, and G.K. Schoolnik. 2001. Regulation of the *Mycobacterium tuberculosis* hypoxic response gene encoding alpha-crystallin. *Proc. Natl. Acad. Sci. USA* **98**:7534–7539.

74. Shi, W., L. A. Basso, D. S. Santos, P. C. Tyler, R. H. Furneaux, J. S. Blanchard, S. C. Almo, and V. L. Schramm. 2001. Structures of purine nucleoside phosphorylase from *Mycobacterium tuberculosis* in complexes with immucillin-H and its pieces. *Biochemistry* **40**:8204–8215.

75. Spek, E. J., T. L. Wright, M. S. Stitt, N. R. Taghizadeh, S. R. Tannenbaum, M. G. Marinus, and B. P. Engelward. 2001. Recombinational repair is critical for survival of *Escherichia coli* exposed to nitric oxide. *J. Bacteriol.* **183**:131–138.

76. Sreevatsan, S., X. Pan, K. E. Stockbauer, N. D. Connell, B. N. Kreiswirth, T. S. Whittam, and J. M. Musser. 1997. Restricted structural gene polymorphism in the *Mycobacterium tuberculosis* complex indicates evolutionary recent global dissemination. *Proc. Natl. Acad. Sci. USA* **94**:9869–9974.

77. Taylor, C. M., M. Beresford, H. A. Epton, D. C. Sigee, G. Shama, P. W. Andrew, and I. S. Roberts. 2002. *Listeria mono-*

cytogenes relA and *hpt* mutants are impaired in surface-attached growth and virulence. *J. Bacteriol.* **184**:621–628.

78. Tsolaki, A. G., A. E. Hirsh, K. DeRiemer, J. A. Enciso, M. Z. Wong, M. Hannan, Y. O. Goguet de la Salmoniere, K. Aman, M. Kaeto-Maeda, and P. M. Small. 2004. Functional and evolutionary genomics of *Mycobacterium tuberculosis*: insights from genomic deletions in 100 strains. *Proc. Natl. Acad. Sci. USA* **101**:4865–4870.

79. Turner, R. J., E. R. Bonner, G. K. Grabner, and R. L. Switzer. 1998. Purification and characterization of *Bacillus subtilis* PyrR, a bifunctional *pyr* mRNA-binding attenuation protein/uracil phosphoribosyl-transferase. *J. Biol. Chem.* **273**:5932–5938.

80. Vaze, M. B., and K. Muniyappa. 1999. RecA protein of *Mycobacterium tuberculosis* possesses pH dependent homologous DNA pairing and strand-exchange activities: implications for allele exchange in mycobacteria. *Biochemistry* **38**:3175–3186.

81. Venkatesh, R., N. Ganesh, N. Guhan, M. S. Reddy, T. Chandrasekhar, and K. Muniyappa. 2002. RecX protein abrogates ATP hydrolysis and strand exchange promoted by RecA: insights into negative regulation of homologous recombination. *Proc. Natl. Acad. Sci. USA* **99**:12091–12096.

82. Venkatesh, J. P. Kumar, P. S. Krishna, R. Majunath, and U. Varshney. 2003. Importance of uracil DNA glycosylase in *Pseudomonas aeruginosa* and *Mycobacterium smegmatis*, G+C-rich bacteria, in mutation prevention, tolerance to acidified nitrite, and endurance in mouse macrophages. *J. Biol. Chem.* **278**:24350–24358.

83. Voskuil, M. I., D. Schnappinger, K. C. Visconti, M. I. Harrell, G. M. Dolganov, D. R. Sherman, and G. K. Schoolnik. 2003. Inhibition of respiration by nitric oxide induces a *Mycobacterium tuberculosis* dormancy program. *J. Exp. Med.* **198**:705–713.

84. Warren, R. M., S. L. Sampson, M. Richardson, G. D. van der Spuy, C. J. Lombard, T. C. Victor, and P. D. van Helden. 2000. Mapping of IS*6110* flanking regions in clinical isolates of *Mycobacterium tuberculosis* demonstrates genome plasticity. *Mol. Microbiol.* **37**:1405–1416.

85. Weller, G. R., B. Kysela, R. Roy, L. M. Tonkin, E. Scanlan, M. Della, S. K. Devine, J. P. Day, A. Wilkinson, F. di Fagagna, K. M. Devine, R. P. Bowater, P. A. Jeggo, S. P. Jackson, and A. J. Doherty. 2002. Identification of a DNA nonhomologous end-joining complex in bacteria. *Science* **297**:1686–1688.

86. Werngren, J., and S. E. Hoffner. 2003. Drug-susceptible *Mycobacterium tuberculosis* Beijing genotype does not develop mutation-conferred resistance to rifampin at an elevated rate. *J. Clin. Microbiol.* **41**:1520–1524.

87. Wheeler, P. R. 1987. Enzymes for purine synthesis and scavenging in pathogenic mycobacteria and their distribution in *Mycobactrium leprae*. *J. Gen. Microbiol.* **133**:3013–3018.

88. Wheeler, P. R. 1987. Biosynthesis and scavenging of purines by pathogenic mycobacteria including *Mycobacterium leprae*. *J. Gen. Microbiol.* **133**:2999–3011.

89. Wheeler, P. R. 1989. Pyrimidine biosynthesis *de novo* in *M. leprae*. *FEMS Microbiol. Lett.* **48**:185–189.

90. Wheeler, P. R. 1990. Biosynthesis and scavenging of pyrimidines by pathogenic mycobacteria. *J. Gen. Microbiol.* **136**:189–201.

91. Yang, F., S. C. Curran, L. S. Li, D. Avarbock, J. D. Graf, M. M. Chua, G. Lu, J. Salem, and H. Rubin. 1997. Characterization of two genes encoding the *Mycobacterium tuberculosis* ribonucleotide reductase small subunit. *J. Bacteriol.* **179**:6408–6415.

92. Yang, F., G. Lu, and H. Rubin. 1994. Isolation of ribonucleotide reductase from *Mycobacterium tuberculosis* and cloning, expression and purification of the large subunit. *J. Bacteriol.* **176**:6738–6743.

93. Yeiser, B., E. D. Pepper, M. F. Goodman, and S. E. Finkel. 2002. SOS-induced DNA polymerases enhance long-term survival and evolutionary fitness. *Proc. Natl. Acad. Sci. USA* **99**:8737–8741.

94. Zaborina, O., X. Li, G. Cheng, V. Kapatral, and A. M. Chakrabarty. 1999. Secretion of ATP-utilizing enzymes, nucleoside diphosphate kinase and ATPase, by *Mycobacterium bovis* BCG: sequestration of ATP from macrophage P2Z receptors? *Mol. Microbiol.* **5**:1333–1343.

95. Zhang, Y., and A. Telenti. 2000. Genetics of drug resistance in *M. tuberculosis*, p. 235–254. *In* G. F. Hatfull and W. R. Jacobs, Jr. (ed.), *Molecular Genetics of Mycobacteria*. ASM Press, Washington, D.C.

Tuberculosis and the Tubercle Bacillus
Edited by Stewart T. Cole et al.
© 2005 ASM Press, Washington, D.C.

Chapter 24

Transport Processes

JEAN CONTENT, MARTINE BRAIBANT, NANCY D. CONNELL, AND JOSE A. AINSA

Numerically, in most prokaryotic genomes, bacterial transporters represent one of the most abundant categories of genes (for instance, about 200 genes, corresponding to about 5% of the *Mycobacterium tuberculosis* genome). Among these, the ATP-binding cassette (ABC) transporters constitute the largest superfamily (about 2.5% of the *M. tuberculosis* genome), which exports or imports very diverse substrates such as ions, amino acids, peptides, drugs, lipids, polysaccharides, antibiotics, and proteins.

Bacterial transporters are therefore very important physiological components required for communication of microorganisms with their environment and for adaptation. Some transporters also contribute to microbial virulence and to drug and potentially multidrug resistance, hence their implication in important public health issues.

This chapter first presents an updated directory of all the predicted mycobacterial transporter superfamilies organized according to the membrane protein Transporter Classification (TC) system, together with their putative function. From among these, a few systems that are experimentally established and physiologically relevant are presented, and their roles in mycobacterial virulence and pathogenicity are examined. Finally, special emphasis is placed on multiple efflux systems in the context of antibiotic resistance.

A DIRECTORY OF MYCOBACTERIAL TRANSPORTERS

We compiled all characterized and putative transport proteins encoded within the *M. tuberculosis* genome. Table 1 summarizes our findings about all transporters identified. According to the Saier classification transport database, these transporters fall into four classes: (i) channels and pores, (ii) electrochemical potential-driven transporters, (iii) primary active transporters, and (iv) transport electron carriers. Additionally, three transporters fall into the category of incompletely characterized transport systems.

Channels and Pores

M. tuberculosis possesses five α-type channel systems belonging to four different families. These transporters usually catalyze facilitated diffusion by passage through a transmembrane aqueous pore consisting of α-helical spanners.

Electrochemical Potential-Driven Transporters

M. tuberculosis possesses 74 secondary transporters, that are driven by electrochemical gradients. They are all included in the subclass of porters (uniporters, symporters, and antiporters) and belong to 21 different families (or superfamilies). The majority of *M. tuberculosis* transporters fall into the major facilitator superfamily (MFS) (26 transporters), the resistance-nodulation-cell division (RND) superfamily (15 transporters), or the amino acid-polyamine-organocation (APC) superfamily (8 transporters). The other families include only one, two, or three transporters.

The MFS is a very large superfamily that includes over a thousand sequenced members. They catalyze uniport, solute:cation (H^+ or Na^+) symport, and solute:H^+ or solute:solute antiport. Members of the RND superfamily catalyze substrate efflux via a H^+ antiport mechanism. The APC superfamily of transport proteins includes members that function as solute:cation symporters and solute:solute antiporters.

(*text continued on page 388*)

Jean Content • Institut Pasteur de Bruxelles B-1180 Brussels, Belgium. **Martine Braibant** • UR86 BioAgresseurs, Santé et Environnement (BASE), INRA de Tours, F-37380 Nouzilly, France. **Nancy D. Connell** • Department of Microbiology and Molecular Genetics, New Jersey Medical School, Newark, NJ 07103. **Jose A. Ainsa** • Departamento de Microbiologia, Facultad de Medicina, Universidad de Zaragoza, 50009-Zaragoza, Spain.

Table 1. Putative transporters encoded by the genome of *M. tuberculosis* H37Rv[a]

Class: channels and pores; subclass: d-type channels

TC no.	Family	Subfamily	ORF[b]	Gene[b]	Predicted function[c]	Known function (reference)
1.A.11.5.1	Chloride channel (ClC)	Not applicable	Rv0143c	—	Cl channel	Not determined
1.A.22.1.2	Large-conductance mechano-sensitive ion channel (MscL)	Not applicable	Rv0985c	*mscL*	Large-conductance mechanosensitive ion channel	Large-conductance ion channel (23, 44, 56, 61)
1.A.23.3.1	Small conductance mechano-sensitive ion channel (MscS)	Not applicable	Rv3104c	—	Small-conductance mechanosensitive ion channel	Not determined
1.A.23.4.1	Small conductance mechano-sensitive ion channel (MscS)	Not applicable	Rv2434c	—	Small-conductance mechanosensitive ion channel	Not determined
1.A.35.3.1	CorA metal ion transporter (MIT) family	Not applicable	Rv1239c	*corA*	Divalent metal ion (Mg^{2+}, Ca^{2+}, Ni^{2+}, etc.) transporter	Not determined

Class: electrochemical potential-driven transporters; subclass: porters (uniporters, symporters, antiporters)

TC no.	Family	Subfamily	ORF[b]	Gene[b]	Predicted function[c]	Known function (reference)
2.A.1.1.1	MFS	Sugar porter (SP) family	Rv3331	*sugI*	Galactose:H$^+$ symporter	Not determined
2.A.1.2.18	MFS	Drug:H$^+$ antiporter-1 (12-spanner) (DHA1) family	Rv0191	—	Lactose and melibiose (and IPTG) efflux pump	Not determined
2.A.1.2.20	MFS	DHA1 family	Rv2456c	—	Fosmomycin resistance protein	Not determined
2.A.1.2.21	MFS	DHA1 family	Rv0849	—	Norfloxacin/enoxacin resistance protein	Not determined
2.A.1.3.1	MFS	DHA2 family	Rv3162c	—	Aminotriazole, 4-nitroquinoline-N-oxide, etc):H$^+$ antiporter (E-value, 0.004)	Not determined
2.A.1.3.7	MFS	DHA2 family	Rv2333c	—	Actinorhodin:H$^+$ antiporter	Not determined
2.A.1.3.11	MFS	DHA2 family	Rv1410c	—	Puromycin:H$^+$ antiporter	Tetracycline and aminoglycoside efflux pump P55 (90)
2.A.1.3.11	MFS	DHA2 family	Rv1634	—	Puromycin:H$^+$ antiporter	Fluoroquinolones efflux protein (37)
2.A.1.3.11	MFS	DHA2 family	Rv2846c	*efpA*	Puromycin:H$^+$ antiporter	Not determined
2.A.1.3.12	MFS	DHA2 family	Rv0783c	*emrB*	Tetracenomycin:H$^+$ antiporter	Not determined
2.A.1.3.12	MFS	DHA2 family	Rv1250	—	Tetracenomycin:H$^+$ antiporter	Not determined
2.A.1.3.12	MFS	DHA2 family	Rv1877	—	Tetracenomycin:H$^+$ antiporter	Not determined
2.A.1.3.12	MFS	DHA2 family	Rv2459	—	Tetracenomycin:H$^+$ antiporter	Not determined
2.A.1.3.12	MFS	DHA2 family	Rv3239c	—	Tetracenomycin:H$^+$ antiporter	Not determined
2.A.1.3.12	MFS	DHA2 family	Rv3728	—	Tetracenomycin:H$^+$ antiporter	Not determined
2.A.1.6.3	MFS	Metabolite:H$^+$ symporter (MHS) family	Rv3476c	*kgtP*	Dicarboxylate:H$^+$ symporter	Not determined
2.A.1.6.6	MFS	MHS family	Rv1200	—	Shikimate:H$^+$ symporter	Not determined

TC no.	Superfamily/class	Family	Rv no.	Gene	Description	Characteristics
2.A.1.8.1	MFS	Nitrate/nitrite porter (NNP) family	Rv0261c	narK3	Nitrite extrusion permease	Not determined
2.A.1.8.1	MFS	NNP family	Rv0267	narU	Nitrite extrusion permease	Not determined
2.A.1.8.1	MFS	NNP family	Rv2329c	narK1	Nitrite extrusion permease	Not determined
2.A.1.8.8	MFS	NNP family	Rv1737c	narK2	NO_2-extrusion, NO_3^-/NO_2^- exchange permease	Not determined
2.A.1.112.2	MFS	Sialate:H⁺ symporter (SHS) family	Rv1902c	nanT	Lactate/pyruvate:H⁺ symporter	Not determined
2.A.1.114.1	MFS	Anion:cation symporter (ACS) family	Rv2994	—	Glucarate porter	Not determined
2.A.1.14.3	MFS	ACS family	Rv1672c	—	Tartrate porter	Not determined
2.A.1.21.1	MFS	Drug:H⁺ antiporter-3 (12-spanner) (DHA3) family	Rv0037c	—	Macrolide (erythromycin, oleandomycin, azythromycin) efflux	Not determined
2.A.1.21.4	MFS	DHA3 family	Rv1258c	—	Multidrug resistance efflux pump	Tetracycline and aminoglycoside efflux protein (1, 39)
2.A.3.1.5	APC superfamily	Amino acid transporter (AAT) family	Rv0522	gabP	β-Alanine/γ-aminobutyrate:H⁺ symporter	L-Arginine/γ-aminobutyrate:H⁺ permease (89)
2.A.3.1.7	APC superfamily	AAT family	Rv1704c	cycA	D-Serine/D-alanine/glycine:H⁺ symporter	Not determined
2.A.3.1.8	APC superfamily	AAT family	Rv0346c	ansP2	Asparagine permease	Not determined
2.A.3.1.8	APC superfamily	AAT family	Rv2127	ansP1	Asparagine permease	Not determined
2.A.3.3.1	APC superfamily	Cationic amino acid (CAT) transporter family	Rv2320c	rocE	High-affinity basic amino acid transporter	Not determined
2.A.3.3.3	APC superfamily	CAT transporter family	Rv3253c	—	Amino acid transporter	Not determined
2.A.3.6.1	APC superfamily	Archeal/bacterial transporter (ABT) family	Rv1979c	—	Cationic amino acid permease	Not determined
2.A.3.6.1	APC superfamily	ABT family	Rv1999c	—	Cationic amino acid permease	Not determined
2.A.4.1.2	Cation diffusion facilitator (CDF) family	Not applicable	Rv2025c	—	Zn^{2+}, Co^{2+} efflux permease	Not determined
2.A.6.4.1	RND superfamily	SecDF family	Rv2586c Rv2587c	secF secD	Secretory accessory protein	Not determined
2.A.6.5.1	RND superfamily	Hydrophobe/amphiphile efflux 2 (HAE2) family	Rv0202c	mmpL11	Antibiotic actinorhodin transport-associated protein	Not determined
2.A.6.5.1	RND superfamily	HAE2 family	Rv0206c	mmpL3	Antibiotic actinorhodin transport-associated protein	Not determined

Continued on following page

Table 1. Continued

TC no.	Family	Subfamily	ORF[b]	Gene[b]	Predicted function[c]	Known function (reference)
2.A.6.5.1	RND superfamily	HAE2 family	Rv1146	mmpL13B	Antibiotic actinorhodin transport-associated protein	Not determined
2.A.6.5.2	RND superfamily	HAE2 family	Rv2942	mmpL7	PDIM lipid exporter	PDIM lipid exporter (20,37)
2.A.6.5.3	RND superfamily	HAE2 family	Rv0402c	mmpL1	Glycopeptidolipid exporter	Not determined
2.A.6.5.3	RND superfamily	HAE2 family	Rv0450c	mmpL4	Glycopeptidolipid exporter	Not determined
2.A.6.5.3	RND superfamily	HAE2 family	Rv0507c	mmpL2	Glycopeptidolipid exporter	Not determined
2.A.6.5.3	RND superfamily	HAE2 family	Rv0676c	mmpL5	Glycopeptidolipid exporter	Not determined
2.A.6.5.3	RND superfamily	HAE2 family	Rv1145	mmpL13A	Glycopeptidolipid exporter	Not determined
2.A.6.5.3	RND superfamily	HAE2 family	Rv1183	mmpL10	Glycopeptidolipid exporter	Not determined
2.A.6.5.3	RND superfamily	HAE2 family	Rv1522c	mmpL12	Glycopeptidolipid exporter	Not determined
2.A.6.5.3	RND superfamily	HAE2 family	Rv1557	mmpL6	Glycopeptidolipid exporter	Not determined
2.A.6.5.3	RND superfamily	HAE2 family	Rv2339	mmpL9	Glycopeptidolipid exporter	Not determined
2.A.6.5.3	RND superfamily	HAE2 family	Rv3823c	mmpL8	Glycopeptidolipid exporter	Not determined (34)
2.A.7.1.2	DMT superfamily	4 TMS small multi-drug resistance (SMR) family	Rv3065	mmr	Small multidrug efflux pump	Multidrug efflux pump (41, 70)
2.A.10.1.1	2-Keto-3-deoxygluconate transporter (KDGT) family	Not applicable	Rv2209	—	2-Keto-3-deoxygluconate:H$^+$ symporter	Not determined
2.A.15.3.2	Betaine/carnitine/choline (BCCT) family	Not applicable	Rv0917	betP	Glycine-betaine/proline-betaine:Na$^+$ symporter	Not determined
2.A.19.1.1	Ca^{2+}:cation (CaCA) family	Not applicable	Rv1607	chaA	Ca^{2+}:H$^+$ antiporter	Not determined
2.A.20.1.2	Inorganic phosphate transporter (pit) family	Not applicable	Rv0545c	pitA	Low-affinity Pi transporter	Not determined
2.A.20.2.4	Inorganic phosphate transporter (pit) family	Not applicable	Rv2281	pitB	Low-affinity P$_i$ transporter	Not determined
2.A.23.1.3	Dicarboxylate/amino acid:cation (Na$^+$ or H$^+$) (DAACS) family	Not applicable	Rv2443	dctA	C$_4$-dicarboxylate transporter	Not determined
2.A.36.3.1	Monovalent cation:proton antiporter 1 (CPA1) family	Not applicable	Rv2287	yjcE	Antiporter (unknown function)	Not determined
2.A.37.1.1	Monovalent cation:proton antiporter 2 (CPA2) family	Not applicable	Rv2692	ceoC	Glutathione-regulated K$^+$ efflux protein	Not determined
2.A.37.1.1	Monovalent cation:proton antiporter 2 (CPA2) family	Not applicable	Rv3200c	—	Glutathione-regulated K$^+$ efflux protein	Not determined

TC no.	Family		Rv no.	Gene	Function	Substrate/value
2.A.37.2.2	Monovalent cation:proton antiporter 2 (CPA2) family	Not applicable	Rv3236c	*kefB*	Na$^+$/H$^+$-K$^+$ antiporter	Not determined
2.A.38.4.2	K$^+$ transporter (TrK) family	Not applicable	Rv3237c	—	High-affinity K$^+$ uptak transporter (E-value, 0.006)	Not determined
2.A.45.2.1	Arsenite-antimonite (ArsB) efflux family	Not applicable	Rv2684	*arsA*	Possible tyrosine transporter	Not determined
2.A.45.2.1	Arsenite-antimonite (ArsB) efflux family	Not applicable	Rv2685	*arsB1*	Possible tyrosine transporter	Not determined
2.A.49.1.3	Ammonium transporter (Amt) family	Not applicable	Rv2920c	*amt*	Ammonium-specific uptake carrier	Not determined
2.A.52.1.1	Ni^{2+}-Co^{2+} transporter (NiCoT) family	Not applicable	Rv2856	*nicT*	High-affinity Ni^{2+} transporter	Not determined
2.A.53.3.1	Sulfate permease (SulP) family	Not applicable	Rv1707	—	Sulfate permease	Not determined
2.A.53.3.1	Sulfate permease (SulP) family	Not applicable	Rv3273	—	Sulfate permease	Not determined
2.A.53.4.1	Sulfate permease (SulP) family	Not applicable	Rv1739c	—	Sulfate transporter	Not determined
2.A.55.3.1	Metal ion (Mn^{2+}-iron) transporter (Nramp) family	Not applicable	Rv0924c	*mntH*	Divalent-cation:H$^+$ symporter	Divalent-cation transporter (1a,10,42)
2.A.59.1.1	Arsenical resistance 3 (Acr3) family	Not applicable	Rv2643	*arsC*	Arsenite transporter	Not determined
2.A.66.1.4	MOP flippase superfamily	Multiantimicrobial extrusion (MATE) family	Rv2836c	*dinF*	DNA damage-inducible protein F (functionally uncharacterized)	Not determined
2.A.75.1.1	L-Lysine exporter (LysE) family	Not applicable	Rv0488	—	L-Lysine exporter	Not determined
2.A.75.1.1	L-Lysine exporter (LysE) family	Not applicable	Rv1986	—	L-Lysine exporter	Not determined

Class: primary active transporters; subclass: P-P bond hydrolysis-driven transporters

TC no.	Family		Rv no.	Gene	Function	Substrate/value
3.A.1.1.3	ABC superfamily	Carbohydrate uptake transporter 1 (CUT1) family	Rv2832c, Rv2833c, Rv2834c, Rv2835c	*ugpC*, *ugpB*, *ugpE*, *ugpA*	Glycerol-phosphate importer	Not determined

Continued on following page

Table 1. *Continued*

TC no.	Family	Subfamily	ORF[b]	Gene[b]	Predicted function[c]	Known function (reference)
3.A.1.1.4	ABC superfamily	CUT1 family	Rv2316	*uspA*	Lactose importer	Not determined
			Rv2317	*uspB*		
			Rv2318	*uspC*		
3.A.1.1.7	ABC superfamily	CUT1 family	Rv1235	*lpqY*	Maltose/trehalose importer	Not determined
			Rv1236	*sugA*		
			Rv1237	*sugB*		
			Rv1238	*sugC*		
3.A.1.1.7	ABC superfamily	CUT1 family	Rv2038c	—	Maltose/trehalose importer	Not determined
			Rv2039c	—		
			Rv2040c	—		
			Rv2041c	—		
3.A.1.2.5	ABC superfamily	CUT2 family	Rv2326c	—	Multiple-sugar importer	Not determined
3.A.1.3.3	ABC superfamily	Polar amino acid uptake transporter (PAAT) family	Rv2563	—	Arginine importer	Not determined
			Rv2564	*glnQ*		
			Rv0411c	*glnH*		
			Rv0072	—		
			Rv0073	—		
3.A.1.5.1	ABC superfamily	Peptide/opine/nickel uptake transporter (PepT) family	Rv3363c	*dppD*	Oligopeptide importer	Not determined
			Rv3364c	*dppC*		
			Rv3365c	*dppB*		
			Rv3366c	*dppA*		
3.A.1.5.1 or 3.A.1.5.3	ABC superfamily	PepT family	Rv1280c	*oppA*	Oligopeptide importer or nickel importer	Peptide importer (49)
			Rv1281c	*oppD*		
			Rv1282c	*oppC*		
			Rv1283c	*oppB*		
3.A.1.6.3	ABC superfamily	Sulfate/tungstate uptake transporter (SulT) family	Rv2397c	*cysA1*	Sulfate importer	Sulfate importer (107)
			Rv2398c	*cysW*		
			Rv2399c	*cysT*		
			Rv2400c	*subI*		
3.A.1.7.1	ABC superfamily	Phosphate uptake transporter (PhoT) family	Rv0820	*pboT*	Phosphate importers	
			Rv0928	*pstS3*		
			Rv0929	*pstC2*		
			Rv0930	*pstA1*		
			Rv0932c	*pstS2*		
			Rv0933	*pstB*		Thermostable ATPase (87)
			Rv0934	*pstS1*		Phosphate-binding protein (24, 27)
			Rv0935	*pstC1*		
			Rv0936	*pstA2*		
3.A.1.8.1	ABC superfamily	Molybdate uptake transporter (MolT) family	Rv1857	*modA*	Molybdate importer	Not determined
			Rv1858	*modB*		
			Rv1859	*modC*		

3.A.1.12.1	ABC superfamily	Quaternary amine uptake transporter (QAT) family	Rv0655	mkl	Glycine betaine/proline importer	Not determined
3.A.1.12.4	ABC superfamily	QAT family	Rv3756c Rv3757c Rv3758c Rv3759c	proZ proW proV proX	Uptake system for choline, L-carnitine, D-carnitine, glycine betaine, crotonobetaine, γ-butyrobetaine, etc.	Not determined
3.A.1.14.4	ABC superfamily	Iron chelate uptake transporter (FeCT) family	Rv0265c	—	Siderophore	Not determined
3.A.1.14.4	ABC superfamily	FeCT family	Rv3041c Rv3044	— fecB	Iron (Fe^{3+}) importer	Not determined
3.A.1.20.1	ABC superfamily	*Brachyspira* iron transporter (BIT) family	Rv1348 Rv1349	— —	Iron transporter	Not determined
3.A.1.102.1	ABC superfamily	Lipooligosaccharide exporter (LOSE) family	Rv1686c Rv1687c	— —	Lipooligosaccharide exporter	Not determined
3.A.1.103.1	ABC superfamily	Lipopolysaccharide exporter (LPSE) family	Rv3781 Rv3783	rfbE rfbD	Lipopolysaccharide exporter	Not determined
3.A.1.105.1	ABC superfamily	Drug exporter 1 (DrugE1) family	Rv2686c Rv2687c Rv2688c	— — —	Daunorubicin, doxorubicin (drug resistance) exporter	Not determined
3.A.1.105.1	ABC superfamily	DrugE1 family	Rv2936 Rv2937 Rv2938	drrA drrB drrC	Daunorubicin, doxorubicin (drug resistance) exporter	Multidrug efflux pump Involved in localization of PDIM (20,21,28)
3.A.1.105.2	ABC superfamily	DrugE1 family	Rv1217c Rv1218c	— —	Oleandomycin (drug resistance) exporter	Not determined
3.A.1.105.2	ABC superfamily	DrugE1 family	Rv1456c Rv1457c Rv1458c	— — —	Oleandomycin (drug resistance) exporter	Not determined
3.A.1.106.1	ABC superfamily	Lipid exporter (LipidE) family	Rv1272c Rv1273c	— —	Lipid exporter	Not determined
3.A.1.120.1	ABC superfamily	Drug resistance ATPase 1 (Drug RA1) family	Rv2477c	—	Macrolide resistance ATPase	Not determined
3.A.1.120.3	ABC superfamily	Drug RA1 family	Rv1473	—	Oleandomycin resistance ATPase	Not determined
3.A.1.120.4	ABC superfamily	Drug RA1 family	Rv1667c Rv1668c	— —	Carbomycin resistance ATPase	Not determined
3.A.1.125.1	ABC superfamily	Lipoprotein translocase (LPT) family	Rv0986 Rv0987	— —	Lipoprotein translocation system	Not determined

Continued on following page

Table 1. *Continued*

TC no.	Family	Subfamily	ORF[b]	Gene[b]	Predicted function[c]	Known function (reference)
3.A.1.201.1	ABC superfamily	Multidrug resistance exporter (MDR) family	Rv0194	—	Broad-specificity multidrug resistance (MDR) efflux pump	Not determined
3.A.1.201.3	ABC superfamily	MDR family	Rv1463	—	Broad-specificity multidrug resistance (MDR) efflux pump	Not determined
3.A.1.203.1	ABC superfamily	Peroxysomal fatty acyl CoA transporter (P-FAT) family	Rv1819c	—	Unknown; homolog of human peroxysomal long-chain fatty acyl (LCFA) transporter	Not determined
3.A.1.204.2	ABC superfamily	Eye pigment precursor transporter (EPP) family	Rv1747	—	Drug resistance transporter	Not determined
3.A.1.?.?	ABC superfamily	Unknown	Rv1620c	cydC	Involved in the assembly of cytochromes	Not determined
			Rv1621c	cydD		
3.A.2.1.1	H$^+$- or Na$^+$-translocating F-type, V-type, and A-type ATPase (F-ATPase) superfamily	Not applicable	Rv1304	atpB	H$^+$-translocating F-type ATPase	Not determined
			Rv1305	atpE		
			Rv1306	atpF		
			Rv1307	atpH		
			Rv1308	atpA		
			Rv1309	atpG		
			Rv1310	atpD		
			Rv1311	atpC		
3.A.3.2.4	P-type ATPase (P-ATPase) superfamily	Not applicable	Rv0107c	ctpI	Ca^{2+}-ATPase (efflux)	Not determined
3.A.3.2.4	P-ATPase superfamily	Not applicable	Rv0425c	ctpH	Ca^{2+}-ATPase (efflux)	Not determined
3.A.3.2.4	P-ATPase superfamily	Not applicable	Rv0908	ctpE	Ca^{2+}-ATPase (efflux)	Not determined
3.A.3.2.4	P-ATPase superfamily	Not applicable	Rv1997	ctpF	Ca^{2+}-ATPase (efflux)	Not determined
3.A.3.5.1	P-ATPase superfamily	Not applicable	Rv0092	ctpA	Cu^{2+}-ATPase (uptake)	Not determined
3.A.3.5.1	P-ATPase superfamily	Not applicable	Rv0103c	ctpB	Cu^{2+}-ATPase (uptake)	Not determined
3.A.3.5.1	P-ATPase superfamily	Not applicable	Rv0969	ctpV	Cu^{2+}-ATPase (uptake)	Not determined
3.A.3.6.1	P-ATPase superfamily	Not applicable	Rv1469	ctpD	Zn^{2+}, Cb^{2+}, Pb^{2+}-ATPase (efflux)	Not determined
3.A.3.6.1	P-ATPase superfamily	Not applicable	Rv1992c	ctpG	Zn^{2+}, Cb^{2+}, Pb^{2+}-ATPase (efflux)	Not determined
3.A.3.6.1	P-ATPase superfamily	Not applicable	Rv3270	ctpC	Zn^{2+}, Cb^{2+}, Pb^{2+}-ATPase (efflux)	Homolog of MtaA (Erdman) putative metal transporter (19)

TC number	Family		ORF[b]	Gene[b]	Function[c]	
3.A.3.6.1	P-ATPase superfamily	Not applicable	Rv3743c	*ctpJ*	Zn^{2+}, Cb^{2+}, Pb^{2+}-ATPase (efflux)	Not determined
3.A.3.7.1	P-ATPase superfamily	Not applicable	Rv1029 Rv1030 Rv1031	*kdpA* *kdpB* *kdpC*	K^{+}-ATPase (uptake)	Not determined
3.A.4.1.1	Arsenite-antimonite (ArsAB) efflux family	Not applicable	Rv3578	*arsB2*	Arsenical resistance efflux pump (membrane component)	Not determined
3.A.4.1.1	ArsAB efflux family	Not applicable	Rv3679	—	Arsenical resistance efflux protein (ATPase component)	Not determined
3.A.4.1.1	ArsAB efflux family	Not applicable	Rv3680	—	Arsenical resistance efflux protein (ATPase component)	Not determined
3.A.5.1.1	Type 2 (general) secretory pathway (IISP) family	Not applicable	Rv2916c Rv3101c Rv3102c	*ffh* *ftsX* *ftsE*	General secretory pathway complex	Not determined Involved in cell division (96)
3.A.5.1.1	IISP family	Not applicable	Rv0638 Rv0732 Rv1440 Rv3240c	*secE1* *secY* *secG* *secA*	General secretory pathway complex	Not determined

Class: transport electron carriers; subclass: transmembrane 2-electron transfer carriers

TC number	Family		ORF[b]	Gene[b]	Function[c]	
5.A.1.4.1	Disulfide-bond oxidoreductase D (DsbD) family	Not applicable	Rv2877c	—	Mercury resistance protein	Not determined

Incompletely characterized transport systems

TC number	Family		ORF[b]	Gene[b]	Function[c]	
9.A.19.2.1	Mg^{2+} transporter-E (MgtE) family	Not applicable	Rv0362	*mgtE*	Mg^{2+} transporter	Not determined
9.B.14.1.1	Putative heme exporter protein (HEP) family	Not applicable	Rv0529	*ccsA*	Cytochrome *c* biogenesis protein	Not determined
9.B.20.1.2	Putative Mg^{2+} transporter C (MgtC) family	Not applicable	Rv1811	*mgtC*	Putative Mg^{2+} transporter	Not determined

[a]See the Appendix for an explanation of the table.
[b]ORF (open reading frame) and gene names are those attributed by Cole et al. (31, 32). — indicates that no name has been attributed by Cole et al. to the predicted transporter gene.
[c]Refers to the function of the representative member of the family present in the Saier database showing the greatest similarity to the *M. tuberculosis* protein. BLASTP E-values above 0.001 are indicated.

Primary Active Transporters

The primary active transporters use a primary source of energy to drive active transport of a solute against a concentration gradient. *M. tuberculosis* transporters of this class are all included in the P—P bond hydrolysis-driven subclass of transporters, which hydrolyze the diphosphate bond of inorganic pyrophosphate, ATP, or another nucleoside triphosphate to drive the transport. *M. tuberculosis* transporters belong to five different families. The majority fall into the ABC superfamily (13) or the P-type ATPase superfamily (12 transporters).

ABC transporters, found in eukaryotes and prokaryotes, constitute a large superfamily of multisubunit permeases that import or export various molecules in response to ATP hydrolysis. Members of the P-type ATPase family catalyze the uptake and/or efflux of cations. They are also driven by ATP hydrolysis.

Transport Electron Carriers

Transport electron carriers are systems that catalyze electron flow across a biological membrane, from donors localized to one side of the membrane to acceptors localized on the other side. One *M. tuberculosis* protein falls into this class of proteins.

FUNCTIONAL UPTAKE TRANSPORTERS

In this section we describe the mycobacterial uptake transporters which have been demonstrated to be functional. Indeed, it is important to consider the gap between the vast knowledge accumulated by genome sequencing and the in silico annotations (13, 32) and the more limited but valuable experimental data that demonstrate functionality or pathophysiological significance of these transporters.

To study the functionality of uptake transporters, multiple approaches have been followed, depending on the system analyzed. The most commonly used is based on knocking out the target gene either by allelic exchange (10, 42, 49, 89) or by transposon insertion mutagenesis (20, 21, 37, 107).

Anion Transporters

Mutagenesis of the CysA-CysW-CysT-SubI putative sulfate importer belonging to the ABC superfamily is exemplary in this respect (107) (Table 1). One *Mycobacterium bovis* BCG methionine auxotroph, selected by screening a library of mutants obtained by transposon mutagenesis, was found to be disrupted within the *cysA* gene encoding the predicted nucleotide-binding subunit of this putative transporter. Prototrophy was fully restored when this

mutation was complemented by expression of the wild-type *cysA* gene from *M. tuberculosis*. Previously, another mutant with a similar phenotype was found to contain a transposon insertion within the *subI* gene, which encodes the predicted high-affinity sulfate-binding subunit of the transporter (62). Both mutants were resistant to the toxicity of the chromate ion (usually transported by sulfate-thiosulphate permeases) and were unable to take up sulfate, suggesting that the ABC transporter is the sole sulfate transporter of *M. bovis* BCG (107). Additional proof that this ABC transporter is functional was obtained by showing that similar K_m and V_{max} values are found in the transporter from the wild-type strain of *M. bovis* BCG and from the *cysA* mutant complemented with the *cysA* gene from *M. tuberculosis*. Sensitivity to classic inhibitors (azide and 1,3-dicyclohexylcarbodiimide) is also characteristic of ABC transporters.

Despite the fact that the sulfate transporter appears to be the sole transporter of sulfate, survival of *cysA* and *subI* mutants in animals was similar to that of wild-type *M. bovis* BCG (107). It may be that mycobacteria incorporate enough methionine from their intracellular host cell replication site to support their growth. Alternatively, sulfate could be incorporated from other putative sulfate transporters whose expression would be induced in vivo. Three other putative sulfate transporters, predicted to belong to the sulfate permease (SulP) family, are indeed encoded by the genome of *M. tuberculosis* (Table 1). Experimental data are needed to determine whether they transport sulfate.

Phosphate is another very important anion, also transported by one or several multisubunit ABC permeases in mycobacteria. On the basis of genomic DNA sequences and their similarity to *Escherichia coli* orthologs, at least three such *M. tuberculosis* phosphate permeases have been described and analyzed (12, 15, 16, 58). In addition, two genes (*pitA* and *pitB*) encoding putative constitutive inorganic phosphate transporters belonging to the inorganic phosphate transporter (pit) family are found in the *M. tuberculosis* complex genomes (Table 1). The reason for these duplications and apparent redundancy is not known. Since phosphate is an essential but often limiting nutrient, it is possible that several inorganic phosphate importers are necessary to allow the survival of *M. tuberculosis* in the different environments to which it is exposed during its infectious cycle (phagosomes, granulomas, caseum, etc.). Otherwise, this feature may help to protect the bacterial genome against accidental loss of very important genes and allow the emergence of newly evolving genes (64).

The functionality of the ABC systems has been investigated by biochemical approaches. Chang et al.

(24) have shown that one of the putative substrate-binding proteins, PstS-1, expressed as a recombinant without signal sequence and purified from *E. coli* inclusion bodies or from a soluble fraction, binds inorganic phosphate in vitro with a K_d of 0.23 μM. The crystal structure of the PstS-1 phosphate receptor bound to phosphate has been determined (103). Sarin et al. (87), on the other hand, have shown that the purified recombinant PstB protein from *M. tuberculosis*, the putative nucleotide binding domain of the transporter, is active in vitro as a thermostable Mg^{2+} dependent ATPase. Interestingly, Collins et al. (33) have shown that PhoT (whose gene is 130 kb from *pstB* in the chromosome) can also function as nucleotide binding domain for the high-affinity phosphate transport in *M. bovis* and is a virulence gene in this species, where the *pstB* gene is frameshifted (46).

An interesting alternative approach consisted of inactivating PstS-1 with a neutralizing monoclonal antibody. The fact that inorganic phosphate uptake by *M. bovis* BCG was reduced to 20% by this very specific immunoglobulin demonstrated that, at least in axenic cultures of *M. bovis* BCG, the PstS-1-containing phosphate permease is functional and represents most of the phosphate uptake system of these bacteria. Unfortunately, no other monoclonal antibodies exerted a similar activity toward the other two putative phosphate-binding subunits PstS-2 and PstS-3 (15).

Amino Acid-Peptide Transporters

Several putative amino acid permeases predicted to belong to the APC or ABC superfamily are encoded by the *M. tuberculosis* genome (Table 1). Seth and Connell have deleted, by allelic exchange, the *M. bovis* BCG homologue of one of them, Rv0522, encoded by *gabP* belonging to the APC superfamily (89). The corresponding knockout strain showed a specific deficit of L-arginine (90%) and γ-aminobutyric acid uptake that was fully compensated in a mutant strain complemented with the wild-type *gabP* gene, demonstrating that Rv0522 is clearly a functional amino acid importer permease in *M. bovis* BCG. Its apparent K_m was estimated at 250 μM for arginine.

On the other hand, a permease belonging to the ABC superfamily encoded by an operon called *oppB-oppC-oppD-oppA* was suspected to function as a peptide importer in *M. bovis* BCG and *M. tuberculosis*. An *M. bovis* BCG strain in which the *oppD* gene was interrupted was obtained by homologous recombination (49). This mutant was shown to resist the toxicity of the tripeptides glutathione and *S*-nitrosoglutathione and displayed a reduced uptake of glutathione compared with that observed in the wild-type strain or in

the *oppD* mutant complemented with a wild-type copy of the operon. In this case also, besides the existence of a functional peptide permease, one other putative permease (Rv3663-Rv3664-Rv3665-Rv3666 encoded by *dppD-dppC-dppB-dppA*) probably plays an additional role in the transport of peptides, which remains to be further explored (Table 1).

Cation Transporter

Natural resistance-associated macrophage protein 1 (Nramp1) has been identified as a critical determinant of susceptibility to infection by intracellular pathogens including mycobacteria (91). It is localized to the membrane of phagosomes and transports divalent cations, including Fe^{2+} and Mn^{2+}. Nramp1 belongs to a family of transporters highly conserved in eukaryotes and prokaryotes.

Analysis of the *M. tuberculosis* genome indicated the presence of a single homologue of Nramp1, Rv0924c, encoded by *mntH* (also called *Mramp* [1a]) (Table 1). *mntH* has been cloned in a plasmid and transcribed into cRNA, which was then injected in *Xenopus laevis* oocytes, where uptake of different cations could be measured. MntH was demonstrated to be an active divalent-cation transporter with a broad specificity, able to transport Zn^{2+} and Fe^{2+}. This uptake is pH dependent, being maximal between pH 5.5 and 6.5, which is compatible with its functioning within intracellular phagosomes. MntH-mediated Zn^{2+} and Fe^{2+} transport is inhibited by an excess of Mn^{2+} and Cu^{2+}, suggesting that MntH may also interact with these two divalent cations.

Based on the finding that both Nramp1 and MntH transport divalent cations, several authors have suggested that mammalian and bacterial transporters may compete for essential metal ions during mycobacterial infections. However both Domenech et al. (42) and Boechat et al. (10) inactivated the *M. tuberculosis mntH* gene by homologous recombination mutagenesis and showed that the virulence of the mutant in mice is not affected. Boechat et al. also suggested that the MntH is mainly an iron transporter since they observed that the growth of the *M. tuberculosis* MntH mutant strain is strongly reduced in an iron depleted medium (10).

Iron transport is considered in chapter 21 of this book.

LARGE-CONDUCTANCE MECHANOSENSITIVE CHANNEL

Many bacterial species utilize membrane tension-gated channel proteins to adapt rapidly to an increase in their cell volume resulting from sudden exposure to a diluted environment ("osmotic down-shock"). When exposed to mechanical pressure, these membrane proteins become open pores that allow the rapid and efficient efflux of several diverse cytoplasmic osmolytes such as some amino acids (e.g., proline), ions (e.g., K^+), sugars (e.g., trehalose), nucleotides (e.g., ATP), and even some small proteins (e.g., thioredoxin) (9). Three channel activities have been found in *E. coli* and several other bacteria: MscL (a mechanosensitive channel of large conductance), MscS (a mechanosensitive channel of smaller conductance) and MscM (a mechanosensitive channel of miniconductance) (76).

The MscL homologue from *M. tuberculosis* has been cloned. After its 3.5-Å crystal structure was determined, suggesting possible gating mechanisms for opening and closing the channel in response to membrane stress, it became one of the best models for the study of mechanosensitive ion channels in prokaryotes (23).

Subsequently, Moe et al. demonstrated by patch clamp analysis that the *M. tuberculosis* MscL protein (Tb-MscL, Rv0985c) is a functional mechanosensitive channel both in *E. coli* spheroplasts overexpressing the native Tb-MscL protein and in azolectin-synthetic proteoliposomes reconstituted with the purified Tb-MscL protein (66). In addition, they showed that the resolubilized Tb-MscL protein crystallized protein reconstituted into azolectin-liposomes was active. In both reconstituted systems, however, the Tb-MscL protein appeared quantitatively different since it required about twice the tension needed to gate the *E. coli* MscL. The authors speculate that this variation might reflect the profound differences existing in the natural membrane environment of the protein in liposomes, in *E. coli* or in the complex, versus the natural lipid environment of the mycobacterial membrane.

Probably for the same reason, the Tb-MscL cannot complement an *mscl yggB* double null strain of *E. coli* from acute osmotic down-shock. Therefore, the role of Tb-MscL in vivo is still unknown, although present data suggest that it could be analogous to the osmoprotection activity observed in other bacteria.

VIRULENCE AND SOLUTE TRANSPORT

Transporters play an essential role in the expression of the virulence phenotype in bacteria. Virulence factors must be exported for interaction with the target host cell, and a number of remarkable examples of this strategy have been recently reviewed (18). Genes encoding transporters have been identified in more general searches for loci required for virulence. For example, a screen for insertion mutational events

in *Listeria monocytogenes* that reduced survival in macrophages identified an arginine transporter (53). A study of genes regulated by iron availability and by the *ideR* locus in *M. tuberculosis* revealed genes encoding transporters as a major class (82).

Amino Acids and Peptides

In particular, the ABC class of peptide transporters, described above, are encoded by key virulence loci in a number of pathogenic bacterial species. In group A streptococci, *dpp* imports essential amino acids and affects protease expression (77). In *Streptococcus pneumoniae*, the oligopeptide permease *opp* controls quorum sensing and pheromone autoinduction (30). In *Staphylococcus aureus*, the largest class of loci affecting survival in multiple infection models is the transporter class (36). Finally, mutants of *Salmonella* resistant to S-nitrosoglutathione map to dipeptide permease (*dpp*) genes and to *rpoS* (38).

As mentioned above, mutations in the *dpp* locus in *M. bovis* BCG (49) and *M. tuberculosis* (V. Venketaraman et al., unpublished data) lead to increased resistance to glutathione and GSNO, compounds toxic to mycobacteria. Survival of the *dpp* mutant in murine macrophages has been measured, and the mutant exhibits a "hypervirulent" phenotype, surviving better than its wild-type parent in both unactivated and activated macrophages. This points to glutathione and/or GSNO as a novel mechanism of innate immunity against mycobacterial infection (100).

An interesting experiment was carried out by Klose and Mekalanos to examine the role of amino acid transport and availability in macrophage survival (54). Two strains of *Salmonella enterica* serovar Typhimurium with single mutations conferring either glutamine auxotrophy or reduced glutamine transport showed no differences in virulence in the mouse compared with that of the wild-type parent. However, when the two mutations were combined in a single strain, the double mutant was attenuated. A similar experiment—that of knocking out synthesis and transport in the same strain—has not yet been performed with *M. tuberculosis*.

However, Pavelka and Jacobs point to similar results by comparing lysine auxotrophs with unmarked deletions in the *lysA* gene (72). *M. smegmatis* and *M. bovis* BCG *lysA* mutants can grow on minimal media with lysine, but *M. tuberculosis lysA* requires a 25-fold-higher concentration of exogenous lysine for colony formation. *M. bovis* BCG and *M. tuberculosis* appear to differ in efficient acquisition of lysine. Furthermore, the *lysA* gene is essential for survival of *M. tuberculosis* H37Rv in immuno-compromised mice (47). The inability of bacterial auxotrophs to survive in vivo is interpreted to indicate that the required compound is not accessible to the organism; an alternative explanation is that transport of the substrate is insufficient. Whether this phenomenon is due to alternative regulation of transport capacity during intracellular growth has not yet been determined for any substrate.

Lipid Transport

A completely different strategy was used by two independent groups, who used the technique of signature-tagged mutagenesis to define mycobacterial genes or functions that are required for the pulmonary growth and development of fully virulent *M. tuberculosis* strains (21, 35). Both groups obtained some attenuated mutants that were affected by transposon insertion either in biosynthesis or in the export of a complex cell wall lipid called phthiocerol dimycocerosate (PDIM), which is found only in pathogenic mycobacteria. These experiments suggest that the synthesis and export of PDIM to the mycobacterial cell wall are essential for the correct replication of *M. tuberculosis* in the lungs. The reason for this is not known. Two distinct lipid transporters seem to be involved: MmpL7 and DrrABC.

MmpL7 (Rv2942) is a 12-transmembrane-domain protein belonging to the RND superfamily. Thirteen other representatives exist in the *M. tuberculosis* genome. The loss of virulence of MmpL7 mutants and their biochemical phenotype (characterized by a normal synthesis of PDIM accompanied by their typical absence on the bacterial cell wall) clearly demonstrates that this transporter is functional and essential for PDIM export (21, 35).

One additional transposon insertion mutant displaying a similar phenotype in terms of virulence (lung tropism) and PDIM distribution was obtained by Camacho et al. (20, 21). In this case, the mutation resides within the *drrC* gene that belongs to the *drrA-drrB-drrC* cluster (Rv2936 to Rv2938) (see also "Exporters and antibiotic resistance" below). This suggests that the DrrABC permease is also functional and implicated in the transport of PDIM to the bacterial cell wall (21) and therefore in the lung tropism and virulence of *M. tuberculosis*.

A challenging question is how these two totally different and nonredundant PDIM transporters cooperate, since both appear to be absolutely required for the transport of PDIM to the bacterial cell wall surface.

Recently, another member of the MmpL family of proteins has been related to the transport of the sulfated glycolipid termed sulfolipid 1 and also to the virulence of *M. tuberculosis* (34).

EXPORTERS AND ANTIBIOTIC RESISTANCE

Most of the drug-resistant isolates of mycobacteria have arisen through the acquisition of chromosomal mutations in genes encoding either drug targets or the drug-activating enzymes (85), which usually confer high levels of resistance. There are also a significant number of low-level-drug-resistant strains in which no mutation can be found. These strains can be regarded as the first step toward the acquisition of chromosomal mutations (and, consequently, higher levels of resistance) as has been described for ethambutol resistance (94). The resistance phenotype in these strains can be explained in several ways: there could be mutations in other (not yet discovered) drug targets, there could be alteration in the permeability of the cell envelope, or the resistance phenotype could be a consequence of the involvement of drug transporters, as has been widely described for other bacterial genera (71).

Drug transporters have become an important part of the drug resistance panorama from many points of view. They decrease the concentration of drugs inside the cell, thereby favoring the acquisition of chromosomal mutations that will eventually confer higher levels of resistance. There are many substances that can selectively inhibit drug transporters and could be used to improve current antituberculosis treatment (101). Finally, because of the low specificity requirements for substrates, drug transporters could easily represent the first line of defense against new antimycobacterial compounds.

Depending on the structure, energy dependence, localization, and other features, membrane transporters have been classified in five different superfamilies (Fig. 1): the ABC superfamily, the MFS, the RND superfamily, the drug/metabolite transporter (DMT) superfamily, and the multidrug/oligosaccharidyl-lipid/polysaccharide (MOP) flippase superfamily. Putative drug transporters belonging to all of these families have been identified in the genome of *M. tuberculosis* H37Rv (32) (Table 1).

ATP-Binding Cassette Superfamily

Several putative *M. tuberculosis* antimicrobial efflux transporters of the ABC superfamily were found to be encoded by the genome of *M. tuberculosis*. Our analysis indicates that they belong to four different families: the drug exporter 1 (DrugE1) family, the drug resistance ATPase 1 (DrugRA1) family, the multidrug resistance family, and the eye pigment precur-

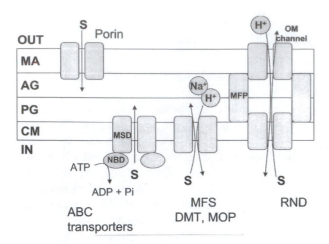

Figure 1. Schematic view of the different types of antibiotic efflux proteins present in *M. tuberculosis*. In the background, the four horizontal bars represent the main layers in the *M. tuberculosis* envelope; the most internal of them is the cell membrane (CM), to which is attached the peptidoglycan (PG) layer, which is also covalently linked to the arabinogalactan (AG). To the latter, mycolic acids (MA) are covalently bound, forming a pseudo-outer membrane, which represents the outer part of the cell wall. Beyond the MA, capsular material is the most external part of the mycobacterial envelope, which has not been represented for simplicity. Several types of proteins participate in the influx or efflux of substrates (S) across the cell envelope. (i) Porins allow S to cross the MA layer by passive diffusion. (ii) The ABC transporters are composed of MSDs, anchored in the CM, and NBDs which hydrolyze ATP, supplying the energy for driving transport. MSD and NBD may be arranged in several combinations. (iii) Transporters of the MFS and the DMT superfamily are proteins located in the CM; they couple the efflux of S with the electrochemical gradient. Similarly, members of the MOP flippase superfamily are predicted to work as substrate:Na^+ antiporters. (iv) Members of the RND superfamily also export substrates by using the electrochemical gradient. In other bacteria, these systems are capable of exporting S directly from the cytoplasm to the external media, due to the presence of membrane fusion proteins (MFP), which bring together the transport protein in the CM and channels in the outer membrane.

sor transporter family (Table 1). Among them, only one transporter (Rv2936-Rv2937-Rv2938) of the DrugE1 family was partially characterized. It is composed of a nucleotide-binding domain (Rv2936) encoded by *drrA* and two membrane-spanning domains (Rv2937 and Rv2938) encoded by *drrB* and *drrC*. The three genes are transcriptionally coupled in a putative operon. When *drrA* and *drrB* are tandemly expressed in *E. coli* or *Mycobacterium smegmatis*, an increased resistance of these cells to several structurally unrelated antibiotics was reported (28). This resistance phenotype could be reversed by verapamil and reserpine, two potent inhibitors of ABC transporters. Surprisingly, the authors did not study the participation of DrrC (Rv2938) in the transport. Since ABC transporters require two hydrophobic membrane-spanning domains and two hydrophilic nucleotide-

binding domains, the reported data suggest that the transporter is able to function as a multidrug efflux pump composed of a homodimer of DrrA (Rv2936) and a homodimer of DrrB (Rv2937). Independently, DrrC was previously identified, by signature-tagged transposon mutagenesis, as a potential virulence factor of *M. tuberculosis*, and, more recently, its physiological role was determined (20, 21). It is involved (putatively in association with DrrA and DrrB) in the translocation of PDIMs into the cell wall of *M. tuberculosis*, thus contributing indirectly in cell envelope architecture and permeability of the bacteria (see also "Virulence and solute transport" above). Recently, using microarray experiments, it has been shown that triclosan can induce the expression of the putative ABC transporter encoded by Rv1686c (6).

Besides the ABC transporters predicted to be antimicrobial efflux transporters, a putative nucleotide-binding domain involved in the uptake of inorganic phosphate in *M. smegmatis* was shown to mediate the efflux of fluoroquinolones (7). The other subunits of this transporter have not yet been studied, and it is not clear whether the gene encoding this nucleotide-binding domain is part of a cluster of genes encoding the other constituents of a multisubunit inorganic-phosphate transporter.

Major Facilitator Superfamily Drug Transporters

Initially, 11 genes encoding putative drug efflux proteins of the MFS were found in the genome of *M. tuberculosis* H37Rv (32). These were Rv0783c, Rv0849, Rv1250, Rv1258c, Rv1410c, Rv1634, Rv1877, Rv2333c, Rv2459, Rv2846c, and Rv2994. Subsequently, a reexamination of the *M. tuberculosis* genome allowed the identification of five other genes (Rv0037c, Rv0191, Rv2456c, Rv3239c, and Rv3728) encoding putative drug efflux pumps of this superfamily (39). In this article, the protein motifs characteristic of the MFS proteins have been redefined to match more precisely those shown by the *M. tuberculosis* proteins.

The first MFS protein of *M. tuberculosis* to be studied was EfpA, encoded by the Rv2846c (*efpA*) gene (43), which is readily expressed by *M. tuberculosis*. The protein shows those motifs characteristic of the MFS members, and homologous genes were detected in several species of mycobacteria. However, no differences could be found in the *efpA* gene from drug-resistant and drug-susceptible strains. In two recent studies, using DNA microarrays, it was found that subinhibitory concentrations of isoniazid and thiolactomycin induced the expression of the *efpA* gene (6, 105).

The *M. tuberculosis* efflux pumps P55, encoded by the Rv1410c gene (90), and Tap, encoded by Rv1258c (39), confer low-level resistance to tetracycline and several aminoglycosides, including the antituberculosis drug streptomycin when expressed in *M. smegmatis*. The Tap protein confers lower resistance levels than does the P55 product. The product of the *M. tuberculosis* Rv1634 gene expressed in *M. smegmatis* was found to confer low-level resistance to several fluoroquinolones (39).

Apart from *M. tuberculosis*, MFS efflux pumps have also been characterized in other mycobacterial species. In the fast-growing species *M. smegmatis*, the *tet(V)* gene encodes an efflux pump that confers low-level resistance to tetracycline and chlortetracycline (40). Also, the LfrA efflux pump from *M. smegmatis* confers low-level resistance to several fluoroquinolones, ethidium bromide, acridine, and some quaternary ammonium compounds (93). Interestingly, homologues of *tet(V)* and *lfrA* genes are absent from the *M. tuberculosis* H37Rv genome. In the saprophytic species *Mycobacterium fortuitum*, the *tap* gene (the orthologue of the *M. tuberculosis* Rv1258c gene) encodes an efflux pump similar to that of *M. tuberculosis*, which confers low-level resistance to tetracycline and aminoglycosides, including streptomycin (1).

Most of these reports describe substrate accumulation experiments to prove that antibiotics are readily exported by these proteins, and these studies also have investigated the effects of ionophores, such as carbonylcyanide *m*-chlorophenylhydrazone (CCCP), and other efflux pump inhibitors, such as reserpine and verapamil, on the resistance levels (1, 39, 40, 90). So far, the *M. smegmatis lfrA* gene has been the only one to be disrupted, resulting in a moderate decrease in resistance to ciprofloxacin, doxorubicin, and rhodamine (86).

Resistance-Nodulation-Cell Division Superfamily

Members of the RND superfamily are composed of 12 transmembrane segments (TMS) with two large loops between TMS 1 and 2 and TMS 7 and 8. They catalyze substrate efflux via an H^+ antiport mechanism. Three of the putative RND transporters encoded by the genome of *M. tuberculosis* (Rv0202c, Rv0206c, and Rv1146) are predicted to belong to the hydrophobe/amphiphile efflux 2 (HAE2) family. They could be implicated in the efflux of antibiotic and in the resistance of *M. tuberculosis* to various drugs. However, none of them was characterized experimentally. Triclosan, a compound that inhibits mycolic acid biosynthesis, induced the expression of the RND protein MmpL6 (6).

Drug/Metabolite Transporter Superfamily

The Rv3065 transporter is the only *M. tuberculosis* protein belonging to the DMT superfamily and to the small multidrug resistance (SMR) family (41, 70). SMR proteins are the smallest multidrug resistance proteins (about 110 amino acids long). They are composed of four transmembrane domains. SMR proteins function as oligomers to extrude various drugs in exchange for protons. Rv3065 is encoded by the *emrE* gene (also named *mmR*) and is similar to EmrE from *E. coli*, the best-characterized member of the SMR family. When expressed in *M. smegmatis* cells, Rv3065 was shown to confer resistance to tetraphenylphosphonium (TPP), erythromycin, ethidium bromide, acriflavine, safranin O, and pyronin Y (41). Studies of the effect of the ionophore CCCP on [^{3}H]TPP intracellular accumulation strongly suggest that the efflux mechanism mediated by Rv3065 uses the proton motive force as the energy source. More recently, Rv3065 was purified, reconstituted into proteoliposomes, and shown to catalyze the uptake of methyl viologen (70). However, the role of this multidrug efflux pump on the resistance of *M. tuberculosis* to various antibiotics has not yet been demonstrated.

Multidrug/Oligosaccharidyl-Lipid/Polysaccharide Flippase Superfamily

One putative *M. tuberculosis* antimicrobial efflux transporter (Rv2836c) belongs to the MOP flippase superfamily and to the multiantimicrobial extrusion (MATE) family. This family is the most recently described family of drug efflux transporters, and only few members were functionally studied (17). Transporters of this family are predicted to adopt a 12-helix structure, and some of them were shown to function by a drug:Na^+ antiport mechanism (26). Rv2836c, encoded by *dinF*, is highly homologous to the functionally uncharacterized DNA damage-inducible protein F of *E. coli* and also to several characterized bacterial efflux transporters of the MATE family (14, 65, 67, 68). Its putative function has not yet been experimentally confirmed.

Transport of Antituberculosis Drugs

Several studies have been performed to identify the potential transporters involved in the uptake and/or efflux of the main antituberculosis drugs.

Rifampin

Accumulation experiments showed that *M. tuberculosis*, *Mycobacterium aurum*, and *M. smegmatis* accumulated rifampin quickly and that steady-state concentrations of this drug increased in the presence of subinhibitory concentrations of either ethambutol (which is known to increase cell wall permeability) or reserpine (an inhibitor of efflux pumps). This suggests that an efflux pump could be involved in the removal of rifampin from cells (75).

Isoniazid

In *M. smegmatis*, which is intrinsically resistant to isoniazid, accumulation levels of this drug increase in the presence of several inhibitory compounds, suggesting the involvement of ATP and/or proton motive force-driven efflux pumps in the uptake of isoniazid (29). Conversely, isoniazid uptake in the naturally sensitive *M. tuberculosis* has been proposed to occur by passive diffusion (4), since inhibitory compounds such as CCCP and arsenate do not have any effect on isoniazid accumulation levels. However, more recently, other authors have shown that reserpine, an efflux pump inhibitor, decreases the isoniazid-induced high-level resistance of *M. tuberculosis*, suggesting the involvement of efflux pumps in isoniazid transport (102). As mentioned above, the transcription of a gene encoding the *efpA* efflux pump was induced on isoniazid treatment (6, 105).

Pyrazinamide

An ATP-dependent transport system seems to be involved in the uptake of pyrazinamide (81), and its failure may cause pyrazinamide resistance. Efflux of pyrazinoic acid (the active derivative of pyrazinamide) has been described recently (109), and its deficiency may be the cause of the unique susceptibility of *M. tuberculosis* to pyrazinamide. Conversely, a very active pyrazinoic acid efflux mechanism is responsible for the natural pyrazinamide resistance of *M. smegmatis*.

Ethambutol

To date, no efflux pump has been related to uptake or efflux of ethambutol.

Streptomycin

As described in the section above, two *M. tuberculosis* efflux pumps have been related to streptomycin resistance (1, 90)

Fluoroquinolones

Several reports have concluded that in *M. smegmatis* and *M. aurum*, the uptake of fluoroquinolones is an energy-independent diffusion process, since in-tracellular accumulation of these antibiotics is not affected by substances such as 2,4-dinitrophenol, Tween 80, ethambutol, and CCCP (35, 104). Similar results have been described for *M. tuberculosis* (74). Other authors isolated a fluoroquinolone-resistant mutant of *M. tuberculosis* in which no mutation could be found in the *gyrAB* genes (55). Since this mutant has a reduced level of uptake of fluoroquinolones, this suggested that efflux pumps were involved in lowering the accumulation levels. Such a suggestion has also been made for *Mycobacterium avium*, because this species shows higher resistance levels to fluoroquinolones than does *M. smegmatis*, whereas the DNA gyrase of both species is equally sensitive to these drugs (51). In fact, several efflux pumps that are capable of transporting fluoroquinolones have been described, as indicated in the previous section (see reference 78 for a review), such as the LfrA MFS efflux pump from *M. smegmatis* (59, 86, 93), the Rv1634 MFS efflux pump from *M. tuberculosis* (39), and the nucleotide-binding domain of a putative *M. smegmatis* ABC transporter involved in inorganic-phosphate transport (3).

REGULATION OF TRANSPORT AND SUBSTRATE SENSORS

In recent years, our knowledge of gene expression and regulation in mycobacteria has progressed notably, and the availability of the *M. tuberculosis* H37Rv and other mycobacterial genomes has provided useful insights into the potential regulatory networks that may operate in these microorganisms.

Regulation of transport processes is an essential component of the adaptive response of mycobacteria to the changing environmental conditions: nutrients, ions, pH, cofactors, drugs, and host defense mechanisms among others. For example, several ABC transporters were induced in *M. smegmatis* on entry into anaerobic stationary phase (69) and also in *M. tuberculosis* under nutrient starvation (5).

We can distinguish two levels of regulation of transport at the molecular level. First, global mechanisms of regulation of gene expression, (such as sigma factors, two-component systems, and transcriptional regulators) contribute to the regulation of transport processes (see chapter 15). Second, every transport system can be controlled specifically by local regulatory mechanisms. For the local regulation, the first event that triggers the activation of the transport regulatory network consists of the detection of a molecule, typically the substrate itself but also some other inducer compounds. Therefore, most of the transport processes rely on such substrate-binding proteins for their regulation.

Although the regulation of transport processes and substrate sensor proteins in mycobacteria is not as well characterized as in other bacterial species, some examples can be outlined.

mar System

The *E. coli mar* operon, involved in multiple antibiotic resistance, has been widely characterized. Basically, the MarR regulator, on binding inducer molecules such as salicylate, activates the transcription of two genes (*marA* and *marB*). In turn, MarA and MarB proteins down-regulate the expression of genes encoding porins and activate the transcription of genes encoding efflux pumps (88). As a result, the bacteria become more resistant to multiple antibiotics. The expression of the *E. coli marA* gene in *M. smegmatis* resulted in an increase of the levels of resistance to several compounds, including the antituberculosis drugs isoniazid, rifampin, and ethambutol, although further studies are needed to characterize the putative transporters involved in this phenotype (63). *M. tuberculosis* has at least two genes similar to the *marA* gene (Rv1931c and Rv3833), and although salicylate does not increase the level of Rv1931c mRNA, it induces resistance to the main antituberculosis drugs (88).

Regulation of Drug Efflux Pumps

For many drug efflux pumps, a local transcriptional regulator is usually encoded in the same locus, for example the QacR regulator of the QacA efflux pump from *S. aureus*, or the TetR regulator of the tetracycline efflux pump TetA. These regulators respond to the concentrations of the substrates transported by the efflux pump (for a recent review, see reference 50). Such systems have not been found yet in mycobacteria, although some efflux pumps are closely associated with putative regulatory proteins, for example the P55 efflux pump and the P27 lipoprotein (8, 90).

Potassium Transport System

Bacteria respond to osmotic stress adjusting the potassium concentration in the cytoplasm. In *M. tuberculosis* (similarly to *E. coli*), the *kpdDE* two-component system detects K^+ limitation, either directly by the sensor histidine kinase KdpD or indirectly through the LprJ and LprF lipoproteins. This signal activates the expression of the *kpdFABC* genes that encode the high-affinity K^+ uptake system (92).

Maltose Transport

Borich et al. (11) have reported the genomic organization of the putative operon involved in maltose transport. Within this operon, the *M. tuberculosis lpqY* gene encodes a product similar to the periplasmic maltose binding protein MalE of *E. coli*.

Iron Transport

Several iron-regulated proteins have been found in *M. tuberculosis* (19). One of them, Irp10, is more abundant under low-iron conditions, and its gene forms an operon with *mtaA*, which encodes a putative metal transport protein. The transcription of both genes is greatly induced under low-iron conditions, suggesting that iron either directly or indirectly regulates its own transport. Readers are referred to chapter 21 for more details.

Phosphate Transport

The phosphate-specific transport system (Pst) of *M. tuberculosis* is composed of three operons, which, in general, include one copy of the ATP-binding protein (PstB), two copies of each of the transmembrane proteins (PstA and PstC), and three copies of the PstS phosphate-binding protein (15, 16, 58). These three PstS proteins are induced under phosphate starvation conditions. Using translation fusions of the *M. tuberculosis pstS1* gene and the reporter *lacZ* gene, two promoters were identified which cause a three- to sixfold increase of the β-galactosidase levels under low-phosphate concentrations in *M. smegmatis* (95). In the latter, the PstS operon appears to be unique and more similar in organization to the one described in *E. coli* (57).

APPENDIX

Genome Sequence Analysis

Table 1 was made by compiling the predicted transport/binding protein-coding genes classified on the Sanger Centre website (http://www.sanger.ac.uk/Projects/M_tuberculosis/Gene_list) and in the Tuberculist database (http://genolist.pasteur.fr/Tuberculist), the predicted transport proteins listed on the Paulsen membrane transport protein analysis website (http://www.biology.ucsd.edu/~ipaulsen/t-transport/index.html), and the ABC transporters and MFS multidrug transporters identified in two recent reviews (13, 39). A total of 210 putative transport proteins were thus identified. Their amino acid sequences were compared to those present in the Saier transport protein database (http://tcdb.ucsd.edu/tcdb/tcclass.php) to predict their putative function and to classify them following the membrane protein TC system (83). The Saier database contains descriptions, TC numbers, and examples of transporters from more than 360 families. Transporters in the database are classified on the basis of five criteria: (i) the transporter class, i.e., channel, carrier (porter), primary active transporter, or group translocator (characterized by V, a number); (ii) the transporter subclass, which in the case of primary active transporters refers to the energy source used to drive transport (characterized by W, a letter); (iii) and (iv) the transporter family and subfamily (or superfamily and family for large families containing more than 1,000 members), which are defined on the basis of sequence similarities (characterized respectively by X and Y, two numbers); and (v) the substrate or range of substrates transported (characterized by Z, a number). The TC number of a particular type of transporter is formed by five numbers or letters (V.W.X.Y.Z) corresponding to the above criteria. The same TC number is given to each transporter (belonging to the same subfamily of a transporter family) that transports the same substrate(s) using the same mechanism, regardless of whether they are orthologs or paralogs.

We compared the predicted *M. tuberculosis* transporter proteins with those of the Saier database by performing BLASTP searches with and without the use of a low-complexity filter. Indeed, it is known that a considerable number of putative transmembrane domains are usually filtered out of a BLASTP search done with a low-complexity filter. Filtering important transmembrane domains of transport proteins may cause the selection of transporter families which are not the most similar to the query sequence. In contrast, BLASTP searches performed without a low-complexity filter may give hits caused by sequence composition bias. To avoid selecting those insignificant hits, we always used the homology assessment program PRSS (73) from the FASTA package (200 random shuffles with a local window of 10 amino acid residues) when the low-complexity filter was not used. PRSS calculates a similarity score between two sequences, compares this similarity score to that obtained after repeatedly shuffling one of the two sequences, and then estimates the probability that the unshuffled score would be obtained by chance. Matches were taken into account only for hits that had a *P* value of 0.0001 or lower.

Among the 210 *M. tuberculosis* putative transporter proteins, 198 proteins gave matches (without filter) with BLAST E-values lower than 0.001 and 2 gave matches with E-values between 0.001 and 0.01. These proteins are listed in Table 1. The last 10 proteins gave no significant matches (E-value, ≥0.01) and were discarded from our analysis. For each protein listed in Table 1, we then verified if the best BLAST match was obtained with the same transporter of the Saier database, whether the low-complexity filter was used or not. When the same transporter

was identified, the *M. tuberculosis* protein acquired its TC number. If different transporters were found, we assigned to the *M. tuberculosis* protein the TC number of the transporter giving the best match when the low-complexity filter was not used; that was done only if the sequence similarity obtained was found to be significant by the PRSS program.

For multisubunit transporters belonging to the large ABC superfamily, the inventory and assembly of the different subunits encoded by the complete genome was previously undertaken (13). Briefly, these subunits, i.e., the nucleotide-binding domains (NBDs), the membrane-spanning domains (MSDs), and the substrate-binding proteins (SBPs), were identified on the basis of their characteristic stretches of amino acids and/or conserved structure. By analysis of transcriptional clusters and searches of homology between the identified subunits and proteins characterized in other organisms, multisubunit transporters were reconstituted and potential substrates were attributed to some of them. We then assigned a TC number to each of these ABC transporters. To this end, each subunit was compared (BLASTP) to the Saier database as described above. When the best BLAST match obtained with each subunit of the ABC transporter identified the same transporter, we assigned the TC number of this transporter to the *M. tuberculosis* ABC transporter. When different subunits of the same transporter were similar to proteins from different TC subcategories (different Y and Z numbers or different Z numbers only), we took into account only the result obtained with the SBP, because these subunits are specific for the transported substrate and very little amino acid sequence similarity occurred between them. If the transporter did not contain any SBP (as is the case for all exporters of this superfamily and some incomplete importers), we took into account the hits obtained with the MSDs rather than those obtained with NBDs. Indeed, it is expected that homologies between NBDs do not significantly influence the assignment of the TC number (particularly the Z number), since they are highly conserved domains, with about 30 to 40% sequence conservation regardless of their substrate specificity. If no MSDs could be attributed to the transporter, matches with NBDs were then taken into account. However, finding substrate specificity for transporters predicted solely on the presence of NBDs (as is the case for Rv0655, Rv2477c, Rv1473, Rv1667c-Rv1668c, and Rv1463) should be considered tentative.

By the above analysis, all of the ABC transporters but two (Rv1620c-Rv1621c and FtsX-FtsE) could be classified into the described subfamilies and potential substrates were attributed to them.

Rv1620c and Rv1621c are two proteins composed of one MSD and one NBD fused in one protein. We previously showed that these proteins are similar to CydC and CydD of *E. coli* and *Bacillus subtilis*, two proteins involved in the export of a component of the assembly of cytochromes that are found in the periplasm or exposed to the external side of the cytoplasmic membrane (79, 80, 106). BLASTP searches made in the Saier database indicate that Rv1620c and Rv1621c belong to different subfamilies, probably because the sequences of CydC and CydD were not introduced into the Saier database. We were therefore unable to assign a complete TC number to this transporter.

FtsX-FtsE, a previously identified ABC transporter that was shown to be involved in cell division, was not further classified in the ABC superfamily (96). Indeed, FtsE of *E. coli* was suspected to participate in the translocation of integral membrane proteins into the inner membrane and therefore was inserted in the type 2 (general) secretory pathway family of the TC system (97). Accordingly, FtsX-FtsE of *M. tuberculosis* was classified in this family (Table 1).

By the present analysis, other ranges of substrates than those assigned in a previous study were attributed to four ABC transporters (13).

The Rv1348-Rv1349 transporter was previously predicted to belong to the family of multidrug tranporters (13). It is now unambiguously classified as an iron transporter, since it shows more similarity to the iron transporters YbtP and YbtQ of *Yersinia pestis* (45) than to multidrug resistance proteins (2, 48). This similarity was not identified by the previous study since the YbtP and YbtQ sequences were not yet released in public databases. These two subunits are therefore probably the components of an iron importer that also contains one of the two previously identified orphan iron-binding proteins, FecB and FecB2 (13).

The Rv0986-Rv0987 transporter was previously shown to be homologous to the putative transporter AttEFG of *Agrobacterium tumefaciens*, which is required for virulence and bacterial attachment to host cells (60). However, BLASTP searches revealed a higher similarity to LolCDE, a newly described ABC transporter of *E. coli,* which mediates the detachment of lipid-modified proteins from membranes (108). Since the homology with LolCDE is higher than that previously observed with AttEFG, we now classified this transporter in the lipoprotein translocase family.

The Rv1272c-Rv1273c transporter was previously predicted to be a multidrug transporter, but the present analysis classified it in the lipid exporter (LipidE) family, composed of a unique member, the lipid flippase MsbA of *E. coli* (13, 110). MsbA corresponds to the best match obtained after a BLASTP search with Rv1272c and Rv1273c against the Saier database (E-value, 3×10^{-80} for Rv1272c and 1×10^{-62} for Rv1273c), but high similarities were also observed to the two multidrug resistance proteins LmrA of *Lactococcus lactis* (E-value, 2×10^{-74} for Rv1272c and 1×10^{-59} for Rv1273c) and HopA of *Lactobacillus brevis* (E-value, 5×10^{-71} for Rv1272c and 5×10^{-61} for Rv1273c). LmrA and HopA belong to the drug exporter 2 (DrugE2) family (84, 99). MsbA is itself highly similar to transporters associated with multidrug resistance, which translocate hydrophobic drugs and lipids, and its structure was used as a model for multidrug resistance ABC transporters (22). The classification of the Rv1272c-Rv1273c transporter in one or the other family is therefore still ambiguous.

Similarly, Rv1819c was previously predicted to be a multidrug transporter but is now classified in the 'peroxysomal fatty acyl-CoA transporter (P-FAT) family,' since it is highly similar to the human peroxysomal long-chain fatty acyl (LCFA) transporter (E-value, 10×10^{-39}) (52). However, it is also homologous to the broad-specificity human multidrug resistance proteins MDR1 (E-value, 1×10^{-11}) and MDR3 (E-value, 2×10^{-15}) of the multidrug resistance exporter family (25, 98). This classification is therefore also hypothetical.

REFERENCES

1a. **Agranoff, D., I. M. Monahan, J. A. Mangan, P. D. Butcher, and S. Krishna.** 1999. *Mycobacterium tuberculosis* expresses a novel pH-dependent divalent cation transporter belonging to the Nramp family. *J. Exp. Med.* **190:**717–724.

1. **Ainsa, J. A., M. C. Blokpoel, I. Otal, D. B. Young, K. A. De Smet, and C. Martin.** 1998. Molecular cloning and characterization of Tap, a putative multidrug efflux pump present in *Mycobacterium fortuitum* and *Mycobacterium tuberculosis.* *J. Bacteriol.* **180:**5836–5843.

2. **Allikmets, R., B. Gerrard, D. Court, and M. Dean.** 1993. Cloning and organization of the *abc* and *mdl* genes of *Escherichia coli*: relationship to eukaryotic multidrug resistance. *Gene* **136:**231–236.

3. **Banerjee, S. K., K. Bhatt, P. Misra, and P. K. Chakraborti.** 2000. Involvement of a natural transport system in the process of efflux-mediated drug resistance in *Mycobacterium smegmatis. Mol. Gen. Genet.* **262:**949–956.

4. **Bardou, F., C. Raynaud, C. Ramos, M. A. Laneelle, and G. Laneelle.** 1998. Mechanism of isoniazid uptake in *Mycobacterium tuberculosis. Microbiology* **144:**2539–2544.

5. **Betts, J. C., P. T. Lukey, L. C. Robb, R. A. McAdam, and K. Duncan.** 2002. Evaluation of a nutrient starvation model of *Mycobacterium tuberculosis* persistence by gene and protein expression profiling. *Mol. Microbiol.* **43:**717–731.

6. **Betts, J. C., A. McLaren, M. G. Lennon, F. M. Kelly, P. T. Lukey, S. J. Blakemore, and K. Duncan.** 2003. Signature gene expression profiles discriminate between isoniazid-, thiolactomycin-, and triclosan-treated *Mycobacterium tuberculosis. Antimicrob. Agents Chemother.* **47:**2903–2913.

7. Bhatt, K., S. K. Banerjee, and P. K. Chakraborti. 2000. Evidence that phosphate specific transporter is amplified in a fluoroquinolone resistant *Mycobacterium smegmatis*. *Eur. J. Biochem.* **267**:4028–4032.

8. Bigi, F., A. Alito, M. I. Romano, M. Zumarraga, K. Caimi, and A. Cataldi. 2000. The gene encoding P27 lipoprotein and a putative antibiotic-resistance gene form an operon in *Mycobacterium tuberculosis* and *Mycobacterium bovis*. *Microbiology* **146**:1011–1018.

9. Blount, P., and P. C. Moe. 1999. Bacterial mechanosensitive channels: integrating physiology, structure and function. *Trends Microbiol.* **7**:420–424.

10. Boechat, N., B. Lagier-Roger, S. Petit, Y. Bordat, J. Rauzier, A. J. Hance, B. Gicquel, and J. M. Reyrat. 2002. Disruption of the gene homologous to mammalian Nramp1 in *Mycobacterium tuberculosis* does not affect virulence in mice. *Infect. Immun.* **70**:4124–4131.

11. Borich, S. M., A. Murray, and E. Gormley. 2000. Genomic arrangement of a putative operon involved in maltose transport in the *Mycobacterium tuberculosis* complex and *Mycobacterium leprae*. *Microbios* **102**:7–15.

12. Braibant, M., L. De Wit, P. Peirs, M. Kalai, J. Ooms, A. Drowart, K. Huygen, and J. Content. 1994. Structure of the *Mycobacterium tuberculosis* antigen 88, a protein related to the *Escherichia coli* PstA periplasmic phosphate permease subunit. *Infect. Immun.* **62**:849–854.

13. Braibant, M., P. Gilot, and J. Content. 2000. The ATP binding cassette (ABC) transport systems of *Mycobacterium tuberculosis*. *FEMS Microbiol. Rev.* **24**:449–467.

14. Braibant, M., L. Guilloteau, and M. S. Zygmunt. 2002. Functional characterization of *Brucella melitensis* NorMI, an efflux pump belonging to the multidrug and toxic compound extrusion family. *Antimicrob. Agents Chemother.* **46**:3050–3053.

15. Braibant, M., P. Lefèvre, L. de Wit, J. Ooms, P. Peirs, K. Huygen, R. Wattiez, and J. Content. 1996. Identification of a second *Mycobacterium tuberculosis* gene cluster encoding proteins of an ABC phosphate transporter. *FEBS Lett.* **394**:206–212.

16. Braibant, M., P. Lefèvre, L. De Wit, P. Peirs, J. Ooms, K. Huygen, A. B. Andersen, and J. Content. 1996. A *Mycobacterium tuberculosis* gene cluster encoding a phosphate transporter, homologous to the *Escherichia coli* Pst system. *Gene* **176**:171–176.

17. Brown, M. H., I. T. Paulsen, and R. A. Skurray. 1999. The multidrug efflux protein NorM is a prototype of a new family of transporters. *Mol. Microbiol.* **31**:394–395.

18. Burns, D. L. 2003. Type IV transporters of pathogenic bacteria. *Curr. Opin. Microbiol.* **6**:29–34.

19. Calder, K. M., and M. A. Horwitz. 1998. Identification of iron-regulated proteins of *Mycobacterium tuberculosis* and cloning of tandem genes encoding a low iron-induced protein and a metal transporting ATPase with similarities to two-component metal transport systems. *Microb. Pathog.* **24**:133–143.

20. Camacho, L. R., P. Constant, C. Raynaud, M. A. Laneelle, J. A. Triccas, B. Gicquel, M. Daffe, and C. Guilhot. 2001. Analysis of the phthiocerol dimycocerosate locus of *Mycobacterium tuberculosis*. Evidence that this lipid is involved in the cell wall permeability barrier. *J. Biol. Chem.* **276**:19845–19854.

21. Camacho, L. R., D. Ensergueix, E. Perez, B. Gicquel, and C. Guilhot. 1999. Identification of a virulence gene cluster of *Mycobacterium tuberculosis* by signature-tagged transposon mutagenesis. *Mol. Microbiol.* **34**:257–267.

22. Chang, G., and C. B. Roth. 2001. Structure of MsbA from

23. Chang, G., R. H. Spencer, A. T. Lee, M. T. Barclay, and D. C. Rees. 1998. Structure of the MscL homolog from *Mycobacterium tuberculosis*: a gated mechanosensitive ion channel. *Science* **282**:2220–2226.

24. Chang, Z., A. Choudhary, R. Lathigra, and F. A. Quiocho. 1994. The immunodominant 38–kDa lipoprotein of *M. tuberculosis* is a phosphate binding protein. *J. Biol. Chem.* **269**: 1956–1958.

25. Chen, C. J., D. Clark, K. Ueda, I. Pastan, M. M. Gottesman, and I. B. Roninson. 1990. Genomic organization of the human multidrug resistance (MDR1) gene and origin of P-glycoproteins. *J. Biol. Chem.* **265**:506–514.

26. Chen, J., Y. Morita, M. N. Huda, T. Kuroda, T. Mizushima, and T. Tsuchiya. 2002. VmrA, a member of a novel class of Na$^+$-coupled multidrug efflux pumps from *Vibrio parahaemolyticus*. *J. Bacteriol.* **184**:572–576.

27. Choudhary, A., M. N. Vyas, N. K. Vyas, Z. Y. Chang, and F. A. Quiocho. 1994. Crystallization and preliminary X-ray crystallographic analysis of the 38–kDa immunodominant antigen of *Mycobacterium tuberculosis*. *Protein Sci.* **3**:2450–2451.

28. Choudhuri, B. S., S. Bhakta, R. Barik, J. Basu, M. Kundu, and P. Chakrabarti. 2002. Overexpression and functional characterization of an ABC (ATP-binding cassette) transporter encoded by the genes *drrA* and *drrB* of *Mycobacterium tuberculosis*. *Biochem. J.* **367**:279–285.

29. Choudhuri, B. S., S. Sen, and P. Chakrabarti. 1999. Isoniazid accumulation in *Mycobacterium smegmatis* is modulated by proton motive force-driven and ATP-dependent extrusion systems. *Biochem. Biophys. Res. Commun.* **256**:682–684.

30. Claverys, J. P., B. Grossiord, and G. Alloing. 2000. Is the Ami-AliA/B oligopeptide permease of *Streptococcus pneumoniae* involved in sensing environmental conditions? *Res. Microbiol.* **151**:457–463.

31. Cole, S. T. 2002. Comparative and functional genomics of the *Mycobacterium tuberculosis* complex. *Microbiology* **148**:2919–2928.

32. Cole, S. T., R. Brosch, J. Parkhill, T. Garnier, C. Churcher, D. Harris, S. V. Gordon, K. Eiglmeier, S. Gas, C. E. Barry III, F. Tekaia, K. Badcock, D. Basham, D. Brown, T. Chillingworth, R. Conner, R. Davies, K. Devlin, T. Feltwell, S. Gentles, N. Hamlin, S. Holroyd, T. Hornsby, K. Jagels, A. Krogh, J. Mclean, S. Moule, L. Murphy, K. Oliver, J. Osborne, M. A. Quail, M.-A. Rajandream, J. Rogers, S. Rutter, K. Seeger, J. Skelton, R. Squares, S. Squares, J. E. Sulston, K. Taylor, S. Whitehead, and B. G. Barrell. 1998. Deciphering the biology of *Mycobacterium tuberculosis* from the complete genome sequence. *Nature* **396**:190–198.

33. Collins, D. M., R. P. Kawakami, B. M. Buddle, B. J. Wards, and G. W. de Lisle. 2003. Different susceptibility of two animal species infected with isogenic mutants of *Mycobacterium bovis* identifies *phoT* as having roles in tuberculosis virulence and phosphate transport. *Microbiology* **149**:3203–3212.

34. Converse, S. E., J. D. Mougous, M. D. Leavell, J. A. Leary, C. R. Bertozzi, and J. S. Cox. 2003. MmpL8 is required for sulfolipid-1 biosynthesis and *Mycobacterium tuberculosis* virulence. *Proc. Natl. Acad. Sci. USA* **100**:6121–6126.

35. Corti, S., J. Chevalier, and A. Cremieux. 1995. Intracellular accumulation of norfloxacin in *Mycobacterium smegmatis*. *Antimicrob. Agents Chemother.* **39**:2466–2471.

36. Coulter, S. N., W. R. Schwan, E. Y. Ng, M. H. Langhorne, H. D. Ritchie, S. Westbrock-Wadman, W. O. Hufnagle, K. R. Folger, A. S. Bayer, and C. K. Stover. 1998. *Staphylococcus*

aureus genetic loci impacting growth and survival in multiple infection environments. *Mol. Microbiol.* **30:**393–404.

37. **Cox, J. S., B. Chen, M. Mcneil, and W. R. Jacobs.** 1999. Complex lipid determine tissue specific replication of *Mycobacterium tuberculosis* in mice. *Nature* **402:**79–83.

38. **De Groote, M. A., D. Granger, Y. Xu, G. Campbell, R. Prince, and F. C. Fang.** 1995. Genetic and redox determinants of nitric oxide cytotoxicity in a *Salmonella typhimurium* model. *Proc. Natl. Acad. Sci. USA* **92:**6399–6403.

39. **De Rossi, E., P. Arrigo, M. Bellinzoni, P. A. Silva, C. Martín, J. A. Aínsa, P. Guglierame, and G. Riccardi.** 2002. The multidrug transporters belonging to major facilitator superfamily in *Mycobacterium tuberculosis*. *Mol. Med.* **8:**714–724.

40. **De Rossi, E., M. C. Blokpoel, R. Cantoni, M. Branzoni, G. Riccardi, D. B. Young, K. A. De Smet, and O. Ciferri.** 1998. Molecular cloning and functional analysis of a novel tetracycline resistance determinant, tet(V), from *Mycobacterium smegmatis*. *Antimicrob. Agents Chemother.* **42:**1931–1937.

41. **De Rossi, E., M. Branzoni, R. Cantoni, A. Milano, G. Riccardi, and O. Ciferri.** 1998. *mmr*, a *Mycobacterium tuberculosis* gene conferring resistance to small cationic dyes and inhibitors. *J. Bacteriol.* **180:**6068–6071.

42. **Domenech, P., A. S. Pym, M. Cellier, C. E. Barry, and S. T. Cole.** 2002. Inactivation of the *Mycobacterium tuberculosis* Nramp orthologue (MntH) does not affect virulence in a mouse model of tuberculosis. *FEMS Microbiol. Lett.* **207:**81–86.

43. **Doran, J. L., Y. Pang, K. E. Mdluli, A. J. Moran, T. C. Victor, R. W. Stokes, E. Mahenthiralingam, B. N. Kreiswirth, J. L. Butt, G. S. Baron, J. D. Treit, V. J. Kerr, P. D. Van Helden, M. C. Roberts, and F. E. Nano.** 1997. *Mycobacterium tuberculosis efpA* encodes an efflux protein of the QacA transporter family. *Clin. Diagn. Lab. Immunol.* **4:**23–32.

44. **Elmore, D. E., and D. A. Dougherty.** 2001. Molecular dynamics simulations of wild-type and mutant forms of the *Mycobacterium tuberculosis* MscL channel. *Biophys. J.* **81:**1345–1359.

45. **Fetherston, J. D., V. J. Bertolino, and R. D. Perry.** 1999. YbtP and YbtQ: two ABC transporters required for iron uptake in *Yersinia pestis*. *Mol. Microbiol.* **32:**289–299.

46. **Garnier, T., K. Eiglmeier, J. C. Camus, N. Medina, H. Mansoor, M. Pryor, S. Duthoy, S. Grondin, C. Lacroix, C. Monsempe, S. Simon, B. Harris, R. Atkin, J. Doggett, R. Mayes, L. Keating, P. R. Wheeler, J. Parkhill, B. G. Barrell, S. T. Cole, S. V. Gordon, and R. G. Hewinson.** 2003. The complete genome sequence of *Mycobacterium bovis*. *Proc. Natl. Acad. Sci. USA* **100:**7877–7882.

47. **Gokulan, K., B. Rupp, M. S. Pavelka, Jr., W. R. Jacobs, Jr., and J. C. Sacchettini.** 2003. Crystal structure of *Mycobacterium tuberculosis* diaminopimelate decarboxylase, an essential enzyme in bacterial lysine biosynthesis. *J. Biol. Chem.* **278:**18588–18596.

48. **Gottesman, M. M., C. A. Hrycyna, P. V. Schoenlein, U. A. Germann, and I. Pastan.** 1995. Genetic analysis of the multidrug transporter. *Annu. Rev. Genet.* **29:**607–649.

49. **Green, R. M., A. Seth, and N. D. Connell.** 2000. A peptide permease mutant of *Mycobacterium bovis* BCG resistant to the toxic peptides glutathione and S-nitrosoglutathione. *Infect. Immun.* **68:**429–436.

50. **Grkovic, S., M. H. Brown, and R. A. Skurray.** 2002. Regulation of bacterial drug export systems. *Microbiol. Mol. Biol. Rev.* **66:**671–701.

51. **Guillemin, I., W. Sougakoff, E. Cambau, V. Revel-Viravau, N. Moreau, and V. Jarlier.** 1999. Purification and inhibition by quinolones of DNA gyrases from *Mycobacterium avium*, *Mycobacterium smegmatis* and *Mycobacterium fortuitum bv. peregrinum*. *Microbiology* **145:**2527–2532.

52. **Kamijo, K., T. Kamijo, I. Ueno, T. Osumi, and T. Hashimoto.** 1992. Nucleotide sequence of the human 70 kDa peroxisomal membrane protein: a member of ATP-binding cassette transporters. *Biochim. Biophys. Acta* **1129:**323–327.

53. **Klarsfeld, A. D., P. L. Goossens, and P. Cossart.** 1994. Five *Listeria monocytogenes* genes preferentially expressed in infected mammalian cells: *plcA, purH, purD, pyrE* and an arginine ABC transporter gene, *arpJ. Mol. Microbiol.* **13:**585–597.

54. **Klose, K. E., and J. J. Mekalanos.** 1997. Simultaneous prevention of glutamine synthesis and high-affinity transport attenuates *Salmonella typhimurium* virulence. *Infect. Immun.* **65:**587–596.

55. **Kocagoz, T., C. J. Hackbarth, I. Unsal, E. Y. Rosenberg, H. Nikaido, and H. F. Chambers.** 1996. Gyrase mutations in laboratory-selected, fluoroquinolone-resistant mutants of *Mycobacterium tuberculosis* H37Ra. *Antimicrob. Agents Chemother.* **40:**1768–1774.

56. **Kochendoerfer, G. G., J. M. Tack, and S. Cressman.** 2002. Total chemical synthesis of a 27 kDa TASP protein derived from the MscL ion channel of *M. tuberculosis* by ketoxime-forming ligation. *Bioconj. Chem.* **13:**474–480.

57. **Kriakov, J., S. Lee, and W. R. Jacobs, Jr.** 2003. Identification of a regulated alkaline phosphatase, a cell surface-associated lipoprotein, in *Mycobacterium smegmatis. J. Bacteriol.* **185:**4983–4991.

58. **Lefèvre, P., M. Braibant, L. De Wit, M. Kalai, D. Röeper, J. Grötzinger, J.-P. Delville, P. Peirs, J. Ooms, K. Huygen, and J. Content.** 1997. Three different putative phosphate transport receptors are encoded by the *Mycobacterium tuberculosis* genome and are present at the surface of *Mycobacterium bovis* BCG. *J. Bacteriol.* **179:**2900–2906.

59. **Liu, J., H. E. Takiff, and H. Nikaido.** 1996. Active efflux of fluoroquinolones in *Mycobacterium smegmatis* mediated by LfrA, a multidrug efflux pump. *J. Bacteriol.* **178:**3791–3795.

60. **Matthysse, A. G., H. A. Yarnall, and N. Young.** 1996. Requirement for genes with homology to ABC transport systems for attachment and virulence of *Agrobacterium tumefaciens. J. Bacteriol.* **178:**5302–5308.

61. **Maurer, J. A., D. E. Elmore, H. A. Lester, and D. A. Dougherty.** 2000. Comparing and contrasting *Escherichia coli* and *Mycobacterium tuberculosis* mechanosensitive channels (MscL). New gain of function mutations in the loop region. *J. Biol. Chem.* **275:**22238–22244.

62. **McAdam, R. A., T. R. Weisbrod, J. Martin, J. D. Scuderi, A. M. Brown, J. D. Cirillo, B. R. Bloom, and W. R. Jacobs.** 1995. In vivo growth characteristics of leucine and methionine auxotrophic mutants of *Mycobacterium bovis* BCG generated by transposon mutagenesis. *Infect. Immun.* **63:**1004–1012.

63. **McDermott, P. F., D. G. White, I. Podglajen, M. N. Alekshun, and S. B. Levy.** 1998. Multidrug resistance following expression of the *Escherichia coli marA* gene in *Mycobacterium smegmatis. J. Bacteriol.* **180:**2995–2998.

64. **Meyer, A.** 2003. Molecular evolution: duplication, duplication. *Nature* **421:**31–32.

65. **Miyamae, S., O. Ueda, F. Yoshimura, J. Hwang, Y. Tanaka, and H. Nikaido.** 2001. A MATE family multidrug efflux transporter pumps out fluoroquinolones in *Bacteroides thetaiotaomicron. Antimicrob. Agents Chemother.* **45:**3341–3346.

66. **Moe, P. C., G. Levin, and P. Blount.** 2000. Correlating a protein structure with function of a bacterial mechanosensitive channel. *J. Biol. Chem.* **275:**31121–31127.

67. Morita, Y., A. Kataoka, S. Shiota, T. Mizushima, and T. Tsuchiya. 2000. NorM of *Vibrio parahaemolyticus* is an Na[+]-driven multidrug efflux pump. *J. Bacteriol.* **182:**6694–6697.

68. Morita, Y., K. Kodama, S. Shiota, T. Mine, A. Kataoka, T. Mizushima, and T. Tsuchiya. 1998. NorM, a putative multidrug efflux protein, of *Vibrio parahaemolyticus* and its homolog in *Escherichia coli. Antimicrob. Agents Chemother.* **42:**1778–1782.

69. Murugasu-Oei, B., A. Tay, and T. Dick. 1999. Upregulation of stress response genes and ABC transporters in anaerobic stationary-phase *Mycobacterium smegmatis. Mol. Gen. Genet.* **262:**677–682.

70. Ninio, S., D. Rotem, and S. Schuldiner. 2001. Functional analysis of novel multidrug transporters from human pathogens. *J. Biol. Chem.* **276:**48250–48256.

71. Paulsen, I. T., and K. Lewis (ed.). 2002. *Microbial Multidrug Efflux.* Horizon Scientific Press, Norwich, United Kingdom.

72. Pavelka, M. S., and W. R. Jacobs. 1999. Comparison of the construction of unmarked deletion mutations in *Mycobacterium smegmatis, Mycobacterium bovis* bacillus Calmette-Guérin, and *Mycobacterium tuberculosis* H37Rv by allelic exchange. *J. Bacteriol.* **181:**4780–4789.

73. Pearson, W. R. 1996. Effective protein sequence comparison. *Methods Enzymol.* **266:**227–258.

74. Piddock, L. J., and V. Ricci. 2001. Accumulation of five fluoroquinolones by *Mycobacterium tuberculosis* H37Rv. *J. Antimicrob. Chemother.* **48:**787–791.

75. Piddock, L. J., K. J. Williams, and V. Ricci. 2000. Accumulation of rifampicin by *Mycobacterium aurum, Mycobacterium smegmatis* and *Mycobacterium tuberculosis. J. Antimicrob. Chemother.* **45:**159–165.

76. Pivetti, C. D., M. R. Yen, S. Miller, W. Busch, Y. H. Tseng, I. R. Booth, and M. H. Saier, Jr. 2003. Two families of mechanosensitive channel proteins. *Microbiol. Mol. Biol. Rev.* **67:**66–85.

77. Podbielski, A., and B. A. Leonard. 1998. The group A streptococcal dipeptide permease (Dpp) is involved in the uptake of essential amino acids and affects the expression of cysteine protease. *Mol. Microbiol.* **28:**1323–1334.

78. Poole, K. 2000. Efflux-mediated resistance to fluoroquinolones in gram-positive bacteria and the mycobacteria. *Antimicrob. Agents Chemother.* **44:**2595–2599.

79. Poole, R. K., F. Gibson, and G. Wu. 1994. The *cydD* gene product, component of a heterodimeric ABC transporter, is required for assembly of periplasmic cytochrome *c* and of cytochrome *bd* in *Escherichia coli. FEMS Microbiol. Lett.* **117:**217–223.

80. Poole, R. K., L. Hatch, M. W. Cleeter, F. Gibson, G. B. Cox, and G. Wu. 1993. Cytochrome *bd* biosynthesis in *Escherichia coli*: the sequences of the *cydC* and *cydD* genes suggest that they encode the components of an ABC membrane transporter. *Mol. Microbiol.* **10:**421–430.

81. Raynaud, C., M. A. Laneelle, R. H. Senaratne, P. Draper, G. Laneelle, and M. Daffe. 1999. Mechanisms of pyrazinamide resistance in mycobacteria: importance of lack of uptake in addition to lack of pyrazinamidase activity. *Microbiology* **145:**1359–1367.

82. Rodriguez, G. M., M. I. Voskuil, B. Gold, G. K. Schoolnik, and I. Smith. 2002. ideR, an essential gene in *Mycobacterium tuberculosis*: role of IdeR in iron-dependent gene expression, iron metabolism, and oxidative stress response. *Infect. Immun.* **70:**3371–3381.

83. Saier, M. H., Jr. 2000. A functional-phylogenetic classification system for transmembrane solute transporters. *Microbiol. Mol. Biol. Rev.* **64:**354–411.

84. Sakamoto, K., A. Margolles, H. W. van Veen, and W. N. Konings. 2001. Hop resistance in the beer spoilage bacterium *Lactobacillus brevis* is mediated by the ATP-binding cassette multidrug transporter HorA. *J. Bacteriol.* **183:**5371–5375.

85. Sander, P., and E. C. Bottger. 1999. Mycobacteria: genetics of resistance and implications for treatment. *Chemotherapy* **45:**95–108.

86. Sander, P., E. De Rossi, B. Boddinghaus, R. Cantoni, M. Branzoni, E. C. Bottger, H. Takiff, R. Rodriquez, G. Lopez, and G. Riccardi. 2000. Contribution of the multidrug efflux pump LfrA to innate mycobacterial drug resistance. *FEMS Microbiol. Lett.* **193:**19–23.

87. Sarin, J., S. Aggarwal, R. Chaba, G. C. Varshney, and P. K. Chakraborti. 2001. B-subunit of phosphate-specific transporter from *Mycobacterium tuberculosis* is a thermostable ATPase. *J. Biol. Chem.* **276:**44590–44597.

88. Schaller, A., Z. Sun, Y. Yang, A. Somoskovi, and Y. Zhang. 2002. Salicylate reduces susceptibility of *Mycobacterium tuberculosis* to multiple antituberculosis drugs. *Antimicrob. Agents Chemother.* **46:**2636–2639.

89. Seth, A., and N. D. Connell. 2000. Amino acid transport and metabolism in mycobacteria: cloning, interruption, and characterization of an L-arginine/gamma-aminobutyric acid permease in *Mycobacterium bovis* BCG. *J. Bacteriol.* **182:** 919–927.

90. Silva, P. E., F. Bigi, M. de la Paz Santangelo, M. I. Romano, C. Martin, A. Cataldi, and J. A. Ainsa. 2001. Characterization of P55, a multidrug efflux pump in *Mycobacterium bovis* and *Mycobacterium tuberculosis. Antimicrob. Agents Chemother.* **45:**800–804.

91. Skamene, E., E. Schurr, and P. Gros. 1998. Infection genomics: Nramp1 as a major determinant of natural resistance to intracellular infections. *Annu. Rev. Med.* **49:**275–287.

92. Steyn, A. J., J. Joseph, and B. R. Bloom. 2003. Interaction of the sensor module of *Mycobacterium tuberculosis* H37Rv KdpD with members of the Lpr family. *Mol. Microbiol.* **47:**1075–1089.

93. Takiff, H. E., M. Cimino, M. C. Musso, T. Weisbrod, R. Martinez, M. B. Delgado, L. Salazar, B. R. Bloom, and W. R. Jacobs. 1996. Efflux pump of the proton antiporter family confers low-level fluoroquinolone resistance in *Mycobacterium smegmatis. Proc. Natl. Acad. Sci. USA* **93:**362–366.

94. Telenti, A., W. J. Philipp, S. Sreevatsan, C. Bernasconi, K. E. Stockbauer, B. Wieles, J. M. Musser, and W. R. Jacobs, Jr. 1997. The *emb* operon, a gene cluster of *Mycobacterium tuberculosis* involved in resistance to ethambutol. *Nat. Med.* **3:**567–570.

95. Torres, A., M. D. Juarez, R. Cervantes, and C. Espitia. 2001. Molecular analysis of *Mycobacterium tuberculosis* phosphate specific transport system in *Mycobacterium smegmatis*. Characterization of recombinant 38 kDa (PstS-1). *Microb. Pathog.* **30:**289–297.

96. Tyagi, J. S., T. K. Das, and A. K. Kinger. 1996. An *M. tuberculosis* DNA fragment contains genes encoding cell division proteins FtsX and FtsE, a basic protein and homologues of PemK and small protein B. *Gene* **177:**59–67.

97. Ukai, H., H. Matsuzawa, K. Ito, M. Yamada, and A. Nishimura. 1998. *ftsE*(Ts) affects translocation of K[+]-pump proteins into the cytoplasmic membrane of *Escherichia coli. J. Bacteriol.* **180:**3663–3670.

98. Van der Bliek, A. M., F. Baas, T. Ten Houte de Lange, P. M. Kooiman, T. Van der Velde-Koerts, and P. Borst. 1987. The human *mdr3* gene encodes a novel P-glycoprotein homologue and gives rise to alternatively spliced mRNAs in liver. *EMBO J.* **6:**3325–3331.

99. van Veen, H. W., K. Venema, H. Bolhuis, I. Oussenko, J. Kok, B. Poolman, A. J. Driessen, and W. N. Konings. 1996. Multidrug resistance mediated by a bacterial homolog of the human multidrug transporter MDR1. *Proc. Natl. Acad. Sci. USA* 93:10668–10672.

100. Venketaraman, V., Y. K. Dayaram, A. G. Amin, R. Ngo, R. M. Green, M. T. Talaue, J. Mann, and N. D. Connell. 2003. Role of glutathione in macrophage control of mycobacteria. *Infect. Immun.* 71:1864–1871.

101. Viveiros, M., C. Leandro, and L. Amaral. 2003. Mycobacterial efflux pumps and chemotherapeutic implications. *Int. J. Antimicrob. Agents* 22:274–278.

102. Viveiros, M., I. Portugal, R. Bettencourt, T. C. Victor, A. M. Jordaan, C. Leandro, D. Ordway, and L. Amaral. 2002. Isoniazid-induced transient high-level resistance in *Mycobacterium tuberculosis*. *Antimicrob. Agents Chemother.* 46:2804–2810.

103. Vyas, N. K., M. N. Vyas, and F. A. Quiocho. 2003. Crystal structure of *M. tuberculosis* ABC phosphate transport receptor: specificity and charge compensation dominated by ion-dipole interactions. *Structure* 11:765–774.

104. Williams, K. J., G. A. Chung, and L. J. Piddock. 1998. Accumulation of norfloxacin by *Mycobacterium aurum* and *Mycobacterium smegmatis*. *Antimicrob. Agents Chemother.* 42:795–800.

105. Wilson, M., J. De Risi, H. H. Kristensen, P. Imboden, S. Rane, P. O. Brown, and G. K. Schoolnik. 1999. Exploring drug-induced alterations in gene expression in *Mycobacterium tuberculosis* by microarray hybridization. *Proc. Natl. Acad. Sci. USA* 96:12833–12838.

106. Winstedt, L., K. Yoshida, Y. Fujita, and C. von Wachenfeldt. 1998. Cytochrome *bd* biosynthesis in *Bacillus subtilis*: characterization of the *cydABCD* operon. *J. Bacteriol.* 180:6571–6580.

107. Wooff, E., S. L. Michell, S. V. Gordon, M. A. Chambers, S. Bardarov, W. R. Jacobs, R. G. Hewinson, and P. R. Wheeler. 2002. Functional genomics reveals the sole sulphate transporter of the *Mycobacterium tuberculosis* complex and its relevance to the acquisition of sulphur in vivo. *Mol. Microbiol.* 43:653–663.

108. Yakushi, T., K. Masuda, S. Narita, S. Matsuyama, and H. Tokuda. 2000. A new ABC transporter mediating the detachment of lipid-modified proteins from membranes. *Nat. Cell Biol.* 2:212–218.

109. Zhang, Y., A. Scorpio, H. Nikaido, and Z. Sun. 1999. Role of acid pH and deficient efflux of pyrazinoic acid in unique susceptibility of *Mycobacterium tuberculosis* to pyrazinamide. *J. Bacteriol.* 181:2044–2049.

110. Zhou, Z., K. A. White, A. Polissi, C. Georgopoulos, and C. R. Raetz. 1998. Function of *Escherichia coli* MsbA, an essential ABC family transporter, in lipid A and phospholipid biosynthesis. *J. Biol. Chem.* 273:12466–12475.

HOST-PATHOGEN INTERACTIONS

IX. PHAGOCYTIC UPTAKE AND INTRACELLULAR SURVIVAL

Chapter 25

Receptor-Mediated Recognition of *Mycobacterium tuberculosis* by Host Cells

MATTHEW J. FENTON, LEE W. RILEY, AND LARRY S. SCHLESINGER

Mycobacterium tuberculosis is an intracellular pathogen of mononuclear phagocytes and is highly adapted to the human host. It has developed multiple strategies to circumvent the normal fate of phagocytosed organisms. During primary lung infection of the human host, *M. tuberculosis* enters and survives in alveolar macrophages (AMs), cells with several unique attributes. While in the alveoli, *M. tuberculosis* bacteria also interact with lung epithelial cells that contribute to the host inflammatory response. Subsequently, bacilli disseminate from the lung and are phagocytosed by a heterogeneous group of tissue macrophages and dendritic cells (DC). This chapter reviews advances in our understanding of the molecular determinants that mediate the interaction of *M. tuberculosis* with host cells such as monocytes/macrophages, epithelial cells, and DC. In this context, it also reviews a family of important regulators of innate immune cell activation, the toll-like receptor (TLR) family.

ENTRY OF *M. TUBERCULOSIS* INTO MONONUCLEAR PHAGOCYTES

M. tuberculosis enters mononuclear phagocytes by receptor-mediated phagocytosis (178), in which several major host cell receptors play a role. These include complement receptors (CRs), the mannose receptor (MR), and type A scavenger receptors (89, 176, 178, 202, 228). The CRs involved are CR1 (CD35) and the leukocyte integrins CR3 (CD11b/CD18) and CR4 (CD11c/CD18) (82). The expression of CRs (particularly CR4) and the MR increases during monocyte differentiation into macrophages, with CR4 and the MR being highly expressed on AMs (139, 197). Fcγ receptors do not play a role in the phagocytosis of *M. tuberculosis* in the absence of specific antibody (178), an important finding for the bacterium since entry via this receptor would be expected to generate a vigorous host response.

M. tuberculosis and Complement Protein C3

Complement activation is important to tuberculosis TB pathogenesis, since the bacteria encounter complement proteins in the alveoli of the lungs (203), during hematogenous dissemination, and in various tissues (126). In these sites, macrophages can secrete complement proteins capable of opsonizing phagocytic particles. The phagocytosis of *M. tuberculosis* by mononuclear phagocytes is enhanced in serum as a result of complement activation that leads to opsonization of bacteria with the C3 activation products C3b and C3bi (177). *M. tuberculosis* cell wall components were shown in early studies to mediate the activation of complement (164, 174). The C3 acceptor molecules on the surface of *M. tuberculosis* are beginning to be defined. The *M. tuberculosis* heparin-binding hemagglutinin (HbhA) is one such potential acceptor (137).

Several mechanisms exist for mediating the opsonization of pathogenic mycobacteria with C3 products, raising the possibility that C3 opsonization varies in form and amount between different tissue sites and during different stages of infection (for example, during primary tuberculosis [TB] infection versus reactivation disease). Apart from issues related to complement protein availability, strain-dependent differences in the composition of *M. tuberculosis* outer "capsular" polysaccharides have been shown to affect C3 deposition to some extent (46). Differences in C3 opsonization would affect the relative involvement of different CRs during entry and might influence the fate of the bacterium.

Matthew J. Fenton • Departments of Medicine, Microbiology, and Immunology, University of Maryland School of Medicine, Baltimore, MD 21201. **Lee W. Riley** • School of Public Health, Division of Infectious Diseases, University of California Berkeley, Berkeley, CA 94720. **Larry S. Schlesinger** • Departments of Medicine and Molecular Virology, Immunology, and Medical Genetics, The Ohio State University, Columbus, Ohio 43210.

Complement activation and C3 deposition on *M. tuberculosis* occur via the alternative complement pathway in high concentrations of nonimmune human serum (178). Mannose-binding lectin (MBL) and its associated serine proteases can activate both classical and alternative complement pathways (reviewed in reference 124). MBL binds to the surface of mycobacteria (93, 161) and may thus mediate the activation of complement, resulting in C3 opsonization of bacteria. Finally, there is evidence that complement protein 2a in serum can cleave C3 independently of the classical complement components C1 and C4b, leading to C3 product deposition on pathogenic mycobacteria, a pathway postulated to be important in tissue sites of infection (184).

In vitro studies have established that human pulmonary cells have the capacity to produce components of the complement cascade. Complement components such as factor B, C2, C4, C3, and C5 are produced by alveolar type II cells, and C2 and factor B are produced by AMs (40, 203). In addition, human C3 gene expression can be induced in the A549 cell line by glucocorticoids (226). Thus, C3 present in the airway could serve as an opsonin for *M. tuberculosis* phagocytosis by AMs even in the absence of an induced inflammatory response.

Complement Receptors

CR3 is the major integrin of phagocytic cells (mononuclear phagocytes and neutrophils) and is also expressed on natural killer (NK) cells and a small set of lymphocytes. In addition to phagocytosis, CR3 mediates stable adhesion of leukocytes to endothelium and the subsequent migration into inflamed organs. These functions are mediated through the binding of several physiological ligands including C3bi (82, 170, 216). The important but less well studied CR4 binds C3bi and serves as a receptor for LPS (23, 96, 115).

CRs play a major role in the phagocytosis of *M. tuberculosis* by human monocytes and macrophages. CR1 and CR3 on human monocytes mediate phagocytosis of the virulent Erdman strain of *M. tuberculosis* (178). Combinations of two monoclonal antibodies against distinct epitopes on the α chain of CR3 reduce the phagocytosis of *M. tuberculosis* by 80%. Monoclonal antibodies against the C3bi-binding epitope of CR3, as well as those against other ligand-binding epitopes, inhibit phagocytosis. Therefore, it is possible that more than one epitope is important in binding *M. tuberculosis* (see below).

The phagocytosis by human monocyte-derived macrophages (MDMs) of two virulent *M. tuberculosis* strains, Erdman and H37Rv, and the attenuated

strain, H37Ra, is enhanced in fresh nonimmune serum relative to that in the absence of serum. Ingestion of these strains occurs in both the presence and absence of serum, and the bacteria are found within phagosomes (176). A combination of monoclonal antibodies against CR1, CR3, and CR4 on MDMs inhibits the phagocytosis of all three strains by nearly 80% in the presence of serum. Although studies using MDMs provide detailed information that is applicable to human AMs, direct examination of AMs provides additional insights. Phagocytosis of *M. tuberculosis* by human AMs is greater than that by monocytes, and CR4 plays a particularly important role (89).

There is evidence for the direct interaction between *M. tuberculosis* surface components and CR3 during phagocytosis based on in vitro studies using human and murine macrophages as well as CR3-transfected Chinese hamster ovary (CHO) cell lines (45, 46, 176, 202). Monoclonal antibodies against CRs significantly inhibit the phagocytosis of bacteria by human macrophages in the absence of serum (176). The binding site for *M. tuberculosis* on CR3 of murine macrophages in the absence of serum was found to be distinct from the C3bi-binding site as determined by monoclonal antibody-blocking experiments (202). Both elicited and activated murine macrophages bound mycobacteria poorly despite expressing CR3. Thus, binding of *M. tuberculosis* did not correlate with expression of CR3, a finding hypothesized by the investigators to be related to the functional state of the binding site on CR3. *M. tuberculosis* binds in nonopsonic fashion to CR3 expressed on CHO cells (45), an interaction mediated by bacterial polysaccharides (46). Binding sites on CR3 for the bacterium (I domain, which recognizes C3bi versus lectin sites) are predicted to affect the cellular response (i.e., ligation of lectin sites leads to cellular activation such as the generation of an oxidative burst [212]) (also see below). In this respect, the host cell response to mycobacterial adherence may also be influenced by the relative involvement of other macrophage receptors, such as the MR, or other CR3-associated receptors, such as CD14 (156).

A recent in vivo study using CR3-deficient mice did not show a difference in bacterial burden or pathology between these animals and their controls (95). However, in that study, intravenous inoculation of bacteria was used rather than the aerosol route, the natural route of infection. Since compartmentalization of the immune response is well established and the lung is unique in this respect, the relative role of the C3-CR3 pathway in TB pathogenesis remains unresolved.

Mannose Receptor

The macrophage MR is a prototypic pattern recognition receptor that binds with high affinity to mannose- and fucose-containing glycoconjugates that are frequently found on the surface of a variety of microbes and are referred to as pathogen-associated molecular patterns (reviewed in reference 130). The MR is a member of a family of C-type lectins that is expressed on MDMs, tissues macrophages, and DC but not monocytes (197–199). AMs demonstrate high MR activity (220). The MR can serve as a molecular link between the innate and adaptive immune responses (199). For example, the MR mediates loading of mycobacterial lipoarabinomannan (LAM) onto CD1 molecules for LAM presentation to T cells (162).

In contrast to CRs, the macrophage MR mediates phagocytosis of the virulent *M. tuberculosis* strains Erdman and H37Rv but not the attenuated H37Ra strain (176, 181). The MR also mediates uptake of other mycobacteria (10). The linear α1-2-linked oligomannosyl "caps" of *M. tuberculosis* cell wall LAM (ManLAM) serve as ligands for the MR during bacterial phagocytosis (100, 181, 182). Subtle differences exist in the ability of LAM from different *M. tuberculosis* strains to bind to the MR, and the inositol phosphate-capped AraLAM from *M. smegmatis* does not bind to this receptor (181). The linear array of the terminal mannosyl units of Erdman LAM may be important in enhancing the affinity of this ligand for the MR by clustering several carbohydrate recognition domains, as described for other glycoconjugates (207). There is not a direct correlation between terminal mannosylation of LAM and virulence. Mycobacteria that vary in virulence in animal models, including *M. tuberculosis* H37Rv, the attenuated H37Ra strain, and *M. bovis* BCG, all contain LAM types with mannosyl caps, although the interior structure of these lipoglycans may differ (104, 163, 218). The ability of these LAM types to interact with the MR also varies (182). Thus, it appears that the precise array, length, and number of caps may be important in determining the interaction with the host cell. The mannose caps of ManLAM have also recently been shown to be recognized by DC-SIGN on DC, a lectin that functions as a bacterial adhesion and pattern recognition receptor (118, 205). Other *M. tuberculosis* surface molecules accessible to the MR are arabinomannans, mannans, and mannoproteins (50, 151). In addition to the LAM-MR interaction, *M. tuberculosis* strains possess their own lectins, some of which are specific for mannans and may be involved in bacterial binding to host cells (80).

The high MR activity on AMs is noteworthy for TB pathogenesis. MR activity is increased by interleukin-4 (IL-4), IL-13, and glucocorticoids and inhibited by gamma interferon (IFN-γ). It has been postulated that induction by these mediators, as well as by transforming growth factor β (TGF-β), produces an alternative activation state of macrophages with many attributes characteristic of AMs (reviewed in reference 78). The phenotypic and molecular characteristics of these macrophages differ considerably from those of classically activated macrophages. For example, alternatively activated macrophages express high levels of pattern recognition receptors, such as the MR and scavenger receptors, but do not display enhanced killing functions toward microbes (13, 138, 201). In this regard, the abundant surfactant-associated protein, surfactant protein A (SP-A), produced in the lungs interacts with macrophages to enhance MR activity (14). Furthermore, nitric oxide (NO) and oxidant production in response to stimuli is reduced in these cells (57, 149). Thus, AMs seem best adapted for removal of small airborne particulates with minimal induction of inflammatory immune responses. While such a cell is suitable for the normal homeostatic needs of the lungs, it might also be an ideal cell for an intracellular pathogen such as *M. tuberculosis*.

There is recent evidence for potential involvement of the MR in mycobacterial infection in humans. A major locus for human susceptibility to *M. leprae* infection has been mapped to chromosome 10p13 (193), the locus of the MR gene (55), and there is a recent report that newly identified variants of the MR are associated with susceptibility to both leprosy and TB (A. V. S. Hill, personal communication).

Other Receptors and Ligands for *M. tuberculosis* Phagocytosis

Although CRs and the MR are the major receptors that mediate phagocytosis on mononuclear phagocytes, it remains possible that other receptors also participate in *M. tuberculosis* phagocytosis, either alone or in conjunction with CRs and/or the MR. CD14 mediates the uptake of nonopsonized *M. tuberculosis* by human microglia, the resident macrophages in the brain (156), and the uptake of *M. bovis* by porcine AMs (103), but not the entry of *M. tuberculosis* into human macrophages (188). Class A scavenger receptors participate in the uptake of nonopsonized *M. tuberculosis* by MDMs (228). Potential *M. tuberculosis* ligands involved in interactions with mononuclear phagocytes and nonprofessional phagocytes include a mammalian cell entry protein (9), a heparin-binding hemagglutinin (133), glucan (46, 54, 186), PE_PGRS proteins (26), phosphatidylinositol mannoside (93), and antigen 85, which is reported to bind to CR3 (88).

Thus, *M. tuberculosis*, a highly host-adapted intracellular pathogen, has evolved to utilize different major host cell receptors to mediate its entry into professional phagocytes. This strategy affords the bacterium greater flexibility for entry, since phagocytes differ in their expression and/or function of these receptors depending on the tissue site, the degree of cell differentiation, and the presence of inflammatory mediators. The involvement of multiple receptor classes in phagocytosis raises the possibility that receptors cooperate to modulate host cell signaling pathways that mediate early host cell responses (see below).

HOST MOLECULES THAT REGULATE PHAGOCYTOSIS OF *M. TUBERCULOSIS*

Regulation of *M. tuberculosis* phagocytosis occurs by several host proteins that vary in their presence and amount in different tissue sites. SP-A, SP-D, MBL, and complement C1q are members of the collectin family of proteins involved in the innate immune response. SP-A enhances the phagocytosis of *M. tuberculosis* through opsonin and nonopsonin mechanisms (53, 73, 154), whereas SP-D reduces the phagocytosis of pathogenic strains of *M. tuberculosis* by binding to LAM on the bacterial surface, thereby inhibiting bacterial interactions with the MR (59, 60). SP-A also enhances CR1 function (210). Differences in the relative concentrations of SP-A and SP-D between individuals, as well as known genetic polymorphisms, raise the possibility that these proteins may play a role in dictating the relative host susceptibility to infection (67). SP-A may be particularly important in influencing *M. tuberculosis* phagocytosis (as well as phagocytosis of other pathogens) in disease states such as alveolar proteinosis or human immunodeficiency virus infection, where SP-A levels are increased (158, 168). There are also genetic polymorphisms of MBL that account for significant variability in its concentration in serum in different populations (113). Elevated concentrations of MBL in the serum of TB patients have been reported, and the associated genetic polymorphisms have been found to correlate with susceptibility to mycobacterial infections (71, 187).

Other host molecules that potentially regulate *M. tuberculosis* phagocytosis include fibronectin through direct and indirect mechanisms (2, 165) and IFN-γ. IFN-γ activation of phagocytes down regulates the expression and/or function of CRs and the MR (135, 223) decreases the adherence of mycobacteria (179, 213). In one study, IFN-γ activation of

macrophages decreased *M. tuberculosis* adherence but led to enhanced intracellular multiplication (52). Inasmuch as several cytokines and inflammatory mediators, such as prostaglandins, influence the surface expression of phagocyte receptors and receptor-mediated phagocytosis, it is likely that these mediators are important in regulating the level of phagocytosis of *M. tuberculosis* and the early host cell response during different stages of disease. In this regard, IL-4 and prostaglandin E_2, two mediators that modulate the host response to mycobacterial infection (reviewed in reference 12), markedly up regulate CR and/or MR expression and function and down regulate phagocyte effector functions (3, 185, 201). Treatment of human monocytes with TGF-β1 is reported to decrease the phagocytosis of H37Ra *M. tuberculosis* but enhance its intracellular growth (90).

Natural antibody to several species of mycobacteria has been found in healthy purified protein derivative-negative persons (11). Natural antibody could play a role in disease pathogenesis for mycobacteria by enhancing C3 deposition onto the bacillus and hence causing greater phagocytosis by mononuclear phagocytes (180). Later in infection with *M. tuberculosis* or during active disease, lysis of bacterially laden macrophages leads to the phagocytosis of *M. tuberculosis* by neighboring macrophages in the presence of high-titer immune antibody. The role of specific antibody in TB pathogenesis and potentially in immune protection is not clear and is probably highly dependent on the nature of the antibody produced. High-titer rabbit antimycobacterial immunoglobulin facilitates the multiplication of BCG in the spleens of mice (68). In an early in vitro study, rabbit antimycobacterial immunoglobulin had no effect on the phagocytosis of *M. tuberculosis* H37Rv by mouse peritoneal macrophages but enhanced phagosome-lysosome (P-L) fusion (8). In a more recent study, an antibody specific for arabinomannan conferred partial protection on mice after a respiratory challenge with *M. tuberculosis* by enhancing the cellular immune response (208). The role of human immune antibody in influencing receptor-mediated phagocytosis and intracellular survival of *M. tuberculosis* by human cells has not been defined. Of interest, the prevention of disseminated forms of TB in childhood has been found to correlate with the production of antibody to LAM (49).

HOST CELL RESPONSES TO PHAGOCYTOSIS OF *M. TUBERCULOSIS*

The mechanisms underlying phagocytosis are complex, culminating in rearrangement of the actin cytoskeleton to engulf the microbe and generation of a variety of biochemical signals (4). There are substantial differences in cellular responses for almost every phagocytic receptor used, and complex interactions between receptors can be expected since a variety of ligands usually coat the microbes. The phagocytic process for *M. tuberculosis* is no exception. Recent literature provides support for the notion that the nature of the receptor-ligand interactions for *M. tuberculosis* can regulate the early host cell response and the fate of the bacterium.

Phagocytosis of many pathogens by professional phagocytes is accompanied by rapid generation of the respiratory burst and P-L fusion (19, 160). For *M. tuberculosis*, the extent of P-L fusion and the microbial determinants involved in this process, during and immediately following phagocytosis, are not well characterized. These early events may be particularly important in the outcome of the primary infection in the lungs, in which the number of bacteria encountering the phagocyte is thought to be very small. These events may depend more on *M. tuberculosis* surface molecules (25, 43, 48, 79, 196) and the receptors utilized (25).

The C3-CR entry pathway for *M. tuberculosis* has long been postulated to provide the bacterium with safe passage into mononuclear phagocytes. CRs are expressed on all mononuclear phagocytes, ensuring access of the bacterium to its intracellular niche. To the potential advantage of the pathogen, ligation of CR3 does not uniformly trigger toxic host cell responses (222) and has been shown to selectively suppress IL-12 production, an important mediator of the cellular immune response to *M. tuberculosis* (123). Data indicate that there is little or no oxidative response to *M. tuberculosis* by nonactivated human macrophages during phagocytosis (S. Wayne, G. Denning, D. J. Kusner, T. M. Kaufman, and L. S. Schlesinger, Abstract, *Clin. Res.* 43:219A, 1995), a result similar to that obtained with *M. kansasii* when using a human myeloid cell line (109).

Several of the adhesion functions of CR3 are attributed to the I (or A) domain within the α subunit of CD11b, which contains the binding sites for several ligands (81). The binding activity of CR3 is not constitutive but is induced by "inside-out signaling" (in response to a variety of soluble and particulate stimuli) that results in a conformational change facilitating receptor function (153, 221). Conversely, CR3, when engaged by some ligands, transduces "outside-in" signals, resulting in certain kinase-dependent cellular effector responses (114). In addition to the I domain, the α subunit of CD11b contains a cation-independent lectin region, which, when ligated generates more potent host responses. Thus, the

binding sites for *M. tuberculosis* on CR3 may affect the host cell response and bacterial fate. The precise nature of the binding sites for *M. tuberculosis* on CR3 is not clear. Phagocytosis of C3-opsonized and nonopsonized *M. tuberculosis* by CR3 on human monocytes and macrophages is inhibited by monoclonal antibodies known to inhibit C3bi particle binding (176, 178), but not by soluble β-glucan (178). Similarly, competitive soluble carbohydrates did not inhibit the binding of *M. kansasii* to CR3 (109). These studies indicate that *M. tuberculosis* binds to the I domain of CR3 potentially via distinct binding sites (L. S. Schlesinger, A. Frist, T. Kaufman, R. R. Ingalls, R. Li, D. T. Golenbock, and M. Arnaout, *Keystone Symp. Macrophage Biol.*, abstr. 223, 1999). However, there is also evidence that capsular polysaccharides of *M. tuberculosis* bind to the lectin region of CR3 (45, 46).

Fundamental differences in the binding interactions to CR3 between C3-opsonized and nonopsonized *M. tuberculosis* are further supported by in vitro studies in which the phagocyte membrane is depleted of cholesterol to ascertain the importance of cholesterol-rich microdomains (rafts). Cholesterol depletion in general results in significant reduction in mycobacterial uptake (72). Cholesterol depletion in neutrophils decreased the uptake of nonopsonic mycobacteria but not of serum-opsonized organisms, indicating that nonopsonic uptake of bacteria via CR3 selectively involves a glycosylphosphatidylinositol-anchored protein in membrane rafts (157). Different molecular mechanisms for binding involving distinct epitopes on CR3 have been found to transduce different cellular responses, depending on the state of bacterial opsonization (108).

Although bacterial viability does not influence the extent of CR3-mediated phagocytosis, it can regulate early host responses during the phagocytic process. Live *M. tuberculosis* but not dead bacteria interfere with host signaling pathways, inhibiting the increase in cytosolic calcium concentration normally seen following CR3-mediated phagocytosis by human macrophages (120), a process more recently found to be mediated by mycobacterial inhibition of the macrophage sphingosine kinase (122). Treatment of the infected cells with a calcium ionophore caused an increase in the intracellular calcium concentration that led to reduced bacterial viability by enhancing P-L fusion. This activity correlated with increased localization of calmodulin and the activated form of calmodulin-dependent protein kinase II to the phagosome; inhibitors of either calmodulin or the kinase could suppress the enhanced fusion, leading to increased bacterial survival (121).

Phospholipase D (PLD) activity is stimulated early in activated leukocytes, producing the major signal transducing molecules phosphatidic acid and diacylglycerol. PLD activity and phosphatidic acid levels increase markedly during the phagocytosis of *M. tuberculosis* by human MDMs in the presence of nonimmune serum (107). The enhanced PLD activity is inhibited by protein tyrosine kinase inhibitors, as well as by 2,3-diphosphoglycerate, a specific competitive inhibitor of PLD. Concomitantly, these inhibitors significantly reduce *M. tuberculosis* phagocytosis. Activation of this signal transduction pathway may therefore play an important role in regulating the phagocytosis of *M. tuberculosis* and in modulating subsequent macrophage functions. The importance of differential activation of signal transduction pathways by pathogenic and nonpathogenic mycobacteria following phagocytosis has recently been reported (171).

The LAM-MR pathway also appears to be preferable for the intracellular pathogen *M. tuberculosis*. MR-dependent phagocytosis is not coupled to activation of the NADPH oxidase (10, 56), and the LAM-MR pathway appears to be important in limiting P-L fusion events (69; B. K. Kang and L. S. Schlesinger, *Keystone Symp. TB Mol. Mech. Immunol. Aspects*, abstr. 211, 1998). ManLAM has recently been found to play a role in retarding phagosomal maturation by interfering with the calmodulin-dependent production of phosphatidylinositol-3-phosphate (PI3P) and its binding effectors on the phagosomal membrane via inhibition of Ca^{2+} fluxes and the PI3-kinase, hVPS34 (70, 219). *M. tuberculosis* LAM is reported to inhibit IL-12 production via the MR by generating a negative signal in the cell (140). Finally, mycobacterial LAM can scavenge toxic oxygen radicals (34, 35), providing another mechanism for enhancing the survival of these bacteria during phagocytosis. Thus, like CRs, involvement of LAM and the MR during *M. tuberculosis* phagocytosis may enhance intracellular survival.

LAM regulates several macrophage effector functions (27, 98), and its ability to suppress or augment host immunologic responses is highly dependent on the mycobacterial species from which it is obtained (36, 61, 172, 225). AraLAM resembles LPS in that it is a potent inducer of proinflammatory mediators, chemokines, and inducible nitric oxide synthase (iNOS) activity. It enhances immediate-early gene expression, is chemotactic for mononuclear phagocytes, scavenges oxygen radicals, and signals phagocytes through CD14 and TLR2 (18, 33, 34, 128, 150, 175, 227). In contrast, *M. tuberculosis* LAM induces proinflammatory mediators poorly, stimulates the anti-inflammatory cytokine TGF-β (47), and regulates phosphatidylinositol-3-OH kinases (69). Differences

in the host cell response to AraLAM and *M. tuberculosis* LAM may relate to the fact that *M. tuberculosis* LAM but not AraLAM binds to the MR. MR-dependent cytokine and Ca^{2+} responses to *M. tuberculosis* LAM have been reported (17, 169), and *M. tuberculosis* LAM can decrease macrophage signaling responses (105, 173). The LAM-MR pathway may also shape the development of the adaptive immune response, as discussed previously (162, 194).

INTERACTION OF *M. TUBERCULOSIS* WITH EPITHELIAL CELLS

The human alveolus, the initial site of infection by inhaled *M. tuberculosis*, consists of type I and type II pneumocytes. It is estimated that an average human male has 28,000 type I and 1,400 type II pneumocytes and 50 to 100 AMs per alveolus (42, 44, 183). Thus, the probability that invading *M. tuberculosis* will encounter alveolar epithelial cells would be expected to be greater than that with AMs. Although experimental animal studies suggest that inhaled *M. tuberculosis* is taken up by AMs after the organism reaches the alveolar space, there is evidence that *M. tuberculosis* can enter type II alveolar epithelial cells in the animal as well as in human hosts (15, 86, 132). However, the clinical relevance or significance of infection of cell types other than macrophages by *M. tuberculosis* is not obvious. Several approaches have been taken to examine this question.

The first approach includes studies that attempted to look for the presence of *M. tuberculosis* in human lung sections that did not contain obvious TB lesions. It is often assumed that in TB, the major site of infection by *M. tuberculosis* is the granulomatous lesion, which develops from infected macrophages that become surrounded by lymphocytes. However, Opie and Aronson reported as early as in 1927 that *M. tuberculosis* could be recovered from necropsy specimens of macroscopically normal lung tissue in nearly 50% of individuals who died of causes other than tuberculosis (147). Phyu et al. have shown that in a murine model of latent tuberculosis, *M. tuberculosis* can be recovered from lung tissue in the absence of any histologic abnormality (159). More recently, Hernandez-Pando et al., using PCR-based methods, compared necropsy lung tissue samples taken from individuals in populations where TB is endemic to those from individuals in a population with low disease prevalence to demonstrate that *M. tuberculosis* can latently infect lungs without eliciting granulomatous lesions (86). They showed that *M. tuberculosis* DNA can be detected in lung tissues of Ethiopian and Mexican individuals who died of causes other than TB whereas no *M. tuberculosis* DNA could be detected in similar lung samples from Norwegian individuals (86). Five (38%) of 13 Ethiopian and 10 (29%) of 34 Mexican necropsy samples were found to contain *M. tuberculosis* DNA. Furthermore, by in situ PCR, the investigators detected the DNA in alveolar and interstitial macrophages, type II pneumocytes, endothelial cells, and fibroblasts (86). These authors suggested that *M. tuberculosis* may indeed be confined to macrophages in classic TB granulomatous lesions because *M. tuberculosis* that enters nonphagocytic cells is killed by the toxic effects of tumor necrosis factor alpha (TNF-α) while the infection of nonphagocytic cells farther away from these lesions or in tissues without such lesions is spared of the TNF-α effect (62, 63). It may be speculated that this cytotoxicity is a consequence of the local diffusion of reactive nitrogen intermediates that may be induced at higher levels by macrophages at these sites with granulomatous lesions whereas cells that do not undergo cytotoxic damage could serve as a sanctuary for *M. tuberculosis*. Nevertheless, the above studies suggest that macrophages are not necessarily the only site of infection with *M. tuberculosis* and that a latent infection is not necessarily confined to histologically abnormal or granulomatous lung tissues.

Another approach to show relevance to pathogenesis of the epithelial cell interaction of *M. tuberculosis* has been to correlate in vitro cell entry and growth characteristics of *M. tuberculosis* strains with their pathogenicity in animal models. The fact that *M. tuberculosis* can enter and replicate inside nonprofessional phagocytes in vitro has been long recognized. Some of the earliest comprehensive studies to examine the growth characteristics of *M. tuberculosis* inside nonphagocytic tissue culture cells were performed by Shepard in the 1950s. He observed that fully virulent strains of *M. tuberculosis* (H37Rv and selected clinical isolates of *M. tuberculosis*) (entered HeLa cells and proliferated inside these cells (189). He found that attenuated *M. tuberculosis* strains, such as H37Ra, R1Rv, and R1Ra, entered the cells but replicated more slowly inside them. He also compared the intracellular growth characteristics of *M. bovis* (Ravenel strain) and BCG, a vaccine strain derived from *M. bovis*, and found that the Ravenel strain replicated significantly more rapidly than did BCG. These observations led Shepard to suggest that the rates of intracellular multiplication of strains of mycobacteria correlated with their reported pathogenicity for mice and guinea pigs (189). He subsequently reported similar observations made by using other nonphagocytic cells, including human amnion and monkey kidney cells (190). A more recent study showed *M. tuberculosis* strain differences in growth

and cell spread in a novel fibroblast microcolony model (30).

Nearly 40 years later, another group of investigators reported that virulent *M. tuberculosis* H37Rv and attenuated *M. bovis* BCG were able to enter A549 human lung epithelial cells in culture but only the virulent strain was cytotoxic (125). Furthermore, they observed that bacterial entry into A549 cells but not into macrophages was increased by intracellular passage of the bacteria in macrophages. They suggested that *M. tuberculosis* therefore may disseminate into the host lymphatics and bloodstream by directly penetrating the alveolar epithelial lining (125).

The tissue culture infection model was further refined by Birkness et al., who described a bilayer model in which a polarized A549 human pneumocyte monolayer was established on the apical side of a microporous membrane and an endothelial cell monolayer was established on the basal side in a transwell apparatus (22). They showed that monocytes added to the lower chamber of the transwell apparatus migrated through the bilayer to the apical surface only when the apical cells were infected with mycobacteria. This suggested a different type of role for epithelial cells in the spread of mycobacteria—that these epithelial cells, when infected with *M. tuberculosis*, may express products that facilitate and enhance the migration of monocytes across endothelial cells to engulf the bacteria.

The above observation was later expanded by Bermudez et al., using a similar transwell tissue culture bilayer model (16). The transwell bilayer was composed of A549 alveolar epithelial cells seeded on one side of a transwell filter membrane and EAhy926 human endothelial cells seeded on the other side of the filter. The investigators first showed that *M. tuberculosis* H37Rv that was passaged in A549 cells was taken up by the endothelial cells with greater efficiency than was the same strain that had not undergone passage in the epithelial cells. *M. tuberculosis* translocated through the bilayer into the lower chamber with an efficiency of 3 to 4% of the inoculum, and monocytes infected with the bacteria crossed the bilayer with greater efficiency when A549 cells were infected. The investigators then showed that infected A549 cells produced increased levels of IL-8 and monocyte chemoattractant protein-1 (MCP-1), chemokines that induce monocyte migration. An antibody against MCP-1 but not against IL-8 inhibited the migration of infected monocytes across the bilayer. The investigators therefore suggested that the infection of alveolar epithelial cells may enhance the migration of infected macrophages, facilitating the dissemination of *M. tuberculosis* within an infected host. Others have indeed shown IL-8 and MCP-1 production by human alveolar epithelial cells when infected with *M. tuberculosis* (112). While all of these studies were performed with cultured cell lines, they provide additional evidence in support of the clinical relevance of epithelial cell infection by *M. tuberculosis*.

Relevant or not, the studies described above demonstrate clearly that *M. tuberculosis* can enter and replicate inside nonprofessional phagocytic cells. The first attempts at characterizing the mechanism of *M. tuberculosis* entry into such cell types were made in the early 1990s. Arruda et al. reported the identification of DNA sequences that conferred on a laboratory strain of *Escherichia coli* the ability to gain entry into HeLa cells (9). The DNA fragment, subsequently named *mce1A*, was found to be part of an operon called *mce1*, which encodes eight putative membrane-associated proteins (41, 209). The *M. tuberculosis* H37Rv genome sequence revealed that the organism contains four homologues of this operon, *mce1*, *mce2*, *mce3*, and *mce4*, each with similar organization of the genes (41). Latex microspheres coated with recombinant Mce1A or its truncated derivative entered HeLa cells, and the cell invasion activity was found to be confined to a 58-amino-acid domain in this protein (37). A 72-amino-acid-fragment called InvX, which incorporated this 58-amino-acid region was expressed in *E. coli* as a fusion to the AIDA (adhesin involved in diffuse adherence) autotransporter translocator (31). This recombinant *E. coli* strain, stably expressing this fusion protein on its surface, entered HeLa cells, and the uptake was demonstrated to be both microfilament and microtubule dependent. The uptake also required the Rho family of GTPases (31). Interestingly, the Mce1A homologue in the *mce2* operon (Mce2A), which is about 67% identical to Mce1A at the deduced amino acid level, is unable to promote the uptake of coated microspheres into HeLa cells (37). Disruption of the *mce1A* homologue in *M. bovis* BCG reduced the ability of this organism to enter HeLa cells (66).

Although the exact function of Mce1A or the *mce1* operon products is not known, Mce1A may mediate the entry of *M. tuberculosis* into alveolar epithelial cells, which in turn may stimulate the expression of chemokines by these cells to attract macrophages and lymphocytes, which ultimately form granulomas. Indeed, there is evidence that infection of BALB/c mice with an *mce1* mutant strain of *M. tuberculosis* is associated with aberrant migration of inflammatory cells to the site of infection in the lungs and reduced expression of IL-8 by A549 cells infected in vitro (192). The mutant actually became hypervirulent in the mouse model of TB, suggesting that its reduced ability to enter epithelial cells enables it to proliferate unchecked extracellularly due

to the reduced migration of macrophages to the site of infection. The activation of these macrophages may also be diminished or delayed due to the aberrant lymphocyte migration, which would further limit the control of *M. tuberculosis* proliferation. Of course, this hypothesis needs confirmation, but all of the studies described above suggest that TB pathogenesis may be more complex than previously thought and that alveolar epithelial cells, or cell types other than macrophages, may play a key role and influence disease outcome after infection with *M. tuberculosis*.

ROLE OF TOLL-LIKE RECEPTOR PROTEINS IN TUBERCULOSIS

Toll-Like Receptor Proteins

Mammalian TLR proteins derive their name from the *Drosophila* Toll protein, to which they have sequence similarity. Toll was originally shown to be critical for dorsal-ventral patterning in fly embryos (200). Generation of adult flies expressing mutant Toll revealed that this transmembrane receptor also served as a critical component of host immunity to fungal infections (110). Toll is a member of a family of related proteins in the fly that are important for host defense against pathogens, most probably because they direct the production of antimicrobial peptides (e.g., defensins). Importantly, the cytoplasmic domain of Toll was found to be homologous to the cytoplasmic domain of the mammalian IL-1 and IL-18 receptors, suggesting that similar receptors might be encoded in the mammalian genome. The ensuing hunt for bona fide mammalian orthologs of *Drosophila* Toll led to the discovery of "hToll" by Medzditov et al. in 1997 (131). These investigators expressed a constitutively active mutant of hToll in THP-1 monocytic leukemia cells and demonstrated that this expression resulted in activation of the transcription factor NF-κB, as well as in the expression of several immune response genes. Following these initial studies, additional mammalian TLR proteins were identified and hToll was subsequently renamed TLR4.

Subsequently, additional mammalian TLR proteins have been identified (reviewed in reference 206). Non-synthetic agonists have been identified for some (TLR2, TLR3, TLR4, TLR5, and TLR9), but not all, of these TLR proteins. TLR2 agonists include a variety of bacterial cell wall products (discussed below). Synthetic poly(I-C) and double-stranded viral RNA have been reported to be TLR3 agonists (5). TLR4 agonists include gram-negative bacterial lipopolysaccharide (LPS), respiratory syncytial virus protein F, and the plant product Taxol (38, 102, 106). Several mammalian proteins (e.g., fibronectin fragments, some heat shock proteins, and β-defensin 2) are also TLR4 agonists (21, 143, 145). Bacterial flagellin has been identified as a TLR5 agonist (83); finally, unmethylated CpG-containing DNA has been identified as a TLR9 agonist (85).

TLR Signal Transduction and TLR-Specific Responses

The sequence similarities between the intracellular domains of Toll, TLR4 (and other mammalian TLR proteins), and the IL-1 and IL-18 receptors suggested that these receptors have a common signal transduction pathway. Subsequent investigation revealed that these receptors do utilize a similar signaling cascade, which culminates in the activation of NF-κB and mitogen-activated protein. In mammals, engagement of TLR4 and the IL-1 receptor leads to the sequential activation of the adapter protein MyD88, the IL-1 receptor-associated kinases, TNF receptor-associated factor-6, and, eventually, the IκB kinase complex (reviewed in reference 146). Recent studies have identified the additional adapter proteins Tollip (29), TIRAP (also called Mal) (64, 94), TRIF (92, 152, 224), and TRAM (65). All 10 known TLR proteins and five known adapter proteins possess a conserved intracellular sequence region that is necessary for signal transduction. This region, known as the TIR (TLR/IL-1 receptor) domain, is thought to mediate protein-protein interactions between the TLR proteins and the adapter proteins.

The existence of a family of TLR proteins, and multiple adapter proteins, suggests that different TLR proteins can induce distinct cellular responses. Numerous investigators have experimentally validated this possibility. For example, engagement of all TLR proteins activates some shared responses (e.g., activation of NF-κB, AP-1, PI3-kinase, and mitogen-activated protein kinases) whereas some responses are TLR specific. One example of a TLR-specific response is the expression and secretion of IFN-γ by activated macrophages and DC (91, 166). IFN-γ is an early-gene product of activated macrophages that exerts potent autocrine and paracrine effects on the cells. IFN-γ secretion is induced following engagement of TLR3 and TLR4 but not TLR2 and TLR5. The binding of IFN-γ to the type I IFN receptor on the same cells that secrete it leads to the autocrine/paracrine activation of the transcription factor STAT1, which is necessary for the expression of STAT1-dependent genes that are not expressed following the engagement of TLR proteins which do not induce IFN-γ expression (215). This is a likely mechanism for some of the TLR-specific patterns of gene expression observed in activated macrophages.

Engagement of the type I IFN receptor by IFN-γ, and the subsequent induction of STAT1 activation, is required for LPS-induced NO production in macrophages (144). Thus, the inability of some TLR2 agonists to induce IFN-γ expression is likely to explain why these TLR2 agonists also fail to induce iNOS gene expression and NO production in macrophages. It should be noted that NO production by *M. tuberculosis*-infected macrophages does not require the TLR adapter protein MyD88 (129). This suggests that *M. tuberculosis*-induced NO production either is TLR independent or utilizes other adapter proteins (e.g., TRAM or TRIF) that function in a TLR-specific manner. Because *M. avium* and *M. bovis* BCG fail to induce NO production by macrophages and do not appear to express a TLR4 agonist, a TLR4-dependent and MyD88-independent pathway may be responsible for NO production in *M. tuberculosis*-infected macrophages. Finally, TLR2 signaling was also found to favor the induction of IL-8 expression, whereas TLR4 signaling was a much stronger inducer of RANTES expression (166). Thus, different patterns of chemokine expression appear to be expressed by macrophages and DC activated via TLR2 versus TLR4, thereby leading to the recruitment of distinct populations of granulocytes to the site of TLR engagement (i.e., infection).

TLR Coreceptors

Some TLR proteins utilize coreceptors that augment TLR-dependent responses and, in some cases, are required for TLR function. For example, both CD14 (58) and the β$_2$-integrin CD11b/CD18 (CR3) (155) augment the responsiveness of cells to the TLR4 agonist gram-negative bacterial LPS. CD14 and CD11b/CD18 are not required for responsiveness to LPS in macrophages, although these TLR4 coreceptors can enhance the sensitivity of cells to LPS by more than 1,000-fold. CD14 is necessary for maximal activation of TLR2 by the mycobacterial AraLAM (128), but it does not promote entry of *M. tuberculosis* into human macrophages (188). CD14 has also been reported to augment TLR2-mediated responses to the 19-kDa lipoprotein antigen (28) but not to viable *M. tuberculosis* (129). The coreceptor MD-2 appears to be absolutely required for activation of TLR4 by LPS and by the plant product Taxol (102, 191). In contrast, MD-2 is not necessary for cellular activation via TLR2, TLR5, or TLR9. Similarly, MD-2 does not appear to mediate the activation of macrophages by intact *M. tuberculosis* (127).

Mycobacterial TLR Agonists

Several mycobacterial products activate mammalian cells in a TLR2-dependent manner. Initially, Means et al. demonstrated that AraLAM purified from rapidly growing mycobacteria could activate mammalian cells in a TLR2-dependent manner (128). ManLAM from *M. tuberculosis* does not appear to be an agonist for TLR2 (129), although this molecule has been reported to possess several distinct biological activities (33, 119, 140). Thus, while mycobacterial lipoglycans can activate cells via CD14 and TLR2, this signaling complex exhibits great specificity, since it is able to distinguish between the closely related lipoglycans ManLAM and AraLAM. As noted above, recognition of ManLAM by DC appears to involve DC-SIGN, a lectin that can discriminate between *Mycobacterium* species through selective recognition of mannose caps on ManLAM (118, 205). Engagement of DC-SIGN leads to suppression of DC maturation through TLR signaling (75). Pathogens, such as *M. tuberculosis*, may use DC-SIGN to both infect DC and down regulate innate immune responses. The molecular mechanism of this down regulation and whether signaling through DC-SIGN leads to the selective suppression of Th1 responses remain to be determined. Consistent with the latter possibility, DC-SIGN expression can be up regulated on MDMs on exposure to the Th2 cytokine IL-13 (195).

Both *M. tuberculosis* and BCG can infect DCs by binding to DC-SIGN, and this binding appears to be mediated by ManLAM in the mycobacterial cell wall. Unlike AraLAM, which is a TLR2 agonist (128), highly purified ManLAM is not a TLR agonist. ManLAM augments LPS-induced IL-10 secretion by human blood monocyte-derived DCs (75), but neither ManLAM nor AraLAM could induce the maturation of these cells in vitro. In contrast, murine splenic DC maturation in vivo by BCG infection was completely dependent on TLR2 expression (M. J. Fenton and M. Armant, unpublished observations). DC maturation induced by LPS and by BCG would be suppressed by exogenous ManLAM, and this suppression could be reversed in the presence of anti-DC-SIGN antibodies, demonstrating that engagement of DC-SIGN down regulated TLR signaling (75).

Subsequent studies have demonstrated that *M. tuberculosis* does possess additional TLR2 agonists. In searching for factors that could contribute to the generation of protective T-cell-mediated immunity, Brightbill et al. purified an IL-12-inducing activity from cell wall-associated *M. tuberculosis* proteins (28). This activity was found to copurify with the 19-kDa lipoprotein antigen of *M. tuberculosis*, and purified lipoprotein mimicked the effect of *M. tuber-culosis* cell wall preparations. Furthermore, using blocking antibodies and reporter gene assays, the 19-kDa lipoprotein was found to activate cells in a TLR2-dependent manner. In addition to the 19-kDa lipoprotein, *M. tuberculosis* has been shown to secrete a distinct factor, termed STF, which activates cells in a TLR2-dependent manner (129). Together, these findings indicate that *M. tuberculosis* is fully capable of expressing multiple factors that can activate cells via TLR2. Furthermore, *M. tuberculosis* is capable of secreting TLR2-activating factors as well as expressing TLR2 agonists on its cell surface.

Given the fact that the TLR protein family recognizes a diverse array of microbial products, it is quite likely that intact *M. tuberculosis* expresses agonists for more than one TLR protein. As anticipated from studies of purified *M. tuberculosis*-derived factors, live *M. tuberculosis* bacilli activate cells via TLR2 (127, 129). However, intact *M. tuberculosis* is also capable of stimulating cells in a TLR4-dependent manner. The TLR4 agonist activity of live *M. tuberculosis* was found to be cell associated and heat labile, thus differing from the secreted heat-stable TLR2 agonist STF. In contrast to *M. tuberculosis*, live *M. avium* and *M. bovis* BCG do not activate cells in a TLR4-dependent manner (84, 111), indicating that mycobacteria differ in their ability to synthesize TLR4 agonists. Although both TLR2 and TLR4 can participate in the activation of macrophages by intact *M. tuberculosis*, the relative contributions of these TLR proteins to cellular responses remain to be completely resolved. The fact that intact *M. avium* and *M. bovis* BCG do not appear to activate macrophages via TLR4 suggests that the TLR4 agonist expressed by *M. tuberculosis* plays a role in virulence. It should be noted that a recent study by Uehori et al. has reported that DC maturation induced by purified BCG peptidoglycan was blocked by 70% by suppression of both TLR2 and TLR4 and by 30 to 40% by suppression of either TLR alone (217). Similar but less profound suppression of DC maturation by BCG cell wall skeletons was also observed. Hence, the presence of BCG peptidoglycan is a minimal requirement for activation of both TLR2 and TLR4 in human DCs, unlike the presence of peptidoglycans of gram-positive bacteria, which activate only TLR2. Additional data presented by these investigators suggest that peptidoglycan receptors other than TLR2 and TLR4 present on human DC are involved in TLR signaling. It remains to be determined whether non-TLR peptidoglycan receptors, such as Nod1 (32, 77), play any role in activation of macrophages and DC by mycobacteria.

Although *M. tuberculosis* expresses multiple TLR agonists, these bacteria are still able to persist and grow in host macrophages. Therefore, it is unclear whether these TLR agonists play any role in regulating the survival of intracellular *M. tuberculosis*. This subject has been addressed in a report by Thoma-Uszynski et al., in which stimulation of infected macrophages by the mycobacterial 19-kDa lipoprotein TLR2 agonist was found to decrease the growth of intracellular *M. tuberculosis* (211). This bacteriostatic activity of the 19-kDa lipoprotein was partially blocked by inhibitors of NO production. A role for NO in the arrest of intracellular *M. tuberculosis* growth by the 19-kDa lipoprotein is supported by the finding that the lipoprotein itself was a potent inducer of NO production by mouse macrophages. Thus, the 19-kDa lipoprotein of *M. tuberculosis* may play a role in the induction of NO-dependent antimicrobial mechanisms in mouse macrophages. Interestingly, the 19-kDa lipoprotein did not induce NO production in human monocytes, although it was still capable of inhibiting the growth of *M. tuberculosis* in these cells.

The role of NO in human responses to mycobacterial infection remains a controversial issue. Nevertheless, TLR2 engagement by the 19-kDa lipoproteins may also play a role in *M. tuberculosis* persistence in macrophages. Harding and colleagues have previously shown that prolonged exposure to the 19-kDa lipoprotein, and other TLR agonists, inhibits class II major histocompatibility complex (MHC) expression and antigen processing (141, 142). TLR2 engagement by the 19-kDa lipoprotein was shown to inhibit IFN-γ-regulated expression of HLA-DR and Fc-γ-RI in human macrophages, resulting in decreased antigen processing and recognition by class II MHC-restricted CD4$^+$ T cells (74). More recently, the capacity of the 19-kDa lipoprotein to inhibit alternate class I MHC antigen processing of mycobacterial antigens was also reported (214). Inhibition of this alternate antigen-processing pathway was shown to be mediated by TLR2 signaling. By inhibiting both class II MHC and alternate class I MHC antigen processing, pathogens that establish prolonged infection of macrophages and DC (such as *M. tuberculosis*) may suppress the adaptive immune response and evade surveillance by both CD4$^+$ and CD8$^+$ T cells, thus promoting chronic infection.

TLR Proteins and Apoptosis

Many bacterial pathogens induce apoptosis of infected cells (136). Shortly after the discovery of mammalian TLR proteins, a synthetic bacterial lipopeptide TLR2 agonist (sBLP, Pam$_3$CysSerLys$_4$) was shown to induce apoptosis in THP-1 cells (6). Moreover, anti-human TLR2 antibodies could block the cytotoxic effect of sBLP, indicating that TLR2 alone could transmit an apoptosis-inducing signal to the THP-1 monocytic cells. The 19-kDa lipoprotein was also reported to induce apoptosis in THP-1 cells and MDMs in a TLR2-dependent manner (116). E5531, a specific antagonist of TLR4, blocked most of the *M. tuberculosis*-induced apoptosis of human AMs (127). This effect was largely secondary to the inhibition of TNF-α secretion, indicating that TLR4 can (at least indirectly) mediate the apoptotic effect of *M. tuberculosis* on AMs. This is also consistent with previous findings of macrophage apoptosis induced by the TLR4 agonist gram-negative bacterial LPS (20).

M. tuberculosis expresses both TLR2 and TLR4 agonists, and while TLR2 activation has been shown to be capable of providing a proapoptotic signal (6), a blockade of TLR4 was sufficient to eliminate almost all *M. tuberculosis*-induced human AM apoptosis (127). This suggests that TLR2 and TLR4 contribute unequally to TLR-mediated induction of apoptosis by *M. tuberculosis*. The mechanism that underlies this inequality remains unknown, although two possibilities exist. First, human AMs may be relatively unresponsive to TLR2 agonists compared with other macrophage populations (97). However, different macrophage populations were found to be similarly responsive to the TLR4 agonist *E. coli* LPS. Second, the expression of proapoptotic factors by *M. tuberculosis*-stimulated macrophages may be selectively induced by cellular activation via TLR4 but not via TLR2.

TLR Proteins and Dendritic Cells

Like macrophages, DC can be infected by *M. tuberculosis* and also respond differently to distinct TLR agonists. The patterns of cytokine and costimulatory-molecule expression on DC during antigen presentation to T cells are a strong determinant of Th commitment (i.e., whether a Th1 or Th2 response is generated following antigen presentation). The responses of human DC to TLR2 and TLR4 agonists were directly compared, and significant differences were reported (166). These differences could have profound implications for the control of innate and acquired immune responses by these TLR proteins. TLR4 (*E. coli* LPS) but not TLR2 (*Staphylococcus aureus* peptidoglycan) agonists stimulated the production of IL-12p70 and IP-10 by DC. Importantly, TLR2 activation led to the induction of IL-12p40 expression but not of IL-12p35 expression. In the absence of IL-12p35, IL-12p40 can homodimerize and antagonizes the activity of IL-12p70 (reviewed in reference 76). Conversely, DC activation via TLR2, but not via TLR4, led to the expression of p19, a novel protein that can heterodimerize with IL-12p40 to form the novel cytokine IL-23. Despite the sequence and subunit similarities, the biological activities of IL-23 do not exactly mimic those of IL-12p70 (148). Thus, while both TLR2 and TLR4 signaling induces IL-12p40 expression, these signaling events differentially induce the expression of the IL-12p40-binding proteins IL-12p35 and p19. This ultimately leads to the preferential induction of either IL-23 (via TLR2) or IL-12p70 (via TLR4) by DC.

TLR Proteins and Antigen Presentation

Cells of the innate immune system are important not only because of their direct effector responses to pathogens but also because of their capacity for antigen presentation to lymphocytes. Much attention has recently been focused on the potential roles of TLR proteins in the maturation and cellular activation of DC, professional antigen-presenting cells that may be most relevant to the development of acquired immunity. Purified TLR2 (87, 134), TLR4 (99), and TLR9 (85) agonists have all been shown to stimulate the maturation and antigen-presenting capacity of DC in vitro. However, the signaling requirements for the induction of DC maturation by these TLR proteins are not identical. As noted above, TLR4 is currently unique among TLR proteins in that it utilizes all four known TLR adapter proteins for signal transduction (64, 94). Prior to the identification of TIRAP/Mal and TRIF, MyD88 knockout mice were used to show that the TLR4 agonist E. coli LPS, but not the TLR9 agonist CpG DNA, could still induce the maturation of MyD88-deficient DC in vitro (99). Presumably, TIRAP/Mal can provide a MyD88-independent signal that is sufficient to stimulate DC maturation. In addition to their capacities to induce DC maturation, TLR2, TLR4, and TLR9 agonists were able to induce the expression of proinflammatory cytokines by DC (85, 99, 134). However, in contrast to the DC maturation response, these cytokine responses were strictly dependent on the expression of MyD88. Thus, microbial agonists for several TLR proteins can activate DC, although cellular maturation and cytokine production appear to have distinct signaling requirements.

Suppression of Antigen Presentation by Mycobacteria

The ability of M. tuberculosis to inhibit the maturation of phagosomes along the endosomal-lysosomal pathway not only aids in the persistence of live M. tuberculosis inside macrophages but also protects the bacilli from lysosomal degradation that could lead to the processing of antigens for presentation in the context of class II MHC. However, recent studies on the regulation of class II MHC-mediated antigen presentation by mycobacterial products have provided insight into how TLR protein signaling may also participate in the evasion of immune surveillance by M. tuberculosis (39, 43, 44, 56, 141, 142). Noss et al. showed that stimulation of macrophages with mycobacterial 19-kDa lipoprotein, a TLR2 agonist, reduced class II MHC mRNA accumulation and surface expression in macrophages (142). This altered expression of class II molecules correlated with decreased presentation of peptide antigens to T-lymphocyte hybridomas. Whole M. tuberculosis and an M. tuberculosis lysate mimicked the suppressive effect observed using purified 19-kDa lipoprotein. It should be noted that this TLR-mediated inhibition of antigen presentation is not an exclusive attribute of TLR2. Gram-negative bacterial LPS and CpG DNA, agonists for TLR4 and TLR9, respectively, were also shown to inhibit the expression of class II MHC molecules (39, 141). Conversely, the processing and presentation of diverse antigens (e.g., HEL, OVA, and RNase) by macrophages could be blocked by M. tuberculosis infection or the addition of exogenous 19-kDa lipoprotein. Lastly, the presentation of mycobacterial antigens (e.g., Ag85B) by M. tuberculosis-infected macrophages could be dramatically suppressed by treatment with exogenous 19-kDa lipoprotein, compared to M. tuberculosis-infected macrophages that received no additional stimulants. Thus, TLR2 activation by mycobacterial agonists may represent an important pathway by which M. tuberculosis can prevent the presentation of its antigens and thus thwart cell-mediated immune responses in vivo.

Paradoxically, TLR proteins appear to mediate both the suppression of antigen presentation and the induction of antimicrobial responses by macrophages. It remains unclear whether TLR-mediated suppression of antigen processing and presentation benefits the pathogen or the host. Harding and colleagues have examined the effects of M. tuberculosis, and the 19-kDa lipoprotein, on class I MHC- and class II-mediated antigen presentation and subsequent generation of cell-mediated immunity to M. tuberculosis (141, 142, 214). Several purified TLR2 agonists and intact M. tuberculosis all suppress antigen processing and presentation by IFN-γ-treated bone marrow-derived murine macrophages in vitro. The kinetics of inhibition of class II MHC expression by TLR agonists was found to be slow, requiring a prolonged (18-h) incubation to manifest substantial suppression. Therefore, an opportunity for the macrophage to process and load antigen onto class II MHC molecules may exist prior to the time when decreased class

II expression actually impairs antigen presentation. Moreover, the decreased synthesis of new class II molecules may effectively stabilize preexisting MHC-antigen complexes on the surface of the antigen-presenting cells. This would result in a population of macrophages and/or DC that present a limited repertoire of bacterial antigens. These antigens would arise from internalized bacilli and would predominate over antigens acquired at later times. Noss et al. refer to this model as the "freeze-frame hypothesis" (142). However, a caveat arises when this model is considered in the context of *M. tuberculosis* uptake by macrophages. *M. tuberculosis* actively inhibits its own destruction by lysosomes by inhibiting phagosomal maturation. This is likely to delay the processing and presentation of mycobacterial antigens. In contrast, TLR activation occurs immediately on, or shortly after, the uptake of *M. tuberculosis* by macrophages. Thus, the bacilli may trigger a TLR-dependent process that leads to the suppression of antigen presentation while simultaneously resisting lysosomal destruction. In the end, it is possible that suppression of class II MHC molecule expression and antigen processing may largely precede the destruction of intracellular *M. tuberculosis*.

Lessons from TLR Knockout Mice

Recently, several laboratories have investigated the roles of TLR2 and TLR4 in host responses to mycobacterial infection. Abel et al. compared the responses of normal C3H/OuJ and TLR4-mutant C3H/HeJ mice to low-dose (50 to 100 CFU/mouse) aerosol infection with *M. tuberculosis* (1). C3H/HeJ mice possess a single point mutation within the intracellular signaling domain of TLR4 (Pro712His) that abrogates receptor function. These investigators found that the TLR4-mutant mice had a reduced capacity to eliminate mycobacteria from the lungs and succumbed to bacterial loads that were sublethal for normal mice (at least for the duration of the experiments). Furthermore, the lungs of these TLR4-mutant mice showed chronic pneumonia, with increased neutrophilic infiltration and reduced macrophage recruitment. Pulmonary expression of TNF-α, IL-12p40, and the chemokine MCP-1 was significantly lower in the TLR4-mutant mice compared to normal controls. Thus, macrophage recruitment and the proinflammatory response to *M. tuberculosis* are impaired in TLR4-mutant mice, resulting in chronic infection and impaired elimination of the bacteria.

Significantly different results were obtained by Reiling et al., who compared the resistance of normal, TLR4-mutant (C3H/HeJ), and TLR2-deficient (TLR2$^{-/-}$) mice to aerosol infection with *M. tuberculosis* (167). Following low-dose aerosol exposure (100 CFU/mouse) to *M. tuberculosis*, both TLR-deficient strains were as resistant as congenic controls to infection. Granuloma formation, macrophage activation, and proinflammatory cytokine secretion in response to low-dose aerosol *M. tuberculosis* infection were found to be identical in normal and TLR-deficient mice. In addition, the absence of the TLR4 coreceptor CD14 did not affect the responses of CD14-deficient mice and of CD14-deficient bone marrow-derived macrophages to *M. tuberculosis* challenge in vivo and in vitro, respectively. In contrast, a high-dose aerosol challenge (2,000 CFU/mouse) revealed that TLR2-deficient but not TLR4-mutant mice were more susceptible than control mice. Furthermore, IL-12p40 levels in the sera of *M. tuberculosis*-infected TLR2$^{-/-}$ mice were diminished, relative to controls, whereas IL-12p40 levels in *M. tuberculosis*-infected TLR4-mutant and normal mice were similar.

IL-12p40 levels in the sera of infected TLR-deficient mice correlated inversely with bacterial load in the organs and ultimately with survival. When cytokine production was examined in vitro, a qualitatively distinct observation was made using MDMs (167). Macrophages from TLR2$^{-/-}$ mice secreted less TNF-α and IL-12p40, following *M. tuberculosis* stimulation in vitro, than did control cells. In contrast, macrophages from TLR4-mutant mice secreted less IL-12p40 following in vitro *M. tuberculosis* stimulation. Interestingly, these *M. tuberculosis*-stimulated mutant macrophages did not secrete significantly less TNF-α than their normal counterparts. Thus, the roles of TLR proteins in cytokine production induced by *M. tuberculosis* differ depending on whether bacterial challenge is performed in vitro or in vivo.

Sugawara et al. have also examined the role of TLR2, as well as TLR6, in the host response to *M. tuberculosis* by using a low-dose aerosol exposure mouse model. They found no contribution of TLR6 to the host response in terms of survival, bacterial loads, histopathology, or selected gene responses (204). In contrast, infected TLR2$^{-/-}$ mice developed granulomatous pulmonary lesions with neutrophil infiltration, which were somewhat larger than those in wild-type mice. Initially, pulmonary expression of iNOS, TNF-α, TGF-β, IL-1β, and IL-2 mRNA was significantly lower than in control mice, whereas IL-6 levels were elevated. No significant differences in cytokine gene expression between TLR2 knockout and wild-type mice were observed 12 weeks after infection.

More recently, Heldwein et al. compared the roles of TLR2 and TLR4 in the host immune response to *M. bovis* BCG (84). Two weeks after intraperitoneal challenge with BCG, few bacilli were present in the lungs of wild-type and TLR4$^{-/-}$ mice whereas bacterial loads were 10-fold higher in the lungs of infected TLR2$^{-/-}$ mice (84). BCG challenge in vitro strongly induced proinflammatory cytokine secretion by macrophages from wild-type and TLR4$^{-/-}$ mice but not from TLR2$^{-/-}$ mice. In contrast, intracellular uptake, intracellular bacterial growth, and suppression of intracellular bacterial growth in vitro by IFN-γ were similar in macrophages from all three mouse strains, suggesting that BCG growth in the lungs of TLR2$^{-/-}$ mice was a consequence of defective adaptive immunity. Antigenic stimulation of splenocytes from infected wild-type and TLR4$^{-/-}$ mice induced T-cell proliferation in vitro, whereas T cells from TLR2$^{-/-}$ mice failed to proliferate. Unexpectedly, activated CD4$^+$ T cells from both TLR-deficient mouse strains secreted less IFN-γ in vitro than did control T cells. A role for TLR4 in the control of bacterial growth and IFN-γ production in vivo was observed only when mice were infected with larger numbers of BCG bacilli. Thus, TLR2 and TLR4 appear to regulate distinct aspects of the host immune response to BCG.

TLR Polymorphisms and Mycobacterial Immunity

Several studies have identified mutations in genes encoding critical components of the host response to tuberculosis (e.g., IFN-γ and IL-12 receptors) that affect the functions of these gene products and increase the susceptibility to infection by *M. tuberculosis* (51). Similarly, two missense mutations affecting the extracellular domain of human TLR4 are associated with hyporesponsiveness to LPS (7) and an increased incidence of septic shock (117). A polymorphism located within the intracellular domains of human TLR2 has been identified (Arg677Trp) and shown to be associated with lepromatous leprosy in a Korean population (101). This human TLR2 mutation was found in 10 of 45 lepromatous leprosy patients but it was not observed in 41 tuberculoid leprosy patients or 45 healthy controls. Subsequent in vitro studies have determined that TLR2 is necessary to mediate macrophage responsiveness to *M. leprae* and that this mutation abrogates the ability of TLR2 to mediate cellular activation by both *M. leprae* and *M. tuberculosis* (24). These investigators also reported that TLR4 is not necessary for the innate immune recognition of irradiated *M. leprae* bacilli.

CONCLUSIONS

Monocytes and macrophages serve as the host cell niche for the highly adapted *M. tuberculosis*. Phagocytosis by these cells involves several major host cell receptors and microbial ligands and is regulated by determinants of the innate immune system. Further regulation is dependent on the tissue site, degree of phagocyte differentiation, and presence of inflammatory mediators. Evidence is accumulating that involvement of specific receptor-binding domains, cooperativity between different receptors, and involvement of specific microbial determinants are important in defining the early host response and microbial fate during and following phagocytosis. The host cell response of *M. tuberculosis* to CR3 is dependent on the precise epitope(s) ligated during entry and the state of bacterial opsonization. The terminal mannose caps of ManLAM, an abundant lipoglycan on the surface of *M. tuberculosis*, are critical microbial ligands for recognition by both macrophages and DC via the MR and DC-SIGN, respectively. In addition, ManLAM regulates several host cell responses and is capable of regulating intracellular trafficking events.

In addition to its binding and uptake by macrophages and DC, it is clear that *M. tuberculosis* interacts with epithelial cells, which contribute to the pathogenesis of disease. In in vitro studies, *M. tuberculosis* enters epithelial cells, a process that involves Mce1A, and bacteria harvested from these cells show enhanced uptake by macrophages. Epithelial cells also contribute to the inflammatory response, regulate cellular migration and recruitment, and appear to participate in bacterial dissemination.

M. tuberculosis ligates different TLR proteins during its interaction with mammalian cells, further refining the host response by the production of cytokines and regulation of apoptosis, antigen presentation, and bacterial survival. The degree to which TLR proteins contribute to the overall innate and adaptive host responses to mycobacterial challenge remains to be fully elucidated. Studies suggest that TLR2 is a major pattern recognition receptor that mediates the activation of macrophages and DC by *M. tuberculosis*, *M. avium*, *M. bovis* BCG, and *M. leprae*. In contrast, expression of a mycobacterial TLR4 agonist has been reported only for *M. tuberculosis*. TLR4 may not be critical for survival in vivo, as determined in the low-dose aerosol infection model of mouse tuberculosis, at least compared to TLR2. High-dose infection models suggest that TLR2 and, to a lesser extent, TLR4 can contribute to survival and host immunity. Nevertheless, both TLR proteins alone appear to contribute less to the host immune response than do inflammatory mediators such as TNF-α and IFN-γ. This probably reflects the natural redundancy in both the numbers of different pattern recognition receptors and the contribution of TLR-independent innate and adaptive immune response pathways that operate in vivo. The finding that a natural TLR2 polymorphism that abolishes receptor function is associated with lepromatous but not tuberculoid leprosy in human populations supports the contention that TLR proteins can measurably affect the host response to mycobacterial infection. Future studies will undoubtedly determine precisely how TLR proteins integrate into innate and adaptive host immune responses in vivo.

REFERENCES

1. Abel, B., N. Thieblemont, V. J. Quesniaux, N. Brown, J. Mpagi, K. Miyake, F. Bihl, and B. Ryffel. 2002. Toll-like receptor 4 expression is required to control chronic *Mycobacterium tuberculosis* infection in mice. *J. Immunol.* 169:3155–3162.

2. Abou-Zeid, C., T. Garbe, R. Lathigra, H. G. Wiker, M. Harboe, G. A. W. Rook, and D. B. Young. 1991. Genetic and immunological analysis of *Mycobacterium tuberculosis* fibronectin-binding proteins. *Infect. Immun.* 59:2712–2718.

3. Abramson, S. L., and J. I. Gallin. 1990. IL-4 inhibits superoxide production by human mononuclear phagocytes. *J. Immunol.* 144:625–630.

4. Aderem, A. 2002. How to eat something bigger than your head. *Cell* 110:5–8.

5. Alexopoulou, L., A. C. Holt, R. Medzhitov, and R. A. Flavell. 2001. Recognition of double-stranded RNA and activation of NF-kappaB by Toll-like receptor 3. *Nature* 413:732–738.

6. Aliprantis, A. O., R.-B. Yang, M. R. Mark, S. Suggett, B. Devaux, J. D. Radolf, G. R. Klimpel, P. Godowski, and A. Zychlinsky. 1999. Cell activation and apoptosis by bacterial lipoproteins through toll-like receptor-2. *Science* 285:736–739.

7. Arbour, N. C., E. Lorenz, B. C. Schutte, J. Zabner, J. N. Kline, M. Jones, K. Frees, J. L. Watt, and D. A. Schwartz. 2000. TLR4 mutations are associated with endotoxin hypo-responsiveness in humans. *Nat. Genet.* 25:187–191.

8. Armstrong, J. A., and P. D. Hart. 1975. Phagosome-lysosome interactions in cultured macrophages infected with virulent tubercle bacilli: reversal of the usual nonfusion pattern and observations on bacterial survial. *J. Exp. Med.* 142:1–16.

9. Arruda, S., G. Bomfim, R. Knights, T. Huima-Byron, and L. W. Riley. 1993. Cloning of an *M. tuberculosis* DNA fragment associated with entry and survival inside cells. *Science* 261:1454–1457.

10. Astarie-Dequeker, C., E. N. N'Diaye, V. Le Cabec, M. G. Rittig, J. Prandi, and I. Maridonneau-Parini. 1999. The mannose receptor mediates uptake of pathogenic and nonpathogenic mycobacteria and bypasses bactericidal responses in human macrophages. *Infect. Immun.* 67:469–477.

11. Bardana, E. J., Jr., J. K. McClatchy, R. S. Farr, and P. Minden. 1973. Universal occurrence of antibodies to tubercle bacilli in sera from non-tuberculous and tuberculous individuals. *Clin. Exp. Immunol.* 13:65–77.

12. Barnes, P. F., R. L. Modlin, and J. J. Ellner. 1994. T-cell responses and cytokines, p. 417–435. *In* B. R. Bloom (ed.), *Tuberculosis: Pathogenesis, Protection, and Control.* ASM Press, Washington, D.C.

13. Becker, S., and E. G. Daniel. 2000. Antagonistic and additive effects of IL-4 and interferon-gamma on human monocytes and macrophages: effects on Fc receptors HLA-D antigens, and superoxide production. *Cell. Immunol.* 129:351–362.

14. Beharka, A. A., C. D. Gaynor, B. K. Kang, D. R. Voelker, F. X. McCormack, and L. S. Schlesinger. 2002. Pulmonary surfactant protein A up-regulates activity of the mannose receptor, a pattern recognition receptor expressed on human macrophages. *J. Immunol.* 169:3565–3573.

15. Bermudez, L. E., and J. Goodman. 1996. *Mycobacterium tuberculosis* invades and replicates within type II alveolar cells. *Infect. Immun.* 64:1400–1406.

16. Bermudez, L. E., F. J. Sangari, P. Kolonoski, M. Petrofsky, and J. Goodman. 2002. The efficiency of the translocation of *Mycobacterium tuberculosis* across a bilayer of epithelial and endothelial cells as a model of the alveolar wall is a consequence of transport within mononuclear phagocytes and invasion of alveolar epithelial cells. *Infect. Immun.* 70:140–146.

17. Bernardo, J., A. M. Billingslea, R. L. Blumenthal, K. F. Seetoo, E. R. Simons, and M. J. Fenton. 1998. Differential responses of human mononuclear phagocytes to mycobacterial lipoarabinomannans: role of CD14 and the mannose receptor. *Infect. Immun.* 66:28–35.

18. Bernier, R., B. Barbeau, M. Olivier, and M. J. Tremblay. 1998. *Mycobcterium tuberculosis* mannose-capped lipoarabinomannan can induce NF-κB-dependent activation of human immunodeficiency virus type 1 long terminal repeat in T cells. *J. Gen. Virol.* 79:1353–1361.

19. Berón, W., C. Alvarez-Dominguez, L. Mayorga, and P. D. Stahl. 1995. Membrane trafficking along the phagocytic pathway. *Trends Cell Biol.* 5:100–104.

20. Bingisser, P., C. Stey, M. Weller, P. Groscurth, and E. Russi. 1996. Apoptosis in human alveolar macrophages is induced by endotoxin and is modulated by cytokines. *Am. J. Respir. Cell Mol. Biol.* 15:64–70.

21. Biragyn, A., P. A. Ruffini, C. A. Leifer, E. Klyushnenkova, A. Shakhov, O. Chertov, A. K. Shirakawa, J. M. Farber, D. M. Segal, J. J. Oppenheim, and L. W. Kwak. 2002. Toll-like receptor 4-dependent activation of dendritic cells by beta-defensin 2. *Science* 298:1025–1029.

22. Birkness, K. A., M. Deslauriers, J. H. Bartlett, E. H. White, C. H. King, and F. D. Quinn. 1999. An in vitro tissue culture bilayer model to examine early events in *Mycobacterium tuberculosis* infection. *Infect. Immun.* 67:653–658.

23. Blackford, J., H. W. Reid, D. J. C. Pappin, F. S. Bowers, and J. M. Wilkinson. 1996. A monoclonal antibody, 3/22, to rabbit CD11c which induces homotypic T cell aggregation: evidence that ICAM-1 is a ligand for CD11c/CD18. *Eur. J. Immunol.* 26:525–531.

24. Bochud, P. Y., T. R. Hawn, and A. Aderem. 2003. Cutting edge: a Toll-like receptor 2 polymorphism that is associated with lepromatous leprosy is unable to mediate mycobacterial signaling. *J. Immunol.* 170:3451–3454.

25. Bouvier, G., A.-M. Benoliel, C. Foa, and P. Bongrand. 1994. Relationship between phagosome acidification, phagosome-lysosome fusion, and mechanism of particle ingestion. *J. Leukoc. Biol.* 55:729–734.

26. Brennan, M. J., G. Delogu, Y. Chen, S. Bardarov, J. Kriakov, M. Alavi, and W. R. Jacobs, Jr. 2001. Evidence that mycobacterial PE-PGRS proteins are cell surface constituents that influence interactions with other cells. *Infect. Immun.* 69:7326–7333.

27. Brennan, P. J., and H. Nikaido. 1995. The envelope of mycobacteria. *Annu. Rev. Biochem.* 64:29–63.

28. Brightbill, H. D., D. H. Libraty, and S. R. Krutzik. 1999. Host defense mechanisms triggered by microbial lipoproteins through toll-like receptors. *Science* 285:732–736.

29. Bulut, Y., E. Faure, L. Thomas, O. Equils, and M. Arditi. 2001. Cooperation of Toll-like receptor 2 and 6 for cellular activation by soluble tuberculosis factor and *Borrelia burgdorferi* outer surface protein A lipoprotein: role of Toll-interacting protein and IL-1 receptor signaling molecules in Toll-like receptor 2 signaling. *J. Immunol.* **167:**987–994.

30. Byrd, T. F., G. M. Green, S. E. Fowlston, and C. R. Lyons. 1998. Differential growth characteristics and streptomycin susceptibility of virulent and avirulent *Mycobacterium tuberculosis* strains in a novel fibroblast-mycobacterium microcolony assay. *Infect. Immun.* **66:**5132–5139.

31. Casali, N., M. Konieczny, M. A. Schmidt, and L. W. Riley. 2002. Invasion activity of a *Mycobacterium tuberculosis* peptide presented by the *Escherichia coli* AIDA autotransporter. *Infect. Immun.* **70:**6846–6852.

32. Chamaillard, M., M. Hashimoto, Y. Horie, J. Masumoto, S. Qiu, L. Saab, Y. Ogura, A. Kawasaki, K. Fukase, S. Kusumoto, M. A. Valvano, S. J. Foster, T. W. Mak, G. Nunez, and N. Inohara. 2003. An essential role for NOD1 in host recognition of bacterial peptidoglycan containing diaminopimelic acid. *Nat. Immunol.* **4:**702–707.

33. Chan, E. D., K. R. Morris, J. T. Belisle, P. Hill, L. K. Remigio, P. J. Brennan, and D. W. H. Riches. 2001. Induction of inducible nitric oxide synthase-NO• by lipoarabinomannan of *Mycobacterium tuberculosis* is mediated by MEK1-ERK, MKK7-JNK, and NF-κB signaling pathways. *Infect. Immun.* **69:**2001–2010.

34. Chan, J., X. Fan, S. W. Hunter, P. J. Brennan, and B. R. Bloom. 1991. Lipoarabinomannan, a possible virulence factor involved in persistence of *Mycobacterium tuberculosis* within macrophages. *Infect. Immun.* **59:**1755–1761.

35. Chan, J., T. Fujiwara, P. Brennan, M. McNeil, S. J. Turco, J.-C. Sibille, M. Snapper, P. Aisen, and B. R. Bloom. 1989. Microbial glycolipids: possible virulence factors that scavenge oxygen radicals. *Proc. Natl. Acad. Sci. USA* **86:**2453–2457.

36. Chatterjee, D., A. D. Roberts, K. Lowell, P. J. Brennan, and I. M. Orme. 1992. Structural basis of capacity of lipoarabinomannan to induce secretion of tumor necrosis factor. *Infect. Immun.* **60:**1249–1253.

37. Chitale, S., S. Ehrt, I. Kawamura, T. Fujimura, N. Shimono, N. Anand, S. Lu, L. Cohen-Gould, and L. W. Riley. 2001. Recombinant *Mycobacterium tuberculosis* protein associated with mammalian cell entry. *Cell Microbiol.* **3:**247–254.

38. Chow, J. C., D. W. Young, D. T. Golenbock, W. J. Christ, and F. Gusovsky. 1999. Toll-like receptor-4 mediates lipopolysaccharide-induced signal transduction. *J. Biol. Chem.* **274:**10689–10692.

39. Chu, R. S., D. Askew, E. H. Noss, A. Tobian, A. M. Krieg, and C. V. Harding. 1999. CpG oligodeoxynucleotides down-regulate macrophage class II MHC antigen processing. *J. Immunol.* **163:**1188–1194.

40. Cole, F. S., W. J. Matthews, Jr., T. H. Rossing, D. J. Gash, N. A. Lichtenberg, and J. E. Pennington. 1983. Complement biosynthesis by human bronchoalveolar macrophages. *Clin. Immunol. Immunopathol.* **27:**153–159.

41. Cole, S. T., R. Brosch, J. Parkhill, T. Garnier, C. Churcher, D. Harris, S. V. Gordon, K. Eiglmeier, S. Gas, C. E. I. Barry, F. Tekaia, K. Badcock, D. Basham, D. Brown, T. Chillingworth, R. Connor, R. Davies, K. Devlin, T. Feltwell, S. Gentles, N. Hamlin, S. Holroyd, T. Hornsby, K. Jagels, A. Krogh, J. McLean, S. Moule, L. Murphy, K. Oliver, J. Osborne, M. A. Quail, M.-A. Rajandream, J. Rogers, S. Rutter, K. Seeger, J. Skelton, R. Squares, S. Squares, J. E. Sulston, K. Taylor, S. Whitehead, and B. G. Barrell. 1998.

Deciphering the biology of *Mycobacterium tuberculosis* from the complete genome sequence. *Nature* **393:**537–544.

42. Crandall, E. D., and K. J. Kim. 1991. Alveolar epithelial barrier properties, p. 273–287. *In* R. J. Crystal and J. B. West (ed.), *The Lung: Scientific Foundations.* Raven Press, New York, N.Y.

43. Crowe, L. M., B. J. Spargo, T. Ioneda, B. L. Beaman, and J. H. Crowe. 1994. Interaction of cord factor (α,α′-trehalose-6,6′-dimycolate) with phospholipids. *Biochim. Biophys. Acta* **1194:**53–60.

44. Crystal, R. J. 1991. Alveolar macrophages, p. 527–538. *In* R. J. Crystal and J. B. West (ed.), *The Lung: Scientific Foundations.* Raven Press, New York, N.Y.

45. Cywes, C., N. L. Godenir, H. C. Hoppe, R. R. Scholle, L. M. Steyn, R. E. Kirsch, and M. R. W. Ehlers. 1996. Nonopsonic binding of *Mycobacterium tuberculosis* to human complement receptor type 3 expressed in Chinese hamster ovary cells. *Infect. Immun.* **64:**5373–5383.

46. Cywes, C., H. C. Hoppe, M. Daffe, and M. R. W. Ehlers. Nonopsonic binding of *Mycobacterium tuberculosis* to complement receptor type 3 is mediated by capsular polysaccharides and is strain dependent. *Infect. Immun.* **65:**4258–4266.

47. Dahl, K. E., H. Shiratsuchi, B. D. Hamilton, J. J. Ellner, and Z. Toossi. 1996. Selective induction of transforming growth factor β in human monocytes by lipoarabinomannan of *Mycobacterium tuberculosis. Infect. Immun.* **64:**399–405.

48. D'Arcy Hart, P., and M. R. Young. 1988. Polyanionic agents inhibit phagosome-lysosome fusion in cultured macrophages. *J. Leukoc. Biol.* **43:**179–182.

49. De Costello, A. M., A. Kumar, V. Narayan, M. S. Akbar, S. Ahmed, C. Abou-Zeid, G. A. W. Rook, J. Stanford, and C. Moreno. 1992. Does antibody to mycobacterial antigens, including lipoarabinomannan, limit dissemination in childhood tuberculosis. *Trans. R. Soc. Trop. Med. Hyg.* **86:**686–692.

50. Dobos, K. M., K. H. Khoo, K. M. Swiderek, P. J. Brennan, and J. T. Belisle. 1996. Definition of the full extent of glycosylation of the 45-kilodalton glycoprotein of *Mycobacterium tuberculosis. J. Bacteriol.* **178:**2498–2506.

51. Dorman, S. E., and S. M. Holland. 2000. Interferon-gamma and interleukin-12 pathway defects and human disease. *Cytokine Growth Factor Rev.* **11:**321–333.

52. Douvas, G. S., D. L. Looker, A. E. Vatter, and A. J. Crowle. 1985. Gamma interferon activates human macrophages to become tumoricidal and leishmanicidal but enhances replication of macrophage-associated mycobacteria. *Infect. Immun.* **50:**1–8.

53. Downing, J. F., R. Pasula, J. R. Wright, H. L. Twigg III, and W. J. Martin, Jr. 1995. Surfactant protein A promotes attachment of *Mycobacterium tuberculosis* to alveolar macrophages during infection with human immunodeficiency virus. *Proc. Natl. Acad. Sci. USA* **92:**4848–4852.

54. Ehlers, M. R. W., and M. Daffe. 1998. Interactions between *Mycobacterium tuberculosis* and host cells: are mycobacterial sugars the key? *Trends Microbiol.* **6:**328–335.

55. Eichbaum, Q., P. Clerc, G. Bruns, F. McKeon, and R. A. B. Ezekowitz. 1994. Assignment of the human macrophage mannose receptor gene (MRC1) to 10p13 by *in situ* hybridization and PCR-based somatic cell hybrid mapping. *Genomics* **22:**656–658.

56. Ezekowitz, R. A. B., R. B. Sim, G. G. MacPherson, and S. Gordon. 1985. Interaction of human monocytes, macrophages, and polymorphonuclear leukocytes with zymosan in vitro. *J. Clin. Investig.* **76:**2368–2376.

57. Fels, A., and Z. A. Cohn. 1986. The alveolar macrophage. *J. Appl. Physiol.* **60:**353–369.

58. Fenton, M. J., and D. T. Golenbock. 1998. LPS-binding proteins and receptors. *J. Leukoc. Biol.* **64:**25–32.

59. Ferguson, J. S., D. R. Voelker, F. X. McCormack, and L. S. Schlesinger. 1999. Surfactant protein D binds to *Mycobacterium tuberculosis* bacili and lipoarrabinomannan via carbohydrate-lectin interactions resulting in reduced phagocytosis of the bacteria by macrophages. *J. Immunol.* **163:**312–321.

60. Ferguson, J. S., D. R. Voelker, J. A. Ufnar, and L. S. Schlesinger. 2002. Surfactant protein D inhibition of human macrophage uptake of *Mycobacterium tuberculosis* is indepenndent of bacterial agglutination. *J. Immunol.* **168:**1309–1314.

61. Fietta, A., C. Francioli, and G. Galdroni Grassi. 2000. Mycobacterial lipoarabinomannan affects human polymorphonuclear and mononuclear phagocyte functions differently. *Haematologica* **85:**11–18.

62. Filley, E. A., H. A. Bull, P. M. Dowd, and G. A. W. Rook. 1992. The effect of *Mycobacterium tuberculosis* on the susceptibility of human cells to the stimulatory and toxic effects of tumour necrosis factor. *Immunology* **77:**505–509.

63. Filley, E. A., and G. A. W. Rook. 1991. Effect of mycobacteria on sensitivity to the cytotoxic effects of tumor necrosis factor. *Infect. Immun.* **59:**2567–2572.

64. Fitzgerald, K. A., E. M. Palsson-McDermott, A. G. Bowie, C. A. Jefferies, A. S. Mansell, G. Brady, E. Brint, A. Dunne, P. Gray, M. T. Harte, D. McMurray, D. E. Smith, J. E. Sims, T. A. Bird, and L. A. O'Neill. 2001. Mal (MyD88-adapter-like) is required for Toll-like receptor-4 signal transduction. *Nature* **413:**78–83.

65. Fitzgerald, K. A., D. C. Rowe, B. J. Barnes, D. R. Caffrey, A. Visintin, E. Latz, B. Monks, P. M. Pitha, and D. T. Golenbock. 2003. LPS-TLR4 signaling to IRF-3/7 and NF-κB involves the Toll adapters TRAM and TRIF. *J. Exp. Med.* **198:**1043–1055.

66. Flesselles, B., N. N. Anand, J. Remani, S. M. Loosmore, and M. H. Klein. 1999. Disruption of the mycobacterial cell entry gene of *Mycobacterium bovis* BCG results in a mutant that exhibits a reduced invasiveness for epithelial cells. *FEMS Microbiol. Lett.* **177:**237–242.

67. Floros, J., H. M. Lin, A. García, M. A. Salazar, X. Guo, S. DiAngelo, M. Montano, J. Luo, A. Pardo, and M. Selman. 2000. Surfactant protein genetic marker alleles identify a subgroup of tuberculosis in a Mexican population. *J. Infect. Dis.* **182:**1473–1478.

68. Forget, A., J. C. Benoit, R. Turcotte, and N. Gusew-Chartrand. 1976. Enhanced activity of anti-mycobacterial sera in experimental *Mycobacterium bovis* (BCG) infection in mice. *Infect. Immun.* **13:**1301–1306.

69. Fratti, R. A., J. M. Backer, J. Gruenberg, S. Corvera, and V. Deretic. 2001. Role of phosphatidylinositol 3-kinase and Rab5 effectors in phagosomal biogenesis and mycobacterial phagosome maturation arrest. *J. Cell Biol.* **154:**631–644.

70. Fratti, R. A., J. Chua, I. Vergne, and V. Deretic. 2003. *Mycobacterium tuberculosis* glycosylated phosphatidylinositol causes phagosome maturation arrest. *Proc. Natl. Acad. Sci. USA* **100:**5437–5442.

71. Garred, P., C. Richter, A. B. Andersen, H. O. Madsen, I. Mtoni, A. Svejgaard, and J. Shao. 1997. Mannan-binding lectin in the sub-Saharan HIV and tuberculosis epidemics. *Scand. J. Immunol.* **46:**204–208.

72. Gatfield, J., and J. Pieters. 2000. Essential role for cholesterol in entry of mycobacteria into macrophages. *Science* **288:**1647–1650.

73. Gaynor, C. D., F. X. McCormack, D. R. Voelker, S. E. McGowan, and L. S. Schlesinger. 1995. Pulmonary surfactant protein A mediates enhanced phagocytosis of *Mycobacterium tuberculosis* by a direct interaction with human macrophages. *J. Immunol.* **155:**5343–5351.

74. Gehring, A. J., R. E. Rojas, D. H. Canaday, D. L. Lakey, C. V. Harding, and W. H. Boom. 2003. The *Mycobacterium tuberculosis* 19-kilodalton lipoprotein inhibits gamma interferon-regulated HLA-DR and Fc gamma R1 on human macrophages through Toll-like receptor 2. *Infect. Immun.* **71:**4487–4497.

75. Geijtenbeek, T. B., S. J. Van Vliet, E. A. Koppel, M. Sanchez-Hernandez, C. M. Vandenbroucke-Grauls, B. Appelmelk, and Y. Van Kooyk. 2003. Mycobacteria target DC-SIGN to suppress dendritic cell function. *J. Exp. Med.* **197:**7–17.

76. Germann, T., E. Rude, F. Mattner, and M. K. Gately. 1995. The IL-12 p40 homodimer as a specific antagonist of the IL-12 heterodimer. *Immunol. Today* **16:**500–501.

77. Girardin, S. E., I. G. Boneca, L. A. Carneiro, A. Antignac, M. Jehanno, J. Viala, K. Tedin, M. K. Taha, A. Labigne, U. Zahringer, A. J. Coyle, P. S. DiStefano, J. Bertin, P. J. Sansonetti, and D. J. Philpott. 2003. Nod1 detects a unique muropeptide from gram-negative bacterial peptidoglycan. *Science* **300:**1584–1587.

78. Goerdt, S., and C. E. Orfanos. 1999. Other functions, other genes: alternative activation of antigen-presenting cells. *Immunity* **10:**137–142.

79. Goren, M. B., P. D. Hart, M. R. Young, and J. A. Armstrong. 1976. Prevention of phagosome-lysosome fusion in cultured macrophages by sulfatides of *Mycobacterium tuberculosis*. *Proc. Natl. Acad. Sci. USA* **73:**2510–2514.

80. Goswami, S., S. Sarkar, J. Basu, M. Kundu, and P. Chakrabarti. 1994. Mycotin: a lectin involved in the adherence of mycobacteria to macrophages. *FEBS Lett.* **355:**183–186.

81. Graves, B. J. 1995. Integrin binding revealed. *Nature Struct. Biol.* **2:**181–183.

82. Harris, E. S., T. M. McIntyre, S. M. Prescott, and G. A. Zimmerman. 2000. The leukocyte integrins. *J. Biol. Chem.* **275:**23409–23412.

83. Hayashi, F., K. D. Smith, A. Ozinsky, T. R. Hawn, E. C. Yi, D. R. Goodlett, J. K. Eng, S. Akira, D. M. Underhill, and A. Aderem. 2001. The innate immune response to bacterial flagellin is mediated by Toll-like receptor 5. *Nature* **410:**1099–1103.

84. Heldwein, K. A., M. D. Liang, T. K. Andresen, K. E. Thomas, A. M. Marty, N. Cuesta, S. N. Vogel, and M. J. Fenton. 2003. TLR2 and TLR4 serve distinct roles in the host immune response against Mycobacterium bovis BCG. *J. Leukoc. Biol.* **74:**277–286.

85. Hemmi, H., O. Takeuchi, T. Kawai, T. Kaisho, S. Sato, H. Sanjo, M. Matsumoto, K. Hoshino, H. Wagner, K. Takeda, and S. Akira. 2000. A Toll-like receptor recognizes bacterial DNA. *Nature* **408:**740–745.

86. Hernandez-Pando, R., M. Jeyanathan, G. Mengistu, D. Aguilar, H. Orozco, M. Harboe, G. A. Rook, and G. Bjune. 2000. Persistence of DNA from *Mycobacterium tuberculosis* in superficially normal lung tissue during latent infection. *Lancet* **356:**2133–2138.

87. Hertz, C. J., S. M. Kiertscher, P. J. Godowski, D. A. Bouis, M. V. Norgard, M. D. Roth, and R. L. Modlin. 2001. Microbial lipopeptides stimulate dendritic cell maturation via toll-like receptor 2. *J. Immunol.* **166:**2444–2450.

88. Hetland, G., and H. G. Wiker. 1994. Antigen 85C on *Mycobacterium bovis* BCG and *M. tuberculosis* promotes monocyte-CR3-mediated uptake of microbeads coated with mycobacterial products. *Immunology* **82:**445–449.

89. Hirsch, C. S., J. J. Ellner, D. G. Russell, and E. A. Rich. 1994. Complement receptor-mediated uptake and tumor

necrosis factor-alpha-mediated growth inhibition of *Mycobacterium tuberculosis* by human alveolar macrophages. *J. Immunol.* **152:**743–753.

90. Hirsch, C. S., T. Yoneda, L. Averill, J. J. Ellner, and Z. Toossi. 1994. Enhancement of intracellular growth of *Mycobacterium tuberculosis* in human monocytes by transforming growth factor-β1. *J. Infect. Dis.* **170:**1229–1237.

91. Hirschfeld, M., J. J. Weis, V. Toshchakov, C. A. Salkowski, M. J. Cody, D. C. Ward, N. Qureshi, S. M. Michalek, and S. N. Vogel. 2001. Signaling by toll-like receptor 2 and 4 agonists results in differential gene expression in murine macrophages. *Infect. Immun.* **69:**1477–1482.

92. Hoebe, K., X. Du, P. Georgel, E. Janssen, K. Tabeta, S. O. Kim, J. Goode, P. Lin, N. Mann, S. Mudd, K. Crozat, S. Sovath, J. Han, and B. Beutler. 2003. Identification of Lps2 as a key transducer of MyD88-independent TIR signalling. *Nature* **424:**743–748.

93. Hoppe, H. C., J. M. De Wet, C. Cywes, M. Daffe, and M. R. Ehlers. 1997. Identification of phosphatidylinositol mannoside as a mycobacterial adhesin mediating both direct and opsonic binding to nonphagocytic mammalian cells. *Infect. Immun.* **65:**3896–3905.

94. Horng, T., G. M. Barton, and R. Medzhitov. 2001. TIRAP: an adapter molecule in the Toll signaling pathway. *Nat. Immunol.* **2:**835–841.

95. Hu, C., T. Mayadas-Norton, K. Tanaka, J. Chan, and P. Salgame. 2000. *Mycobacterium tuberculosis* infection in complement receptor 3-deficient mice. *J. Immunol.* **165:**2596–2602.

96. Ingalls, R. R., and D. T. Golenbock. 1995. CD11c/CD18, a transmembrane signaling receptor for lipopolysaccharide. *J. Exp. Med.* **181:**1473–1479.

97. Jones, B. W., T. K. Means, K. A. Heldwein, M. A. Keen, P. J. Hill, J. T. Belisle, and M. J. Fenton. 2001. Different toll-like receptor agonists induce distinct macrophage responses. *J. Leukoc. Biol.* **69:**1036–1044.

98. Juffermans, N. P., A. Verbon, J. T. Belisle, P. J. Hill, P. Speelman, S. J. H. Van Deventer, and T. Van der Poll. 2000. Mycobacterial lipoarabinomannan induces an inflammatory response in the mouse lung. A role for interleukin-1. *Am. J. Respir. Crit. Care Med.* **162:**486–489.

99. Kaisho, T., O. Takeuchi, T. Kawai, K. Hoshino, and S. Akira. 2001. Endotoxin-induced maturation of MyD88-deficient dendritic cells. *J. Immunol.* **166:**5688–5694.

100. Kang, B. K., and L. S. Schlesinger. 1998. Characterization of mannose receptor-dependent phagocytosis mediated by *Mycobacterium tuberculosis* lipoarabinomannan. *Infect. Immun.* **66:**2769–2777.

101. Kang, T. J., and G. T. Chae. 2001. Detection of Toll-like receptor 2 (TLR2) mutation in the lepromatous leprosy patients. *FEMS Immunol. Med. Microbiol.* **31:**53–58.

102. Kawasaki, K., S. Akashi, R. Shimazu, T. Yoshida, K. Miyake, and M. Nishijima. 2000. Mouse toll-like receptor 4.MD-2 complex mediates lipopolysaccharide-mimetic signal transduction by Taxol. *J. Biol. Chem.* **275:**2251–2254.

103. Khanna, K. V., C. S. Choi, G. Gekker, P. K. Peterson, and T. W. Molitor. 1996. Differential infection of porcine alveolar macrophage subpopulations by nonopsonized *Mycobacterium bovis* involves CD14 receptors. *J. Leukoc. Biol.* **60:**214–220.

104. Khoo, K.-H., A. Dell, H. R. Morris, P. J. Brennan, and D. Chatterjee. 1995. Inositol phosphate capping of the nonreducing termini of lipoarabinomannan from rapidly growing strains of *Mycobacterium. J. Biol. Chem.* **270:**12380–12389.

105. Knutson, K. L., Z. Hmama, P. Herrera-Velit, R. Rochford, and N. E. Reiner. 1997. Lipoarabinomannan of *Mycobacterium tuberculosis* promotes portein tyrosine dephosphorylation and inhibition of mitogen-activated protein kinase in human mononuclear phagocytes. *J. Biol. Chem.* **273:**645–652.

106. Kurt-Jones, E. A., L. Popova, L. Kwinn, L. M. Haynes, L. P. Jones, R. A. Tripp, E. E. Walsh, M. W. Freeman, D. T. Golenbock, L. J., Anderson, and R. W. Finberg. 2000. Pattern recognition receptors TLR4 and CD14 mediate response to respiratory syncytial virus. *Nat. Immunol.* **1:**398–401.

107. Kusner, D. J., C. F. Hall, and L. S. Schlesinger. 1996. Activation of phospholipase D is tightly coupled to the phagocytosis of *Mycobacterium tuberculosis* or opsonized zymosan by human macrophages. *J. Exp. Med.* **184:**585–595.

108. Le Cabec, V., S. Carreno, A. Moisand, C. Bordier, and I. Maridonneau-Parini. 2002. Complement receptor 3 (CD11b/CD18) mediates type I and type II phagocytosis during nonopsonic and opsonic phagocytosis, respectively. *J. Immunol.* **169:**2003–2009.

109. Le Cabec, V., C. Cols, and I. Maridonneau-Parini. 2000. Nonopsonic phagocytosis of zymosan and *Mycobacterium kansasii* by CR3 (CD11b/CD18) involves distinct molecular determinants and is or is not coupled with NADPH oxidase activation. *Infect. Immun.* **68:**4736–4745.

110. Lemaitre, B., E. Nicolas, L. Michaut, J. M. Reichhart, and J. A. Hoffmann. 1996. The dorsoventral regulatory gene cassette spatzle/Toll/cactus controls the potent antifungal response in *Drosophila* adults. *Cell* **86:**973–983.

111. Lien, E., T. J. Sellati, A. Yoshimura, T. H. Flo, G. Rawadi, R. W. Finberg, J. D. Carroll, T. Espevik, R. R. Ingalls, J. D. Radolf, and D. T. Golenbock. 1999. Toll-like receptor 2 functions as a pattern recognition receptor for diverse bacterial products. *J. Biol. Chem.* **574:**33419–33425.

112. Lin, Y., M. Zhang, and P. F. Barnes. 1998. Chemokine production by a human alveolar epithelial cell line in response to *Mycobacterium tuberculosis. Infect. Immun.* **66:**1121–1126.

113. Lipscombe, R. J., D. W. Beatty, M. Ganczakowski, E. A. Goddard, T. Jenkins, Y. L. Lau, A. B. Spurdle, M. Sumiya, J. A. Summerfield, and M. W. Turner. 1996. Mutations in the human mannose-binding protein gene: frequencies in several population groups. *Eur. J. Hum. Genet.* **4:**13–19.

114. Loftus, J. C., J. W. Smith, and M. H. Ginsberg. 1994. Integrin-mediated cell adhesion: the extracellular face. *J. Biol. Chem.* **269:**25235–25238.

115. Loike, J. D., B. Sodeik, L. Cao, S. Leucona, J. I. Weitz, P. A. Detmers, S. D. Wright, and S. C. Silverstin. 1991. CD11c/CD18 on neutrophils recognizes a domain at the N terminus of the Aα chain of fibrinogen. *Proc. Natl. Acad. Sci. USA* **88:**1044–1048.

116. Lopez, M., L. M. Sly, Y. Luu, D. Young, H. Cooper, and N. E. Reiner. 2003. The 19-kDa *Mycobacterium tuberculosis* protein induces macrophage apoptosis through Toll-like receptor-2. *J. Immunol.* **170:**2409–2416.

117. Lorenz, E., J. P. Mira, K. L. Cornish, N. C. Arbour, and D. A. Schwartz. 2000. A novel polymorphism in the toll-like receptor 2 gene and its potential association with staphylococcal infection. *Infect. Immun.* **68:**6398–6401.

118. Maeda, N., J. Nigou, J. L. Herrmann, M. Jackson, A. Amara, P. H. Lagrange, G. Puzo, B. Gicquel, and O. Neyrolles. 2003. The cell surface receptor DC-SIGN discriminates between *Mycobacterium* species through selective recognition of the mannose caps on lipoarabinomannan. *J. Biol. Chem.* **278:**5513–5516.

119. Maiti, D., A. Bhattacharyya, and J. Basu. 2001. Lipoarabinomannan from *Mycobacterium tuberculosis* promotes

macrophage survival by phosphorylating Bad through a phosphatidylinositol 3-kinase/Akt pathway. *J. Biol. Chem.* **276:**329–333.

120. Malik, Z. A., G. D. Denning, and D. J. Kusner. 2000. Inhibition of CA^{2+} signaling by *Mycobacterium tuberculosis* is associated with reduced phagosome-lysosome fusion and increased survival within human macrophages. *J. Exp. Med.* **191.**287–302.

121. Malik, Z. A., S. S. Iyer, and D. J. Kusner. 2001. *Mycobacterium tuberculosis* phagosomes exhibit altered calmodulin-dependent signal transduction: contribution to inhibition of phagosome-lysosome fusion and intracellular survival in human macrophages. *J. Immunol.* **166:**3392–3401.

122. Malik, Z. A., C. R. Thompson, S. Hashimi, B. Porter, S. S. Iyer, and D. J. Kusner. 2003. Cutting edge: *Mycobacterium tuberculosis* blocks Ca^{2+} signaling and phagosome maturation in human macrophages via specific inhibition of sphingosine kinase. *J. Immunol.* **170:**2811–2815.

123. Marth, T., and B. L. Kelsall. 1997. Regulation of interleukin-12 by complement receptor 3 signaling. *J. Exp. Med.* **185:**1987–1995.

124. Matsushita, M. 1996. The lectin pathway of the complement system. *Microbiol. Immunol.* **40:**887–893.

125. McDonough, K. A., and Y. Kress. 1995. Cytotoxicity for lung epithelial cells is a virulence-associated phenotype of *Mycobacterium tuberculosis*. *Infect. Immun.* **63:**4802–4811.

126. McPhaden, A. R., and K. Whaley. 1993. Complement biosynthesis by mononuclear phagocytes. *Immunol. Res.* **12:**213–232.

127. Means, T. K., B. W. Jones, A. B. Schromm, B. A. Shurtleff, J. A. Smith, J. Keane, D. T. Golenbock, S. N. Vogel, and M. J. Fenton. 2001. Differential effects of a toll-like receptor antagonist on *Mycobacterium tuberculosis*-induced macrophage responses. *J. Immunol.* **166:**4074–4082.

128. Means, T. K., E. Lien, A. Yoshimura, S. Wang, D. T. Golenbock, and M. J. Fenton. 1999. The CD14 ligands lipoarabinomannan and lipopolysaccharide differ in their requirement for toll-like receptors. *J. Immunol.* **163:**6748–6755.

129. Means, T. K., S. Wang, E. Lien, A. Yoshimura, D. T. Golenbock, and M. J. Fenton. 1999. Human toll-like receptors mediate cellular activation by *Mycobacterium tuberculosis*. *J. Immunol.* **163:**3920–3927.

130. Medzhitov, R., and C. Janeway, Jr. 2000. Innate immunity. *N. Engl. J. Med.* **343:**338–344.

131. Medzhitov, R., P. Preston-Hurlburt, and C. A. Janeway, Jr. 1997. A human homologue of the *Drosophia* Toll protein signals activation of adaptive immunity. *Nature* **388:**394–397.

132. Mehta, P. K., C. H. King, E. H. White, J. J. Murtagh, Jr., and F. D. Quinn. 1996. Comparison of in vitro models for the study of *Mycobacterium tuberculosis* invasion and intracellular replication. *Infect. Immun.* **64:**2673–2679.

133. Menozzi, F. D., R. Bischoff, E. Fort, M. J. Brennan, and C. Locht. 1998. Molecular characterization of the mycobacterial heparin-binding hemagglutinin, a mycobacterial adhesin. *Proc. Natl. Acad. Sci. USA* **95:**12625–12630.

134. Michelsen, K. S., A. Aicher, M. Mohaupt, T. Hartung, S. Dimmeler, C. J. Kirschning, and R. R. Schumann. 2001. The role of toll-like receptors (TLRs) in bacteria-induced maturation of murine dendritic cells (DCS). Peptidoglycan and lipoteichoic acid are inducers of DC maturation and require TLR2. *J. Biol. Chem.* **276:**25680–25686.

135. Mokoena, T., and S. Gordon. 1987. Human macrophage activation: modulation of mannosyl, fucosyl receptor activity in vitro by lymphokines, gamma and alpha interferons, and dexamethasone. *J. Clin. Investig.* **75:**624–631.

136. Moss, J. E., A. O. Aliprantis, and A. Zychlinsky. 1999. The regulation of apoptosis by microbial pathogens. *Int. Rev. Cytol.* **187:**203–259.

137. Mueller-Ortiz, S. L., A. R. Wanger, and S. J. Norris. 2001. Mycobacterial protein HbhA binds human complement component C3. *Infect. Immun.* **69:**7501–7511.

138. Munder, M., K. Eichmann, and M. Modolell. 1998 Alternative metabolic states in murine macrophages reflected by the nitric oxide synthase/arginase balance: competitive regulation by CD4$^+$ T cells correlates with Th1/Th2 phenotype. *J. Immunol.* **160:**5347–5354.

139. Myones, B. L., J. G. Dalzell, N. Hogg, and G. D. Ross. 1988. Neutrophil and monocyte cell surface p150,955 has iC3b-receptor (CR4) activity resembling CR3. *J. Clin. Investig.* **82:**640–651.

140. Nigou, J., C. Zelle-Rieser, M. Gilleron, M. Thurnher, and G. Puzo. 2001. Mannosylated liparabinomannans inhibit IL-12 production by human dendritic cells: evidence for a negative signal delivered through the mannose receptor. *J. Immunol.* **166:**7477–7485.

141. Noss, E. H., C. V. Harding, and W. H. Boom. 2000. *Mycobacterium tuberculosis* inhibits MHC class II antigen processing in murine bone marrow macrophages. *Cell. Immunol.* **201:**63–74.

142. Noss, E. H., R. K. Pai, T. J. Sellati, J. D. Radolf, J. Belisle, D. T. Golenbock, W. H. Boom, and C. V. Harding. 2001. Toll-like receptor 2-dependent inhibition of macrophage class II MHC expression and antigen processing by 19-kDa lipoprotein of *Mycobacterium tuberculosis*. *J. Immunol.* **167:**910–918.

143. Ohashi, K., V. Burkart, S. Flohe, and H. Kolb. 2000. Cutting edge: heat shock protein 60 is a putative endogenous ligand of the toll-like receptor-4 complex. *J. Immunol.* **164:**558–561.

144. Ohmori, Y., and T. A. Hamilton. 2001. Requirement for STAT1 in LPS-induced gene expression in macrophages. *J. Leukoc. Biol.* **69:**598–604.

145. Okamura, Y., M. Watari, E. S. Jerud, D. W. Young, S. T. Ishizaka, J. Rose, J. C. Chow, and J. F. Strauss III. 2001. The extra domain A of fibronectin activates Toll-like receptor 4. *J. Biol. Chem.* **276:**10229–10233.

146. O'Neill, L. A. 2002. Signal transduction pathways activated by the IL-1 receptor/toll-like receptor superfamily. *Curr. Top. Microbiol. Immunol.* **270:**47–61.

147. Opie, E. L., and J. D. Aronson. 1927. Tubercle bacilli in latent tuberculous lesions and in lung tissue without tuberculous lesions. *Arch. Pathol. Lab. Med.* **4:**1–21.

148. Oppmann, B., R. Lesley, B. Blom, J. C. Timans, Y. Xu, B. Hunte, F. Vega, N. Yu, J. Wang, K. Singh, F. Zonin, E. Vaisberg, T. Churakova, M. Liu, D. Gorman, J. Wagner, S. Zurawski, Y. Liu, J. S. Abrams, K. W. Moore, D. Rennick, R. Waal-Malefyt, C. Hannum, J. F. Bazan, and R. A. Kastelein. 2000. Novel p19 protein engages IL-12p40 to form a cytokine, IL-23, with biological activities similar as well as distinct from IL-12. *Immunity* **13:**715–725.

149. Oren, R., A. E. Farnham, K. Saito, E. Milofsky, and M. L. Karnovsky. 1963. Metabolic patterns in three types of phagocytizing cells. *J. Cell Biol.* **17:**487–501.

150. Orr, S. L., and P. Tobias. 2000. LPS and LAM activation of the U373 astrocytoma cell line: differential requirement for CD14. *J. Endotoxin Res.* **6:**215–222.

151. Ortalo-Magné, A., M.-A. Dupont, A. Lemassu, A. B., Andersen, P. Gounon, and M. Daffé. 1995. Molecular composition of the outermost capsular material of the tubercle bacillus. Microbiology **141:**1609–1620.

152. Oshiumi, H., M. Matsumoto, K. Funami, T. Akazawa, and T. Seya. 2003. TICAM-1, an adaptor molecule that partici-

pates in Toll-like receptor 3-mediated interferon-beta induction. *Nat. Immunol.* **4:**161–167.

153. O'Toole, T. E., Y. Katagiri, R. J. Faull, K. Peter, R. Tamura, V. Quaranta, J. C. Loftus, S. J. Shattil, and M. H. Ginsberg. 1994. Integrin cytoplasmic domains mediate inside-out signal transduction. *J. Cell Biol.* **124:**1047–1059.

154. Pasula, R., J. F. Downing, J. R. Wright, D. L. Kachel, T. E. Davis, Jr., and W. J. Martin, Jr. 1997. Surfactant protein A (SP-A) mediates attachment of *Mycobacterium tuberculosis* to murine alveolar macrophages. *Am. J. Respir. Cell Mol. Biol.* **17:**209–217.

155. Perera, P. Y., T. N. Mayadas, O. Takeuchi, S. Akira, M. Zaks-Zilberman, S. M. Goyert, and S. N. Vogel. 2001. CD11b/CD18 acts in concert with CD14 and toll-like receptor (TLR) 4 to elicit full lipopolysaccharide and taxol-inducible gene expression. *J. Immunol.* **166:**574–581.

156. Peterson, P. K., G. Gekker, S. Hu, W. S. Sheng, W. R., Anderson, R. J. Ulevitch, P. S. Tobias, K. V. Gustafson, T. W. Molitor, and C. C. Chao. 1995. CD14 receptor-mediated uptake of nonopsonized *Mycobacterium tuberculosis* by human microglia. *Infect. Immun.* **63:**1598–1602.

157. Peyron, P., C. Bordier, E. N. N'Diaye, and I. Maridonneau-Parini. 2000. Nonopsonic phagocytosis of *Mycobacterium kansasii* by human neutrophils depends on cholesterol and is mediated by CR3 associated with glycosylphosphatidylinositol-anchored proteins. *J. Immunol.* **165:**5186–5191.

158. Phelps, D. S., and R. M. Rose. 1991. Increased recovery of surfactant protein A in AIDS-related pneumonia. *Am. Rev. Respir. Dis.* **143:**1072–1075.

159. Phyu, S., T. Mustafa, T. Hofstad, R. Nilsen, R. Fosse, and G. Bjune. 1998. A mouse model for latent tuberculosis. *Scand. J. Infect. Dis.* **30:**59–68.

160. Pitt, A., L. S. Mayorga, P. D. Stahl, and A. L. Schwartz. 1992. Alterations in the protein composition of maturing phagosomes. *J. Clin. Investig.* **90:**1978–1983.

161. Polotsky, V. Y., J. T. Belisle, K. Mikusova, R. A. B. Ezekowitz, and K. A. Joiner. 1997. Interaction of human mannose-binding protein with *Mycobacterium avium*. *J. Infect. Dis.* **175:**1159–1168.

162. Prigozy, T. I., P. A. Sieling, D. Clemens, P. L. Stewart, S. M. Behar, S. A. Porcelli, M. B. Brenner, R. L. Modlin, and M. Kronenberg. 1997. The mannose receptor delivers lipoglycan antigens to endosomes for presentation to T cells by CD1b molecules. *Immunity* **6:**187–197.

163. Prinzis, S., D. Chatterjee, and P. J. Brennan. 1993. Structure and antigenicity of lipoarabinomannan from *Mycobacterium bovis* BCG. *J. Gen. Microbiol.* **139:**2649–2658.

164. Ramanathan V. D., J. Curtis, and J. L. Turk. 1980. Activation of the alternative pathway of complement by mycobacteria and cord factor. *Infect. Immun.* **29:**30–35.

165. Ratliff, T. L., R. McCarthy, W. B. Telle, and E. J. Brown. 1993. Purification of a mycobacterial adhesion for fibronectin. *Infect. Immun.* **61:**1889–1894.

166. Re, F., and J. L. Strominger. 2001. Toll-like receptor 2 (TLR2) and TLR4 differentially activate human dendritic cells. *J. Biol. Chem.* **276:**37692–37699.

167. Reiling, N., C. Holscher, A. Fehrenbach, S. Kroger, C. J. Kirschning, S. Goyert, and S. Ehlers. 2002. Cutting edge: Toll-like receptor (TLR)2- and TLR4-mediated pathogen recognition in resistance to airborne infection with *Mycobacterium tuberculosis*. *J. Immunol.* **169:**3480–3484.

168. Reyes, J. M., and P. B. Putong. 1980. Association of pulmonary alveolar lipoproteinosis with mycobacterial infection. *Am. J. Clin. Pathol.* **74:**478–485.

169. Riedel, D. D., and S. H. E. Kaufmann. 2000. Differential tolerance induction by lipoarabinomannan and lipopolysac-

charide in human macrophages. *Microbes Infect.* **2:**463–471.

170. Rieu, P., T. Ueda, I. Haruta, C. P. Sharma, and M. A. Arnaout. 1994. The A-domain of b2 integrin CR3 (CD11b/CD18) is a receptor for the hookworm-derived neutrophil adhesion inhibitor NIF. *J. Cell Biol.* **127:**2081–2091.

171. Roach, S. K., and J. S. Schorey. 2002. Differential regulation of the mitogen-activated protein kinases by pathogenic and nonpathogenic mycobacteria. *Infect. Immun.* **70:**3040–3052.

172. Roach, T. I. A., C. H. Barton, D. Chatterjee, and J. M. Blackwell. 1993. Macrophage activation: lipoarabinomannan from avirulent and virulent strains of *Mycobacterium tuberculosis* differentially induces the early genes c-*fos*, KC, JE, and tumor necrosis factor-alpha. *J. Immunol.* **150:**1886–1896.

173. Rojas, M., L. F. Garcia, J. Nigou, G. Puzo, and M. Olivier. 2000. Mannosylated lipoarabinomannan antagonizes *Mycobacterium tuberculosis*-induced macrophage apoptosis by altering Ca^{+2}-dependent cell signaling. *J. Infect. Dis.* **182:**240–251.

174. Rourke, F. J., S. S. Fan, and M. S. Wilder. 1979. Anticomplementary activity of tuberculin: relationship to platelet aggregation and lytic response. *Infect. Immun.* **23:**160–167.

175. Savedra, R., Jr., R. L. Delude, R. R. Ingalls, M. J. Fenton, and D. T. Golenbock. 1996. Mycobacterial lipoarabinomannan recognition requires a receptor that shares components of the endotoxin signaling system. *J. Immunol.* **157:**2549–2554.

176. Schlesinger, L. S. 1993. Macrophage phagocytosis of virulent but not attenuated strains of *Mycobacterium tuberculosis* is mediated by mannose receptors in addition to complement receptors. *J. Immunol.* **150:**2920–2930.

177. Schlesinger, L. S. 1998. *Mycobacterium tuberculosis* and the complement system. *Trends Microbiol.* **6:**47–49.

178. Schlesinger, L. S., C. G. Bellinger-Kawahara, N. R. Payne, and M. A. Horwitz. 1990. Phagocytosis of *Mycobacterium tuberculosis* is mediated by human monocyte complement receptors and complement component C3. *J. Immunol.* **144:**2771–2780.

179. Schlesinger, L. S., and M. A. Horwitz. 1991. Phagocytosis of *Mycobacterium leprae* by human monocyte-derived macrophages is mediated by complement receptors CR1(CD35), CR3(CD11b/CD18), and CR4(CD11c/CD18), and interferon gamma activation inhibits complement receptor function and phagocytosis of this bacterium. *J. Immunol.* **147:**1983–1994.

180. Schlesinger, L. S., and M. A. Horwitz. 1994. A role for natural antibody in the pathogenesis of leprosy: antibody in nonimmune serum mediates C3 fixation to the *Mycobacterium leprae* surface and hence phagocytosis by human mononuclear phagocytes. *Infect. Immun.* **62:**280–289.

181. Schlesinger, L. S., S. R. Hull, and T. M. Kaufman. 1994. Binding of the terminal mannosyl units of lipoarabinomannan from a virulent strain of *Mycobacterium tuberculosis* to human macrophages. *J. Immunol.* **152:**4070–4079.

182. Schlesinger, L. S., T. M. Kaufman, S. Iyer, S. R. Hull, and L. K. Marciando. 1996. Differences in mannose receptor-mediated uptake of lipoarabinomannan from virulent and attenuated strains of *Mycobacterium tuberculosis* by human macrophages. *J. Immunol.* **157:**4568–4575.

183. Schneeberger, E. E. 1991. Alveolar type I cells, p. 229–234. In R. J. Crystal and J. B. West (ed.), The Lung: Scientific Foundations. Raven Press, New York, N. Y.

184. Schorey, J. S., M. C. Carroll, and E. J. Brown. 1997. A macrophage invasion mechanism of pathogenic mycobacteria. *Science* **277:**1091–1093.

185. Schreiber, S., S. L. Perkins, S. L. Teitelbaum, J. Chappel, P. D. Stahl, and J. S. Blum. 1993. Regulation of mouse bone marrow macrophage mannose receptor expression and activation by prostaglandin E and IFN-gamma. *J. Immunol.* **151:**4973–4981.

186. Schwebach, J. R., A. Glatman-Freeman, L. Gunther-Cummins, Z. Dai, J. B. Robbins, R. Schneerson, and A. Casadevall. 2002. Glucan is a component of the *Mycobacterium tuberculosis* surface that is expressed in vitro and in vivo. *Infect. Immun.* **70:**2566–2575.

187. Selvaraj, P., P. R. Narayannan, and A. M. Reetha. 1999. Association of functional mutant homozygotes of the mannose binding protein gene with susceptibility to pulmonary tuberculosis in India. *Tubercle Lung Dis.* **79:**221–227.

188. Shams, H., B. Wizel, D. L. Lakey, B. Samten, R. Vankayalapati, R. H. Valdivia, R. L. Kitchens, D. E. Griffith, and P. F. Barnes. 2003. The CD14 receptor does not mediate entry of *Mycobacterium tuberculosis* into human mononuclear phagocytes. *FEMS Immunol. Med. Microbiol.* **36:**63–69.

189. Shepard, C. C. 1957. Growth characteristics of tubercle bacilli and certain other mycobacteria in HeLa cells. *J. Exp. Med.* **105:**39–48.

190. Shepard, C. C. 1958. A comparison of the growth of selected mycobacteria in HeLa, monkey kidney, and human amnion cells in tissue culture. *J. Exp. Med.* **107:**237–246.

191. Shimazu, R., S. Akashi, H. Ogata, Y. Nagai, K. Fukudome, K. Miyake, and M. Kimoto. 1999. MD-2, a molecule that confers lipopolysaccharide responsiveness on Toll-like receptor 4. *J. Exp. Med.* **189:**1777–1782.

192. Shimono, N., L. Morici, N. Casali, S. Cantrell, B. Sidders, S. Ehrt, and L. W. Riley. 2003. Hypervirulent mutant of *Mycobacterium tuberculosis* resulting from disruption of the *mce1* operon. *Proc. Natl. Acad. Sci. USA* **100:**15918–15923.

193. Siddiqui, M. R., S. Meisner, K. Tosh, K. Balakrishnan, S. Ghei, S. E. Fisher, M. Golding, N. P. S. Narayan, T. Sitaraman, U. Sengupta, R. Pitchappan, and A. V. S. Hill. 2001. A major susceptibility locus for leprosy in India maps to chromosome 10p13. *Nat. Genet.* **27:**439–441.

194. Sieling, P. A., D. Chatterjee, S. A. Porcelli, T. I. Prigozy, R. J. Mazzaccaro, T. Soriano, B. R. Bloom, M. B. Brenner, M. Kronenberg, P. J. Brennan, and R. L. Modlin. 1995. CD1-restricted T cell recognition of microbial lipoglycan antigens. *Science* **269:**227–230.

195. Soilleux, E. J., L. S. Morris, G. Leslie, J. Chehimi, Q. Luo, E. Levroney, J. Trowsdale, L. J. Montaner, R. W. Doms, D. Weissman, N. Coleman, and B. Lee. 2002. Constitutive and induced expression of DC-SIGN on dendritic cell and macrophage subpopulations in situ and in vitro. *J. Leukoc. Biol.* **71:**445–457.

196. Spargo, B. J., L. M. Crowe, T. Ioneda, B. L. Beaman, and J. H. Crowe. 1991. Cord factor (α,α-trehalose 6,6'-dimycolate) inhibits fusion between phospholipid vesicles. *Proc. Natl. Acad. Sci. USA* **88:**737–740.

197. Speert, D. P., and S. C. Silverstein. 1985. Phagocytosis of unopsonized zymosan by human monocyte-derived macrophages: maturation and inhibition by mannan. *J. Leukoc. Biol.* **38:**655–658.

198. Stahl, P. D. 1990. The macrophage mannose receptor: current status. *Am. J. Respir. Cell Mol. Biol.* **2:**317–318.

199. Stahl, P. D., and R. A. Ezekowitz. 1998. The mannose receptor is a pattern recognition receptor involved in host defense. *Curr. Opin. Immunol.* **10:**50–55.

200. Stein, D., S. Roth, E. Vogelsang, and C. Nusslein-Volhard. 1991. The polarity of the dorsoventral axis in the *Drosophila* embryo is defined by an extracellular signal. *Cell* **65:**725–735.

201. Stein, M., S. Keshav, N. Harris, and S. Gordon. 1992. Interleukin 4 potently enhances murine macrophage mannose receptor activity: a marker of alternative immunologic macrophage activation. *J. Exp. Med.* **176:**287–292.

202. Stokes, R. W., I. D. Haidl, W. A. Jefferies, and D. P. Speert. 1993. Mycobacteria-macrophage interactions: macrophage phenotype determines the nonopsonic binding of *Mycobacterium tuberculosis* to murine macrophages. *J. Immunol.* **151:**7067–7076.

203. Strunk, R. C., D. M. Eidlen, and R. J. Mason. 1988. Pulmonary alveolar type II epithelial cells synthesize and secrete proteins of the classical and alternative complement pathways. *J. Clin. Investig.* **81:**1419–1426.

204. Sugawara, I., H. Yamada, C. Li, S. Mizuno, O. Takeuchi, and S. Akira. 2003. Mycobacterial infection in TLR2 and TLR6 knockout mice. *Microbiol. Immunol.* **47:**327–336.

205. Tailleux, L., O. Schwartz, J. L. Herrmann, E. Pivert, M. Jackson, A. Amara, L. Legres, D. Dreher, L. P. Nicod, J. C. Gluckman, P. H. Lagrange, B. Gicquel, and O. Neyrolles. 2003. DC-SIGN is the major *Mycobacterium tuberculosis* receptor on human dendritic cells. *J. Exp. Med.* **197:**121–127.

206. Takeda, K., T. Kaisho, and S. Akira. 2003. Toll-like receptors. *Annu. Rev. Immunol.* **21:**335–376.

207. Taylor, M. E., K. Bezouska, and K. Drickamer. 1992. Contribution to ligand binding by multiple carbohydrate-recognition domains in the macrophage mannose receptor. *J. Biol. Chem.* **267:**1719–1726.

208. Teitelbaum, R., A. Glatman-Freedman, and B. Chen. 1998. A mAb recognizing a surface antigen of *Mycobacterium tuberculosis* enhances host survival. *Proc. Natl. Acad. Sci. USA* **95:**15688–15693.

209. Tekaia, F., S. V. Gordon, T. Garnier, R. Brosch, B. G. Barrell, and S. T. Cole. 1999. Analysis of the proteome of *Mycobacterium tuberculosis* in silico. *Tubercle Lung Dis.* **79:**329–342.

210. Tenner, A. J., S. L. Robinson, J. Borchelt, and J. R. Wright. 1989. Human pulmonary surfactant protein (SP-A), a protein structurally homologous to C1q, can enhance FcR- and CR1-mediated phagocytosis. *J. Biol. Chem.* **264:**13923–13928.

211. Thoma-Uszynski, S., S. Stenger, O. Takeuchi, M. Ochoa, M. Engele, P. Sieling, P. Barnes, M. Rollinghoff, P. Bolcskei, M. Wagner, S. Akira, M. Norgard, J. Belisle, P. Godowski, B. Bloom, and R. Modlin. 2001. Induction of direct antimicrobial activity through mammalian Toll-like receptors. *Science* **291:**1544–1547.

212. Thornton, B. P., V. Vetvicka, M. Pitman, R. C. Goldman, and G. D. Ross. 1996. Analysis of the sugar specificity and molecular location of the b-glucan-binding lectin site of complement receptor type 3 (CD11b/CD18). *J. Immunol.* **156:**1235–1246.

213. Toba, H., J. T. Crowford, and J. J. Ellner. 1989. Pathogenicity of *Mycobacterium avium* for human monocytes: absence of macrophage activating factor activity of gamma interferon. *Infect. Immun.* **57:**239–244.

214. Tobian, A. A., N. S. Potter, L. Ramachandra, R. K. Pai, M. Convery, W. H. Boom, and C. V. Harding. 2003. Alternate class I MHC antigen processing is inhibited by Toll-like receptor signaling pathogen-associated molecular patterns: *Mycobacterium tuberculosis* 19-kDa lipoprotein, CpG DNA, and lipopolysaccharide. *J. Immunol.* **171:**1413–1422.

215. Toshchakov, V., B. W. Jones, P. Y. Perera, K. Thomas, M. J. Cody, S. Zhang, B. R. Williams, J. Major, T. A. Hamilton, M. J. Fenton, and S. N. Vogel. 2002. TLR4, but not TLR2, mediates IFN-beta-induced STAT1alpha/beta-

dependent gene expression in macrophages. *Nat. Immunol.* 3:392-398.

216. Ueda, T., P. Rieu, J. Brayer, and M. A. Arnaout. 1994. Identification of the complement iC3b binding site in the β2 integrin CR3 (CD11b/CD18). *Proc. Natl. Acad. Sci. USA* 91: 10680–10684.

217. Uehori, J., M. Matsumoto, S. Tsuji, T. Akazawa, O. Takeuchi, S. Akira, T. Kawata, I. Azuma, K. Toyoshima, and T. Seya. 2003. Simultaneous blocking of human Toll-like receptors 2 and 4 suppresses myeloid dendritic cell activation induced by *Mycobacterium bovis* bacillus Calmette-Guérin peptidoglycan. *Infect. Immun.* 71:4238–4249.

218. Venisse, A., J.-M. Berjeaud, P. Chaurand, M. Gilleron, and G. Puzo. 1993. Structural features of lipoarabinomannan from *Mycobacterium bovis* BCG. Determination of molecular mass by laser desorption mass spectrometry. *J. Biol. Chem.* 268:12401–12411.

219. Vergne, I., J. Chua, and V. Deretic. 2003. Tuberculosis toxin blocking phagosome maturation inhibits a novel Ca^{2+}/calmodulin-PI3K hVPS34 cascade. *J. Exp. Med.* 198:653–659.

220. Wileman, T. E., M. R. Lennartz, and P. D. Stahl. 1986. Identification of the macrophage mannose receptor as a 175-kDa membrane protein. *Proc. Natl. Acad. Sci. USA* 83:2501–2505.

221. Williams, M. J., P. E. Hughes, T. E. O'Toole, and M. H. Ginsberg. 1994. The inner world of cell adhesion: integrin cytoplasmic domains. *Trends Cell Biol.* 4:109–112.

222. Wilson, C. B., V. Tsai, and J. S. Remington. 1980. Failure to trigger the oxidative metabolic burst by normal macrophages: possible mechanism for survival of intracellular pathogens. *J. Exp. Med.* 151:328–346.

223. Wright, S. D., P. A. Detmers, M. T. C. Jong, and B. C. Meyer. 1986. Inteferon-gamma depresses binding of ligand by C3b and C3bi receptors on cultured human monocytes, an effect reversed by fibronectin. *J. Exp. Med.* 163:1245–1259.

224. Yamamoto, M., S. Sato, H. Hemmi, K. Hoshino, T. Kaisho, H. Sanjo, O. Takeuchi, M. Sugiyama, M. Okabe, K. Takeda, and S. Akira. 2003. Role of adaptor TRIF in the MyD88-independent toll-like receptor signaling pathway. *Science* 301:640–643.

225. Yoshida, A., and Y. Koide. 1997. Arabinofuranosyl-terminated and mannosylated lipoarabinomannans from *Mycobacterium tuberculosis* induce different levels of interleukin-12 expression in murine macrophages. *Infect. Immun.* 65: 1953–1955.

226. Zach, T. L., L. D. Hill, V. A. Herrman, M. P. Leuschen, and M. K. Hostetter. 1992. Effect of glucocorticoids on C3 gene expression by the A549 human pulmonary epithelial cell line. *J. Immunol.* 148:3964–3969.

227. Zhang, Y., M. Doerfler, T. C. Lee, B. Guillemin, and W. N. Rom. 1993. Mechanisms of stimulation of interleukin-1beta and tumor necrosis factor-alpha by *Mycobacterium tuberculosis* components. *J. Clin. Investig.* 91:2076–2083.

228. Zimmerli, S., S. Edwards, and J. D. Ernst. 1996. Selective receptor blockade during phagocytosis does not alter the survival and growth of *Mycobacterium tuberculosis* in human macrophages. *Am. J. Respir. Cell Mol. Biol.* 15:760–770.

Tuberculosis and the Tubercle Bacillus
Edited by Stewart T. Cole et al.
© 2005 ASM Press, Washington, D.C.

Chapter 26

Mycobacterium tuberculosis: the Indigestible Microbe

DAVID G. RUSSELL

Mycobacterium tuberculosis survives within the phagocytes of its host, yet these cells are key to the effective control of the infection. Their ambivalent role as both "saint and sinner" in this infection is dictated by the interplay between the bacterium and the immunoresponsive macrophage (51). Over the past decade, our appreciation of the subtleties of this interaction has expanded considerably as many groups have focused their research on clarifying this dialogue.

ARRIVING AT A FUNCTIONAL DEFINITION OF THE *M. TUBERCULOSIS*-CONTAINING VACUOLE

M. *tuberculosis* gains entry to the macrophage through the ligation of receptors that activate phagocytosis. While the majority of studies indicate that the bacilli favor complement receptors, which are benign because they trigger minimal superoxide production, experimental data suggest that the identity of receptors occupied impact little on the subsequent survival of the bacteria (71), although differential use of receptors may affect the invasion of different phagocyte populations

Following phagocytosis, the bacteria continue to reside within a membrane-bound vacuole of host origin (Fig. 1). The seminal studies of D'Arcy Hart in the early 1970s described how the absence of fusion with lysosomes correlated with viability of the infecting bacteria (3, 4, 8) (Fig. 2). The capacity of M. *tuberculosis* bacilli to regulate the fusigenicity of their vacuoles is a characteristic that is shared by other pathogenic *Mycobacterium* spp., including M. *bovis*, M. *avium*, M. *paratuberculosis*, and M. *leprae*, and data from these species have contributed to our current understanding of the nature of this compartment.

In 1986, Frehel and colleagues observed transient delivery of lysosomal tracers to vacuoles containing M. *avium* and suggested that these vacuoles

had access to early endosomal compartments (26). Then in 1991 Crowle et al. reported that the vacuoles containing M. *avium* and M. *tuberculosis* were less acidic than neighboring lysosomes (15). Sturgill-Koszycki et al. used excitation ratio fluorometry to measure the pH of these vacuoles and reported it to be pH 6.2 to 6.3 (62). They also isolated the bacterium-containing vacuoles and reported them to be deficient in the proton ATPase complexes responsible for the acidification of phagosomes.

In 1996, several studies were published that permitted a much fuller understanding of the functional profile of the compartments in which live M. *tuberculosis* reside. These vacuoles were shown to be highly dynamic and readily accessible to glycosphingolipids from the macrophage plasmalemma (52). They had a paucity of proton-ATPase complexes and a profile of endosomal contituents consistent with the maturation of their phagosomes being arrested at a point that retained fusion with early endosomes (61). Consequently, markers of the recycling endosomal system, namely, the transferrin receptor and its cargo, could be shown to traffic through the bacterium-containing compartments (12, 61). Although certain "lysosomal" markers, such as cathepsin D, could be detected in these compartments, careful analysis of the hydrolase revealed that it was in a high-molecular-weight, unprocessed form (61, 64). These data indicated that the enzyme had not passed through an acidic environment and had therefore originated from the synthetic pathway of the cell, presumably through delivery from the trans-Golgi network. Most researchers in this field now work under the assumption that the vacuoles containing pathogenic *Mycobacterium* spp. are phagosomes that are blocked in their normal maturation process (10, 16, 17, 51, 53, 66). The membrane-trafficking pathways that intersect with the bacterium-containing vacuoles are shown in Fig. 3. Current research interest is now focused on three specific areas. (i) Exactly where is the point of arrest in the

---

David G. Russell • Microbiology and Immunology, College of Veterinary Medicine, Cornell University, Ithaca, NY 14853.

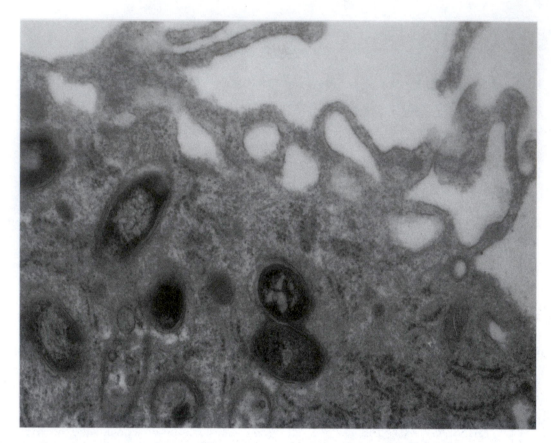

Figure 1. Electron micrograph of a murine macrophage infected 4 days previously with *M. tuberculosis*. The bacteria reside in membrane-bound vacuoles, many of which remain in tight association with the surface of the bacteria.

maturation process? (ii) How does the bug do this? (iii) What are the implications throughout the course of the infection?

EXACTLY WHERE IS THE POINT OF ARREST IN THE PHAGOSOME MATURATION PROCESS?

Small GTPases, or Rab proteins, have been implicated in regulating the fusion capacity of endosomal vesicles during their differentiation or maturation through the endosomal-lysosomal continuum. The early endosomal GTPase Rab5 has been found to associate stably with vacuoles containing pathogenic *Mycobacterium* bacilli (13, 68). The retention of Rab5 indicates arrest at an extremely early phase in the maturation process. Indeed, manipulation of Rab5 through the use of permanently membrane-bound mutated forms of the protein generates vacuoles that are stable and exhibit homotypic fusion with early endosomes. Mouse coronin I (TACO) has also been reported to associate stably with *Mycobacterium* vacuoles, although its role in the regulation of

maturation and its impact on bacterial survival are the subject of conflicting reports (23, 58).

The regulation of membrane fusion in endosome biogenesis at this stage of the differentiation process is still debated hotly in the cell biology literature, although the major "players" have been identified (9, 60). In essence, Rab5 binds Vps34, a class III phosphatidylinositol 3-kinase that generates phosphatidylinositol 3-phosphate (PI 3-P) on the cytosolic face of the vacuole. PI 3-P, in turn, acts as an acceptor for the early endosomal antigen EEA1, which also complexes with Rab5. EEA1 binds calmodulin, and this step in the process is sensitive to inhibitors of Ca^{2+}/calmodulin activity (37, 44). EEA1, acquisition and accumulation are necessary for the accumulation of Rab7, the small GTPase that is enriched on lysosomes.

There are three bodies of data that describe potential points of intercession by the bacterium. These bodies of data actually have several common features and need not be mutually exclusive. All three data sets focus on the role of calmodulin in phagosome biogenesis and maturation.

In the first series of studies, Malik et al. reported that *M. tuberculosis* blocked the normal calmodulin-

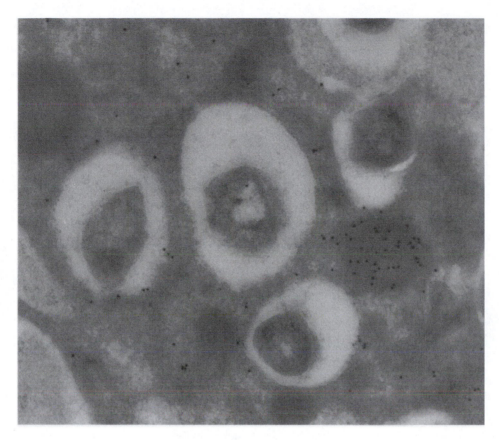

Figure 2. Immunoelectron micrograph of a murine macrophage infected 4 days previously with *M. avium*, demonstrating that the bacterium-containing phagosomes show minimal interaction with dense lysosomal compartments loaded with biotinylated, mannosylated bovine serum albumin. The infected macrophages were incubated with biotinylated mannosylated bovine serum albumin for 45 min, rinsed, and fixed. The biotinylated, mannosylated bovine serum albumin was detected by incubation of the sections with streptavidin/antistreptavidin and 18-nm-diameter gold particles with conjugated secondary antibody, as detailed previously (70).

dependent signal transduction that was observed in the maturation of phagosomes containing inert particles or dead bacteria (40, 41). The treatment of infected macrophages with the calcium ionophore induced an elevation in cytosolic [Ca^{2+}] that led to the recruitment of calmodulin, activation of calmodulin-dependent kinase II, and enhanced maturation of the bacterium-containing vacuole. These authors went on to show that the blockage in Ca^{2+}-mediated signaling was due to an inhibition of sphingosine kinase activity exhibited by live but not dead bacteria (42). Moreover, treatment of macrophages with the competitive inhibitor dihydrosphingosine inhibited the normal maturation of phagosomes containing dead bacteria.

In the second series, Fratti et al. showed that while *M. bovis* BCG-containing phagosomes acquired Rab5 and accumulated Vps34, they failed to bind the PI 3-P-binding protein EEA1 (24). Vergne et al. suggested that the lack of binding was due to the absence of PI 3-P on the cytosolic face of the vac-

uole as a result of the bacterium interfering with the kinase activity of Vps34 (67). They proposed that this suppression of kinase activity was due to the bacterium interfering with the Ca^{2+}/calmodulin activation of Vps34 activity and went on to demonstrate that Vps34 activity was depressed by the bacterial lipidoglycan lipoarabinomannan (LAM) (25, 67). This model is diagrammed in Fig. 4A.

Although the involvement of calmodulin and calmodulin-dependent kinase II has been observed by several groups, there is still some debate about its mode of action. Corvera and colleagues have also studied the activity of calmodulin in the modulation of Vps34 and EEA1 in model phagosomes and reported that calmodulin did not affect Vps34 kinase activity but instead blocked EEA1 binding to PI 3-P (37). These data imply that the *M. tuberculosis*-containing phagosomes may fail to bind EEA1 and yet could possess PI 3-P on their cytosolic face. This latter scenario is detailed in Fig. 4B and is consistent with the experiments of B. A. Butcher and D. G. Russell (unpublished data), who have shown

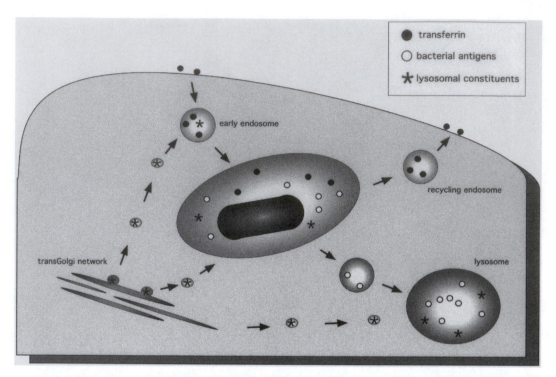

Figure 3. Diagram illustrating the major intracellular trafficking pathways that intersect with the vacuoles containing live, virulent *M. tuberculosis* bacilli. These vacuoles are accessed by the recycling endosomal system, as evidenced by their acquisition of transferrin. Components of the bacteria released into the bacterium-containing vacuoles traffic out of the vacuoles and coalesce in dense lysosomal compartments. Finally, the bacterium-containing vacuoles, in common with most endosomal-lysosomal stages, show intersection with delivery vesicles derived from the *trans*-Golgi network of the host cell.

that *M. tuberculosis*-containing phagosomes bind green fluorescent protein::2XFYVE, a fusion construct consisting of green fluorescent protein fused to the PI 3-P-binding domain from EEA1 that binds the phosphoinositide but is not regulated by calmodulin (27, 28). These researchers went on to demonstrate by thin-layer

chromatography analysis that isolated *M. tuberculosis*-containing vacuoles did contain PI 3-P, although it should be noted these biochemical data do not address the accessibility of the lipid.

Despite the apparent discontinuity of the current data, there is actually a great deal of agreement

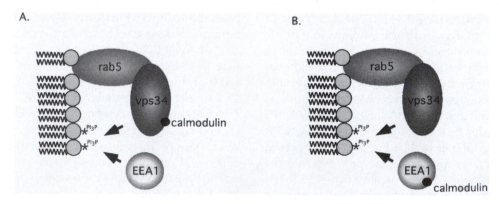

Figure 4. Diagram illustrating the contrasting regulatory pathways proposed to control EEA1 binding to phagosomes. (A) Vergne et al. reported that activity of vps34, a PI 3-kinase, was regulated by calmodulin (67). They suggested that the bacterial cell wall lipid LAM suppresses the [Ca^{2+}] flux required to activate vps34 and that therefore no PI 3-P is generated in the membranes of the bacterium-containing phagosomes that fail to acquire EEA1. This model would predict a direct correlation between PI 3-P presence and EEA1 binding. (B) In contrast, Lawe et al. failed to observe any modulation of vps34 activity by calmodulin but found that EEA1 binding was dependent on Ca^{2+}/calmodulin activation through the IQ domain and other calmodulin-responsive domains (37). This latter model predicts that PI 3-P presence does not necessarily correspond to EEA1 acquisition.

between the laboratories on the following basic observations. The point of arrest in phagosome maturation is at the accumulation of EEA1. This process is modulated by compounds that affect Ca^{2+}/calmodulin and class III PI 3-kinase activity. Moreover, the regulatory pathways evoked are not mutually exclusive, because they could function on both Vps34 and EEA1.

There are additional data that imply that PIs are not the only lipid moieties capable of regulating the maturation of phagosomes. Malik and colleagues demonstrated that the Ca^{2+}/calmodulin-mediated regulation of phagosome-lysosome fusion was accompanied by an elevation in sphingosine kinase activity and that inhibition of the macrophage sphingosine kinase blocked the maturation of the phagosome (42). In another recent study by Anes et al., it was demonstrated that the sphingosine 1-phosphate content of the phagosome membrane influenced actin polymerization on isolated phagosomes and that arrested, *M. tuberculosis*-containing phagosomes were deficient in actin nucleation (2). These investigators went on to show that certain lipids added exogenously to infected cells could drive the maturation of the *M. tuberculosis*-containing vacuole. However it is unclear if this "whole-cell" phenomenon was achieved through a comparable mechanism, because certain lipids, such as sphingosine 1-phosphate, function both as a primary messenger and as a ligand for activation receptors such as the endothelial differentiation gene (EDG) receptor family (31, 32, 35). Clearly, the role played by lipids in influencing the passage of the phagosome through the cell deserves much more attention than has been paid to date.

HOW DOES THE BUG DO THIS?

The mechanism by which pathogenic *Mycobacterium* spp. arrest the normal maturation process of their phagosomes has been the subject of several studies over the past few years.

Initially it was proposed that ammonia production from the bacterial urease was responsible for arresting the maturation process, and, indeed, studies showed that blockage of proton ATPase activity with bafilomycin delayed endosome differentiation (29). However, *M. bovis* BCG, in which the urease gene was disrupted, demonstrated minimal survival phenotype in either macrophages in culture or in mice, and on closer examination the rates of phagosome-lysosome fusion were unaltered (D. G. Russell, unpublished observations).

There is a significant body of literature that implicates cell wall lipidoglycans in modulating membrane fusion capacity. Older studies report that the additon of cord factor, trehalose dimycolate (TDM), to artificial membrane bilayers severely impairs their capacity to fuse with one another (14, 30, 59).

More recently, it was reported that LAM-bearing particles exhibited a markedly reduced progression through the endosome-lysosome continuum. Fratti et al. observed that LAM-coated beads behaved similarly to viable *M. bovis* BCG in that these particles resided in vacuoles that failed to recruit EEA1 (25). In addition, Vergne et al. reported that LAM was actually inhibitory to Vps34 activity and that this inhibition was achieved by blocking the Ca^{2+}/calmodulin activity that accompanies normal progression of phagosomes (67). A role for LAM in blocking the rise in cytosolic $[Ca^{2+}]$ associated with phagocytosis would also be consistent with the observations by Malik et al. (41, 42). Indrigo et al. reported that another bacterial cell wall lipidoglycan, TDM, was also capable of blocking the maturation of phagosomes containing latex beads coated with the bacterial lipid (36). In an intriguing series of experiments, they demonstrated that *M. tuberculosis* bacilli that were extracted with petroleum ether to remove TDM were impaired for arresting phagosome maturation and for survival but that this defect could be reversed by reconstituting these bacilli with exogenous TDM.

The complex oligosaccharides of several intracellular pathogens have been implicated in modulating the fusigenicity of phagosomes, ranging from the lipophosphoglycan of *Leishmania* to the lipooligosaccharide of *Listeria* (1, 18, 19). In these cases, the modulation is transient and delays rather than arrests the maturation process. It has been proposed that this behavior buys the pathogen time to upregulate the expression of genes that are necessary for the stable parasitization of the host cell. It is therefore important to establish if the effects of LAM or TDM on vacuolar maturation are enduring or represent a strategy that is enhanced by other bacterial factors. Although an imperfect experiment, it remains puzzling why dead bacilli are delivered to the lysosome if LAM or TDM were the sole mediator(s) of inhibition.

WHAT ARE THE IMPLICATIONS THROUGHOUT THE COURSE OF THE INFECTION?

While the arrest of phagosome maturation is a fascinating question in cell biology, it has broad implications that evolve during the course of the infection. The macrophage is both an antigen-presenting cell and an immune-effector cell capable of killing *M. tuberculosis* if given the correct stimuli.

The nature of the environment in which the bacterium finds itself is becoming clearer from expression-profiling data that are accumulating from real-time PCR studies and microarray analysis (57, 63). In brief, the environment(s) inside the macrophage induces genes associated with a range of stress responses from iron and oxygen limitation and cell wall damage to an enforced metabolic shift to anaerobic metabolism and utilization of fatty acids as a carbon source. The subtle and not so subtle influence of the host immune system on this environment was demonstrated previously through the regulated expression and dependence on isocitrate lyase (ICL1), the gating enzyme into the glyoxylate pathway (33, 34, 43). The attenuated phenotype of an *icl1*-deficient mutant was detectable only in activated macrophages or in an immunocompetent host. These data suggested that macrophage activation altered the intraphagosomal environment, requiring a metabolic shift in carbon utilization. The data regarding ICL1 expression in human infections are more complex and highlight some of the caveats associated with the use of mice as a model for infection (22, 63). In situ reverse transcription-PCR from human granulomas demonstrate that ICL1 expression is detected in bacteria inside macrophages at the periphery of the granuloma but not in the majority of bacilli at the center of the structure. While this is consistent with the "immune pressure" theory of anapleurotic metabolism, it does indicate that the bacterial population is more diverse in a real host with an effective transmission cycle.

ANTIGEN PRESENTATION AND THE INFECTED MACROPHAGE

The *M. tuberculosis*-containing vacuole remains a dynamic intracellular compartment that continues to fuse with other vesicles and therefore retains the potential to interface with the antigen-sampling and presentation machinery of the host cell. Clemens and Horwitz reported the detection of major histocompatibility complex (MHC) class II molecules in infected macrophages analyzed by immunoelectron microscopy (11). However, these macrophages were treated with gamma interferon to increase MHC expression levels and hence facilitate detection. Studies of resting macrophages infected with *M. bovis* BCG demonstrated that while MHC class II molecules were detectable in early phagosomes following infection, their levels diminished over time and they were undetectable in the *Mycobacterium*-containing vacuoles after 48 h (65). Moreover the MHC class II molecules detected at

early time points were present as sodium dodecyl sulfate-stable complexes; this infers that they are already peptide loaded and therefore came from the cell surface during phagosome formation. In this study, Ullrich et al. went on to confirm that treatment of macrophages with gamma interferon rendered the *Mycobacterium*-containing vacuoles accessible to MHC class II molecules and also H-2M molecules, inferring that activation of the macrophage relocated the pathogen into the antigen-sampling and processing pathway of the cell (65). The capacity of these MHC molecules to sample and present bacterial antigens was demonstrated functionally by Ramachandra et al. (49), who demonstrated the successful formation of MHC-bacterial antigen complexes within the endosomal continuum of activated, infected macrophages.

Macrophages express low levels of CD1 molecules, which present nontraditional antigens such as bacterial lipids. The presentation of such molecules is exhibited predominantly by dendritic cells. It has been shown recently that dendritic cells will present bacterial lipids acquired through internalization of vesicles derived from the apoptotic death of infected bystander macrophages (54, 56).

It is inferred that, in resting macrophages, the bacilli are sequestered outside the normal antigen presentation pathway of the infected cells, a suggestion made previously by Pancholi et al. (48). However, this would be a simplification of the situation, because everything that is secreted by the intracellular bacterium has the capacity to enter into the antigen-processing pathway. The most abundant of the released antigens appear to be the bacterial cell wall lipids. Analysis of the bulk flow of these moieties by immunoelectron microscopy and density gradient electrophoresis of infected cells demonstrates that the lipids traffic, with no obvious selectivity, to the multivesicular lysosomes in the macrophage (5–7). When infected with *M. bovis* BCG, these lipids include mycoside B, trehalose monomycolate, TDM, PI mannosides, cardiolipin, and phosphatidylethanolamine (50). The lysosomal compartments in which the lipids coalesce are capable of exocytic release of their internal vesicles to the external milieu. Biochemical analysis of the resulting vesicles show that they contain bacterial lipids and proteins, such as members of the Ag85 complex as well as the lipids listed above, and are highly enriched for MHC class II molecules (6, 7). Similar membrane vesicles from dendritic cells are functional presenters of bacterial antigen capable of stimulating T cells directly, although a role in eliciting a cellular immune response through cross-priming has also been demonstrated (56).

ACTIVATION OF HOST MACROPHAGES

Appropriately activated macrophages are capable of killing *M. tuberculosis*. This response is well documented for the murine system and is reproduced readily in vitro; however, activation of human macrophages to the same level has not been achieved reproducibly in culture. It is, however, important to note that human macrophages isolated from sites of infection are highly activated and produce nitric oxide readily (46, 47).

Macrophages activated by gamma interferon prior to infection deliver the bacteria to acidic, hydrolytically competent lysosomes (55, 69). Although the data are persuasive that killing requires inducible nitric oxide synthase (iNOS)/NOS2 expression, it is unlikely that the killing would be as effective without delivery of the bacteria to this environment (38). Recent analysis of activated macrophages has led to the identification of LRG-47, a novel GTPase that is expressed on exposure of macrophages to gamma interferon (39). LRG-47$^{-/-}$ mice are exquisitely sensitive to infection by *M. tuberculosis* despite expression of NOS2, indicating that reactive nitrogen intermediate-mediated killing is insufficient in the absence of LRG-47 activity. Experiments with infected macrophages have shown the LRG-47 drives increased maturation of the *M. tuberculosis*-containing phagosomes, and the authors speculate that this may be achieved through increased recruitment of H-ATPase complexes (39).

DICHOTOMY OF THE IMMUNE RESPONSE

Clearly, the bacilli have a vested interest in avoiding delivery to an acidic, hydrolytic environment, and they appear to employ multiple strategies to bypass this fate. Many infectious agents try to avoid induction of a protective immune response through suppressing antigen presentation, exhibiting antigenic variation, or minimizing the exposure of immunogens. Although such strategies have been evoked for *M. tuberculosis*, it is clear that, as the infection progresses, the host does develop a strong immune response that maintains the granuloma and restricts dissemination of the disease during the latent, asymptomatic phase of infection. It is, however, intriguing that, while the bacterium may need to avoid the induction or effector phase of an immune response at the localized level of the individual infected macrophage, it is dependent ultimately on a robust immune response for effective transmission (20, 21, 45). Successful transmission relies on the differentiation of the granuloma into a caseating, necrotic structure that spills bacteria into

the lung and induces a productive cough. This "reprogramming" of the granuloma appears to rely on the progressive nature of the immune response to infection.

CONCLUDING REMARKS

The success of *M. tuberculosis* as a pathogen hinges on its ability to either modulate or respond to its host cell, the macrophage, throughout the changing phases of the infection in its host. This interplay is complex and is expressed at levels ranging from intracellular environments to the granulomatous foci. Our appreciation of the plasticity of this dialogue is only now emerging through the unprecedented technological advances that have occurred over the past few years. This is a great time to be working in this field!

Acknowledgments. D.G.R. is supported by grants from the U.S. Public Health Service from the National Institute of Allergy and Infectious Diseases and The National Heart, Lung, and Blood Institute.

REFERENCES

1. **Alvarez-Dominguez, C., A. M. Barbieri, W. Beron, A. Wandinger-Ness, and P. D. Stahl.** 1996. Phagocytosed live *Listeria monocytogenes* influences Rab5-regulated in vitro phagosome-endosome fusion. *J. Biol. Chem.* **271:**13834–13843.
2. **Anes, E., M. P. Kuhnel, E. Bos, J. Moniz-Pereira, A. Habermann, and G. Griffiths.** 2003. Selected lipids activate phagosome actin assembly and maturation resulting in killing of pathogenic mycobacteria. *Nat. Cell Biol.* **5:**793–802.
3. **Armstrong, J. A., and P. D. Hart.** 1975. Phagosome-lysosome interactions in cultured macrophages infected with virulent tubercle bacilli. Reversal of the usual nonfusion pattern and observations on bacterial survival. *J. Exp. Med.* **142:**1–16.
4. **Armstrong, J. A., and P. D. Hart.** 1971. Response of cultured macrophages to *M. tuberculosis* with observations of fusion of lysosomes with phagosomes. *J. Exp. Med.* **134:**713–740.
5. **Beatty, W. L., E. R. Rhoades, H. J. Ullrich, D. Chatterjee, J. E. Heuser, and D. G. Russell.** 2000. Trafficking and release of mycobacterial lipids from infected macrophages. *Traffic* **1:**235–247.
6. **Beatty, W. L., and D. G. Russell.** 2000. Identification of mycobacterial surface proteins released into subcellular compartments of infected macrophages. *Infect. Immun.* **68:**6997–7002.
7. **Beatty, W. L., H. J. Ullrich, and D. G. Russell.** 2001. Mycobacterial surface moieties are released from infected macrophages by a constitutive exocytic event. *Eur. J. Cell. Biol.* **80:**31–40.
8. **Brown, C. A., P. Draper, and P. D. Hart.** 1969. Mycobacteria and lysosomes: a paradox. *Nature* **221:**658–60.
9. **Christoforidis, S., H. M. McBride, R. D. Burgoyne, and M. Zerial.** 1999. The Rab5 effector EEA1 is a core component of endosome docking. *Nature* **397:**621–625.
10. **Clemens, D. L.** 1996. Characterization of the *Mycobacterium tuberculosis* phagosome. *Trends Microbiol.* **4:**113–118.
11. **Clemens, D. L., and M. A. Horwitz.** 1995. Characterization of the *Mycobacterium tuberculosis* phagosome and evidence that

phagosomal maturation is inhibited. *J. Exp. Med.* **181**:257–270.

12. Clemens, D. L., and M. A. Horwitz. 1996. The *Mycobacterium tuberculosis* phagosome interacts with early endosomes and is accessible to exogenously administered transferrin. *J. Exp. Med.* **184**:1349–1355.

13. Clemens, D. L., B. Y. Lee, and M. A. Horwitz. 2000. Deviant expression of Rab5 on phagosomes containing the intracellular pathogens *Mycobacterium tuberculosis* and *Legionella pneumophila* is associated with altered phagosomal fate. *Infect. Immun.* **68**:2671–2684.

14. Crowe, L. M., B. J. Spargo, T. Ioneda, B. L. Beaman, and J. H. Crowe. 1994. Interaction of cord factor (α, α′-trehalose-6,6′-dimycolate) with phospholipids. *Biochim. Biophys. Acta* **1194**:53–60.

15. Crowle, A. J., R. Dahl, E. Ross, and M. H. May. 1991. Evidence that vesicles containing living, virulent *Mycobacterium tuberculosis* or *Mycobacterium avium* in cultured human macrophages are not acidic. *Infect. Immun.* **59**:1823–1831.

16. de Chastellier, C., and L. Thilo. 1998. Modulation of phagosome processing as a key strategy for *Mycobacterium avium* survival within macrophages. *Res. Immunol.* **149**:699–702.

17. Deretic, V., and R. A. Fratti. 1999. *Mycobacterium tuberculosis* phagosome. *Mol. Microbiol.* **31**:1603–1609.

18. Dermine, J. F., S. Scianimanico, C. Prive, A. Descoteaux, and M. Desjardins. 2000. *Leishmania* promastigotes require lipophosphoglycan to actively modulate the fusion properties of phagosomes at an early step of phagocytosis. *Cell Microbiol.* **2**:115–126.

19. Desjardins, M., and A. Descoteaux. 1997. Inhibition of phagolysosomal biogenesis by the *Leishmania* lipophosphoglycan. *J. Exp. Med.* **185**:2061–2068.

20. Doenhoff, M. J. 1998. Granulomatous inflammation and the transmission of infection: schistosomiasis—and TB too? *Immunol. Today* **19**:462–467.

21. Doenhoff, M. J. 1997. A role for granulomatous inflammation in the transmission of infectious disease: schistosomiasis and tuberculosis. *Parasitology* **115**(Suppl.):S113–S125.

22. Fenhalls, G., L. Stevens, L. Moses, J. Bezuidenhout, J. C. Betts, P. van Helden, P. T. Lukey, and K. Duncan. 2002. In situ detection of *Mycobacterium tuberculosis* transcripts in human lung granulomas reveals differential gene expression in necrotic lesions. *Infect. Immun.* **70**:6330–6338.

23. Ferrari, G., H. Langen, M. Naito, and J. Pieters. 1999. A coat protein on phagosomes involved in the intracellular survival of mycobacteria. *Cell* **97**:435–447.

24. Fratti, R. A., J. M. Backer, J. Gruenberg, S. Corvera, and V. Deretic. 2001. Role of phosphatidylinositol 3-kinase and Rab5 effectors in phagosomal biogenesis and mycobacterial phagosome maturation arrest. *J. Cell Biol.* **154**:631–644.

25. Fratti, R. A., J. Chua, I. Vergne, and V. Deretic. 2003. *Mycobacterium tuberculosis* glycosylated phosphatidylinositol causes phagosome maturation arrest. *Proc. Natl. Acad. Sci. USA* **100**:5437–5442.

26. Frehel, C., C. de Chastellier, T. Lang, and N. Rastogi. 1986. Evidence for inhibition of fusion of lysosomal and prelysosomal compartments with phagosomes in macrophages infected with pathogenic *Mycobacterium avium*. *Infect. Immun.* **52**:252–262.

27. Gaullier, J. M., E. Ronning, D. J. Gillooly, and H. Stenmark. 2000. Interaction of the EEA1 FYVE finger with phosphatidylinositol 3-phosphate and early endosomes. Role of conserved residues. *J. Biol. Chem.* **275**:24595–24600.

28. Gaullier, J. M., A. Simonsen, A. D'Arrigo, B. Bremnes, H. Stenmark, and R. Aasland. 1998. FYVE fingers bind PtdIns(3)P. *Nature* **394**:432–433.

29. Gordon, A. H., P. D. Hart, and M. R. Young. 1980. Ammonia inhibits phagosome-lysosome fusion in macrophages. *Nature* **286**:79–80.

30. Goren, M. B., P. D'Arcy Hart, M. R. Young, and J. A. Armstrong. 1976. Prevention of phagosome-lysosome fusion in cultured macrophages by sulfatides of *Mycobacterium tuberculosis*. *Proc. Natl. Acad. Sci. USA* **73**:2510–2514.

31. Graeler, M., and E. J. Goetzl. 2002. Activation-regulated expression and chemotactic function of sphingosine 1-phosphate receptors in mouse splenic T cells. *FASEB J.* **16**:1874–1878.

32. Graler, M. H., and E. J. Goetzl. 2002. Lysophospholipids and their G protein-coupled receptors in inflammation and immunity. *Biochim. Biophys. Acta* **1582**:168–174.

33. Honer zu Bentrup, K., A. Miczak, D. L. Swenson, and D. G. Russell. 1999. Characterization of activity and expression of isocitrate lyase in *Mycobacterium avium* and *Mycobacterium tuberculosis*. *J. Bacteriol.* **181**:7161–7167.

34. Honer zu Bentrup, K., and D. G. Russell. 2001. Mycobacterial persistence: adaptation to a changing environment. *Trends Microbiol.* **9**:597–605.

35. Hornuss, C., R. Hammermann, M. Fuhrmann, U. R. Juergens, and K. Racke. 2001. Human and rat alveolar macrophages express multiple EDG receptors. *Eur. J. Pharmacol.* **429**:303–308.

36. Indrigo, J., R. L. Hunter, Jr., and J. K. Actor. 2003. Cord factor trehalose 6,6′-dimycolate (TDM) mediates trafficking events during mycobacterial infection of murine macrophages. *Microbiology* **149**:2049–2059.

37. Lawe, D. C., N. Sitouah, S. Hayes, A. Chawla, J. V. Virbasius, R. Tuft, K. Fogarty, L. Lifshitz, D. Lambright, and S. Corvera. 2003. Essential role of Ca^{2+}/calmodulin in early endosome antigen-1 localization. *Mol. Biol. Cell* **14**:2935–2945.

38. MacMicking, J. D., R. J. North, R. LaCourse, J. S. Mudgett, S. K. Shah, and C. F. Nathan. 1997. Identification of nitric oxide synthase as a protective locus against tuberculosis. *Proc. Natl. Acad. Sci. USA* **94**:5243–5248.

39. MacMicking, J. D., G. A. Taylor, and J. D. McKinney. 2003. Immune control of tuberculosis by IFN-gamma-inducible LRG-47. *Science* **302**:654–659.

40. Malik, Z. A., G. M. Denning, and D. J. Kusner. 2000. Inhibition of Ca^{2+} signaling by *Mycobacterium tuberculosis* is associated with reduced phagosome-lysosome fusion and increased survival within human macrophages. *J. Exp. Med.* **191**:287–302.

41. Malik, Z. A., S. S. Iyer, and D. J. Kusner. 2001. *Mycobacterium tuberculosis* phagosomes exhibit altered calmodulin-dependent signal transduction: contribution to inhibition of phagosome-lysosome fusion and intracellular survival in human macrophages. *J. Immunol.* **166**:3392–3401.

42. Malik, Z. A., C. R. Thompson, S. Hashimi, B. Porter, S. S. Iyer, and D. J. Kusner. 2003. Cutting edge: *Mycobacterium tuberculosis* blocks Ca^{2+} signaling and phagosome maturation in human macrophages via specific inhibition of sphingosine kinase. *J. Immunol.* **170**:2811–2815.

43. McKinney, J. D., K. Honer zu Bentrup, E. J. Munoz-Elias, A. Miczak, B. Chen, W. T. Chan, D. Swenson, J. C. Sacchettini, W. R. Jacobs, Jr., and D. G. Russell. 2000. Persistence of *Mycobacterium tuberculosis* in macrophages and mice requires the glyoxylate shunt enzyme isocitrate lyase. *Nature* **406**:735–738.

44. Mills, I. G., S. Urbe, and M. J. Clague. 2001. Relationships between EEA1 binding partners and their role in endosome fusion. *J. Cell Sci.* **114**:1959–1965.

45. Moreira, A. L., L. Tsenova, M. H. Aman, L. G. Bekker, S. Freeman, B. Mangaliso, U. Schroder, J. Jagirdar, W. N. Rom, M. G. Tovey, V. H. Freedman, and G. Kaplan. 2002.

Mycobacterial antigens exacerbate disease manifestations in *Mycobacterium tuberculosis*-infected mice. *Infect. Immun.* **70:**2100–2107.

46. **Nathan, C.** 2002. Inducible nitric oxide synthase in the tuberculous human lung. *Am. J. Respir. Crit. Care Med.* **166:**130–131.

47. **Nathan, C., and M. U. Shiloh.** 2000. Reactive oxygen and nitrogen intermediates in the relationship between mammalian hosts and microbial pathogens. *Proc. Natl. Acad. Sci. USA* **97:**8841–8848.

48. **Pancholi, P., A. Mirza, N. Bhardwaj, and R. M. Steinman.** 1993. Sequestration from immune CD4$^+$ T cells of mycobacteria growing in human macrophages. *Science* **260:**984–986.

49. **Ramachandra, L., E. Noss, W. H. Boom, and C. V. Harding.** 2001. Processing of *Mycobacterium tuberculosis* antigen 85B involves intraphagosomal formation of peptide-major histocompatibility complex II complexes and is inhibited by live bacilli that decrease phagosome maturation. *J. Exp. Med.* **194:**1421–1432.

50. **Rhoades, E. R., F.-F. Hsu, J. B. Torrelles, J. Turk, D. Chatterjee, and D. G. Russell.** 2003. Identification and macrophage activating activity of glycolipids released from intracellular *Mycobacterium* spp. *Mol. Microbiol.* **48:**875–888.

51. **Russell, D. G.** 2001. *Mycobacterium tuberculosis*: here today, and here tomorrow. *Nat. Rev. Mol. Cell Biol.* **2:**569–577.

52. **Russell, D. G., J. Dant, and S. Sturgill-Koszycki.** 1996. *Mycobacterium avium*- and *Mycobacterium tuberculosis*-containing vacuoles are dynamic, fusion-competent vesicles that are accessible to glycosphingolipids from the host cell plasmalemma. *J. Immunol.* **156:**4764–4773.

53. **Russell, D. G., H. C. Mwandumba, and E. E. Rhoades.** 2002. *Mycobacterium* and the coat of many lipids. *J. Cell Biol.* **158:**421–426.

54. **Schaible, U. E., K. Hagens, K. Fischer, H. L. Collins, and S. H. Kaufmann.** 2000. Intersection of group I CD1 molecules and mycobacteria in different intracellular compartments of dendritic cells. *J. Immunol.* **164:**4843–4852.

55. **Schaible, U. E., S. Sturgill-Koszycki, P. H. Schlesinger, and D. G. Russell.** 1998. Cytokine activation leads to acidification and increases maturation of *Mycobacterium avium*-containing phagosomes in murine macrophages. *J. Immunol.* **160:**1290–1296.

56. **Schaible, U. E., F. Winau, P. A. Sieling, K. Fischer, H. L. Collins, K. Hagens, R. L. Modlin, V. Brinkmann, and S. H. Kaufmann.** 2003. Apoptosis facilitates antigen presentation to T lymphocytes through MHC-I and CD1 in tuberculosis. *Nat. Med.* **9:**1039–1046.

57. **Schnappinger, D., S. Ehrt, M. I. Voskuil, Y. Liu, J. A. Mangan, I. M. Monahan, G. Dolganov, B. Efron, P. D. Butcher, C. Nathan, and G. K. Schoolnik.** 2003. Transcriptional adaptation of *Mycobacterium tuberculosis* within macrophages: insights into the phagosomal environment. *J. Exp. Med.* **198:**693–704.

58. **Schuller, S., J. Neefjes, T. Ottenhoff, J. Thole, and D. Young.** 2001. Coronin is involved in uptake of *Mycobacterium bovis* BCG in human macrophages but not in phagosome maintenance. *Cell Microbiol.* **3:**785–793.

59. **Spargo, B. J., L. M. Crowe, T. Ioneda, B. L. Beaman, and J. H. Crowe.** 1991. Cord factor (α, α'-trehalose-6,6'-dimycolate) inhibits fusion between phospholipid vesicles. *Proc. Natl. Acad. Sci. USA* **88:**737–740.

60. **Stenmark, H., and D. J. Gillooly.** 2001. Intracellular trafficking and turnover of phosphatidylinositol 3-phosphate. *Semin. Cell Dev. Biol.* **12:**193–199.

61. **Sturgill-Koszycki, S., U. E. Schaible, and D. G. Russell.** 1996. *Mycobacterium*-containing phagosomes are accessible to early endosomes and reflect a transitional state in normal phagosome biogenesis. *EMBO. J.* **15:**6960–6968.

62. **Sturgill-Koszycki, S., P. H. Schlesinger, P. Chakraborty, P. L. Haddix, H. L. Collins, A. K. Fok, R. D. Allen, S. L. Gluck, J. Heuser, and D. G. Russell.** 1994. Lack of acidification in *Mycobacterium* phagosomes produced by exclusion of the vesicular proton-ATPase. *Science* **263:**678–681.

63. **Timm, J., F. A. Post, L. G. Bekker, G. B. Walther, H. C. Wainwright, R. Manganelli, W. T. Chan, L. Tsenova, B. Gold, I. Smith, G. Kaplan, and J. D. McKinney.** 2003. Differential expression of iron-, carbon-, and oxygen-responsive mycobacterial genes in the lungs of chronically infected mice and tuberculosis patients. *Proc. Natl. Acad. Sci. USA* **100:**14321–14326.

64. **Ullrich, H. J., W. L. Beatty, and D. G. Russell.** 1999. Direct delivery of procathepsin D to phagosomes: implications for phagosome biogenesis and parasitism by *Mycobacterium.* *Eur. J. Cell Biol.* **78:**739–748.

65. **Ullrich, H. J., W. L. Beatty, and D. G. Russell.** 2000. Interaction of *Mycobacterium avium*-containing phagosomes with the antigen presentation pathway. *J. Immunol.* **165:**6073–6080.

66. **Vergne, I., J. Chua, and V. Deretic.** 2003. *Mycobacterium tuberculosis* phagosome maturation arrest: selective targeting of PI3P-dependent membrane trafficking. *Traffic* **4:**600–606.

67. **Vergne, I., J. Chua, and V. Deretic.** 2003. Tuberculosis toxin blocking phagosome maturation inhibits a novel Ca^{2+}/calmodulin-PI3K hVPS34 cascade. *J. Exp. Med.* **198:**653–659.

68. **Via, L. E., D. Deretic, R. J. Ulmer, N. S. Hibler, L. A. Huber, and V. Deretic.** 1997. Arrest of mycobacterial phagosome maturation is caused by a block in vesicle fusion between stages controlled by *rab5* and *rab7*. *J. Biol. Chem.* **272:**13326–13331.

69. **Via, L. E., R. A. Fratti, M. McFalone, E. Pagan-Ramos, D. Deretic, and V. Deretic.** 1998. Effects of cytokines on mycobacterial phagosome maturation. *J. Cell Sci.* **111:**897–905.

70. **Xu, S., A. Cooper, S. Sturgill-Koszycki, T. van Heyningen, D. Chatterjee, I. Orme, P. Allen, and D. G. Russell.** 1994. Intracellular trafficking in *Mycobacterium tuberculosis* and *Mycobacterium avium*-infected macrophages. *J. Immunol.* **153:**2568–2578.

71. **Zimmerli, S., S. Edwards, and J. D. Ernst.** 1996. Selective receptor blockade during phagocytosis does not alter the survival and growth of *Mycobacterium tuberculosis* in human macrophages. *Am. J. Respir. Cell Mol. Biol.* **15:**760–770.

Chapter 27

Intracellular Models of *Mycobacterium tuberculosis* Infection

JOHN CHAN, RICHARD F. SILVER, BEATE KAMPMANN, AND ROBERT S. WALLIS

Intracellular models of *Mycobacterium tuberculosis* infection have proven to be invaluable tools to address diverse questions in mycobacterial research. In the hands of basic-science researchers, they have helped shape our understanding of mycobacterial pathogenesis at the cellular level, identifying host defense mechanisms against intracellular infection and mycobacterial strategies to counter these defenses. At the same time, these models have also been studied by clinical researchers as potential correlates of human protection against tuberculosis, particularly as immunity is lost due to human immunodeficiency virus (HIV) infection or is augmented following vaccination with *M. bovis* BCG. These parallel investigations have yielded important insights into aspects of cellular mycobacterial immunity that are shared among mammalian species, as well as those that appear to be unique to human hosts and that may contribute to the distinctive characteristics of human tuberculosis. This chapter begins with an analysis of basic host-pathogen interactions in the infected murine macrophage. We then describe two models in which infected human monocytes interact with lymphocytes and other cells to generate antimycobacterial activity. Lastly, we summarize clinical trials in which these models were used to analyze the effects of BCG vaccination and other immunologic interventions.

HOST AND MICROBIAL STRATEGIES TARGETING THE MACROPHAGE

Macrophages constitute a major component of cell-mediated immunity to *M. tuberculosis* (13, 59). The best-studied macrophage antimycobacterial mechanisms are those mediated by (i) the production of nitric oxide (NO) and related reactive nitrogen intermediates (RNI) and (ii) phagolysosomal fusion. In each instance, mycobacterial strategies have evolved to counter these mechanisms.

Nitric Oxide and Reactive Nitrogen Intermediates

NO and related RNI are antimycobacterial effector molecules that are generated by nitric oxide synthase 2 (NOS2). This enzyme is induced in macrophages by both exogenous stimuli (such as microbial products) and the cytokines produced by activated T lymphocytes (such as gamma interferon [IFN-γ] and tumor necrosis factor [TNF-α]). The antimycobacterial effects of RNI are readily apparent in cultures of murine macrophage (13, 15, 28, 59). The in vivo significance of these in vitro observations has been subsequently established in murine experimental tuberculosis models by using NOS inhibitors or animals in which the *nos2* gene had been inactivated (14). These animal data clearly establish that RNI are essential for the control of tuberculosis in both the acute and persistent phases of infection (39, 60, 82).

Nonetheless, the role of nitrogen oxides in the control of human tuberculous infection remains controversial. This controversy originates, in large part, from the lack of a satisfactory in vitro human system that consistently shows induction of NOS2 and production of RNI in order to demonstrate antimycobacterial effects and from the lack of human genetic diseases involving *nos2*. Several studies provide indirect evidence supporting a role of RNI in human antimycobacterial defenses. Individuals with genetic defects in the intracellular signaling pathways of interleukin 12 (IL-12) are highly susceptible to disseminated mycobacterial infection (1, 27) or IFN-γ (33, 51, 68); in mice, these pathways are essential for production of RNI. Similarly, certain polymorphisms of the receptor of vitamin D have been linked to human susceptibility to tuberculosis (6); in human

John Chan • Department of Microbiology & Immunology, Albert Einstein College of Medicine, Bronx, NY 10461. Richard F. Silver • Department of Medicine, Case Western Reserve University, Cleveland, OH 44106. Beate Kampmann • Department of Pediatrics, Imperial College, London SW7 2AZ, United Kingdom. Robert S. Wallis • Department of Medicine UMDNJ—New Jersey Medical School, Newark, NJ 07103.

macrophage-like cell lines, these regulate the expression of *nos2* and the ability to limit intracellular *M. tuberculosis* growth (77). This indirect evidence, however, should be interpreted with caution due to the pleiotropic effects of cytokines and vitamins.

The most compelling evidence for a role of RNI in human defenses against *M. tuberculosis* comes from studies of lung macrophages. Rich et al. reported that alveolar macrophages from healthy individuals generate NO on infection with *M. tuberculosis* and that the ability of these macrophages to control the growth of intracellular bacilli correlates with NO production (76). Separate studies by Choi et al., Nicholson et al., and Wang et al., reported increased NOS2 expression in the lungs of patients with active pulmonary tuberculosis (18, 69, 100). In some of these studies, the increases resolved with treatment, indicating that they represented a response to infection. Nozaki et al. have similarly reported that the ability of pulmonary macrophages to control the growth of *M. bovis* BCG was NOS2 dependent (71). These studies provide substantial evidence that RNI plays an important role in the control of *M. tuberculosis* infection in humans, particularly in lung macrophages; however, further discussion of some of this controversy appears later in this chapter.

Evading the Toxic Effects of Reactive Nitrogen Intermediates

The potent antimycobacterial effects of RNI notwithstanding, *M. tuberculosis* has a unique ability to persist in the infected host, sometimes reactivating to cause disease decades after the primary infection (38). These observations suggest that the tubercle bacillus possesses means by which the antimycobacterial effects of RNI can be evaded. Clinical isolates of *M. tuberculosis* vary in their susceptibility to acidified nitrite (72); relatively resistant isolates are apparently more virulent in a guinea pig experimental tuberculosis model. This is perhaps the first evidence that RNI resistance mechanisms exist in the tubercle bacillus. Soon thereafter, it was reported that DNAs from a highly RNI-resistant *M. tuberculosis* isolate conferred resistance to toxic nitrogen oxides on otherwise susceptible heterologous hosts including *Escherichia coli* and *M. smegmatis* (35). This study led to the identification of the first *M. tuberculosis* RNI resistance gene, *nox1*. A similar approach has identified yet another RNI resistance-conferring allele of *M. tuberculosis*—the *noxR3* gene (79). The precise mechanisms by which these two genes mediate RNI resistance are presently unknown.

The availability of the complete *M. tuberculosis* strain H37Rv genome sequence (22) has allowed the bioinformatics identification of *M. tuberculosis* homologues of genes known to protect other bacteria against oxidative stress. This approach has helped identify alkyl hydroperoxide reductase subunit C (AhpC), a known oxidative stress protein in *E. coli* and *Salmonella enterica* serovar Typhimurium (49, 91, 93), as yet another *M. tuberculosis* component that protects against RNI toxicity (16). This study has shown that *M. tuberculosis* AhpC can protect the highly RNI-susceptible *ahpC*-disrupted strain of *S. enterica* serovar Typhimurium, as well as human cells, against the toxic effects of nitrogen oxides (16). Biochemical analysis of the wild-type and mutant AhpC proteins has shown that this peroxiredoxin has the ability to catabolize peroxynitrite anion (ONOO$^-$) (9), a potent oxidant formed by the reaction between NO and superoxide anion (O$_2^-$), two free radical species generated by activated macrophages (5). Further investigation of the biochemistry of AhpC revealed that this peroxiredoxin forms a complex with dihydrolipoamide dehydrogenase (Lpd), dihydrolipoamide succinyltransferase (SucB), and the thioredoxin-like AhpD. This complex is able to carry out peroxidase and peroxynitrite activity in the presence of NADH (10). Complementation studies using an *E. coli* mutant with disruption of the peptide methionine sulfoxide reductase (*msrA*) gene have revealed an enzymatic basis for ONOO$^-$ resistance (90). The Δ*msrA E. coli* mutant is hypersusceptible to the toxic effects of nitrite and GSNO, two compounds that can form peroxynitrite anion intracellularly under aerobic conditions. This susceptibility can be reversed by complementation with the *M. tuberculosis msrA* gene (90). MsrA catalyzes the reduction of methionine sulfoxide (Met-O), formed by the reaction of ONOO$^-$ and the methionine (Met) residue of proteins. Thus, *M. tuberculosis* MsrA may play a significant role in resistance to ONOO$^-$ toxicity by converting Met-O, whose presence in polypeptides can be detrimental to the host, to Met (90). Clearly, *M. tuberculosis* possesses means by which the toxic effects of ONOO$^-$ can be evaded. Indeed, in vitro studies have shown that virulent *M. tuberculosis* is relatively resistant to OONO$^-$ compared to the generally avirulent *M. smegmatis* and *M. bovis* BCG strains, which are highly susceptible (103). It will be of interest to evaluate the aforementioned anti-ONOO$^-$ activities in these relatively avirulent mycobacterial species.

In a different line of investigation, Ouellet et al. have demonstrated that BCG *glbN*, which encodes one of the two truncated hemoglobins in this species as well as in *M. tuberculosis*, may play an important role in mycobacterial resistance to RNI. A BCG mutant with disruption of *glbN* exhibits reduced capacity to metabolize NO during the stationary phase of growth (75). The *glbN* mutant also displays diminished aerobic respiration, compared to wild-type BCG, when subjected to NO stress. These results support a role for mycobacterial *glbN* in resistance to the toxic effect of RNI.

Recent microarray analyses have demonstrated that RNI can regulate *M. tuberculosis* gene expression in vitro (74, 98). Genes that are up-regulated by RNI may contribute to persistence (74, 98). In vivo studies using a murine experimental tuberculosis model involving *nos2*-deficient mice have provided evidence suggesting that RNI regulate *M. tuberculosis* gene expression in vivo (74). These studies also revealed that there is a remarkable overlap between the RNI-inducible regulon and that previously reported to be regulated by hypoxia; both nitrosative stress and anaerobicity up-regulate the expression of the same putative two-component regulatory response system (74, 98). Together, the results of these studies suggest that (i) RNI are capable of regulating *M. tuberculosis* gene expression in vivo, (ii) the reactive nitrogen species up-regulate genes that may promote mycobacterial survival in the infected host, and (iii) nitrosative stress and hypoxia may regulate mycobacterial gene expression by a common signal transduction pathway.

In summary, accumulating evidence strongly suggests that *M. tuberculosis* is well equipped with anti-RNI activities. Whether these RNI-detoxifying mechanisms promote the persistence of the tubercle bacillus in the host remains to be determined. Given the existence of multiple and maybe redundant mechanisms by which *M. tuberculosis* can evade RNI toxicity, proof of the relevance of these in vitro observations in the host might not be straightforward. Finally, the recent demonstration that RNI regulate the expression of *M. tuberculosis* genes that may be conducive to survival in the host suggests the possibility that reactive nitrogen species may serve as a danger signal that plays a role in promoting mycobacterial persistence.

Phagolysosomal Fusion

After undergoing phagocytosis, bacteria are internalized by macrophages into a vesicle called the phagosome (Fig. 1). The microbe-containing phagosome then matures to form the phagolysosome. This process subjects the ingested bacteria to attack by hydrolytic enzymes of the lysosomes (3, 25, 53), whose activity is optimal at acidic pH. As a result, phagolysosomal fusion can lead to the killing and elimination of ingested bacteria and therefore represents a potent antimicrobial mechanism of phagocytes. Phagolysosomal fusion is a highly complex process involving the interactions of phagosomes with various endocytic compartments (30, 31, 97). These interactions result in extensive remodeling of the phagosomal membrane. Emerging experimental evidence strongly suggest that *M. tuberculosis* has evolved mechanisms to evade the antimicrobial activity of the lysosomal enzymes by intercepting the process involved in the maturation of the bacillus-containing phagosome into a phagolysosome, as well as to modulate the intraphagosomal environment, thereby promoting persistence (29, 44, 80, 81). An example of the modulation of the intravesicular environment by the tubercle bacillus is its ability to exclude phagosomal vacuolar H$^+$-ATPases (75, 83, 92, 102); by so doing, *M. tuberculosis* may be better able to persist in the otherwise hostile acidic environment (66, 73) within the phagosome.

In the 1970's, D'Arcy Hart and colleagues posited that the ability of *M. tuberculosis* to disrupt phagolysosomal fusion is a virulence attribute (2, 46).

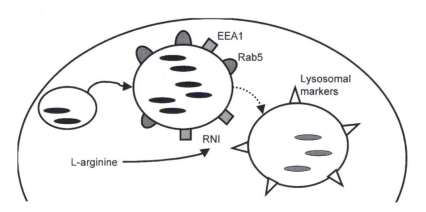

Figure 1. After phagocytosis, the tubercle bacillus is subject to attack by reactive radicals including various reactive nitrogen intermediates (RNI) and the hydrolytic enzymes of the lysosome. *M. tuberculosis* has evolved sophisticated means by which these potent antimicrobial activities of macrophages can be evaded.

Their electron microsopy studies, together with the use of lysosomal tracers to localize lysosomes, demonstrated that while phagosomes of macrophages containing live bacilli of the virulent H37Rv strain of *M. tuberculosis* fail to fuse with lysosomes, those harboring dead ones were able to do so (2, 46). This observation was later confirmed by various laboratories using reagents that enable the tagging of molecules expressed on the surface of various endocytic compartments (29, 44, 80, 81). Although live bacilli are able to interfere with the maturation of phagosomes, these vesicles are not completely insulated from the extraphagosomal environment, since existing evidence supports an active interaction between *M. tuberculosis*-containing phagosomes and various intracellular compartments (29, 44, 80, 81). In addition, this interaction can be modulated by IFN-γ, which promotes maturation of the *M. tuberculosis*-containing phagosome through LRG-47 (a member of a 47-kDa guanosine triphosphatase [GTPase] family) (61). This may represent an IFN-γ-dependent, NO-independent mechanism for control of intracellular mycobacterial replication.

Recent studies have elucidated the biochemical and molecular basis for the arrest of maturation of phagosomes containing live *M. tuberculosis*. This line of investigation has been fostered by the characterization of the events involved in the trafficking of intracellular vesicles, particularly that of the endocytic pathway (30, 31, 97). Several studies have examined the critical role of compartment-specific SNARE proteins (for "soluble *N*-ethylmaleimide-sensitive factor-attachment protein receptor") in mediating membrane fusion between transport and target vesicles (50). Membrane fusion between two compartments requires the pairing of the transport vesicle SNAREs with that on the target vesicles. The formation of the SNARE complex is supported by tethering proteins. By virtue of their ability to tether transport and target vesicles at specific SNARE-independent sites within a cellular compartment, the tethering proteins can provide target specificity. The Rab family of small GTP-binding proteins have also been identified as playing an important role in regulating intervesicular fusion (104). These GTPases can interact with tethering molecules. Finally, SNAREs, components of the tethering complexes, and Rab proteins have been shown to be involved in phagolysosomal biogenesis (reviewed in reference 97).

It is becoming clear that *M. tuberculosis* can interfere with the tethering and fusion machinery involved in phagolysosomal biogenesis. The kinetics of the recruitment and exclusion of Rab5 and Rab7, GTPases that are associated with early and late endosomes, respectively, has been a focus of investigation

(20, 21, 40, 96). It has been demonstrated that aberrant retention of Rab5 is associated with the arrest maturation of bacillus-containing phagosomes (20, 40, 96). Biochemical analysis of intracellular vesicles has provided evidence that the BCG-containing phagosomes of macrophages of the J774 murine cell line are deficient in Rab7 recruitment (96). The results of an independent study that took an immunoelectron microscopy approach revealed that abundant Rab7 is associated with *M. tuberculosis*-containing phagosomes of HeLa cells overexpressing this GTPase (21). These phagosomes, despite the presence of apparently abundant Rab7, are deficient in acquiring lysosome-associated membrane glycoprotein 1, a sign of maturation arrest. This observation is in agreement with the results of studies examining HeLa cells expressing a constitutively active (GTP-bound) Rab7 mutant (21). While the discrepant Rab7 data generated by the two independent studies (21, 96) may simply be due to the differences in the experimental models employed (including mycobacteria strains, host cells, and methods of analysis), they could also imply that *M. tuberculosis* disruption of the maturation of phagosomes involves multiple mechanisms. Nevertheless, these results support the possibility that *M. tuberculosis* may interfere with phagosomal biogenesis at a point where Rab5 and Rab7 regulate the evolution of the bacillus-containing phagosomes (96).

Elucidation of the chemistry of the cell wall of the tubercle bacillus has been a most important area of tuberculosis research that helps advance our understanding of the bacterium-host interactions. In searches of specific mycobacterial components that may interfere with phagosome maturation, it has been shown that mannosylated lipoarabinomannan (ManLAM), a complex *M. tuberculosis* glycolipid, attenuates the activity of hVPS34, a phosphatidylinositol 3(OH) kinase (PI3-K), as well as inhibiting the recruitment of early endosome autoantigen 1 (EEA1), a tethering molecule (40). EEA1 interacts with SNAREs and has been implicated in endosome-endosome fusion and vesicular trafficking between the *trans*-Golgi network (TGN) (a major biosynthetic and organelle sorting compartment) and endosomes (19, 65, 86, 87). Significantly, it has been shown in experiments with an in vitro latex bead system that both EEA1 and the PI3-K hVPS34 are Rab5 effectors that participate in the normal maturation of phagosomes (40). It is thought that in this process (58, 70), hVPS34 produces phosphatidylinositide 3-phosphate [PI(3)P], which plays an important role in the recruitment of EEA1. The EEA1 recruitment is mediated through the interaction of PI(3)P with the FYVE domain of the autoantigen. As a result, *M. tuberculosis* ManLAM may contribute to the maturation arrest of bacillus-containing phagosomes by virtue of its ability to attenuate hVPS34 and to inhibit EEA1 recruitment, suggesting that the interference occurs at a point close to Rab5 recruitment (40).

To further address the mechanisms by which *M. tuberculosis* ManLAM interferes with phagosomal maturation, phagosomes of J774 mouse macrophages containing fluorescent BCG- or ManLAM-coated beads were analyzed (43). This study revealed that phagosomes containing ManLAM-coated beads are deficient in the acquisition of the SNARE protein syntaxin 6 and show diminished accumulation of cathepsin D. The majority of syntaxin 6 in J774 macrophages colocalizes with furin, a TGN marker, and cathepsin D apparently originates in the TGN (43). These results therefore suggest that bacillus-containing phagosomes may be deficient in their interactions with the TGN. This notion is supported by experimental data showing that the Golgi-disrupting agent brefeldin A attenuates the acquisition of syntaxin 6 and cathepsin D by latex bead-containing J774 phagosomes (43). Using the PI3-K inhibitor wortmannin and an EEA1-inhibitory antibody as probes, the ability of ManLAM to inhibit TGN-phagosome trafficking has been linked to the ability of this complex *M. tuberculosis* glycolipid to adversely affect PI3-K activity and to attenuate EEA1 recruitment (40, 43). Collectively, these results suggest that syntaxin 6, PI3-K, and EEA1 play important roles in the trafficking of lysosomal components, such as cathepsin D, from the TGN to the phagosomes. Thus, it has been proposed that *M. tuberculosis* ManLAM may be able to arrest the maturation of phagosomes in infected macrophages by targeting syntaxin 6 acquisition, PI3-K signaling, and EEA1 recruitment, thereby promoting persistence (43). With respect to the SNARE proteins, there is evidence that syntaxin 6 is not the sole SNARE targeted by *M. tuberculosis* to disrupt phagosome maturation. It has been reported that mycobacterium-containing phagosomes are associated with an aberrant form of cellubrevin, a SNARE protein involved in phagosomal maturation (41). These data suggest that modification of cellubrevin by the tubercle bacillus might yet be another means by which *M. tuberculosis* disrupts phagosomal maturation.

It has been demonstrated previously that *M. tuberculosis* can block the fusion of phagosomes and lysosomes by inhibiting Ca^{2+} signaling (55, 62–64). Evidence exists that the tubercle bacillus interferes with Ca^{2+} signaling by down-regulating calmodulin-dependent signal transduction (63) and inhibiting sphingosine kinase (64). By directly testing the role of ManLAM on Ca^{2+}/calmodulin-dependent signaling, a recent study has provided evidence that the ability

of *M. tuberculosis* to block phagosome maturation may be due to the ability of LAM from virulent tubercle bacilli, but not that from the avirulent and rapidly growing *M. smegmatis*, to interfere with a Ca^{2+}/calmodulin–PI3-K hVPS34 signaling pathway that is required for the production of PI3P on phagosomes (95). Finally, a recent study designed to examine BCG-containing phagosomes of murine J774 macrophages has revealed that the stress-induced p38 mitogen-activated protein kinase (MAPK) may play a role in modulating phagosome biogenesis (42). Signaling through p38 MAPK has been reported to be associated with exclusion of EEA1 from endocytic membranes, and this protein kinase is also activated in *M. tuberculosis*-infected cells. Examination of BCG-containing J774 phagosomes has shown that inhibition of p38 MAPK activity is associated with enhanced recruitment of phagosomal EEA1 as well as markers of late endocytic vesicles, the latter being a sign of phagosome maturation (42). Thus, cellular p38 MAPK activation during tuberculous infection may adversely affect phagosome maturation, thereby promoting persistence.

Before leaving this section, the role of coronin 1 in mycobacterial persistence, controversy notwithstanding, is worthy of discussion. It has been recently proposed that a mechanism by which the tubercle bacillus may prevent phagosomal maturation is by retention on the bacillus-containing phagosomes of coronin 1, also known as TACO (for "tryptophan-aspartate-rich coat protein") (37). Coronin 1 is a 43-kDa WD repeat host protein first identified in *Dictyostelium discoideum* (26). A mutant of *D. discoideum* coronin 1 is found to be abnormal in phagocytosis, cytokinesis, and locomotion (26). Organelle electrophoresis and metabolic labeling studies have provided evidence that phagosomes of J774 macrophages containing live BCG bacilli are associated with TACO retention. This phenomenon is not apparent in macrophages infected with dead BCG bacilli. Studies using an immunohistochemical and confocal-microscopy approach yielded similar results. While Kupffer cells, hepatic macrophages that do not express TACO, are able to rapidly degrade ingested BCG bacilli, cells of a TACO-negative melanoma cell line, when transfected with TACO, display decreased killing of the bacilli as well as attenuated phagolysosomal fusion. Therefore, the apparent resistance of the liver to the tubercle bacillus may be due to the inability of *M. tuberculosis* to block phagosome maturation due to the lack of TACO in Kupffer cells. Based on these results, it has been speculated that TACO retention by mycobacterium-containing phagosomes enables *M. tuberculosis* to disrupt phagosome maturation, thereby shielding the phagocytized bacilli from the toxic effect of the lysosomes and consequently promoting persistence (37). However, results of a recent study have revealed that the TACO retention phenomenon is observed in phagosomes containing clumped bacilli while those with dispersed organisms are not associated with retention of this host protein (84). This observation therefore at once challenges the role of TACO retention in the arrest of the maturation of mycobacterium-containing phagosomes and raises the intriguing possibility that clumping may be a virulence attribute of *M. tuberculosis* (84). Direct evidence for TACO retention by *M. tuberculosis*-containing phagosomes in mycobacterial persistence in the host remains to be demonstrated.

Clearly, the tubercle bacillus has evolved a wide array of mechanisms by which the antimicrobial activity of the lysosomes can be evaded. There is, however, evidence that these evasive strategies could be overcome by the host. For example, it has been shown that maturation arrest exhibited by phagosomes containing *M. avium* (another pathogenic mycobacterium) in unstimulated macrophages (45) is not apparent when the host cells are immunologically activated by agents such as IFN-γ and lipopolysaccharide (83). Indeed, the IFN-γ-inducible 47-kDa LRG-47 was critical in host defense against *M. tuberculosis* in a murine experimental tuberculosis model involving mice deficient in LRG-47; the antimycobacterial activity of this GTPase has been linked to its ability to promote the maturation of bacillus-containing phagosomes (61). These observations underscore that complexity of the interaction between *M. tuberculosis* and the host.

MODELS OF T-CELL-DEPENDENT INTRACELLULAR KILLING

Two general models have been described to study the effects of interactions of infected monocytes (or monocyte-derived macrophages) with other types of cells on the control of intracellular mycobacterial growth. In the first, monocytes are infected with *M. tuberculosis* as an adherent monolayer, extracellular bacilli are removed by washing, and lymphocytes (or other cells) are added to the cultures. The advantages of this model are that the infection ratio can be accurately measured and the effects of specific added cell populations (whether monoclonal, polyclonal, or heterogeneous) can be readily determined. Its disadvantages are that adherence may affect phagocytosis and other cellular interactions requiring direct cell contact and that its time and labor requirements make it difficult to incorporate in clinical trials.

The second model uses heparinized blood rather than isolated mononuclear cells and is performed with the cells in suspension, with constant mixing, rather than as a monolayer. Cultures are infected by adding mycobacteria at a very low infection ratio (fewer than 1 CFU per 5 monocytes). Phagocytosis is highly efficient, so that removal of extracellular bacilli is not required (99). Isolated monocytes in suspension show increased capacity to kill *M. smegmatis* via non-RNI-dependent mechanisms (4); this may account for the greater capacity for restriction of growth of this model compared to that of monocytes plus T cells. Two methods have been described to assess mycobacterial viability in the completed whole-blood cultures. The studies by Kampmann et al. were performed using BCG containing a luciferase reporter phage construct, and viability was assessed as light production (52); those by Cheon et al. used time to positivity after inoculation into BACTEC (17). The results obtained using the two methods to assess viability are generally correlated. The resulting simplicity of the whole-blood model makes it amenable for use in field studies and clinical trials. The luciferase readout is particularly rapid and inexpensive; this advantage is partially offset by the requirement for log-phase bacterial cells as the inoculum (frozen cells cannot be used). The BACTEC readout permits studies of virulence of any mycobacterial isolate, using frozen stocks; this is offset by its cost. The complexity of the cellular interactions in the whole-blood model is potentially both a disadvantage and a strength. For example, at early time points after inoculation, bacilli are mainly contained within neutrophils; at later time points, they are visible mainly in monocytes. Specific studies have not yet been performed to examine this transition. However, the ingestion by monocytes of mycobacterium-containing neutrophil apoptotic bodies may contribute to this process, both in vitro and in vivo. The complexity of the whole-blood model may be valuable in mimicking cellular interactions as they occur early in granuloma formation in vivo.

MECHANISMS FOR CELLULAR CONTROL OF MYCOBACTERIAL GROWTH IN HUMAN MACROPHAGES

In vitro studies of the control of growth of *M. tuberculosis* within human cells have been largely modeled on the work of Crowle, who utilized 7-day cultures of *M. tuberculosis*-infected monocytes to identify components of immune T-cell supernatants that mediated the control of intracellular growth (23). These studies, in sharp contrast to those carried out with murine systems, showed that IFN-γ itself does not activate human monocytes to control intracellular *M. tuberculosis* (34). This observation has since been confirmed by several other investigators (7, 78, 85). The inability of these human in vitro systems to demonstrate significant cytokine-mediated killing of *M. tuberculosis* led to skepticism about the biological relevance of the model. Subsequently, however, vitamins D and A were shown to be active in human defenses against *M. tuberculosis* in the model (24, 78). Other studies have also suggested a role for TNF-α in inhibiting the growth of avirulent *M. tuberculosis* within human phagocytes (47). However, the magnitude of these effects was significantly reduced compared to that of IFN-γ in the murine system, despite ample evidence that T cells in these models recognize mycobacterial antigens and undergo appropriate proliferation, cytokine production, and cytotoxicity.

Faced with this apparent paradox, several research groups have examined the effects of cytotoxic mechanisms on the viability of intracellular *M. tuberculosis*. Malloy et al., for example, have demonstrated that ATP-induced apoptosis of monocytes infected with *M. bovis* BCG resulted in killing of the intracellular bacilli. In contrast, monocyte lysis resulting from treatment with H_2O_2 resulted in the release of viable BCG bacilli from infected cells (67). These findings inspired further investigation of both the mechanisms of ATP-induced killing of intracellular mycobacteria and the correlations between the ability of various lymphocyte populations to mediate lytic and apoptotic death of infected monocytes and their capacity to kill intracellular mycobacteria.

ATP-Mediated Killing

The ability of ATP to mediate killing of intracellular BCG was confirmed by Lammas et al. (56). Kusner and Adams subsequently extended these observations to show that ATP also mediated the killing of virulent strains of *M. tuberculosis* (54). Studies using receptor-specific agonists (benxoylbenzoic ATP) and antagonists (oxidized ATP and others) demonstrated that the antimycobacterial effects of ATP were mediated by P2X7 (formerly P2Z) purinergic receptors (56). Further studies have indicated that ATP serves to reverse the arrested phagosome-lysosome fusion that is characteristic of mycobacterial infection. Induction of phospholipid D production and increased intracellular calcium concentrations both result from P2X7 activation and independently serve to facilitate phagosomal maturation, resulting in killing of intracellular *M. tuberculosis* (55). These investigations of ATP-induced killing of *M. tuberculosis* serve to confirm the central role of inhibition of phagosome-lysosome fusion in successful parasitization of human

phagocytes by *M. tuberculosis* and could eventually lead to the development of novel antimicrobial agents in tuberculosis treatment. However, the relevance of ATP-mediated bacterial killing to in vivo immune-mediated activation of infected phagocytes remains unclear, since studies by Canaday et al. indicate that the concentration of ATP released by *M. tuberculosis*-specific cytotoxic T cells is several orders of magnitude lower than that needed to mediate the inhibition of intracellular mycobacterial growth (11).

Lymphocyte-Mediated Killing of Intracellular *M. tuberculosis*: CD4 and CD8 T Cells

The lack of convincing effects of the cytokines produced by T cells on intracellular *M. tuberculosis* growth has led several investigators to examine other mechanisms requiring direct cell contact. Silver et al. established a model of low-level infection of human monocytes with virulent *M. tuberculosis* H37Rv in order to optimize conditions for observing the ability of soluble mediators to activate the killing of intracellular bacilli. Toward this end, an infection model was developed with *M. tuberculosis* H37Rv, using a 1:1 multiplicity of infection, resulting in consistent infection with fewer than five bacilli per cell. Nonetheless, high concentrations of exogenous TNF-α had no impact on the intracellular growth of *M. tuberculosis* in this model, and recombinant IFN-γ mediated only a modest reduction in intracellular growth. In contrast, the addition of unsorted peripheral blood lymphocytes to infected monocytes reduced intracellular growth 10-fold over a 1-week assay. Transferred supernatants of cocultures were considerably less effective at mediating killing than were the lymphocytes themselves. Lymphocytes treated with the protein synthesis inhibitor emetine retained a significant capacity to mediate intracellular killing, further emphasizing the importance of direct cell-to-cell contact in lymphocyte-mediated killing of intracellular *M. tuberculosis*. The participation of CD4 T cells in the inhibition of intracellular *M. tuberculosis* growth is restricted mainly to cultures of tuberculin skin test reactors. Lymphocyte-mediated CD4-independent mechanisms (such as those involving NK cells) are evident regardless of skin test status; this has been shown in both the whole-blood and monocyte-plus-lymphocyte infection models (85, 94).

Subsequent studies evaluated the roles of specific cytotoxic mechanisms and cell-cell interactions in mediating the killing of intracellular *M. tuberculosis* by several human lymphocyte populations. Canaday et al. demonstrated killing of *M. tuberculosis* antigen-specific CD4$^+$ and CD8$^+$ short-term cell lines (12). Both CD4$^+$ and CD8$^+$ lines displayed cytotoxicity to infected monocytes. Furthermore, for both types of lines, cytotoxicity was mediated predominantly by granule release rather than FasL-dependent mechanisms. Killing of intracellular *M. tuberculosis* could not be linked to either mechanism of cytotoxicity, however. Specifically, blocking of FasL-Fas interactions with specific antibody, as well as blocking of perforin function with concanamycin A, each significantly reduced the cytotoxicity of CD4$^+$ and CD8$^+$ T-cell lines to infected target cells but did not inhibit lymphocyte-mediated killing of intracellular *M. tuberculosis*.

Because of its role in stimulating cell-mediated immune responses, the interaction of the CD4$^+$ T-cell surface molecule CD40L (CD154) with CD40 on infected monocytes was also investigated as a possible pathway for activation of killing of the intracellular organisms. Again, however, effective inhibition of this pathway had no effect on the ability of either unsorted peripheral blood lymphocytes or antigen-specific short-term CD4$^+$ T-cell lines to mediate the killing of *M. tuberculosis* (57).

Natural Killer Cells

NK cells have the capacity to kill intracellular *M. tuberculosis*, whether these cells are isolated from PPD-positive or PPD-negative subjects. Although NK cells were initially identified by their ability to lyse target cells through perforin-mediated mechanisms, inhibition of NK cell granule release (by addition of the calcium chelator EGTA) had no effect on the ability of NK cells to mediate the killing of intracellular *M. tuberculosis*. NK cell-mediated apoptosis of infected MN was observed in this system, but both apoptosis and killing of *M. tuberculosis* were again found to be independent of the FasL-Fas interactions (8). Thus, an additional possibility remained that NK cells mediate the killing of intracellular *M. tuberculosis* by Fas-independent apoptotic pathways.

CD1-Restricted T Cells

The finding that mice deficient in β_2-microglobulin have a markedly impaired ability to contain infection with *M. tuberculosis* also led to interest in presentation of *M. tuberculosis* antigens by the nonclassical CD1-dependent pathway, since β_2-microglobulin is a component of the CD1 complex. Stenger et al. evaluated the ability of cytotoxic CD1-restricted T cells to mediate the killing of intracellular *M. tuberculosis* (89). CD1-restricted clones were developed by incubating peripheral blood mononuclear cells (PBMC) with *M. tuberculosis* extract in the presence of granulocyte-macrophage colony-stimulating

factor and IL-4, in order to increase the expression of CD1 on antigen-presenting cells. The resulting clones were found to express two surface phenotypes, which correlated with two distinct pathways of cytotoxicity. The cytotoxicity of CD4$^-$ CD8$^-$ (double-negative [DN]) T cells to *M. tuberculosis*-infected macrophages was Fas dependent, whereas CD4$^-$ CD8$^+$ CD1-restricted T cells lysed infected cells by granule-dependent mechanisms. The FasL-dependent cytotoxicity mediated by DN CD1-restricted T-cell lines was not associated with killing of intracellular *M. tuberculosis*. In contrast, pretreatment of CD1-restricted CD8$^+$ T cells with strontium, which induces degranulation, eliminated the capacity of these cells to kill intracellular organisms.

Both the granule-dependent cytotoxicity, as mediated by CD1-restricted CD8$^+$ T cells, and the Fas/FasL-dependent cytotoxicity of DN CD1-restricted T cells result in macrophage apoptosis via caspase-dependent pathways. Subsequent studies using the pan-caspase inhibitor *N*-benzoylcarbonyl-Val-Ala-Asp-fluoromethylketone (ZVAD-FMK) indicated that the killing of intracellular *M. tuberculosis* by CD1-restricted CD8$^+$ T cells was independent of target cell apoptosis.

Granulysin

Further studies have demonstrated that granulysin, a component of cytotoxic granules, itself has the capacity to kill extracellular *M. tuberculosis*, and they have suggested a mechanism of killing based on the adherence of granulysin to the cell wall, resulting in increased permeability. Granulysin alone was unable to alter the viability of intracellular *M. tuberculosis*. It was postulated that granulysin is itself unable to pass through intact cell membranes to allow its interaction with intracellular organisms. Addition of perforin, which permeabilizes target cell membranes, did not itself reduce the viability of intracellular *M. tuberculosis*. However, incubation of infected macrophages with a combination of perforin and granulysin did result in bacterial killing. These findings suggest the possibility these two components of cytotoxic granules work in synchrony to mediate the killing of intracellular *M. tuberculosis*, with perforin serving to permeabilize cell membranes so that granulysin may gain entry into infected macrophages and kill the organism. This concept of bacterial killing resulting from direct antimicrobial effects of lymphocyte products represents a significant paradigm shift from the traditional view that cell-mediated immunity is maintained by the ability of lymphocytes to activate the inherent killing mechanisms of infected mononuclear phagocytes.

Gamma-Delta T Cells

Dieli et al. demonstrated that human gamma-delta ($\gamma\delta$) T-cell clones had the ability to kill both extracellular and intracellular *M. tuberculosis* (32). The authors then demonstrated that the addition of antiperforin antibodies blocked $\gamma\delta$ T-cell-mediated killing of intracellular but not extracellular *M. tuberculosis*. Subsequently, *M. tuberculosis*-specific $\gamma\delta$ T-cell clones were treated with strontium to release the contents of cytotoxic granules. The supernatants of strontium-treated cells had the capacity to mediate the killing of intracellular *M. tuberculosis*. Immunoadsorption of these supernatants with antigranulysin antibodies eliminated their capacity to mediate bacterial killing (32).

The findings regarding $\gamma\delta$ T cells are thus consistent with the above hypothesis that perforin serves to permeabilize *M. tuberculosis*-infected phagocytes, allowing the entry of the antimicrobial component granulysin, and they provide the first direct link between products of a specific lymphocyte population and killing of *M. tuberculosis*. It is unclear why similar studies of CD4 and CD8 T cells, as well as NK cells, have thus far failed to link granule release and activity with killing of *M. tuberculosis* despite involving similar methods. The more clear-cut linkage of lymphocyte activity with mycobacterial killing demonstrated with $\gamma\delta$ T cells and CD1-restricted T cells may in part reflect the use of clones (as opposed to short-term T-cell lines) in these studies, which may lead to selection for more narrowly defined immunologic functions. In any case, the relevance of CD1-restricted T cells and $\gamma\delta$ T cells to protective immunity remains uncertain, and there is no evidence that the mechanism of granulysin-mediated bacterial killing explains the antimycobacterial actions of other lymphocyte subsets whose role in protective immunity is better established. This lack of clear definition of mechanisms of lymphocyte-mediated killing in some assays had led to concern that killing in these systems may be an artifact of the culture system (101). However, the observation that killing, as measured in several distinct in vitro assays, is enhanced following BCG vaccination suggests that these assays are biologically relevant (17, 48). Further studies to correlate specific functions of *M. tuberculosis*-reactive lymphocytes with killing of intracellular *M. tuberculosis* will clarify the significance of these observations.

STUDIES OF CLINICAL POPULATIONS

Several studies have examined the ability to control intracellular mycobacterial replication in human populations varying in tuberculosis risk or protection. The goals of these studies have been both to explore the potential role of these models as correlates of protection against tuberculosis (36) and to determine the clinical significance of the various mechanisms for intracellular killing described above.

The ability to control the growth of intracellular mycobacteria in the whole-blood model is superior in tuberculin reactors than in nonreactors (Table 1) (52); this is consistent with the protection afforded by tuberculin reactivity against exogenous reinfection with *M. tuberculosis* (88). The ability of tuberculin reactors to control growth could be blocked by antibodies to IFN-γ or TNF-α and could be inhibited by methylprednisolone or pentoxifylline (17, 52). Control of intracellular BCG growth improves after BCG vaccination of neonates (52a) and after repeated BCG vaccination of adults (17, 48). Studies comparing age-matched cohorts of HIV-infected and uninfected children from South Africa demonstrated an association between low CD4 cell counts, low IFN-γ production, and impaired ability to regulate the growth of BCG in blood from HIV-infected children (94). Impaired control of infection was not reconstituted by the addition of exogenous IFN-γ but, in a small cohort, improved following initiation of antiretroviral therapy (B. Eley, G. N. Tena, and B. Kampmann, *Durban S. Afr. AIDS Conf.*, abstr. T1-S4-A24, 2003).

These findings indicate an overall correlation of whole-blood bactericidal activity with protection

Table 1. Immune control of mycobacterial growth in the blood of tuberculosis patients and healthy volunteers[a]

Subjects	Δlog CFU of mycobacterial strain:			
	H37Ra	BCG	H37Rv	Clinical
Healthy PPD⁻ persons	$+0.25 \pm 0.2$	$+0.15 \pm 0.2$	$+0.5 \pm 0.2$	$+1.0 \pm 0.1$
Healthy PPD⁺ persons	-0.27 ± 0.2	-0.25 ± 0.4	$+0.5 \pm 0.2$	$+0.9 \pm 0.1$
TB patients	-0.54 ± 0.5			$+0.13 \pm 0.3$

[a]Positive values indicate growth; negative values indicate killing. TB patients were studied after completion of chemotherapy, using their own isolates. Patients showed superior killing of H37Ra compared to controls ($P < 0.01$ for all). Patients contained the growth of their own clinical isolate as readily as controls did that of the attenuated strain H37Ra.

against tuberculosis, despite the apparent inability of the model to generate RNI. Additional studies are warranted to determine the accuracy of the model to reflect mycobacterial immunity in individuals and to determine the relative contributions of antimycobacterial mechanisms expressed therein to control of replication.

REFERENCES

1. Altare, F., A. Durandy, D. Lammas, J. F. Emile, S. Lamhamedi, F. Le Deist, P. Drysdale, E. Jouanguy, R. Doffinger, F. Bernaudin, O. Jeppsson, J. A. Gollob, E. Meinl, A. W. Segal, A. Fischer, D. Kumararatne, and J. L. Casanova. 1998. Impairment of mycobacterial immunity in human interleukin-12 receptor deficiency. *Science* **280:**1432–1435.

2. Armstrong, J. A., and P. D. Hart. 1971. Response of cultured macrophages to *Mycobacterium tuberculosis*, with observations on fusion of lysosomes with phagosomes. *J. Exp. Med.* **134:**713–740.

3. Bainton, D. F. 1981. The discovery of lysosomes. *J. Cell Biol.* **91:**66s–76s.

4. Barker, K., H. Fan, C. Carroll, G. Kaplan, J. Barker, W. Hellmann, and Z. A. Cohn. 1996. Nonadherent cultures of human monocytes kill *Mycobacterium smegmatis*, but adherent cultures do not. *Infect. Immun.* **64:**428–433.

5. Beckman, J. S., and W. H. Koppenol. 1996. Nitric oxide, superoxide, and peroxynitrite: the good, the bad, and ugly. *Am. J. Physiol.* **271:**C1424–C1437.

6. Bellamy, R., C. Ruwende, T. Corrah, K. P. McAdam, H. C. Whittle, and A. V. Hill. 1998. Variations in the NRAMP1 gene and susceptibility to tuberculosis in West Africans. *N. Engl. J. Med.* **338:**640–644.

7. Bonecini-Almeida, M. G., S. Chitale, I. Boutsikakis, J. Geng, H. Doo, S. He, and J. L. Ho. 1998. Induction of in vitro human macrophage anti-*Mycobacterium tuberculosis* activity: requirement for IFN-gamma and primed lymphocytes. *J. Immunol.* **160:**4490–4499.

8. Brill, K. J., Q. Li, R. Larkin, D. H. Canaday, D. R. Kaplan, W. H. Boom, and R. F. Silver. 2001. Human natural killer cells mediate killing of intracellular *Mycobacterium tuberculosis* H37Rv via granule-independent mechanisms. *Infect. Immun.* **69:**1755–1765.

9. Bryk, R., P. Griffin, and C. Nathan. 2000. Peroxynitrite reductase activity of bacterial peroxiredoxins. *Nature* **407:**211–215.

10. Bryk, R., C. D. Lima, H. Erdjument-Bromage, P. Tempst, and C. Nathan. 2002. Metabolic enzymes of mycobacteria linked to antioxidant defense by a thioredoxin-like protein. *Science* **295:**1073–1077.

11. Canaday, D. H., R. Beigi, R. F. Silver, C. V. Harding, W. H. Boom, and G. R. Dubyak. 2002. ATP and control of intracellular growth of mycobacteria by T cells. *Infect. Immun.* **70:**6456–6459.

12. Canaday, D. H., R. J. Wilkinson, Q. Li, C. V. Harding, R. F. Silver, and W. H. Boom. 2001. CD4$^+$ and CD8$^+$ T cells kill intracellular *Mycobacterium tuberculosis* by a perforin and Fas/Fas ligand-independent mechanism. *J. Immunol.* **167:**2734–2742.

13. Chan, J., and J. Flynn. 1999. Nitric oxide in *Mycobacterium tuberculosis* infection, p. 281–310. *In* F. Fang (ed.), *Nitric Oxide and Infection*. Plenum Publishing Corp., New York, N.Y.

14. Chan, J., K. Tanaka, D. Carroll, J. Flynn, and B. R. Bloom. 1995. Effects of nitric oxide synthase inhibitors on murine infection with *Mycobacterium tuberculosis*. *Infect. Immun.* **63:**736–740.

15. Chan, J., Y. Xing, R. S. Magliozzo, and B. R. Bloom. 1992. Killing of virulent *Mycobacterium tuberculosis* by reactive nitrogen intermediates produced by activated murine macrophages. *J. Exp. Med.* **175:**1111–1122.

16. Chen, L., Q. W. Xie, and C. Nathan. 1998. Alkyl hydroperoxide reductase subunit C (AhpC) protects bacterial and human cells against reactive nitrogen intermediates. *Mol. Cell* **1:**795–805.

17. Cheon, S. H., B. Kampmann, A. G. Hise, M. Phillips, H. Y. Song, K. Landen, Q. Li, R. Larkin, J. J. Ellner, R. F. Silver, D. F. Hoft, and R. S. Wallis. 2002. Bactericidal activity in whole blood as a potential surrogate marker of immunity after vaccination against tuberculosis. *Clin. Diagn. Lab. Immunol.* **9:**901–907.

18. Choi, H. S., P. R. Rai, H. W. Chu, C. Cool, and E. D. Chan. 2002. Analysis of nitric oxide synthase and nitrotyrosine expression in human pulmonary tuberculosis. *Am. J. Respir. Crit. Care Med.* **166:**178–186.

19. Christoforidis, S., H. M. McBride, R. D. Burgoyne, and M. Zerial. 1999. The Rab5 effector EEA1 is a core component of endosome docking. *Nature* **397:**621–625.

20. Clemens, D. L., B. Y. Lee, and M. A. Horwitz. 2000. Deviant expression of Rab5 on phagosomes containing the intracellular pathogens *Mycobacterium tuberculosis* and *Legionella pneumophila* is associated with altered phagosomal fate. *Infect. Immun.* **68:**2671–2684.

21. Clemens, D. L., B. Y. Lee, and M. A. Horwitz. 2000. *Mycobacterium tuberculosis* and *Legionella pneumophila* phagosomes exhibit arrested maturation despite acquisition of Rab7. *Infect. Immun.* **68:**5154–5166.

22. Cole, S. T., R. Brosch, J. Parkhill, T. Garnier, C. Churcher, D. Harris, S. V. Gordon, K. Eiglmeier, S. Gas, C. E. Barry, F. Tekaia, K. Badcock, D. Basham, D. Brown, T. Chillingworth, R. Connor, R. Davies, K. Devlin, T. Feltwell, S. Gentles, N. Hamlin, S. Holroyd, T. Hornsby, K. Jagels, A. Krogh, J. McLean, S. Moule, L. Murphy, K. Oliver, J. Osborne, M. A. Quail, M.-A. Rajandream, J. Rogers, S. Rutter, K. Seeger, J. Skelton, R. Squares, S. Squares J. E. Sulston, K. Taylor, S. Whitehead, and B. G. Barrell. 1998. Deciphering the biology of *Mycobacterium tuberculosis* from the complete genome sequence. *Nature* **393:**537–544.

23. Crowle, A. 1981. Preliminary demonstration of human tuberculoimmunity in vitro. *Infect. Immun.* **31:**453–464.

24. Crowle, A., E. R. Ross, and M. H. May. 1987. Inhibition by 1,25-(OH)$_2$ vitamin D$_3$ of the multiplication of virulent tubercle bacilli in cultured human macrophages. *Infect. Immun.* **55:**2945–2950.

25. De Duve, C., and R. Wattiaux. 1966. Functions of lysosomes. *Annu. Rev. Physiol.* **28:**435–492.

26. de Hostos, E. L. 1999. The coronin family of actin-associated proteins. *Trends Cell Biol.* **9:**345–350.

27. de Jong, R., F. Altare, I. A. Haagen, D. G. Elferink, T. Boer, V. van Breda, P. J. Kabel, J. M. Draaisma, J. T. van Dissel, F. P. Kroon, J. L. Casanova, and T. H. Ottenhoff. 1998. Severe mycobacterial and *Salmonella* infections in interleukin-12 receptor-deficient patients. *Science* **280:**1435–1438.

28. Denis, M. 1991. Killing of *Mycobacterium tuberculosis* within human monocytes: activation by cytokines and calcitriol. *Clin. Exp. Immunol.* **84:**200–206.

29. Deretic, V., and R. A. Fratti. 1999. *Mycobacterium tuberculosis* phagosome. *Mol. Microbiol.* **31:**1603–1609.

30. Desjardins, M. 1995. Biogenesis of phagolysosomes: the "kiss and run" hypothesis. *Trends Cell Biol.* **5:**183–186.

31. Desjardins, M., L. A. Huber, R. G. Parton, and G. Griffiths.

1994. Biogenesis of phagolysosomes proceeds through a sequential series of interactions with the endocytic apparatus. *J. Cell Biol.* **124**:677–688.

32. Dieli, F., M. Troye-Blomberg, S. E. Farouk, G. Sirecil, and A. Salerno. 2001. Biology of gammadelta T cells in tuberculosis and malaria. *Curr. Mol. Med.* **1**:437–446.

33. Dorman, S. E., and S. M. Holland. 1998. Mutation in the signal-transducing chain of the interferon-gamma receptor and susceptibility to mycobacterial infection. *J. Clin. Investig.* **101**:2364–2369.

34. Douvas, G. S., D. L. Looker, A. E. Vatter, and A. J. Crowle. 1985. Gamma interferon activates human macrophages to become tumoricidal and leishmanicidal but enhances replication of macrophage-associated mycobacteria. *Infect. Immun.* **50**:1–8.

35. Ehrt, S., M. U. Shiloh, J. Ruan, M. Choi, S. Gunzburg, C. Nathan, Q. Xie, and L. W. Riley. 1997. A novel antioxidant gene from *Mycobacterium tuberculosis*. *J. Exp. Med.* **186**:1885–1896.

36. Ellner, J. J., C. S. Hirsch, and C. C. Whalen. 2000. Correlates of protective immunity to *Mycobacterium tuberculosis* in humans. *Clin. Infect. Dis.* **30**(Suppl. 3):S279–S282.

37. Ferrari, G., H. Langen, M. Naito, and J. Pieters. 1999. A coat protein on phagosomes involved in the intracellular survival of mycobacteria. *Cell* **97**:435–447.

38. Flynn, J. L., and J. Chan. 2001. Immunology of tuberculosis. *Annu. Rev. Immunol.* **19**:93–129.

39. Flynn, J. L., C. A. Scanga, K. E. Tanaka, and J. Chan. 1998. Effects of aminoguanidine on latent murine tuberculosis. *J. Immunol.* **160**:1796–1803.

40. Fratti, R. A., J. M. Backer, J. Gruenberg, S. Corvera, and V. Deretic. 2001. Role of phosphatidylinositol 3-kinase and Rab5 effectors in phagosomal biogenesis and mycobacterial phagosome maturation arrest. *J. Cell Biol.* **154**:631–644.

41. Fratti, R. A., J. Chua, and V. Deretic. 2002. Cellubrevin alterations and *Mycobacterium tuberculosis* phagosome maturation arrest. *J. Biol. Chem.* **277**:17320–17326.

42. Fratti, R. A., J. Chua, and V. Deretic. 2003. Induction of p38 mitogen-activated protein kinase reduces early endosome autoantigen 1 (EEA1) recruitment to phagosomal membranes. *J. Biol. Chem.* **278**:46961–46967.

43. Fratti, R. A., J. Chua, I. Vergne, and V. Deretic. 2003. *Mycobacterium tuberculosis* glycosylated phosphatidylinositol causes phagosome maturation arrest. *Proc. Natl. Acad. Sci. USA* **100**:5437–5442.

44. Fratti, R. A., I. Vergne, J. Chua, J. Skidmore, and V. Deretic. 2000. Regulators of membrane trafficking and *Mycobacterium tuberculosis* phagosome maturation block. *Electrophoresis* **21**:3378–3385.

45. Frehel, C., C. De Chastellier, T. Lang, and N. Rastogi. 1986. Evidence for inhibition of fusion of lysosomal and prelysosomal compartments with phagosomes in macrophages infected with pathogenic *Mycobacterium avium*. *Infect. Immun.* **52**:252–262.

46. Hart, P. D., J. A. Armstrong, C. A. Brown, and P. Draper. 1972. Ultrastructural study of the behavior of macrophages toward parasitic mycobacteria. *Infect. Immun.* **5**:803–807.

47. Hirsch, C. S., J. J. Ellner, D. G. Russell, and E. A. Rich. 1994. Complement receptor-mediated uptake and tumor necrosis factor-alpha-mediated growth inhibition of *Mycobacterium tuberculosis* by human alveolar macrophages. *J. Immunol.* **152**:743–753.

48. Hoft, D. F., S. Worku, B. Kampmann, C. C. Whalen, J. J. Ellner, C. S. Hirsch, R. B. Brown, R. Larkin, Q. Li, H. Yun, and R. F. Silver. 2002. Investigation of the relationships between immune-mediated inhibition of mycobacterial growth and other potential surrogate markers of protective *Mycobacterium tuberculosis* immunity. *J. Infect. Dis.* **186**:1448–1457.

49. Jacobson, F. S., R. W. Morgan, M. F. Christman, and B. N. Ames. 1989. An alkyl hydroperoxide reductase from *Salmonella typhimurium* involved in the defense of DNA against oxidative damage. Purification and properties. *J. Biol. Chem.* **264**:1488–1496.

50. Jahn, R., and T. C. Sudhof. 1999. Membrane fusion and exocytosis. *Annu. Rev. Biochem.* **68**:863–911.

51. Jouanguy, E., S. Lamhamedi-Cherradi, D. Lammas, S. E. Dorman, M. C. Fondaneche, S. Dupuis, R. Doffinger, F. Altare, J. Girdlestone, J. F. Emile, H. Ducoulombier, D. Edgar, J. Clarke, V. A. Oxelius, M. Brai, V. Novelli, K. Heyne, A. Fischer, S. M. Holland, D. S. Kumararatne, R. D. Schreiber, and J. L. Casanova. 1999. A human IFNGR1 small deletion hotspot associated with dominant susceptibility to mycobacterial infection. *Nat. Genet.* **21**:370–378.

52. Kampmann, B., P. O. Gaora, V. A. Snewin, M. P. Gares, D. B. Young, and M. Levin. 2000. Evaluation of human antimycobacterial immunity using recombinant reporter mycobacteria. *J. Infect. Dis.* **182**:895–901.

52a. Kampmann, B., G. Tena, S. Mzazi, D. Young, B. Eley, and M. Levin. Novel human in vitro system to evaluate antimycobacterial vaccines. *Infect. Immun.*, in press.

53. Kornfeld, S. 1987. Trafficking of lysosomal enzymes. *FASEB J.* **1**:462–468.

54. Kusner, D. J., and J. Adams. 2000. ATP-induced killing of virulent *Mycobacterium tuberculosis* within human macrophages requires phospholipase D. *J. Immunol.* **164**:379–388.

55. Kusner, D. J., and J. A. Barton. 2001. ATP stimulates human macrophages to kill intracellular virulent *Mycobacterium tuberculosis* via calcium-dependent phagosome-lysosome fusion. *J. Immunol.* **167**:3308–3315.

56. Lammas, D., C. Stober, C. J. Harvey, N. Kendrick, S. Panchalingam, and D. S. Kumararatne. 1997. ATP-induced killing of mycobacteria by human macrophages is mediated by purinergic P2Z (P2X7) receptors. *Immunity* **7**:433–444.

57. Larkin, R., C. D. Benjamin, Y. M. Hsu, Q. Li, L. Zukowski, and R. F. Silver. 2002. CD40 ligand (CD154) does not contribute to lymphocyte-mediated inhibition of virulent *Mycobacterium tuberculosis* within human monocytes. *Infect. Immun.* **70**:4716–4720.

58. Lawe, D. C., V. Patki, R. Heller-Harrison, D. Lambright, and S. Corvera. 2000. The FYVE domain of early endosome antigen 1 is required for both phosphatidylinositol 3-phosphate and Rab5 binding. Critical role of this dual interaction for endosomal localization. *J. Biol. Chem.* **275**:3699–3705.

59. MacMicking, J., Q. W. Xie, and C. Nathan. 1997. Nitric oxide and macrophage function. *Annu. Rev. Immunol.* **15**:323–350.

60. MacMicking, J. D., R. J. North, R. LaCourse, J. S. Mudgett, S. K. Shah, and C. F. Nathan. 1997. Identification of nitric oxide synthase as a protective locus against tuberculosis. *Proc. Natl. Acad. Sci. USA* **94**:5243–5248.

61. MacMicking, J. D., G. A. Taylor, and J. D. McKinney. 2003. Immune control of tuberculosis by IFN-gamma-inducible LRG-47. *Science* **302**:654–659.

62. Malik, Z. A., G. M. Denning, and D. J. Kusner. 2000. Inhibition of Ca^{2+} signaling by *Mycobacterium tuberculosis* is associated with reduced phagosome-lysosome fusion and increased survival within human macrophages. *J. Exp. Med.* **191**:287–302.

63. Malik, Z. A., S. S. Iyer, and D. J. Kusner. 2001. *Mycobacterium tuberculosis* phagosomes exhibit altered calmodulin-dependent signal transduction: contribution to inhibition of phagosome-lysosome fusion and intracellular survival in human macrophages. *J. Immunol.* **166**:3392–3401.

64. Malik, Z. A., C. R. Thompson, S. Hashimi, B. Porter, S. S. Iyer, and D. J. Kusner. 2003. Cutting edge: *Mycobacterium tuberculosis* blocks Ca^{2+} signaling and phagosome maturation in human macrophages via specific inhibition of sphingosine kinase. *J. Immunol.* **170**:2811–2815.

65. McBride, H. M., V. Rybin, C. Murphy, A. Giner, R. Teasdale, and M. Zerial. 1999. Oligomeric complexes link Rab5 effectors with NSF and drive membrane fusion via interactions between EEA1 and syntaxin 13. *Cell* **98**:377–386.

66. Mellman, I., R. Fuchs, and A. Helenius. 1986. Acidification of the endocytic and exocytic pathways. *Annu. Rev. Biochem.* **55**:663–700.

67. Molloy, A., P. Laochumroonvorapong, and G. Kaplan. 1994. Apoptosis, but not necrosis, of infected monocytes is coupled with killing of intracellular bacillus Calmette-Guérin. *J. Exp. Med.* **180**:1499–1509.

68. Newport, M. J., C. M. Huxley, S. Huston, C. M. Hawrylowicz, B. A. Oostra, R. Williamson, and M. Levin. 1996. A mutation in the interferon-gamma-receptor gene and susceptibility to mycobacterial infection. *N. Engl. J. Med.* **335**:1941–1949.

69. Nicholson, S., M. G. Bonecini-Almeida, J. R. Lapa e Silva, C. Nathan, Q. W. Xie, R. Mumford, J. R. Weidner, J. Calaycay, J. Geng, N. Boechat, C. Linhares, W. Rom, and J. L. Ho. 1996. Inducible nitric oxide synthase in pulmonary alveolar macrophages from patients with tuberculosis. *J. Exp. Med.* **183**:2293–2302.

70. Nielsen, E., S. Christoforidis, S. Uttenweiler-Joseph, M. Miaczynska, F. Dewitte, M. Wilm, B. Hoflack, and M. Zerial. 2000. Rabenosyn-5, a novel Rab5 effector, is complexed with hVPS45 and recruited to endosomes through a FYVE finger domain. *J. Cell. Biol.* **151**:601–612.

71. Nozaki, Y., Y. Hasegawa, S. Ichiyama, I. Nakashima, and K. Shimokata. 1997. Mechanism of nitric oxide-dependent killing of *Mycobacterium bovis* BCG in human alveolar macrophages. *Infect. Immun.* **65**:3644–3647.

72. O'Brien, L., J. Carmichael, D. B. Lowrie, and P. W. Andrew. 1994. Strains of *Mycobacterium tuberculosis* differ in susceptibility to reactive nitrogen intermediates in vitro. *Infect. Immun.* **62**:5187–5190.

73. Ohkuma, S., and B. Poole. 1978. Fluorescence probe measurement of the intralysosomal pH in living cells and the perturbation of pH by various agents. *Proc. Natl. Acad. Sci. USA* **75**:3327–3331.

74. Ohno, H., G. Zhu, V. P. Mohan, D. Chu, S. Kohno, W. R. Jacobs, Jr., and J. Chan. 2003. The effects of reactive nitrogen intermediates on gene expression in *Mycobacterium tuberculosis*. *Cell Microbiol.* **5**:637–648.

75. Ouellet, H., Y. Ouellet, C. Richard, M. Labarre, B. Wittenberg, J. Wittenberg, and M. Guertin. 2002. Truncated hemoglobin HbN protects *Mycobacterium bovis* from nitric oxide. *Proc. Natl. Acad. Sci. USA* **99**:5902–5907.

76. Rich, E. A., M. Torres, E. Sada, C. K. Finegan, B. D. Hamilton, and Z. Toossi. 1997. *Mycobacterium tuberculosis* (MTB)-stimulated production of nitric oxide by human alveolar macrophages and relationship of nitric oxide production to growth inhibition of MTB. *Tubercle Lung Dis.* **78**:247–255.

77. Rockett, K. A., R. Brookes, I. Udalova, V. Vidal, A. V. Hill, and D. Kwiatkowski. 1998. 1,25-Dihydroxyvitamin D_3 induces nitric oxide synthase and suppresses growth of *Mycobacterium tuberculosis* in a human macrophage-like cell line. *Infect. Immun.* **66**:5314–5321.

78. Rook, G., J. Steele, M. Ainsworth, and B. R. Champion. 1986. Activation of macrophages to inhibit proliferation of *Mycobacterium tuberculosis*: comparison of the effects of recombinant interferon gamma on human monocytes and murine peritoneal macrophages. *Immunology* **59**:333–338.

79. Ruan, J., G. St John, S. Ehrt, L. Riley, and C. Nathan. 1999. noxR3, a novel gene from *Mycobacterium tuberculosis*, protects *Salmonella typhimurium* from nitrosative and oxidative stress. *Infect. Immun.* **67**:3276–3283.

80. Russell, D. G. 2001. *Mycobacterium tuberculosis*: here today, and here tomorrow. *Nat. Rev. Mol. Cell Biol.* **2**:569–577.

81. Russell, D. G., H. C. Mwandumba, and E. E. Rhoades. 2002. *Mycobacterium* and the coat of many lipids. *J. Cell Biol.* **158**:421–426.

82. Scanga, C. A., V. P. Mohan, K. Tanaka, D. Alland, J. L. Flynn, and J. Chan. 2001. The inducible nitric oxide synthase locus confers protection against aerogenic challenge of both clinical and laboratory strains of *Mycobacterium tuberculosis* in mice. *Infect. Immun.* **69**:7711–7717.

83. Schaible, U. E., S. Sturgill-Koszycki, P. H. Schlesinger, and D. G. Russell. 1998. Cytokine activation leads to acidification and increases maturation of *Mycobacterium avium*-containing phagosomes in murine macrophages. *J. Immunol.* **160**:1290–1296.

84. Schuller, S., J. Neefjes, T. Ottenhoff, J. Thole, and D. Young. 2001. Coronin is involved in uptake of *Mycobacterium bovis* BCG in human macrophages but not in phagosome maintenance. *Cell Microbiol.* **3**:785–793.

85. Silver, R. F., Q. Li, W. H. Boom, and J. J. Ellner. 1998. Lymphocyte-dependent inhibition of growth of virulent *Mycobacterium tuberculosis* H37Rv within human monocytes: requirement for $CD4^+$ T cells in purified protein derivative-positive, but not in purified protein derivative-negative, subjects. *J. Immunol.* **160**:2408–2417.

86. Simonsen, A., J. M. Gaullier, A. D'Arrigo, and H. Stenmark. 1999. The Rab5 effector EEA1 interacts directly with syntaxin-6. *J. Biol. Chem.* **274**:28857–28860.

87. Simonsen, A., R. Lippe, S. Christoforidis, J. M. Gaullier, A. Brech, J. Callaghan, B. H. Toh, C. Murphy, M. Zerial, and H. Stenmark. 1998. EEA1 links PI(3)K function to Rab5 regulation of endosome fusion. *Nature* **394**:494–498.

88. Stead, W. W. 1981. Tuberculosis among elderly persons: an outbreak in a nursing home. *Ann. Intern. Med.* **94**:606–610.

89. Stenger, S., R. J. Mazzaccaro, K. Uyemura, S. Cho, P. F. Barnes, J. P. Rosat, A. Sette, M. B. Brenner, S. A. Porcelli, B. R. Bloom, and R. L. Modlin. 1997. Differential effects of cytolytic T cell subsets on intracellular infection. *Science* **276**:1684–1687.

90. St. John, G., N. Brot, J. Ruan, H. Erdjument-Bromage, P. Tempst, H. Weissbach, and C. Nathan. 2001. Peptide methionine sulfoxide reductase from *Escherichia coli* and *Mycobacterium tuberculosis* protects bacteria against oxidative damage from reactive nitrogen intermediates. *Proc. Natl. Acad. Sci. USA* **98**:9901–9906.

91. Storz, G., M. F. Christman, H. Sies, and B. N. Ames. 1987. Spontaneous mutagenesis and oxidative damage to DNA in *Salmonella typhimurium*. *Proc. Natl. Acad. Sci. USA* **84**:8917-8921.

92. Sturgill-Koszycki, S., P. H. Schlesinger, P. Chakraborty, P. L. Haddix, H. L. Collins, A. K. Fok, R. D. Allen, S. L. Gluck, J. Heuser, and D. G. Russell. 1994. Lack of acidification in *Mycobacterium phagosomes* produced by exclusion of the vesicular proton-ATPase. *Science* **263**:678–681.

93. Tartaglia, L. A., G. Storz, M. H. Brodsky, A. Lai, and B. N. Ames. 1990. Alkyl hydroperoxide reductase from *Salmonella typhimurium*. Sequence and homology to thioredoxin reductase and other flavoprotein disulfide oxidoreductases. *J. Biol. Chem.* **265:**10535–10540.

94. Tena, G. N., D. B. Young, B. Eley, H. F. Henderson, M. Nicol, M. Levin, and B. Kampmann. 2003. Failure to control growth of mycobacteria in blood from children infected with HIV, and its relationship to T cell function. *J. Infect. Dis.* **187:**1544–1551.

95. Vergne, I., R. A. Fratti, P. J. Hill, J. Chua, J. Belisle, and V. Deretic. 2004. *Mycobacterium tuberculosis* phagosome maturation arrest: mycobacterial phosphatidylinositol analog phosphatidylinositol mannoside stimulates early endosomal fusion. *Mol. Biol. Cell* **15:**751–760.

96. Via, L. E., D. Deretic, R. J. Ulmer, N. S. Hibler, L. A. Huber, and V. Deretic. 1997. Arrest of mycobacterial phagosome maturation is caused by a block in vesicle fusion between stages controlled by *rab5* and *rab7*. *J. Biol. Chem.* **272:**13326–13331.

97. Vieira, O. V., R. J. Botelho, and S. Grinstein. 2002. Phagosome maturation: aging gracefully. *Biochem. J.* **366:**689–704.

98. Voskuil, M. I., D. Schnappinger, K. C. Visconti, M. I. Harrell, G. M. Dolganov, D. R. Sherman, and G. K. Schoolnik. 2003. Inhibition of respiration by nitric oxide induces a *Mycobacterium tuberculosis* dormancy program. *J. Exp. Med.* **198:**705–713.

99. Wallis, R. S., M. Palaci, S. Vinhas, A. G. Hise, F. C. Ribeiro, K. Landen, S. H. Cheon, H. Y. Song, M. Phillips, R. Dietze, and J. J. Ellner. 2001. A whole blood bactericidal assay for tuberculosis. *J. Infect Dis.* **183:**1300–1303.

100. Wang, C. H., C. Y. Liu, H. C. Lin, C. T. Yu, K. F. Chung, and H. P. Kuo. 1998. Increased exhaled nitric oxide in active pulmonary tuberculosis due to inducible NO synthase upregulation in alveolar macrophages. *Eur. Respir. J.* **11:**809–815.

101. Warwick-Davies, J., J. Dhillon, L. O'Brien, P. W. Andrew, and D. B. Lowrie. 1994. Apparent killing of *Mycobacterium tuberculosis* by cytokine-activated human monocytes can be an artefact of a cytotoxic effect on the monocytes. *Clin. Exp. Immunol.* **96:**214–217.

102. Xu, S., A. Cooper, S. Sturgill Koszycki, T. van Heyningen, D. Chatterjee, I. Orme, P. Allen, and D. G. Russell. 1994. Intracellular trafficking in *Mycobacterium tuberculosis* and *Mycobacterium avium*-infected macrophages. *J. Immunol.* **153:**2568–2578.

103. Yu, K., C. Mitchell, Y. Xing, R. S. Magliozzo, B. R. Bloom, and J. Chan. 1999. Toxicity of nitrogen oxides and related oxidants on mycobacteria: *M. tuberculosis* is resistant to peroxynitrite anion. *Tubercle Lung Dis.* **79:**191–198.

104. Zerial, M., and H. McBride. 2001. Rab proteins as membrane organizers. *Nat. Rev. Mol. Cell Biol.* **2:**107–117.

Tuberculosis and the Tubercle Bacillus
Edited by Stewart T. Cole et al.
© 2005 ASM Press, Washington, D.C.

Chapter 28

Dendritic Cells in Host Immunity to *Mycobacterium tuberculosis*

Marc Mendelson, Willem Hanekom, and Gilla Kaplan

Since their identification by Steinman and Cohn over 30 years ago (86), dendritic cells (DCs) have been shown to play a central role in the initiation and control of the protective host immune response to pathogens (Fig. 1) (88). DCs contribute to the host's ability to distinguish pathogens from self-antigens, to the induction of both primary and secondary T-cell activation and thus to the control of immunity to the pathogen, to determination of the nature of the T-cell helper response (e.g., either Th1 or Th2) (59), and to the establishment of tolerance to foreign antigens when necessary. DCs, which arise from bone marrow precursors, are released into the blood and then traffic to peripheral organs such as the lungs (16). In the blood, various DCs subsets and DCs precursors are found, including myeloid CD11c$^+$ DCs (mDCs), CD123$^+$ plasmacytoid DCs (pDCs), and monocyte precursors of tissue DCs. In peripheral organs, where predominantly mDCs and Langerhans DCs are found, the cells play a central role in the induction and control of immune responses to microbial antigens. In contrast, pDCs, found predominantly in the blood, play an important role in the early immune response to viral infections by secreting large amounts of alpha interferon (IFN-α) (84). In addition, pDCs may contribute to the induction of protective immunity to microbial pathogens (29).

Although as yet incompletely defined, DCs are clearly involved in induction of the protective immune response of humans to infection with *Mycobacterium tuberculosis*. Following inhalation of *M. tuberculosis* into the lungs, the bacilli are phagocytosed by pulmonary alveolar macrophages. The pathogen resides and replicates within cellular phagosomes, where its ability to subvert acidification and fusion with the late endosomal compartments contribute to its survival (90). Control of microbial growth by the phagocyte is dependent on activation of the infected macrophages with cytokines, including IFN-γ, produced predomi-

nantly by antigen-specific T cells and natural killer (NK) cells (28). Pulmonary DCs may play a central role in orchestrating the lung protective immune response, since these cells line the epithelial surface and reside in the pulmonary interstitium (83). Also, at times of tissue inflammation, such as that induced by pathogen entry, an increase in the recruitment of blood DC precursors to the lungs has been noted (5). These DCs recognize and capture antigens, including those of *M. tuberculosis* (85). Antigen capture is followed by morphologic, phenotypic, and functional changes in the DCs, facilitating optimal development of the adaptive immune response. DCs present antigen to lymphocytes in the context of classical major histocompatibility complex (MHC) molecules (4), as well as nonclassical molecules such as CD1 (38), and control the lymphocyte response by cellular contact and by cytokine production. In response, lymphocytes differentiate, proliferate, execute various effector functions (which may involve peripheral tolerance), and may develop into memory cells. Recent advances in the understanding of the interactions between DCs and *M. tuberculosis* and how these interactions affect the course of immune activation and induction of protection against infection are reviewed.

M. TUBERCULOSIS UPTAKE AND REPLICATION WITHIN DCs

DCs bind antigens via surface C-type lectins and Fcγ/Fcε receptors. Phagocytosis of particulate material and intact organisms occurs by receptor-mediated endocytosis (23, 25, 51, 77, 81, 93). The same receptors may also be involved in phagocytosis of cell debris following apoptosis and necrosis (1, 2, 70, 80) and in uptake of extracellular solutes by macropinocytosis (81). Endocytosis of *M. tuberculosis* occurs via a specialized C-type lectin known as DC-associated

Marc Mendelson and Gilla Kaplan • Laboratory of Mycobacterial Immunity and Pathogenesis, Public Health Research Institute, International Center for Public Health, Newark, NJ 07103. **Willem Hanekom** • Departments of Pediatrics and of Microbiology and Immunology, University of Miami School of Medicine, Miami, FL 33136.

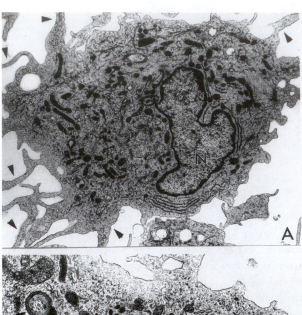

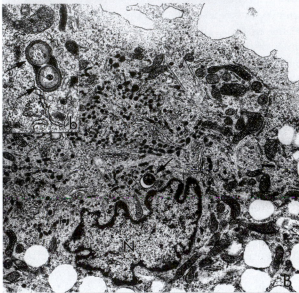

Figure 1. (A) Electron micrograph of an in vitro-matured monocyte-derived DC showing the characteristic dendritic processes (arrows). (B) Monocyte-derived DC infected with *M. tuberculosis* (arrow), with a higher-magnification view (insert) showing replicating *M. tuberculosis* bacilli (arrows).

ICAM-3 nongrabbing integrin, or DC-SIGN (34, 92). DC-SIGN interacts with mannose-capped lipoarabinomannan (Man-LAM) of the *M. tuberculosis* cell wall, specifically binding dimeric and trimeric mannose residues (26, 34, 92). Nonpathogenic environmental mycobacteria, such as *M. smegmatis*, lack a mannose cap on their LAM and therefore cannot interact with DC-SIGN. Because DC-SIGN-mediated entry is associated with specific DC activation (see below), it follows that the type of LAM present on the surface of a mycobacterial species is likely to determine the nature of the immune response induced.

M. tuberculosis binding of DC-SIGN is associated with targeting of the pathogen to lysosome-associated membrane protein 1 (LAMP-1)-containing compartments within the cell (34, 92). LAMP-1$^+$ compartments within DCs can mature to late endosomes/lysosomes, facilitating antigen processing and presentation, as is evidenced by Man-LAM presentation to T cells via CD1b (23, 76). Following DC-SIGN interaction with Man-LAM, the receptor expression is down-regulated on the DC surface (34). Uptake of *M. tuberculosis* by murine and human DCs has been demonstrated by a number of studies carried out both in vitro (10, 31, 35, 40, 41, 44, 89) and in vivo (52). Following uptake by murine bone marrow-derived DCs, virulent *M. tuberculosis* appears to replicate within the cells. However, the extent of replication is dependent on the maturation status of the cell (10): when DCs are first activated by IFN-γ and lipopolysaccharide (LPS), mycobacterial growth is inhibited, although the organisms are probably not killed. Similarly, following intravenous infection of mice with *M. bovis* BCG, mycobacterial growth could not be shown in splenic DCs, suggesting that the DCs inhibited the growth of this nonpathogenic mycobacterium (52). Studies of *M. tuberculosis* replication within human DCs have yielded conflicting results. Tailleux et al. showed that monocyte-derived immature DCs (Mo-iDCs) failed to support the replication of *M. tuberculosis* (91). In contrast, Fortsch et al. demonstrated growth of *M. tuberculosis* within Mo-iDCs (31). Addition of interleukin-10 (IL-10) to Mo-iDCs cultures resulted in reversion of the cell phenotype into macrophage-like cells and inhibition of mycobacterial growth. Our own studies in vitro have shown that Mo-iDCs support replication of the *M. tuberculosis* clinical strains CDC 1551 and HN878 (mean 1.5-log-unit growth) over a 6-day period (M. Mendelson, unpublished data).

TOLL-LIKE RECEPTOR RECOGNITION OF *M. TUBERCULOSIS*

Mammalian Toll-like receptors (TLR) comprise a family of 11 currently identified proteins that recognize pathogen-associated molecular patterns common to different groups of organisms, including *M. tuberculosis* (102). Blood DCs and in vitro-generated Mo-iDCs express a number of different TLRs, including TLR2 and TLR4 (50, 54, 96). Purified *M. tuberculosis* antigens, such as the 19-kDa lipoprotein, bind to TLR2 (12), whereas intact *M. tuberculosis* bacilli appear to interact with both TLR2 and TLR4 and possibly with other TLRs (68, 69, 103). Studies of the interactions between TLRs and *M. tuberculosis* have been carried out predominantly with human monocytes or macrophages. For example, blocking TLR2 on Mo-iDCs resulted in inhibition of *M. tuberculosis*

19-kDa lipoprotein-induced IL-12 production in vitro (95). *M. tuberculosis* 19-kDa lipoprotein also acts as a maturation stimulus for Mo-iDCs in a TLR2-dependent manner (42).

Recent studies have shown that the immunologic outcome of infection with a particular pathogen may be determined by the balance of TLR and C-type lectin receptor interactions. For example, concurrent engagement of Dectin-1 and TLR2 by different ligands of the yeast cell wall component zymosan leads to collaborative induction of an inflammatory response (32). Thus, the generation of a protective immune response by the human host to *M. tuberculosis* is likely to be the result of a combination of stimulatory and inhibitory signals generated by the interaction with pattern recognition receptors such as TLR2/TLR4 and C-type lectins such as DC-SIGN. Binding of Man-LAM to DC-SIGN induces the production of the anti-inflammatory cytokine IL-10 (34), whereas production of proinflammatory IL-12, tumor necrosis factor alpha (TNF-α), and IL-6 was observed following binding of *M. tuberculosis* antigens such as the 19-kDa lipoprotein (68, 69, 103).

EFFECT OF *M. TUBERCULOSIS* ON DENDRITIC CELL MATURATION

Following capture and internalization of antigens, the DCs may undergo phenotypic and functional changes termed maturation, thought to be critical for enabling the induction of conventional T-cell effector immunity. Once matured, DCs migrate efficiently from peripheral tissues to T-cell areas within regional lymph nodes, where immune activation takes place. Homing to T-cell areas requires up-regulation of the chemokine receptor CCR7, rendering the DCs sensitive to the chemokines CCL19 and CCL21 (18, 39, 58, 106). Direct evidence of the transport of *M. tuberculosis* from the lungs to regional lymph nodes in vivo within infected DCs has recently been reported. *M. tuberculosis*-infected bone marrow-derived DCs instilled into the trachea of BALB/c mice were shown to up-regulate CCR7 mRNA expression and migrate to regional mediastinal lymph nodes (9). Moreover, these cells were capable of stimulating a Th1 immune response. Although full maturation of DCs and stimulation of Th1 immunity following antigen capture is one possible scenario in response to invading pathogens, it is important to note that DCs that have remained immature, regardless of whether antigen has been captured, may also migrate to lymph nodes. These cells preferentially home to non-T-cell areas and may be involved in the expansion of regulatory T (Tr) cells and the induction of tolerance (48).

DC maturation is associated with up-regulation of MHC class I and II via increased synthesis and transport to the cell membrane and with decreased degradation of these molecules. In addition, costimulatory molecules such as CD80 (B7.1) and CD86 (B7.2) are transported to the cell surface along with MHC class II, where T-cell receptor triggering is enhanced by the formation of membrane microdomains (100). Engagement of costimulatory molecules by CD28 expressed on the surface of the T cells leads to recruitment of membrane rafts containing kinases and adapters to the immunological synapse, thus amplifying by up to 100-fold the signaling process started by T-cell receptor engagement (59). Lastly, maturation of DCs is associated with the production of the Th1-polarizing cytokine IL-12, which is crucial for optimal stimulation of T-cell responses (85). The importance of this cytokine in regulating the immune response is highlighted by the observation that individuals with germ line mutations in genes of the IL-12 receptor and signaling pathway (that result in defective activity) have an increased risk of contracting mycobacterial diseases, including tuberculosis (13).

How does *M. tuberculosis* affect DC maturation and subsequent immune responses? For the pathogen, a selective advantage would be gained if it could subvert DC maturation, thereby preventing or delaying the induction of specific, conventional effector immunity. Indeed, a number of other microorganisms have developed strategies to subvert DC maturation. These include viruses such as vaccinia virus which inhibits DC maturation by secretion of cytokine receptor homologues that bind to the cells and induce DC apoptosis (24). The protozoan *Plasmodium falciparum* inhibits the maturation of iDCs indirectly, via erythrocyte adhesion to DCs, which is dependent on pathogen-induced expression of the variable antigen PfEMP-1 on the surface of the infected erythrocytes (104). *Trypanosoma cruzi*, on the other hand, produces soluble factors that inhibit DC maturation (105). *M. tuberculosis* has also been shown to subvert DC maturation. Infection of Mo-iDCs with virulent *M. tuberculosis* leads to down-regulation of surface CD1 expression, thereby reducing the ability of the cells to present mycobacterial lipid antigens (89). Furthermore, infection of Mo-iDCs with the laboratory strain *M. tuberculosis* H37Rv in the presence of a "maturation cocktail" of cytokines that induce full DC maturation, i.e., TNF-α, IL-1β, and prostaglandin E$_2$ was reported by us to inhibit the expression of phenotypic markers of DC maturation (40). These DCs failed to induce allogeneic T-cell proliferation (40). Geijtenbeek et al. (34) also demonstrated that *M. tuberculosis* cell wall components may inhibit phenotypic maturation induced by LPS, a powerful maturation stimulus. In the later study, Man-LAM binding to DC-SIGN in the presence of LPS resulted in reduced surface expression of costimulatory molecules through a mechanism involving Man-LAM induction of IL-10 production. In contrast, another antigen, *M. tuberculosis* 19-kDa lipoprotein, has been reported to stimulate DC maturation in vitro (42) without inducing IL-10 production (95). In contrast, several other studies have demonstrated that *M. tuberculosis* infection of DCs in vitro is associated with some phenotypic maturation (41, 42, 60, 99).

Recent studies from our laboratory have suggested that different clinical isolates of *M. tuberculosis* may vary in the degree to which they affect DC maturation. In our studies, the effects of two clinical isolates, CDC 1551 and HN878, are being compared. CDC 1551 induces increased surface expression of phenotypic markers of DC maturation, increased IL-12 production, and enhanced DC-induced allogeneic lymphoproliferation and autologous T-cell activation compared with HN878 (Mendelson, unpublished). Interestingly, the clinical isolate HN878 has recently been identified as a member of the W-Beijing family of *M. tuberculosis* isolates (G. Kaplan, unpublished data), a family of strains shown to be more virulent in mice than strains from other family groups (61). Infection of mice with CDC 1551 is associated with enhanced protective immunity and prolonged survival compared to infection with HN878 (63, 64). Thus, W-Beijing strains may be more virulent in part because of their inability to stimulate optimal DC maturation.

Taken together, our results and those of others suggest that the effects of *M. tuberculosis* on DC maturation are as yet not fully defined. However, it is of interest that failure to induce an optimal effector immune response may be one potential mechanism of increasing pathogen survival. Given the role of immature DCs in inducing tolerance and the prominence of IL-10 in this process, it is tempting to speculate that *M. tuberculosis*, or certain strains of *M. tuberculosis*, may induce limited conventional DC maturation and reduced or delayed effector immunity while activating a prominent Tr-cell response. This possibility needs to be confirmed in further investigations.

ROLE OF *M. TUBERCULOSIS*-EXPOSED DCs IN STIMULATION OF ADAPTIVE IMMUNE RESPONSES

As discussed above, DCs regulate the adaptive immune response to *M. tuberculosis* by stimulating the activation and proliferation of naive and memory T cells in regional lymph nodes. The adaptive immune response to *M. tuberculosis* involves the generation of effector functions of a number of T-cell subsets (11a, 28) including CD4$^+$ and CD8$^+$ T cells, $\gamma\delta$ T cells, and CD1-restricted T cells. The homing of antigen-loaded DCs and circulating T cells to the T-cell areas of regional lymph nodes, in response to CCL19 and CCL21 (30, 78), positions the cells optimally for DC–T-cell interaction. T-cell differentiation and proliferation proceed in areas of DC–T-cell clusters (65), and antigen-specific T cells have been shown to efficiently bind DCs in culture and in vivo (45–47, 65). It is hypothesized that TCRs on resting T cells within these clusters "scan" the surface of DCs for MHC-bound peptide (87). This is achieved via loose binding of DC-SIGN to ICAM-3, expressed on the surface of resting T cells (33). Priming is enhanced by the presence of costimulatory molecules, DC-derived cytokines such as IL-12 and IL-18, and small molecular growth enhancers such as cysteine (3). Activated T-cell blasts leave the regional lymph nodes, trafficking to sites of inflammation such as the lungs. Migration is aided by the alteration of ligand expression, with down-regulation of CCR7 and L-selectin (CD62) and up-regulation of a number of ligands such as CD44 and P-selectin glycoprotein ligand (87). This directs cells to inflamed tissue, where activated T cells are capable of recognizing and reacting to cell surface antigen expressed by a number of different cells, including, most importantly in the case of *M. tuberculosis*, the infected alveolar macrophage.

Macrophage activation, leading to improved control of *M. tuberculosis* replication, is dependent on two principal cytokine signals, IFN-γ and TNF-α. IFN-γ is produced early in the immune response to *M. tuberculosis* by NK T cells, in response to lipid and glycolipid antigen presented in the context of CD1 (22), and by $\gamma\delta$ cells, in response to pyrophosphate, nucleotide, and alkylamine antigens (11). Once the adaptive immune response is induced, IFN-γ is produced predominantly by Th1-polarized CD4$^+$ and CD8$^+$ T cells. DCs induce the maturation of Th cells into IFN-γ-producing Th1 cells through the secretion of a number of Th1-polarizing cytokines, including IL-12, IL-18, IL-23, and probably IFN-α (21, 53, 55). Consequently, Th1 cells, primed and expanded in response to *M. tuberculosis* antigen presented by DCs in regional lymph nodes, circulate to the site of infection such as the lung, where they release IFN-γ, activating the infected macrophage to control the replication of the bacilli. TNF-α is secreted by CD4$^+$ T cells and by macrophages in an autocrine manner (97). It is a key cytokine involved in the maintenance of granuloma architecture (62), the regulation of chemokine secretion and chemokine receptor expression (which together direct incoming cells to the site of infection) and the control of macrophage activation (27). Together, IFN-γ and TNF-α induce macrophage activation, which is associated with stimulation of inducible nitric oxide synthase, reactive nitrogen intermediates, and oxidative effector molecules (101a).

IN VIVO STUDIES OF THE ROLE OF DENDRITIC CELLS IN TUBERCULOSIS

Despite increasing knowledge about the interaction between *M. tuberculosis* and DCs in vitro, relatively little is known about the sequence of events during infection with *M. tuberculosis* in vivo. Studies with rats have documented that, at birth, only very small numbers of DCs, expressing low levels of surface MHC class II, are present in the airway wall (71). Furthermore, recent studies have shown that mature DCs are not constitutively expressed in the tracheobronchial mucosa of infants within the first year of life, although an increase in their numbers is triggered by infectious stimuli (98). Since neonates and infants younger than 1 year are particularly prone to severe disseminated forms of tuberculosis, it is tempting to speculate that the reduced capacity to control infection with *M. tuberculosis* at this age may in part be a result of quantitative and qualitative differences in respiratory tract DCs.

The importance of chemokine secretion and the expression of chemokine receptors involved in cellular recruitment of DCs to sites of infection during active tuberculosis (TB) has also been emphasized. Homing of DCs to the lungs is orchestrated by local secretion of chemokines and expression of chemokine receptors on the incoming DCs. Blood myeloid CD11c$^+$ DC precursors have been shown to express CCR2, which directs DCs to the lungs in response to monocyte chemoattractant protein 1 (MCP-1) (82). Indeed, CCR2 knockout mice infected with *M. tuberculosis* rapidly succumb to progressive infection, with 90% death by day 24 (73). In addition, DC recruitment to regional draining lymph nodes was reduced in these mice, indicating a defect in normal trafficking of DCs in the absence of CCR2 expression. In contrast to CCR2 knockouts, studies of MCP-1 knockout mice showed that control of *M. tuberculosis* infection was only partially attenuated, suggesting that other ligands such as MCP-2, MCP-3, and MCP-5 may compensate for the lack of MCP-1. A number of other studies with mice have confirmed that DCs are recruited from blood to the site of infection within 3 days of aerosol infection with *M. tuberculosis* (36, 49, 72). During steady state, constitutive turnover of lung DCs was found to be on the order of 3 days, as determined by radiation chimera studies

(43, 67). However, during acute inflammation, rapid recruitment of DC precursors and stimulation of DC migration resulted in cellular turnover of 36 to 48 h. Immunohistochemical studies of mice injected intravenously with purified protein derivative (PPD)-coated Sepharose beads have shown that 1 day after injection, DCs were located in close proximity to the beads. By day 3, DCs were distributed throughout the granuloma, adjacent to lymphocytes, increasing the likelihood of cell-cell contact and local stimulation of infiltrating T cells (49). Hence, recruitment of blood DCs to the granuloma may enhance the immune response to *M. tuberculosis* by increasing T-cell stimulation. Once chronic *M. tuberculosis* infection has been established, total DC numbers in the lungs appear to be reduced and costimulatory molecules on the surface of lung DCs are up-regulated (36). This may have important implications for persistence of *M. tuberculosis* infection during active disease.

Studies of human peripheral blood DCs have demonstrated a reduction in the numbers of circulating CD11c$^+$ mDCs in the blood of patients with active disease compared to that in age-matched healthy controls (101). Concomitant with this reduction in the number of circulating DCs was the histological finding that cells that are positive for fascin (an actin-bundling protein restricted to mature DCs, Reed-Sternberg cells of Hodgkin's disease, and Epstein-Barr virus-infected B cells [74]) can be found in granulomas from patients with active tuberculosis. The accumulation of such cells in the lymphocyte areas of the granuloma suggests that they may have been recruited from blood in response to *M. tuberculosis* infection. It remains possible, however, that fascin$^+$ cells represent monocytes that have undergone differentiation to Mo-iDC and matured further in the tissues in response to *M. tuberculosis* and the local cytokine milieu.

We have recently initiated studies to compare the number and function of blood DCs in human immunodeficiency virus-seronegative adults with various clinical presentations of TB. Our preliminary studies show that pulmonary tuberculosis is associated with a reduction in the number of CD11c$^+$ mDCs in the blood. This is associated with functional impairment expressed as a reduced ability of CD11c$^+$ mDCs to produce IL-12 in response to stimulation with virulent *M. tuberculosis* in vitro (Mendelson, unpublished). In contrast, patients with pleural TB maintain both normal levels of cells and optimal functional responses of blood DCs, similar to those exhibited by healthy laboratory volunteers. Our results may help to explain in part the long-known observation that, prior to the regular use of antimycobacterial chemotherapy, tuberculous pleural effusions were associated with better prognosis and greater likelihood of spontaneous resolution than was pulmonary disease (79). Furthermore, since pleural tuberculosis is associated with the production of high levels of IFN-γ and TNF-α from CD4$^+$ T cells (7, 8), preservation of the numbers and function of blood DCs available to migrate to the pleura and stimulate T cells in situ may be an important factor in determining the natural history of the disease.

DENDRITIC CELLS IN THE DEVELOPMENT OF NEW ANTITUBERCULOSIS VACCINES

The central role of DCs in the regulation of cellular immunity provides a rationale for manipulating DC function in vaccine development. DCs have natural adjuvant properties; i.e., their presence increases a given T-cell response to antigen. When used in vaccines, DCs can induce a broad range of T- and B-cell immunity (6). This property of the cells is particularly attractive for designing new vaccines to prevent pulmonary TB. DC-based vaccines for clinical use are manufactured by pulsing autologous monocyte-derived DCs with specific antigens ex vivo and maturing the cells with cytokine cocktails (15). Such vaccines have been used in patients to treat or prevent cancers, with some success. Many variables associated with clinical DC vaccination for cancers have been optimized, resulting in protocols that facilitate the induction of broad CD4$^+$ and CD8$^+$ T-cell immunity. This contrasts, for example, with induction of preferential CD4$^+$ T-cell immunity by novel protein subunit TB vaccines. So far, DC vaccination technology is in its infancy and may appear cumbersome or impractical. However, the field is advancing rapidly (6), and our understanding of DC biology may be particularly useful for vaccination strategies in which DCs are preferentially targeted to the lungs (see below).

Results of mouse studies of DC-based vaccination against TB are encouraging. A single intravenous vaccination with PPD-pulsed DCs was shown to induce long-lived immunity, measured by IFN-γ production after in vitro incubation of lymph node or spleen cells with PPD (19). In another study, intraperitoneal immunization with DCs, pulsed with virulent M. tuberculosis and then irradiated, resulted in induction of both T- and B-cell immunity (94). Protection against a subsequent intravenous virulent M. tuberculosis challenge was superior to that afforded by BCG alone. In another study, peptides corresponding to the amino termini of eight M. tuberculosis proteins and initiating with formyl-methionine residues were synthesized (20). These peptides, shown to bind to the mouse nonclassical MHC class I molecule H-2M3a, were used to pulse DCs, which were then injected into normal mice. Induction of specific cytotoxic T-cell immunity was demonstrated, as well as retardation of M. tuberculosis growth following an aerosol challenge. McShane et al. immunized mice intravenously with DCs pulsed with a CD4$^+$ T-cell-restricted epitope, a CD8$^+$ T-cell-restricted epitope, or both epitopes of a secretory protein of M. tuberculosis antigen 85A (66). Interestingly, on subsequent intravenous challenge with virulent M. tuberculosis, copresentation of both epitopes was required for protection, which was equal to that afforded by BCG. A mucosal DC vaccination approach in mice has also been assessed: DCs were first harvested from the lungs, pulsed with antigen 85, and then administered intranasally (37). After vaccination, splenic cells were able to produce IFN-γ following ex vivo incubation with M. tuberculosis-pulsed DCs. However, lung histological examination revealed a florid inflammatory response with infiltration of numerous macrophages, DCs, and specific CD4$^+$ and CD8$^+$ T cells. These vaccinated mice were not more resistant to an aerosol challenge of virulent M. tuberculosis than were controls, suggesting that not all enhanced immune responses in the lungs are advantageous to the host. These studies have greatly enhanced our knowledge about DC vaccination against TB. However, DC vaccination variables, such as DC differentiation/maturation status and route of delivery, which have subsequently emerged as critical for the success of vaccines, have not been investigated and should be evaluated in future studies (15). For example, vaccination with specifically matured antigen-pulsed DCs may be superior in inducing effector T-cell immunity compared with the use of immature antigen-pulsed DCs, which may even induce tolerance (17). Additionally, intradermal DC vaccine delivery, rather than intravenous delivery, may be associated with better specific skin DC targeting and therefore greater success. Vaccines that specifically target DC function in vivo, whether as a TB subunit, DNA, or other vaccine, may be a more practical vaccination strategy for the prevention of TB. For example, targeting of antigens to the appropriate DC subset may be important in determining the nature of the protective immune response induced (6, 75).

Since a number of T-cell subsets have been implicated in the protective immune response to TB, it is assumed that an ideal candidate vaccine must target as many T-cell subsets as possible. DC vaccination may accomplish this goal. In addition, strategies used to protect DCs from apoptosis, thereby increasing their life span and efficiency of antigen presentation to the T cells, may be beneficial. Indeed, when the anti-apoptotic protein Bcl-x$_L$ was cotransfected into DCs with human papillomavirus DNA, vaccine responses in mice were enhanced, giving rise to potent specific cytotoxic T-cell and Th1 immunity (14, 56, 57). Similar approaches to TB vaccination should be evaluated.

CONCLUSION

Our understanding of the interaction of *M. tuberculosis* with DCs and the subsequent chain of events that determine the outcome of infection remains incompletely defined. However, recent advances in our knowledge have identified exciting new areas of study. Of particular interest is the pivotal role of the

DC receptor DC-SIGN, involved in the capture and internalization of *M. tuberculosis*. As such, DC-SIGN represents a new candidate for the study of gene polymorphisms that may alter the course of natural infection. In addition, the factors which decide the overall pattern of response following binding of *M. tuberculosis* to DC-SIGN in vivo need to be defined. Despite a number of reports of stimulation of DC maturation by *M. tuberculosis*, recent studies suggest that the organism may also subvert the normal maturation process. We hypothesize that one of the factors determining the outcome of infection is the exact nature of the infecting strain and the balance between its ability to stimulate and its ability to inhibit DC

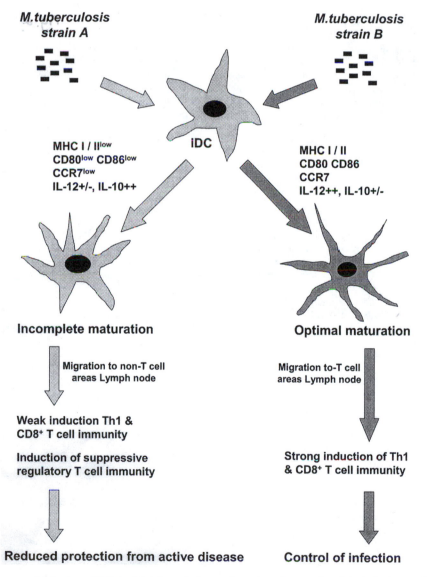

Figure 2. The outcome of infection of DCs by *M. tuberculosis* may depend on the capacity of the infecting strain to induce DC maturation. In the figure, infection with strain A induces suboptimal DC maturation, thereby inducing a weak Th1 response. The immature state of the infected DC augments the action of Tr cells, allowing active disease and subsequent persistence. Strain B, in contrast, induces optimal DC maturation and a strong Th1 response, leading to control of the infection and reducing the chance of active disease.

maturation. According to this hypothesis, suboptimal DC maturation by a specific infecting strain may induce a weak Th1 response and poor protective immunity. In addition, since iDCs are known to induce peripheral tolerance (88), incomplete DC maturation induced by the infecting strain may result in the stimulation of a Tr-cell response, resulting in further suppression of effector immunity (Fig. 2). In contrast, a strain capable of imparting a strong maturation stimulus, with the same or a lesser degree of inhibition, would induce a robust effector response, with efficient control of infection.

REFERENCES

1. Albert, M. L., S. F. Pearce, L. M. Francisco, B. Sauter, P. Roy, R. L. Silverstein, and N. Bhardwaj. 1998. Immature dendritic cells phagocytose apoptotic cells via $\alpha v \beta 5$ and CD36, and cross-present antigens to cytotoxic T-lymphocytes. *J. Exp. Med.* **188**:1359–1368.

2. Albert, M. L., B. Sauter, and N. Bhardwaj. 1998. Dendritic cells acquire antigen from apoptotic cells and induce class I-restricted CTLs. *Nature* **392**:86–89.

3. Angelini, G., S. Gardella, M. Ardy, M. R. Ciriolo, G. Filomeni, F. Trapani, F. Clarke, R. Sitia, and A. Rubartelli. 2002. Antigen-presenting dendritic cells provide the reducing extracellular microenvironment required for T lymphocyte activation. *Proc. Natl. Acad. Sci. USA* **99**:1491–1496.

4. Banchereau, J., and R. L. Steinman. 1998. Dendritic cells and control of immunity. *Nature* **392**:245–252.

5. Banchereau, J., F. Briere, C. Caux, J. Davoust, S. Lebecque, Y. J. Yiu, B. Pulendran, and K. Palucka. 2000. Immunobiology of dendritic cells. *Annu. Rev. Immunol.* **18**:767–811.

6. Banchereau, J., S. Paczesny, P. Blanco, L. Bennett, V. Pascual, J. Fay, and A. K. Palucka. 2003. Dendritic cells: controllers of the immune system and a new promise for immunotherapy. *Ann. N.Y. Acad. Sci.* **987**:180–187.

7. Barnes, P. F., S. J. Fong, P. J. Brennan, P. E. Twomey, A. Mazumder, and R. L. Modlin. 1990. Local production of tumour necrosis factor and IFN-γ in tuberculous pleuritis. *J. Immunol.* **145**:149–151.

8. Barnes, P. F., S. D. Mistry, C. L. Cooper, C. Pirmez, T. H. Rea, and R. L. Modlin. 1989. Compartmentalization of a CD4+ T lymphocyte subpopulation in tuberculous pleuritis. *J. Immunol.* **142**:1114–1119.

9. Bhatt, K., S. P. Hickman, and P. Salgame. 2004. A new approach to modeling early lung immunity in murine tuberculosis. *J. Immunol.* **172**:2748–2751.

10. Bodnar, K. A., N. V. Serbina, and J. A. Flynn. 2001. Fate of *Mycobaterium tuberculosis* within murine dendritic cells. *Infect. Immun.* **69**:800–809.

11. Boom, W. H. 1999. γδ T cells and *Mycobacterium tuberculosis*. *Microbes Infect.* **1**:187–195.

11a. Boom, W. H., D. H. Canaday, S. A. Fulton, A. J. Gehring, R. E. Rojas, and M. Torres. 2003. Human immunity to *M. tuberculosis*: T cell subsets and antigen processing. *Tuberculosis* **83**:98–106.

12. Brightbill, H. D., D. H. Libraty, S. R. Krutzik, R. B. Yang, J. T. Belisle, J. R. Bieharski, M. Maitland, M. V. Norgard, S. E. Plevy, S. T. Smale, D. M. Caraday. S. A. Fulton, W. H. Boom, A. J. Gehring, R. E. Rojas, and M. Torres. 1999. Host defense mechanism triggered by microbial lipoprtoteins through Toll-like receptors. *Science* **285**:732–736.

13. Caragol, I., M. Raspall, C. Fieschi, J. Feinberg, M. N. Larrosa, M. Hernandez, C. Figueras, J.-M. Bertran, J.-L. Casanova, and T. Espanol. 2003. Clinical tuberculosis in 2 of 3 siblings with interleukin-12 receptor β1 deficiency. *Clin. Infect. Dis.* **37**:302–306.

14. Chen, C. H., T. L. Wang, C. F. Hung, Y. Yang, R. A. Young, D. M. Pardoll, and T. C. Wu. 2000. Enhancement of DNA vaccine potency by linkage of antigen gene to an HSP70 gene. *Cancer Res.* **60**:1035–1042.

15. Cranmer, L. D., K. T. Trevor, and E. M. Hersh. 2003. Clinical applications of dendritic cell vaccination in the treatment of cancer. *Cancer Immunol. Immunother.* **53**:275–306.

16. Del Hoyo, G. M., P. Martin, H. H. Vargas, S. Ruiz, C. F. Arlas, and C. Ardavin. 2002. Characterization of a common precursor population for dendritic cells. *Nature* **415**:1043–1047.

17. Dhodapkar, M. V., R. M. Steinman, J. Krasovsky, C. Munz, and N. Bhardwaj. 2001. Antigen-specific inhibition of effector T-cell function in humans after injection of immature dendritic cells. *J. Exp. Med.* **193**:233–238.

18. Dieu, M. C., B. Vandervliet, A. Vicari, J. M. Bridon, E. Oldham, S. Ait-Yahia, F. Briere, A. Zlotnik, S. Lebecque, and C. Caux. 1998. Selective recruitment of immature and mature dendritic cells by distinct chemokines expressed in different anatomic sites. *J. Exp. Med.* **188**:373–386.

19. Dillon, S. M., J. F. Griffin, D. N. Hart, J. D. Watson, and M. A. Baird. 1998. A long-lasting interferon-gamma response is induced to a single inoculation of antigen-pulsed dendritic cells. *Immunology* **95**:132–140.

20. Dow, S. W., A. Roberts, J. Vyas, J. Rodgers, R. R. Rich, I. Orme, and T. A. Potter. 2000. Immunization with f-Met peptides induces immune reactivity against *Mycobacterium tuberculosis*. *Tubercle Lung Dis.* **80**:5–13.

21. Ebner, S., G. Ratzinger, B. Kroshbacher, M. Schmuth, A. Weiss, D. Reider, R. A. Kroczek, M. Herold, C. Heufler, P. Fritsch, and N. Romani. 2001. Production of interleukin-12 by human monocyte derived dendritic cells is optimal when the stimulus is given at the onset of maturation and is further enhanced by interleukin-4. *J. Immunol.* **166**:633–641.

22. Emoto, M., Y. Emoto, and I. B. Buchwalow. 1999. Induction of IFN-gamma-producing CD4+ natural killer T cells by *Mycobacterium bovis* bacillus Calmette Guérin. *Eur. J. Immunol.* **29**:650–659.

23. Enering, A. J., M. Cella, D. Fluitsma, M. Brockhaus, E. C. Hoefsmit, A. Lanzavecchia, and J. Pieters. 1997. The mannose receptor functions as a high capacity and broad specificity antigen receptor in human dendritic cells. *Eur. J. Immunol.* **27**:2417–2425.

24. Engelmayer, J., M. Larsson, M. Subklewe, A. Chahroudi, W. I. Cox, R. M. Steinman, and N. Bhardwaj. 1999. Vaccinia virus inhibits the maturation of human dendritic cells: A novel mechanism of immune evasion. *J. Immunol.* **163**:6762–6768.

25. Fanger, N. A., K. Wardwell, L. Shen, T. F. Tedder, and P. M. Guyre. 1996. Type I (CD64) and type II (CD32) Fc γ receptor-mediated phagocytosis by human blood dendritic cells. *J. Immunol.* **157**:541–548.

26. Figdor, C. G., Y. van Kooyk, and G. J. Adema. 2002. C-type lectin receptors on dendritic cells and Langerhans cells. *Nat. Rev. Immunol.* **2**:77–84.

27. Flesch, I. E., and S. H. Kaufmann. 1992. Role of cytokines in tuberculosis. *Immunobiology* **189**:316–339.

28. Flynn, J. L., and J. Chan. 2001. Immunology of tuberculosis. *Annu. Rev. Immunol.* **19**:93–129.

29. Fonteneau, J. F., M. Gilliet, M. Larsson, I. Dasilva, C. Munz, Y.-J. Liu, and N. Bhardwaj. 2003. Activation of influenza virus-specific CD4$^+$ and CD8$^+$ T cells: a new role for plasmacytoid dendritic cells in adaptive immunity. *Blood* 101:3520–3526.

30. Forster, R., A. Schubel, D. Breitfield, E. Kremmer, I. Renner-Muller, E. Wolf, and M. Lipp. 1999. CCR7 coordinates the primary immune response by establishing functional microenvironments in secondary lymphoid organs. *Cell* 99:23–33.

31. Fortsch, D., M. Rollinghoff, and S. Stenger. 2000. IL-10 converts human dendritic cells into macrophage-like cells with increased antibacterial activity against virulent *Mycobacterium tuberculosis*. *J. Immunol.* 165:978–987.

32. Gantner, B. N., R. M. Simmons, S. J. Canavera, S. Akira, and D. M. Underhill. 2003. Collaborative induction of inflammatory responses by Dectin-1 and Toll-like receptor 2. *J. Exp. Med.* 197:1107–1117.

33. Geijtenbeek, T. B. H., R. Torensma, S. J. van Vliet, G. C. van Duijnhoven, G. J. Adema, Y. van Kooyk, and C. G. Figdor. 2000. Identification of DC-SIGN, a novel dendritic cell-specific ICAM-3 receptor that supports primary immune responses. *Cell* 100:575–585.

34. Geijtenbeek, T. B. H., S. L. van Vliet, E. A. Koppel, M. Sanchez-Hernandez, M. J. E. Vandenbroucke-Grauls, B. Appelmelk, and Y. van Kooyk. 2003. Mycobacteria target DC-SIGN to suppress dendritic cell function. *J. Exp. Med.* 197:7–17.

35. Giacomini, E., E. Iona, L. Ferroni, M. Miettinen, L. Fattorini, G. Orefici, I. Julkunen, and E. M. Coccia. 2001. Infection of human macrophages and dendritic cells with *Mycobacterium tuberculosis* induces a differential cytokine gene expression that modulates T-cell response. *J. Immunol.* 166:7033–7041.

36. Gonzalez-Juarrero, M., T. S. Shim, A. Kipnis, A. P. Junqueira-Kipnis, and I. Orme. 2003. Dynamics of macrophage cell populations during murine pulmonary tuberculosis. *J. Immunol.* 171:3128–3135.

37. Gonzalez-Juarrero, M., J. Turner, R. J. Basaraba, J. T. Belisle, and I. M. Orme. 2002. Florid pulmonary inflammatory responses in mice vaccinated with Antigen-85 pulsed dendritic cells and challenged by aerosol with *Mycobacterium tuberculosis*. *Cell Immunol.* 220:13–19.

38. Gumperz, J. E., and M. B. Brenner. 2001. CD1-specific T cells in microbial immunity. *Curr. Opin. Immunol.* 13:471–478.

39. Gunn, M. D., K. Tangemann, C. Tam, J. G. Cyster, S. D. Rosen, and L. T. Williams. 1998. A chemokine expressed in lymphoid high endothelial venules promotes the adhesion and chemotaxis of naive T lymphocytes. *Proc. Natl. Acad. Sci. USA* 95:258–263.

40. Hanekom, W. A., M. Mendillo, C. Manca, P. A. Haslett, M. R. Siddiqui, C. Barry III, and G. Kaplan. 2002. *Mycobacterium tuberculosis* inhibits maturation of human monocyte-derived dendritic cells in vitro. *J. Infect. Dis.* 188:257–266.

41. Henderson, R. A., S. C. Watkins, and J. A. Flynn. 1997. Activation of human dendritic cells following infection with *Mycobacterium tuberculosis*. *J. Immunol.* 159:635–433.

42. Hertz, C. J., S. M. Kiertscher, P. J. Godowski, D. A. Bouis, M. V. Norgard, M. D. Roth, and R. L. Modlin. 2001. Microbial lipopeptides stimulate dendritic cell maturation via Toll-like receptor 2. *J. Immunol.* 166:2444–2450.

43. Holt, P. G., S. Haining, D. J. Nelson, and J. S. Sedgwick. 1994. Origin of steady-state turnover of class II MHC-bearing dendritic cells in the epithelium of the conducting airways. *J. Immunol.* 153:256–261.

44. Inaba, K., M. Inaba, M. Naito, and R. M. Steinman. 1993. Dendritic cell progenitors phgocytose particulates, including bacillus Calmette-Guérin organisms, and sensitize mice to mycobacterial antigens. *J. Exp. Med.* 178:479–488.

45. Inaba, K., and R. M. Steinman. 1985. Protein-specific helper T lymphocyte formation initiated by dendritic cells. *Science* 229:475–479.

46. Inaba, K., and R. M. Steinman. 1984. Resting and sensitized T lymphocytes exhibit distinct stimulatory (antigen-presenting cell) requirements for growth and lymphokine release. *J. Exp. Med.* 160:1717–1735.

47. Ingulli, E., A. Mondino, A. Khoruts, and M. K. Jenkins. 1997. In vivo detection of dendritic cell antigen presentation to CD4$^+$ T cells. *J. Exp. Med.* 185:2133–2141.

48. Iwashiro, M., R. J. Messer, K. E. Peterson, I. M. Stromnes, T. Sugie, and K. J. Hasenkrug. 2001. Immunosuppression by CD4$^+$ regulatory T cells induced by chronic retroviral infection. *Proc. Natl. Acad. Sci USA* 98:9226–9230.

49. Iyonaga, K., K. M. McCarthy, and E. S. Schneeberger. 2002. Dendritic cells and the recruitment of a granulomatous immune response in the lung. *Am. J. Respir. Cell Mol. Biol.* 26:671–679.

50. Jarrossay, D., G. Napolitani, M. Colonna, F. Sallusto, and A. Lanzavecchia, A. 2001. Specialization and complementarity in microbial molecule recognition by human myeloid and plasmacytoid dendritic cells. *Eur. J. Immunol.* 31:3388–3393.

51. Jiang, W., W. L. Swiggard, C. Heufler, M. Peng, A. Mirza, R. M. Steinman, and M. C. Nussenzweig. 1995. The receptor DEC-205 expressed by dendritic cells and thymic epithelial cells is involved in antigen processing. *Nature* 375:151–155.

52. Jiao, X., R. Lo-Man, P. Guermonprez, L. Fiette, E. Deriaud, S. Burgaud, B. Gicquel, N. Winter, and C. Leclerc. 2002. Dendritic cells are host cells for mycobacteria in vivo that trigger innate and acquired immunity. *J. Immunol.* 168:1294–1301.

53. Kadowaki, N., S. Antoneko, J. Y. Lau, and Y. J. Liu. 2000. Natural interferon-α/β-producing cells link innate and adaptive immunity. *J. Exp. Med.* 192:219–226.

54. Kadowaki, N., S. Ho, S. Antonenko, R. de Waal Malefyt, R. A. Kastelein, F. Bazan, and J. Yong-Liu. 2001. Subsets of human dendritic cells express different toll-like receptors and respond to different microbial antigens. *J. Exp. Med.* 194:863–869.

55. Kalinski, P., J. H. Schuitemaker, C. M. Hilkens, E. A. Wierenga, and M. L. Kapsenberg. 1999. Final maturation of dendritic cells is associated with impaired responsiveness to IFN-gamma and to bacterial IL-12 inducers: decreased ability of mature dendritic cells to produce IL-12 during the interaction with Th cells. *J. Immunol.* 162:3231–3236.

56. Kim, T. W., C. F. Hung, D. Boyd, J. Juang, L. He, J. W. Kim, J. M. Hardwick, and T. C. Wu. 2003. Enhancing DNA vaccine potency by combining a strategy to prolong dendritic cell life with intracellular targeting strategies. *J. Immunol.* 171:2970–2976.

57. Kim, T. W., C. F. Hung, M. Ling, J. Juang, L. He, J. M. Hardwick, S. Kumar, and T. C. Wu. 2003. Enhancing DNA vaccine potency by coadministration of DNA encoding anti-apoptotic proteins. *J. Clin. Investig.* 112:109–117.

58. Kriehumber, E., S. Breiteneder-Gerleff, M. Groeger, T. W. Kim, C. F. Hung, D. Boyd, J. Juang, L. He, J. W. Kim, J. M. Hardwick, and T. C. Wu. 2001. Isolation and characterization of dermal lymphatic and blood endothelial cells reveal stable and functionally specialized cell lineages. *J. Exp. Med.* 194:797–808.

59. Lanzavecchia, A., and F. Sallusto. 2001. Regulation of T-cell immunity by dendritic cells. *Cell* 106:263–266.

60. Latchumanan, V. K., B. Singh, P. Sharma, and K. Natarajan. 2002. *Mycobacterium tuberculosis* antigens induce the differentiation of dendritic cells from bone marrow. *J. Immunol.* 169:6856–6864.

61. Lopez, B., D. Aguilar, H. Orozco, M. Burger, C. Espitia, V. Ritacco, L. Barrera, K. Kremer, R. Hernandez-Pando, K. Huygen, and D. van Soolingen. 2003. A marked difference in pathogenesis and immune response induced by different *Mycobacterium tuberculosis* genotypes. *Clin. Exp. Immunol.* 133:30–37.

62. Lukas, N. W., S. W. Chensue, R. M. Strieter, V. K. Latchumanan, B. Singh, P. Sharma, and K. Natajaran. 1994. Inflammatory granuloma formation is mediated by TNF-alpha-inducible intercellular adhesion molecule-1. *J. Immunol.* 152:5883–5889.

63. Manca, C., L. Tsenova, C. E. Barry III, A. Bergtold, S. Freeman, P. A. Haslett, P. Musser, V. H. Freedman, and G. Kaplan. 1999. *Mycobacterium tuberculosis* CDC1551 induces a more vigorous host repsonse in vivo and in vitro, but is not more virulent than other clinical isolates. *J. Immunol.* 162:6740–6746.

64. Manca, C., L. Tsenova, A. Bergtold, S. Freeman, M. Tovey, J. M. Musser, C. E. Barry III, V. H. Freedman, and G. Kaplan. 2001. Virulence of a *Mycobacterium tuberculosis* clinical isolate in mice is determined by failure to induce Th1 type immunity and is associated with induction of IFN α/β. *Proc. Natl. Acad. Sci. USA* 98:5752–5757.

65. Matsuno, K., T. Ezaki, S. Kudo, and Y. Uehara. 1996. A life stage of particle-laden rat dendritic cells in vivo: their terminal division, active phagocytosis and translocation from the liver to hepatic lymph. *J. Exp. Med.* 183:1865–1878.

66. McShane, H., S. Behboudi, N. Goonetilleke, R. Brookes, and A. V. Hill. 2002. Protective immunity against *Mycobacterium tuberculosis* induced by dendritic cells pulsed with both CD8+- and CD4+-T-cell epitopes from antigen 85A. *Infect. Immun.* 70:1623–1626.

67. McWilliam, A. S., D. Nelson, J. A. Thomas, and P. G. Holt. 1994. Rapid dendritic cell recruitment is a hallmark of the acute inflammatory response at mucosal surfaces. *J. Exp. Med.* 179:1331–1336.

68. Means, T. K., B. W. Jones, A. B. Schromm, B. A. Shurtleff, J. A. Smith, J. Keane, D. T. Golenbrock, S. N. Vogel, and M. J. Fenton. 2001. Differential effects of a Toll-like receptor antagonist on *Mycobacterium tuberculosis*-induced macrophage responses. *J. Immunol.* 166:4074–4082.

69. Means, T. K., S. Wang, E. Lien, A. Yoshimura, D. T. Golenbock, and M. J. Fenton. 1999. Human Toll-like receptors mediate cellular activation by *Mycobacterium tuberculosis*. *J. Immunol.* 163:3920–3927.

70. Moll, H. 1993. Epidermal Langerhans cells are critical for immunoregulation of cutaneous leishmaniasis. *Immunol. Today* 14:383–387.

71. Nelson, D. J., and P. G. Holt. 1995. Defective regional immunity in the respiratory tract of neonates is attributable to hyporesponsiveness of local dendritic cells to activation signals. *J. Immunol.* 155:3517–3524.

72. Peters, W., and J. D. Ernst. 2003. Mechanisms of cell recruitment in the immune response to *Mycobacterium tuberculosis*. *Microbes Infect.* 5:151–158.

73. Peters, W., H. M. Scott, H. F. Chambers, J. L. Flynn, I. F. Charo, and J. D. Ernst. 2001. Chemokine receptor 2 serves an early and essential role in resistance to *Mycobacterium tuberculosis*. *Proc. Natl. Acad. Sci. USA* 98:7958–7963.

74. Pinkus, G., S. Pinkus, J. L. Langhoff, E. Matsumura, F. Yamashiro, S. Mosialos, and J. W. Said. 1997. Fascin, a sensitive new marker for Reed-Sternberg cells of Hodgkin's disease. Evidence for a dendritic or B cell derivation. *Am. J. Pathol.* 150:543–562.

75. Pope, M. 2003. Dendritic cells as a conduit to improve HIV vaccines. *Curr. Mol. Med.* 3:229–242.

76. Prigozy, T. I., P. A. Sieling, D. Clemens, P. L. Stewart, S. M. Behar, S. A. Porcelli, M. B. Brenner, R. L. Modlin, and M. Kronenberg. 1997. The mannose receptor delivers lipoglycan antigens to endosomes for presentation to T cells by CD1b molecules. *Immunity* 6:187–197.

77. Reis e Sousa, C., P. D. Stahl, and J. M. Austyn. 1993. Phagocytosis of antigens by Langerhans cells in vitro. *J. Exp. Med.* 178:509–19.

78. Robbiani, D. F., R. A. Finch, D. Jager, W. A. Muller, A. C. Sartorelli, and G. J. Randolph. 2000. The leukotriene C4 transporter MRP1 regulates CCL19 (MIP3beta, ELC)-dependent mobilization of dendritic cells to lymph nodes. *Cell* 103:757–768.

79. Roper, W. H., and J. J. Waring. 1955. Primary serofibrinous pleural effusion in military personnel. *Am. Rev. Tuberc.* 71:616–634.

80. Rubartelli, A., A. Poggi, and M. R. Zocchi. 1997. The selective engulfment of apoptotic bodies by dendritic cells is mediated by the α(v)β3 integrin and requires intracellular and extracellular calcium. *Eur. J. Immunol.* 27:1893–1900.

81. Sallusto, F., M. Cella, C. Danieli, and A. Lanzavecchia. 1995. Dendritic cells use macropinocytosis and the mannose receptor to concentrate antigen to the MHC class II compartment. Downregulation by cytokines and bacterial products. *J. Exp. Med.* 182:389–400.

82. Sallusto, F., P. Schaerli, P. Loetscher, P. Schaniel, D. Lenig, C. R. Mackay, S. Qin, and A. Lanzavecchia. 1998. Rapid and coordinated switch in chemokine receptor expression during dendritic cell maturation. *Eur. J. Immunol.* 28:2760–2769.

83. Sertl, K., T. Takemura, E. Tschachler, V. J. Ferrans, M. A. Kaliner, and E. M. Shevach. 1986. Dendritic cells with antigen-presenting capability reside in airway epithelium, lung parenchyma, and visceral pleura. *J. Exp. Med.* 163:436–451.

84. Siegal, F. P., M. Kadowaki, P. A. Shodell, P. A. Fitzgerald-Bocarsly, K. Shah, S. Ho, S. Antonenko, and Y. J. Liu. 1999. The nature of the peripheral type I interferon-producing cells in human blood. *Science* 284:1835–1839.

85. Steinman, R. M. 2001. Dendritic cells and the control of immunity: enhancing the efficiency of antigen presentation. *Mt. Sinai J. Med.* 68:106–166.

86. Steinman, R. M., and Z. A. Cohn. 1973. Identification of a novel cell type in peripheral lymphoid organs of mice. I. Morphological, quantitation, tissue distribution. *J. Exp. Med.* 137:1142–1162.

87. Steinman, R. M., and T. M. Moran. 2004. Dendritic cells, p. 269–284. *In* W. M. Rom and S. M. Garay (ed.), *Tuberculosis*. Lippincott Williams & Wilkins, Philadelphia, Pa.

88. Steinman, R. M., and M. C. Nussenzweig. 2002. Avoiding horror autotoxicus: the importance of dendritic cells in peripheral T-cell tolerance. *Proc. Natl. Acad. Sci. USA* 99:351–358.

89. Stenger, S., K. R. Niazi, and R. L. Modlin, 1998. Downregulation of CD1 on antigen-presenting cells by infection with *Mycobacterium tuberculosis*. *J. Immunol.* 161:3582–3588.

90. Sturgill-Koszycki, S., P. H. Schlesinger, P. Chakraborty, P. L. Haddix, H. L. Collins, A. K. Fok, R. D. Allen, S. L. Gluck, J. Heuser, and D. G. Russell. 1994. Lack of acidification in *Mycobacterium phagosomes* produced by exclusion of the vesicular proton-ATPase. *Science* 263:678–681.

91. Tailleux, L., O. Neyrolles, S. Honore-Bouakline, E. Perret,

F. Sanchez, J.-P. Abastado, P. H. Lagrange, J. C. Gluckman, M. Rosenzwajg, and J.-L. Herrman. 2003. Constrained intracellular survival of *Mycobacterium tuberculosis* in human dendritic cells. *J. Immunol.* **170:**1939–1948.

92. Tailleux, L., O. Schwartz, J. L. Herrmann, E. Pivert, M. Jackson, A. Amara, L. Legres, D. Dreher, L. P. Nicod, J. C. Gluckman, P. H. Lagrange, B. Gicquel, and O. Neyrolles. 2003. DC-SIGN is the major *Mycobacterium tuberculosis* receptor on human dendritic cells. *J. Exp. Med.* **197:**121–127.

93. Tan, M. C., A. M. Mommaas, J. W. Drijfhout, R. Jordens, J. J. Onderwater, D. Verwoerd, A. A. Mulder, A. N. van der Heiden, D. Scheidegger, L. C. Oomen, T. H. Ottenhoff, A. Tulp, J. J. Neefjes, and F. Koning. 1997. Mannose receptor-mediated uptake of antigens strongly enhances HLA class II-restricted antigen presentation by cultured dendritic cells. *Eur. J. Immunol.* **27:**2426–2435.

94. Tascon, R. E., C. S. Soares, S. Ragno, E. Stavropoulos, E. M. Hirst, and M. J. Colston. 2000. *Mycobacterium tuberculosis*-activated dendritic cells induce protective immunity in mice. *Immunology* **99:**473–480.

95. Thoma-Uszynski, S., S. M. Kiertscher, M. T. Ochoa, D. A. Bouis, M. V. Norgard, K. Miyake, P. J. Godowski, M. D. Roth, and R. L. Modlin. 2000. Activation of Toll-like receptor 2 on human dendritic cells triggers induction of IL-12, but not IL-10. *J. Immunol.* **165:**3804–3810.

96. Thoma-Uszynski, S., S. Stenger, O. Takeuchi, M. T. Ochoa, M. Engele, P. A. Sieling, P. F. Barnes, P. Rollinghoff, P. L. Bolcskei, M. Wagner, S. Akira, M. V. Norgard, J. T. Belisle, P. J. Godowski, B. R. Bloom, and R. L. Modlin. 2001. Induction of direct antimicrobial activity through mammalian Toll-like receptors. *Science* **291:**1544–1547.

97. Thurnher, M., R. Ramoner, G. Gastl, C. Radmayr, G. Bock, M. Herold, H. Klocker, and G. Bartsch. 1997. Bacillus Calmette Guérin mycobacteria stimulate human blood dendritic cells. *Int. J. Cancer* **70:**128–134.

98. Tschernig, T., A. S. Debertin, F. Paulsen, W. J. Kleemann, and R. Pabst. 2001. Dendritic cells in the mucosa of the human trachea are not regularly found in the first year of life. *Thorax* **56:**427–431.

99. Tsuji, S., M. Matsumoto, O. Takeuchi, S. Akira, I. Azuma, A. Hayashi, K. Toyoshima, and T. Seya. 2000. Maturation of human dendritic cells by cell wall skeleton of *Mycobacterium bovis* bacillus Calmette-Guérin: involvement of Toll-like receptors. *Infect. Immun.* **68:**6883–6890.

100. Turley, S. J., K. Inaba, W. S. Garrett, M. Ebersold, J. Unternaehrer, R. M. Steinman, and I. Mellman. 2000. Transport of peptide-MHC class II complexes in developing dendritic cells. *Science* **288:**522–527.

101. Uehira, K., R. Amakawa, T. Ito, K. Tajima, S. Naitoh, Y. Ozaki, T. Shimizu, K. Yamaguchi, Y. Uemura, H. Kitajima, S. Yonezu, and S. Fukuhara. 2002. Dendritic cells are decreased in blood and accumulated in granuloma in tuberculosis. *Clin. Immunol.* **105:**296–303.

101a. Ulrichs, T., and S. H. E. Kaufmann. 2004. Cell mediated immune response, p. 251–262. *In* W. M. Rom and S. M. Garay (ed.), *Tuberculosis*. Lippincott Williams & Wilkins, Philadelphia, Pa.

102. Underhill, D., and A. Ozinsky. 2002. Toll-like receptors: key mediators of microbe detection. *Curr. Opin. Immunol.* **14:**103–110.

103. Underhill, D., A. Ozinsky, K. D. Smith, and A. Aderem. 1999. Toll-like receptor-2 mediates mycobacteria-induced proinflammatory signaling in macrophages. *Proc. Natl. Acad. Sci. USA* **96:**14459–14463.

104. Urban, B. C., D. J. Ferguson, A. Pain, N. Wilcox, M. Plebanski, J. M. Austyn, and D. J. Roberts. 1999. *Plasmodium falciparum*-infected erythrocytes modulate the maturation of dendritic cells. *Nature* **400:**73–77.

105. Van Overtvelt, L., N. Vanderheyde, V. Verhasselt, J. Ismaili L. de Vos, M. Goldman, F. Willems, and B. Vray. 1999. *Trypanosoma cruzi* infects human dendritic cells and prevents their maturation: inhibition of cytokines, HLA-DR and costimulatory molecules. *Infect. Immun.* **67:**4033–4040.

106. Willimann, K., D. F. Legler, M. Loetscher, R. S. Roos, M. B. Delgado, I. Clark-Lewis, M. Baggiolini, and B. Moser. 1998. The chemokine SLC is expressed in T-cell areas of lymph nodes and mucosal lymphoid tissues and attracts activated T cells via CCR7. *Eur. J. Immunol.* **6:**2025–2034.

X. HOST IMMUNE RESPONSES AND ANTIGENIC VARIATION

Tuberculosis and the Tubercle Bacillus
Edited by Stewart T. Cole et al.
© 2005 ASM Press, Washington, D.C.

Chapter 29

CD8 T Cells in Tuberculosis

STEFAN H. E. KAUFMANN AND JOANNE L. FLYNN

The now-classical concept of self-restricted antigen recognition by T cells, as originally formulated by Peter Doherty and Rolf Zinkernagel, did not simply explain how microbial pathogens residing within host cells are recognized by T lymphocytes (10, 52). The concept went one step further in proposing a division of tasks for the two principal antigen-presenting molecules, the major histocompatibility complex (MHC) class II (MHC II) and MHC I gene products. Generally, the MHC II molecules are responsible for presentation of bacterial antigens whereas the MHC I antigens are specialized in presenting viral antigens. Teleologically, this made sense for two reasons. First, bacteria preferentially reside in phagosomal compartments, which are readily accessed by MHC II molecules, whereas viruses reside in the cytosolic compartment, which is surveyed by MHC I molecules. Second, viruses can infect virtually all host cells and all host cells express MHC I molecules, whereas bacteria are found primarily in macrophages, which belong to the small group of professional antigen-presenting cells (APC) expressing MHC II. This differential tissue distribution allows for scanning of all host cells by MHC I-restricted T cells and for focusing of MHC II-restricted T cells on macrophages, the major habitat of intracellular bacterial pathogens.

Since then, it has been realized that this concept—like most biological principles—is not as strict as originally envisaged. Additional antigen-presenting molecules exist, most of which share with MHC I molecules the surface expression of a heavy chain with β_2-microglobulin (β_2m) (20). Some of these elements are encoded within the MHC gene locus and therefore are termed nonclassical MHC Ib molecules as opposed to the classical MHC Ia molecules. Others are encoded outside of the MHC and hence are called MHC I-like molecules. These restriction elements present antigens to small but distinct T-cell populations often subsumed as unconventional T cells. More-

over, it was found that the tasks of different T cells are separated by a confluent rather than a strict line. Thus, some intracellular bacteria, e.g., *Listeria monocytogenes*, egress from the phagosome into the cytosol, where their antigens are treated like viral antigens and presented via MHC I (37). Other intracellular microbes are controlled by both MHC I- and MHC II-restricted T cells, although they remain in the phagosomal compartment. The best-known member of this group is *Mycobacterium tuberculosis* (37). In this chapter, we focus on CD8 T cells, with an emphasis on the MHC Ia-restricted T cells in tuberculosis, but we also touch on the unconventional CD8 T cells restricted by β_2m-associated nonclassical MHC Ib or MHC I-like molecules.

THE T-CELL SYSTEM

Dichotomous systems are often used to render complex systems more comprehensible. We use this approach in briefly describing the position of CD8 T cells in the context of the lymphocyte system (Fig. 1).

The lymphocyte system comprises B cells, which secrete antibodies, and T cells, which recognize their antigens via a cell-bound T-cell receptor (TCR). A minor population of T cells express a TCR composed of a γ and δ chain, whereas the vast majority of T cells use an α/β TCR. In humans, γ/δ T cells recognize nonproteinaceous ligands, typically containing phosphate, without the need for any known presentation molecule (19). In contrast, antigen recognition by α/β T cells depends strictly on presentation of antigens by specialized molecules. In the overwhelming number of cases, classical MHC molecules are responsible for presentation. The MHC II molecules present antigens to CD4 T cells, whereas CD8 T cells are stimulated by MHC I-presented antigens. A minor population of T cells recognize antigens presented by

Stefan H. E. Kaufmann • Department of Immunology, Max-Planck-Institute for Infection Biology, D-10117 Berlin, Germany.
JoAnne L. Flynn • Department of Molecular Genetics and Biochemistry, University of Pittsburgh School of Medicine, Pittsburgh, PA 15213.

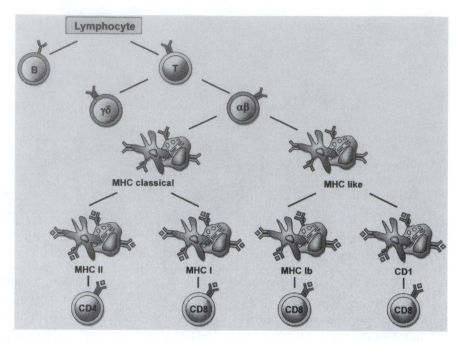

Figure 1. Dichotomous view of the T-lymphocyte system, showing the major T-cell populations. Frequently, the MHC II-restricted CD4 T cells and the MHC I-restricted CD8 T cells are termed "conventional T cells" whereas the γ/δ T cells and the MHC Ib and CD1-restricted T cells are often subsumed under the term "unconventional T cells."

surface molecules that share some characteristics with the classical MHC molecules. These are the non-classical MHC Ib molecules and the CD1 molecules (Fig. 1). The CD1 molecules present glycolipids and hence—like the γ/δ T cells—mitigate the dogma that T cells are exclusively restricted by MHC-peptide complexes.

Although the T cells which recognize mycobacterial glycolipids in the context of group I CD1 molecules are not only CD8$^+$ but also double negative and sometimes even CD4$^+$, they are considered in this chapter where appropriate. In contrast, the T cells that recognize glycolipids in the context of group II CD1 molecules are consistently CD8$^-$ and hence are largely ignored here.

A ROLE FOR CD8 T CELLS IN TUBERCULOSIS?

Although MHC II-restricted CD4 T cells are central mediators of the immune response to tuberculosis, increasing evidence, mostly from experiments with the mouse system but more recently also from experiments with the human system, emphasizes an important role for CD8 T cells in immunity to this pathogen (8). In early studies performed with the mouse model, using T-cell-depleting antibodies, it could be shown that CD4 and CD8 T-cell depletion exacerbates tuberculosis (21). Reciprocally, adoptive transfer of selected CD4 T cells and of CD8 T cells both conferred protec-

tive activity against tuberculosis (21). Because of the chronicity of *M. tuberculosis* infection, both T-cell depletion experiments and adoptive transfer experiments suffer from inherent drawbacks.

The availability of gene knockout (KO) mice with distinct immune deficiencies therefore represented a major step forward in the identification of T cells crucial for protection against tuberculosis. The first genetically engineered mouse mutants available for the study of immune responses to tuberculosis were those deficient in β_2m, i.e., mice that are unable to surface-express MHC I and therefore are also devoid of functional CD8 T cells. These mice were quite susceptible to tuberculosis (14). However, as mentioned above, β_2m is responsible not only for surface expression of classical MHC Ia but also for that of nonclassical MHC Ib and the MHC I-like molecules, notably CD1. Moreover, recent evidence suggests a primary role of β_2m in iron uptake (38). Thus, markedly exacerbated tuberculosis, as seen in β_2m KO mice, could not be associated unequivocally with MHC Ia-restricted CD8 T cells.

Additional experiments using mice deficient in TAP (transporter associated with antigen processing), CD8, or the classical MHC Ia heavy chain, however, provided formal proof for a role of CD8 T cells in protection against experimental tuberculosis of mice (5, 34, 46). At the same time, however, these experiments revealed that additional mechanisms must have been responsible for the severe disease exacerbation in β_2m KO mice. Indeed, it is now clear that β_2m KO mice suffer from a multitude of defects, which all contribute to the marked susceptibility to tuberculosis, including iron overload and participation of T cells restricted by MHC Ib or MHC I-like molecules.

The group I CD1 molecules do not exist in mice and therefore cannot account for such effects (18, 39); in contrast, the group II CD1 molecules (CD1d) are present in mice. However, CD1d KO mice do not differ from controls with respect to susceptibility to tuberculosis (5). Hence, they do not represent essential elements of protection against tuberculosis. However, tentative evidence provides a role for this T-cell population in the immune response to *M. tuberculosis*, notably in the formation of granulomatous lesions (2, 50).

MAJOR ANTIGEN-PRESENTING CELLS: MACROPHAGES AND DC

Although macrophages represent the major habitat for *M. tuberculosis*, dendritic cells (DC) harbor this pathogen as well. Both cell types are professional APC; i.e., they are endowed with the capacity to stimulate an antigen-specific response in naive T cells. Generally speaking, macrophages have a superior phagocytic and degradative activity over DC whereas DC are better equipped for T-cell priming and stimulation due to the abundant surface expression of MHC and costimulatory molecules and their potent capacity to produce T-cell-stimulating cytokines (4). DC are also well equipped for glycolipid presentation because, in contrast to macrophages, they express all members of the CD1 family (31). Importantly, DC can capture an antigen at the site of infection and transport it to draining lymph nodes, where T-cell stimulation takes place. Therefore, DC are important transit cells between the primary lesion and the draining lymph node of the Ghon complex. As described below, evidence is accumulating that a mechanism exists allowing antigen transport from infected macrophages to bystander DC. This mechanism seems to combine the advantages of both cells, i.e., the potent capacity of macrophages to degrade microbes and that of DC to present microbial antigens in the most efficacious way.

FATE OF CD8 T-CELL ANTIGENS: FROM PROTEIN TO PEPTIDE

MHC Ia

In recent years, there have been numerous reports of classically restricted mycobacterium-specific CD8 T cells induced by *M. tuberculosis* infection in mice and humans (24). Extensive analyses have elucidated the conventional pathway for processing and presentation of protein antigens by MHC I molecules (1, 29). The MHC I heavy chain comprises three domains, of which the α1 and α2 domains form a groove that can accommodate peptides of 8 to 9 amino acids (aa). The grooves in different MHC haplotypes differ and therefore bind distinct peptides.

The peptides are anchored to the groove via distinct aa anchor residues, which define peptides as epitopes for a given MHC haplotype. Typically, the peptides destined for MHC I binding are generated in the cytoplasm, from where they are transported into the endoplasmic reticulum (ER) by means of TAP. Before this, the proteins are degraded by proteasomes, large multimolecular complexes which form a cylinder (Fig. 2). Passage of proteins through this proteolytic cylinder results in degradation of proteins into peptides. The proteasome generates the carboxy-terminal end of a precursor peptide of up to 15 aa. In the ER, a recently identified protease termed ER aminopeptidase 1 (ERAP-1) further trims the peptide to its final

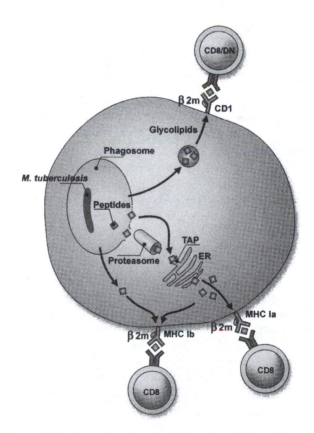

Figure 2. The β_2m-dependent T cells in tuberculosis and the respective antigen-processing pathways. The β_2m-dependent T cells comprise classical MHC Ia-restricted CD8 T cells, nonclassical MHC Ib-restricted CD8 T cells, and the group I CD1-restricted CD8 T cells. The last of these T-cell populations sometimes is double negative (DN) or even CD4+.

length of 8 to 9 aa from the amino terminus (12). Peptides are loaded onto the MHC I molecules, which are then transported to the cell surface. The loading of MHC I molecules by appropriate peptides is promoted by numerous molecules located within the ER, including calnexin, calreticulin, oxidoreductase, and tapasin. The whole processing pathway is under the control of gamma interferon (IFN-γ), which converts the proteasome into a more active immunoproteasome and upregulates the expression of TAP, ERAP-1, and surface MHC I. These findings together suggest that presentation of antigenic peptides is defined not only by the type of amino acids, which determine the anchoring of the peptide in the MHC cleft, but also by the cleavage sites, which allow production of the appropriate precursor and the final peptide by the proteasome and ERAP-1, respectively. Programs have been developed which allow prediction of dominant epitopes for a given MHC haplotype based on the amino acid motif responsible for anchoring, the amino acid sequence determining the cleavage site, or both. Application of these prediction programs will promote the identification of dominant CD8 T-cell epitopes of *M. tuberculosis*.

MHC Ib

The murine MHC Ib molecule H2-M3 presents short *N*-formylmethionine (*N*-fMet) peptides. *N*-fMet represents a signal sequence for bacterial proteins and hence is characteristic of bacterial proteins and absent from mammalian proteins. Only the mitochondrial proteins are *N* formylated due to their prokaryotic origin. All bacteria initiate protein synthesis by means of the *N*-fMet signal sequence. Probably processing and presentation are similar to these for MHC Ia molecules, although TAP-independent processing occurs frequently (Fig. 2) (25). Two recent studies have revealed stimulation of MHC Ib-restricted CD8 T cells by *N*-fMet peptides from *M. tuberculosis* and shown that immunization with such peptides can induce a protective immune response (7, 11). *N*-fMet peptides, which are recognized by human T cells, have been described previously. However, it appears that in humans these peptides are presented by MHC II to CD4 T cells (33).

Human CD8 T cells specific for *M. tuberculosis* antigens presented by MHC Ib molecules exist (16, 26). Processing of these antigens is proteasome dependent but does not require TAP-dependent transport through the ER. Although there are some similarities to the presentation of *N*-fMet peptides by H2-M3, evidence supporting a direct relationship between the two types of CD8 T-cell stimulation does not exist. Rather, the majority of antigens from *M. tuberculosis*

recognized by CD8 T cells are presented in the context of HLA-E, at least in some latently infected individuals. HLA-E is a monomorphic nonclassical MHC Ib molecule. It appears that this presentation involves a proteasome-independent pathway and thus has some similarity to the murine H2-M3 pathway.

GLYCOLIPID PRESENTATION BY GROUP I CD1 MOLECULES TO CD8 T CELLS

Although encoded outside of the MHC, the CD1 molecules have several similarities to MHC I, including the following: (i) they are noncovalently associated with β$_2$m on the cell surface, and (ii) the CD1 heavy chain comprises three domains, of which the first two form a narrow and deep cleft that accommodates lipid tails of glycolipids (18, 39). The CD1 molecules, however, are nonpolymorphic, and hence antigens must be highly conserved, at least with regard to the lipid tail which is accommodated in the hydrophobic cleft of the CD1 molecule. Abundant cell wall glycolipids of mycobacteria are presented by group I CD1 molecules to T cells. These include phosphatidylinositol mannosides, lipoarabinomannan, mycolic acids, and hexosyl-1-phosphoisoprenoids. Recently, phosphatidylinositol mannosides have been identified as the first mycobacterial antigens presented by the group II CD1 molecule, CD1d (13a).

The group I CD1 molecules are localized in different intracellular compartments. The intracellular distribution of CD1a resembles that of MHC I; CD1b is found mostly in late endosomal/lysosomal vesicles; CD1c is found both on the cell surface and in early endosomes. CD1-restricted T cells with self-reactivity have been described, and evidence has been presented that these T cells regulate DC maturation (44, 51). Hence, CD1-restricted T cells could play a role in the induction of T-cell responses by DC.

FATE OF ANTIGENS FOR CD8 T CELLS: FROM PHAGOSOME TO MHC I

Despite earlier claims that *M. tuberculosis* can leave the phagosome, it is now generally accepted that *M. tuberculosis* and the vaccine strain *M. bovis* BCG are "phagosomal inhabitants." *M. tuberculosis* arrests the phagosome at an early maturation stage by counteracting its acidification (17). According to what has been said above, therefore, the question arises how antigens from *M. tuberculosis* can be introduced to MHC Ia. In principle, the following options need to be considered.

1. Some MHC I molecules are retained in early phagosomes, where *M. tuberculosis* preferentially resides. Hence, antigen loading of MHC I could occur directly in this compartment.
2. The extensive exchange between phagosomes and endosomes could allow antigen loading of vacuolar MHC I molecules.
3. *M. tuberculosis* persists within host cells for long periods, during which the vacuolar membrane may become leaky, thus allowing antigen exchange with the cytosolic compartment. The leakiness can be increased by pore formation by mycobacterial lysins and phospholipases.
4. Excretion of the phagosomal cargo can result in MHC I peptide loading by regurgitation.
5. Apoptosis induced by *M. tuberculosis* results in the formation of apoptotic vesicles, which can be taken up by bystander APC. Antigenic cargo transported within these vesicles can thus be presented by MHC I molecules on bystander APC.

The last two options allow for cross-priming, i.e., transfer of antigens from infected macrophages to more proficient APC, such as DC (39a). This transfer is not restricted to CD8 T cells but can also promote CD4 T-cell stimulation.

Although it appears that different pathways lead to antigen presentation for CD8 T cells, the formation of apoptotic blebs is a potent mechanism both for glycolipid presentation by group I CD1 molecules and for peptide presentation by MHC I molecules (Fig. 3). The encounter of macrophages and DC with mycobacteria suppresses both antigen presentation and effector functions in these cells (30, 48). Cross-priming allows antigen transfer from suppressed or deactivated cells to more proficient APC and effector cells, i.e., mature DC or immigrant monocytes, respectively. The host immune response could therefore benefit from separating the cell responsible for antigen presentation from the infected cell. Ultimately, the actual infected macrophage (or DC) needs to be recognized by CD8 T cells if these cells are to play a role in host defense.

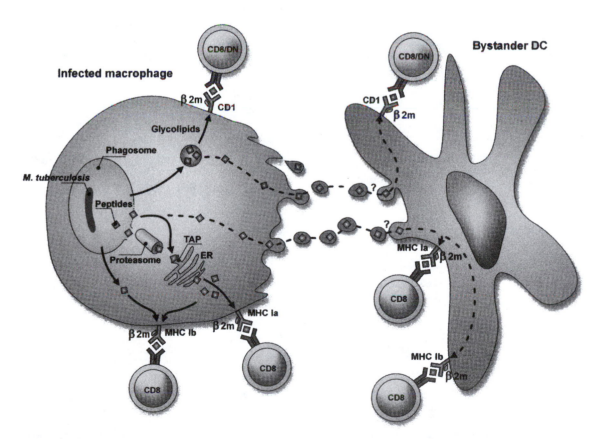

Figure 3. Cross-priming as a mechanism of efficient stimulation of β₂m-dependent T cells. Macrophages infected with *M. tuberculosis* undergo apoptosis, leading to the formation of apoptotic blebs. These apoptotic blebs carry antigenic cargo derived from *M. tuberculosis* from infected cells to bystander DC, which are better equipped for antigen-specific T-cell stimulation.

FUNCTIONS OF CD8 T CELLS

The possible functions of CD8 T cells in the control of tuberculosis include cytokine production, macrophage activation, killing of infected cells, and killing of *M. tuberculosis* (Fig. 4). CD8 T cells are often referred to as cytotoxic T lymphocytes (CTL) due to their ability to kill host cells. However, not all CD8 T cells are CTL. The actual function of CD8 T cells in this infection has not been clearly dissected. It is likely that both the cytokine-producing and cytotoxic functions are important in the immune response, but perhaps at different stages of infection.

CD8 T cells that respond to *M. tuberculosis* antigens in the lungs can produce IFN-γ and tumor necrosis factor alpha (TNF-α) (42). IFN-γ is a key molecule in the protective response to *M. tuberculosis*, due, at least in part, to the macrophage-activating properties of this cytokine. Macrophage activation is essential in the control of *M. tuberculosis*, and in vitro, CD8 T cells can activate macrophages to produce reactive nitrogen intermediates, such as nitric oxide, and kill *M. tuberculosis*. In the mouse system, CD8 T cells contribute less to IFN-γ production in the lungs than CD4 T cells do (42). The number of CD8 T cells in mouse lungs during acute infection that have the potential to produce IFN-γ in response to *M. tuberculosis* antigens is ~25 to 30% smaller than that of CD4 T cells. The kinetics of priming of CD8 T cells seems to be delayed compared to that of CD4 T cells.

TNF-α production by CD8 T cells may also be important in the control of *M. tuberculosis* infection. This cytokine is key for survival of mice infected with *M. tuberculosis* and participates in macrophage activation as well as granuloma formation and maintenance. It has recently been shown to be important in human tuberculosis as well, in that patients being treated for various inflammatory diseases with anti-TNF-α antibodies have a much higher than expected incidence of tuberculosis (22). TNF-α is produced by macrophages as well as T cells in tuberculosis, and contributions by each cell type may be important in the control of the infection.

There are also reports of interleukin-4 (IL-4)-producing CD8 T cells in human infection (45). In patients with tuberculosis, the number of IFN-γ-producing CD8 T cells in the peripheral blood is decreased while the number of IL-4-producing CD8 T cells is increased. However, this may be due to a selective recruitment of IFN-γ-producing *M. tuberculosis*-specific cells to the lungs during active disease. The significance of these "Tc2" cell types in control or exacerbation of infection is not clear. In situ hybridization studies of human lung sections from non-healing tuberculosis patients show IL-4 producing T cells in some granulomas (13), although it is not clear which types of T cells are produced.

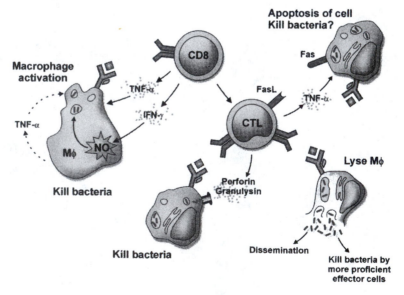

Figure 4. CD8 T-cell functions. CD8 T cells can activate macrophages via the release of cytokines, including IFN-γ and TNF-α, which induce phagolysosome fusion and reactive nitrogen intermediate (such as nitric oxide) production to kill intracellular *M. tuberculosis*. CD8 T cells can also act as CTL and lyse infected macrophages. This lysis can occur in the context of a granuloma, where released mycobacteria can be taken up and killed by activated macrophages. Perforin can mediate lysis but also enables granule-associated proteins, such as granulysin and granzymes, to enter the infected macrophage. Granulysin can directly kill intracellular *M. tuberculosis*. Finally, CD8 T cells can cause apoptosis of infected macrophages through a Fas/Fas-ligand- or TNF-α-mediated pathway.

In addition to the cytokine-producing potential of CD8 T cells in response to *M. tuberculosis* antigens, these cells can be cytotoxic. CD8 T cells recognizing antigen in the context of MHC I on the surface of macrophages can specifically lyse those macrophages (6, 9, 40), indicating that these cells could be recognized and killed in vivo. Perforin is a protein that is present in the cytotoxic granules of CD8 T cells and forms a pore in the target cell for the delivery of other granule proteins, such as granzymes. Lysis of infected macrophages is a perforin-dependent phenomenon (40, 49) whose outcome is not completely clear. Lysis may cause bacilli to be released from the infected cell. Although this would seem at first glance to be a mechanism for dissemination of bacteria, it may in fact be a strategy to release bacteria from macrophages that are incapable of being properly activated. In the context of a granuloma, releasing bacteria may be a means of facilitating uptake by other, more activated macrophages in the vicinity.

Perforin-mediated cytoxicity can also lead to apoptosis (programmed cell death) of the macrophage rather than to lysis. In this case, bacteria may not be released by the macrophage. Apoptosis could also be induced via Fas ligand on activated CD8 T cells binding to Fas on infected macrophages. It is not clear what role apoptosis plays in the control of *M. tuberculosis* infection, particularly in vivo. Although most evidence suggests that apoptosis would inhibit the intracellular bacteria (3), there are data suggesting that Fas ligand-induced apoptosis has little effect on *M. tuberculosis* (49).

An important mechanism used by CD8 T cells that directly relates to killing of intracellular *M. tuberculosis* is the production of a granule-associated protein, granulysin (47). Granulysin is a saposin-like protein (SAPLIP) that interacts with lipid membranes and activates lipid-degrading enzymes. This molecule enters infected macrophages via the perforin pore and can directly kill intracellular bacteria. CD8 T cells that produce granulysin are toxic to intracellular mycobacteria, while cytotoxic cells that do not produce granulysin will lyse the macrophages but do not affect intracellular bacilli. Purified granulysin kills *M. tuberculosis* in the absence of macrophages, but the perforin pore is required for entry of this molecule into the infected cells. Granulysin has been found only in human CD8 T cells, and there appears to be no mouse homolog protein. Therefore, it is not possible to directly test the importance of this molecule in the control of tuberculosis in a murine model. Since granulysin production by CD8 T cells is potentially very important in killing intracellular *M. tuberculosis*, CD8 T cells in mice are lacking a crucial effector function. Therefore, it is not possible to ascertain the true contribution of the CD8 T-cell subset by using the current mouse models.

The relative contribution of cytokine production or perforin-mediated lysis by CD8 T cells to controlling the infection is currently unknown. There are studies supporting a major role for cytokine (IFN-γ) secretion by these cells, while other studies indicate that cytotoxic function may be more important. However, recent data obtained with the mouse model indicate that the function of CD8 T cells in tuberculosis may depend on the stage of the infection (J. L. Flynn, unpublished studies). Cytotoxicity seems to peak early in the infection and then decline to very low levels. Cytokine secretion also peaks during early infection but remains at a relatively high level during the chronic phase of infection. There are probably different signals from the antigen-presenting cells or in the environment of the infected lung that regulate whether CD8 T cells are cytotoxic or cytokine producing or both. One could envision that a tight control of the function of these cells is necessary to limit immunopathology and subsequent lung damage.

MEMORY CD8 T CELLS

The memory response to *M. tuberculosis* in the lungs is weak compared to that of some viral infections. A model that has been used to study memory responses is infection of mice followed by antimycobacterial drug treatment beginning 4 weeks after infection. Mice are treated for 2 months and rested for 2 to 3 months prior to challenge. Following secondary aerosol challenge, the numbers of T cells in the lungs do not increase substantially until 2 weeks postinfection, although an increase in the activation state of T cells in the lungs can be observed 1 week after challenge. However, the memory response induced by a prior *M. tuberculosis* infection or by most vaccine preparations leads to only an approximately 10-fold reduction in bacterial numbers, and even this reduction is not sustained for long. Therefore, the robustness and efficacy of the memory T-cell response to *M. tuberculosis* challenge could be improved, and enhancing this response might lead to better protection.

A CD8 T-cell memory response is observed in the lungs following *M. tuberculosis* challenge (41). Measurement of IFN-γ production and activation markers clearly shows an enhanced response by CD8 T cells in "immune" mice compared to naive mice after aerosol challenge. However, by 3 weeks after the challenge, the response in the naive mice is similar to that in the "immune" mice. The overall levels of CD8 T cells responding to the secondary infection are not especially high. The cytotoxic potential of these cells remains to be investigated.

The relatively weak T-cell memory response in the lungs may be due to the chronic nature of the infection, although in mice treated for 2 months with two antimycobacterial drugs, the bacterial numbers are negligible or nonexistent (35). The relatively low challenge dose may not provide adequate migration signals to the memory T cells in a rapid fashion, leading to a slower memory response in the lungs. Various studies have demonstrated that humans latently infected with *M. tuberculosis* have a high circulating frequency of CD8 T cells recognizing *M. tuberculosis* antigens, including ESAT-6 and CFP10 (23, 27). These studies support the notion that a long-lived CD8 T-cell memory response is induced following infection. Single-cell analysis, by tetramer staining and IFN-γ-based enzyme-linked immunospot assay, indicates that the frequency of *M. tuberculosis*-specific CD8 T-cell responses induced by infection is in the same range as that seen in viral infections. However, the expression of such memory responses in the lungs following reexposure may be weak, as was observed in the mouse model. Further studies with animal models are necessary to determine the factors limiting memory responses in the lungs and to develop strategies to improve the recall response.

CD8 T CELLS IN VIVO

CD8 T cells specific for mycobacterial antigens are primed in the lung-draining lymph nodes within 2 weeks of aerosol infection in the mouse and can be found at low levels in the lungs beginning at 2 weeks postinfection. The numbers of CD8 T cells increase up to 4 weeks postinfection, and then the response contracts slightly as the bacterial numbers come under control. However, the CD8 T-cell response is maintained at a relatively high level during chronic infection. The numbers of CD8 T cells in the murine lungs are about 30 to 50% smaller than those of CD4 T cells. In the nonhuman primate model of tuberculosis, CD4 and CD8 T cells are present in approximately equal proportions in the lungs and granulomas. CD8 T cells have been reported to be present in human tuberculous granulomas as well (32). It was reported that CD8 T cells in the mouse model are found primarily in the periphery of the granuloma while the CD4 T cells are more evenly distributed throughout the granuloma (15). However, the structures of the granulomas in mice are very different from those in humans, with lymphocytic clusters and macrophage sheets rather than lymphocytes arranged in a circular fashion around centrally located macrophages.

CD4 AND CD8 T CELLS: DIFFERENT ROLES FOR DIFFERENT CELLS?

One confusing aspect of tuberculosis immunology involves the specific roles of the different immune components in protection or pathology. It has been clearly demonstrated that both CD4 and CD8 T cells can produce IFN-γ as well as TNF-α. However, both subsets seem to be important for control of infection. This suggests that there are unique functions of CD4 and CD8 T cells in protection. In chronically infected mice, there is an ongoing CD4 and CD8 T-cell response, with IFN-γ produced by each subset. Depletion of CD4 T cells in these mice by using anti-CD4 antibody causes an increase in the numbers of CD8 T cells in the lungs and an increased production of IFN-γ from these cells (36). This results in wild-type IFN-γ levels in the lungs of CD4-T-cell-depleted mice. In addition, these mice have wild-type levels of nitric oxide synthase 2 and reactive nitrogen intermediates in the macrophages in the lungs. However, despite these compensatory mechanisms, the mice succumb to the infection. These data and the results of studies with acute models of infection indicate that CD4 T cells play additional roles in protection, apart from IFN-γ production and macrophage activation.

CD4 T cells are necessary for a long-lived and functional CD8 T-cell response in certain other infectious-disease models, including virus and parasite diseases. CD4-T-cell-deficient mice have increased numbers of CD8 T cells producing IFN-γ, and so it appears that CD4 T cells are not necessary for priming CD8 T cells or cytokine production. However, the cytotoxic activity of CD8 T cells does seem to depend on CD4 T cells (43). CD8 T cells from the lungs of CD4$^{-/-}$ mice are deficient in the ability to specifically lyse infected macrophages. The mechanism by which CD4 T cells influence the function of CD8 T cells in tuberculosis remains unknown, although it appears that the environment of the lung is important.

CD4 and CD8 T cells may also participate at different times in the infection. There are data supporting roles for CD4 and CD8 T cells in control of acute and chronic or latent infection. The factors dictating which subset is participating in the immune response at a particular time, or which function is important during a specific stage of infection, could include the cytokine milieu of the lungs, the nature of the APC, the status of the granuloma, the activation state of the T cells, and the number of bacteria present. The cytokine environment of the lungs could be modulated by the pathology induced by the infection. In situations with extensive immunopathology, IL-10 levels are higher, and this may affect T-cell or APC function. The APC may play a major role in determining the contribution of each subset. For example, heavily infected macrophages may present more antigen to CD8 T cells and less to CD4 T cells, due to inhibition of MHC II presentation (28). There may also be differences in responses depending on the APC encountered, for example, DC or macrophages in the lungs. It remains to be seen how and when each response is important and how to modulate the responses to provide optimum protection in the lungs.

In summary, CD8 T cells that recognize mycobacterial antigens on macrophages or DC are induced following *M. tuberculosis*. The available data support a role for CD8 T cells in the control of tuberculosis. The processing and presentation of antigens to these cells involve both classical and nonclassical pathways and molecules, and so the potential repertoire of antigens recognized by CD8 T cells is quite large. These cells probably participate in the protective response via cytokine production and cytotoxic activity. Given the potential for effective immune responses mediated by CD8 T cells, more researchers are using strategies that include the induction of CD8 T cells in vaccine candidates for tuberculosis. The results of these studies may provide important data on the ability of CD8 T cells to contribute to protection against this disease.

Acknowledgments. The work of S.H.E.K. on tuberculosis receives financial support from DFG (priority program "Novel vaccination strategies" KA 573/4-2), EC (Cluster on TB Vaccine Development), and BMBF (Competence networks "Genomics of Pathogenic Bacteria," "Bacterial Proteomics," Proteomics of Membrane-Bound Proteins," "Structural Genomics of *M. tuberculosis*"). J.L.F. receives support from the National Institutes of Health (NIAID and NHLBI) (grants AI37859, AI47485, AI40310, AI50732, HL71241, and HL68526) and the American Lung Association (CI-016-N).

REFERENCES

1. Antoniou, A. N., S. J. Powis, and T. Elliott. 2003. Assembly and export of MHC class I peptide ligands. *Curr. Opin. Immunol.* 15:75–81.
2. Apostolou, I., Y. Takahama, C. Belmant, T. Kawano, M. Huerre, G. Marchal, J. Cui, M. Taniguchi, H. Nakauchi, J. J. Fournie, P. Kourilsky, and G. Gachelin. 1999. Murine natural killer T(NKT) cells [correction of natural killer cells] contribute to the granulomatous reaction caused by mycobacterial cell walls. *Proc. Natl. Acad. Sci. USA* 96:5141–5146.
3. Balcewicz-Sablinska, M. K., J. Keane, H. Kornfeld, and H. G. Remold. 1998. Pathogenic *Mycobacterium tuberculosis* evades apoptosis of host macrophages by release of TNF-R2, resulting in inactivation of TNF-α. *J. Immunol.* 161:2636–2641.
4. Banchereau, J., and R. M. Steinman. 1998. Dendritic cells and the control of immunity. *Nature* 392:245–252.
5. Behar, S. M., C. C. Dascher, M. J. Grusby, C. R. Wang, and M. B. Brenner. 1999. Susceptibility of mice deficient in CD1D or TAP1 to infection with *Mycobacterium tuberculosis*. *J. Exp. Med.* 189:1973–1980.
6. Cho, S., V. Mehra, S. Thoma-Uszynski, S. Stenger, N. Serbina, R. Mazzaccaro, J. L. Flynn, P. F. Barnes, S. South-

wood, E. Celis, B. R. Bloom, R. L. Modlin, and A. Sette. 2000. Antimicrobial activity of MHC class I restricted CD8+ T cells in human tuberculosis. *Proc. Natl. Acad. Sci. USA* 97:12210–12215.
7. Chun, T., N. V. Serbina, D. Nolt, B. Wang, N. M Chiu, J. L. Flynn, and C.-R. Wang. 2001. Induction of M3-restricted cytotoxic T lymphocyte responses by N-formylated peptides derived from *Mycobacterium tuberculosis*. *J. Exp. Med.* 193:1213–1220.
8. Collins, H. L., and S. H. E. Kaufmann. 2001. Aquired immunity against bacteria, p. 207–221. *In* S. H. E. Kaufmann, A. Sher and R. Ahmed (ed.), *Immunology of Infectious Diseases*. ASM Press, Washington, D.C.
9. De Libero, G., I. Flesch, and S. H. E. Kaufmann. 1988. Mycobacteria-reactive Lyt-2+ T-cell lines. *Eur. J. Immunol.* 18:59–66.
10. Doherty, P. C. 1997. The Nobel Lectures in Immunology. The Nobel Prize for Physiology or Medicine, 1996. Cell mediated immunity in virus infections. *Scand. J. Immunol.* 46:527–540.
11. Dow, S. W., A. Roberts, J. Vyas, J. Rodgers, R. R. Rich, I. Orme, and T. A. Potter. 2000. Immunization with f-Met peptides induces immune reactivity against *Mycobacterium tuberculosis*. *Tubercle Lung Dis.* 80:5–13.
12. Falk, K., and O. Rotzschke. 2002. The final cut: how ERAP1 trims MHC ligands to size. *Nat. Immunol.* 3:1121–1122.
13. Fenhalls, G., A. Wong, J. Bezuidenhout, P. van Helden, P. Bardin, and P. T. Lukey. 2000. In situ production of gamma interferon, interleukin-4, and tumor necrosis factor alpha mRNA in human lung tuberculous granuloma. *Infect. Immun.* 68:2827–2836.
13a. Fischer, K., E. Scotet, M. Niemeyer, H. Koebernick, J. Zerrahn, S. Maillet, R. Hurwitz, M. Kursar, M. Bonneville, S. H. E. Kaufmann, and U. E. Schaible. 2004. Mycobacterial phosphatidyl-inositol mannoside is a natural antigen for CD1d-restricted T cells. *Proc. Natl. Acad. Sci. USA* 101:10685–10690.
14. Flynn, J. L., M. M. Goldstein, K. J. Triebold, B. Koller, and B. R. Bloom. 1992. Major histocompatibility complex class I-restricted T cells are required for resistance to *Mycobacterium tuberculosis* infection. *Proc. Natl. Acad. Sci. USA* 89:12013–12017.
15. Gonzalez-Juarrero, M., O. C. Turner, J. Turner, P. Marietta, J. V. Brooks, and I. M. Orme. 2001. Temporal and spatial arrangement of lymphocytes within lung granulomas induced by aerosol infection with *Mycobacterium tuberculosis*. *Infect. Immun.* 69:1722–1728.
16. Heinzel, A. S., J. E. Grotzke, R. A. Lines, D. A. Lewinsohn, A. L. McNabb, D. N. Streblow, V. M. Braud, H. J. Grieser, J. T. Belisle, and D. M. Lewinsohn. 2002. HLA-E-dependent presentation of Mtb-derived antigen to human CD8+ T cells. *J. Exp. Med.* 196:1473–1781.
17. Hess, J., U. Schaible, B. Raupach, and S. H. Kaufmann. 2000. Exploiting the immune system: toward new vaccines against intracellular bacteria. *Adv. Immunol.* 75:1–88.
18. Joyce, S., and L. Van Kaer. 2003. CD1-restricted antigen presentation: an oily matter. *Curr. Opin. Immunol.* 15:95–104.
19. Kaufmann, S. H. 1996. Gamma/delta and other unconventional T lymphocytes: what do they see and what do they do? *Proc. Natl. Acad. Sci. USA* 93:2272–2279.
20. Kaufmann, S. H. 2001. How can immunology contribute to the control of tuberculosis? *Nat. Rev. Immunol.* 1:20–30.
21. Kaufmann, S.H. 1993. Immunity to intracellular bacteria. *Annu. Rev. Immunol.* 11:129–163.
22. Keane, J., S. Gershon, R. P. Wise, E. Mirabile-Levens, J. Kasznica, W. D. Schwieterman, J. N. Siegel, and M. M. Braun. 2001. Tuberculosis associated with infliximab, a tumor necrosis factor alpha-neutralizing agent. *N. Engl. J. Med.* 345:1098–1104.

23. Lalvani, A., R. Brookes, R. Wilkinson, A. Malin, A. Pathan, P. Andersen, H. Dockrell, G. Pasvol, and A. Hill. 1998. Human cytolytic and interferon gamma-secreting CD8+ T lymphocytes specific for *Mycobacterium tuberculosis*. *Proc. Natl. Acad. Sci. USA* 95:270–275.

24. Lazarevic, V., and J. Flynn. 2002. CD8+ T cells in tuberculosis. *Am. J. Respir. Crit. Care Med.* 166:1116–1121.

25. Lenz, L. L., and M. J. Bevan. 1996. H2-M3-restricted presentation of *Listeria monocytogenes* antigens. *Immunol. Rev.* 151:107–121.

26. Lewinsohn, D., M. Alderson, A. Briden, S. Riddell, S. Reed, and K. Grabstein. 1998. Characterization of human CD8+ T cells reactive with *Mycobacterium tuberculosis*-infected antigen presenting cells. *J. Exp. Med.* 187:1633–40.

27. Lewinsohn, D. M., L. Zhu, V. J. Madison, D. C. Dillon, S. P. Fling, S. G. Reed, K. H. Grabstein, and M. R. Alderson. 2001. Classically restricted human CD8+ T lymphocytes derived from *Mycobacterium tuberculosis*-infected cells: definition of antigen specificity. *J. Immunol.* 166:439–446.

28. Noss, E. H., R. K. Pai, T. J. Sellati, J. D. Radolf, J. Belisle, D. T. Golenbock, W. H. Boom, and C. V. Harding. 2001. Toll-like receptor 2-dependent inhibition of macrophage class II MHC expression and antigen processing by 19-kDa lipoprotein of *Mycobacterium tuberculosis*. *J. Immunol.* 167:910–918.

29. Pamer, E., and P. Cresswell. 1998. Mechanisms of MHC class I-restricted antigen processing. *Annu. Rev. Immunol.* 16:323–358.

30. Pancholi, P., A. Mirza, N. Bhardwaj, and R. M. Steinman. 1993. Sequestration from immune CD4+ T cells of mycobacteria growing in human macrophages. *Science* 260:984–986.

31. Porcelli, S. A., and R. L. Modlin. 1999. The CD1 system: antigen-presenting molecules for T-cell recognition of lipids and glycolipids. *Annu. Rev. Immunol.* 17:297–329.

32. Randhawa, P. S. 1990. Lymphocyte subsets in granulomas of human tuberculosis: an in situ immunofluorescence study using monoclonal antibodies. *Pathology* 22:153–155.

33. Ristori, G., C. Montesperelli, M. T. Fiorillo, L. Battistini, A. Chersi, R. Sorrentino, G. Borsellino, A. Perna, D. Tramonti, S. Cannoni, M. P. Perrone, F. Giubilei, P. Riccio, M. Salvetti, and C. Buttinelli. 2001. T-cell response to N-formylated peptides in humans. *Eur. J. Immunol.* 31:2762–2770.

34. Rolph, M. S., B. Raupach, H. H. Kobernick, H. L. Collins, B. Perarnau, F. A. Lemonnier, and S. H. Kaufmann. 2001. MHC class Ia-restricted T cells partially account for β2-microglobulin-dependent resistance to *Mycobacterium tuberculosis*. *Eur. J. Immunol.* 31:1944–1949.

35. Scanga, C. A., V. P. Mohan, H. Joseph, K. Yu, J. Chan, and J. Flynn. 1999. Reactivation of latent tuberculosis: variations on the Cornell murine model. *Infect. Immun.* 67:4531–4538.

36. Scanga, C. A., V. P. Mohan, K. Yu, H. Joseph, K. Tanaka, J. Chan, and J. L. Flynn. 2000. Depletion of CD4+ T cells causes reactivation of murine persistent tuberculosis despite continued expression of IFN-γ and NOS2. *J. Exp. Med.* 192:347–358.

37. Schaible, U. E., H. L. Collins, and S. H. Kaufmann. 1999. Confrontation between intracellular bacteria and the immune system. *Adv. Immunol.* 71:267–377.

38. Schaible, U. E., H. L. Collins, F. Priem, and S. H. Kaufmann. 2002. Correction of the iron overload defect in β2-microglobulin knockout mice by lactoferrin abolishes their increased susceptibility to tuberculosis. *J. Exp. Med.* 196:1507–1513.

39. Schaible, U. E., and S. H. Kaufmann. 2000. CD1 and CD1-restricted T cells in infections with intracellular bacteria. *Trends Microbiol.* 8:419–425.

39a. Schaible, U. E., F. Winau, P. A. Sieling, K. Fischer, H. L. Collins, K. Hagens, R. L. Modlin, V. Brinkmann, and S. H. E. Kaufmann. 2003. Apoptosis facilitates antigen presentation to T-lymphocytes through MHC-I and CD1 in tuberculosis. *Nat. Med.* 9:1039–1046.

40. Serbina, N. V., C.-C. Liu, C. A. Scanga, and J. L. Flynn. 2000. CD8+ cytotoxic T lymphocytes from lungs of *M. tuberculosis* infected mice express perforin in vivo and lyse infected macrophages. *J. Immunol.* 165:353–363.

41. Serbina, N. V., and J. L. Flynn. 2001. CD8 T cells participate in the memory response to *Mycobacterium tuberculosis*. *Infect. Immun.* 69:4320–4328.

42. Serbina, N. V., and J. L. Flynn. 1999. Early emergence of CD8+ T cells primed for production of type 1 cytokines in the lungs of *Mycobacterium tuberculosis*-infected mice. *Infect. Immun.* 67:3980–3988.

43. Serbina, N. V., V. Lazarevic, and J. L. Flynn. 2001. CD4+ T cells are required for the development of cytotoxic CD8+ T cells during *Mycobacterium tuberculosis* infection. *J. Immunol.* 167:6991–7000.

44. Shamshiev, A., A. Donda, T. I. Prigozy, L. Mori, V. Chigorno, C. A. Benedict, L. Kappos, S. Sonnino, M. Kronenberg, and G. De Libero. 2000. The αβ T cell response to self-glycolipids shows a novel mechanism of CD1b loading and a requirement for complex oligosaccharides. *Immunity* 13:255–264.

45. Smith, S. M., M. R. Klein, A. S. Malin, J. Sillah, K. P. McAdam, and H. M. Dockrell. 2002. Decreased IFN-gamma and increased IL-4 production by human CD8+ T cells in response to *Mycobacterium tuberculosis* in tuberculosis patients. *Tuberculosis* 82:7–13.

46. Sousa, A. O., R. J. Mazzaccaro, R. G. Russell, F. K. Lee, O. C. Turner, S. Hong, L. Van Kaer, and B. R. Bloom. 1999. Relative contributions of distinct MHC class I-dependent cell populations in protection to tuberculosis infection in mice. *Proc. Natl. Acad. Sci. USA* 97:4204–4208.

47. Stenger, S., D. A. Hanson, R. Teitelbaum, P. Dewan, K. R. Niazi, C. J. Froelich, T. Ganz, S. Thoma-Uszynski, A. Melian, C. Bogdan, S. A. Porcelli, B. R. Bloom, A. M. Krensky, and R. L. Modlin. 1998. An antimicrobial activity of cytotoxic T cells mediated by granulysin. *Science* 282:121–125.

48. Stenger, S., K. R. Niazi, and R. L. Modlin. 1998. Down-regulation of CD1 on antigen presenting cells by infection with *Mycobacterium tuberculosis*. *J. Immunol.* 161:3582–3588.

49. Stenger, S., R. Mazzaccaro, K. Uyemura, S. Cho, P. Barnes, J. Rosat, A. Sette, M. Brenner, S. Porcelli, B. Bloom, and R. Modlin. 1997. Differential effects of cytolytic T cell subsets on intracellular infection. *Science* 276:1684–1687.

50. Szalay, G., U. Zugel, C. H. Ladel, and S. H. Kaufmann. 1999. Participation of group 2 CD1 molecules in the control of murine tuberculosis. *Microbes Infect.* 1:1153–1157.

51. Vincent, M. S., D. S. Leslie, J. E. Gumperz, X. Xiong, E. P. Grant, and M. B. Brenner. 2002. CD1-dependent dendritic cell instruction. *Nat. Immunol.* 3:1163–1168.

52. Zinkernagel, R. M. 1997. The Nobel Lectures in Immunology. The Nobel Prize for Physiology or Medicine, 1996. Cellular immune recognition and the biological role of major transplantation antigens. *Scand. J. Immunol.* 46:421–36.

Chapter 30

CD1 and Tuberculosis

CHRISTOPHER C. DASCHER AND MICHAEL B. BRENNER

The primary task of the immune system is the recognition of foreign antigens in the host, a situation which typically signals the presence of an infectious microorganism. The critical role of antigen presentation to T cells by the host immune system following tuberculosis infection is well known. Previously, the presentation of peptides generated from *Mycobacterium tuberculosis* proteins by the major histocompatibility complex (MHC) class I and II (MHC I and MHC II) antigen presentation pathways was thought to be the only means by which T cells could recognize foreign antigens. The CD1 gene family adds yet a third antigen-presenting pathway for the stimulation of antigen-specific T cells. The CD1 genes in humans encode a family of nonpolymorphic cell surface glycoproteins that are related to the MHC I family but have structurally diverged to serve a unique function in antigen presentation. Unlike MHC, the CD1 proteins have evolved the capacity to present lipids and glycolipids to T cells in a manner that is analogous to the paradigm established for peptide presentation by the MHC. Moreover, a number of lipid antigens that are presented to T cells by CD1 have been derived from *M. tuberculosis* and other mycobacterial species. These include mycolic acid and lipoarabinomannan, which represent some of the most abundant lipid molecules in the mycobacterial cell wall. The T cells that recognize these lipid antigens have important antimicrobial effector functions including cytolytic activity, production of inflammatory cytokines, and release of the antimicrobial molecule granulysin, which may contribute to host defense against tuberculosis. This chapter reviews the immunobiology of CD1 and its potentially important role in the immune response to *M. tuberculosis* infection.

CD1 GENES AND EXPRESSION

The CD1 genes in humans encode a small family of glycoproteins that are distantly related to the MHC I protein family (Fig. 1) (40). However, the CD1 locus is present on human chromosome 1 and is therefore genetically unlinked to the MHC locus on chromosome 6 (13). There are five CD1 genes, designated CD1A, CD1B, CD1C, CD1D, and CD1E. These five genes code for the distinct CD1 isoforms that are relatively nonpolymorphic between individuals (34, 42). Based on homology of the amino acid sequences of the five isoforms, the CD1 family can be subdivided into three groups. The group 1 CD1 is composed of the CD1a, CD1b, and CD1c isoforms, while group 2 is composed of the single CD1d isoform (12). The CD1e isoform is of intermediate homology and has recently been proposed to form a third CD1 group (group 3) (1). Evidence for CD1 genes or proteins has been found in all mammals where it has been looked for. Moreover, each of the CD1 isoforms has significant homology to orthologous isoforms across a range of mammalian species. Interestingly, mice and rats have only the group 2 (CD1d) isoforms while primates and other mammals have all three CD1 groups (11). Comparative genomic analysis between mice and humans strongly suggests that the group 1 CD1 isoforms were deleted in mice at some point during their evolution (19). Taken together, these data suggest that the CD1 genes arose early in mammalian evolution and have been conserved as a distinct gene family across a wide evolutionary timescale.

The CD1 isoforms are expressed as heterodimeric glycoproteins on the cell surface with a CD1-encoded heavy chain that is noncovalently linked to the invariant β_2-microglobulin light chain. The overall structure of the CD1 proteins resembles MHC I in having three extracellular domains, $\alpha1$, $\alpha2$, and $\alpha3$, with the $\alpha1$ and $\alpha2$ domains forming the antigen binding pocket and the $\alpha3$ domain being membrane proximal and associated with the β_2-microglobulin light chain. Unlike MHC I, which is expressed on all somatic cells in the body, the CD1 proteins are ex-

Christopher C. Dascher and Michael B. Brenner • Division of Rheumatology, Immunology and Allergy, Brigham and Women's Hospital and Harvard Medical School, Boston, MA 02115.

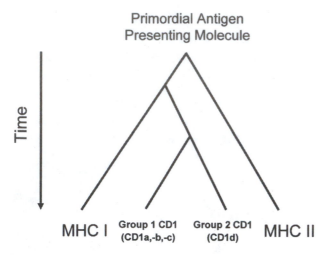

Figure 1. Hypothetical evolution of CD1 and the MHC. There are five distinct CD1 genes in humans that are unlinked to the MHC locus. These are divided into two groups based on sequence homology. Analysis of protein sequence data shows that CD1 diverged from the MHC family early in vertebrate evolution. The divergence of MHC I and MHC II is estimated at approximately 250 million to 300 million years ago. CD1 and MHC I share many structural features and thus probably have a common ancestor. However, the exact time of the divergence of CD1 and MHC I is difficult to estimate since both gene families are under strong selective pressure. So far, CD1 genes have been found only in placental mammals.

pressed primarily on professional antigen-presenting cells found in both lymphoid and nonlymphoid tissues in a distribution comparable to that of MHC II (Table 1). These include lymph node dendritic cells (DC), B cells, epidermal Langerhans' cells, and dermal DC (reviewed in references 7 and 57). Peripheral blood monocytes are typically group 1 CD1 negative but upregulate the group 1 CD1 isoforms following cytokine stimulation and differentiation into immature DC (14). Importantly, CD1 is expressed on DC within granulomas from patients with both *M. tuberculosis* and *M. leprae* infections, although the role of DC in granuloma formation and maintenance is unclear (65, 78). In contrast to the more restricted expression of group 1 CD1 isoforms, the group 2 (CD1d) isoform is expressed on virtually all lymphoid and myeloid cells but at significantly lower levels relative to the group 1 CD1 isoforms (25). In addition, CD1d does not appear to be upregulated on DC following cytokine stimulation (14, 25). Hence, the CD1 isoforms are widely expressed throughout the immune system on cells involved primarily with antigen presentation in both normal tissue and tuberculous granulomas.

CD1 PROTEIN STRUCTURE

Insights into the structure of CD1 and its ability to bind lipid antigens have been greatly enhanced by the solution of the human CD1a and CD1b and mouse CD1d crystal structures (27, 83, 84). These structures reveal critical differences between the antigen binding domains of MHC I and CD1. Like MHC I, the antigen binding groove of CD1 is formed by the α1 and α2 domains, with two antiparallel α-helices forming the sides of the groove and a β-pleated sheet forming the floor (Fig. 2a and b). However, the CD1 groove is deeper and the opening formed by the α-helices is narrower than in MHC I (Fig. 2c). In addi-

Table 1. Antigen-presenting pathways for T cells

Characteristic	Pathway			
	CD1		MHC	
	Group 1 (CD1a to CD1c)	Group 2 (CD1d)	Class I	Class II
Antigens	Lipid and glycolipids[a]	Lipid and glycolipids[b]	Peptides	Peptides
Antigen loading	Recycling endosomes, late endosomes, lysosomes	Late endosomes, lysosomes	Endoplasmic reticulum	Late endosomes, lysosomes
Cellular expression	Professional APC[c] (DC, Langerhans' cells, B cells)	Most leukocytes (B cells, macrophages, DC)	All somatic cells	Professional APC (DC, Langerhans' cells, B cells)
Polymorphism	Limited	Limited	High	High
T-cell phenotype	CD4, CD8, DN	CD4, DN	CD8	CD4
TCR	αβ and γδ	αβ (invariant TCR-α)	αβ	αβ
Implicated in tuberculosis	Yes	Yes[d]	Yes	Yes

[a]Many of the group 1 CD1 antigens are derived from *Mycobacterium* species, although a number of autoreactive T cells have been found. This suggests that group 1 CD1 isoforms can react to self-lipids as well.
[b]To date, no lipids derived from bacteria or other pathogens have been described for CD1d. However, a number of endogenous self-lipids have been described.
[c]APC, antigen-presenting cells.
[d]The CD1d knockout mice do not show any significant differences in survival or bacterial burden compared to wild-type animals on infection with virulent *M. tuberculosis*. However, pharmacologic stimulation of CD1d-restricted NKT cells at the time of infection with the lipid antigen αGC does improve morbidity and mortality (see the text).

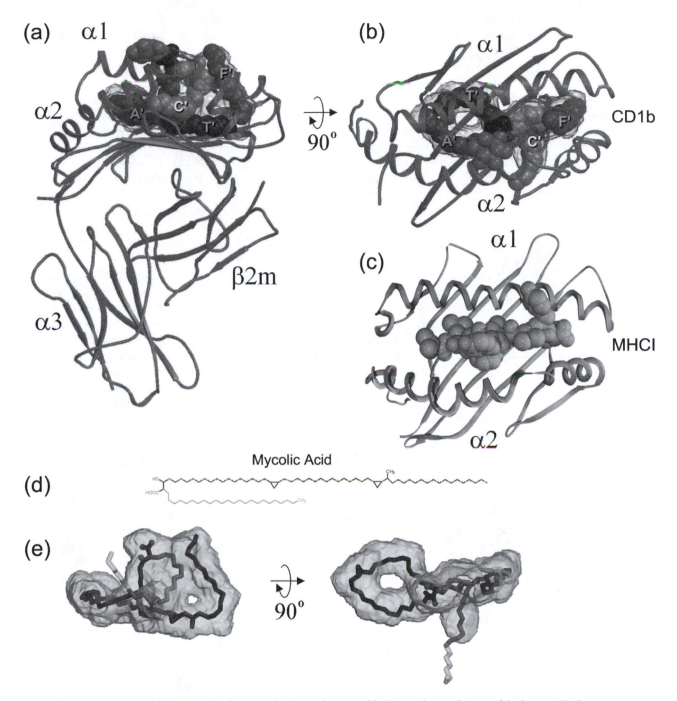

Figure 2. Structure of the human CD1b protein-lipid complex. (a and b) Two orthogonal views of the human CD1b structure from the side (a) and from the top (b) of the structure with bound phosphatidylinositol in the antigen binding pocket. The internal cavity that forms the antigen binding pocket is shown as a transparent surface, and the various channels are indicated as A′, C′, F′, and T′. (c) Structure of human HLA-A2, with the human T-cell leukemia virus type 1 Tax peptide (space filling) in the antigen binding groove shown for comparison to CD1b (22). (d) Structure of *M. tuberculosis* mycolic acid with the meromycolate chain (dark) and the shorter alpha chain (light) and carboxylate groups. (e) Hypothetical model of mycolic acid as it would appear folded into the CD1b protein. The left-hand orthogonal view corresponds to the orientation of the CD1b protein in panel a, and the right hand view corresponds to the orientation in b. In this model, the C_{60} long meromycolate chain (dark) is fully contained within channels A′, T′ and F′, a superchannel of ca. 70 Å. The shorter C_{25} alkyl chain (light) is lodged in the C′ channel. The crystal structure provides no guidance to how to model the end of the C_{25} chain in the mycolic acid, and this part of the model is therefore indicated by an extended gray chain. Panels a, b, and e reprinted from reference 27 with permission from the authors and publisher. © 2002 Nature Publishing Group.

tion, the helical ends of the CD1 antigen binding domain are closed off, resulting in the formation of an enclosed "pocket" with a small opening along the upper face of the protein. Importantly, the residues that line the pocket are largely hydrophobic, which makes it electrostatically neutral and hence ideal for binding hydrophobic acyl chains.

Comparison of the crystal structures of murine CD1d and human CD1b reveal several important differences between the two isoforms that could be relevant to lipid antigen binding (26). The CD1d antigen binding pocket is a relatively open volume, unobstructed by the side chains lining the groove, whereas the CD1b antigen binding pocket is composed of a series of channels that snake through the internal volume to form the antigen binding domain. Interestingly, the CD1b protein has a hole along the lateral face, which can allow lipid acyl chains to protrude from the side of the protein and which is not present in either CD1a or CD1d (Fig. 2a). This feature could allow longer acyl chains to be bound, which otherwise could not be accommodated within the space of the internal channels. It is predicted that long acyl chains either pass continuously through several channels or exit via the C' channel. These features may be of particular relevance for *M. tuberculosis* lipids, such as mycolic acid, that can have acyl chains in excess of 80 carbons (C_{80}) in

length, or they may result in the binding of lipids containing multiple acyl chains (Fig. 2d and e). Taken together, these structural data provide independent validation for the specialized function of CD1 in presenting lipid and glycolipid antigens to T cells.

CD1 LIPID AND GLYCOLIPID ANTIGENS FROM *M. TUBERCULOSIS*

Porcelli et al. identified the first antigen-specific CD1-restricted T-cell line that recognized a mycobacterial antigen presented by CD1b (56). Biochemical purification of the bioactive component from *M. tuberculosis* by Beckman et al. revealed the remarkable finding that the antigen was mycolic acid, a major lipid found in the mycobacterial cell wall (4). This was the first example of a bacterial lipid antigen that could be presented by CD1 and recognized by antigen-specific T cells. Subsequent studies have identified a number of lipid antigens from *M. tuberculosis* and other mycobacterial species that are presented by CD1 to specific T cells (Fig. 3). These include lipoarabinomannan, phosphatidylinositol mannoside (PIM), glucose monomycolate, didehydroxymycobactin, sulfoglycolipid, and mannosyl-β_1-phosphodolichol (29, 49–51, 64). Most of these molecules are constituents

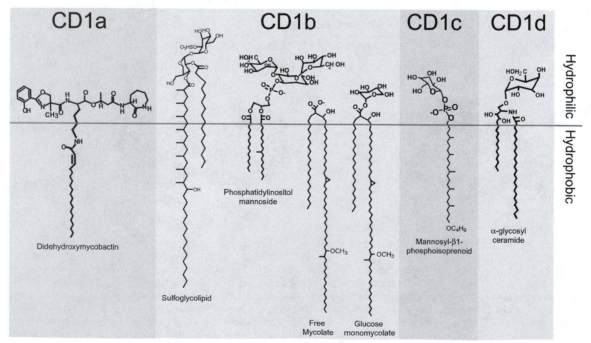

Figure 3. Structures of known CD1 lipid antigens. The first six lipid molecules are derived from *Mycobacterium* species and are presented by either CD1a, CD1b, or CD1c. The αGC (far right) is derived from the marine sponge *Agelas mauritanius*. All of the molecules have a common structural motif, which is a hydrophobic acyl chain linked to a hydrophilic head group such as a simple sugar or carboxylate group. Both structural and functional data support a model in which the hydrophobic acyl chain is anchored into the CD1 binding groove and the hydrophilic head group is exposed to the aqueous environment and interacts with the TCR. While the αGC is not known to exist in bacteria or mammalian tissues, it is a ligand for CD1d and a potent stimulator of CD1d-restricted NK T cells. Lipid structures courtesy of Branch Moody, Brigham and Women's Hospital.

of mycobacterial cell walls and are found only in *Mycobacterium* or other closely related bacterial genera. The presence of CD1-restricted T cells specific for several of the most abundant mycobacterial lipids suggests that CD1 is likely to play a role in the host response to *M. tuberculosis* infection.

There are a range of molecular lipid classes that have been identified as CD1-presented T-cell antigens, including fatty acids, glycolipids, phospholipids, and lipopeptides. Examination of the various CD1-presented lipid and glycolipid antigens identified thus far suggests the existence of a common structural motif. Specifically, these lipid antigens have one or two hydrophobic acyl chains linked to a hydrophilic head group such as a simple sugar or carboxyl group. These data suggest a model in which the hydrophobic lipid tails are anchored into the CD1 pocket with the hydrophilic head group of the lipid projecting through the top of the pocket, thus being exposed to the solvent and accessible for recognition by the T cell receptor (TCR) (58). This model is strongly supported by the data on the human CD1b crystal structure, which was cocrystallized with two self-lipid molecules: phosphatidylinositol and ganglioside GM_2 (33, 63). In phosphatidylinositol, the lipid tails are anchored into the antigen binding pocket and the hydrophilic inositol ring protrudes from the top and is exposed to the aqueous environment (Fig. 2a) (27). Functional studies by Moody et al. demonstrated that the length of the lipid acyl chains of glucose monomycolate could be varied with minimal loss of T-cell activity (49). In contrast, T-cell activity was extremely sensitive to modifications in the carbohydrate portion of the antigen. Similarly for mycolic acids, substitution of the carboxylate group abolished T-cell recognition, indicating the importance of the hydrophilic head group in T-cell recognition (30). Proof that lipid antigen recognition is TCR mediated was provided by transfection of cloned TCR genes isolated from a single lipid-reactive CD1-restricted T-cell, which then conferred antigen specificity to the transfectant (31). Moreover, mutagenesis of key amino acids in the CDR3 loops of the TCR that were predicted to interact with the CD1b-antigen complex abrogated antigen recognition (30). Thus, both structural and functional data support a model of lipid antigen presentation by CD1, which, while analogous to MHC, has evolved the unique ability to bind microbial lipids and glycolipids and present them for recognition by TCRs.

CD1 AND THE INTRACELLULAR ENVIRONMENT

For efficient antigen presentation to occur, the antigens (lipids) and antigen-presenting molecules

(CD1) must intersect in an intracellular compartment. A number of studies have addressed the unique mechanisms of CD1 lipid antigen uptake, loading, and presentation. With respect to antigen uptake, the precise mechanisms for the CD1 pathway are still unclear. Receptor-mediated endocytosis of LAM by the mannose receptor and subsequent colocalization of LAM and CD1b in late endosomes and lysosomes have been demonstrated (59). However, specific receptors or serum proteins that bind other CD1 lipid and glycolipid antigens have not been identified. Nevertheless, the necessity for antigen uptake into endosomes has been shown for most of the mycobacterial lipid antigens. This is supported by the observation that chemical fixation of the APC prior to addition of the lipid antigen eliminates T-cell recognition, especially for lipids with long acyl chains. The sphingolipid activator proteins have been implicated in loading antigens into both CD1b and CD1d, thus defining the first accessory molecules that are required for efficient presentation of at least a subset of lipid antigens (82, 85). However, evidence for lipid antigen loading of CD1 at or near the cell surface has also been described (10, 47). To date, antigen processing in the form of breaking down mycobacterial lipids has not been demonstrated, although some structures with large carbohydrate head groups (e.g., LAM) probably require cleavage to a size suitable for CD1 loading or interaction with the TCR (64).

One of the hallmarks of *M. tuberculosis* bacteria is the capacity to survive within the intracellular environment. This has important consequences for antigens produced by bacteria in situ since mycobacterial lipids may traffic differently from proteins in infected cells. *M. tuberculosis* has evolved the capacity to replicate inside antigen-presenting cells and to minimize contact with late endosomes and lysosomes. In addition, cells infected with *M. tuberculosis* inhibit MHC II transport and processing, thus subverting this vital pathway of antigen presentation (39). In contrast, cells infected with live *M. bovis* BCG actively traffic lipids out of the bacterial phagosome, where they localize in both early and late endosomes and, in some cases, are also released from the cell as exocytic vesicles that are taken up by adjacent uninfected cells (2). Some of these lipids (e.g., PIM2) have macrophage-activating activity, in addition to being CD1 antigens (60). Several studies have shown that CD1-restricted T cells are able to respond to cells infected with virulent *M. tuberculosis* (41, 70). Thus, lipid molecules presented by CD1 may provide an alternate source of antigens for presentation by infected APCs that might otherwise evade immune surveillance.

The unique chemical properties of lipid molecules, in contrast to peptides, suggest that the mechanisms for lipid antigen processing and loading into CD1 are probably different from those for peptide loading into MHC. An important observation made by Mukherjee et al. was that the length of a lipid acyl chain may be a critical factor in determining where a particular lipid is localized once it is taken up by a cell and enters the endosomal network (52). This may have important consequences for lipid antigen presentation, given the wide range of acyl chain lengths found in mycobacterial lipids. For example, the short-chain form (C_{32}) of glucose monomycolate, a CD1b-presented antigen, can be added to live or fixed cells, where it can be presented to T cells within minutes, consistent with surface loading of the antigen (47). In contrast, long-chain (C_{80}) glucose monomycolate requires several hours for maximal T-cell activity, is sensitive to endosomal acidification blockers, and cannot be presented by fixed cells (47). Thus, the biophysical properties of the lipid antigens may influence the endosomal compartments where a particular antigen is loaded into CD1.

The potentially distinct distribution of lipids into particular endosomal compartments presents a challenge to the CD1 antigen presentation system. However, the multiple CD1 isoforms found in many animal species may have evolved as an adaptation to the capacity of lipids to distribute broadly within the cell. Support for this hypothesis comes from the appreciation that each of the CD1 isoforms traffics to different subcompartments within the endosomal system (reviewed in references 48 and 75). All of the CD1 isoforms are thought to be assembled with β_2M in the endoplasmic reticulum (9, 43, 76). They then traffic to the plasma membrane and follow a major pathway of internalization from the cell surface into endosomes (Fig. 4). The CD1a isoform then traffics mainly to early and recycling endosomes (73); CD1b traffics from the cell surface through late endosomes and lysosomes and can be colocalized with MHC II in specialized lysosomes known as MIIC (73, 74); CD1c is distributed broadly through early and late endosomes (10, 77); and human CD1d traffics from the plasma membrane through early endosomes to late endosomes but only partially colocalizes in lysosomes (72, 77). This differential trafficking may allow the multiple CD1 isoforms to sample antigens from distinct compartments along the endosomal pathway (19, 48, 62). The molecular basis for these distinct intracellular trafficking routes is largely accounted for by short endosomal sorting motifs in the cytoplasmic tails of the CD1 isoforms that serve as binding sites for adapter proteins (16, 24, 48, 72). In addition to distinct sorting characteristics, different structural features of the $\alpha 1$ and $\alpha 2$ antigen binding domains among the CD1 isoforms permit binding of

lipids with specific physical properties such as the different lengths of the lipid tails (27). Thus, the different CD1 isoforms may have evolved antigen binding domains adapted for binding different classes of lipids in addition to having cytoplasmic tails that impart the capacity to sample these antigens from a broad range of intracellular compartments.

EFFECTOR FUNCTIONS OF CD1-RESTRICTED T CELLS

The group 1 CD1-restricted T-cell lines described thus far include examples belonging to all of the major phenotypic T-cell subsets, including $CD4^- CD8^- \alpha\beta TCR^+$, $CD4^+ CD8^- \alpha\beta TCR^+$, $CD4^- CD8^+ \alpha\beta TCR^+$, and $\gamma\delta TCR^+$ T cells (6, 26, 55, 56, 61). Examples of CD1-restricted T-cell lines specific for mycobacterial lipid antigens have been found for each of the group 1 CD1 (CD1a, CD1b, and CD1c) isoforms (3, 4, 49, 61, 64). Functionally, the CD1-restricted T cells have characteristics consistent with a proinflammatory phenotype, a critical feature for proper control of M. tuberculosis and other intracellular infections (Fig. 5). For example, the M. tuberculosis-specific CD1-restricted T cells all express high levels of gamma interferon (IFN-γ) and have cytolytic activity, including the capacity to lyse infected cells. In addition, some subsets of CD1-restricted T cells, including the $CD4^+$, $CD8^+$, and $\gamma\delta^+$ T-cell subsets, express high levels of the antimicrobial peptide granulysin (28, 54, 68–70). These data demonstrate that CD1-restricted T cells have important effector functions including cytokine secretion, cytolytic activity, and the capacity to directly kill intracellular M. tuberculosis. Thus, the CD1-restricted T cells have several antimicrobial effector functions that may contribute to the host immune response to M. tuberculosis infection.

The data gathered thus far indicate that the group 1 CD1 isoforms (CD1a, CD1b, and CD1c) are largely involved in foreign antigen presentation while CD1d-restricted T cells serve a more immunomodulatory function. While this functional dichotomy has been based on strong data for both CD1 groups, recent evidence suggests that the picture is more complex than first appreciated. While the group 1 CD1-restricted T cells specific for mycobacterial lipid antigens share many features with MHC-restricted effector T cells, the long-standing phenomenon of self-reactivity in this population has only begun to be addressed (80, 81). Vincent et al. have recently shown that self-reactive group 1 CD1-restricted T cells can potentiate DC maturation and induce their production of interleukin-12 (IL-12), thus potentially influencing the subsequent adaptive immune response to infection

T Cell Adaptive Immunity

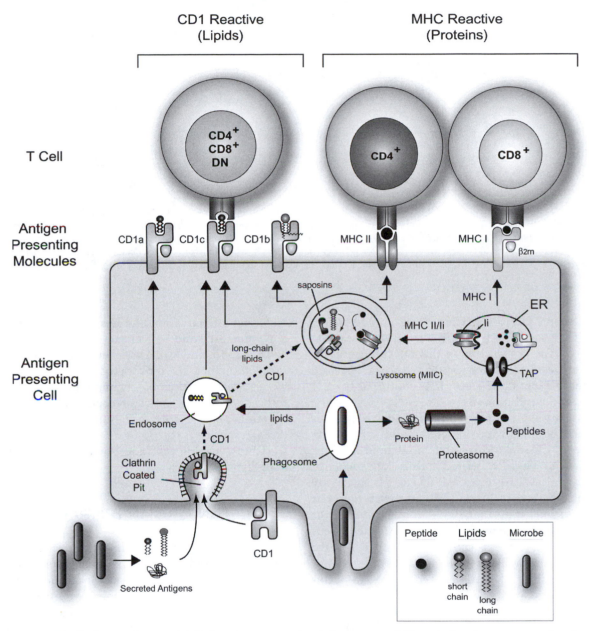

Figure 4. T-cell adaptive immunity. Multiple antigen presentation pathways are available to the host immune system for stimulation of T cells. A model antigen-presenting cell, such as a DC, is able to take up pathogens or pathogen-derived molecules from the surrounding extracellular environment. Live organisms are able to prevent maturation of the phagosome and hence prevent interaction with lysosomes and subsequent killing. The bacilli may survive and grow within the phagosome environment and thus evade immune surveillance. Some evidence exists for secretion of *M. tuberculosis* proteins into the cytosol, where they could be processed for presentation by MHC I. Lipid antigens with different structures may partition into different intracellular compartments. For example, short-chain lipids may traffic to recycling endosomes, where they would be accessible to CD1a, while long-chain lipids may traffic to lysosomes for loading and presentation by CD1b. Dashed lines represent the main-line sequence of endosomal maturation. Lipids may be transported out of the phagosome containing live organisms to then enter the antigen presentation pathway for CD1 and MHC II. Likewise, secreted antigens or lipids shed from extracellular bacteria are taken up by endocytosis and enter the endosomal network. Each of the CD1 molecules traffics through the endocytic system in a unique pattern. The CD1a isoform samples recycling endosomes, while CD1b samples late endosomes and lysosomes. The CD1c isoform samples both of these compartments. Together, the CD1 antigen presentation system is able to survey most of the intracellular environment for potential antigenic lipid molecules and to transport these to the cell surface for T-cell recognition.

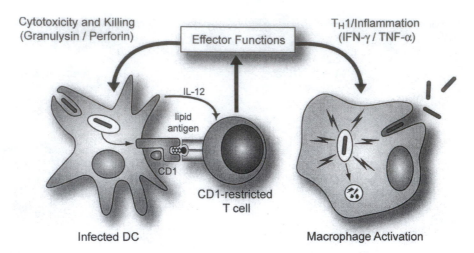

Figure 5. Effector functions of CD1-restricted T cells. T cells reactive to lipids presented by CD1 on the cell surface secrete high levels of proinflammatory cytokines including IFN-γ and tumor necrosis factor alpha (TNF-α), both critical for containment of *M. tuberculosis* infections and granuloma formation. Furthermore, activation of macrophages increases the killing of ingested bacilli. The CD1-restricted T cells release perforin and granulysin, which have direct bactericidal effects on *M. tuberculosis*. The CD1-restricted T cells are also cytolytic and have the capacity to kill infected host cells in a CD1-dependent manner.

(81). Group 2 CD1d-restricted T cells could also mediate IL-12 secretion but only after antigen stimulation (81). The in vivo role of this novel function for CD1-restricted T cells remains to be shown, but these data suggest that these T cells may contribute to early events during infection (81).

In contrast to the array of mycobacterial lipids that have been shown to be presented by the CD1a, CD1b, or CD1c isoforms, bacterial lipid antigens presented by CD1d-restricted T cells have remained elusive while CD1d-restricted T cells that recognize self-lipids have been found (33). However, there are now data indicating that PIM4, an *M. tuberculosis* phospholipid, is recognized by CD1d-restricted T cells (S. Kaufmann, personal communication). This is the first demonstration of a foreign bacterial lipid antigen presented by CD1d. However, the extent of this type of foreign lipid reactivity by the group 2 CD1d-restricted T cell subset has not been assessed. Recent in vitro data obtained by Brigl and coworkers showed that CD1d-restricted T cells potently produced IFN-γ when exposed to IL-12 (8). This cytokine production requires the recognition of CD1d-presented self-lipids but not exogenous microbial antigens. These data suggest a model in which CD1d-restricted T cells become activated in response to self-lipids presented by CD1d in combination with IL-12 production in response to signals of a live infection, possibly through Toll-like receptors (Fig. 5). However, this model does not formally exclude the possibility that CD1d can present foreign antigens to T cells in vivo.

Overall, the CD1d-restricted T cells have been implicated in a range of immunological phenomena including inflammation and host defense, as well as autoimmunity and cancer (reviewed in references 7, 18, 32, 46, and 80). These data support the initial speculation that CD1d-restricted T cells have evolved to carry out a predominantly immunoregulatory role rather than foreign antigen recognition and that this function plays a role in a number of infectious-disease models (18, 35, 66). However, data on CD1d-restricted T cells and human tuberculosis remain limited.

CD1 AND HUMAN TUBERCULOSIS

CD1-restricted T-cell lines that recognize mycobacterial lipid antigens examined thus far have been derived from peripheral blood mononuclear cells of normal donors with unknown exposure histories. More recently, several studies have found evidence for CD1-restricted T-cell responses linked to exposure to *M. tuberculosis* (29, 50, 79). To examine the role of CD1-restricted T-cells in tuberculosis, Moody et al. examined a set of healthy people who recently had a conversion of their skin test to purified protein derivative (PPD) because of contact with patients with active pulmonary tuberculosis (50). In these studies, proliferative responses from peripheral blood mononuclear cells to the known lipid antigen mannosyl-β₁-phosphodolichol (Fig. 3) were assessed and compared to those for matched PPD-negative subjects. A significant increase in CD1c-restricted T-cell proliferation was observed in the tuberculosis group compared to the PPD-negative control group.

Additional studies by Ulrichs et al. have demonstrated the presence of CD1-restricted T-cell responses to lipid antigen in response to *M. tuberculosis* infection. In these studies, asymptomatic patients with a recent PPD conversion showed significant CD1-dependent T-cell responses to a lipid extract of *M. tuberculosis* and to purified glucose monomycolate (79). Interestingly, patients with clinically active pulmonary tuberculosis showed no significant response to lipid antigens or whole bacterial sonicates. However, T-cell responses were detected 2 weeks after initiation of antituberculosis chemotherapy (79). These data are consistent with results of previous studies that found that patients with active pulmonary tuberculosis exhibit a generalized transforming growth factor β-mediated suppression of T-cell responses, in contrast to asymptomatic PPD-positive household contacts (38). Taken together, the results of these studies provide the first evidence that microbial lipid antigens are presented by CD1 in vivo and that CD1-restricted lipid antigen-specific T cells are generated during the natural course of *M. tuberculosis* infection in humans.

The persistence of CD1-restricted T-cell responses to mycobacterial lipid antigens, suggesting T-cell memory, has also been demonstrated. In a recent study, Kawashima et al. found that healthy adults who had been BCG vaccinated and were PPD positive had detectable CD1-restricted T-cell responses compared to matched PPD-negative controls (45). Interestingly, the CD1-restricted T cells were predominantly of the $CD8^+$ $\alpha\beta TCR^+$ phenotype. This is in contrast to the data obtained from patients with active tuberculosis, for whom the predominant CD1-restricted T cells were $CD4^+$ (79). Further analysis of this phenotypic difference may provide insights into the nature of the T-cell response during the acute phase of a natural tuberculosis infection, compared to the long-term T-cell memory responses generated by BCG vaccination. Together, these data clearly document the presence of CD1-restricted T cells in humans exposed to live mycobacteria, either by natural infection with *M. tuberculosis* or by BCG vaccination. Further studies are needed to define the relative contribution of CD1-restricted T cells to the overall cell-mediated immune response following *M. tuberculosis* infection.

CD1 AND ANIMAL MODELS OF TUBERCULOSIS

Small-animal models of tuberculosis continue to provide a useful tool for examining the role of CD1 in the immune response to *M. tuberculosis* infection. These models have also been used to evaluate the potential application of lipid antigens as vaccine components. It is essential to note that the human CD1-restricted T cells specific for mycobacterial lipid antigens are restricted to one of the group 1 CD1 isoforms (either CD1a, CD1b, or CD1c). Most of the animal species examined thus far have CD1 genes that vary in both number and isoform type between species. These factors must be appreciated when selecting an appropriate animal model. Guinea pigs were developed as an alternative CD1 animal model system because they were found to express homologs of the human group 1 CD1 isoforms, including CD1b and CD1c (20, 37). Using this model, Hiromatsu et al. have shown that immunization of guinea pigs with lipid antigens from *M. tuberculosis* is capable of inducing CD1-restricted T-cell recall responses in vivo (36). Furthermore, lipid-immunized guinea pigs challenged with virulent *M. tuberculosis* via aerosol administration exhibit reduced pulmonary pathology compared to negative control animals (21). These data are consistent with the observations from the studies of human tuberculosis patients, cited above, that point to the capacity of CD1-restricted T cells to be primed and persist in vivo. It is worth noting that one of the potential advantages of incorporating lipid antigens into a subunit vaccine is the virtual absence of polymorphisms of the CD1 genes between individuals in the human population (34). This overcomes one of the inherent problems of protein-only vaccines that rely on the highly polymorphic host MHC. Therefore, the potential exists for lipid antigens to be incorporated into subunit vaccines for tuberculosis and other infectious diseases. These data also support the development of live-attenuated vaccines that retain the native lipid components of the pathogen.

The CD1d-restricted T cells influence the Th1/Th2 phenotypic profile of T cells in some infectious-disease models (reviewed in references 18, 32, and 66). Therefore, although mycobacterial lipids presented by CD1d have not been described, it was of interest to examine the potential role of CD1d in tuberculosis. Because mice have only the single CD1d isoform, they are useful for evaluating the role of CD1d-restricted cells in tuberculosis and other disease models but not for evaluating the group 1 CD1 isoforms typically associated with mycobacterial lipid antigen presentation. In data from several laboratories, control of bacterial replication and survival were not impaired in CD1D knockout mice infected with virulent *M. tuberculosis* by either the intravenous or aerosol route (5, 23, 67). These data would suggest that this subset of T cells either is not critical or is compensated for during infection in the murine model of tuberculosis.

While CD1D knockout mice did not exhibit overt differences in morbidity or mortality from those of wild-type mice following *M. tuberculosis* infection, pharmacologic stimulation of CD1d-restricted T cells during infection was able to alter the course of disease. The lipid α-galactosylceramide (αGC) is derived from a marine sponge and, while not a physiological antigen in mammals, is a potent activator of CD1d-restricted T cells (Fig. 3) (44). Treatment of mice with αGC at the time of *M. tuberculosis* infection leads to improved survival of animals and reduced bacterial load in the lungs but not the spleen (17). Therefore, while elimination of the CD1d antigen presentation pathway in knockout mice does not alter the outcome of *M. tuberculosis* infection, the pharmacologic stimulation of CD1d-restricted T cells at the time of infection can provide a beneficial effect on the clinical outcome of disease. Similar results of αGC treatment have been found in other infectious-disease models, suggesting a common mechanism of action, although this has not been clearly established (reviewed in reference 18). One possible explanation may be the rapid burst of proinflammatory cytokines (e.g., IFN-γ) that occurs following the activation of CD1d-restricted T cells by αGC administration to mice (15, 53). This early cytokine stimulation may then serve to modulate the subsequent adaptive immune response or trigger other accessory cells, such as NK cells, necessary for optimal immune responses (71). Further study of this phenomenon should provide insight into the mechanism of protection induced by CD1d-restricted T-cell stimulation in tuberculosis.

CONCLUSION

M. tuberculosis bacilli possess one of the more unusual cell walls in the bacterial kingdom, with many of the lipid molecules being unique to this genus. Therefore, it should not be a surprise that the host immune system has evolved a mechanism to exploit the distinctive molecular signatures of this pathogen. In the context of the immune system, it is likely that CD1-restricted T cells represent two separate components along the spectrum of the host immune responses. The group 1 CD1 antigen presentation system has many of the features typically associated with adaptive immunity, including specific foreign antigen recognition by diverse T cells with the capacity for immunological memory. On the other hand, the group 2 CD1d-restricted T cells appear to recognize self-lipids and play a role in the early immune response, perhaps serving as a bridge between the immediate innate immune response and the delayed adaptive immune responses. However, it is likely that future studies will reveal overlaps between these dual roles. Important questions that remain to

be addressed include a better understanding of the precise role of lipid antigens and CD1 in the natural history of human tuberculosis. A more thorough understanding of how CD1 antigen presentation fits into the overall host immune response to infection may lead to novel interventional therapies and improved vaccine formulations for tuberculosis and other infectious diseases.

Acknowledgments. We thank Stephan Gadola and Vincenzo Cerundolo for kindly supplying the CD1b crystal structure figures, Branch Moody for supplying the lipid structure files, and Jenny Gumperz for assistance with Fig. 5. We also thank Manfred Brigl, Alissa Chackerian, Sam Behar, John Higgins, and Carme Roura-Mir for critical review of the manuscript.

REFERENCES

1. Angenieux, C., J. Salamero, D. Fricker, J. P. Cazenave, B. Goud, D. Hanau, and H. de La Salle. 2000. Characterization of CD1e, a third type of CD1 molecule expressed in dendritic cells. *J. Biol. Chem.* 275:37757–37764.
2. Beatty, W. L., E. R. Rhoades, H. J. Ullrich, D. Chatterjee, J. E. Heuser, and D. G. Russell. 2000. Trafficking and release of mycobacterial lipids from infected macrophages. *Traffic* 1:235–247.
3. Beckman, E. M., A. Melian, S. M. Behar, P. A. Sieling, D. Chatterjee, S. T. Furlong, R. Matsumoto, J. P. Rosat, R. L. Modlin, and S. A. Porcelli. 1996. CD1c restricts responses of mycobacteria-specific T cells. Evidence for antigen presentation by a second member of the human CD1 family. *J. Immunol.* 157:2795–2803.
4. Beckman, E. M., S. A. Porcelli, C. T. Morita, S. M. Behar, S. T. Furlong, and M. B. Brenner. 1994. Recognition of a lipid antigen by CD1-restricted αβ+ T cells. *Nature* 372:691–694.
5. Behar, S. M., C. C. Dascher, M. J. Grusby, C. R. Wang, and M. B. Brenner. 1999. Susceptibility of mice deficient in CD1D or TAP1 to infection with *Mycobacterium tuberculosis*. *J. Exp. Med.* 189:1973–1980.
6. Bendelac, A., R. D. Hunziker, and O. Lantz. 1996. Increased interleukin 4 and immunoglobulin E production in transgenic mice overexpressing NK1 T cells. *J. Exp. Med.* 184:1285–1293.
7. Brigl, M., and M. B. Brenner. 2003. CD1: antigen presentation and T cell function. *Annu. Rev. Immunol.* 22:817–890.
8. Brigl, M., L. Bry, S. C. Kent, J. E. Gumperz, and M. B. Brenner. 2003. Mechanism of CD1d-restricted natural killer T cell activation during microbial infection. *Nat. Immunol.* 4:1230–1237.
9. Briken, V., R. M. Jackman, S. Dasgupta, S. Hoening, and S. A. Porcelli. 2002. Intracellular trafficking pathway of newly synthesized CD1b molecules. *EMBO. J.* 21:825–834.
10. Briken, V., R. M. Jackman, G. F. Watts, R. A. Rogers, and S. A. Porcelli. 2000. Human CD1b and CD1c isoforms survey different intracellular compartments for the presentation of microbial lipid antigens. *J. Exp. Med.* 192:281–288.
11. Calabi, F., and A. Bradbury. 1991. The CD1 system. *Tissue Antigens* 37:1–9.
12. Calabi, F., J. M. Jarvis, L. Martin, and C. Milstein. 1989. Two classes of CD1 genes. *Eur. J. Immunol.* 19:285–292.
13. Calabi, F., and C. Milstein. 1986. A novel family of human major histocompatibility complex-related genes not mapping to chromosome 6. *Nature* 323:540–543.
14. Cao, X., M. Sugita, N. Van Der Wel, J. Lai, R. A. Rogers, P. J. Peters, and M. B. Brenner. 2002. CD1 molecules efficiently

present antigen in immature dendritic cells and traffic independently of MHC class II during dendritic cell maturation. *J. Immunol.* **169:**4770–4777.

15. Carnaud, C., D. Lee, O. Donnars, S. H. Park, A. Beavis, Y. Koezuka, and A. Bendelac. 1999. Cutting edge: Cross-talk between cells of the innate immune system: NKT cells rapidly activate NK cells. *J. Immunol.* **163:**4647–4650.

16. Cernadas, M., M. Sugita, N. Van Der Wel, X. Cao, J. E. Gumperz, S. Maltsev, G. S. Besra, S. M. Behar, P. J. Peters, and M. B. Brenner. 2003. Lysosomal localization of murine CD1d mediated by AP-3 is necessary for NK T cell development. *J. Immunol.* **171:**4149–4155.

17. Chackerian, A., J. Alt, V. Perera, and S. M. Behar. 2002. Activation of NKT cells protects mice from tuberculosis. *Infect. Immun.* **70:**6302–6309.

18. Dascher, C. C., and M. B. Brenner. 2003. CD1 antigen presentation and infectious disease, p. 164–182. *In* H. Herwald (ed.), *Host Response Mechanisms in Infectious Disease*, vol. 10. S. Karger, Basel, Switzerland.

19. Dascher, C. C., and M. B. Brenner. 2003. Evolutionary constraints on CD1 structure: insights from comaprative genomic analysis. *Trends Immunol.* **24:**412–418.

20. Dascher, C. C., K. Hiromatsu, J. W. Naylor, P. P. Brauer, K. A. Brown, J. R. Storey, S. M. Behar, E. S. Kawasaki, S. A. Porcelli, M. B. Brenner, and K. P. LeClair. 1999. Conservation of a CD1 multigene family in the guinea pig. *J. Immunol.* **163:**5478–5488.

21. Dascher, C. C., K. Hiromatsu, X. Xiong, C. M. Morehouse, G. F. Watts, G. Liu, D. N. McMurray, K. P. LeClair, S. Porcelli, and M. B. Brenner. 2003. Immunization with a mycobacterial lipid vaccine improves pulmonary pathology in the guinea pig model of tuberculosis. *Int. Immunol.* **15:**915–925.

22. Ding, Y. H., K. J. Smith, D. N. Garboczi, U. Utz, W. E. Biddison, and D. C. Wiley. 1998. Two human T cell receptors bind in a similar diagonal mode to the HLA-A2/Tax peptide complex using different TCR amino acids. *Immunity* **8:**403–411.

23. D'Souza, C. D., A. M. Cooper, A. A. Frank, S. Ehlers, J. Turner, A. Bendelac, and I. M. Orme. 2000. A novel nonclassic β$_2$-microglobulin-restricted mechanism influencing early lymphocyte accumulation and subsequent resistance to tuberculosis in the lung. *Am. J. Respir. Cell Mol. Biol.* **23:**188–193.

24. Elewaut, D., A. P. Lawton, N. A. Nagarajan, E. Maverakis, A. Khurana, S. Honing, C. A. Benedict, E. Sercarz, O. Bakke, M. Kronenberg, and T. I. Prigozy. 2003. The adaptor protein AP-3 is required for CD1d-mediated antigen presentation of glycosphingolipids and development of Vα14i NKT cells. *J. Exp. Med.* **198:**1133–1146.

25. Exley, M., J. Garcia, S. B. Wilson, F. Spada, D. Gerdes, S. M. Tahir, K. T. Patton, R. S. Blumberg, S. Porcelli, A. Chott, and S. P. Balk. 2000. CD1d structure and regulation on human thymocytes, peripheral blood T cells, B cells and monocytes. *Immunology* **100:**37–47.

26. Faure, F., S. Jitsukawa, C. Miossec, and T. Hercend. 1990. CD1c as a target recognition structure for human T lymphocytes: analysis with peripheral blood gamma/delta cells. *Eur. J. Immunol.* **20:**703–706.

27. Gadola, S. D., N. R. Zaccai, K. Harlos, D. Shepherd, J. C. Castro-Palomino, G. Ritter, R. R. Schmidt, E. Y. Jones, and V. Cerundolo. 2002. Structure of human CD1b with bound ligands at 2.3 Å, a maze for alkyl chains. *Nat. Immunol.* **3:**721–726.

28. Gansert, J. L., V. Kiessler, M. Engele, F. Wittke, M. Rollinghoff, A. M. Krensky, S. A. Porcelli, R. L. Modlin, and S. Stenger. 2003. Human NKT cells express granulysin and exhibit antimycobacterial activity. *J. Immunol.* **170:**3154–3161.

29. Gilleron, M., S. Stenger, Z. Mazorra, F. Wittke, S. Mariotti, G. Bohmer, J. Prandi, L. Mori, G. Puzo, and G. De Libero. 2004. Diacylated sulfoglycolipids are novel mycobacterial antigens stimulating CD1-restricted T cells during infection with *Mycobacterium tuberculosis. J. Exp. Med.* **199:**649–659.

30. Grant, E. P., E. M. Beckman, S. M. Behar, M. Degano, D. Frederique, G. S. Besra, I. A. Wilson, S. A. Porcelli, S. T. Furlong, and M. B. Brenner. 2002. Fine specificity of TCR complementarity-determining region residues and lipid antigen hydrophilic moieties in the recognition of a CD1–lipid complex. *J. Immunol.* **168:**3933–3940.

31. Grant, E. P., M. Degano, J. P. Rosat, S. Stenger, R. L. Modlin, I. A. Wilson, S. A. Porcelli, and M. B. Brenner. 1999. Molecular recognition of lipid antigens by T cell receptors. *J. Exp. Med.* **189:**195–205.

32. Gumperz, J. E., and M. B. Brenner. 2001. CD-specific T cells in microbial immunity. *Curr. Opin. Immunol.* **13:**471–478.

33. Gumperz, J. E., C. Roy, A. Makowska, D. Lum, M. Sugita, T. Podrebarac, Y. Koezuka, S. A. Porcelli, S. Cardell, M. B. Brenner, and S. M. Behar. 2000. Murine CD1d-restricted T cell recognition of cellular lipids. *Immunity* **12:**211–221.

34. Han, M., L. I. Hannick, M. DiBrino, and M. A. Robinson. 1999. Polymorphism of human CD1 genes. *Tissue Antigens* **54:**122–127.

35. Hansen, D. S., M. A. Siomos, L. Buckingham, A. A. Scalzo, and L. Schofield. 2003. Regulation of murine cerebral malaria pathogenesis by CD1d-restricted NKT cells and the natural killer complex. *Immunity* **18:**391–402.

36. Hiromatsu, K., C. C. Dascher, K. P. LeClair, M. Sugita, S. T. Furlong, M. B. Brenner, and S. A. Porcelli. 2002. Induction of CD1-restricted immune responses in guinea pigs by immunization with mycobacterial lipid antigens. *J. Immunol.* **169:**330–339.

37. Hiromatsu, K., C. C. Dascher, M. Sugita, C. Gingrich-Baker, S. M. Behar, K. P. LeClair, M. B. Brenner, and S. A. Porcelli. 2002. Characterization of guinea-pig group 1 CD1 proteins. *Immunology* **106:**159–172.

38. Hirsch, C. S., R. Hussain, Z. Toossi, G. Dawood, F. Shahid, and J. J. Ellner. 1996. Cross-modulation by transforming growth factor beta in human tuberculosis: suppression of antigen-driven blastogenesis and interferon gamma production. *Proc. Natl. Acad. Sci. USA* **93:**3193–3198.

39. Hmama, Z., R. Gabathuler, W. A. Jefferies, G. de Jong, and N. E. Reiner. 1998. Attenuation of HLA-DR expression by mononuclear phagocytes infected with *Mycobacterium tuberculosis* is related to intracellular sequestration of immature class II heterodimers. *J. Immunol.* **161:**4882–4893.

40. Hughes, A. L. 1991. Evolutionary origin and diversification of the mammalian CD1 antigen genes. *Mol. Biol. Evol.* **8:**185–201.

41. Jackman, R. M., S. Stenger, A. Lee, D. B. Moody, R. A. Rogers, K. R. Niazi, M. Sugita, R. L. Modlin, P. J. Peters, and S. A. Porcelli. 1998. The tyrosine-containing cytoplasmic tail of CD1b is essential for its efficient presentation of bacterial lipid antigens. *Immunity* **8:**341–351.

42. Jones, D. C., C. M. Gelder, T. Ahmad, I. A. Campbell, M. C. Barnardo, K. I. Welsh, S. E. Marshall, and M. Bunce. 2001. CD1 genotyping of patients with *Mycobacterium malmoense* pulmonary disease. *Tissue Antigens* **58:**19–23.

43. Kang, S. J., and P. Cresswell. 2002. Calnexin, calreticulin, and ERp57 cooperate in disulfide bond formation in human CD1d heavy chain. *J. Biol. Chem.* **277:**44838–44844.

44. Kawano, T., J. Cui, Y. Koezuka, I. Toura, Y. Kaneko, K. Motoki, H. Ueno, R. Nakagawa, H. Sato, E. Kondo, H. Koseki, and M. Taniguchi. 1997. CD1d-restricted and TCR-mediated activation of vα14 NKT cells by glycosylceramides. *Science* **278:**1626–1629.

45. Kawashima, T., Y. Norose, Y. Watanabe, Y. Enomoto, H. Narazaki, E. Watari, S. Tanaka, H. Takahashi, I. Yano, M. B. Brenner, and M. Sugita. 2003. Cutting edge: Major CD8 T cell response to live bacillus Calmette-Guérin is mediated by CD1 molecules. *J. Immunol.* **170:**5345–5348.

46. Kronenberg, M., and L. Gapin. 2002. The unconventional lifestyle of NKT cells. *Nat. Rev. Immunol.* **2:**557–568.

47. Moody, D. B., V. Briken, T. Y. Cheng, C. Roura-Mir, M. R. Guy, D. H. Geho, M. L. Tykocinski, G. S. Besra, and S. A. Porcelli. 2002. Lipid length controls antigen entry into endosomal and nonendosomal pathways for CD1b presentation. *Nat. Immunol.* **3:**435–442.

48. Moody, D. B., and S. A. Porcelli. 2003. Intracellular pathways of CD1 antigen presentation. *Nat. Rev. Immunol.* **3:**11–22.

49. Moody, D. B., B. B. Reinhold, M. R. Guy, E. M. Beckman, D. E. Frederique, S. T. Furlong, S. Ye, V. N. Reinhold, P. A. Sieling, R. L. Modlin, G. S. Besra, and S. A. Porcelli. 1997. Structural requirements for glycolipid antigen recognition by CD1b-restricted T cells. *Science* **278:**283–286.

50. Moody, D. B., T. Ulrichs, W. Muhlecker, D. C. Young, S. S. Gurcha, E. Grant, J. P. Rosat, M. B. Brenner, C. E. Costello, G. S. Besra, and S. A. Porcelli. 2000. CD1c-mediated T-cell recognition of isoprenoid glycolipids in *Mycobacterium tuberculosis* infection. *Nature* **404:**884–888.

51. Moody, D. B., D. C. Young, T. Y. Cheng, J. P. Rosat, C. Roura-Mir, P. B. O'Connor, D. M. Zajonc, A. Walz, M. J. Miller, S. B. Levery, I. A. Wilson, C. E. Costelo, M. B. Brenner. 2004. T-cell activation by lipopeptide antigens. *Science* **303:**527–531.

52. Mukherjee, S., T. T. Soe, and F. R. Maxfield. 1999. Endocytic sorting of lipid analogues differing solely in the chemistry of their hydrophobic tails. *J. Cell Biol.* **144:**1271–1284.

53. Nieuwenhuis, E. E., T. Matsumoto, M. Exley, R. A. Schleipman, J. Glickman, D. T. Bailey, N. Corazza, S. P. Colgan, A. B. Onderdonk, and R. S. Blumberg. 2002. CD1d-dependent macrophage-mediated clearance of *Pseudomonas aeruginosa* from lung. *Nat. Med.* **8:**588–593.

54. Ochoa, M. T., S. Stenger, P. A. Sieling, S. Thoma-Uszynski, S. Sabet, S. Cho, A. M. Krensky, M. Rollinghoff, E. Nunes Sarno, A. E. Burdick, T. H. Rea, and R. L. Modlin. 2001. T-cell release of granulysin contributes to host defense in leprosy. *Nat. Med.* **7:**174–179.

55. Porcelli, S., M. B. Brenner, J. L. Greenstein, S. P. Balk, C. Terhorst, and P. A. Bleicher. 1989. Recognition of cluster of differentiation 1 antigens by human CD4⁻CD8⁻ cytolytic T lymphocytes. *Nature* **341:**447–450.

56. Porcelli, S., C. T. Morita, and M. B. Brenner. 1992. CD1b restricts the response of human CD4⁻8⁻ T lymphocytes to a microbial antigen. *Nature* **360:**593–597.

57. Porcelli, S. A. 1995. The CD1 family: a third lineage of antigen-presenting molecules. *Adv. Immunol.* **59:**1–98.

58. Porcelli, S. A., and M. B. Brenner. 1997. Antigen presentation: mixing oil and water. *Curr. Biol.* **7:**R508–R511.

59. Prigozy, T. I., P. A. Sieling, D. Clemens, P. L. Stewart, S. M. Behar, S. A. Porcelli, M. B. Brenner, R. L. Modlin, and M. Kronenberg. 1997. The mannose receptor delivers lipoglycan antigens to endosomes for presentation to T cells by CD1b molecules. *Immunity* **6:**187–197.

60. Rhoades, E., F. Hsu, J. B. Torrelles, J. Turk, D. Chatterjee, and D. G. Russell. 2003. Identification and macrophage-activating activity of glycolipids released from intracellular *Mycobacterium bovis* BCG. *Mol. Microbiol.* **48:**875–888.

61. Rosat, J. P., E. P. Grant, E. M. Beckman, C. C. Dascher, P. A. Sieling, D. Frederique, R. L. Modlin, S. A. Porcelli, S. T. Furlong, and M. B. Brenner. 1999. CD1-restricted microbial lipid antigen-specific recognition found in the CD8⁺ αβ T cell pool. *J. Immunol.* **162:**366–371.

62. Roura-Mir, C., and D. B. Moody. 2003. Sorting out self and microbial lipid antigens for CD1. *Microbes Infect.* **5:**1137–1148.

63. Shamshiev, A., A. Donda, I. Carena, L. Mori, L. Kappos, and G. De Libero. 1999. Self glycolipids as T-cell autoantigens. *Eur. J. Immunol.* **29:**1667–1675.

64. Sieling, P. A., D. Chatterjee, S. A. Porcelli, T. I. Prigozy, R. J. Mazzaccaro, T. Soriano, B. R. Bloom, M. B. Brenner, M. Kronenberg, P. J. Brennan, and R. L. Modlin. 1995. CD1-restricted T cell recognition of microbial lipoglycan antigens. *Science* **269:**227–230.

65. Sieling, P. A., D. Jullien, M. Dahlem, T. F. Tedder, T. H. Rea, R. L. Modlin, and S. A. Porcelli. 1999. CD1 expression by dendritic cells in human leprosy lesions: correlation with effective host immunity. *J. Immunol.* **162:**1851–1588.

66. Skold, M., and S. M. Behar. 2003. Role of CD1d-restricted NKT cells in microbial immunity. *Infect. Immun.* **71:**5447–5455.

67. Sousa, A. O., R. J. Mazzaccaro, R. G. Russell, F. K. Lee, O. C. Turner, S. Hong, L. Van Kaer, and B. R. Bloom. 2000. Relative contributions of distinct MHC class I-dependent cell populations in protection to tuberculosis infection in mice. *Proc. Natl. Acad. Sci. USA* **97:**4204–4208.

68. Spada, F. M., E. P. Grant, P. J. Peters, M. Sugita, A. Melian, D. S. Leslie, H. K. Lee, E. van Donselaar, D. A. Hanson, A. M. Krensky, O. Majdic, S. A. Porcelli, C. T. Morita, and M. B. Brenner. 2000. Self-recognition of CD1 by γ/δ T cells: implications for innate immunity. *J. Exp. Med.* **191:**937–948.

69. Stenger, S., D. A. Hanson, R. Teitelbaum, P. Dewan, K. R. Niazi, C. J. Froelich, T. Ganz, S. Thoma-Uszynski, A. Melian, C. Bogdan, S. A. Porcelli, B. R. Bloom, A. M. Krensky, and R. L. Modlin. 1998. An antimicrobial activity of cytolytic T cells mediated by granulysin. *Science* **282:**121–125.

70. Stenger, S., R. J. Mazzaccaro, K. Uyemura, S. Cho, P. F. Barnes, J. P. Rosat, A. Sette, M. B. Brenner, S. A. Porcelli, B. R. Bloom, and R. L. Modlin. 1997. Differential effects of cytolytic T cell subsets on intracellular infection. *Science* **276:**1684–1687.

71. Stetson, D. B., M. Morhrs, R. L. Reinhardt, J. L. Baron, Z. Wang, L. Gapin, M. Kronenberg, and R. M. Locksley. 2003. Costitutive cytokine mRNAs mark natural killer (NK) and NK T cells poised for rapid effector functrion. *J. Exp. Med.* **198:**1069–1076.

72. Sugita, M., X. Cao, G. F. Watts, R. A. Rogers, J. S. Bonifacino, and M. B. Brenner. 2002. Failure of trafficking and antigen presentation by CD1 in AP-3-deficient cells. *Immunity* **16:**697–706.

73. Sugita, M., E. P. Grant, E. van Donselaar, V. W. Hsu, R. A. Rogers, P. J. Peters, and M. B. Brenner. 1999. Separate pathways for antigen presentation by CD1 molecules. *Immunity* **11:**743–752.

74. Sugita, M., R. M. Jackman, E. van Donselaar, S. M. Behar, R. A. Rogers, P. J. Peters, M. B. Brenner, and S. A. Porcelli. 1996. Cytoplasmic tail-dependent localization of CD1b antigen-presenting molecules to MIICs. *Science* **273:**349–352.

75. Sugita, M., P. J. Peters, and M. B. Brenner. 2000. Pathways for lipid antigen presentation by CD1 molecules: nowhere for intracellular pathogens to hide. *Traffic* **1:**295–300.

76. Sugita, M., S. A. Porcelli, and M. B. Brenner. 1997. Assembly and retention of CD1b heavy chains in the endoplasmic reticulum. *J. Immunol.* **159:**2358–2365.

77. Sugita, M., N. van Der Wel, R. A. Rogers, P. J. Peters, and M. B. Brenner. 2000. CD1c molecules broadly survey the endocytic system. *Proc. Natl. Acad. Sci. USA* **97:**8445–8450.

78. Uehira, K., R. Amakawa, T. Ito, K. Tajima, S. Naitoh, Y. Ozaki, T. Shimizu, K. Yamaguchi, Y. Uemura, H. Kitajima, S. Yonezu, and S. Fukuhara. 2002. Dendritic cells are decreased in blood and accumulated in granuloma in tuberculosis. *Clin. Immunol.* **105:**296–303.

79. Ulrichs, T., D. B. Moody, E. Grant, S. H. Kaufmann, and S. Porcelli. 2003. T-cell responses to CD1–presented lipid antigens in humans with *Mycobacterium tuberculosis* infection. *Infect. Immun.* **71:**3076–3087.

80. Vincent, M. S., J. E. Gumperz, and M. B. Brenner. 2003. Understanding the function of CD1-restricted T cells. *Nat. Immunol.* **4:**517–523.

81. Vincent, M. S., D. S. Leslie, J. E. Gumperz, X. Xiong, E. P. Grant, and M. B. Brenner. 2002. CD1-dependent dendritic cell instruction. *Nat. Immunol.* **3:**1163–1168.

82. Winau, F., V. Schwierzeck, R. Hurwitz, N. Remmel, P. A. Siel-ing, R. L. Modlin, S. A. Porcelli, V. Brinkmann, M. Sugita, K. Sandhoff, S. H. Kaufmann, and U. E. Schaible. 2004. Saposin C is required for lipid presentation by human CD1b. *Nat. Immunol.* **5:**169–174.

83. Zajonc, D. M., M. A. Elsliger, L. Teyton, and I. A. Wilson. 2003. Crystal structure of CD1a in complex with a sulfatide self antigen at a resolution of 2.15 Å. *Nat. Immunol.* **4:**808–815.

84. Zeng, Z., A. R. Castano, B. W. Segelke, E. A. Stura, P. A. Peterson, and I. A. Wilson. 1997. Crystal structure of mouse CD1: an MHC-like fold with a large hydrophobic binding groove. *Science* **277:**339–345.

85. Zhou, D., C. Cantu III, Y. Sagiv, N. Schrantz, A. B. Kulkarni, X. Qi, D. J. Mahuran, C. R. Morales, G. A. Grabowski, K. Benlagha, P. Savage, A. Bendelac, and L. Teyton. 2004. Editing of CD1d-bound lipid antigens by endosomal lipid transfer proteins. *Science* **303:**523–527.

Tuberculosis and the Tubercle Bacillus
Edited by Stewart T. Cole et al.
© 2005 ASM Press, Washington, D.C.

Chapter 31

Th1 and Th2 Cytokines in the Human Immune Response to Tuberculosis

PETER F. BARNES AND RAMAKRISHNA VANKAYALAPATI

T cells contribute to defense against infectious agents by producing specific patterns of cytokines, which can be broadly divided into Th1 cytokines, including gamma interferon (IFN-γ) and interleukin-2 (IL-2), and Th2 cytokines, including IL-4, IL-5, IL-10, and IL-13. Mononuclear phagocytes produce IL-12, IL-10, and IL-18, which strongly influence the T-cell cytokine response. IL-12 is a potent stimulus for T cells to secrete IFN-γ, whereas IL-10 inhibits the production of IL-12 and favors the development of cells that produce Th2 cytokines. IL-18 acts synergistically with IL-12 to enhance T-cell production of IFN-γ. However, in the absence of IL-12, IL-18 can induce Th2 responses by eliciting the production of IL-4, IL-5, and IL-13 by T cells and IL-13 by natural killer (NK) cells (16, 44).

Immune defenses against *Mycobacterium tuberculosis* are mediated primarily by T cells, and IFN-γ is essential for protective immunity. Mice with a targeted deletion of the IFN-γ gene are highly susceptible to tuberculosis, and patients with IL-12 deficiency or with defective receptors for IFN-γ or IL-12 experience severe infections with *M. bovis* BCG and other mycobacteria (1, 23). Although genetic defects that markedly limit the activity of IFN-γ clearly enhance susceptibility to mycobacterial disease, the contribution of defective Th1 cytokine production to development of tuberculosis in persons without these genetic defects is uncertain. In the past decade, a wealth of data has accumulated on the cytokine response in persons infected with *M. tuberculosis*. However, many results are conflicting, in part because ethical and logistical constraints do not permit manipulation of some critical experimental factors. We review these data below, present a hypothesis that reconciles most published findings, outline potential mechanisms for cytokine dysregulation in human tuberculosis, and speculate on the feasibility of modulating the cytokine response to improve the treatment of tuberculosis.

CYTOKINE RESPONSE AT THE SITE OF DISEASE

Investigators have studied cytokine production and mRNA expression in bronchoalveolar lavage fluid (2, 24, 29, 36) and in lung tissue (10) from patients with pulmonary tuberculosis, pleural fluid from those with tuberculous pleuritis (4, 42, 46), and lymph nodes from patients with tuberculous lymphadenitis (20). These studies demonstrate that the local inflammatory response is dominated by IFN-γ and the Th1 initiator cytokines IL-12 and IL-18, compared to findings from a variety of control groups, including persons with inactive tuberculosis, nontuberculous infections, and noninfectious inflammatory conditions. In contrast, increased amounts of IL-4 protein or mRNA were not detected in patients with tuberculosis (2, 4, 10, 20, 24, 36). IL-10 expression is enhanced at the site of disease in tuberculosis (4, 20, 30), but this is not a reliable marker of human Th2 cells, since T-cell clones from the lungs of tuberculosis patients produce both IFN-γ and IL-10, similar to other human Th1 cells (11).

Why does the prominent Th1 cytokine response at the site of disease not protect against the development of tuberculosis? One possibility is that macrophages fail to respond to IFN-γ, perhaps because *M. tuberculosis* inhibits signal transduction by IFN-γ in macrophages, preventing the downstream effects that eliminate mycobacteria (37). Alternatively, IFN-γ may be produced too late in the course of infection to prevent progressive disease. During the critical host-pathogen interactions in the early phases of infection, IFN-γ levels may be low in patients who

Peter F. Barnes • Center for Pulmonary and Infectious Disease Control, Department of Medicine, and Department of Microbiology and Immunology, The University of Texas Health Center at Tyler, Tyler, TX 75708. *Ramakrishna Vankayalapati* • Center for Pulmonary and Infectious Disease Control and Department of Microbiology and Immunology, The University of Texas Health Science Center at Tyler, Tyler, TX 75708.

subsequently develop tuberculosis whereas these levels may be elevated in persons who become healthy tuberculin reactors. Ethical and logistical considerations have precluded extensive investigation of the early local cytokine response to *M. tuberculosis* infection. Only one study evaluated bronchoalveolar lavage fluid cells from persons who were presumably recently infected with *M. tuberculosis* (tuberculin-positive healthy household contacts of persons with sputum smear-positive tuberculosis) and those who were probably infected in the remote past (healthy tuberculin reactors without recent exposure to tuberculosis). The frequency of cells producing IFN-γ in response to *M. tuberculosis* antigens was significantly higher in persons with recent infection, emphasizing that the cytokine response changes with time (29).

SYSTEMIC CYTOKINE RESPONSE

Studies of the systemic cytokine response can be divided into studies evaluating circulating cytokine levels or mRNA of unstimulated blood cells and those investigating cytokine production by blood cells stimulated with *M. tuberculosis* antigens in vitro.

Cytokine Production and mRNA Expression in Blood

Conflicting findings have been reported regarding the balance of Th1 and Th2 cytokines in the blood of tuberculosis patients. Four groups found that concentrations of IFN-γ were increased in tuberculosis patients compared to those in healthy contacts of these patients (8, 41, 43, 45). Others noted that peripheral blood mononuclear cells (PBMC) of tuberculosis patients had reduced expression of IFN-γ mRNA (32) and decreased expression of soluble lymphocyte activation gene 3 (19), which is a putative marker of Th1 cells. These last two studies are less definitive because evaluation of mRNA expression may not accurately reflect protein levels and because soluble lymphocyte activation gene 3 and IFN-γ production are not always regulated in parallel (28). Furthermore, concentrations in serum of IL-18, which enhances *M. tuberculosis*-induced IFN-γ production by human peripheral blood lymphocytes (42), are also increased in tuberculosis patients, and levels of IL-18 parallel those of IFN-γ (45). Therefore, the preponderance of evidence indicates that systemic Th1 cytokine levels are elevated in tuberculosis patients.

Most studies suggest that Th2 cytokines are also upregulated in the blood of tuberculosis patients. IL-10 levels in serum are high (8, 41, 43), and mRNA expression of IL-4 and IL-13 is increased in PBMC

of tuberculosis patients (32). The most convincing evidence for enhanced systemic expression of Th2 cytokines in tuberculosis is provided by a large study of 414 tuberculosis patients and 828 healthy controls from The Gambia and Guinea. This study showed that plasma immunoglobulin E and macrophage-derived chemokine levels, both of which are strongly associated with Th2 responses, were markedly elevated in tuberculosis patients (19). However, serum IL-4 concentrations have been reported to be increased in only one study (8) but unchanged in two others (4, 43). IL-4 may be difficult to detect in serum because it is rapidly bound to its receptor. Taken together, these studies indicate that the systemic Th2 response is enhanced in tuberculosis patients compared to healthy controls.

Cytokine Production by Peripheral Blood Cells Stimulated with Mycobacterial Antigens

Many publications have examined the cytokine response by PBMC of tuberculosis patients and of healthy tuberculin reactors stimulated with mycobacterial antigens. Most investigators have reported that PBMC of tuberculosis patients show decreased *M. tuberculosis*-induced IFN-γ production (5, 14, 20, 38, 48). Findings regarding monokine secretion have been more variable. Tuberculosis patients have been reported to have normal (41, 46, 47) or reduced (34) production of IL-12 and reduced (42) or increased (34) secretion of IL-18. IL-10 production was found to be increased in tuberculosis patients in some studies (14, 34, 38) and unchanged in others (4, 13, 20, 41). These inconsistencies may reflect differences in patient populations. For example, greater IL-10 production may be found in populations that include a higher percentage of anergic patients, because these individuals show a higher proportion of IL-10-producing T cells (6). In addition, because IL-10, IL-12, and IL-18 are produced by monocytes in response to mycobacterial antigens, the variable percentage of monocytes in PBMC of tuberculosis patients may result in differential production of these monokines.

Studies in which enzyme-linked immunosorbent assay (ELISA) was used to measure IL-4 levels in cell culture supernatants have consistently shown that mycobacterial antigen-stimulated PBMC from tuberculosis patients and from healthy tuberculin reactors produce extremely low or undetectable levels of IL-4 (4, 13, 14, 20, 38). In striking contrast, studies using the enzyme-linked immunospot assay or immunolabeling to detect intracellular cytokine-producing cells have demonstrated an increased number of IL-4-producing T cells in PBMC isolated from tuberculosis patients and stimulated with mycobacterial antigens or mitogens, compared to findings in PBMC from healthy tuberculin reactors (5, 33, 35, 40). The most likely explanation for these findings is that IL-4 is rapidly bound to responding cells and is therefore not present in sufficient quantities for detection by ELISA whereas methods that detect intracellular cytokines or individual cytokine-secreting cells, which are generally more sensitive than ELISA, permit the identification of IL-4-producing cells. An alternative possibility is that the number of IL-4-producing cells is larger in tuberculosis patients but they produce less IL-4 per cell, resulting in equivalent IL-4 levels. This is unlikely since there is no precedent for this scenario in other experimental systems.

HYPOTHESIS FOR CYTOKINE DYSREGULATION IN HUMAN TUBERCULOSIS

For tuberculosis patients, we can summarize the many studies cited above as follows: (i) there is enhanced production of IFN-γ and IL-10, but not IL-4, at the site of disease; (ii) systemic levels of IFN-γ, IL-10, and IL-4 are elevated; (iii) *M. tuberculosis*-stimulated peripheral blood T cells produce reduced amounts of IFN-γ and increased amounts of IL-4. Are the high systemic levels of IFN-γ due to leakage of this cytokine from the site of disease or to systemic upregulation of the Th1 response? We think that the former explanation is more likely because tuberculosis patients with advanced disease have the highest serum IL-18 and IFN-γ levels (43, 45) and also have the most marked inflammatory response and the highest Th1 cytokine concentrations at the diseased site (39). In addition, it is difficult to reconcile a systemic increase in the Th1 response with the reduced capacity of peripheral blood T cells to produce IFN-γ in response to *M. tuberculosis*.

The most parsimonious hypothesis to explain the different findings regarding the Th1/Th2 cytokine balance in human tuberculosis is that the local cytokine response is dominated by the production of IFN-γ and of IL-10, the latter secreted by macrophages and by Th1 cells that produce IFN-γ and IL-10. These cytokines leak from tissue sites into the circulation, resulting in elevated levels of IFN-γ and IL-10 in serum. Although IL-4 is not produced at the site of disease, there is systemic upregulation of the Th2 response and a high frequency of IL-4-secreting T cells, resulting in increased IL-4 production in blood. The enhanced systemic Th2 response and sequestration of IFN-γ-producing cells at the site of disease result in decreased *M. tuberculosis*-induced IFN-γ production by peripheral blood T cells from tuberculosis patients. The central elements of this hypothesis are shown in Fig. 1.

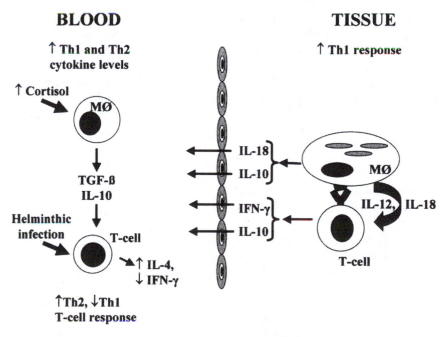

Figure 1. Cytokine production in human tuberculosis. At the tissue sites of disease, macrophages produce cytokines that favor the production of Th1 cells. Cytokines such as IL-10, IL-18, and IFN-γ leak into the systemic circulation, resulting in high levels in serum. In the blood, monocytes produce TGF-β and IL-10, which favor the development of Th2 cells, resulting in systemic production of IL-4. Elevated cortisol levels and helminthic infections probably contribute to these effects. Mφ, macrophage.

MECHANISMS THAT MAY ENHANCE THE SYSTEMIC Th2 RESPONSE AND DAMPEN THE Th1 RESPONSE

Helminthic Infection

Helminthic infections and tuberculosis are both common in developing nations, and current or prior helminthic infections can strongly bias mycobacterial antigen-elicited cytokine production toward a Th2 response (22). Some of the variability in the Th2 response found in tuberculosis patients may result in part from the differential prevalence of helminthic infections in the populations studied. Among patients from Holland and the United States, where helminthic infections are uncommon, IL-4 levels in the serum of tuberculosis patients were not elevated (4, 43). In contrast, among patients from Argentina and from Africa, where helminthic infection is more common, increased levels of IL-4 and markers of IL-4 production were found in the serum of tuberculosis patients (8, 19). In most developing countries, helminthic infection is probably more common in tuberculosis patients than in healthy controls, since both diseases are associated with crowding and poverty. In the only study to address this issue, current or prior helminthic infection was present in 48% of tuberculosis patients compared to 27% of healthy controls (19). Although helminthic infections may bias the antimycobacterial response toward the production of Th2 cytokines, this is unlikely to fully account for upregulation of the systemic Th2 response in tuberculosis. One study of more than 400 tuberculosis patients found that enhanced IL-4 production resolved after successful antituberculosis therapy but not in cases of treatment failure, suggesting that uncontrolled tuberculosis itself is associated with an enhanced systemic Th2 response (19).

Immunosuppressive Monokines

Monocytes from tuberculosis patients produce increased amounts of transforming growth factor β (TGF-β) (13, 14), which downregulates costimulatory molecules on antigen-presenting cells, such as CD40, CD80, and CD86 (25), and reduces IL-12 receptor expression on M. tuberculosis-stimulated T cells (47), decreasing their capacity to produce IFN-γ in response to IL-12. Neutralization of TGF-β either with naturally occurring inhibitors or with antibodies enhances M. tuberculosis-induced IFN-γ production (12). IL-10 is another monokine that can inhibit Th1 responses. IL-10 concentrations in the serum of tuberculosis patients are elevated (8, 41, 43), reducing the capacity of PBMC to produce IFN-γ in response to M. tuberculosis (41). This is probably mediated through the ability of IL-10 to inhibit macrophage production of IL-12 and expression of costimulatory molecules (25), as well as by decreasing IL-12 receptor expression on T cells (47).

The reasons for systemic upregulation of TGF-β and IL-10 in tuberculosis patients are uncertain. An intriguing possibility is that altered corticosteroid metabolism results in increased conversion of cortisone to cortisol, which in turn can enhance the production of TGF-β and IL-10 by monocytes (3).

Apoptosis

Peripheral blood T cells from tuberculosis patients show increased spontaneous and M. tuberculosis-induced apoptosis, as well as increased release of soluble Fas, compared to the results of parallel studies with healthy controls (15). These abnormalities were most marked in patients with severe disease, and there is a strong inverse correlation between the extent of apoptosis and the capacity of PBMC to produce IFN-γ in response to M. tuberculosis (15). Enhanced apoptosis and disproportionate elimination of IFN-γ-producing cells could result from upregulation of the systemic Th2 response, since IL-4 enhances TNF-α-induced apoptosis of M. tuberculosis-reactive T cells (31) and since activated Th1 cells are more susceptible to Fas/Fas ligand-mediated apoptosis than are activated Th2 cells (49).

CD40 Ligand Expression

The capacity of M. tuberculosis-stimulated T cells to produce IFN-γ is modulated by signaling through CD40 on antigen-presenting cells and CD40 ligand on T cells. CD40 ligand expression is reduced in peripheral blood T cells from tuberculosis patients, and soluble CD40 ligand trimer increased M. tuberculosis-induced IFN-γ secretion by PBMC from tuberculosis patients (27). In addition, CD40 ligand expression increased after successful antituberculosis therapy, paralleling the restoration of IFN-γ production. The reduced CD40 ligand expression in tuberculosis patients may be due to the effects of IL-4, which inhibits sustained expression of CD40 ligand by T cells (18). It is less likely to be mediated by IL-10 and TGF-β, since these cytokines reduce CD40 expression on antigen-presenting cells (25) and CD40 expression in PBMC is increased in tuberculosis patients (27).

Defects in IFN-γ Promoter Activity

Little is known about the transcription factors that bind to the IFN-γ promoter under physiologic conditions in human infectious disease, and the intracellular signaling pathways that result in decreased M. tuberculosis-induced IFN-γ secretion by T cells from tuberculosis patients are largely unexplored. Activation-specific expression of IFN-γ by T cells is controlled in part by binding of the transcription factor cyclic AMP response element-binding proteins (CREB) to the IFN-γ promoter. We recently found that freshly isolated T cells from tuberculosis patients have low IFN-γ promoter activity coupled with markedly reduced expression of CREB (26). Transient transfection of Jurka cells with a dominant-negative CREB repressor plasmid downregulated IFN-γ promoter activity, suggesting that reduced expression of CREB in tuberculosis patients decreases IFN-γ promoter activity and IFN-γ production (26). Experiments should be performed to characterize these defects in intracellular signaling and to determine if they are mediated in part by the enhanced systemic Th2 response.

IS CYTOKINE DYSREGULATION THE CAUSE OR EFFECT OF TUBERCULOSIS?

Dysregulation of the systemic Th1 and Th2 cytokine responses may be a secondary effect of tuberculosis, since tuberculosis commonly results in malnutrition, which in turn is associated with enhanced Th2 and reduced Th1 cytokine responses (21). On the other hand, it is equally plausible that persons who mount a weak Th1 or dominant Th2 response to mycobacterial infection are predisposed to progression of *M. tuberculosis* infection to disease. Distinguishing these possibilities is central to our understanding of the pathogenesis of tuberculosis. Unfortunately, because immunologic studies of tuberculosis patients are performed only relatively late in the course of disease, it has not been possible to resolve this critical issue. It may not be feasible to address this question by studies of humans because it would require followup of a huge cohort of recently infected persons, coupled with serial determinations of their cytokine responses and clinical evaluations to detect tuberculosis at an early stage. Because it is strongly recommended that persons with recent *M. tuberculosis* infection receive treatment with isoniazid to prevent the development of tuberculosis, ethical constraints would make it difficult to conduct such a study. These investigations may be feasible in primates, but the large number of animals involved would make such an investigation extremely costly.

THERAPEUTIC MODULATION OF THE CYTOKINE RESPONSE

Because Th1 cytokines contribute to effective immunity to *M. tuberculosis*, modulating the cytokine response may improve the treatment of tuberculosis patients. On the other hand, Th1 cytokines have the potential to cause excessive inflammation and immunopathology, since the highest local and systemic levels of Th1 cytokines are found in patients with the most severe tuberculosis (39, 43, 45). Therefore, caution is mandatory when using this approach.

Standard antituberculosis therapy results in rapid bacillary elimination in patients with drug-susceptible tuberculosis, and most problems that arise during the initial phase of therapy are due to continued local and systemic inflammation. In this setting, agents that enhance the Th1 response are unlikely to provide clinical benefit. Patients with prolonged fever and tissue inflammation respond well to corticosteroids (9), and there is limited scope for more specific measures to reduce the production of Th1 cytokines.

In patients with multidrug-resistant tuberculosis, the efficacy of antituberculosis agents is suboptimal and modulation of the cytokine response is more likely to play a role in therapy. Intradermal administration of IL-2, in combination with antituberculosis agents, reduced the sputum bacillary burden in five of eight patients with multidrug-resistant tuberculosis (17). Local administration of cytokines is theoretically more appealing than systemic therapy, since the former approach is likely to result in fewer side effects. Administration of IFN-γ by aerosol yielded favorable clinical and microbiologic effects in five patients with multidrug-resistant tuberculosis (7). These preliminary studies demonstrated that IFN-γ and IL-2 can be safely administered and provide short-term benefits. However, durable responses or cure have not yet been documented. Inhibition of the Th2 response by neutralization of IL-10 or TGF-β may provide an alternative or complementary means of enhancing the Th1 response, but it has not yet been studied in experiments with tuberculosis patients.

In the past decade, our knowledge about the general features of the human cytokine response to tuberculosis has advanced significantly. Nevertheless, the host and microbial factors that contribute to the variability in cytokine production between individual tuberculosis patients remain largely undefined. A more comprehensive understanding of these factors, in combination with methods to deliver cytokines to specific cells or tissue sites, is necessary before we can fulfill the potential promise of modulating the cytokine response to treat selected patients.

Acknowledgments. This work was supported in part by the National Institutes of Health (grant AI44935), the Potts Memorial Foundation, the Cain Foundation for Infectious Disease Research, and the Center for Pulmonary and Infectious Disease Control. P. F. B. holds the Margaret E. Byers Cain Chair for Tuberculosis Research.

REFERENCES

1. Altare, F., A. Durandy, D. Lammas, J.-F. Emile, S. Lamhamedi, F. Le Deist, P. Drysdale, E. Jouanguy, R. Doffinger, F. Bernaudin, O. Jeppsson, J. A. Gollob, E. Meinl, A. W. Segal, A. Fischer, D. Kumurante, and J.-L. Casanova. 1998. Impairment of mycobacterial immunity in human interleukin-12 receptor deficiency. *Science* 280:1432–1435.

2. Aubert-Pivert, E. M., F. M. Chedevergne, G. M. Lopez-Ramirez, J. H. Colle, P. L. Scheinmann, B. M. Gicquel, and J. M. de Blic. 2000. Cytokine transcripts in pediatric tuberculosis: a study with bronchoalveolar cells. *Tubercle Lung Dis.* 80:249–258.

3. Baker, R. W., B. R. Walker, R. J. Shaw, J. W. Honour, D. S. Jessop, S. L. Lightman, A. Zumla, and G. A. W. Rook. 2000. Increased cortisol:cortisone ratio in acute pulmonary tuberculosis. *Am. J. Respir. Crit. Care Med.* 162:1641–1647.

4. Barnes, P. F., S. Lu, J. S. Abrams, E. Wang, M. Yamamura, and R. L. Modlin. 1993. Cytokine production at the site of disease in human tuberculosis. *Infect. Immun.* 61:3482–3489.

5. Bhattacharyya, S., R. Singla, A. B. Dey, and H. K. Prasad. 1999. Dichotomy of cytokine profiles in patients and high-risk healthy subjects exposed to tuberculosis. *Infect. Immun.* 67:5597–5603.

6. Boussiotis, V.A., E. Y. Tsai, E. J. Yunis, S. Thim, J. C. Delgado, C. C. Dascher, A. Berezovskaya, D. Rousset, J.-M. Reynes, and A. E. Goldfeld. 2000. IL-10-producing T cells suppress immune responses in anergic tuberculosis patients. *J. Clin. Investig.* 105:1317–1325.

7. Condos, R., W. N. Rom, and N. W. Schluger. 1997. Treatment of multidrug-resistant pulmonary tuberculosis with interferon-gamma via aerosol. *Lancet* 349:1513–1515.

8. Dlugovitzky, D., A. Torres-Morales, L. Rateni, M. A. Farroni, C. Largacha, O. Molteni, and O. Bottasso. 1997. Circulating profile of Th1 and Th2 cytokines in tuberculosis patients with different degrees of pulmonary involvement. *FEMS Immunol. Med. Microbiol.* 18:203–207.

9. Dooley, D. P., J. L. Carpenter, and S. Rademacher. 1997. Adjunctive corticosteroid therapy for tuberculosis: a critical reappraisal of the literature. *Clin. Infect. Dis.* 25:872–887.

10. Fenhalls, G., L. Stevens, J. Bezuidenhout, G. E. Amphlett, K. Duncan, P. Bardin, and P. T. Lukey. 2002. Distribution of IFN-γ, IL-4 and TNF-α protein and CD8 T cells producing IL-12p40 mRNA in human lung tuberculous granulomas. *Immunology* 105:325–335.

11. Gerosa, F., C. Nisii, S. Righetti, R. Micciolo, M. Marchesini, A. Cazzadori, and G. Trinchieri. 1999. CD4+ T-cell clones producing both interferon-γ and interleukin-10 predominate in bronchoalveolar lavages of active pulmonary tuberculosis patients. *Clin. Immunol.* 92:224–234.

12. Hirsch, C. S., J. J. Ellner, R. Blinkhorn, and Z. Toossi. 1997. In vitro restoration of T-cell responses in tuberculosis and augmentation of monocyte effector function against *Mycobacterium tuberculosis* by natural inhibitors of transforming growth factor β. *Proc. Natl. Acad. Sci. USA* 94:3926–3931.

13. Hirsch, C. S., R. Hussain, Z. Toossi, G. Dawood, F. Shahid, and J. J. Ellner. 1996. Cross-modulation by transforming growth factor β in human tuberculosis: suppression of antigen-driven blastogenesis and interferon γ production. *Proc. Natl. Acad. Sci. USA* 93:3193–3198.

14. Hirsch, C. S., Z. Toossi, C. Othieno, J. L. Johnson, S. K. Schwander, S. Robertson, R. S. Wallis, K. Edmonds, A. Okwera, R. Mugerwa, P. Peters, and J. J. Ellner. 1999. Depressed T-cell interferon-γ responses in pulmonary tuberculosis: analysis of underlying mechanisms and modulation with therapy. *J. Infect. Dis.* 180:2069–2073.

15. Hirsch, C. S., Z. Toossi, G. Vanham, J. L. Johnson, P. Peters, A. Okwera, R. Mugerwa, P. Mugyenyi, and J. J. Ellner. 1999. Apoptosis and T-cell hyporesponsiveness in pulmonary tuberculosis. *J. Infect. Dis.* 179:945–953.

16. Hoshino, T., R. H. Wiltrout, and H. A. Young. 1999. IL-18 is a potent coinducer of IL-13 in NK and T cells: a new potential role for IL-18 in modulating the immune response. *J. Immunol.* 162:5070–5077

17. Johnson, B.J., L.G. Bekker, R. Rickman, S. Brown, M. Lesser, S. Ress, P. Willcox, L. Steyn, and G. Kaplan. 1997. rhuIL-2 adjunctive therapy in multidrug resistant tuberculosis: a comparison of two treatment regimens and placebo. *Tubercle Lung Dis.* 78:195–203.

18. Lee, B. O., L. Haynes, S. M. Eaton, S. L. Swain, and T. D. Randall. 2002. The biological outcome of CD40 signaling is dependent on the duration of CD40 ligand expression: reciprocal regulation by interleukin (IL)-4 and IL-12. *J. Exp. Med.* 196:693–704.

19. Lienhardt, C., A. Azzurri, A. Amedel, K. Fielding, J. Sillah, O. Y. Sow, B. Bah, A. Beneglano, A. Diallo, R. Manetti, K. Manneh, P. Gustafson, S. Bennett, M. M. D'Elios, K. McAdam, and G. Del Prete. 2002. Active tuberculosis in Africa is associated with reduced Th1 and increased Th2 activity *in vivo*. *Eur. J. Immunol.* 32:1605–1613.

20. Lin, Y., M. Zhang, F. M. Hofman, J. Gong, and P. F. Barnes. 1996. Absence of a prominent Th2 cytokine response in human tuberculosis. *Infect. Immun.* 64:1351–1356.

21. Lord, G. M., G. Matarese, J. K. Howard, R. J. Baker, S. R. Bloom, and R. I. Lechler. 1998. Leptin modulates the T-cell immune response and reverses starvation-induced immunosuppression. *Nature* 394:897–901.

22. Malhotra, I., P. Mungai, A. Wamachi, J. Kioko, J. H. Ouma, J. W. Kazura, and C. L. King. 1999. Helminth- and bacillus Calmette-Guérin-induced immunity in children sensitized in utero to filariasis and schistosomiasis. *J. Immunol.* 162:6843–6848.

23. Ottenhoff, T. H. M., D. Kumararatne, and J.-L. Casanova. 1998. Novel human immunodeficiencies reveal the essential role of type-I cytokines in immunity to intracellular bacteria. *Immunol. Today* 19:491–494.

24. Robinson, D. S., S. Ying, I. K. Taylor, A. Wangoo, D. M. Mitchell, A. B. Kay, Q. Hamid, and R. J. Shaw. 1994. Evidence for a Th1-like bronchoalveolar T-cell subset and predominance of interferon-gamma gene activation in pulmonary tuberculosis. *Am. J. Respir. Crit. Care Med.* 149:989–993.

25. Rojas, R. E., K. N. Balaji, A. Subramanian, and W. H. Boom. 1999. Regulation of human CD4+ αβ T-cell-receptor-positive (TCR+) and γδ TCR+ T-cell responses to *Mycobacterium tuberculosis* by interleukin-10 and transforming growth factor β. *Infect. Immun.* 67:6461–6472.

26. Samten, B., P. Ghosh, A. Yi, S. E. Weis, D. L. Lakey, R. Gonsky, U. Pendurthi, B. Wizel, Y. Zhang, M. Zhang, J. Gong, M. Fernandez, H. Safi, R. Vankayalapati, H. A. Young, and P. F. Barnes. 2002. Reduced expression of nuclear cyclic adenosine 5′-monophospate response element-binding proteins and IFN-γ promoter function in disease due to an intracellular pathogen. *J. Immunol.* 168:3520–3526.

27. Samten, B., E. K. Thomas, J.-H. Gong, and P. F. Barnes. 2000. Depressed CD40 ligand expression contributes to reduced gamma interferon production in human tuberculosis. *Infect. Immun.* 68:3002–3006.

28. Scala, E., M. Carbonari, P. Del Porto, M. Cibati, T. Tedesco, A. M. Mazzone, R. Paganelli, and M. Fiorilli. 1998. Lymphocyte activation gene-3 (LAG-3) expression and IFN-γ production are variably coregulated in different human T lymphocyte subpopulations. *J. Immunol.* 161:489–493.

29. Schwander, S. K., M. Torres, C. C. Carranza, D. Escobedo, M. Tary-Lehmann, P. Anderson, Z. Toossi, J. J. Ellner, E. A. Rich, and E. Sada. 2000. Pulmonary mononuclear cell responses to antigens of *Mycobacterium tuberculosis* in healthy household contacts of patients with active tuberculosis and healthy controls from the community. *J. Immunol.* **165:**1479–1485.

30. Schwander, S. K., M. Torres, E. Sada, C. Carranza, E. Ramos, M. Tary-Lehmann, R. S. Wallis, J. Sierra, and E. A. Rich. 1998. Enhanced responses to *Mycobacterium tuberculosis* antigens by human alveolar lymphocytes during active pulmonary tuberculosis. *J. Infect. Dis.* **178:**1434–1445.

31. Seah, G. T., and G. A. W. Rook. 2001. IL-4 influences apoptosis of mycobacterium-reactive lymphocytes in the presence of TNF-α. *J. Immunol.* **167:**1230–1237.

32. Seah, G. T., G. M. Scott, and G. A. W. Rook. 2000. Type 2 cytokine gene activation and its relationship to extent of disease in patients with tuberculosis. *J. Infect. Dis.* **181:**385–389.

33. Smith, S. M., M. R. Klein, J. Sillah, K. P. W. J. McAdam, and H. M. Dockrell. 2002. Decreased IFN-γ and increased IL-4 production by human CD8⁺ T cells in response to *Mycobacterium tuberculosis* in tuberculosis patients. *Tuberculosis* **82:**7–13.

34. Song, C.-H., H.-J. Kim, J.-K. Park, J.-H. Lim, U.-O. Kim, J.-S. Kim, T.-H. Paik, K.-Y. Kim, J.-W. Suhr, and E.-K. Jo. 2000. Depressed interleukin-12 (IL-12), but not IL-18, production in response to a 30- or 32-kilodalton mycobacterial antigen in patients with active pulmonary tuberculosis. *Infect. Immun.* **68:**4477–4484.

35. Surcel, H.-M., M. Troye-Blomberg, S. Paulie, G. Andersson, C. Moreno, G. Pasvol, and J. Ivanyi. 1994. Th1/Th2 profiles in tuberculosis, based on the proliferation and cytokine responses of blood lymphocytes to mycobacterial antigens. *Immunology* **81:**171–176.

36. Taha, R. A., T. C. Kotsimbos, Y. Song, D. Menzies, and Q. Hamid. 1997. IFN-γ and IL-12 are increased in active compared with inactive tuberculosis. *Am. J. Respir. Crit. Care Med.* **155:**1135–1139.

37. Ting, L.-M., A.C. Kim, A. Cattamanchi, and J. D. Ernst. 1999. *Mycobacterium tuberculosis* inhibits IFN-γ transcriptional responses without inhibiting activation of STAT1. *J. Immunol.* **163:**3898–3906.

38. Torres, M., T. Herrera, H. Villareal, E. A. Rich, and E. Sada. 1998. Cytokine profiles for peripheral blood lymphocytes from patients with active pulmonary tuberculosis and healthy household contacts in response to the 30-kilodalton antigen of *Mycobacterium tuberculosis*. *Infect. Immun.* **66:**176–180.

39. Tsao, T. C. Y., C. C. Huang, W.-K. Chiou, P.-Y. Yang, M.-J. Hsieh, and K.-C. Tsao. 2002. Levels of interferon-γ and interleukin-2 receptor-α for bronchoalveolar lavage fluid and serum were correlated with clinical grade and treatment of pulmonary tuberculosis. *Int. J. Tuberc. Lung Dis.* **6:**720–727.

40. van Creve, R., F. Karyadi, F. Preyers, M. Leenders, B.-J. Kullberg, R. H. H. Nelwan, and J. W. M. van der Meer. 2000. Increased production of interleukin 4 by CD4⁺ and CD8⁺ T cells from patients with tuberculosis is related to the presence of pulmonary cavities. *J. Infect Dis.* **181:**1194–1197.

41. Vankayalapati, R., B. Wizel, S. E. Weis, P. Klucar, H. Shams, B. Samten, and P. F. Barnes. 2003. Serum cytokine concentrations do not parallel *Mycobacterium tuberculosis*-induced cytokine production in patients with tuberculosis. *Clin. Infect. Dis.* **36:**24–28.

42. Vankayalapati, R., B. Wizel, S. E. Weis, B. Samten, W. M. Girard, and P. F. Barnes. 2000. Production of interleukin-18 in human tuberculosis. *J. Infect. Dis.* **182:**234–239.

43. Verbon, A., N. Juffermans, S. J. H. van Deventer, P. Speelman, H. Van Deutekom, and T. van der Poll. 1999. Serum concentrations of cytokines in patients with active tuberculosis and after treatment. *Clin. Exp. Immunol.* **115:**110–113.

44. Wild, J. S., A. Sigounas, N. Sur, M. S. Siddiqui, R. Alam, M. Kurimoto, and S. Sur. 2000. IFN-γ-inducing factor (IL-18) increases allergic sensitization, serum IgE, Th2 cytokines, and airway eosinophilia in a mouse model of allergic asthma. *J. Immunol.* **164:**2701–2710.

45. Yamada, G., N. Shijubo, K. Shigehara, H. Okamura, M. Kurimoto, and S. Abe. 2000. Increased levels of circulating interleukin-18 in patients with advanced tuberculosis. *Am. J. Respir. Crit. Care Med.* **161:**1786–1789.

46. Zhang, M., M. K. Gately, E. Wang, J. Gong, S. F. Wolf, S. Lu, R. L. Modlin, and P. F. Barnes. 1994. Interleukin-12 at the site of disease in tuberculosis. *J. Clin. Investig.* **93:**1733–1739.

47. Zhang, M., J.-H. Gong, D. H. Presky, W. Xue, and P. F. Barnes. 1999. Expression of the IL-12 receptor β1 and β2 subunits in human tuberculosis. *J. Immunol.* **162:**2441–2447.

48. Zhang, M., Y. Lin, D. V. Iyer, J. Gong, J. S. Abrams, and P. F. Barnes. 1995. T-cell cytokine responses in human infection with *Mycobacterium tuberculosis*. *Infect. Immun.* **63:**3231–3234.

49. Zhang, X., T. Brunner, L. Carter, R. W. Dutton, P. Rogers, L. Bradley, T. Sato, J. C. Reed, D. Green, and S. L. Swain. 1997. Unequal death in T helper cell (Th)1 and Th2 effectors: Th1, but not Th2, effectors undergo rapid Fas/FasL-mediated apoptosis. *J. Exp. Med.* **185:**1837–1849.

Tuberculosis and the Tubercle Bacillus
Edited by Stewart T. Cole et al.
© 2005 ASM Press, Washington, D.C.

Chapter 32

Role of Antibody-Mediated Immunity in Host Defense against *Mycobacterium tuberculosis*

AHARONA GLATMAN-FREEDMAN AND ARTURO CASADEVALL

For many decades, the dominant view in the field of mycobacterial immunology has been that host defense against *Mycobacterium tuberculosis* relies exclusively on cell-mediated immunity. A role for antibodies in either protection against *M. tuberculosis* infection or in the pathogenesis of tuberculosis, has been generally discounted (1, 18, 26). This view emerged as a result of several factors: the difficulty involved in demonstrating natural protective antibody responses to *M. tuberculosis*, the theory that an immune response to a particular pathogen was primarily cell mediated or antibody mediated, and the notion that host defense against intracellular pathogens was the function of cell-mediated immunity.

In search of new solutions to the overwhelming problem of tuberculosis, investigators set out several years ago to evaluate the help that can be offered by antibody-mediated immunity in host defense against *M. tuberculosis*, with the possibility that it may lead to the development of a novel and effective vaccine strategy.

EXPERIENCE WITH SERUM THERAPY

In the late 19th century and the beginning of the 20th century, a substantial amount of experimentation was performed in an attempt to identify an effective serum against tuberculosis. These studies were inspired by the successful development of serum therapy of several infectious diseases including those caused by *Streptococcus pneumoniae*, *Neisseria meningitidis*, group A streptococcus, and several toxin-producing microorganisms (11). Serum therapy entailed the administration of animal or human sera for the treatment of an infectious disease. Most sera were obtained from animals immunized with a specific pathogen and consequently could be considered immune sera. The active component of serum therapy was antibody.

We identified about a dozen investigative sources reporting the generation and use of immune sera against tuberculosis (reviewed in reference 34). Most studies reported some benefit following the administration of serum but lacked suitable controls by present-day standards. The efficacy of many studies is difficult to evaluate because the reports contained little detail regarding the diagnostic criteria used or the preparation, administration, and specific effect of the serum. Comparisons between the studies are difficult because different antigens were used by the individual investigators for the preparation of antituberculosis sera (reviewed in reference 34). The most detailed studies were reported by Paul Paquin and Carl Fisch, and both described favorable effects following serum administration. Their reports were noteworthy for the degree of detail provided and the level of scientific rigor. Below we provide detailed descriptions of those investigations since the original sources are often not immediately available.

Paul Paquin

Paul Paquin reported the efficacy of serum therapy against experimental tuberculosis between 1895 and 1998 (34, 67, 70). The serum was prepared by immunizing horses with tuberculin and *M. tuberculosis* over 2 to 6 months (34, 67, 70) and administered to patients by hypodermic injections. The initial group receiving serum consisted of 22 patients with pulmonary tuberculosis for whom the diagnosis was confirmed by the presence of tubercle bacilli in sputum specimens. After approximately 2 months of

Aharona Glatman-Freedman • Division of Infectious Diseases, Department of Pediatrics, Children's Hospital at Montefiore, Albert Einstein College of Medicine, 1300 Morris Park Ave., Bronx, NY 10461. **Arturo Casadevall** • Division of Infectious Diseases, Departments of Medicine and of Microbiology and Immunology, Albert Einstein College of Medicine, 1300 Morris Park Ave., Bronx, NY 10461.

therapy, improvement was reported for 82% of the patients. The improvement was manifested by decreased cough, clearance of pulmonary infiltrates, reduction in hemoptysis, improved appetite, weight gain, reduction in sputum bacillary load, and increase in lung vital capacity (67, 68). Six months after initiation of serum therapy, all the patients remained alive and more than half were discharged from the hospital (67). Patients from a different tuberculosis ward within the same hospital, who received no serum, served as controls. During the initial 4 months of the study, more than 30 deaths were reported in the control group compared to none in the group receiving serum therapy. To assure the medical community that the improvement observed was due to serum therapy rather than to placebo effect, Paquin reported that almost all patients were initially reluctant to accept the new treatment and most were treated against their will. After achieving initial improvement, the treatment was interrupted for 2 weeks and symptoms reemerged; reinstitution of serum therapy resulted in renewed efficacy (67).

In 1897, Paquin published the results of long-term follow-up of patients treated with his serum (69). Of the 252 patients available to follow-up, 57 (23%) had recovered (40 of them had been monitored for 1 to 3 years after receiving serum therapy and were still alive and well), 76 (30%) had shown improvements in their condition and were able to carry out daily activities, 80 (32%) showed improvement to a lesser extent, 3 (1%) experienced clinical recovery without changes in cavitary lesions, and 36 (14%) had died. These results are interesting, considering that the mortality from untreated tuberculosis is approximately 50% (19). Supporting studies reporting on the efficacy of Paquin's serum in treating patients with pulmonary tuberculosis were published by other investigators (38, 73, 92). Several small studies reported less favorable results (31, 51, 97).

Carl Fisch

In 1897 Carl Fisch published the results of animal experiments performed with immune horse serum (31). The serum was prepared by immunizing horses with two types of tuberculin and aqueous extracts of the growth medium (31, 34). The first experiment examined the efficacy of serum administered before infection with M. tuberculosis. Seven guinea pigs were included in the experiment: three received multiple injections of serum over a 30-day period followed by challenge with a lethal dose of tubercle bacilli, and four served as controls (two receiving serum alone and two receiving tubercle bacilli alone). The animals receiving serum (with or without challenge with tubercle

bacilli) remained healthy for 7 weeks and gained weight. Necropsy performed 6 weeks after infection of one of the animals receiving both serum and tubercle bacilli showed no signs of disease. The two animals receiving tubercle bacilli without serum died 21 and 24 days after challenge and had characteristic tuberculous lesions (31). Fisch also found that the effect of the serum administered prior to infection was dose dependent (a higher dose was more effective).

A second experiment examined the effect of simultaneous administration of serum and tubercle bacilli. Tubercle bacilli were mixed with various volumes of serum, and the suspensions were then administered subcutaneously or intraperitoneally. Eleven animals receiving suspensions containing 0.25 to 1 ml of serum remained alive 2.5 months after challenge and gained weight. Of three animals that received suspensions containing only 0.1 ml of serum, two died after 37 and 54 days and the third was reported to have a "large infiltration" (organ not specified) and had lost weight. Controls, consisting of three animals receiving M. tuberculosis alone and three animals inoculated with a mixture containing immune serum from another source (made by Paquin), died 16 to 29 days after inoculation.

Fisch also examined whether serum administered after infection had a beneficial effect. Three groups of 6 guinea pigs each were used (18 animals). The groups received serum starting on day 4, 7, or 10 after challenge; serum was then administered on alternate days for the following 4 weeks and once a week thereafter. The animals from all three groups remained alive 2.5 months after challenge. Signs of illness such as ulcers or fever were reportedly reversed by serum treatment, and the tuberculin test was negative in three animals tested after 6 weeks of treatment. Two additional animals receiving serum therapy starting 10 days after challenge demonstrated signs of resolving disease on necropsy. Of three animals injected with serum starting on day 14 after challenge, two developed signs of illness and one died 7 weeks after the challenge. Controls that received tubercle bacilli only (three animals) or were treated with serum made by Paquin (three animals) died 20 to 28 days after infection. Fisch concluded that his immune serum both protected against and cured tuberculosis.

Fisch also performed two small studies with monkeys and demonstrated that monkeys receiving serum therapy survived longer than the controls did (reviewed in reference 34).

Outcome of Serum Therapy Studies

Although the studies by Paquin and Fisch were detailed and rigorous by the standards of their time, most other studies lacked suitable controls, reported little detail, and used different antituberculosis sera (reviewed in reference 34). Despite the limitations of these studies, some common themes emerged in the experience with serum therapy for tuberculosis. Serum therapy appeared to be more effective in patients with early and localized tuberculosis than in those with long-standing, chronic cases (40, 44, 45, 56, 58, 97). Furthermore, long periods of therapy were often required in order to achieve a sustained beneficial effect (40, 67, 68, 95).

The challenges encountered in the development of serum therapy for tuberculosis were in contrast to the successful development of serum therapy for pneumococcal pneumonia and other infectious diseases (reviewed in reference 10). The inability of different investigators to generate effective antituberculosis sera in a consistent manner was probably the most important factor in shaping the scientific view that antibody-mediated immunity has little or no effect on the outcome of *M. tuberculosis* infection. However, the majority of published experiments did provide some evidence for efficacy of serum therapy against *M. tuberculosis*. Unfortunately, the lack of appropriate controls, the minimal descriptions in many reports, and the lack of knowledge of the antibody titer in the sera made the experience of serum therapy inconclusive with regard to the efficacy of antibody in protection against tuberculosis. Serum therapy for tuberculosis was disappointing because a consistently effective serum formulation was never developed.

Serum therapy studies were highly controversial. In 1903, Alexander Marmorek, who studied the effect of serum therapy in animals and humans, was forced to resign from his position at the Pasteur Institute due to disagreements over the value of serum therapy against tuberculosis (58). Albert Calmette and Edward L. Trudeau also performed experiments with immune serum (8, 100, 101) and reported overall negative results. Their powerful influence in the field of tuberculosis undoubtedly played a role in the overall trend toward abandoning the use of serum therapy for tuberculosis.

STUDIES WITH POLYCLONAL ANTIBODIES

Little effort to develop serum therapy for tuberculosis occurred after the 1920s. However, continued advances in immunology and microbiology led to a new period in the study of antibody against *M. tuberculosis*. This period started in the 1930s and was characterized by the fact that virtually all studies done with immune sera included a measurement of antibody concentration. The development of methods for fractionation of sera allowed investigators to study the effect of antibody-containing fractions. Interest emerged in the usefulness of serological studies for the diagnosis of tuberculosis and prediction of outcome. During this period, there was also a marked shift in interest from antibody-mediated to cell-mediated immunity against *M. tuberculosis*. As a result, the literature on antibody studies was spotty and was spread over several decades. The literature continued to provide evidence both for and against the importance of antibody-mediated immunity in tuberculosis; hence, the role of antibodies in protection against tuberculosis has always been uncertain and somewhat controversial.

To establish the role of antibody-mediated immunity against microbial pathogens, one of several criteria needs to be fulfilled: (i) direct correlation between immunity to infection and the presence of specific serum antibody; (ii) demonstration that administration of specific antibody mediates protection against the pathogen in question; and/or (iii) demonstration of an association between susceptibility to infection and an antibody-mediated immunity disorder. Supportive data for a role of antibodies in host defense can be provided by in vitro studies demonstrating that specific antibody inhibits the pathogen's growth, prevents infection in tissue culture, neutralizes a toxin elaborated by the pathogen, serves as an opsonin, promotes antibody-dependent cellular cytotoxicity, and/or triggers the complement cascade. Many of these parameters of antibody efficacy were used in studies with *M. tuberculosis* (reviewed in reference 34).

The literature on studies of antibody-mediated immunity against *M. tuberculosis* can be divided into several general categories: serological studies, passive antibody studies, animal studies, in vitro studies, and human studies (reviewed in reference 34). Passive antibody experiments were performed with animals, and human studies consisted mainly of serological experiments that attempted to correlate the presence of antibodies with the outcome of infection. Several studies of humans examined the effect of antibody on skin test reactivity (reviewed in reference 34).

Serological Studies

Serological studies can provide evidence for the importance of antibody-mediated immunity against a pathogen when a correlation can be established between the presence of a specific antibody and reduced susceptibility to disease. Numerous studies have attempted to find an association between the presence of antibodies to *M. tuberculosis* and the occurrence of clinical disease. Correlation between antibody titers and improved outcome of tuberculosis has been described by some investigators (15, 21, 24, 80, 87, 89, 91), but not by others (47, 52, 71), for both human and animal studies. Some studies demonstrating a correlation between antibodies and improved outcome also provided evidence for differences in antibody efficacy depending on the target antigen. Overall, the results suggested that antibodies to mycobacterial polysaccharide(s) may affect the course of infection (15, 21, 24, 87, 89, 91). Immunoglobulin G (IgG) antibodies to lipoarabinomannan (LAM) were associated with protection against dissemination in one study (21). Of special interest are the results of serological studies of human immunodeficiency virus (HIV)-positive patients. HIV-positive patients have higher rates of tuberculosis (94), a situation that is thought to be due to their impaired cellular immunity. However, since some studies (4, 22) have documented abnormalities in the antibody response to mycobacterial antigens in HIV-positive patients, such a deficit may contribute to their susceptibility to aggressive tuberculosis infection.

Animal Studies

Overall, animal experiments showed inconsistent results as well. However, the 20th century advances in technology allowed investigators to examine the effects of different fractions of serum or body fluid. Studies done by Zitrin and Wasz-Höckert (110) as well as by Tsuji et al. (102) showed that certain serum or body fluid fractions were beneficial in prolonging survival or affecting mycobacterial growth in animals. Zitrin and Wasz-Höckert (110) administered human serum or its fractions obtained from tuberculosis patients to mice. They demonstrated that serum gamma globulin fractions had a protective effect. However, they also found that fractions containing alpha and beta globulins from the same patients had a protective effect as well. The alpha- and beta-globulin fractions are not known to contain antibodies; however, it is worth noting that both alpha- and beta-globulin fractions of normal serum were reported to have an inhibitory effect on the growth of Cryptococcus neoformans (76). Some investigators, who did not demonstrate antibody-mediated protection, considered the possibility that antibodies important for protection may have been missing from their preparations (74, 75). A disease-enhancing effect of antibodies on Mycobacterium bovis BCG infection was found in a study by Forget et al. (32).

Another approach to demonstrating a role for antibody-mediated immunity is to assess the outcome of infection in a host deficient in antibody produc-

tion. Tuberculosis in humans has not been associated with defects in humoral immunity, but we are not aware of studies that have systematically tried to make a correlation between antibody deficits and the prevalence of clinical disease. The availability of mouse strains with defective humoral immunity provides a means of studying the problem experimentally. At least three studies have been done with B-cell-deficient mice, and they have produced different results. Vordermeier et al. found that B-cell-deficient (μ-chain knockout) mice challenged with M. tuberculosis H37Rv intravenously, had significantly higher organ CFU compared to non-B-cell-deficient controls (105). However, mortality was not increased in the B-cell-deficient mice. On the other hand, studies by Johnson et al. reported no differences in CFU or tissue histopathological findings between B-cell-deficient mice and controls challenged with M. tuberculosis H37Rv via the aerosol route (100 to 1000 bacilli per mouse) (43). A third study examined the outcome of B-cell-deficient mice infected with M. tuberculosis CDC 1551 via the aerosol route (delivering 50 to 100 bacilli per mouse) (6) and found no difference in lung CFU between B-cell-deficient mice and controls. However, B-cell-deficient mice had less severe granuloma formation and reduced CFU in liver and spleen. When the B-cell-deficient mice were reconstituted with naïve B cells before infection, pulmonary granuloma as well as liver and spleen CFU were similar to those in wild-type mice. In contrast, administration of immune serum containing M. tuberculosis-specific antibodies did not have such effect. Hence, one of the three studies reported a worse outcome for experimental M. tuberculosis infection in B-cell-deficient mice. In interpreting the results of studies with B-cell-deficient mice, it is important to consider some limitations of the model. First, a comparison between B-cell-deficient and wild-type mice may not show a large difference if the wild-type mice make primarily nonprotective antibodies. Second, B cells have other functions in host immunity apart from making immunoglobulins, including antigen presentation and cytokine production. Third, some B-cell-deficient mice have been reported to make small amounts of IgA (54).

In Vitro Studies

In vitro studies that demonstrate microbicidal or microbistatic effects can suggest potential mechanisms by which antibodies may exert their effects against M. tuberculosis. Several studies have reported that immune sera could enhance cellular function against M. tuberculosis by the promotion of phagosome-lysosome fusion (2) and increased killing of the pathogen (17).

Other studies have reported direct effects of antibodies on *M. tuberculosis*, such as neutralization, agglutination, bacteriostasis, and bacteriolysis (5, 27, 90). In several studies, these antimycobacterial effects have been associated with the gamma-globulin fraction of immune sera (27, 90, 110). Antibodies to mycobacterial polysaccharide appeared to mediate an indirect effect in one study by binding to the free polysaccharide and inhibiting its immunoregulatory effect (88). In vitro studies, like in vivo studies, have provided evidence both for and against the ability of antibody-mediated immunity to modify the course of infection (reviewed in reference 34).

Conclusions from Studies with Polyclonal Antibodies

The literature on antibody-mediated effects against *M. tuberculosis* is extensive and spans over 100 years of investigation. Despite a considerable amount of work, the most striking aspect of the literature is the degree to which studies attributing an effect to specific antibodies are contradicted by studies showing no effect. Although studies showing an effect of antibodies against *M. tuberculosis* outnumber those that report negative results, this effect may reflect a bias in the publication of positive results. Nevertheless, the literature is often contradictory and is not internally consistent. The paradox is enhanced by the fact that the quality of studies showing positive and negative results is comparable, suggesting that the problem is inherent to the system being studied or to the method being applied to investigate the problem. One possible explanation for the inconsistent results is variation in the quality and quantity of serum antibodies elicited by the various immunization protocols. Polyclonal antibodies present in serum are heterogeneous in terms of antigen specificity, affinity, isotype, and function, and they can be present in various concentrations in different preparations. In this respect, antibodies that are protective, nonprotective, or disease enhancing may be present in various proportions in different preparations, giving rise to different study results.

STUDIES WITH MONOCLONAL ANTIBODIES

Monoclonal antibody (MAb) technology, described for the first time in the 1970s, allowed the selection of individual antibodies with particular antigen specificities. This method resulted in the availability of homogeneous populations of antibodies, each specific for a particular antigenic determinant (epitope), in large quantities. Furthermore, it can provide reagents of particular isotype, affinity, and function.

Use of MAbs to clarify the role of humoral immunity has previously been found useful for *C. neoformans*, *Candida albicans*, and other pathogens (reviewed in references 9, 33, and 34). In parallel with the observation made with *M. tuberculosis*, the role of antibody-mediated immunity to *C. neoformans* was uncertain while polyclonal antibody preparations were used (reviewed in reference 34). The use of MAbs directed to *C. neoformans* capsular glucuronoxylomannan, on the other hand, enabled the identification of individual MAbs that had protective, nonprotective or disease-enhancing effects on the course of *C. neoformans* infection (reviewed in reference 34). Furthermore, the function of MAbs was found to be reliant on isotype (62, 63, 66, 81, 108), epitope specificity (61, 65), and concentration (61, 65). We hypothesized that a similar complexity in antibody response to *M. tuberculosis* may account for the variable results reported, and we proceeded to study the problem using MAbs.

Effect of Monoclonal Antibodies on Survival

The first study describing a beneficial effect of MAb on the course of *M. tuberculosids* infection was performed with MAb 9d8 (Table 1), an IgG3 antibody that recognizes arabinomannan (AM) exclusively (98). *M. tuberculosis* Erdman strain, preincubated with MAb 9d8, was administered via the intratracheal route to mice. Mice receiving *M. tuberculosis* coated with MAb 9d8 survived significantly longer than did the controls (98) (Color Plate 9). Prolongation of survival was achieved with several strains of mice, including gamma interferon and major histocompatibility complex class II-deficient mice (98). Enhanced survival was observed without a concomitant reduction of CFU. However, there were significant changes in the histological response to *M. tuberculosis* infection in the lungs of antibody-treated mice that were interpreted as indicative of an enhanced granulomatous response (98) (Color Plate 9). An example of a similar dichotomy between CFU and histopathological findings was also observed with *C. neoformans*, where antibody prolonged survival and enhanced inflammation but did not affect CFU, at least in the early phase of infection (30). It is of interest that another MAb which recognizes the mycobacterial surface, MAb 5c11, an IgM antibody that recognizes both LAM and AM, did not have a protective effect on the course of *M. tuberculosis* infection in the same model (98). Hence, this study established that protective and nonprotective antibodies existed for *M. tuberculosis*.

Table 1. Effect of MAbs on various aspects of mycobacterial infection

Antibody	Isotype	Target antigen	Nature of antigen	Challenge	Experimental model	Biological effects	Reference
9d8	IgG3	AM	Polysaccharide	*M. tuberculosis*	Mouse	Enhanced survival; enhanced granulomatous formation	98
MBS43	IgG2b	MPB83	Lipoglyco-protein	*M. bovis*	Mouse	Enhanced survival; reduced lesion size; reduced overall lung pathology	Chambers et al., Abstract, 2000; 12a
5c11	IgM	LAM	Lipopolysac-charide	LAM	Mouse	Enhanced serum clearance; reduced spleen uptake; increased liver uptake	35
TBA61	IgA	16-kDa α-crystallin	Protein	*M. tuberculosis*	Mouse	Reduced lung CFU in early stages of infection	107a
4057D2	IgG3	HBHA	Glycoprotein	*M. bovis* BCG, *M. tuberculosis*	Mouse	Reduced spleen CFU	72
3921E4	IgG2a	HBHA	Glycoprotein	*M. bovis* BCG, *M. tuberculosis*	Mouse	Reduced spleen CFU	72
KT10	IgM	MAb KT4	MAb to killer toxin	*M. tuberculosis*	In vitro	Growth inhibition	20

Enhanced survival was also observed in experiments performed with *Mycobacterium bovis*, using MAb MBS43 (Table 1), an IgG2b antibody directed to MPB83 (107), a lipoglycoprotein associated with the surface of *M. bovis* (106). Administration of *M. bovis* preincubated with MAb MBS43 to BALB/c mice via the intravenous route resulted in prolonged survival compared to controls (12a; M. A. Chambers, A. O. Whelan, K. Lloyd, K. Jahans, A. Glatman-Freedman, and R. G. Hewinson, *Third Int. Conf. Mycobacterium bovis*, abstract, 2000). Prolonged survival was associated with reduction of lesion size and decreased pathology in the lungs (Chambers et al., Abstract, 2000).

The studies demonstrating a beneficial effect of MAbs on the course of *M. tuberculosis* infection have been criticized on the grounds that antibody and mycobacteria were mixed before administration into the lungs via a nonphysioloical route (intratracheal or intravenous). It is important to consider this experimental approach in the context of accepted methods in the humoral-immunity field. Studies using similar methods established the beneficial role of antibodies against several important pathogens such as *S. pneumoniae* and *N. meningitidis* by incubating antibody and microorganisms before infection (reviewed in references 10 and 33). In addition, those pathogens were injected intratracheally, intravenously, or intra-

dermally, using niches that are not usually exposed to these pathogens or bypassing the physiological pathways (reviewed in references 10 and 33). Aggregation of mycobacteria was thought by some critics to be responsible for the study results; however, the effect observed cannot be attributed to antibody-induced aggregation since antibody-treated and control mice had comparable CFU 24 h after infection (98). Overall, although nonphysiological, the experiments using such models were instrumental in demonstrating the usefulness of antibodies against several pathogens.

Effect of Monoclonal Antibody on Antigen Clearance

Seibert and colleagues suggested in 1956, following their studies with rabbits, that antibodies to mycobacterial polysaccharide could be indirectly protective (88). They suggested that by binding to free mycobacterial polysaccharide, antibodies could allow "other" natural antimicrobial agents to exert their protective effect against mycobacteria (88). Polysaccharides of many pathogens have been implicated in virulence (reviewed in reference 7). Polysaccharides and polysaccharide-containing fractions constitute an important part of the mycobacterial surface (23), and the mannose-capped mycobacterial lipopolysaccharide

LAM (ManLAM) has been implicated in the immunopathogenesis of tuberculosis (64).

To evaluate the effect of antibody on the fate of free polysaccharide in mice, purified ManLAM and MAb 5c11, a LAM binding IgM MAb (Table 1), were used. In the absence of MAb 5c11, purified ManLAM, administered intravenously, was taken up by the spleen marginal-zone macrophages and to a lesser degree by the liver. Administration of MAb 5c11 prior to the administration of ManLAM enhanced the clearance of ManLAM from the circulation and modified its deposition in tissues. In the presence of MAb 5c11, ManLAM was directed toward the hepatobiliary system, where bile and bile salts caused a reduction in its immunoreactivity (35). The effect of MAb 5c11 on the clearance of ManLAM was very rapid; only 10 min was required for MAb 5c11 to pass from the circulation to the bile and to lower the concentration of ManLAM in the serum significantly. In addition to demonstrating the effect of antibody on the fate of free mycobacterial polysaccharide, this study suggested that liver and bile salts might play a part in defense against mycobacterial infection by inactivating mycobacterial polysaccharides, especially in the presence of specific antibody. A criticism of this study is that it does not correlate this effect with alteration of the outcome of infection. However, the fact that antibody can alter antigen trafficking suggests that it may have an effect on the course of infection. Immunomodulatory effects were exerted by several mycobacterial fractions such as LAM (64, 96) and trehalose-6,6′-dimycolate (cord factor) (79). It is thus possible that altering the pharmacokinetics of such mycobacterial fractions could contribute to the overall protection against *M. tuberculosis*. However, the effect of MAb on a single mycobacterial antigen may not suffice to affect the course of experimental infection. To observe a significant biological effect, it may be necessary to alter the pharmacokinetics of several mycobacterial fractions. The importance of the LAM clearance study (35) is that it provides a proof of principle for the concept that antibody may play a part in affecting the pharmacokinetics of mycobacterial antigens and thus potentially aid in protection against tuberculosis.

Effect of Monoclonal Antibodies on Early Stages of Infection

Cell-mediated immunity is thought to confer protection against *M. tuberculosis* by controlling the replication of mycobacteria after establishment of infection. Antibodies, on the other hand, can potentially affect the fate of mycobacteria in the early stages of infection.

When administered intranasally, MAb TBA61, an IgA antibody to the 16-kDa α-crystallin antigen of *M. tuberculosis* (29), led to a reduction in lung CFU 9 days after challenge with *M. tuberculosis* intranasally or via aerosol (107a) (Table 1). The MAb was effective in both polymeric and monomeric forms. The effect of MAb TBA61 was short-lived, and no differences in CFU between the experimental and control groups were noted on day 28 after challenge (107a).

Despite the short duration of the protective effect provided by MAb TBA61, this study suggested a role for IgA in protection against tuberculosis and showed that antibody may affect the course of mycobacterial infection in its early stages. This study also demonstrated the importance of timing in the administration of certain antibodies. Both pre- and post-infection doses of MAb were necessary to achieve a statistically significant reduction of CFU mediated by MAb TBA61 (107a).

Effect of Monoclonal Antibodies on Mycobacterial Dissemination

M. tuberculosis can disseminate to pulmonary lymph nodes and distal organs such as the spleen, liver, and central nervous system. Dissemination is thought to occur either via entry into alveolar macrophages or via interaction with epithelial cells (72). Heparin binding hemagglutinin adhesin (HBHA), a surface-exposed glycoprotein, is involved in the binding of *M. tuberculosis* to epithelial cells (72). The growth of *M. tuberculosis* and *M. bovis* BCG in which the *hbha* gene, encoding HBHA, is disrupted was reduced in the spleens but not in the lungs of mice (72) compared to that of wild-type strains, suggesting that HBHA plays a role in mycobacterial dissemination.

The effect of antibodies on mycobacterial dissemination was examined by using MAbs 4057D2 (an IgG3 antibody) and 3921E4 (an IgG2a antibody) directed to HBHA (59) (Table 1). Intranasal administration of mycobacteria coated with anti-HBHA MAbs to mice was associated with reduced CFU in the spleen but not in the lungs (72). These results indicate that anti-HBHA antibodies can interfere with mycobacterial dissemination. In this regard, an earlier study had reported an association between a low titer of serum IgG to LAM and an increased likelihood of disseminated tuberculosis in young children (21).

Effect of Killer Toxin-Like Antibodies on *M. tuberculosis*

An interesting application of antibodies that bind mycobacterial cells but are not elicited by mycobacterial epitopes was described by Conti et al. (20).

Both human natural antibodies and murine MAbs representing the internal image of a killer toxin originating from the yeast *Pichia anomala* were tested against *M. tuberculosis*. The killer toxin itself is inactive at physiological temperatures; however, killer toxin-like anti-idiotypic antibodies can mimic the activity of killer toxin at these temperatures. These antibodies work by binding to a putative receptor found in taxonomically unrelated microorganisms. The killer toxin-like antibodies were demonstrated to bind the surface of *M. tuberculosis*, and when incubated with a multidrug-resistant *M. tuberculosis* isolate, they caused a reduction in growth and CFU (20) (Table 1). These studies established that certain antibodies can mediate a direct effect against *M. tuberculosis*.

POTENTIAL MECHANISMS FOR ANTIBODY-MEDIATED IMMUNITY AGAINST *M. TUBERCULOSIS*

Although several studies in recent years support a role for antibody in host defense against *M. tubercu-*

losis, the mechanisms of antibody-mediated immunity against this pathogen are essentialy unknown. Several mechanisms by which certain antibodies could modify the outcome of infection are plausible (Fig. 1).

Interference with Adhesion

Adhesion of microbes to host tissues is a significant step in the colonization of the host and the establishment of infection. Antibodies to surface determinants of *M. tuberculosis* could interfere with the adhesion of mycobacteria to host cells. A study by Venisse et al. demonstrated that ManLAM from *M. bovis* BCG can bind to macrophages and granulocytes (104). Binding occurred either via the mannose receptors of macrophages or via mannan binding proteins in the serum, allowing selective uptake of mannosylated bacteria by granulocytes. Schlesinger et al. demonstrated that ManLAM from *M. tuberculosis* Erdman binds human macrophages via mannose receptors (84), and that preincubation of *M. tuberculosis* Erdman with MAb CS-40, a LAM binding MAb

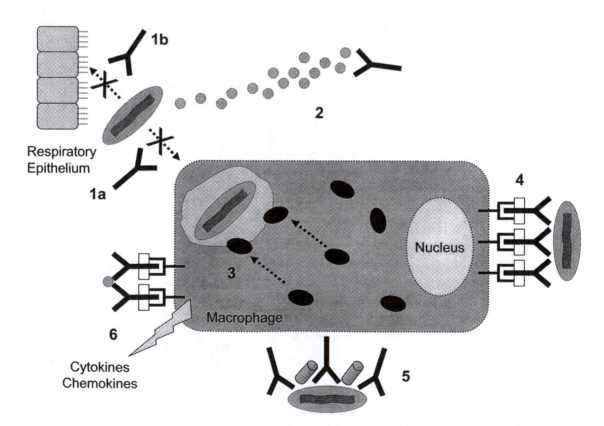

Figure 1. Schematic representation of a proposed mechanism for antibody-mediated immunity to *M. tuberculosis*. 1, Interference with adhesion to macrophages (1a) or respiratory epithelium (1b); 2, neutralization or clearance of mycobacterial antigens or toxins; 3, promotion of phagosome-lysosome fusion; 4, opsonization via Fc receptor; 5, complement activation; 6, effect on signal transduction with release of cytokines and chemokines.

(14), inhibited mycobacterial adherence (84). Also for *Mycobacterium leprae* and *Mycobacterium w,* specific antibody was shown to prevent attachment to macrophages and granulocytes (3, 16).

MAbs to HBHA, a surface-exposed glycoprotein involved in the binding of *M. tuberculosis* to epithelial cells (59), provide an interesting example in this regard (72). Intranasal administration of mycobacteria coated with the anti-HBHA MAbs 4057D2 (an IgG3 antibody) and 3921E4 (an IgG2a antibody) to mice was associated with reduced CFU in the spleen but not in the lungs (72), suggesting that anti-HBHA antibodies interfered with mycobacterial dissemination and thus with the outcome of infection, possibly by preventing adhesion to the epithelial cells.

Promotion of Phagosome-Lysosome Fusion

M. tuberculosis infection of phagocytic cells is thought to be associated with interference of phagosome-lysosomal fusion (2). Lysosomes contain microbicidal substances that could potentially kill or inhibit *M. tuberculosis*, and interference with phagosome-lysosomal fusion is a mechanism that can permit *M. tuberculosis* to survive and replicate inside macrophages. Armstrong and D'Arcy Hart demonstrated that antibody-mediated phagocytosis of mycobacteria promoted phagosome-lysosome fusion (2). This phenomenon, if it occurs in vivo, could enhance the microbicidal function of phagocytic cells.

Toxin Neutralization

The ability of antibodies to bind and neutralize harmful microbial products is a classic function of antibody-mediated immunity. Mycobacterial infection is associated with the release of microbial products that could potentially affect host immune function. Studies done in the preantibiotic era demonstrated that immune sera could protect experimental animals against the toxic effects of mycobacterial antigen preparations (25, 31, 46, 55, 103). This phenomenon was presumably due to the antibodies found in the immune sera, which bound to and neutralized mycobacterial toxins. ManLAM, a surface mycobacterial lipopolysaccharide, has been implicated in the immunopathogenesis of tuberculosis (64). Hence, antibodies directed to LAM that promote the clearance of this antigen may be beneficial to the host. In this regard, we have shown that a LAM binding MAb was able to enhance the clearance of LAM (35) from the serum. Specific antibody was also found to neutralize the toxic effects of cord factor (48, 49), which is known to exert important immunoregulatory effects on the innate and adaptive immune system (79).

Effect of Antibody on Cytokine Expression

An additional potential mechanism for antibody is the promotion of cytokine release through Fc receptor cross-linking. Hussain et al. examined the effect of antibodies to purified protein derivative (PPD) on modulation of the expression of tumor necrosis factor alpha (TNF-α) by monocytes (41). TNF-α is a proinflammatory cytokine involved in the host response to *M. tuberculosis* and the immunopathology of tuberculosis (13, 28, 41, 50, 77, 93). The secretion of TNF-α by PPD-stimulated monocytes from PPD skin test-negative donors was enhanced in the presence of heat-inactivated serum obtained from patients with pulmonary tuberculosis (41). TNF-α secretion directly correlated with the concentration in serum of IgG1 to PPD (Table 1), and adsorption of IgG1 from the serum samples led to reduction of TNF-α secretion (41). In another study by the same group, done with monocytes stimulated by protein fractions containing secreted antigens of *M. tuberculosis*, the investigators demonstrated that the presence of antigen-specific IgG1 was accompanied by enhanced production of the proinflammatory cytokines TNF-α and interleukin-6 and decreased production of the down-regulatory cytokine interleukin-10 (42). These studies suggest a potential role for certain antibodies in mediating a biological effect through cytokine release. They also imply that antibody specificity and subclass can be significant in mediating a specific biological effect in the context of mycobacterial infection.

Complement Activation

M. tuberculosis is not lysed by complement; however, it can use the complement system for cell entry. It can enter mononuclear phagocytes via complement receptors CR1, CR3, and CR4, and the complement system plays an important role in opsonization of mycobacteria prior to cell entry (reviewed in reference 82). Phagocytosis of *M. tuberculosis* by macrophages is enhanced in the presence of complement as a result of complement activation which leads to opsonization of the bacterium with the C3 products C3b and C3bi. Schlesinger and Horwitz demonstrated that natural antibody can mediate C3 fixation to *M. leprae* phenolic glycolipid-1 (PGL-1) through the classical complement pathway (83). Hetland et al. found that IgG directed to LAM from the serum of tuberculosis patients or rabbits can mediate classical complement activation induced by mycobacteria (39). It is therefore possible that antibody could alter the magnitude and fate of *M. tuberculosis* phagocytosis by mononuclear macrophages via the complement system and in this way could modify the outcome of *M. tuberculosis* infection to either the benefit or detriment of the host.

Other Mechanisms

Antibodies are multifunctional molecules that can play multiple roles in enhancing host defense and protection against pathogens (Fig. 1). In addition to the above-mentioned mechanisms, antibodies can serve as opsonins, mediate antibody-dependent cellular cytotoxicity, and possibly enhance antigen presentation. Antibodies may exert their effect independently or enhance and redirect cellular immune mechanisms against *M. tuberculosis*. An example of enhancement of cellular immunity by antibody was demonstrated by a study from our group showing that prolonged survival mediated by antibody was associated with improved granulomatous formation (98).

To date, none of the mechanisms discussed in this section have been directly associated with modifying the course of *M. tuberculosis* infection, but they remain potential mechanisms by which antibody-mediated immunity could affect the outcome of *M. tuberculosis* infection.

PROSPECTS FOR ANTIBODY-BASED VACCINES

The BCG vaccine, which has been used since the early 1920s, has been shown to protect children against disseminated tuberculosis. It does not, however, prevent pulmonary tuberculosis (12), which is the most common and contagious form of tuberculosis. In recent years major efforts have been directed toward the development of new vaccine candidates against *M. tuberculosis*. The vaccine candidates under development include live attenuated, subunit, and DNA vaccines (reviewed in reference 19). BCG and most vaccines in development are thought to confer protection to the host by enhancing cell-mediated immunity and controlling the replication of mycobacteria after the establishment of infection. This mechanism of protection differs from that of most vaccines presently used in humans, which confer protection by eliciting protective antibody responses that are thought to eliminate the infecting inoculum (78). *M. tuberculosis* is a facultative intracellular pathogen for which cell-mediated immunity is considered the primary immune response. For many decades, the predominant scientific view has been that antibodies play little or no role in the defense against *M. tuberculosis* infection. The observations summarized in this chapter challenge this dogma, and studies using MAbs provide supportive evidence for the view that

some antibodies to *M. tuberculosis* can be useful to the host. These developments could, in theory, be exploited for the development of a novel vaccine strategy against *M. tuberculosis*, based on eliciting a protective antibody response.

Vaccines presently used in humans belong to one of three main categories: inactivated, live attenuated, and subunit vaccines. The majority of these vaccines are thought to provide protection by eliciting protective antibody responses (78). Antibody responses, in turn, are used as surrogate markers to measure vaccine immunogenicity. Among the most successful antibacterial vaccines are the polysaccharide subunit vaccines. They include the *Haemophilus influenzae* type B vaccine, the *Streptococcus pneumoniae* vaccine, and, more recently the *Salmonella enterica* serovar Typhi and meningococcal serogroup C conjugate vaccines (57, 99). These vaccines contain the capsular polysaccharides of these pathogens, which, when used by themselves, are poorly immunogenic and elicit a T-cell-independent antibody response (53). However, conjugation of the polysaccharides to a protein carrier results in vaccines that elicit a T-cell-dependent antibody response to the polysaccharide antigen, allowing their use in young children, who do not develop effective T-cell-independent antibody responses (53). The *S. enterica* serovar Typhi conjugate vaccine provides a precedent for a polysaccharide conjugate vaccine that confers protection against a facultative intracellular pathogen by eliciting a protective antibody response. Polysaccharide conjugate vaccines offer several advantages: absence of virulence due to revertant strains or host immunosuppression, consistency in production, and a predictable immune response.

The primary consideration in attempting to develop a vaccine that will confer protection by eliciting a protective antibody response to *M. tuberculosis* is whether a protective antibody response can be elicited and, if so, which antigens should be chosen as components of such vaccine.

Studies using MAbs directed to AM and to the carbohydrate portion of LAM (35, 98) suggest that polysaccharide antigens, in particular, could elicit a protective antibody response. It is also worth noting that both MBP83 (the target for the protective MAb MBS43) (60) and HBHA (the target for MAbs 4057D2 and 3921E4) (72) are glycosylated.

To date, several polysaccharide conjugate vaccine candidates have been described, including vaccine candidates consisting of a LAM-derived oligosaccharide conjugated to tetanus toxoid (Fig. 2) or cross-reactive mutant (CRM197) diphtheria toxoid (37). LAM-derived oligosaccharides were also conjugated to antigen 85B (Ag85B) or a 75-kDa protein of *M. tuberculosis* (36). Our group has been studying vaccine candidates consisting of the capsular polysaccharides AM (34a) and glucan (86) conjugated to recombinant *Pseudomonas aeruginosa* exoprotein A (rEPA). These vaccine candidates were found to be immunogenic in animals, eliciting IgG responses (34a, 36, 37, 86). Vaccine candidates consisting of LAM-derived oligosaccharides were recently shown to enhance survival and prevent weight loss in mice infected intranasally or intravenously and guinea pigs infected by aerosol challenge with a virulent strain of *M. tuberculosis* (36). Our group demonstrated that mice immunized with an AM-rEPA conjugate vaccine had reduced organ CFU 7 days after infection with *M. tuberculosis* Erdman or *M. bovis* BCG, suggesting a beneficial effect of the polysaccharide conjugate vaccine. Interestingly, the effect was noted only early after infection, prior to the development of effective

cell-mediated immunity (34a). Although the effect was modest, the ability of the AM-rEPA conjugate vaccine to modify the course of infection provides encouragement for the continued investigation of this class of vaccines.

MAbs directed to HBHA provide an example of a beneficial effect provided by antibodies to a protein antigen (72), suggesting that protein antigens should also be considered candidates for developing vaccines that elicit a protective antibody response. Preliminary results showed that a vaccine candidate consisting of HBHA induced high antigen-specific antibody serum titers and led to CFU reduction in the lungs and spleens of mice infected with *M. tuberculosis* Erdman. The impact on CFU reduction was similar to that achieved by immunization with BCG (M. Parra, T. Pickett, G. Delogu, K. Pethe, F. D. Menozzi, C. Locht,

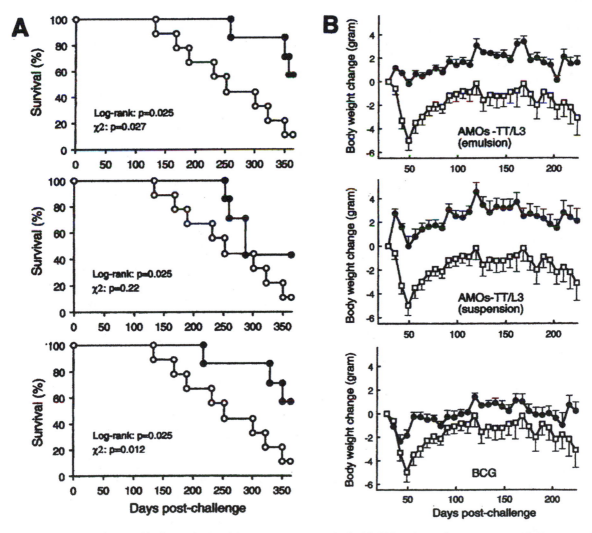

Figure 2. Survival (A) and body weight (B) of C57BL/6 mice immunized with AM conjugated to tetanus toxoid (TT) in L3 adjuvant emulsion (top panels) or suspension (middle panels), as compared to mice immunized with BCG (bottom panels) and infected intranasally with *M. tuberculosis* (10^5 CFU). Black symbols represent mice immunized with AM conjugate vaccine or BCG, and open symbols represent controls. Adapted from reference 36. © 2003 with permission from Elsevier.

and M. J. Brennan, *Fourth World Congr. Tuberculosis*, abstract, 2002). Since the administration of MAbs to HBHA was associated with a reduction of mycobacterial CFU in the spleen of mice infected intranasally (72), it is possible that the HBHA candidate vaccine can confer protection, at least in part, by inducing a beneficial antibody response.

The principal goal for a vaccine strategy against *M. tuberculosis* that relies on eliciting an antibody response is to prevent the development of disease, possibly by eliminating or containing the infecting inoculum. This approach differs from that of BCG and most other vaccines currently under investigation, which are thought to provide protection by enhancing cell-mediated immunity that controls mycobacterial replication after the establishment of tissue infection. Antibodies elicited by a vaccine may confer protection by one of several mechanisms, such as (i) opsonization of mycobacteria and promotion of phagocytosis and killing by alveolar macrophages, (ii) prevention of mycobacterial adherence and penetration into cells, (iii) neutralization of mycobacterial virulence factors, (iv) clearance of mycobacterial antigens, and (v) modification of the inflammatory responses by promoting changes in cytokine release through Fc receptor cross-linking (reviewed in reference 34).

Whether antibodies induced by a vaccine could function separately or in conjunction with cellular immunity is unclear. In this regard, the potential for antibodies to enhance the cell-mediated immune response was implied by our study demonstrating that MAb-treated mice demonstrated improved granuloma formation (98). Cell-mediated immunity may be important in eliminating mycobacteria that have escaped neutralization by antibody or modifying the activity of antibodies. It has been previously shown that the effect of antibody can depend on the host T cells (109). In the case of *C. neoformans*, for instance, it was demonstrated that in the absence of CD4$^+$ T cells or gamma interferon, protective MAbs were not effective. On the other hand, disease-enhancing MAbs became protective in mice depleted of CD8$^+$ lymphocytes (109). Hence, future studies will have to carefully examine the dependence of antibody-mediated efficacy against *M. tuberculosis* on T-cell function in hosts with deficient T-cell function.

SUMMARY

The available data strongly suggest that certain antibodies can favorably affect the course of infection if they are present at the time and site of mycobacterial infection (12a, 35, 72, 98). Although the effect of natural antibodies on the course of *M. tuberculosis* infection is unclear, the available evidence indicates that it is feasible to generate protective antibodies to *M. tuberculosis*. However, the conditions for optimal antibody function against mycobacterial infections is poorly understood. In this regard, the importance of antibody specificity, isotype, delivery, affinity, and concentration, as well as the need to use several antibodies, must be carefully explored. The surface of *M. tuberculosis* is dynamic, as shown, for example, by the changes in expression of AM over time (85); it is conceivable that different types of antibodies may be required at different stages of infection and disease. The presence of antibodies at the site of infection, prior to *M. tuberculosis* entry into cells, may be of particular importance to the fate of infection. This can potentially be accomplished by antibody passage from serum to the respiratory tract or by induction of mucosal antibodies by vaccination. In this respect, an IgG1 MAb to *C. neoformans* administered intraperitoneally was found in bronchoalveolar washings and protected mice against intratracheal infection with *C. neoformans* (30). In addition, IgG MAbs to surface proteins of *M. tuberculosis*, administered intravenously, were found in lung lavage fluid of mice shortly after administration (29). Overall, the evidence demonstrates that MAbs can have a beneficial effect on different aspects of mycobacterial infection such as prolongation of survival (12a, 98), CFU reduction (107a), prevention of dissemination (72), and clearance of polysaccharide (35). These data suggest a potential advantage of using several MAbs to optimize the beneficial effect of antibody-mediated immunity on the course of infection. This concept may be of particular importance with respect to the modulation experienced by the mycobacterial surface during growth (85).

The progress made in recent years is encouraging and should stimulate interest in evaluating the mechanisms by which antibodies may contribute to host defense against *M. tuberculosis*. Antibodies may also be important in immunocompromised hosts with poor cell-mediated immunity. The evidence that antibodies can, in certain circumstances, modify the outcome of *M. tuberculosis* infection to benefit the host suggests that it may be possible to identify conditions that will magnify protection. The future challenges are to systematically dissect the conditions required for optimal antibody-mediated immunity against *M. tuberculosis* and to develop vaccine candidates that will work by eliciting protective antibody responses.

REFERENCES

1. **Andersen, P.** 1997. Host responses and antigens involved in protective immunity to *Mycobcterium tuberculosis*. *Scand. J. Immunol.* **45**:115–131.

2. **Armstrong, J. A., and P. D. Hart.** 1975. Phagosome-lysosome interactions in cultured macrophages infected with virulent tubercle bacilli. *J. Exp. Med.* **142:**1–16.

3. **Band, H., S. Sinha, and G. P. Talwar.** 1987. Inhibition of interaction of mycobacteria with Schwann cells by antimycobacterial antibodies. *J. Neuroimmunol.* **14:**235–239.

4. **Barrera, L., I. de Kantor, V. Ritacco, A. Reniero, B. Lopez, J. Benetucci, M. Beltran, O. Libonatti, E. Padula, J. Castagnino, and L. Gonzalez Montaner.** 1992. Humoral response to *Mycobacterium tuberculosis* in patients with human immunodeficiency virus infection. *Tubercle Lung Dis.* **73:**187–191.

5. **Bluhm, I.** 1952. The influence of immune and normal human serum on the respiration of tubercle bacilli. *Acta Med. Scand. Suppl.* **275:**1–28.

6. **Bosio, C. M., D. Gardner, and K. L. Elkins.** 2003. Infection of B cell-deficient mice with CDC 1551, a clinical isolate of *Mycobacterium tuberculosis*: delay in dissemination and development of lung pathology. *J. Immunol.* **164:**6417–6425.

7. **Buttery, J., and E. R. Moxon.** 2002. Capsulate bacteria and the lung. *Br. Med. Bull.* **61:**63–80.

8. **Calmette, A.** 1923. Passive immunity: attempts at antituberculous serotherapy, p. 603–612. In *Tubercle Bacillus Infection and Tuberculosis in Man and Animals.* The Williams & Wilkins Co., Baltimore, Md.

9. **Casadevall, A.** 2003. Antibody-mediated immunity against intracellular pathogens: two-dimentional thinking comes full circle. *Infect. Immun.* **71:**4225–4228.

10. **Casadevall, A., and M. D. Scharff.** 1994. Serum therapy revisited: animal models of infection and development of passive antibody therapy. *Antimicrob. Agents Chemother.* **38:**1695–1702.

11. **Casadevall, A., and M. D. Scharff.** 1995. Return to the past: the case for antibody-based therapies in infectious diseases. *Clin. Infect. Dis.* **21:**150–161.

12. **Centers for Disease Control and Prevention.** 1996. The role of BCG vaccine in the prevention and control of tuberculosis in the United States. A joint statement by the Advisory Council for the Elimination of Tuberculosis and the Advisory Committee on Immunization Practices. *Morb. Mortal. Wkly. Rep.* **45:**1–18.

12a. **Chambers, M. A., D. Gavier-Widén, and R. G. Hewinson.** 2004. Antibody bound to the surface antigen MPB83 of *Mycobacterium bovis* enhances survival against high dose and low dose challenge. *FEMS Immunol. Med. Microbiol.* **41:**93–100.

13. **Chan, J., and S. H. E. Kaufmann.** 1994. Immune mechanism of protection, p. 389–415. In B. R. Barry (ed.), *Tuberculosis. Pathogenesis, Protection, and Control.* ASM Press, Washington, D.C.

14. **Chatterjee, D., K. Lowell, B. Rivoire, M. R. McNeil, and P. J. Brennan.** 1992. Lipoarabinomannan of *Mycobacterium tuberculosis*. Capping with mannosyl residues in some strains. *J. Biol. Chem.* **267:**6234–6239.

15. **Choucroun, N.** 1949. Precipitin test for carbohydrate antibodies in human tuberculosis. *Am. Rev. Tuberc.* **59:**710–712.

16. **Choudhury, A., N. F. Mistry, and N. H. Antia.** 1989. Blocking of *Mycobacterium leprae* adherence to dissociated Schwann cells by anti-mycobacterial antibodies. *Scand. J. Immunol.* **30:**505–509.

17. **Clawson, B. J.** 1936. The destruction of tubercle bacilli within phagocytes in vitro. *J. Infect. Dis.* **58:**64–69.

18. **Collins, F. M.** 1991. Antituberculous immunity: new solutions to an old problem. *Rev. Infect. Dis.* **13:**940–950.

19. **Collins, H. L., and S. H. E. Kaufmann.** 2001. Prospects for better tuberculosis vaccines. *Lancet Infect. Dis.* **1:**21–28.

20. **Conti, S., F. Fanti, W. Magliani, M. Gerloni, D. Bertolotti, A. Salati, A. Cassone, and L. Polonelli.** 1998. Mycobactericidal activity of human natural, monoclonal, and recombinant yeast killer toxin-like antibodies. *J. Infect. Dis.* **177:**807–811.

21. **Costello, A. M., A. Kumar, V. Narayan, M. S. Akbar, S. Ahmed, C. Abou-Zeid, G. A. W. Rook, J. Stanford, and C. Moreno.** 1992. Does antibody to mycobacterial antigens, including lipoarabinomannan, limit dissemination in childhood tuberculosis? *Trans. R. Soc. Trop. Med. Hyg.* **86:**686–692.

22. **Da Costa, C. T. K. A., S. Khanolkar-Young, A. M. Elliott, K. M. A. Wasunna, and K. P. W. J. McAdam.** 1993. Immunoglobulin G subclass responses to mycobacterial lipoarabinomannan in HIV-infected and non-infected patients with tuberculosis. *Clin. Exp. Immunol.* **91:**25–29.

23. **Daffe, M., and P. Draper.** 1998. The envelope layers of mycobacteria with reference to their pathogenicity. *Adv. Microb. Physiol.* **39:**131–203.

24. **Daniel, T. M., M. J. Oxtoby, E. M. Pinto, and E. S. Moreno.** 1981. The immune spectrum in patients with pulmonary tuberculosis. *Am. Rev. Respir. Dis.* **123:**556–559.

25. **De Schweinitz, E. A. and M. Dorset.** 1897. Some products of the tuberculosis bacillus and the treatment of experimental tuberculosis with antitoxic serum. *N. Y. Med. J.* **66:**105–111.

26. **Dunlap, N. E., and D. E. Briles.** 1993. Immunology of tuberculosis. *Med. Clin. North Am.* **77:**1235–1251.

27. **Emmart, E. W., and F. B. Seibert.** 1945. The effect of tuberculous and sensitized sera and serum fractions on the development of tubercles in the chorio-allantoic membrane of the chick. *J. Immunol.* **50:**143–160.

28. **Engele, M., E. Stossel, K. Castiglione, N. Schwerdtner, M. Wagner, P. Bolcskei, M. Rollinghoff, and S. Stenger.** 2002. Induction of TNF in human alveolar macrophages as a potential evasion mechanism of virulent *Mycobacterium tuberculosis*. *J. Immunol.* **168:**1328–1337.

29. **Falero-Diaz, G., S. Challacombe, D. Rahman, M. Mistry, G. Douce, G. Dougan, A. Acosta, and J. Ivanyi.** 2000. Transmission of IgA and IgG monoclonal antibodies to mucosal fluids following intranasal or parenteral delivery. *Int. Arch. Allergy Immunol.* **122:**143–150.

30. **Feldmesser, M., and A. Casadevall.** 1997. Effect of serum IgG1 to *Cryptococcus neoformans* glucuronoxylomannan on murine pulmonary infection. *J. Immunol.* **158:**790–799.

31. **Fisch, C.** 1897. The antitoxic and bactericidal properties of the serum of horses treated with Koch's new tuberculin. *JAMA* **29:**882–889.

32. **Forget, A., J. C. Benoit, R. Turcotte, and N. Gusew-Chartrand.** 1976. Enhancement activity of anti-mycobacterial sera in experimental *Mycobacterium bovis* (BCG) infection in mice. *Infect. Immun.* **13:**1301–1306.

33. **Glatman-Freedman, A.** 2003. Advances in antibody-mediated immunity against *Mycobacterium tuberculosis*: implications for a novel vaccine strategy. *FEMS Immunol. Med. Microbiol.* **39:**9–16.

34. **Glatman-Freedman, A., and A. Casadevall.** 1998. Serum therapy for tuberculosis revisited: reappraisal of the role of antibody-mediated immunity against *Mycobacterium tuberculosis*. *Clin. Microbiol. Rev.* **11:**514–532.

34a. **Glatman-Freedman, A., A. Casadevall, Z. Dai, W. R. Jacobs, Jr., A. Li, S. L. Morris, J. A. Navoa, S. Piperdi, J. B. Robbins, R. Schneerson, J. R. Schwebach, and M. Shapiro.** 2004. Antigenic evidence of prevalence and diversity of *Mycobacterium tuberculosis* arabinomannan. *J. Clin. Microbiol.* **42:**3225–3231.

35. **Glatman-Freedman, A., A. J. Mednick, N. Lendvai, and A. Casadevall.** 2000. Clearance and organ distribution of *Mycobacterium tuberculosis* lipoarabinomannan (LAM) in the presence and absence of LAM-binding IgM. *Infect. Immun.* **68:**335–341.

36. Hamasur, B., M. Haile, A. Pawlowski, U. Schroder, A. Williams, G. Hatch, G. Hall, P. Marsh, G. Kallenius, and S. B. Svenson. 2003. *Mycobacterium tuberculosis* arabino-mannan-protein conjugates protect against tuberculosis. *Vaccine* **21**:4081–4093.

37. Hamasur, B., G. Kallenius, and S. B. Svenson. 1999. Synthesis and immunologic characterization of *Mycobacterium tuberculosis* lipoarabinomannan specific oligosaccharide-protein conjugates. *Vaccine* **17**:2853–2861.

38. Hayden, A. M. 1896. Report of results and recoveries obtained by the use of anti-tubercle serum. *JAMA* **26**:965–966.

39. Hetland, G., H. G. Wiker, K. Hogasen, B. Hamasur, S. B. Svenson, and M. Harboe. 1998. Involvement of antilipoarabinomannan antibodies in classical complement activation in tuberculosis. *Clin. Diagn. Lab. Immunol.* **5**:211–218.

40. Holmes, A. M. 1899. A further report on the use of "antiphthisic serum T.R." (Fisch) in tuberculosis. *JAMA* **33**:886–888.

41. Hussain, R., H. Shiratsuchi, J. J. Ellner, and R. S. Wallis. 2000. PPD-specific IgG1 antibody subclass upregulate tumor necrosis factor expression in PPD-stimulated monocytes: possible link with disease pathogenesis in tuberculosis. *Clin. Exp. Immunol.* **119**:449–455.

42. Hussain, R., H. Shiratsuchi, M. Phillips, J. J. Ellner, and R. S. Wallis. 2001. Opsonizing antibodies (IgG1) upregulate monocyte proinflammatory cytokines tumour necrosis factor-alpha (TNF-α) and IL-6 but not anti-inflammatory cytokine IL-10 in mycobacterial antigen-stimulated monocytes—implications for pathogenesis. *Clin. Exp. Immunol.* **123**:210–218.

43. Johnson, C. M., A. M. Cooper, A. A. Frank, C. B. C. Bonorino, L. J. Wysoki, and I. M. Orme. 1997. *Mycobacterium tuberculosis* aerogenic rechallenge infections in B cell-deficient mice. *Tubercle Lung. Dis.* **78**:257–261.

44. Josset, A. 1924. Les conditions de succes de la serotherapie antituberculeuse chez l'homme. *Bull. Mem. Soc. Medi. Hop. Paris* **40**:923–939.

45. Josset, A. 1924. Seize année de serotherapie antituberculeuse. *Bull. Mem. Soc. Med. Hop. Paris* **40**:777–781.

46. Josset, A. 1924. Resultats experimentaux de la serotherapie antituberculeuse. *Bull. Mem. Soc. Hop. Paris* **40**:826–831.

47. Kardito, T., and J. M. Grange. 1980. Immunological and clinical features of smear-positive pulmonary tuberculosis in East Java. *Tubercle* **61**:231–238.

48. Kato, M. 1972. Antibody formation to trehalose-6,6'-dimycolate (cord factor) of *Mycobacterium tuberculosis*. *Infect. Immun.* **5**:203–212.

49. Kato, M. 1974. Further study on neutralization of biochemical activity of cord factor by anti-cord factor antibody. *Infect. Immun.* **10**:277–279.

50. Kisich, K. O., M. Higgins, G. Diamond, and L. Heifets. 2002. Tumor necrosis factor alpha stimulates killing of *Mycobacterium tuberculosis* by human neutrophils. *Infect. Immun.* **70**:4591–4599.

51. Lemen, J. R. 1898. Three years of serum therapy in tuberculosis. *N. Y. Med. J.* **67**:672–677.

52. Lenzini, L., P. Rottoli, and L. Rottoli. 1977. The spectrum of human tuberculosis. *Clin. Exp. Immunol.* **27**:230–237.

53. Lesinski, G. B. and M. A. Westerink. 2001. Vaccines against polysaccharide antigens. *Curr. Drug Targets Infect. Disorders* **1**:325–334.

54. Macpherson, A. J. S., A. Lamarre, K. McCoy, G. R. Harriman, B. Odermatt, G. Dougan, H. Hengartner, and R. M. Zinkernagel. 2001. IgA production without mu or delta chain expression in developing B cells. *Nat. Immunol.* **2**:625–631.

55. Maragliano, C. 1896. Le serum antituberculeux et son antitoxine. *Rev. Tuberc.* **1896**:131–138.

56. Maragliano, E. 1896. Premiere statistique du traitement de la tuberculose par la serum Maragliano. *Rev. Tuberc.* **1896**:156–157.

57. Marchant, C. D. and M. L. Kumar. 2002. Immunizations, p. 232–262. *In* H. B. Jenson and R. S. Baltimore (ed.), *Pediatric Infectious Diseases: Principles and Practices*. The W. B. Saunders Co., Philadelphia, Pa.

58. Marmorek, A. 1903. Antituberculous serum and "vaccine." *Lancet* **ii**:1642–1645.

59. Menozzi, F. D., J. H. Rouse, M. Alavi, M. Laude-Sharp, J. Muller, R. Bischoff, M. J. Brennan, and C. Locht. 1996. Identification of a heparin-binding hemagglutinin present in mycobacteria. *J. Exp. Med.* **184**:993–1001.

60. Michell, S. L., A. O. Whelan, P. R. Wheeler, M. Panico, R. L. Easton, A. T. Etienne, S. M. Haslam, A. Dell, H. R. Morris, A. J. Reason, J. L. Herrmann, D. B. Young, and R. G. Hewinson. 2003. The MPB83 antigen from *Mycobacteium bovis* contains O-linked mannose and (1→3) mannobiose moieties. *J. Biol. Chem.* **278**:16423–16432.

61. Mukherjee, J., G. Nussbaum, M. D. Scharff, and A. Casadevall. 1995. Protective and nonprotective monoclonal antibodies to *Cryptococcus neoformans* originating from one B cell. *J. Exp. Med.* **181**:405–409.

62. Mukherjee, J., M. D. Scharff, and A. Casadevall. 1992. Protective murine monoclonal antibodies to *Cryptococcus neoformans*. *Infect. Immun.* **60**:4534–4541.

63. Mukherjee, S., S. C. Lee, and A. Casadevall. 1995. Antibodies to *Cryptococcus neoformans* glucuronoxylomannan enhance antifungal activity of murine macrophages. *Infect. Immun.* **63**:573–579.

64. Nigou, J., M. Gilleron, M. Rojas, L. F. Garcia, M. Thurnher, and G. Puzo. 2002. Mycobacterial lipoarabinomannans: modulators of dendritic cell function and the apoptotic response. *Microbes Infect.* **4**:945–953.

65. Nussbaum, G., W. Cleare, A. Casadevall, M. D. Scharff, and P. Valdom. 1997. Epitope location in the *Cryptococcus neoformans* capsule is a determinant of antibody efficacy. *J. Exp. Med.* **185**:685–694.

66. Nussbaum, G., R. Yuan, A. Casadevall, and M. D. Scharff. 1996. Immunoglobulin G3 blocking antibodies to the fungal pathogen *Cryptococcus neoformans*. *J. Exp. Med.* **183**:1905–1909.

67. Paquin, P. 1895. The treatment of tuberculosis by injections of immunized blood serum. *JAMA* **24**:842–845.

68. Paquin, P. 1895. Anti tubercle serum. *JAMA* **24**:341–346.

69. Paquin, P. 1897. Further report of cases treated with anti-tubercle serum. *JAMA* **29**:98–99.

70. Paquin, P. 1898. How we treat consumption today. *JAMA* **30**:294–299.

71. Peterson, J. C., R. Langercranz, S. I. Rollof, and J. Lind. 1952. Tuberculin hemmagglutination studies in active tuberculosis infections, benign and virulent. *Acta Paediatr.* **41**:57–73.

72. Pethe, K., S. Alonso, F. Biet, G. Delogu, M. J. Brennan, C. Locht, and F. D. Menozzi. 2001. The heparin-binding haemagglutinin of *M. tuberculosis* is required for extrapulmonary dissemination. *Nature* **412**:190–194.

73. Prioleau, W. H. 1898. Antitubercle serum (Paquin) in tuberculosis. *JAMA* **31**:687–688.

74. Raffel, S. 1946. The relationship of acquired resistance, allergy, antibodies and tissue reactivities to the components of the tubercle bacillus. *Am. Rev. Tuberc.* **54**:564–573.

75. Reggiardo, Z., and G. Middlebrook. 1974. Failure of passive serum transfer of immunity against aerogenic tuberculosis in rabbits. *Proc. Soc. Exp. Biol. Med.* **145**:173–175.

76. Reiss, F., G. Szilagyi, and E. Mayer. 1975. Immunological studies of anticryptococcal factor of normal human serum. *Mycopathologia* 55:175–178.

77. Roach, D. R., A. G. Bean, C. Demangel, M. P. France, H. Briscoe, and W. J. Britton. 2002. TNF regulates chemokine induction essential for cell recruitment, granuloma formation, and clearance of mycobacterial infection. *J. Immunol.* 168:4620–4627.

78. Robbins, J. B., R. Schneerson, and S. C. Szu. 1996. Hypothesis: how licenced vaccines confer protective immunity. *Adv. Exp. Med. Biol.* 397:169–182.

79. Ryll, R., Y. Kumazawa, and I. Yano. 2001. Immunological properties of trehalose dimycolate (cord factor) and other mycolic acid-containing glycolipids—a review. *Microbiol. Immunol.* 45:801–811.

80. Sanchez-Rodriguez, C., C. Estrada-Chavez, J. Garcia-Vigil, F. Laredo-Sanchez, J. Halabe-Cherem, A. Pereira-Suarez, and R. Mancilla. 2002. An IgG antibody response to the antigen 85 complex is associated with good outcome in Mexican Totonaca Indians with pulmonary tuberculosis. *Int. J. Tuberc. Lung Dis.* 6:706–712.

81. Sanford, J. E., D. M. Lupan, A. M. Schlageter, and T. R. Kozel. 1990. Passive immunization against *Cryptococcus neoformans* with an isotype-switch family of monoclonal antibodies reactive with cryptococcal polysaccharide. *Infect. Immun.* 58:1919–1923.

82. Schlesinger, L. S. 1998. *Mycobacterium tuberculosis* and the complement system. *Trends Microbiol.* 6:47–49.

83. Schlesinger, L. S., and M. A. Horwitz. 1991. Phenolic glycolipid-1 of *Mycobacterium leprae* binds complement component C3 in serum and mediates phagocytosis by human monocytes. *J. Exp. Med.* 174:1031–1038.

84. Schlesinger, L. S., S. R. Hull, and T. M. Kaufman. 1994. Binding of the terminal mannosyl units of lipoarabinomannan from a virulent strain of *Mycobacterium tuberculosis* to human macrophages. *J. Immunol.* 152:4070–4079.

85. Schwebach, J. R., A. Casadevall, R. Schneerson, Z. Dai, X. Wang, J. B. Robbins, and A. Glatman-Freedman. 2001. Expression of a *Mycobacterium tuberculosis* arabinomannan antigen in vitro and in vivo. *Infect. Immun.* 69:5671–5678.

86. Schwebach, J. R., A. Glatman-Freedman, L. Gunter-Cummins, Z. Dai, J. R. Robbins, R. Schneerson, and A. Casadevall. 2002. Glucan is a component of the *Mycobacterium tuberculosis* surface that is expressed in vitro and in vivo. *Infect. Immun.* 70:2566–2575.

87. Seibert, F. B. 1956. The significance of antigen-antibody reactions in tuberculosis. *J. Infect. Dis.* 99:76–83.

88. Seibert, F. B. 1958. The interplay of an immune substance with tuberculopolysaccharide and its antibody in tuberculosis. *J. Infect. Dis.* 103:52–60.

89. Seibert, F. B., E. E. Miller, U. Buseman, M. V. Seibert, E. Soto-Figueroa, and L. Fry. 1956. The significance of antibodies to tuberculoprotein and polysaccharide in resistance to tuberculosis. *Am. Rev. Tuberc. Pulm. Dis.* 73:547–562.

90. Seibert, F. B., and J. W. Nelson. 1943. Proteins of tuberculin. *J. Am. Chem. Soc.* 65:272–278.

91. Seibert, F. B., and M. V. Seibert. 1957. Relationship between immunity and circulating antibodies, complement and tuberculopolysaccharide in tuberculosis. *J. Infect. Dis.* 101:109–118.

92. Shropshire, L. L. 1896. A limited experience with the Paul Paquin antitubercle serum. *N. Y. Med. J.* 63:15–16.

93. Smith, S., D. Liggitt, E. Jeromsky, X. Tan, S. J. Skerrett, and C. B. Wilson. 2002. Local role for tumor necrosis factor alpha in the pulmonary inflammatory response to *Mycobacterium tuberculosis* infection. *Infect. Immun.* 70:2082–2089.

94. Snider, D. E., M. Raviglione, and A. Kochi. 1994. Global burden of tuberculosis, p. 3–11. *In* B. R. Bloom (ed.), *Tuberculosis. Pathogenesis, Protection, and Control.* ASM Press, Washington, D.C.

95. Spahlinger, H. 1922. Note on the treatment of tuberculosis. *Lancet* i:5–8.

96. Strohmeier, G. R., and M. J. Fenton. 1999. Roles of lipoarabinomannan in the pathogenesis of tuberculosis. *Microbes Infect.* 1:709–717.

97. Stubbert, J. E. 1898. Some statistics upon sero-therapy in tuberculosis. *Trans. Am. Climatol. Assoc.* 14:214–230.

98. Teitelbaum, R., A. Glatman-Freedman, B. Chen, J. B. Robbins, E. Unanue, A. Casadevall, and B. R. Bloom. 1998. A mAb recognizing a surface antigen of *Mycobacterium tuberculosis* enhances host survival. *Proc. Natl. Acad. Sci. USA* 95:15688–15693.

99. Trotter, C. L., M. E. Ramsay, and E. B. Kaczmarski. 2002. Meningococcal serogroup C conjugate vaccination in England and Wales: coverage and initial impact of the campaign. *Commun. Dis. Public Health* 5:220–225.

100. Trudeau, E. L., and E. R. Baldwin. 1898. Experimental studies on the preparation and effects of antitoxins for tuberculosis. *Am. J. Med. Sci.* 116:692–707.

101. Trudeau, E. L., and E. R. Baldwin. 1899. Experimental studies on the preparation and effects of antitoxins for tuberculosis. *Am. J. Med. Sc.* 117:56–76.

102. Tsuji, S., K. Ito, and S. Oshima. 1957. The role of humoral factors in native and acquired resistance to tuberculosis. *Am. Rev. Tuberc. Pulm. Dis.* 76:90–102.

103. Vallee, H. 1909. Sur le proprietes du serum du cheval hyperimmunise contre la tuberculose a l'aide de bacilles humains virulents. *C. R. Hebd. Seances Soc. Biol.* 67:700–702.

104. Venisse, A., J. J. Fournie, and G. Puzo. 1995. Mannosylated lipoarabinomannan interacts with phagocytes. *Eur. J. Biochem.* 231:440–447.

105. Vordermeier, H. M., N. Venkataprasad, D. P. Harris, and J. Ivanyi. 1996. Increase of tuberculous infection in the organs of B cell-deficient mice. *Clin. Exp. Immunol.* 106:312–316.

106. Wiker, H. G., K. P. Lyashchenko, A. M. Aksoy, K. A. Lightbody, J. M. Pollock, S. V. Komissarenko, S. O. Bobrovnik, I. N. Kolesnikova, L. O. Mykhalsky, M. L. Gennaro, and M. Harboe. 1998. Immunochemical characterization of the MPB70/80 and MPB83 proteins of *Mycobacterium bovis*. *Infect. Immun.* 66:1445–1452.

107. Wiker, H. G., S. Nagai, R. G. Hewinson, W. P. Russell, and M. Harboe. 1996. Heterogenenous Expression of related MBP 70 and MPB 83 proteins distinguish various substrains of *Mycobacterium bovis* BCG and *Mycobacterium tuberculosis* H37Rv. *Scand. J. Immunol.* 43:374–380.

107a. Williams, A., R. Reljic, I. Naylor, S. O. Clark, G. Falero-Diaz, M. Singh, S. Challacombe, P. O. Marsh, and J. Ivanyi. 2004. Passive protection with immunoglobulin A antibodies against tuberculous early infection of the lung. *Immunology* 111:328–333.

108. Yuan, R., A. Casadevall, G. Spira, and M. D. Scharff. 1995. Isotype switching from IgG3 to IgG1 converts a nonprotective murine antibody to *Cryptococcus neoformans* into a protective antibody. *J. Immunol.* 154:1810–1816.

109. Yuan, R. R., A. Casadevall, J. Oh, and M. D. Scharff. 1997. T cells cooperate with passive antibody to modify *Cryptococcus neoformans* infection in mice. *Proc. Natl. Acad. Sci. USA* 94:2483–2488.

110. Zitrin, C. M., and O. Wasz-Höckert. 1957. Preliminary experiments on passive transfer of protective humoral antibodies in tuberculosis. *Am. Rev. Tuberc. Pulm. Dis.* 76:256–262.

Tuberculosis and the Tubercle Bacillus
Edited by Stewart T. Cole et al.
© 2005 ASM Press, Washington, D.C.

Chapter 33

The PE and PPE Multigene Families of Mycobacteria

MICHAEL J. BRENNAN, NICO C. GEY VAN PITTIUS, AND CLARA ESPITIA

Epidemiologists searching for new molecular tools to compare strains and to differentiate between species of mycobacteria first recognized an abundance of genes containing the repetitive sequences -CGGCGGCAA- and -GCCGGTGTTG- within the genomes of pathogenic mycobacteria (22, 39). In this genomic era, we now recognize that the redundant polymorphic GC-rich repetitive sequence (PGRS) present in *Mycobacterium tuberculosis* and other mycobacteria belongs to the subfamily of PE_PGRS genes present in the PE multigene family (18). The other class of repetitive sequences, the major polymorphic tandem repeat (MPTR) (37), is found in the genes belonging to the PPE multigene family. The PE and PPE gene families are two copious multigene families of unknown function, comprising around 10% of the genome of *M. tuberculosis* and containing 100 and 70 members, respectively, in the genome of the laboratory strain H37Rv. The reason for the extensive genomic redundancy in the PE and PPE families remains a mystery but is also a focus for interesting scientific debate and speculation (7, 9, 16). The preservation of these extensive gene families implies that they are critical for the survival of *M. tuberculosis* and other mycobacteria at some stage in the life cycle of these organisms.

In this chapter, we review what is known about the expression, function, and immunological response to the PE, PE_PGRS, and PPE genes. Table 1 includes a list of the currently recognized PE, PE_PGRS, and PPE genes found in the laboratory strain *M. tuberculosis* H37Rv (18) and in the *M. tuberculosis* clinical isolate CDC 1551 (31). For the *M. tuberculosis* H37Rv strains, both the original Rv numbers and the more recently revised gene numbers based on the reannotation of the PE, PE_PGRS, and PPE gene families (12) are provided. An effort has been made to accurately compare the corresponding genes found in the genomes

of both *M. tuberculosis* H37Rv and *M. tuberculosis* CDC 1551, but because of continuing reevaluation of the genomes, the websites http://genolist.pasteur.fr/Tuberculist/and http://www.tigr.org/should be consulted for more complete information.

PE MULTIGENE FAMILY

The decoding of the genome of the *M. tuberculosis* laboratory strain H37Rv identified almost 100 novel genes distributed throughout the genome, encoding proteins with significant homology within the first ~100 amino acids. Typically this domain has a Pro-Glu (PE) sequence at residues 8 and 9 relative to the N terminus, which has been used to name this group of genes (Fig. 1A). About 37 of these genes (PE genes) consist of open reading frames (ORFs) whose products average ~110 amino acids in size, with some as small as 28 amino acids (Rv3018A) and others as large as 588 amino acids (Rv0151c). A large subfamily of genes, ~63 in *M. tuberculosis* H37Rv, encode products with a novel Gly-Ala rich domain linked to the PE domain containing numerous repeats of -GGA- and -GGN- residues. The polymorphic GC-rich repetitive sequence (PGRS) acronym has been used to describe this Gly-Ala rich domain, and so the name "PE_PGRS" is used for members of this subfamily (18). Remarkably, the largest of these genes, *Rv3508*, encodes a protein of 1,901 amino acids, containing 960 glycine residues and 88 -GGAGGX- repeats. A few members of this family also exist which contain heterogeneous sequences linked to PE or PE_PGRS sequences (Fig. 1A). An example of this has been noted by Adindla and Guruprasad (3), who have identified AB-type repeats at the C termini of the products of two PE_PGRS genes (Rv0978c and

---

Michael J. Brennan • Center for Biologics Evaluation and Research, Food and Drug Administration, Bldg. 29, Rm. 503, 29 Lincoln Dr. (HFM-431), Bethesda, MD 20892. **Nico C. Gey van Pittius** • US/MRC Centre for Molecular and Cellular Biology, Department of Medical Biochemistry, Faculty of Health Sciences, Stellenbosch University, P.O. Box 19063/Francie van Zijl Drive, Tygerberg 7505, South Africa. **Clara Espitia** • Departamento de Inmunología, Instituto de Investigaciones Biomédicas, Universidad Nacional Autónoma de México, Apartado Postal 7022804510, México D.F., México.

Table 1. PE, PE_PGRS, and PPE genes present in *M. tuberculosis* strains H37Rv and CDC 1551[a]

H37Rv gene	PE, PE_PGRS, or PPE no.	CDC 1551 gene	H37Rv gene	PE, PE_PGRS, or PPE no.	CDC 1551 gene
Rv0151	PE1	*MT0160*	*Rv1441c*	PE_PGRS26	*MT1486*
Rv0152c	PE2	*MT0161*	*Rv1450c*	PE_PGRS27	*MT1497.1*
Rv0159c	PE3	*MT0168*	*Rv1452c*	PE_PGRS28	*MT1499*
Rv0160c	PE4	*MT0169*	*Rv1468c*	PE_PGRS29	*MT1514.1*
Rv0285	PE5	*MT0298*	*Rv1651c*	PE_PGRS30	*MT1689*
Rv0335c	PE6	*MT0349*	*Rv1759c*	wag22	*MT1807*
Rv0916c	PE7/MTB10	*MT0941*	*Rv1768*	PE_PGRS31	*MT1818*
Rv1040c	PE8	*MT1069*	*Rv1803c*	PE_PGRS32	*MT1853*
Rv1088	PE9	*MT1119*	*Rv1818c*	PE_PGRS33	*MT1866*
Rv1089	PE10	*MT1120*	*Rv1840c*	PE_PGRS34	*MT1888*
Rv1169c	PE11	*MT1206*	*Rv1983*	PE_PGRS35	*MT2036*
Rv1172c	PE12	*MT1209*	*Rv2098c*[b]	PE_PGRS36	*MT2159*
Rv1195	PE13	*MT1233*	*Rv2126c*	PE_PGRS37	*MT2185.1*
Rv1214c	PE14	*MT1252*	*Rv2162c*	PE_PGRS38	*MT2220*
Rv1386	PE15	*MT1430*	*Rv2340*	PE_PGRS39	*MT2404*
Rv1430	PE16	*MT1474*	*Rv2371*	PE_PGRS40	*MT2440*
Rv1646	PE17	*MT1684*	*Rv2396*	PE_PGRS41	*MT2467.1*
Rv1788	PE18	*MT1837*	*Rv2487c*	PE_PGRS42	*MT2561*
Rv1791	PE19	*MT1840*	*Rv2490c*	PE_PGRS43	*MT2564*
Rv1806	PE20	*MT1855*	*Rv2591*	PE_PGRS44	*MT2668.1*
Rv2099c[b]	PE21	*MT2159*	*Rv2615c*	PE_PGRS45	*MT2690*
Rv2107	PE22	*MT2166*	*Rv2634c*	PE_PGRS46	*MT2712*
Rv2328	PE23	*MT2390*	*Rv2741*	PE_PGRS47	*MT2812*
Rv2408	PE24	*MT2481*	*Rv2853*	PE_PGRS48	*MT2919*
Rv2431c	PE25	*MT2506*	*Rv3344c*	PE_PGRS49	*MT3448*
Rv2519	PE26	*MT2595*	*Rv3345c*	PE_PGRS50	*MT3449*
Rv2769c	PE27	*MT2839*	*Rv3367*	PE_PGRS51	*MT3476*
Rv3018A	PE27A	ND	*Rv3388*	PE_PGRS52	*MT3495*
Rv3020c[d]	PE28	*MT3105*	*Rv3507*	PE_PGRS53	*MT3612*
Rv3022A	PE29	*MT3106.1*	*Rv3508*	PE_PGRS54	*MT3612.1*
Rv3097c	PE30	*MT3181*	*Rv3511*	PE_PGRS55	*MT3615.1*[c]
Rv3477	PE31	*MT3581*	*Rv3512*	PE_PGRS56	*MT3615.1*[c]
Rv3622c	PE32	*MT3724*	*Rv3514*	PE_PGRS57	*MT3615.3*
Rv3650	PE33	*MT3752*	*Rv3590c*	PE_PGRS58	*MT3696*
Rv3746c	PE34	*MT3854*	*Rv3595c*	PE_PGRS59	*MT3701*
Rv3872	PE35	*MT3986*	*Rv3652*	PE_PGRS60	ND
Rv3893c	PE36	*MT4008*	R3653	PE_PGRS61	*MT3756*
Rv0109	PE_PGRS1	*MT0118*	*Rv3812*	PE_PGRS62	*MT3920*
Rv0124	PE_PGRS2	*MT0132*	*Rv0096*	PPE1	*MT0105*
Rv0278c	PE _PGRS3	*MT0291*	*Rv0256c*	PPE2	*MT0269*
Rv0279c	PE_PGRS4	ND	*Rv0280*	PPE3	*MT0292*
Rv0297	PE_PGRS5	*MT0311*	*Rv0286*	PPE4	*MT0299*
Rv0532	PE_PGRS6	*MT0556*	*Rv0304c*	PPE5	*MT0318*[c]
Rv0578c	PE_PGRS7	*MT0607*	*Rv0305c*	PPE6	*MT0318*[c]
Rv0742	PE_PGRS8	*MT0768*	*Rv0354c*	PPE7	*MT0369*
Rv0746	PE_PGRS9	*MT0772.1*	*Rv0355c*	PPE8	*MT0370*
Rv0747	PE_PGRS10	*MT772.5*	*Rv0387c*	Rv0387c	*MT0400*[c]
Rv0754	PE_PGRS11	*MT0778*	*Rv0388c*	PPE9	*MT0400*[c]
Rv0832	PE_PGRS12	*MT0854*	*Rv0442c*	PPE10	*MT0458*
Rv0833	PE_PGRS13	*MT0854.1*	*Rv0453*	PPE11	*MT0469*
Rv0834c	PE_PGRS14	*MT0855*	*Rv0755c*	PPE12	*MT0779*
Rv0872c	PE_PGRS15	*MT0894*	*Rv0878c*	PPE13	*MT0901*
Rv0977	PE_PGRS16	*MT1004*	*Rv0915c*	PPE14/MTB41	*MT0940*
Rv0978c	PE_PGRS17	*MT1006.1*	*Rv1039c*	PPE15	*MT1068*
Rv0980c	PE_PGRS18	*MT1008*	*Rv1135c*	PPE16	*MT1168*
Rv1067c	PE_PGRS19	*MT1096.1*	*Rv1168c*	PPE17	*MT1205*
Rv1068c	PE_PGRS20	*MT1097*	*Rv1196*	PPE18/mtb39a	*MT1234*
Rv1087	PE_PGRS21	*MT1118.1*	*Rv1361c*	PPE19/mtb39b	*MT1406*
Rv1091	PE_PGRS22	*MT1123*	*Rv1387*	PPE20	*MT1431*
Rv1243c	PE_PGRS23	*MT1280.1*	*Rv1548c*	PPE21	*MT1599*
Rv1325c	PE_PGRS24	*MT1367*	*Rv1705c*	PPE22	*MT1745*
Rv1396c	PE_PGRS25	*MT1440.1*	*Rv1706c*	PPE23	*MT1746*

Table 1. *Continued*

H37Rv gene	PE, PE_PGRS, or PPE no.	CDC 1551 gene	H37Rv gene	PE, PE_PGRS, or PPE no.	CDC 1551 gene
Rv1753c	PPE24	*MT1796*	*Rv3021c*	PPE47	*MT3106c*
Rv1787	PPE25	*MT1836*	*Rv3022c*	PPE48	*MT3106c*
Rv1789	PPE26	*MT1838*	*Rv3125c*	PPE49	*MT3209*
Rv1790	PPE27	*MT1839*	*Rv3135*	PPE50	ND
Rv1800	PPE28	*MT1849*	*Rv3136*	PPE51	*MT3221*
Rv1801	PPE29	*MT1850*	*Rv3144c*	PPE52	*MT3231*
Rv1802	PPE30	*MT1851*	*Rv3159c*	PPE53	*MT3247*
Rv1807	PPE31	*MT1856*	ND	ND	*MT3248*
Rv1808	PPE32	*MT1856.1*	*Rv3343c*	PPE54	*MT3447*
Rv1809	PPE33	*MT1857*	*Rv3347c*	PPE55	*MT3453*
Rv1917c	PPE34	*MT1968*	*Rv3350c*	PPE56	*MT3458*
Rv1918c	PPE35	*MT1969*	*Rv3425*	PPE57	ND
Rv2108	PPE36	*MT2167*	*Rv3426*	PPE58	ND
Rv2123	PPE37/irg2	*MT2182.1*	*Rv3429*	PPE59	*MT3533*
Rv2352c	PPE38	*MT2419*	*Rv3478*	PPE60/mtb39c	*MT3582*
ND	ND	*MT2422*	*Rv3532*	PPE61	*MT3636*
Rv2353c	PPE39	*MT2423*	*Rv3533c*	PPE62	*MT3637*
Rv2356c	PPE40	*MT2425*	*Rv3539*	PPE63	*MT3643*
Rv2430c	PPE41	*MT2505*	*Rv3558*	PPE64	*MT3663*
Rv2608	PPE42	*MT2683*	*Rv3621c*	PPE65	*MT3723*
Rv2768c	PPE43	*MT2838*	*Rv3738c*	PPE66	*MT3844c*
Rv2770c	PPE44	*MT2840*	*Rv3739c*	PPE67	*MT3844c*
Rv2892c	PPE45	*MT2959*	*Rv3873*	PPE68	*MT3987*
Rv3018c	PPE46	*MT3098*	*Rv3892c*	PPE69	*MT4007*
Rv3018c	PPE46	*MT3101*			

[a]Sequences were analyzed using website servers from the Pasteur Institute (http://genolist.pasteur.fr/TubercuList), The Institute for Genomic Research (http://www.tigr.org), the National Center for Biotechnology Information (http://www.ncbi.nlm.nih.gov/BLAST/), Genome-Entrez (http://www.ncbi.nlm.nih.gov/PMGifs/Genomes/prokdata.html), and DNAMAN software. The table shows corresponding PE, PE_PGRS, and PPE genes found in the genomes of *M. tuberculosis* H37Rv and *M. tuberculosis* CDC 1551 and includes the revised numbering system for the annotation of the PE, PE_PGRS, and PPE genes (12). Where the identification of corresponding genes is inconclusive, due to frameshift mutations and gene duplications, these are indicated as ND (not determined).

[b]The frameshift mutation giving rise to PE *Rv2099c* and PE_PGRS *Rv2098c* has been authenticated by the presence of a single intact orthologue of this ancestral gene in the genome of *M. tuberculosis* CDC 1551, namely, MT2159.

[c]The frameshift mutation giving rise to these Rv genes have been authenticated by the presence of a single intact orthologue of the ancestral gene occurring in the genome of *M. tuberculosis* CDC 1551, which results in the assignment of the identical gene in CDC 1551.

[d]*Rv3020c* has been annotated incorrectly as a member of the PE gene family and belongs to the ESAT-6 gene family.

Rv0980c), similar to AB repeats found in surface antigens in *Methanosarcina mazei*. In comparison, the *M. tuberculosis* CDC 1551 genome has 35 PE genes and 60 PE_PGRS genes (Table 1) (31). The origin and evolution of these redundant genes remains unclear and is presently subject to "the chicken or the egg" arguments. For instance, it can be argued that since the PE genes exist as small ORFs, they expanded into PE_PGRS genes (62). Conversely, the PE genes could have arisen from preexisting PE_PGRS genes through genetic duplication of the PE domain. As more becomes known about the presence of these genes in other mycobacterial species and about the localization and function of the specific domains found in the PE and PE_PGRS proteins, this puzzle will probably be solved. Nevertheless, the fact that only certain mycobacterial species contain PE and PE_PGRS genes (see below) and the failure to find similar genes in other organisms make the investigation of this fascinating mycobacterial gene family intriguing.

PE_PGRS GENES

Molecular hybridization studies using a specific PGRS probe (55), as well as genomic sequencing, indicate that PE_PGRS genes exist not only in *M. tuberculosis* but also in *Mycobacterium marinum*, *Mycobacterium gordonae*, *Mycobacterium kansasii*, *Mycobacterium bovis*, and probably *Mycobacterium smegmatis*. (46, 55). They have not been found in *Mycobacterium avium*, *Mycobacterium abscessus*, *Mycobacterium chelonae*, *Mycobacterium flavescens*, *Mycobacterium fortuitum*, *Mycobacterium simiae*, *Mycobacterium terrae*, *Mycobacterium xenopi*, *Mycobacterium microti*, *Mycobacterium gastri*, or *Mycobacterium szulgai*. *Mycobacterium leprae* has a number of PE_PGRS pseudogenes but no intact ORFs. It has been noted that the lack of intact PE and PE_PGRS as well as PPE genes in the *M. leprae* genome contributes significantly to its smaller genome size (19). Comparison of the numerous PE_PGRS genes found

A

~110 aa

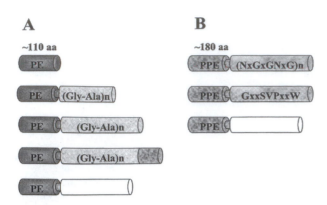

B

~180 aa

Figure 1. Schematic showing the most typical members of the PE and PPE multi-gene families. (A) In addition to ORFs encoding simple PE proteins, these sequences are present as N-terminal domains of more complex genes. The predominant subfamily consists of the PE_PGRS gene products in which the PGRS domain can vary in size but is typically composed of Gly-Ala repetitive sequences. A few PE_PGRS gene products contain atypical sequences at the C-terminus, and a few PE genes are also linked to other non-PGRS sequences, including one, *Rv3097c* that encodes a putative lipase (18). (B) The predominant subfamily of the PPE gene family consists of the PPE-MPTR genes, where the MPTR domain can vary in size but is typically composed of AsnXGlyXGlyAsnXGly repetitive sequences. The second most dominant subfamily is the PPE-SVP subfamily, containing the motif GlyXXSerValProXXTrp at around position 350 in the amino acid (aa) sequence. Other atypical members also exist.

within strains of *M. tuberculosis* shows that both the PE and PGRS domains are very homogenous, but polymorphisms occur particularly within the PGRS domain, which is highly GC rich and contains the repetitive glycine-rich sequences. Perhaps more interestingly, this sequence variation in the PGRS region also extends to interspecies and interstrain comparisons of genes. Following the sequencing of the *M. tuberculosis* H37Rv genome, Cole et al. (18) pointed out that the gene in *M. bovis* BCG Pasteur corresponding to Rv 0746 differs by the deletion of 29 codons and the insertion of 46 codons within the PGRS domain. BCG vaccine strains completely lack certain PE_PGRS genes (as well as PE and PPE genes) found in *M. tuberculosis* H37Rv (6). The sequencing of the *M. tuberculosis* CDC 1551 genome has shown that the PE_PGRS genes are among the most variable in this *M. tuberculosis* strain when insertions in ORFs are compared with those of *M. tuberculosis* H37Rv (31). Comparative analysis also demonstrates that in a head-to-head comparison of homologous genes in the two *M. tuberculosis* genomes, the PGRS regions can contain both insertions and deletions. For example, as seen in Fig. 2A, the PE_PGRS gene *MT1866* in *M. tuberculosis* CDC 1551 contains a 30-codon deletion and a 3-codon insertion within the PGRS domain compared to the corresponding *Rv1818c* gene found

in *M. tuberculosis* H37Rv. It is apparent, as proposed by Poulet and Cole (46), that strand slippage during replication occurs frequently in the GC-rich PGRS region. A brief survey of the many PE_PGRS genes in both the *M. tuberculosis* H37Rv and *M. tuberculosis* CDC 1551 genomes illustrates the remarkable variability that occurs within the Gly-Ala repetitive PGRS domain. It seems most likely that the numerous PE_PGRS genes serve as a pool of genetic variation and possibly antigenic diversity for mycobacteria. It remains to be determined whether these genetic alterations help certain mycobacteria survive under selective pressures, such as dramatic changes in environment, including survival within granulomas (47), or an attack by the immune system of the human host.

A potential role for PE-PGRS proteins in altering the antigenic profile of the organism implies that these proteins are exposed to the host immune system. In fact, there is increasing evidence to suggest that certain PE_PGRS proteins are found at the cell surface of mycobacteria. Antisera raised against DNA vaccines expressing PE_PGRS protein have been shown to recognize surface antigens on mycobacteria (4, 8). Fluorescence microscopy of *M. smegmatis* expressing the PE_PGRS Rv1818c gene fused to enhanced green fluorescent protein (EGFP) suggests that this protein may be localized to the bacterial cell surface (Fig. 3) (25). Investigation of a BCG transposon mutant specifically lacking the PE_PGRS gene *Rv1818c* has implicated the product of this gene in bacterium-bacterium interactions as well as in bacterium-macrophage cell interactions (8) and suggests that the Rv1818c protein may function as a surface adhesin. Also, certain PE_PGRS proteins bind to fibronectin (1, 29), suggesting that interactions of mycobacteria with host cells and the extracellular matrix could be mediated through interactions of PE_PGRS proteins with fibronectin. Taken together, this evidence suggests that at least some of the PE_PGRS proteins are intercalated into the mycobacterial cell wall, where they are positioned to interact with other cells as well as the immune system. Other glycine-rich proteins, such as the fibrous proteins found in silk (36) and in plant cell walls (65), are noted for their elasticity and tensile strength. The similarity of the glycine-rich PGRS domain to these proteins suggests that PE_PGRS proteins could also be part of the structural foundation of the mycobacterial cell wall.

Expression of PE_PGRS genes has been inferred from the reaction of serum antibodies from *M. tuberculosis*-infected animals or human patients with recombinant PE_PGRS proteins (24, 29, 59). The presence of cross-reactive epitopes within the repetitive PGRS domain, however, prohibits the use of this antiserum for experiments demonstrating that specific

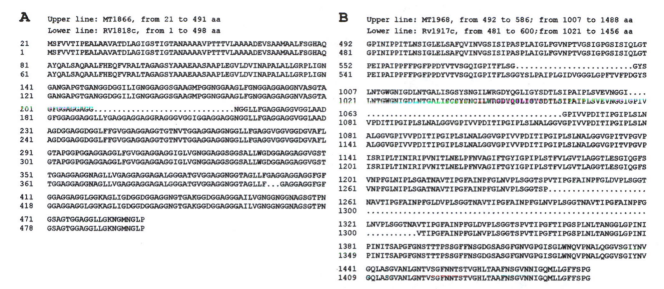

A
```
Upper line: MT1866, from 21 to 491 aa
Lower line: RV1818c, from 1 to 498 aa

21   MSFVVTIPEALAAVATDLAGIGSTIGTANAAAAVPTTTVLAAAADEVSAAMAALFSGHAQ
1    MSFVVTIPEALAAVATDLAGIGSTIGTANAAAAVPTTTVLAAAADEVSAAMAALFSGHAQ

81   AYQALSAQAALFHEQFVRALTAGAGSYAAAEAASAAPLEGVLDVINAPALALLGRPLIGN
61   AYQALSAQAALFHEQFVRALTAGAGSYAAAEAASAAPLEGVLDVINAPALALLGRPLIGN

141  GANGAPGTGANGGDGGILIGNGGAGGSGAAGMPGGNGGAAGLFGNGGAGGAGGNVASGTA
121  GANGAPGTGANGGDGGILIGNGGAGGSGAAGMPGGNGGAAGLFGNGGAGGAGGNVASGTA

201  GFGGAGGAGG..............................NGGLLFGAGGAGGVGGLAAD
181  GFGGAGGAGGLLYGAGGAGGAGGRAGGGVGGIGGAGGAGGNGGLLFGAGGAGGVGGLAAD

231  AGDGGAGGDGGLFFGVGGAGGAGGTGTNVTGGAGGAGGNGGLLFGAGGVGGVGGDGVAFL
241  AGDGGAGGDGGLFFGVGGAGGAGGTGTNVTGGAGGAGGNGGLLFGAGGVGGVGGDGVAFL

291  GTAPGGPGGAGGAGGLFGVGGAGGAGGIGLVGNGGAGGSGGSALLWGDGGAGGAGGVGST
301  GTAPGGPGGAGGAGGLFGVGGAGGAGGIGLVGNGGAGGSGGSALLWGDGGAGGAGGVGST

351  TGGAGGAGGNAGLLVGAGGAGGAGALGGGATGVGGAGGNGGTAGLLFGAGGAGGAGGFGF
361  TGGAGGAGGNAGLLVGAGGAGGAGALGGGATGVGGAGGNGGTAGLLF...GAGGAGGFGF

411  GGAGGAGGLGGKAGLIGDGGDGGAGGNGTGAKGGDGGAGGGAILVGNGGNGGNAGSGTPN
418  GGAGGAGGLGGKAGLIGDGGDGGAGGNGTGAKGGDGGAGGGAILVGNGGNGGNAGSGTPN

471  GSAGTGGAGGLLGKNGMNGLP
478  GSAGTGGAGGLLGKNGMNGLP
```

B
```
Upper line: MT1968, from 492 to 586; from 1007 to 1488 aa
Lower line: Rv1917c, from 481 to 600; from 1021 to 1456 aa

492  GPINIPPITLNSIGLELSAFQVINVGSISIPASPLAIGLFGVNPTVGSIGPGSISIQLGT
481  GPINIPPITLNSIGLELSAFQVINVGSISIPASPLAIGLFGVNPTVGSIGPGSISIQLGT

552  PEIPAIPPFFPGFPPDYVTVSGQIGPITFLSG....................GYS
541  PEIPAIPPFFPGFPPDYVTVSGQIGPITFLSGGYSLPAIPLGIDVGGGLGPFTVFPDGYS

1007 LNTGWGNIGDLNTGALISGSYSNGILWRGDYQGLIGYSDTLSIPAIPLSVEVNGGI....
1021 LNTGWGNIGDLNTGALISGSYSNGILWNGDVQGLIGYSDTLSIPAIPLSVEVNGGIGPIV

1063 ..................................GPIVVPDITIPGIPLSLN
1081 VPDITIPGIPLSLNALGGVGPIVVPDITIPGIPLSLNALGGVGPIVVPDITIPGIPLSLN

1081 ALGGVGPIVVPDITIPGIPLSLNALGGVGPIVVPDITIPGIPLSLNALGGVGPITVPGVP
1141 ALGGVGPIVVPDITIPGIPLSLNALGGVGPIVVPDITIPGIPLSLNALGGVGPITVPGVP

1141 ISRIPLTINIRIPVNITLNELPFNVAGIFTGYIGPIPLSTFVLGVTLAGGTLESGIQGFS
1201 ISRIPLTINIRIPVNITLNELPFNVAGIFTGYIGPIPLSTFVLGVTLAGGTLESGIQGFS

1201 VNPFGLNIPLSGATNAVTIPGFAINPFGLNVPLSGGTSPVTIPGFAINPFGLDVPLSGGT
1261 VNPFGLNIPLSGATNAVTIPGFAINPFGLNVPLSGGTSP....................

1261 NAVTIPGFAINPFGLDVPLSGGTNAVTIPGFAINPFGLNVPLSGGTNAVTIPGFAINPFG
1300 ....................................................

1321 LNVPLSGGTNAVTIPGFAINPFGLDVPLSGGTSPVTIPGFTIPGSPLNLTANGGLGPINI
1300 ..........VTIPGFAINPFGLNVPLSGGTSPVTIPGFTIPGSPLNLTANGGLGPINI

1381 PINITSAPGFGNSTTTPSSGFFNSGDGSASGFGNVGPGISGLWNQVPNALQGGVSGIYNV
1349 PINITSAPGFGNSTTTPSSGFFNSGDGSASGFGNVGPGISGLWNQVPNALQGGVSGIYNV

1441 GQLASGVANLGNTVSGFNNTSTVGHLTAAFNSGVNNIGQMLLGFFSPG
1409 GQLASGVANLGNTVSGFNNTSTVGHLTAAFNSGVNNIGQMLLGFFSPG
```

Figure 2. A comparison of the amino acid products of the corresponding PE_PGRS and PPE-MPTR genes in two *M. tuberculosis* genomes shows both deletions and insertions within the repetitive domains. (A) Amino acid (aa) sequence encoded by the *Rv1818c* PE_PGRS gene from *M. tuberculosis* H37Rv, compared with the amino acid sequence encoded by the corresponding gene, *MT1866*, found in the clinical *M. tuberculosis* isolate CDC 1551. A 33-codon deletion in *MT1866* within the PGRS domain accounts for the loss of four -GGAGGX- repeats. *MT1866* also contains an -AGG- insert compared with the *Rv1818c* PE_PGRS gene. (B) Amino acid (aa) sequence encoded by the *Rv1917c* PPE gene from *M. tuberculosis* H37Rv, aligned to the amino acid sequence encoded by the corresponding gene, *MT1968*, found in the clinical *M. tuberculosis* isolate CDC 1551. There are three insertions/deletions present in the MPTR regions of these genes, corresponding to differences of 25, 46, and 92 amino acids, respectively.

PE_PGRS proteins are expressed in vivo. A review of the studies that have provided evidence for the expression of specific PE_PGRS as well as PE and PPE genes is shown in Table 2. Banu et al. (4) have found, using reverse transcription-PCR (RT-PCR), that 10 different PE_PGRS genes are expressed by *M. tuberculosis* H37Rv in culture. Recent studies, also using

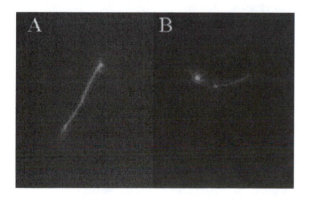

Figure 3. Fluorescence microscopy of transformed *M. smegmatis* cells expressing PE_PGRS protein (A) or PE protein (B) as fusions with EGFP. The full-length PE_PGRS and PE domain of the *Rv1818c* gene (24) were fused to EGFP and transformed into *M. smegmatis* using the pMV206 vector (25). These observations suggest that the PE_PGRS-GFP protein is uniformly distributed throughout the cell wall while the PE-GFP protein is more localized to defined, possibly polar regions within the cell wall. We are grateful to Giovanni Delogu for permission to use his unpublished data.

RT-PCR (32) (a summary of the results is given in Table 2), show that differential expression of specific PE_PGRS genes occurs when clinical isolates of *M. tuberculosis* grown in vitro are compared. A few studies suggest that the regulation of expression of PE_PGRS genes also occurs within the host. In vivo expression of two PE_PGRS genes (*M. marinum* genes corresponding to *Rv1651c* and *Rv3812*) has been associated with virulence and with the presence of pathogenic *M. marinum* in granulomatous tissue (47). Investigations using microarray techniques have indicated that the expression of a number of PE_PGRS genes may be controlled by iron-dependent regulatory systems (53), nutrient starvation (5) or acidic environments (30) (Table 2). Use of recombinase-based in vivo expression technology (RIVET) has indicated that the PE_PGRS gene *Rv0834c* is upregulated under conditions of low pH (58). To date, however, there has been no careful analysis of native PE_PGRS proteins purified from *M. tuberculosis* or other mycobacteria, and it is unknown, for instance, whether these proteins contain posttranslational modifications.

The PGRS region of the PE_PGRS genes has significant homology to the Gly-Ala repeat region of the Epstein-Barr virus nuclear antigen, EBNA1, a protein that is critical for the persistence of the virus in infected human B cells (27). Although EBNA1 is a major target

Table 2. Evidence for expression of PE, PE_PGRS, and PPE genes

Gene no.	Method of identification	Reference(s)
PE genes		
Rv0285	Microarray (downregulated)[c], microarray (R1)[d]	5, 53
Rv0335c	Microarray (upregulated)[c]	5
Rv1169c	Microarray (upregulated)[c], microarray (I1)[d], microarray (upregulated)[g]	5, 30, 53
Rv1172c	RT-PCR[b], microarray (upregulated, hspR)[f]	32, 61
Rv1195	Microarray (downregulated)[c], microarray (I1)[d]	5, 53
Rv1386	Microarray (downregulated)[c]	5
Rv1791	Microarray (upregulated, hspR/hrcA)[f]	61
Rv2431c	Microarray (downregulated)[c]	5
Rv3020c	Microarray (downregulated)[c]	5
Rv3477	Microarray (upregulated)[c]	5
Rv3872	Microarray (downregulated)[c]	5
PE_PGRS genes		
Rv0279c	Microarray (I1)[d]	53
Rv0578c	RT-PCR[b]	32
Rv0834c	RIVET[e]	58
Rv0872c	Microarray (upregulated)[c]	5
Rv0980c	RT-PCR[a]	4
Rv1067c	RT-PCR[a]	4
Rv1068c	RT-PCR[a]	4
Rv1243c	RT-PCR[a]	4
Rv1325c	RT-PCR[a]	4
Rv1396c	RT-PCR[a]	4
Rv1441c	RT-PCR[a]	4
Rv1818c	RT-PCR[a]	4
Rv1983	RT-PCR[a]	4
Rv2162c	RT-PCR[a]	4
Rv2741	Microarray (R2)[d]	53
Rv3367	Microarray (upregulated)[c]	5
Rv3508	Microarray (upregulated, hspR)[f]	61
Rv3652	RT-PCR[b]	32
Rv3718c	GFP/SacB[h]	63
PPE genes		
Rv0286 (as well as the *M. avium* orthologue of Rv0286)	Microarray (downregulated)[c], microarray (R1)[d], SCOTS[i]	5, 38, 53
Rv0354c	Microarray (downregulated)[c]	5
M. avium orthologue of Rv0453	SCOTS[i]	38
Rv0755c	RAP-PCR[j]	51
Rv0915c (MTB41)	T-cell expression cloning[k]	60
Rv1039	Microarray (upregulated)[c]	5
Rv1168c	Microarray (upregulated)[c]	5
Rv1196 (MTB39a)	Microarray (downregulated)[c], T-cell expression cloning[l]	5, 28
Rv1361c (MTB39b)	Microarray (downregulated)[c], T-cell expression cloning[l]	5, 28
Rv1387	Microarray (downregulated)[c], microarray (downregulated)[g]	5, 30
Rv1801	Microarray (upregulated)[c]	5
M. avium orthologue of Rv1802	SCOTS[i]	38
Rv1808	Microarray (upregulated)[c]	5
Rv1809	Microarray (upregulated)[c]	5
MT1968 (Rv1917c)	Microarray (downregulated)[g], RT-PCR[m]	30, 56
Rv2123/irg2	Microarray (R1)[d]	52, 53
Rv2430c	Microarray (downregulated)[c]	5
Rv2770c	mRNA differential-display assay[n]	50
Rv3136	Microarray (downregulated)[c]	5
Rv3159c	Microarray (downregulated)[c]	5
Rv3478 (MTB39c)	Microarray (downregulated)[c], T-cell expression cloning[l]	5, 28

[a] Gene expression determined by RT-PCR (4).

[b] Gene expression determined by RT-PCR (32).

[c] Gene expression either upregulated or downregulated in response to nutrient starvation as determined by microarray analysis (5).

[d] Gene expression regulated by IdeR and iron as determined by microarray analysis. R1, IdeR and iron-repressed genes; I1, IdeR-independent, iron induced genes; R2, IdeR-independent, iron-repressed genes (53).

[e] Acid-inducible gene expression determined by recombinase-based in vivo expression technology (RIVET) (58).

[f] Gene expression in heat shock regulator mutants, *hspR*, Hsp70 regulator mutant of *Mtb*, *hspR/hrcA*, Hsp70 regulator and repressor double mutant of *Mtb* (61).

[g] Gene expression either upregulated or downregulated in response to the acidic conditions found inside the macrophage as determined by microarray analysis (30).

[h] *Mtb* genes expressed within host cells identified using fluorescence induction and sucrose counterselection (63).

[i] *M. avium* genes expressed during growth in human macrophages detected by selective capture of transcribed sequences (SCOTS) (38).

[j] Genes differentially expressed between attenuated *M. tuberculosis* H37Ra and virulent H37Rv identified by RNA arbitrarily primed differential display PCR (RAP-PCR) (51).

[k] Genes expressing antigens involved with the early control of tuberculosis, identified using direct T-cell expression cloning (60).

[l] Expression screening of a genomic *M. tuberculosis* library with tuberculosis patient sera (28).

[m] Gene expression in liquid cultures of *M. tuberculosis* by RT-PCR (56).

[n] Genes differentially expressed between attenuated *M. tuberculosis* H37Ra and virulent H37Rv identified by mRNA differential display (DD) (50).

for a humoral immune response, studies have suggested that it is invisible to recognition by cytotoxic T lymphocytes because the Gly-Ala repeat domain prevents proteasome-dependent processing and antigen presentation through the major histocompatibility complex class I pathway (40, 41). The fact that the PGRS domain contains Gly-Ala repeats similar to those in EBNA1 suggests that PE_PGRS proteins could have a parallel inhibitory effect on proteasome-dependent processes within host cells. Indeed, it has been demonstrated that when the PE_PGRS gene is fused to EGFP and intracellular degradation rates are monitored by fluorescence microscopy, intracellular processing of the PE_PGRS protein is limited compared with that of other mycobacterial protein-EGFP fusions (7). This resistance to degradation is dependent on the presence of the PGRS domain, since it does not occur with PE-EGFP fusions. The expression of PE_PGRS genes by *M. tuberculosis* within antigen-presenting cells could result in the inhibition of processing and presentation of PE_PGRS proteins and other mycobacterial antigens through the major histocompatibility complex class I pathway. Limiting antigen presentation could restrict the development of an effective immune response to these mycobacterial components and provide a mechanism by which *M. tuberculosis* evades an effective host immune response. This may be an important requirement for an organism such as *M. tuberculosis*, which can persist in a latent state for many years (20), and is supported by the finding that while a DNA vaccine construct expressing a PE_PGRS protein does not protect mice against an *M. tuberculosis* aerosol challenge (24), a PE DNA vaccine does elicit effective immunity in this tuberculosis challenge model (T. Pickett and M. J. Brennan, unpublished observations). This observation is compatible with the idea that PE sequences that are part of PE_PGRS proteins may be processed differently from PE proteins alone. More extensive investigation of this potentially important immunomodulatory function of PE_PGRS proteins is needed.

PE GENES

Although we understand little about the PE_PGRS gene subfamily and their proteins, we know even less about the expression, localization, and function of the more diminutive proteins encoded by the PE genes. As noted in Fig. 4, PE genes are highly homologous both within strains (compare H37Rv with CDC 1551), within species (compare *M. avium* PE with others), and when found as the PE domain within the PE_PGRS subfamily of genes (compare the PE domain found in PE_PGRS *Rv1818c*). A significant number of encoded amino acid residues are conserved within the PE domain, with the PE genes from *M. leprae* being the least homologous within this group. Interestingly, there is enough diversity within these genes to account for the existence of more than 30 PE genes in *M. tuberculosis* and *M. bovis* (18, 31, 33, 35). *M. avium*, which appears to lack PE_PGRS genes, has at least one PE gene, which is most similar to *Rv1788* (http://www.tigr.org/), while *M. leprae* has about four intact PE genes (19). In contrast to the PE_PGRS genes that contain multiple insertions and deletions and encode amino acid substitutions, there are few interstrain differences when the corresponding PE genes from H37Rv and CDC 1551 are compared. One PE gene, *Rv3018A*, is absent in the CDC 1551

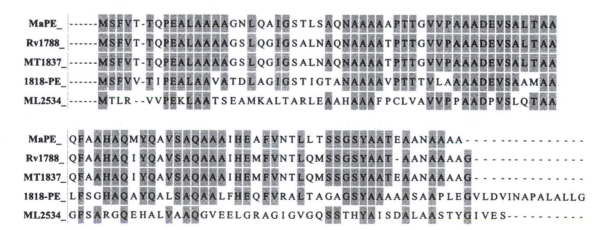

Figure 4. Multiple alignment of the amino acid sequence encoded by PE genes from *M. avium* (MaPE), *M. tuberculosis* H37Rv (PE gene *Rv1788*), *M. tuberculosis* CDC 1551 (PE gene *MT1837*), part of the PE domain of the PE_PGRS *Rv1818c* gene from *M. tuberculosis* H37Rv (1818-PE), and *M. leprae* (PE gene ML2534). Conserved amino acids are shaded, and alignment was performed using the Clustal W sequence alignment provided by Computational Molecular Biology at the National Institutes of Health (http://www.molbio.info.nih.gov/molbio/).

genome (Table 1), although it seems clear that this gene is only a fragment of a previously existing gene that has been deleted in a precursor of both strains. One PE gene, *Rv3097c*, contains a sequence at the 3′ end which encodes a polypeptide with a predicted esterase/lipase activity (18). Since this is the only PE gene with a predicted function, this unique gene may have been created by a fusion event between a PE gene and a gene encoding an enzyme with this activity.

Evidence for expression of a limited number of PE genes has resulted from RT-PCR studies and from microarray analysis of the expression of mycobacterial genes under changing environmental conditions (Table 2). The expression of Rv1169c by *M. tuberculosis* is influenced by both the presence of iron (53) and the pH of the environment (30), while the expression of three PE genes, *Rv0285*, *Rv0916c*, and *Rv1195*, is affected by the mycobacterial metal-dependent regulator, the IdeR protein (53). Also, Flores and Espitia (32) have demonstrated, using RT-PCR, that the PE gene *Rv1172c* is expressed by three *M. tuberculosis* strains as well as by *Mycobacterium canetti*. One PE gene, *Rv3872*, is found in the RD1 region of difference that is missing in all strains of BCG (42) and has been associated with the virulence phenotype of *M. tuberculosis*. While there are some data to show that guinea pigs can elicit antibodies to recombinant *Rv3872* protein (10), there is no evidence to suggest that *Rv3872* is a virulence factor. There is, however, some evidence to suggest that a cellular response is produced in *M. bovis*-infected cattle against the PE protein encoded by *Rv3872* (13). A PPE gene sits adjacent to *Rv3872* in the RD1 region, and it has been noted that PE and PPE genes commonly occur as neighbors throughout the genome (N. C. Gey van Pittius, S. L. Sampson, H. Lee, Y. Kim and P. D. van Helden, *Keystone Symp. Tuberc. Integrating Host Pathog. Biol.*, abstr. 417, 2003; M. Strong, P. Mallick, S. Wang, and D. Eisenberg, *Keystone Symp. Tuberc. Integrating Host Pathog. Biol.*, abstr. 455, 2003). The implication of this observation remains unclear (see below). So far, there is no evidence to suggest that a humoral immune response is induced by PE proteins expressed in vivo. Studies with mice indicate that following immunization with PE_PGRS DNA vaccines, antibodies are produced only to the PGRS domain (24), and antibodies in sera from *M. tuberculosis*-infected human patients are directed toward the repetitive PGRS domains within the PE_PGRS proteins (29, 59). Also, a small serological study of tuberculosis patients and *M. tuberculosis*-infected individuals from southern India indicates that there is no antibody response to PE proteins in these groups (V. Dheenadhayalan, R. Pitchappan, and M. J.

Brennan, unpublished observations). Careful study of the expression and characterization of a PE protein, as well as the immunological response to this family of proteins, awaits further investigation.

The function of the PE proteins as well as the PE domain present within the PE_PGRS proteins remains unclear. As part of the PE_PGRS protein, the PE sequence may be found at the cell surface and could play a role in bacterium-bacterium or bacterium-host interactions mediated by PE_PGRS proteins (7). The PE polypeptide could "anchor" the protein in the cell wall, allowing the antigenically variable PGRS domain access to the extracellular environment. It is also possible that, together with PE_PGRS proteins, individual PE proteins form a protein complex at the surface or within mycobacteria much like that observed for fimbriae (2). In fact, investigations using GFP fusion proteins suggest that PE protein may be localized to defined polar regions in the bacterial cell wall (Fig. 3) (25). This observation is compatible with the formation of complex surface structures. Another possibility is that PE polypeptides function similarly to the "PEST" (proline [P], glutamic acid [E], serine [S], and threonine [T]) sequences found in some eukaryotic proteins (54) and in the pore-forming listeriolysin O protein of the intracellular pathogen *Listeria monocytogenes* (23). In general, the PEST sequence is thought to target proteins for degradation and inactivation (48). This hypothesis provides a degree of irony, since the PGRS domain, as discussed above, may inhibit degradation.

The observation that many PE-PPE gene pairs exist in the *M. tuberculosis* genome (Gey van Pittus et al., *Keystone Symp.*, 2003; Strong, *Keystone Symp.*, 2003) and that homologous PE sequences are part of the N-terminal domain of PE_PGRS genes suggests that the PE sequence could play a role in the expression of both PPE and PE_PGRS genes or in the secretion or transport of PPE or PE_PGRS proteins to certain compartments within the bacterium. A mechanism regulating the systematic secretion of different PPE or PE_PGRS proteins to the bacterial surface would expose these highly polymorphic domains to the host immune system, where they could serve as a continuous "change of clothes" for the mycobacterial organism. This diversity would be a significant advantage for the tubercle bacillus, which often needs to persist unnoticed for long periods within the human host. In this scenario, one could imagine how this transport function for PE would occur in PE_PGRS proteins, but it is less clear how it might occur for the distinct, albeit adjacent, PPE genes. A possible clue may come from investigation of the *recA* gene of *M. tuberculosis*. Colston and Davis (21) have shown that the structure of the mature RecA protein of

M. tuberculosis and *M. leprae* results from a very unusual process of protein splicing. A 440-amino-acid region of the translated protein is excised, and the N- and C-terminal domains are then religated. In a similar fashion, the PE and PPE neighbors could be transcribed and translated together (in fact, there is some suggestion from expression data that certain PE-PPE pairs are cotranscribed [Table 2]. The posttranslational splicing could result in a mature PE_PPE protein much like the proteins encoded by PE_PGRS genes.

PPE MULTIGENE FAMILY

The PPE gene family is second only to the PE genes in the numbers of closely related genes found within the genome of *M. tuberculosis*. The putative protein products of the PPE genes range in size from 77 to 3,300 amino acids and, much like the protein products of the PE family, contain a highly conserved N-terminal domain of around 180 amino acids, with a proline-proline-glutamic acid (PPE) motif at positions 7 to 9 (18). The PPE family can be divided into three subgroups based on homology and the presence of specific sequence motifs within the C-terminal domains (Fig. 1B). The members of the largest subfamily, containing the MPTR (34), are rich in asparagine and glycine; these amino acids are present in the multiple repeats of the MPTR motif signature sequence, AsnXGlyXGlyAsnXGly (17, 62). This repeat motif is encoded by a consensus repeat sequence, GCCGGT-GTTG, separated by 5-bp spacers (17). Another prominent set of gene products within the PPE family, the PPE-SVP (Ser-Val-Pro) subgroup, are characterized by the single motif GlyXXSerValProXXTrp, which occurs near position 350 in the amino acid sequence. Other gene products containing a homologous PPE N-terminal domain exist, but they generally have no consistent sequence homology within the C-terminal region (34). The C-terminal domains of the products of members of the PPE gene family are of variable size; within the MPTR subgroup, this region can encode more than 3000 amino acid residues (18). These domains also contain repeat sequences of different copy numbers (34) and often have extensive polymorphisms in the different *M. tuberculosis* complex strains. As suggested for PE_PGRS genes, this widespread variation suggests that duplication events, probably due to strand slippage during replication, have commonly occurred in the history of the organism (18). Similar to the PE genes, there is a great paucity of information regarding the expression, function, and immunogenicity of the proteins encoded by the numerous PPE genes.

There is accumulating experimental evidence from a number of investigations, using different methods, to indicate that certain PPE genes are expressed (Table 2). Probably the earliest evidence for in vivo expression of a PPE gene comes from the investigation of the serine-rich antigen of *M. leprae* (64), which is one of the major antigens recognized by leprosy patients. More recent investigations by Rivera-Marrero et al. (51), using RAP-PCR, have identified genes that are differentially expressed when attenuated (H37Ra) and virulent (H37Rv and Erdman) laboratory strains of *M. tuberculosis* are compared. This study showed increased expression of the PPE gene MTV041.29 (Rv0755c) in H37Ra relative to the virulent H37Rv strain. In the following year, Rindi et al. (50) demonstrated the differential expression of the PPE gene Rv2770c in *M. tuberculosis* H37Rv when compared to H37Ra. More recently, T-cell expression cloning has resulted in the identification of two PPE antigens, MTB41 (Rv0915c) and MTB39A (Rv1196) (28, 60). These antigens are effective immunogens in animal models of tuberculosis and may be potentially useful as diagnostic aids and/or vaccines for tuberculosis. The MTB39A antigen is a component of a promising subunit vaccine against tuberculosis (49), while MTB41 expressed from a DNA vaccine confers protection against infection with *M. tuberculosis* comparable to that afforded by BCG (60). Hou et al. (38) employed a SCOTS method (for "selective capture of transcribed sequences") to identify cDNA molecules that represent genes expressed by *M. avium* during growth within human macrophages. Of the 46 genes that were identified, 3 belong to the PPE family (orthologues of *Rv0453*, *Rv1802*, and *Rv0286*), indicating that, at least in *M. avium*, the corresponding PPE proteins are expressed (38). Importantly, several studies using microarray analysis have also suggested that expression of PPE genes within mycobacteria may be regulated by specific changes in environmental conditions (Table 2). Rodriguez et al. (52) have found that the PPE gene *Rv2123* is upregulated under low-iron conditions, leading to the hypothesis that it may encode a siderophore involved in iron uptake. Further work by this group (53) confirmed this gene was an iron- and IdeR-repressed gene, along with another PPE gene, Rv0286.

Because of their highly polymorphic C-terminal domains (14, 15, 18, 34), PPE genes may serve as a source of antigenic variation for mycobacteria. In support of this hypothesis, sequence variation has been observed between the orthologues of PPE genes in an in silico comparative analysis of the genomes of *M. tuberculosis* H37Rv and *M. bovis* (35). Although the genome sequence of *M. bovis* is >99.9% identical at the nucleotide level to that of *M. tuberculosis*, the loci showing the greatest degree of variation are found within the PPE genes, as well as the PE genes. The PPE-MPTR protein Rv1917c has been the focus of an extensive investigation (56) and has been found to be expressed in liquid cultures of *M. tuberculosis* H37Rv, to be localized in the cell wall, and to be at least partly exposed on the cell surface of mycobacteria. This has significance with regard to a possible function in antigenic variation, since the *Rv1917c* gene was found to be highly polymorphic in comparisons of clinical isolates of *M. tuberculosis* (56), *M. bovis* (44), and the *M. tuberculosis* laboratory strains H37Rv and CDC 1551 (Fig. 2B). These findings are in agreement with the generally accepted idea that genes that encode cell wall or secreted proteins show the greatest variation because of their role in the interaction with the host immune system (35; T. Garnier, K. Eiglmeier, S. V. Gordon, J. C. Camus, M. Pryor-Stinear, M. H. Mansoor, L. Keating, P. W. Wheeler, J. Parkhill, B. Barrell, S. T. Cole, and R. G. Hewinson, *Keystone Symp. Tuberc. Integrating Host Pathog. Biol.*, abstr. 131, 2003).

Although there has been some progress, the function(s) of the PPE proteins remains vague. In addition to a possible role in antigenic variation, it has been postulated that PPE proteins could function as storage proteins for the rare amino acid asparagine, since asparagines are preferred nitrogen sources of *M. tuberculosis* (15, 62). In fact, the abundance of asparagines in the PPE proteins is remarkable, given the relative scarcity of this amino acid in the proteome of *M. tuberculosis*. Other investigations have suggested that the members of the PPE gene family may be involved in the pathogenesis of mycobacterial diseases. In one case, a transposon mutant containing an insertion in the PPE gene *Rv3018c* is attenuated for growth in macrophages (11). Also, using microarray analysis and real-time RT-PCR to analyze the transcriptional response of *M. tuberculosis* to low pH in vitro, Fisher et al. (30) found that 81 genes were differentially expressed. Two PPE genes, *Rv1387* and *MT1968* (*Rv1917c*), were repressed more than twofold; and conversely, one PE gene, Rv1169c, was induced. Since these conditions may be encountered in human macrophages, these results suggest that PPE genes could be differentially regulated within host cells.

SUMMARY

The role of the polymorphic PE and PPE genes in mycobacterial antigenic variation requires not only a careful analysis of the genomic polymorphisms in these genes but also an examination of the immuno-dominant domains within the encoded proteins. For example, investigation of the immune response to PE_PGRS proteins suggests that the PGRS domain, the site of common polymorphisms, contains a predominant B-cell epitope (24). Antisera raised against one recombinant PE_PGRS protein can cross-react with other PE_PGRS proteins but not with all of them (4). Taken together, these findings suggest that, although Gly-Ala repeats probably contribute to the B-cell epitope, other specific amino acids or protein conformations must occur that result in antibody specificity. There is some suggestion from hydrophobicity profiles of predicted PE_PGRS proteins that they may traverse the bacterial cell surface, exposing multiple antigenic domains. As observed for polymorphic neisserial porin proteins (43), presentation of specific antigenic domains could then result in antigenic (strain) diversity, which would have important implications for diagnosis and vaccine development as well as for the immune response of the host to pathogenic mycobacteria. In addition, at least two PPE proteins, MTB39A (Rv1196) and MTB41 (Rv0915), contain a dominant T-cell epitope and elicit an effective T-cell response (28, 60). Comparison with other PPE proteins will be important for our understanding of immune reactions and the role of this family of genes in antigenic diversity.

It is interesting that in a recent study by Sassetti et al. (57), where genes required for in vitro growth of *M. tuberculosis* were identified by high-density mutagenesis, only three PE genes (*Rv0285*, *Rv0335c* and *Rv1169c*) and six PPE genes (*Rv0286*, *Rv0755c*, *Rv1753c*, *Rv3018c*, *Rv3135*, and *Rv3343c*) were shown to be required for in vitro growth. Since 52 PE and 31 PPE genes were shown to be nonessential for in vitro growth of *M. tuberculosis* H37Rv, one interpretation of this finding is that most PE (including PE_PGRS) and PPE genes are nonessential for the growth of mycobacteria. This suggests that these two families are required for functions other than the normal cellular growth processes and may be required only when the organism encounters "unfriendly" environments, including that of the human host. In this chapter, we have reviewed evidence indicating that the expression of a large number of genes belonging to the PE and PPE families can be regulated under different environmental conditions (Table 2). This could be explained by the fact that the high mobility and duplication rates of the PE and PPE genes have caused them to be inserted into different genomic positions downstream of a variety of promoters or within regulatory operons. However, a more intriguing hypothesis is that a number of these genes are specifically regulated to assist the organism in adapting to environmental conditions, as first suggested by the work of Ramakrishnan et al. (47). As mentioned above, interpretation of the importance of the PE and PPE multigene families is complicated by the finding that there are only a few potentially functional members of the PE and PPE gene families (57) and no intact PE_PGRS genes found in the genome of *M. leprae* (although 30 pseudogenes were detected [19]). However, we cannot escape the fact that the PE and PPE gene families may encode >4% of the total proteins in certain mycobacterial organisms including *M. tuberculosis*, which implies that they most probably fulfill an important function(s) related to the survival of mycobacteria within different environmental niches. The exploration of this hypothesis will likely prove to be of great importance to scientists and clinicians interested in the pathogenesis of tuberculosis and other mycobacterial diseases.

Acknowledgments. We are especially grateful to Thames Pickett, V. Dheenadhyalan, Javier Flores, and Giovanni Delogu for sharing unpublished data and for comments on the manuscript.

ADDENDUM

A number of recent publications have explored the expression and immunological response to PE and PPE genes found in ESAT6/CFP10 gene clusters in mycobacteria (see, for example, references 26 and 45).

REFERENCES

1. Abou-Zeid, C., T. Garbe, R. Lathigra, H. G. Wiker, M. Harboe, G. A. Rook, and D. B. Young. 1991. Genetic and immunological analysis of *Mycobacterium tuberculosis* fibronectin-binding proteins. *Infect. Immun.* 59:2712–2718.

2. Abraham, S. N., A. B. Jonsson, and S. Normark. 1998. Fimbriae-mediated host-pathogen cross-talk. *Curr. Opin. Microbiol.* 1:75–81.

3. Adindla, S., and L. Guruprasad. 2003. Sequence analysis corresponding to the PPE and PE proteins in *Mycobacterium tuberculosis* and other genomes. *J. Biosci.* 28:169–179.

4. Banu, S., N. Honore, B. Saint-Joanis, D. Philpott, M. C. Prevost, and S. T. Cole. 2002. Are the PE-PGRS proteins of *Mycobacterium tuberculosis* variable surface antigens? *Mol. Microbiol.* 44:9–19.

5. Betts, J. C., P. T. Lukey, L. C. Robb, R. A. McAdam, and K. Duncan. 2002. Evaluation of a nutrient starvation model of *Mycobacterium tuberculosis* persistence by gene and protein expression profiling. *Mol. Microbiol.* 43:717–731.

6. Behr, M. A., M. A. Wilson, W. P. Gill, H. Salamon, G. K. Schoolnik, S. Rane, and P. M. Small. 1999. Comparative genomics of BCG vaccines by whole-genome DNA microarray. *Science* 284:1520–1523.

7. Brennan, M. J., and G. Delogu. 2002. The PE multigene family: a "molecular mantra" for mycobacteria. *Trends Microbiol.* 10:246–249.

8. Brennan, M. J., G. Delogu, Y. Chen, S. Bardarov, J. Kriakov, M. Alavi, and W. R. Jacobs, Jr. 2001. Evidence that mycobacterial PE_PGRS proteins are cell surface constituents that influence interactions with other cells. *Infect. Immun.* 69:7326–7333.

9. Brosch, R., A. S. Pym, S. V. Gordon, and S. T. Cole. 2001.The evolution of mycobacterial pathogenicity: clues from comparative genomics. *Trends Microbiol.* 9:452–458.

10. Brusasca, P. N., R. Colangeli, K. P. Lyashchenko, X. Zhao, M. Vogelstein, J. S. Spencer, D. N. McMurray, and M. L. Gennaro. 2001. Immunological characterization of antigens encoded by the RD1 region of the *Mycobacterium tuberculosis* genome. *Scand. J. Immunol.* 54:448–452.

11. Camacho, L. R., D. Ensergueix, E. Perez, B. Gicquel, and C. Guilhot. 1999. Identification of a virulence gene cluster of *Mycobacterium tuberculosis* by signature-tagged transposon mutagenesis. *Mol. Microbiol.* 34:257–267.

12. Camus, J. C., M. J. Pryor, C. Medigue, and S. Cole. 2002. Reannotation of the genome sequence of *Mycobacterium tuberculosis* H37Rv. *Microbiology* 148:2967–2973.

13. Cockle, P. J., S. V. Gordon, A. Lalvani, B. M. Buddle, R. G. Hewinson, and M. Vordermeier. 2002. Identification of novel *Mycobacterium tuberculosis* antigens with potential as diagnostic reagents or subunit vaccine candidates by comparative genomics. *Infect. Immun.* 70:6996–7003.

14. Cole, S. T. 1998. Comparative mycobacterial genomics. *Curr. Opin. Microbiol.* 1:567–571

15. Cole, S. T. 1999. Learning from the genome sequence of *Mycobacterium tuberculosis* H37Rv. *FEBS Lett.* 452:7–10

16. Cole, S. T. 2002. Comparative and functional genomics of the *Mycobacterium tuberculosis* complex. *Microbiology* 148:2929–2928.

17. Cole, S. T., and B. G. Barrell. 1998. Analysis of the genome of *Mycobacterium tuberculosis* H37Rv. *Novartis. Found. Symp.* 217:160–172

18. Cole, S. T., R. Brosch, J. Parkhill, T. Garnier, C. Churcher, D. Harris, S. V. Gordon, K. Eiglmeier, S. Gas, C. E. Barry III, F. Tekaia, K. Badcock, D. Basham, D. Brown, T. Chillingworth, R. Connor, R. Davies, K. Devlin, T. Feltwell, S. Gentles, N. Hamlin, S. Holroyd, T. Hornsby, K. Jagels, A. Krosh, J. McLean, S. Moule, L. Murphy, K. Oliver, J. Osborne, M. A. Quail, M.-A. Rajandream, J. Rogers, S. Rutter, K. Seager, J. Skelton, R. Squares, S. Squares, J. E. Sulston, K. Taylor, S. Whitehead, and B. G. Barrell. 1998. Deciphering the biology of *Mycobacterium tuberculosis* from the complete genome sequence. *Nature* 393:537–544.

19. Cole, S. T., K. Eiglmeier, J. Parkhill, K. D. James, N. R. Thomson, P. R. Wheeler, N. Honore, T. Garnier, C. Churcher, D. Harris, K. Mungall, D. Basham, D. Brown T, Chillingworth, R. Connor, R. M. Davies, K. Devlin, S. Duthoy, T. Feltwell, A. Fraser, N. Hamlin, S. Holroyd, T. Hornsby, K. Jagels, C. Lacroix, J. Maclean, S. Moule, L. Murphy, K. Oliver, M. A. Quail, M.-A. Rajandream, K. M. Rutherford, S. Rutter, K. Seeger, S. Simon, M. Simmonds, J. Skelton, R. Squares, S. Squares, K. Stevens, K. Taylor, S. Whitehead, J. R. Woodward, and B. G Barrell. 2001. Massive gene decay in the leprosy bacillus. *Nature* 409:1007–1011.

20. Collins, F. M. 1993. Tuberculosis: the return of an old enemy. *Crit. Rev. Microbiol.* 19:1–16.

21. Colston, M. J., and E. O. Davis. 1994. Homologous recombination, DNA repair, and mycobacterial *recA* genes, p. 217–226. *In* B. R. Bloom (ed.), *Tuberculosis: Pathogenesis, Protection and Control.* ASM Press, Washington, DC.

22. Cousins, D., S. Williams, E. Liebana, A. Aranaz, A. Bunschoten, J. Van Embden, and T. Ellis. 1998. Evaluation of four DNA typing techniques in epidemiological investigations of bovine tuberculosis. *J. Clin. Microbiol.* 36:68–178.

23. Decatur, A. L., and D. A. Portnoy. 2000. A PEST-like sequence in listeriolysin O essential for *Listeria monocytogenes* pathogenicity. *Science* 290:992–995.

24. Delogu, G., and M. J. Brennan. 2001. Comparative immune response to PE and PE_PGRS antigens of *Mycobacterium tuberculosis*. *Infect. Immun.* 69:5606–5611.

25. Delogu, G., C. Pusceddu, A. Bua, G. Fadda, M. J. Brennan, and S. Zanetti. 2004. Rv1818c-encoded PE_PGRS protein of *Mycobacterium tuberculosis* is surface exposed and influences bacterial cell structure. *Mol. Microbiol.* **52:**725–733.

26. Demangel, C., P. Brodin, P. J. Cockle, R. Brosch, L. Majlessi, C. Leclerc, and S. T. Cole. 2004. Cell envelope protein PPE68 contributes to *Mycobacterium tuberculosis* RD1 immunogenecity independently of a 10-kilodalton culture filtrate protein and ESAT-6. *Infect. Immun.* **72:**2170–2176.

27. Dillner, J., L. Sternas, B. Kallin, H. Alexander, B. Ehlin-Henriksson, H. Jornvall, G. Klein, and R. Lerner. 1984. Antibodies against a synthetic peptide identify the Epstein-Barr virus-determined nuclear antigen. *Proc. Natl. Acad. Sci. USA* **81:**4652–4656.

28. Dillon, D. C., M. R. Alderson, C. H. Day, D. M. Lewinsohn, R. Coler, T. Bement, A. Campos-Neto, Y. A. Skeiky, I. M. Orme, A. Roberts, S. Steen, W. Dalemans, R. Badaro, and S. G. Reed. 1999. Molecular characterization and human T-cell responses to a member of a novel *Mycobacterium tuberculosis* mtb39 gene family. *Infect. Immun.* **67:**2941–2950.

29. Espitia, C., J. P. Laclette, M. Mondragon-Palomino, A. Amador, J. Campuzano, A. Martens, M. Singh, R. Cicero, Y. Zhang, and C. Moreno. 1999. The PE-PGRS glycine-rich proteins of *Mycobacterium tuberculosis*: a new family of fibronectin-binding proteins? *Microbiology* **145:**3487–3495.

30. Fisher, M. A., B. B. Plikaytis, and T. M. Shinnick. 2002. Microarray analysis of the *Mycobacterium tuberculosis* transcriptional response to the acidic conditions found in phagosomes. *J. Bacteriol.* **184:**4025–4032.

31. Fleischmann, R. D., D. Alland, J. A. Eisen, L. Carpenter, O. White, J. Peterson, R. DeBoy, R. Dodson, M. Gwinn, D. Haft, E. Hickey, J. F. Kolonay, W. C. Nelson, L. A. Umayam, M. Ermolaeva, S.L. Salzberg, A. Delcher, T. Utterback, J. Weidman, H. Khouri J. Gill, A. Mikula, W. Bishai, W. R. Jacobs, Jr., J. C. Venter, and C. M. Fraser. 2002. Whole-genome comparison of *Mycobacterium tuberculosis* clinical and laboratory strains. *J. Bacteriol.* **184:**5479–5490.

32. Flores, J., and C. Espitia. 2003. Differential expression of PE and PE-PGRS genes in *Mycobacterium tuberculosis* strains. *Gene* **318:**75–81.

33. Gordon, J. E., R. B. Brosch, A. Billault, T. Farnier, K. Eiglmeier, and S. T. Cole. 1999. Identification of variable regions in the genomes of tubercle bacilli using bacterial artificial chromosome arrays. *Mol. Microbiol.* **32:**643–655.

34. Gordon, S. V., K. Eiglmeier, R. Brosch, T. Garnier, N. Honore, B. Barrell, and S. T. Cole. 1999. Genomics of *Mycobacterium tuberculosis* and *Mycobacterium leprae*, p. 93–109. *In* C. Ratledge and J. Dale (ed.), *Mycobacteria: Molecular Biology and Virulence*. Blackwell Science Ltd., Oxford, United Kingdom.

35. Gordon, S. V., K. Eiglmeier, T. Garnier, R. Brosch, J. Parkhill, B. Barrell, S. T. Cole, and R. G. Hewinson. 2001. Genomics of *Mycobacterium bovis*. *Tuberculosis* **81:**157–163.

36. Hayashi, C. Y., and R. V. Lewis. 2000. Molecular architecture and evolution of a modular spider silk protein gene. *Science* **287:**1477–1479.

37. Hermans, P. W. M., D. van Soolingen, and J. D. A. van Embden. 1992. Characterization of a major polymorphic tandem repeat in *Mycobacterium tuberculosis* and its potential use in the epidemiology of *Mycobacterium kansasii* and *Mycobacterium gordonae*. *J. Bacteriol.* **174:**4157–4165.

38. Hou, J. Y., J. E. Graham, and J. E. Clark-Curtiss. 2002. *Mycobacterium avium* genes expressed during growth in human macrophages detected by selective capture of transcribed sequences (SCOTS). *Infect. Immun.* **70:**3714–3726.

39. Kremer, K., D. van Soolingen, R. Frothingham, W. H. Haas, P. W. Hermans, C. Martin, P. Palittapongarnpim, B. B. Plikaytis, L. W. Riley, M. A. Yakrus, J. M. Musser, and J. D. van Embden. 1999. Comparison of methods based on different molecular epidemiological markers for typing of *Mycobacterium tuberculosis* complex strains: interlaboratory study of discriminatory power and reproducibility. *J. Clin. Microbiol.* **37:**2607–2618.

40. Levitskaya, J., M. Coram, V. Levitsky, S. Imreh, P. M. Steigerwald-Mullen, G. Klein, M. G. Kurilla, and M. G. Masucci. 1995. Inhibition of antigen processing by the internal repeat region of the Epstein-Barr virus nuclear antigen-1. *Nature* **375:**685–688.

41. Levitskaya, J., A. Sharipo, A. Leonchiks, A. Ciechanover, and M. G. Masucci. 1997. Inhibition of ubiquitin/proteasome-dependent protein degradation by the Gly-Ala repeat domain of the Epstein-Barr virus nuclear antigen 1. *Proc. Natl. Acad. Sci. USA* **94:**12616–12621.

42. Lewis, K. N., R. Liao, K. M. Guinn, M. J. Hickey, S. Smith, M.-A. Behr, and D. R. Sherman. 2003. Deletion of RD1 from *Mycobacterium tuberculosis* mimics Bacille Calmette-Guérin attenuation. *J. Infect. Dis.* **187:**117–123.

43. McKnew, D. L., F. Lynn, J. M. Zenilman, and M. C. Bash. 2003. Porin variation among clinical isolates of *Neisseria gonorrhoeae* over a 10-year period, as determined by Por variable region typing. *J. Infect. Dis.* **187:**1213–1222.

44. O'Brien, R., O. Flynn, E. Costello, D. O'Grady, and M. Rogers. 2000. Identification of a novel DNA probe for strain typing *Mycobacterium bovis* by restriction fragment length polymorphism analysis. *J. Clin. Microbiol.* **38:**1723–1730.

45. Okkels, L. M., I. Brock, F. Follmann, E. M. Agger, S. M. Anend, T. H. M. Ottenhoff, F. Oftung, I. Rosenkrands, and P. Anderson. 2003. PPE protein (Rv3873) from DNA segment RD1 of *Mycobacterium tuberculosis*: strong recognition of both specific T-cell epitopes and epitopes conserved within the PPE family. *Infect. Immun.* **71:**6116–6123.

46. Poulet, S., and S. T. Cole. 1995. Characterization of the highly abundant polymorphic GC-rich-repetitive sequence (PGRS) present in *Mycobacterium tuberculosis*. *Arch. Microbiol.* **163:** 87–95.

47. Ramakrishnan, L., N. A. Federspiel, and S. Falkow. 2000. Granuloma-specific expression of mycobacterium virulence proteins from the glycine-rich PE-PGRS family. *Science* **288:**1436–1439.

48. Rechsteiner, M., and S. W. Rogers. 1996. PEST sequences and regulation by proteolysis. *Trends Biochem. Sci.* **267:**267–271.

49. Reed, S. G., M. R. Alderson, W. Dalemans, Y. Lobet, and Y. A. W. Skeiky. 2003. Prospects for a better vaccine against tuberculosis. *Tuberculosis* **83:**213–219.

50. Rindi, L., N. Lari, and C. Garzelli. 1999. Search for genes potentially involved in *Mycobacterium tuberculosis* virulence by mRNA differential display. *Biochem. Biophys. Res. Commun.* **258:**94–101.

51. Rivera-Marrero, C. A., M. A. Burroughs, R. A. Masse, F. O. Vannberg, D. L. Leimbach, J. Roman, and J. J. Murtagh, Jr. 1998. Identification of genes differentially expressed in *Mycobacterium tuberculosis* by differential display PCR. *Microb. Pathog.* **25:**307–316.

52. Rodriguez, G. M., B. Gold, M. Gomez, O. Dussurget, and I. Smith. 1999. Identification and characterization of two divergently transcribed iron regulated genes in *Mycobacterium tuberculosis*. *Tubercle Lung Dis.* **79:**287–298.

53. Rodriguez, G. M., M. I. Voskuil, B. Gold, G. K. Schoolnik, and I. Smith. 2002. *ideR*, an essential gene in *Mycobacterium tuberculosis*: role of IdeR in iron-dependent gene expression,

iron metabolism, and oxidative stress response. *Infect. Immun.* **70:**3371–3381.

54. Rogers, S., R. Wells, and M. Rechsteiner. 1986. Amino acid sequences common to rapidly degraded proteins: the PEST hypothesis. *Science* **234:**364–368.

55. Ross, B. C., K. Raios, K. Jackson, and B. Dwyer. 1992. Molecular cloning of a highly repeated DNA element from *Mycobacterium tuberculosis* and its use as an epidemiological tool. *J. Clin. Microbiol.* **30:**942–946.

56. Sampson, S. L., P. Lukey, R. M. Warren, P. D. van Helden, M. Richardson, and M. J. Everett. 2001. Expression, characterization and subcellular localization of the *Mycobacterium tuberculosis* PPE gene Rv1917c. *Tuberculosis* **81:**305–317.

57. Sassetti, C. M., D. H. Boyd, and E. J. Rubin. 2003. Genes required for mycobacterial growth defined by high density mutagenesis. *Mol. Microbiol.* **48:**77–84.

58. Saviola, B., S. C. Woolwine, and W. R. Bishai. 2003. Isolation of acid-inducible genes of *Mycobacterium tuberculosis* with the use of recombinase-based in vivo expression technology. *Infect. Immun.* **71:**1379–1388.

59. Singh, K. K., X. Zhang, A. S. Patibandla, P. Chien, Jr., and S. Laal. 2001. Antigens of *Mycobacterium tuberculosis* expressed during preclinical tuberculosis: serological immunodominance of proteins with repetitive amino acid sequences. *Infect. Immun.* **69:**4185–4191.

60. Skeiky, Y. A., P. J. Ovendale, S. Jen, M. R. Alderson, D. C. Dillon, S. Smith, C. B. Wilson, I. M. Orme, S. G. Reed, and A. Campos-Neto. 2000. T cell expression cloning of a *Mycobacterium tuberculosis* gene encoding a protective antigen associated with the early control of infection. *J. Immunol.* **165:**7140–7149.

61. Stewart, G. R., L. Wernisch, R. Stabler, J. A. Mangan, J. Hinds, K. G. Laing, D. B. Young, and P. D. Butcher. 2002. Dissection of the heat-shock response in *Mycobacterium tuberculosis* using mutants and microarrays. *Microbiology* **148:**3129–3138.

62. Tekaia, F., S. V. Gordon, T. Garnier, R. Brosch, B. G. Barrell, and S. T. Cole. 1999. Analysis of the proteome of *Mycobacterium tuberculosis in silico*. *Tubercle Lung Dis.* **79:**329–342.

63. Triccas, J. A., F. X. Berthet, V. Pelicic, and B. Gicquel. 1999. Use of fluorescence induction and sucrose counterselection to identify *Mycobacterium tuberculosis* genes expressed within host cells. *Microbiology* **145:**2923–2930.

64. Vega-Lopez, F., L. A. Brooks, H. M. Dockrell, K. A. De Smet, J. K. Thompson, R. Hussain, and N. G. Stoker. 1993. Sequence and immunological characterization of a serine-rich antigen from *Mycobacterium leprae*. *Infect. Immun.* **61:**2145–2153.

65. Ye, Z. H., Y. R. Song, A. Marcus, and J. E. Varner. 1991. Comparative localization of three classes of cell wall proteins. *Plant J.* **1:**175–183.

XI. ANIMAL MODELS

Chapter 34

Mycobacterium marinum and Fish and Frog Models of Infection

MICHELE TRUCKSIS, CHRISTOPHER L. PRITCHETT, AND RENATE REIMSCHUESSEL

Mycobacterium marinum is a natural pathogen of poikilothermic organisms including fish and frogs (10, 29). In these animals it causes a chronic granulomatous disease that in fish is referred to as fish tuberculosis due to its similar histologic appearance to human tuberculosis (30). *M. marinum* has been heralded in the past few years as a surrogate model organism for analysis of *Mycobacterium tuberculosis* pathogenesis (4, 9, 13, 16, 18, 25).

MYCOBACTERIUM MARINUM

In addition to *M. marinum*, *Mycobacterium fortuitum* and *Mycobacterium chelonae* subsp. *abscessus* can cause natural infection of poikilothermic animals including fish (6, 7, 8, 27). Our laboratory examined the relative virulence of these three *Mycobacterium* species in the goldfish and found that *M. marinum* was the most virulent (26; our unpublished results). Because of these findings, we have pursued the use of *M. marinum* as a surrogate model organism. The utility of *M. marinum* as a surrogate model organism lies in its close genetic relationship to the *M. tuberculosis* complex organisms and the parallel mechanisms used by these pathogens to counter the defense mechanisms of their hosts. *M. marinum* is closely related to *M. tuberculosis*, as shown by DNA-DNA hybridization and 16S rDNA analysis (28). In addition, studies in our laboratory examining putative virulence genes in *M. marinum* showed that of 36 genes analyzed, 33 have an *M. tuberculosis* gene homologue (our unpublished results). Of these 33 gene products, 21 have greater than 50% identity in protein sequence between the two species (our unpublished results). The similarity is less striking at the nucleotide level, suggesting that although function (protein sequence) is preserved between *M. marinum*

and *M. tuberculosis*, codon usage may vary (our unpublished results).

The parallels in proteomics are translated into parallels in mechanisms used by the *Mycobacterium* species in surviving within the host. The organisms persist inside macrophages within the host. Both *M. marinum* and *M. tuberculosis* are able to arrest the lysosomal maturation pathway (4, 13, 23). Although the exact mechanism used by these mycobacteria is not known, it is known that the bacteria reside in early lysosomes and these lysosomes containing the mycobacteria do not acquire the vacuolar ATPases that cause acidification of lysosomes after they fuse with endosomal compartments (4, 23). Therefore, both *M. marinum* and *M. tuberculosis* can survive within macrophages by inhibiting acidification of the phagosome and preventing maturation of the phagolysosome.

From a practical perspective, *M. marinum* is a more attractive organism to study than *M. tuberculosis* because it grows significantly faster than *M. tuberculosis*, having a generation time of 4 h (10) compared to 20 h for *M. tuberculosis*. Additionally, although it is a human pathogen, *M. marinum* can be grown in a standard microbiology laboratory. The route of infection with *M. marinum* is by direct inoculation through the skin, not via aerosol. The normal route of infection for *M. tuberculosis* is, in contrast, the aerosol route, therefore this organism requires biocontainment in a biosafety level 3 facility.

Finally, from the viewpoint of the host, *M. marinum* infection in its natural hosts displays the characteristic immune hallmarks of giant-cell formation and granuloma formation that are seen in human tuberculosis. The development of two animal models, the goldfish, *Carassius auratus* (25), and the leopard frog, *Rana pipiens* (18), has provided the first natural-infection models for the study of mycobacterial pathogenesis.

Michele Trucksis • Division of Infectious Diseases & Immunology, University of Massachusetts Medical School, Worcester, MA 01605. **Christopher L. Pritchett** • Biology Department, Northeastern State University, Tahlequah, OK 74464. **Renate Reimschuessel** • Center for Veterinary Medicine, Food and Drug Administration, Laurel, MD 20857.

A FISH MODEL

Natural Infection

M. marinum was first isolated in freshwater fish by Bataillon et al. in 1897 (5) and from a saltwater aquarium by Aronson in 1926 (2). It is now known to infect more than 150 species of fish (15) and is an occasional zoonotic human pathogen, with transmission occurring through direct skin inoculation (32) but not via an aerosol. The natural route of infection in fish is unknown; however, many investigators think it occurs either via ingestion of water or contaminated food containing the organism followed by invasion via the gastrointestinal tract or via inoculation after trauma to the epidermis (31). Dissemination of the organism throughout the animal may result from invasion or phagocytosis of either mononuclear cells or tissue macrophages. Cannibalism of infected fish by healthy fish may also contribute to transmission of the disease. In natural infections, the infected fish population first develops an asymptomatic infection that, after months to years, results in progressively symptomatic disease, emaciation, and deaths (30). The disease is a particularly difficult problem in aquaculture facilities and "fish farms," where high densities of fish facilitate the spread of the infection and may also result in stress-induced immunosuppression, making the animals more susceptible to infection. Historically, mycobacterial species have been a serious problem in salmonids (20), with recent surveys showing over 25% of some northeastern Pacific coast hatchery salmonids to be infected (1). Mycobacteriosis is also a problem for other food fish such as striped bass, tilapia, and European sea bass (11, 14, 23). The economic impact of infection is due to both increased mortality in fish stocks and decreased reproductive performance.

Carassius auratus, the Goldfish Model of Mycobacterial Infection

Unlike the traditional animal models used to study experimental tuberculosis infection, the introduction of the goldfish, *C. auratus* (Fig. 1), as an animal model to study mycobacterial pathogenesis is recent (25). A thorough review of the technical aspects of infecting the fish with *M. marinum* is given in reference 21. This chapter describes the highlights of the model, details its use to date, and discusses its potential future use.

In the initial description of the model (25), the fish were inoculated intraperitoneally through the lateral abdominal musculature. This route was chosen because it hastens the course of infection. Attempts to

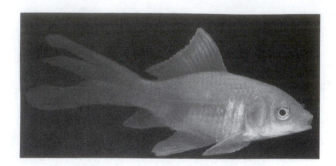

Figure 1. The goldfish, *Carassius auratus*.

infect fish through submersion in water containing *M. marinum* failed to result in disease even after 6 months of follow-up (our unpublished results), suggesting that if this is the natural route of infection, the disease may not be clinically apparent until years after exposure. Following intraperitoneal inoculation, the organisms can be isolated from the peritoneal cavity in some animals even as late as 16 weeks postinoculation. However, the numbers of organisms isolated from a peritoneal wash in most animals is several log units below the number isolated in the same animals from homogenates of liver, spleen, or kidney. The organisms are capable of systemic dissemination from the peritoneal cavity within 1 week of inoculation.

The growth rate of *M. marinum* in fish organs is similar in the organs most often studied, the liver, spleen, and kidneys. The CFU of organisms plateaus by 8 weeks postinoculation and remains at this level for at least 16 weeks (25).

The goldfish develop infection after inoculation with as few as 600 CFU of *M. marinum* via the intraperitoneal route. This low dose results in as great an immune response and corresponding disease as is seen with an inoculation dose of 10^7 CFU (Table 1).

Response to infection in goldfish

A relevant observation about the fish model is the similarity of the fish host response to *M. marinum* infection and the human host response to *M. tuberculosis* infection. In both hosts, the mycobacteria disseminate soon after infection. This is evidenced in humans by the delayed hypersensitivity reaction to purified protein derivative and in goldfish by isolation of viable mycobacteria from retroperitoneal organs (such as the trunk kidney) as soon as 1 week postinoculation. Despite the infection, both humans and fish appear well during the early stages.

In the fish, an initial acute inflammatory response in the peritoneal cavity is present by 2 weeks

Table 1. Minimal infectious dose of *M. marinum*

Inoculum (CFU/animal)	No. positive/total no.[a]	
	Fish model[b]	Frog model[c]
10^6	1/2	4/4
10^5	2/2	3/4
10^4	2/2	4/4
10^3	ND[d]	0/4
10^2	2/2	0/4
10^1	ND	0/2

[a]Number of granuloma-positive animals at 8 weeks postinoculation/total number of animals.
[b]Data from reference 25.
[c]Data from reference 18.
[d]ND, not done.

postinoculation. At earlier times (1 week), only a minority of animals show any inflammation. The acute inflammatory response in the peritoneal cavity is characterized by an accumulation of lymphocytes, macrophages, as well as degenerating cells and bacteria. This acute inflammatory response is followed by a chronic inflammatory response, which begins about 2 weeks postinoculation and progresses until the animal dies, often from secondary bacterial or parasitic infections after progressive wasting. The animal's vital organs are often riddled with granulomas. The chronic inflammatory response is characterized initially by epithelial macrophages, sometimes appearing foamy, and occasional giant cells. These then aggregate to form early granulomas. As the granulomas mature, the epithelioid macrophages condense and fibroblasts surround the granuloma, forming a prominent capsule. The granulomatous response is time dependent, not dose dependent, with a mature granulomatous reaction occurring by 8 weeks postinoculation. The morphology of the granulomas varies and includes necrotizing, nonnecrotizing, and caseous granulomas. The presence of caseous granulomas (Fig. 2), as seen in human tuberculosis, parallels that of granulomas seen in the guinea pig and rabbit models of tuberculosis. Thus, *M. marinum* and the goldfish model provide a surrogate model for studying *M. tuberculosis* and can be used to address questions of pathogenesis including invasion, survival, latency and the host pathological response.

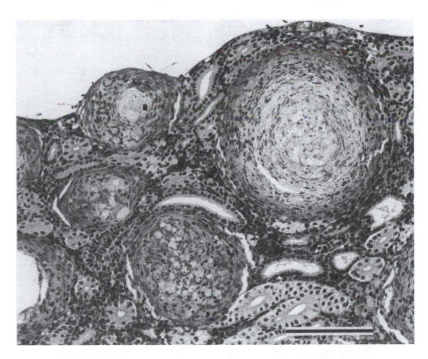

Figure 2. Histopathology of the kidney of a fish infected 8 weeks earlier with *M. marinum* ATCC 927. The kidney is replaced by granulomas of different morphologies located in the interstitium. The large granuloma (upper right) has a very prominent fibroblastic capsule surrounding a core of large, foamy epithelioid macrophages and minimal necrotic debris. The smaller granuloma bulging from the surface of the kidney (upper left) contains a caseous necrotic core surrounded by epithelioid macrophages which are encircled by an irregular ring of fibroblasts. The necrotic center contains a small focus of melanin, a pigment which accumulates in some goldfish macrophages. The other two granulomas (lower left) contain large epithelioid macrophages with either a foamy, eosinophilic cytoplasm or a pale yellow-orange cytoplasm containing ceroid. These granulomas are enveloped by fibroblasts, ranging from multiple to a single cell layer thick, and represent some of the earlier stages of granuloma formation. The section was stained with hematoxylin and eosin stain. Bar, 80 μm.

Applications of the goldfish model to mycobacterial pathogenesis

Identification of avirulent mutants. Our laboratory has applied signature-tagged mutagenesis to the goldfish model of mycobacterial pathogenesis to identify putative virulence genes of *M. marinum*. In a screen of 1,000 mutants, we identified 33 which appeared to be attenuated for survival in the fish. In an in vitro model using fish monocytes as a model for mycobacterial host-pathogen interactions, El-Etr et al. have found that fish monocytes can differentiate between pathogenic and nonpathogenic mycobacterial species (13). Thus the fish model, as well as monocytes derived from fish, can differentiate between virulent and avirulent strains of *Mycobacterium* and can then be used as a screening tool to identify virulence factors in *Mycobacterium* species.

Vaccine challenge model. Our laboratory has also demonstrated that the goldfish model can be used as a vaccine challenge model (21). In a proof-of-principle experiment, wild-type *M. marinum* was used as a vaccine strain to immunize naïve goldfish. At 4 weeks postinfection, the animals were challenged with 50% lethal dose of *M. marinum*. Vaccinated fish were significantly protected from death compared to the unvaccinated control animals (70% survival in vaccinated animals versus 20% survival in nonvaccinated animals). This established that protective immunity develops following *M. marinum* infection and makes feasible the development of rationally attenuated live vaccine strains, which could then be evaluated in the goldfish model.

A Zebrafish Model

The mouse model remains the most widely used model to study tuberculosis infection. Part of its appeal is the ability to use specific-gene-disrupted mice to examine particular host factors responsible for controlling or developing disease due to *M. tuberculosis* infection. Transgenic goldfish are not yet available. However, another natural fish host for *M. marinum* infection, the zebrafish, *Danio rerio*, has emerged as a popular biomedical model organism. In February 2001 the Sanger Institute started sequencing the genome of the zebrafish, and in 2003 a whole-genome preliminary assembly database was made public (http://www.sanger.ac.uk/Projects/D_rerio/). The zebrafish information network (http://zfin.org) has a wide array of transgenic and mutant strains available, making this fish species an appealing model host (24).

Zebrafish develop the characteristic granulomatous inflammatory host response to natural infection with *M. marinum* (Fig. 3) (24). In fact, infection in established zebrafish colonies occurs and can be devastating if it is not controlled (3). Recently, Davis et al. (12) described the use of *M. marinum* infection of zebrafish embryos to study the early stages of granuloma formation. These studies showed that the interaction of *Mycobacterium* and macrophage alone can initiate granuloma-like formation.

The availability of the entire zebrafish genome, the numbers of transgenic or mutant strains currently available, and the fact that *Mycobacterium* infection of the zebrafish represents a natural infection model mean that efforts to further develop this species as a mycobacterial pathogenesis model system are worthwhile.

A FROG MODEL

Natural Infection

Natural infection of reptiles and amphibians with *M. marinum* has not been systematically stud-

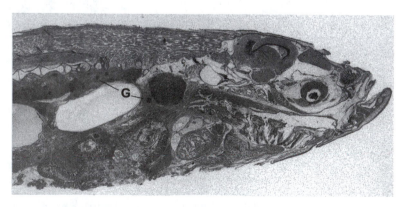

Figure 3. Sagittal section of a whole zebrafish with mycobacteriosis. G, granulomas in the kidney and viscera due to the bacterial infection. Reprinted from M. L. Kent, J. M. Spitsbergen, J. M. Matthews, J. W. Fournie, and M. Westerfield, 2002, *Diseases of Zebrafish in Research Facilities* (http://www.zfin.org) with permission.

ied. Pathologic lesions consistent with *Mycobacterium* infection have been described, and when infection occurs, lesions are found throughout the body, demonstrating that the infection is systemic (19). Infection usually occurs in debilitated animals, or in the case of captive animals, those receiving inappropriate husbandry (23a).

Experimental Infection

Studies with *M. marinum* by Clark and Shepard (10) found that ectothermic animals, such as reptiles and amphibians, were more likely to develop disseminated infection than localized disease. They inoculated several species of frogs with *M. marinum* and found that all were susceptible, dying between 4 and 69 days postinoculation. Postmortem examination revealed acid-fast organisms in phagocytes or small infiltrates consistent with *M. marinum* infection. Tadpoles, the developmental stage of the frog, were also susceptible to *M. marinum* infection. Interestingly, Clark and Shepard (10) demonstrated that *M. marinum* is transmissible to tadpoles through contaminated water or from cohabitation in aquaria with infected fish.

Rana pipiens, the Frog Model of Mycobacterial Infection

The frog model was developed by Ramakrishnan and Falkow (16), who found that *M. marinum* caused a chronic tuberculosis-like illness in the leopard frog, *R. pipiens* (Fig. 4), that was rarely lethal (16). Leopard frogs were inoculated intraperitoneally with three strains of *M. marinum* at doses of 10^6 to 10^7 CFU. Following intraperitoneal inoculation, one of the strains, *M. marinum* M, disseminated, as evidenced by pronounced granuloma formation in the liver, kidneys, spleen, and pleural lining of the lungs by 7 weeks postinoculation. Although few organisms were visualized by microscopy, *M. marinum* M was

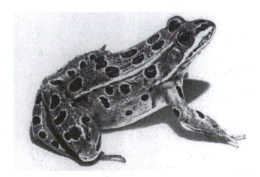

Figure 4. The leopard frog, *Rana pipiens*. Courtesy of Robert N. Fischer, U.S. Geological Survey, San Diego, Calif. (http://www.werc.usgs.gov/fieldguide/).

cultured from the liver, spleen, kidneys, and lungs of all infected frogs (16, 18).

The growth rate of *M. marinum* M in the liver, spleen, and kidneys of frogs inoculated with 10^6 CFU was examined. *M. marinum* was isolated from the organs by 2 weeks after inoculation. There was no significant change in CFU over the course of the experiment, which continued for 58 weeks (18).

The minimum infectious dose of *M. marinum* in the frog was determined in a series of experiments in which groups of frogs were inoculated with 2.3×10^1 to 2.3×10^6 CFU (18) (Table 1). Although *M. marinum* could be isolated from the animals at each dose and the number of organisms recovered increased with higher-titer inocula, only doses of 10^4 CFU or higher induced granuloma formation.

Response to infection in frogs

Granuloma formation following inoculation was time and dose dependent. No granulomas were seen at 2 weeks, but loose aggregates of macrophages or small granulomas were visible by 4 weeks. By 6 weeks, well-formed granulomas were present in the majority of frogs, and this progressed so that after 8 weeks (Fig. 5) all frogs examined had well-formed granulomas. Granulomas consisting of epithelioid macrophages with relatively few *M. marinum* organisms were identified (18). No caseating granulomas were reported.

Fulminant disease in immunosuppressed *M. marinum*-infected frogs

The course of human tuberculosis is dependent in part on the immuno competence of the host. Patients chronically treated with corticosteroids, such as those with chronic rheumatic diseases, asthma, or solid-organ transplants, are more susceptible to infection with *M. tuberculosis* and more likely to reactivate a latent *M. tuberculosis* infection. To determine if altering the immuno competence of the frog would change the course of *M. marinum* disease in the frog model, frogs were treated with hydrocortisone at a dose shown to suppress cellular immunity (18). An acute disease was elicited in hydrocortisone-treated frogs, with five of seven frogs dying within 19 weeks after receiving an intraperitoneal dose of 10^7 CFU of *M. marinum* strain M. Intense peritoneal inflammation, liver abscesses, and numerous acid-fast bacilli were seen on necropsy, but only poorly formed granulomas were observed. This fulminant disease following steroid-induced immunosuppression is consistent with the more fulminant disease seen in natural infection in debilitated or stressed captive animals (23a).

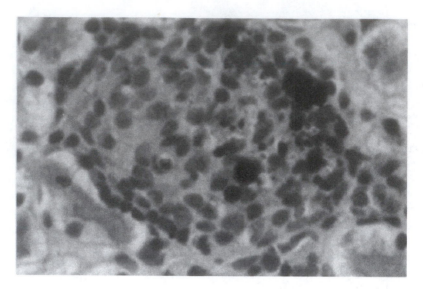

Figure 5. Lesions produced in *M. marinum*-infected frogs. Sections from livers 8 weeks postinfection show typical granulomas during infection with *M. marinum*. The sections were stained with hematoxylin and eosin. Magnification, ×400. Reprinted from reference 18.

Applications of the frog model to mycobacterial pathogenesis

Identification of granuloma- and/or macrophage-specific gene expression. Ramakrishnan et al. used the frog model of mycobacterial pathogenesis to identify genes which are specifically expressed in the granuloma in infected frogs or in M. marinum-infected macrophages (17). These two environments are the preferred niches within the host where the organism is thought to persist. Using differential fluorescence induction, promoter trap libraries were screened in macrophages or in granulomas of infected frogs. The majority of promoters identified were activated in both environments, but some promoters were found which showed specific granuloma expression. The studies identified members of the PE/PE-PGRS and PPE families of proteins (proteins of unknown function containing glycine-rich repeats) as specifically expressed in both macrophages and granulomas (17). Subsequent studies with a mutant with a specific disruption in mag24 confirmed that the mutant was attenuated in virulence. The mag24 mutant produced ill-defined granulomas and failed to persist in the host to the same magnitude degree as the wild-type parental strain (17). These studies and further screens have uncovered bacterial determinants that may contribute to the unusual property of persistence typical of mycobacterium infections.

Additional studies by Chan et al. (9) using differential fluorescence induction to conduct a survey of *M. marinum* gene expression in granulomas of infected frogs determined that *M. marinum* is metaboli-cally active in frog granulomas. Many gene promoters involved in metabolic pathways were expressed in the logarithmic phase in vitro cultures as well as in the granulomas of frogs. Thus, the frog model has been used to dissect the complex pattern of *M. marinum* gene expression in the granuloma, the site most likely to harbor *M. marinum* during the latent stage of infection. This insight may be used to design more effective drugs to eradicate latent tuberculosis infection.

SUMMARY

In summary, the fish and frog models of mycobacterial infection offer an opportunity to examine the interaction of a *Mycobacterium* species, *M. marinum*, with its host in natural infection models. The advantages lie in the both the organism and the hosts. *M. marinum* compares favorably with *M. tuberculosis* both in the pathogenic mechanisms it utilizes to induce disease in its host and in its genetic makeup. It also offers the advantages of having a much shorter generation time and being a less severe biohazard in the laboratory compared to *M. tuberculosis*. The advantages in using the fish and the frog are that these models reflect a natural-infection model and, in comparison to other animal models, have a low cost. The greatest disadvantage is the lack of available reagents to examine cytokine profiles in response to infection and the fact that these animals are not inbred. However, with the availability of zebrafish strains and the release of the zebrafish genome, a more sophisticated natural-infection model may be possible.

REFERENCES

1. Arakawa, C. K., and J. L. Fryer. 1984. Isolation and characterization of a new subspecies of *Mycobacterium chelonei* from salmonid fish. *Helgol. Meersunters.* 37:329–342.

2. Aronson, J. D. 1926. Spontaneous tuberculosis in salt water fish. *J. Infect. Dis.* 39:315–320.

3. Astrofsky, K. M., M. D. Schrenzel, R. A. Bullis, R. M. Smolowitz, and J. G. Fox. 2000. Diagnosis and management of atypical *Mycobacterium* spp. infections in established laboratory zebrafish (*Brachydanio rerio*) facilities. *Comp. Med.* 50:666–672.

4. Barker, L. P., K. M. George, S. Falkow, and P. L. C. Small. 1997. Differential trafficking of live and dead *Mycobacterium marinum* organisms in macrophages. *Infect. Immun.* 65:1497–1504.

5. Bataillon, E., L. Dubard, and L. Terre. 1897. Un noveau type de tuberculose. *C. R. Seances Soc. Biol. Fil.* 4:446–449.

6. Belas, R., P. Faloon, and A. Hannaford. 1995. Potential applications of molecular biology to the study of fish mycobacteriosis. *Annu. Rev. Fish Dis.* 5:133–173.

7. Bragg, R. R., H. F. Huchzermeyer, and M. A. Hanisch. 1990. *Mycobacterium fortuitum* isolated from three species of fish in South Africa. *Onderstepoort J. Vet. Res.* 57:101–102.

8. Bruno, D. W., J. Griffiths, C. G. Mitchell, B. P. Wood, Z. J. Fletcher, F. A. Drobniewski, and T. S. Hastings. 1998. Pathology attributed to *Mycobacterium chelonae* infection among farmed and laboratory-infected Atlantic salmon *Salmo salar*. *Dis. Aquat. Org.* 33:101–109.

9. Chan, K., T. Knaak, L. Satkamp, O. Humbert, S. Falkow, and L. Ramakrishnan. 2002. Complex pattern of *Mycobacterium marinum* gene expression during long-term granulomatous infection. *Proc. Natl. Acad. Sci. USA* 99:3920–3925.

10. Clark, H. F., and C. C. Shepard. 1963. Effect of environmental temperatures on infection with *Mycobacterium marinum* (Balnei) of mice and a number of poikilothermic species. *J. Bacteriol.* 86:1057–1069.

11. Colorni, A., M. Ankaous, A. Diamant, and W. Knibb. 1993. Detection of mycobacteriosis in fish using the polymerase chain reaction technique. *Bull. Eur. Assoc. Fish Pathol.* 13:195–198.

12. Davis, J. M., H. Clay, J. L. Lewis, N. Ghori, P. Herbomel, and L. Ramakrishnan. 2002. Real-time visualization of *Mycobacterium*-macrophage interactions leading to initiation of granuloma formation in zebrafish embryos. *Immunity* 17:693–702.

13. El-Etr, S. H., L. Yan, and J. D. Cirillo. 2001. Fish monocytes as a model for mycobacterial host-pathogen interaction. *Infect. Immun.* 69:7310–7317.

14. Hedrick, R. P., T. McDowell, and J. Groff. 1987. Mycobacteriosis in cultured striped bass from California. *J. Wild. Dis.* 23:391–395.

15. Nigrelli, R. F., and H. Vogel. 1963. Spontaneous tuberculosis in fishes and in other cold-blooded vertebrates with special reference to *Mycobacterium fortuitum* Cruz from fish and human lesions. *Zoologica* 48:131–144.

16. Ramakrishnan, L., and S. Falkow. 1994. *Mycobacterium marinum* persists in cultured mammalian cells in a temperature-restricted fashion. *Infect. Immun.* 62:3222–3229.

17. Ramakrishnan, L., N. A. Federspiel, and S. Falkow. 2000. Granuloma-specific expression of *Mycobacterium* virulence proteins from the glycine-rich PE-PGRS family. *Science* 288:1436–1439.

18. Ramakrishnan, L., R. H. Valdivia, J. H. McKerrow, and S. Falkow. 1997. *Mycobacterium marinum* causes both long-term subclinical infection and acute disease in the leopard frog (*Rana pipiens*). *Infect. Immun.* 65:767–773.

19. Reichenbach-Klinke, H., and E. Elkan. 1965. Infectious diseases, p. 220–233, *In* H. Reichenbach-Klinke and E. Elkan (ed.), *The Principal Diseases of Lower Vertebrates*. Academic Press, Inc., New York, N.Y.

20. Ross, A. J., and H. E. Johnson. 1962. Studies on transmission of mycobacterial infections in chinook salmon. *Prog. Fish-Cult.* 24:147–149.

21. Ruley, K. M., R. Reimschuessel, and M. Trucksis. 2002. Goldfish as an animal model system for mycobacterial infection. *Methods Enzymol.* 358:29–39.

22. Russell, D. G. 2001. *Mycobacterium tuberculosis*: here today, and here tomorrow. *Nat. Rev. Mol. Cell Biol.* 2:569–577.

23. Sakanari, J. A., C. A. Reilly, and M. Moser. 1983. Tubercular lesions in Pacific Coast populations of striped bass. *Trans. Am. Fish. Soc.* 112:565–566.

23a. Siegmund, O. H. 1973. *The Merck Veterinary Manual*. Merck & Co., Rahway, N.J.

24. Sprague, J., E. Doerry, S. Douglas, and M. Westerfield. 2001. The Zebrafish Information Network (ZFIN): a resource for genetic, genomic, and developmental research. *Nucleic Acids Res.* 29:87–90.

25. Talaat, A., R. Reimschuessel, S. S. Wasserman, and M. Trucksis. 1998. Goldfish, *Carassius auratus*, a novel animal model for the study of *Mycobacterium marinum* pathogenesis. *Infect. Immun.* 66:2938–2942.

26. Talaat, A. M., M. Trucksis, A. S. Kane, and R. Reimschuessel. 1999. Pathogenicity of *Mycobacterium fortuitum* and *Mycobacterium smegmatis* to goldfish, *Carassius auratus*. *Vet. Microbiol.* 66:151–164.

27. Teska, J. D., L. E. Twerdok, J. Beaman, M. Curry, and R. A. Finch. 1997. Isolation of *Mycobacterium abscessus* from Japanese Medaka. *J. Aquat. Anim. Health* 9:234–238.

28. Tonjum, T., D. B. Welty, E. Jantzen, and P. L. Small. 1998. Differentiation of *Mycobacterium ulcerans*, *M. marinum*, and *M. haemophilum*: mapping of their relationships to *M. tuberculosis* by fatty acid profile analysis, DNA-DNA hybridization, and 16S rRNA gene sequence analysis. *J. Clin. Microbiol.* 36:918–925.

29. Travis, W. D., L. B. Travis, G. D. Roberts, D. W. Su, and L. W. Weiland. 1985. The histological spectrum in *Mycobacterium marinum* infection. *Arch. Pathol. Lab. Med.* 109:1109–1113.

30. van Duijn, C. 1981. Tuberculosis in fishes. *J. Small Anim. Pract.* 22:391–411.

31. Walker, C. 2000. Fish diseases, p. 1.12–1.14. *In* M. Westerfield (ed.), *The Zebrafish Book. A Guide for the Laboratory Use of Zebrafish (Danio rerio)*, 4th ed. University of Oregon Press, Eugene.

32. Woods, G. L., and J. A. Washington. 1987. Mycobacteria other than *Mycobacterium tuberculosis*: review of microbiologic and clinical aspects. *J. Infect. Dis.* 9:275–294.

Chapter 35

Experimental Infection Models of Tuberculosis in Domestic and Wild Animals

BRYCE M. BUDDLE, JOHN M. POLLOCK, AND R. GLYN HEWINSON

Tuberculosis in domestic and wild animals presents a wide spectrum of disease manifestations. In species such as cattle, the disease progresses very slowly and is usually confined to the primary disease complex, the lungs and associated lymph nodes, while in species such as the Australian brushtail possum (*Trichosurus vulpecula*), the disease rapidly becomes disseminated. The different animal species vary markedly in the number of bacilli found within lesions, in the resulting necrosis, fibrosis, and calcification, and in the degree of tuberculin sensitivity (39). This spectrum of disease is also seen in human tuberculosis, where the disease is usually contained but becomes disseminated in infants and immunocompromised individuals. Domestic and wild animals experimentally infected with tuberculosis can serve as useful models of the disease in humans since these animals are outbred and are natural hosts of the disease. In addition, the disease outcome in these animals can be influenced by genetic and environmental factors. In both domestic and wild animals, tuberculosis is caused almost entirely by *Mycobacterium bovis* and is known as bovine tuberculosis. Sequencing of the genomes of *M. bovis* and *M. tuberculosis* has revealed that the majority of their genes are identical. Strikingly, the genome sequence of *M. bovis* is >99.95% identical to that of *M. tuberculosis*, but deletion of genetic information has led to a reduced genome size. There are no genes unique to *M. bovis*, highlighting the fact that differential gene expression may be the key to the host tropisms of human and bovine bacilli. *M. bovis* has a remarkably broad host range including humans, nonhuman primates, and domestic livestock (cattle, goats, farmed deer, farmed Asiatic buffaloes, camels, and llamas) as well as numerous wild animal species (11). Wildlife can serve as a reservoir of disease for domestic animals, and species which act as maintenance hosts of

the disease are the brushtail possum in New Zealand, the badger in the United Kingdom and Ireland, white-tailed deer and bison in North America, and the African buffalo in Africa.

Over the past 10 years, there has been a resurgence in research on bovine tuberculosis due to the sharp rise in the incidence of the disease in countries such as the United Kingdom and to the continuing problem of wildlife reservoirs in countries such as New Zealand. Research efforts have focused on gaining an understanding of the pathogenesis of the disease and developing improved diagnostic tests and vaccines for disease control. Experimental models of the disease in cattle, deer, possums, and ferrets have been important in enhancing progress in these areas. An advantage of working on bovine tuberculosis, compared to human tuberculosis, is that experimentally induced disease is studied in the natural host, which allows for more meaningful screening of vaccines and accurate estimates of the sensitivity and specificity of diagnostic tests. In this chapter, we focus principally on experimental infection of cattle since this model has many features that make it appealing as a model for the human disease (Table 1). The experimental infection models of deer, possums, ferrets and badgers add to our understanding of tuberculosis and are compared to those in cattle.

PATHOGENESIS OF EXPERIMENTAL INFECTION OF CATTLE WITH *M. BOVIS*

Models of bovine tuberculosis in cattle have been established to provide essential information for the development of new strategies of disease control, including improved methods for diagnosis and vaccination. Additionally, since these models represent

Bryce M. Buddle • AgResearch, Wallaceville Animal Research Centre, P.O. Box 40063, Upper Hutt, New Zealand. John M. Pollock • Veterinary Sciences Division, Department of Agriculture and Rural Development for Northern Ireland, Belfast BT4 3SD, United Kingdom. R. Glyn Hewinson • TB Research Group, Department of Bacterial Diseases, VLA Weybridge, Addlestone, Surrey KT15 3NB, United Kingdom.

Table 1. Use of cattle as a model for tuberculosis of humans

Advantages

Cattle are natural hosts of tuberculosis, with infection acquired predominantly via the respiratory route

Clinical disease may take years to develop

The disease has similar pathology (marked granulomatous reaction) and immune responses (predominantly cellular) to tuberculosis in humans

A large array of immunological reagents are available

Kinetics of the immune response can be readily followed, leading to the identification of immune correlates of protection and disease

Calves are immunologically competent at birth, allowing for neonatal vaccination

Calves become sensitized to antigens of environmental mycobacteria at a young age

BCG has variable efficacy in cattle, which provides an opportunity to detect vaccines that are better than BCG

Candidate vaccines that show promise in laboratory models can be tested in a natural host under a variety of environmental conditions before progressing to clinical trials

Accurate assessment of the sensitivity and specificity of diagnostic tests in cattle is possible, with verification of the infection status following slaughter

Disadvantages

The model uses *M. bovis* and not *M. tuberculosis*

There is no cavitation of the lungs

The model is relatively expensive

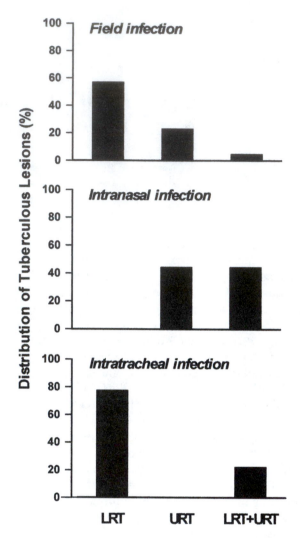

Figure 1. Effect of route of infection on lesion distribution in bovine tuberculosis. Data represent percentages of animals with tuberculous lesions detected in the major lymph nodes of the lower respiratory tract (LRT) (bronchial/mediastinal), of the upper respiratory tract (URT) (retropharyngeal/submaxillary), and of both of these regions (LRT and URT) following field infection ($n = 2,886$) (24) and experimental infection by the intranasal or intratracheal route ($n = 9$ for both).

tuberculosis in a natural host, they offer great potential for advancing our knowledge of the pathogenesis and immunology of mycobacterial diseases in general.

The aerogenous route is considered the most important for natural infection of cattle with *M. bovis*. Therefore, recent models have focused on infection via the respiratory tract, often intranasally or intratracheally. Intranasal infection involves the instillation of defined doses of *M. bovis* into the posterior nasal passages via a cannula (22). Intratracheal infection involves the use of a longer cannula to introduce *M. bovis* into the trachea (2).

It has become clear that the process of infection has a profound effect on the resulting pathological changes, as summarized in Fig. 1. For example, in natural, field cases of bovine tuberculosis in Northern Ireland, most tuberculous lesions are detected in the lymph nodes associated with the lungs but a significant number are also detected in the lymph nodes of the upper respiratory tract. Recent experimental infections have shown that intranasal infection leads to predominant pathology of the lymph nodes associated with the upper respiratory tract while intratracheal infection leads to pathology of both the lymph nodes associated with the upper and lower tracts and the lungs themselves. While these differences are not absolute, as indicated by the proportion of animals with lesions in both regions, the apparent

polarizing effects of these models have led to investigation of alternative models. These include infection by contact with previously infected animals (8), infection via the tonsils (27), and infection by exposure to infectious aerosol (25).

Results from these models have indicated that the number of mycobacteria contained in the infecting inoculum has a profound effect on pathology. For example, in intranasal infection, low doses (10^2 to 10^3 CFU) result in disease only in some of the animals, whereas higher doses (10^6 to 10^7 CFU) infect all calves and produce fulminant, progressive disease in some individuals (as reviewed in reference 21). Of relevance to disease transmission, it has been shown that cattle with tuberculosis shed *M. bovis* in nasal secretions and that shedding is most likely 80 to 100 days after natural infection (23). Recent experiments using a range of infective experimental doses delivered intranasally have shown that the frequency of shedding, as well as the ultimate pathology, is influenced by the initial infecting dose (J. M. Pollock, unpublished observations). Together, these findings indicate that the route and dose of infection are essential factors in any study of tuberculosis pathogenesis and mycobacterial virulence.

Understanding of the pathological processes associated with tuberculosis has been increased by recent studies using the bovine intranasal-infection model (reviewed in reference 21). Sequential postmortem examinations of calves infected with *M. bovis* have shown that upper respiratory tract and lung granulomas can be detected as early as 14 days postinfection. It has also been shown that development of specific in vitro cellular immune responses is linked temporally to formation of these early granulomas. This observation is consistent with concepts of immunopathogenesis as a fundamental mechanism in tuberculosis. Further investigation of the cellular architecture of the granuloma has shown that T cells are a key component and that γδ T cells are among the first to become involved (7).

IMMUNE RESPONSES IN EXPERIMENTAL INFECTION OF CATTLE

In common with the human disease, it has been found that cell-mediated immune responses predominate in early bovine tuberculosis and that the development of an antibody response is often associated with advanced stages of infection (17, 31). Studies of the kinetics of antibody responses in experimental bovine tuberculosis have characterized a number of antigenic targets (18). One observation with implications for the general principles of antituberculosis immunity was that the specific antigenic targets are not consistent and vary depending on the animal and the time postinfection.

Because of the recent focus on cell-based immune responses as readouts for diagnostic tests (e.g., the gamma interferon [IFN-γ] test) or as effectors in the logical development of vaccines, there has been increased study of the role of T cells in bovine tuberculosis. Experimental models of infection have suggested a time-based progression in the involvement of different types of T-cell as the disease progresses (32). Initial involvement of γδ T cells was indicated by a rapid decrease in peripheral numbers of these cells within days of infection. This change was subse-

quently linked to increasing numbers of these cells in the lungs within the first weeks of infection (7). Following initial involvement of γδ T cells, the kinetic study showed that αβ T cells (CD4 and then CD8 T cells) became involved. All of these cell types express a range of surface activation molecules in the context of bovine tuberculosis (46). As regards functional capabilities, CD4 T cells are dominant producers of IFN-γ, while CD8 cells can also produce this cytokine and have the greatest potential to lyse *M. bovis*-infected macrophages (reviewed in reference 31).

There has been recent interest in innate immune responses in tuberculosis. In the bovine disease, there is evidence that γδ T cells play a role in early responses, prior to the development of normal characteristics of acquired responsiveness, such as in vitro lymphocyte proliferation (7, 32). Recent observations that these cells become activated in response to *M. bovis* infection, respond predominantly to protein antigens and synthetic peptides derived from such proteins (35), as well as to nonprotein antigens, and play an apparent role in the induction of Th1-biased responses, have led to the proposal that γδ T cells play an important role in innate responses to tuberculosis (33). Interestingly, bovine γδ T cells also suppress or modulate other (αβ) T-cell populations, perhaps by secreting transforming growth factor β (TGF-β) (35).

DEVELOPMENT OF IMPROVED VACCINES FOR CONTROL OF TUBERCULOSIS

Use of an effective tuberculosis vaccine for cattle would be highly desirable in the countries that cannot control bovine tuberculosis by using the conventional "test and slaughter" strategy, whereby animals giving a positive skin reaction to tuberculin are identified as infected and slaughtered. Over the past 10 years, the intratracheal infection model in cattle has been used to optimize vaccination strategies, evaluate new vaccines, and gain an understanding of the immune processes involved in protection and disease. Vaccination of 5- to 8-month-old calves with one or two doses of BCG (10^4 to 10^6 CFU) significantly reduced the proportion of animals with macroscopic tuberculous lesions and pathological scores compared with nonvaccinated animals, although complete protection has not been seen (reviewed in reference 4). In one study, calves naturally sensitized to environmental mycobacteria prior to BCG vaccination were not protected against challenge while those with a similar genetic background, but not sensitized, were protected (5). These findings concur with results from many human trials, where exposure to environmental mycobacteria is thought to be a contributing factor in the failure of BCG to protect against pulmonary tuberculosis (13). Sequential infections with environmental mycobacteria and BCG may induce a varied response. Experimental infection of calves with *Mycobacterium avium* has been shown to prime immune responses to a subsequent BCG vaccination, but the responses were biased toward antigens of *M. avium* (16). However, the influence of *M. avium* infection on the protective efficacy of BCG against *M. bovis* infection has yet to be determined in this system.

The time at which BCG is administered to infants may be critical for achieving optimum protection. Factors such as the state of maturity of the immune system at birth and exposure to environmental mycobacteria may influence the optimal timing of BCG vaccination. Calves can serve as a useful model to improve vaccination strategies for neonates. A recent study has shown that vaccination of calves at birth or 6 weeks of age induced a high level of protection against challenge with virulent *M. bovis* at 4 months of age (6). Since the calves were responding to environmental mycobacterial antigens at 6 weeks of age, the results indicated that the responsiveness to these antigens at 6 weeks of age did not adversely influence the development of protection induced by BCG vaccination. In contrast, animals in the same study that were vaccinated at birth and revaccinated at 6 weeks had significantly less protection than those vaccinated only at birth. The kinetics of the immune responses suggested that these young calves cleared the initial BCG infection more slowly than older animals and that revaccination before the initial BCG infection is cleared may trigger an inappropriate immune response.

A range of different types of tuberculosis vaccines, including attenuated *M. bovis* vaccine strains, DNA vaccines, and protein vaccines, have been evaluated in the cattle vaccination/challenge model. Vaccination of 5- to 6-month-old calves with either of two auxotrophic strains of *M. bovis* induced protection against challenge with *M. bovis* (5). In that study, the calves were naturally sensitized to environmental mycobacteria prior to vaccination and a 10-fold-lower dose of BCG vaccine was ineffective in inducing protective immunity. DNA (MPB70 or MPB83) vaccines that induced protection in a small-animal model were shown to induce CD4[+] T-cell responses but not a tuberculin skin response in cattle (42). Failure to induce skin test reactivity is considered a desirable characteristic since vaccination would not compromise the use of the skin test for the diagnosis of bovine tuberculosis. However, in a subsequent challenge experiment, these vaccines did not induce protection, and boosting with MPB70 protein predominantly enhanced the humoral responses without improving protection (49). Vaccination intramuscularly and in-

tradermally with DNA vaccines encoding Hsp65, Hsp70, and Apa also failed to induce protection, but a combination of priming with two doses of these DNA vaccines and boosting with BCG vaccine produced an encouraging result. Vaccination with DNA prime/BCG boost resulted in significant improvement in six pathological and microbiological characteristics of protection, while BCG alone induced improvement in only two of these characteristics (36). Results of trials using tuberculosis protein vaccines have been disappointing since vaccines that induce some protection in mice have not induced protection or strong cellular responses in cattle (47, 48). The identification of appropriate adjuvants capable of inducing strong cellular immune responses in cattle is a major factor limiting progress in the development of effective protein vaccines.

IDENTIFICATION OF IMMUNOLOGICAL CORRELATES OF PROTECTION AND DISEASE

The kinetics of immune responses to vaccination and subsequent challenge can be readily measured in cattle and provides insights into possible correlates of protection and disease. IFN-γ released from bovine purified protein derivative (PPD)-stimulated whole-blood cultures is a convenient measure of the antigen-specific production of this cytokine in large numbers of animals following vaccination and challenge. It is well recognized that IFN-γ is crucial for the activation of macrophage effector function and control of mycobacterial infections. Subcutaneous vaccination of 5- to 6-month-old calves with 10^4 to 10^6 CFU of BCG induces a rapid rise in IFN-γ responses after 2 weeks, but these responses fall by 5 to 8 weeks after vaccination (Fig. 2). IFN-γ responses to bovine PPD after vaccination but prior to challenge do not provide an indication of which BCG-vaccinated animals will be protected from disease, while responses after challenge correlate with disease severity and protective efficacy. By 17 to 21 weeks after challenge, BCG-vaccinated animals that are not protected have significantly higher responses than do BCG-vaccinated animals that are protected (Fig. 2, $P < 0.05$). Furthermore, IFN-γ responses of the *M. bovis*-infected, nonvaccinated animals rise faster after challenge than the corresponding responses of infected animals from the BCG-vaccinated group, indicating that IFN-γ responses after challenge can specify different degrees of protection.

ESAT-6-specific IFN-γ production in cattle after challenge with *M. bovis* is also a useful correlate of disease severity in vaccination trials and is particularly useful since ESAT-6 is not expressed by BCG (41).

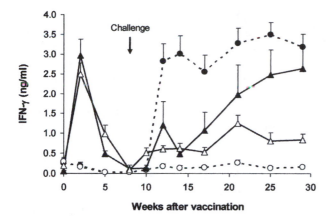

Figure 2. Effect of BCG vaccination and subsequent challenge of calves with *M. bovis* on IFN-γ released from whole-blood cultures stimulated with bovine PPD. All calves were challenged with 10^3 CFU of *M. bovis* intratracheally at 8 weeks after vaccination. The tuberculous-lesion status of calves after *M. bovis* challenge is as follows: ●, nonvaccinated calves that developed lesions (*n* = 10); ○, nonvaccinated calves with no lesions (*n* = 6); ▲, BCG-vaccinated calves that developed lesions (*n* = 6); △, BCG-vaccinated calves with no lesions (*n* = 24). IFN-γ levels are presented as mean concentration; error bars represents standard error of the mean.

IFN-γ responses to ESAT-6 can serve as a predictor of both vaccine efficacy and disease severity, as shown in Fig. 3. It should be noted that the animals in these experiments were at a relatively early stage of disease and were asymptomatic at the time of postmortem examination. This is not the case for human patients, who usually present at the clinic with mani-

fest symptoms of tuberculosis. Therefore, immune responses in the bovine model are more likely to be akin to those observed in human contacts that eventually progress to clinical tuberculosis. This is consistent with the results of a recent study that demonstrated a strong association between in vitro IFN-γ responsiveness to ESAT-6 and later progression to clinical tuberculosis in healthy human household contacts. Contacts who remained healthy during the time of observation generally either responded weakly to ESAT-6 or did not respond at all (12).

DEVELOPMENT OF IMPROVED DIAGNOSTICS

Defining more specific reagents for the detection of tuberculosis infection or for differentiating between vaccinated and infected individuals is a priority for research in both human and veterinary medicine. The experimental-infection model in cattle has been particularly useful for defining antigen candidates, since the kinetics of the immune response can be readily measured and results can be validated in the field when naturally infected animals are killed and their infection status is verified at postmortem examination. Although the tuberculin skin test is routinely used for detection of *M. bovis*-infected cattle in the field, the whole-blood IFN-γ test is increasingly being used as an ancillary test for confirming tuberculosis, due to its relatively high sensitivity (30). Over the past few years, large numbers of mycobacterial antigens have been screened in the IFN-γ test against blood samples from experimentally infected cattle. The aim has been to identify antigens more specific than tuberculin PPD and to differentiate between vaccinated animals and those infected with *M. bovis*.

BCG vaccination sensitizes animals to tuberculin PPD-based diagnostic tests. Therefore, the development of differential diagnostic assays has concentrated on antigens whose genes are deleted or underexpressed in BCG but strongly expressed in virulent *M. bovis*. The most encouraging results have been obtained with two antigens, ESAT-6 and CFP-10, that are recognized frequently by tuberculous cattle but are not recognized by BCG-vaccinated cattle (3, 44). Animals that were BCG vaccinated but still developed disease following challenge with *M. bovis* responded to either recombinant ESAT-6 or an ESAT-6/CFP-10-derived peptide cocktail in the IFN-γ assay. In contrast, BCG-vaccinated animals without signs of disease (i.e., those that were fully protected) did not respond to these antigens (41). Both antigens also improved the specificity of the IFN-γ test compared to PPD in nonvaccinated, naturally

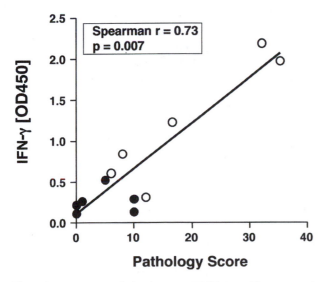

Figure 3. Positive correlation between ESAT-6-specific IFN-γ and disease severity. IFN-γ was released from whole-blood cultures stimulated with ESAT-6 at 11 weeks after *M. bovis* infection. Responses of individual cattle are shown in relation to the severity of disease observed at the postmortem examination: ●, BCG vaccinated calves; ○, nonvaccinated calves. OD450, optical density at 450 nm. Reprinted from reference 41, with permission.

infected animals, although the sensitivity of the test decreased when these antigens were used (29, 30, 40, 43, 44).

USE OF COMPARATIVE GENOMICS TO IDENTIFY DIAGNOSTIC ANTIGENS

The identification of further specific antigens is clearly required to close the sensitivity gap between tuberculin and a cocktail of ESAT-6 and CFP-10. The rapid advance in mycobacterial genomics means that the genome sequences of *M. tuberculosis*, *M. bovis*, and BCG Pasteur have now been largely elucidated. Sequence information about the genomes of *M. avium* and *M. paratuberculosis* is also becoming available. Systematic comparative genome analysis can therefore be performed to identify potentially specific antigens that either can distinguish between vaccination and infection or are more species specific than tuberculin. Since *M. bovis* has greater than 99.9% DNA identity to *M. tuberculosis*, antigens identified in cattle after *M. bovis* infection will have almost identical amino acid sequences to their *M. tuberculosis* counterparts and can therefore be directly tested in humans. Recently, cattle models of *M. bovis* infection and BCG vaccination were used to identify highly immunogenic antigens from three genomic regions deleted in BCG Pasteur (RD1, RD2, and RD14) that could be useful as specific diagnostic reagents. Pools of overlapping peptides spanning 13 of these open reading frames were tested in *M. bovis*-infected, BCG-vaccinated, and nonvaccinated environmentally sensitized control cattle. Almost all antigens were recognized in infected cattle but with widely different responder frequencies that varied between 0 and 86%, suggesting a clear hierarchy of immunodominance among mycobacterial antigens. In particular, six antigens showed promise as diagnostic antigens (i.e., Rv1983, Rv1986, Rv3872, Rv3873, Rv3878, and Rv3879) (9, 20). Importantly, a number of antigens have been identified, which are recognized by *M. bovis*-infected cattle, that do not respond to ESAT-6 and/or CFP-10 and are therefore likely to improve the overall sensitivity (20).

Antigen mining using comparative genomics has been facilitated by the use of synthetic peptides to identify epitopes that are recognized in a major histocompatibility complex-promiscuous manner among cattle breeds. For ESAT-6, such epitopes were readily identified in *M. bovis*-infected cattle and could be formulated into peptide cocktails that gave equivalent responses to the recombinant form of the protein (44). With respect to the relevance of this approach to human diagnostics, a striking overlap has been observed between ESAT-6-derived peptide determinants most frequently recognized in cattle and the epitope specificity of published human ESAT-6-specific responses. For example, the T-cell repertoire of both humans and cattle is strongly directed toward an epitope(s) within the N-terminal portion (residues 1 to 16) of ESAT-6 (45). This suggests the existence of similar immunodominant epitopes within mycobacterial antigens that are recognized by humans and cattle. Consistent with this hypothesis is the recent finding that a virtual-matrix-based human prediction program could identify peptides that were recognized by $CD4^+$ T cells from *M. bovis*-infected cattle. In this study, 73% of the experimentally defined peptides from 10 *M. bovis* antigens that were recognized by bovine T cells contained motifs predicted by the program. Moreover, three of five peptides from the mycobacterial antigen Rv3019c that were predicted to contain HLA-DR-restricted epitopes were recognized by T cells from *M. bovis*-infected cattle (45). These results reinforce the relevance of the bovine model to human tuberculosis research and suggest that bioinformatics might be used to increase the efficiency of epitope screening and selection in humans and cattle.

EXPERIMENTAL TUBERCULOSIS INFECTION OF OTHER DOMESTIC AND WILD ANIMALS

Deer

Deer naturally infected with *M. bovis* develop tuberculous lesions similar to those found in cattle, although they may be more severe. The lesions are found predominantly in the lungs and the thoracic and retropharyngeal lymph nodes. An intratonsillar challenge model has been developed in deer by inoculating 10^2 CFU of *M. bovis* into the tonsillar crypt (14). The resulting lesions are found predominantly in the retropharyngeal lymph nodes, mimicking lesions commonly seen in the natural disease. This model has been used to study pathogenesis (26), the heritability of resistance to tuberculosis (19), and the development of improved vaccination strategies (15). To investigate the heritable basis for resistance and susceptibility of deer to tuberculosis, a large group of farmed red deer stags were challenged with *M. bovis* and, following slaughter, were categorized into resistant or susceptible phenotypes (19). Offspring bred from six of these stags by artificial insemination of stored semen were similarly challenged. The offspring showed a pattern of response to *M. bovis* challenge similar to those of their sires, providing evidence of a strong genetic basis for resistance to tuberculosis, with an estimated heritability of 0.48. Selection lines of resistant and susceptible animals now provide opportunities to study mechanisms of resistance. In separate vaccination-challenge studies, a single dose of BCG vaccine (10^6 CFU) administered subcutaneously to 6- to 12-month-old animals induced significant protection against disease (presence of lesions) but not against infection (isolation of *M. bovis*) (15), while two doses of BCG 8 weeks apart induced significant protection against infection and disease. No protection was induced when animals were vaccinated with two doses of heat-killed BCG (5×10^7 CFU) in an oil adjuvant.

Possums

Lesions in possums naturally infected with *M. bovis* are most frequently found in the lungs and superficial lymph nodes. Experimental-infection models have been established in possums by intratracheal inoculation of very low doses (10 to 100 CFU) of *M. bovis* or by exposing anesthetised possums to an aerosol of *M. bovis* in an aerosol-generating chamber. Lesions are characterized by extensive necrosis, infiltration of large numbers of neutrophils, numerous acid-fast bacilli, and a limited granulomatous reaction (28). Delivery of BCG vaccine by a variety of routes including subcutaneous injection, intranasal spray, and instillation into the gastrointestinal tract has resulted in a significant level of protection against a challenge with *M. bovis* (reviewed in reference 4). Vaccination of recently captured possums with BCG does not prevent animals from developing tuberculous lesions from a subsequent challenge, although it does result in a reduction in the severity of disease. A recent BCG vaccination field trial involving the capture and release of possums has produced more encouraging results. In an area where bovine tuberculosis is endemic, 50% of possums from a total population of 300 possums were vaccinated with BCG by both intranasal spray and conjunctival instillation (10). The BCG vaccine had an efficacy of 69% in preventing the development of clinical tuberculous lesions. A cost-effective way of delivering vaccine to wild possums is required, and an oral-bait tuberculosis vaccine is a possibility. Although BCG cultures delivered orally or intragastrically were relatively ineffective, BCG delivered intraduodenally or intragastrically with an antacid medication induced protection against an experimental challenge (4). These encouraging results demonstrate that BCG could be effective if it was protected from degradation in the stomach. BCG encapsulated in a lipid matrix has been fed to possums and has resulted in significant protection against an experimental aerosol challenge with *M. bovis* (1).

The very high susceptibility of possums to *M. bovis* infection and the limited protection of possums

against experimentally induced infection provide opportunities to identify tuberculosis vaccines that are more effective than BCG. In one study, killed *M. vaccae* mixed with live BCG and administered intranasally induced significantly greater protection than did BCG alone (37). In another study, vaccination with two newly derived attenuated *M. bovis* strains induced a higher degree of protection than that seen with BCG (4).

Ferrets

Lesions in ferrets naturally infected with *M. bovis* are found most commonly in the mesenteric and head lymph nodes, indicating that in New Zealand, the principal route is probably from consumption of *M. bovis*-infected possum carcasses. An experimental-infection model has been established by feeding ferrets with meat laced with high doses (10^6 CFU) of *M. bovis* (34). Ferrets orally vaccinated with live BCG incorporated into dietary meat were partially protected against oral challenge with virulent *M. bovis*.

Badgers

The natural route of infection of badgers with tuberculosis is thought to be via aerosol and through bite wounds. A bite wound model has been established by using intradermal inoculation with 10^3 CFU *M. bovis*. In a preliminary study, badgers vaccinated with 10^6 CFU of BCG by the intradermal route lived longer and shed fewer bacilli than did nonvaccinated control animals after being challenged intradermally with *M. bovis* (38). An intratracheal challenge model is under development in the Republic of Ireland (E. P. Gormley and L. A. L. Corner, personal communication).

CONCLUDING REMARKS

The study of experimentally induced tuberculosis models in animals other than laboratory animals (mice, guinea pigs, and rabbits) can greatly expand our knowledge of tuberculosis. Although the mouse model has been very important in gaining an understanding of the pathogenesis of tuberculosis, studies of species such as cattle are valuable since the disease more closely mimics that seen in humans and the kinetics of the disease can be readily studied. Factors which contribute to the relevance of the cattle model in this situation include its status as a natural host for the disease and an outbred species, as well as the influence of environmental factors on the development of the disease. Unlike human vaccine trials, cattle and deer can be experimentally challenged, which results in a reproducible disease and in trials that can be completed within a relatively short time. Neonatal calves are a useful model for testing vaccines in infants since they are immunocompetent at birth and become naturally sensitized to environmental mycobacteria at a young age. Finally, one of the major advantages of studying infection by a pathogen in a natural host amenable to experimentation is that the kinetics of the immune response can be monitored by repeated blood sampling after infection and can be related to the development of pathology and disease. Such an approach facilitates the identification of diagnostic antigens and immune correlates of protection and disease. In addition, results obtained using experimental infections can be validated in the field because naturally infected animals can be killed and their infection status can be verified at postmortem examination.

Acknowledgments. We express our appreciation to Margot Skinner, Des Collins, Geoff de Lisle, Jim McNair, and Martin Vordermeier for critical reading of the manuscript and for making helpful suggestions.

REFERENCES

1. **Aldwell, F. E., D. Keen, N. Parlane, M. A. Skinner, G. W. de Lisle, and B. M. Buddle.** 2003. Oral vaccination with *Mycobacterium bovis* BCG in a lipid formulation induces resistance to pulmonary tuberculosis in possums. *Vaccine* **22:**70–76.

2. **Buddle, B. M., G. W. de Lisle, A. Pfeffer, and F. E. Aldwell.** 1995. Immunological responses and protection against *Mycobacterium bovis* in calves vaccinated with a low dose of BCG. *Vaccine* **13:**1123–1130.

3. **Buddle, B. M., N. A. Parlane, D. L. Keen, F. E. Aldwell, J. M. Pollock, K. Lightbody, and P. Andersen.** 1999. Differentiation between *Mycobacterium bovis* BCG-vaccinated and *M. bovis*-infected cattle by using recombinant mycobacterial antigens. *Clin. Diagn. Lab. Immunol.* **6:**1–5.

4. **Buddle, B. M., M. A. Skinner, D. N. Wedlock, D. M. Collins, and G. W. de Lisle.** 2002. New generation vaccines and delivery systems for control of bovine tuberculosis in cattle and wildlife. *Vet. Immunol. Immunopathol.* **87:**177–185.

5. **Buddle, B. M., B. J. Wards, F. E. Aldwell, D. M. Collins, and G. W. de Lisle.** 2002. Influence of sensitisation to environmental mycobacteria on subsequent vaccination against bovine tuberculosis. *Vaccine* **20:**1126–1133.

6. **Buddle, B. M., D. N. Wedlock, N. A. Parlane, L. A. L. Corner, G. W. de Lisle, and M. A. Skinner.** 2003. Revaccination of neonatal calves with *Mycobacterium bovis* BCG reduced the level of protection against tuberculosis induced by a single vaccination. *Infect. Immun.* **71:** 6411–6419.

7. **Cassidy, J. P., D. G. Bryson, M. M. Gutiérrez Cancela, F. Forster, J. M. Pollock, and S. D. Neill.** 2001. Lymphocyte subtypes in experimentally induced early stage bovine tuberculosis lesions. *J. Comp. Pathol.* **124:**46–51.

8. **Cassidy, J. P., D. G. Bryson, J. M. Pollock, R. T. Evans, F. Forster, and S. D. Neill.** 1999. Lesions in cattle exposed to *Mycobacterium bovis*-inoculated calves. *J. Comp. Pathol.* **121:**321–337.

9. **Cockle, P. J., S. V. Gordon, A. Lalvani, B. M. Buddle, R. G. Hewinson, and H. M. Vordermeier.** 2002. Identification of novel *Mycobacterium tuberculosis* antigens with potential as diagnostic reagents or subunit vaccine candidates by comparative genomics. *Infect. Immun.* **70:**6996–7003.

10. **Corner, L. A., S. Norton, B. M. Buddle, and R. S. Morris.** 2002. The efficacy of bacilli Calmette-Guérin vaccine in wild brushtail possums (*Trichosurus vulpecula*). *Res. Vet. Sci.* **73:**145–152.

11. **de Lisle, G. W., C. G. Mackintosh, and R. G. Bengis.** 2001. *Mycobacterium bovis* in free-living and captive wildlife, including farmed deer. *Rev. Sci. Tech. Off. Int. Epizool.* **20:**86–111.

12. **Doherty, T. M., A. Demissie, J. Olobo, D. Wolday, S. Britton, T. Eguale, P. Ravn, and P. Andersen.** 2002. Immune responses to the *Mycobacterium tuberculosis*-specific antigen ESAT-6 signal subclinical infection among contacts of tuberculosis patients. *J. Clin. Microbiol.* **40:**704–706.

13. **Fine, P. E. M.** 1995. Variation in protection by BCG: implications of and for heterologous immunity. *Lancet* **346:**1339–1345.

14. **Griffin, J. F. T., C. G. Mackintosh, and G. S. Buchan.** 1995. Animals models of protective immunity in tuberculosis to evaluate candidate vaccines. *Trends Microbiol.* **3:**418–424.

15. **Griffin, J. F. T., C. G. Mackintosh, L. Slobbe, A. J. Thomson, and G. S. Buchan.** 1999. Vaccine protocols to optimise the protective efficacy of BCG. *Tubercle Lung Dis.* **79:**135–143.

16. **Howard, C. J., L. S. Kwong, B. Villarreal-Ramos, P. Sopp, and J. C. Hope.** 2002. Exposure to *Mycobacterium avium* primes the immune system of calves for vaccination with *Mycobacterium bovis* BCG. *Clin. Exp. Immunol.* **130:**190–195.

17. **Lenzini, L., P. Rottoli, and L. Rottoli.** 1977. The spectrum of human tuberculosis. *Clin. Exp. Immunol.* **27:**230–237.

18. **Lyashchenko, K. P., J. M. Pollock, R. Colangeli, and M. L. Gennaro.** 1998. Diversity of antigen recognition by serum antibodies in experimental bovine tuberculosis. *Infect. Immun.* **66:**5344–5349.

19. **Mackintosh, C. G., T. Qureshi, K. Waldrup, R. E. Labes, K. G. Dodds, and J. F. T. Griffin.** 2000. Genetic resistance to experimental infection with *Mycobacterium bovis* in red deer (*Cervus elaphus*). *Infect. Immun.* **68:**1620–1625.

20. **Mustafa, A. S., P. J. Cockle, F. Shaban, R. G. Hewinson, and H. M. Vordermeier.** 2002. Immunogenicity of *Mycobacterium tuberculosis* RD1 region gene products in infected cattle. *Clin. Exp. Immunol.* **130:**37–42.

21. **Neill, S. D., D. G. Bryson, and J. M. Pollock.** 2001. Pathogenesis of tuberculosis in cattle. *Tuberculosis* **81:**79–86.

22. **Neill, S. D., J. Hanna, J. J. O'Brien, and R. M. McCracken.** 1988. Excretion of *Mycobacterium bovis* by experimentally infected cattle. *Vet. Rec.* **123:**340–343.

23. **Neill, S. D., J. J. O'Brien, and J. Hanna.** 1991. A mathematical model for *Mycobacterium bovis* excretion from tuberculous cattle. *Vet. Microbiol.* **28:**103–109.

24. **Neill, S. D., J. M. Pollock, D. B. Bryson, and J. Hanna.** 1994. Pathogenesis of *Mycobacterium bovis* infection in cattle. *Vet. Microbiol.* **40:**41–52.

25. **Palmer, M. V., W. R. Waters, and D. L. Whipple.** 2002. Aerosol delivery of virulent *Mycobacterium bovis* to cattle. *Tuberculosis* **82:**275–282.

26. **Palmer, M. V., W. R. Waters, and D. L. Whipple.** 2002. Lesion development in white-tailed deer (*Odocoileus virginianus*) experimentally infected with *Mycobacterium bovis*. *Vet. Pathol.* **39:**334–340.

27. **Palmer, M. V., D. L. Whipple, J. C. Rhyan, C. A. Bolin, and D. A. Saari.** 1999. Granuloma development in cattle after intratonsilar inoculation with *Mycobacterium bovis*. *Am. J. Vet. Res.* **60:**310–315.

28. Pfeffer, A., B. M. Buddle, and F. E. Aldwell. 1994. Tuberculosis in the brushtail possum (*Trichosurus vulpecula*) after intratracheal inoculation with low dose of *Mycobacterium bovis*. *J. Comp. Pathol.* 111: 353–363.

29. Pollock, J. M., and P. Andersen. 1997. The potential of the ESAT-6 antigen secreted by virulent mycobacteria for specific diagnosis of tuberculosis. *J. Infect. Dis.* 175:1251–1254.

30. Pollock, J. M., B. M. Buddle, and P. Andersen. 2001. Towards more accurate diagnosis of bovine tuberculosis using defined antigens. *Tuberculosis* 81:65–69.

31. Pollock, J. M., and S. D. Neill. 2002. *Mycobacterium bovis* infection and tuberculosis in cattle. *Vet. J.* 163:115–127.

32. Pollock, J. M., D. A. Pollock, D. G. Campbell, R. M. Girvin, A. D. Crockard, S. D. Neill, and D. P. Mackie. 1996. Dynamic changes in circulating and antigen responsive T-cell subpopulations post-*Mycobacterium bovis* infection in cattle. *Immunology* 87:236–241.

33. Pollock, J. M., and M. D. Welsh. 2002. The WC1$^+$ γδ T-cell population in cattle: a possible role in resistance to intracellular infection. *Vet. Immunol. Immunopathol.* 89:105–114.

34. Qureshi, T., R. E. Labes, M. L. Cross, J. F. T. Griffin, and C. G. Mackintosh. 1999. Partial protection against oral challenge with *Mycobaterium bovis* in ferrets (*Mustela furo*) following oral vaccination with BCG. *Int. J. Tuberc. Lung Dis.* 3:1025–1033.

35. Rhodes, S. G., R. G. Hewinson, and H. M. Vordermeier. 2001. Antigen recognition and immunomodulation by γδ T cells in bovine tuberculosis. *J. Immunol.* 166: 5604–5610.

36. Skinner, M. A., B. M. Buddle, D. N. Wedlock, D. L. Keen, G. W. de Lisle, R. E. Tascon, J. C. Ferraz, D. B. Lowrie, P. J. Cockle, H. M. Vordermeier, and R. G. Hewinson. 2003. A DNA prime-BCG boost vaccination strategy in cattle induces protection against bovine tuberculosis. *Infect. Immun.* 71:4901–4907.

37. Skinner, M. A., D. L. Keen, N. A. Parlane, G. F. Yates, and B. M. Buddle. 2002. Increased protection against bovine tuberculosis in the brushtail possum (*Trichosurus vulpecula*) when BCG is administered with killed *Mycobacterium vaccae*. *Tuberculosis* 82:15–22.

38. Stuart, F. A., K. H. Mahmood, J. L. Stanford, and D. G. Pritchard. 1988. Development of diagnostic tests for, and vaccination against, tuberculosis in badgers. *Mammal Rev.* 18: 74–75.

39. Thoen, C. O. 1994. Tuberculosis in wild and domestic animals, p. 157–162. *In* B. R. Bloom, (ed.), *Tuberculosis: Pathogenesis, Protection, and Control.* ASM Press, Washington, D.C.

40. van Pinxteren, L. A., P. Ravn, E. M. Agger, J. Pollock, and P. Andersen. 2000. Diagnosis of tuberculosis based on the two specific antigens ESAT-6 and CFP10. *Clin. Diagn. Lab. Immunol.* 7:155–160.

41. Vordermeier, H. M., M. A. Chambers, P. J. Cockle, A. O. Whelan, J. Simmons, and R. G. Hewinson. 2002. Correlation of ESAT-6-specific gamma interferon production with pathology in cattle following *Mycobacterium bovis* BCG vaccination against experimental bovine tuberculosis. *Infect. Immun.* 70: 3026–3032.

42. Vordermeier, H. M., P. J. Cockle, A. O. Whelan, S. Rhodes, M. A. Chambers, D. Clifford, K. Huygen, R. Tascon, D. Lowrie, M. J. Colston, and R. G. Hewinson. 2000. Effective DNA vaccination of cattle with the mycobacterial antigens MPB83 and MPB70 does not compromise the specificity of the comparative intradermal tuberculin skin test. *Vaccine* 19:1246–1255.

43. Vordermeier, H. M., P. J. Cockle, A. O. Whelan, S. Rhodes, and R. G. Hewinson. 2000. Toward the development of diagnostic assays to discriminate between *Mycobacterium bovis* infection and bacille Calmette-Guérin vaccination in cattle. *Clin. Infect. Dis.* 30(Suppl. 3):S291–298.

44. Vordermeier, H. M., A. Whelan, P. J. Cockle, L. Farrant, N. Palmer, and R. G. Hewinson. 2001. Use of synthetic peptides derived from the antigens ESAT-6 and CFP-10 for differential diagnosis of bovine tuberculosis in cattle. *Clin. Diagn. Lab. Immunol.* 8:571–578.

45. Vordermeier, M., A. O. Whelan, and R. G. Hewinson. 2003. Recognition of mycobacterial epitopes by T cells across mammalian species and use of a program that predicts human HLA-DR binding peptides to predict bovine epitopes. *Infect. Immun.* 71:1980–19887.

46. Waters, W. R., T. E. Rahner, M. V. Palmer, D. Cheng, B. J. Nonnecke, and D. L. Whipple. 2003. Expression of L-selectin (CD62L), CD44, and CD25 on activated bovine T cells. *Infect. Immun.* 71:317–326.

47. Wedlock, D. N., B. Vesosky, M. A. Skinner, G. W. de Lisle, I. M. Orme, and B. M. Buddle. 2000. Vaccination of cattle with *Mycobacterium bovis* culture filtrate proteins and interleukin-2 against bovine tuberculosis. *Infect. Immun.* 68:5809–5815.

48. Wedlock, D. N., D. L. Keen, F. E. Aldwell, P. Andersen, and B. M. Buddle. 2002. Effect of adjuvants on immune responses of cattle vaccinated with culture filtrate proteins from *Mycobacterium tuberculosis*. *Vet. Immunol. Immunopathol* 86:79–88.

49. Wedlock, D. N., M. A. Skinner, N. A. Parlane, H. M. Vordermeier, R. G. Hewinson, G. W. de Lisle, and B. M. Buddle. 2003. Vaccination of cattle with DNA vaccines encoding the mycobacterial antigens MPB70 and MPB83: protein boosting induces antibody and does not enhance vaccine efficacy. *Tuberculosis* 83:339–349.

Tuberculosis and the Tubercle Bacillus
Edited by Stewart T. Cole et al.
© 2005 ASM Press, Washington, D.C.

Chapter 36

Animal Models of Tuberculosis

JoAnne L. Flynn, Andrea M. Cooper, and William Bishai

Tuberculosis is primarily a human disease, although most mammals, as well as birds and fish, are susceptible to infection with mycobacteria. However, studying tuberculosis in human subjects, although ultimately important and necessary, can be very challenging. An experimental-infection model allows the researcher the luxury of timing infections and end points and varying the dose, route, and strain of infection. Although in vitro experiments are also valuable for many studies, an animal model is essential for truly understanding a disease, as well as designing new and effective preventions and treatments. With an animal model, one can test a wide range of treatment options, vary doses and timing of drugs, and try vaccines or other treatments that might not be allowed in studies of the human population. Testing of drugs or vaccines in animal models prior to studies in the human population are essential to avoid safety problems in the field. In addition, the ability to manipulate the animal host affords the possibility of addressing mechanisms of resistance and susceptibility, contributing to our overall understanding of an infectious disease.

Tuberculosis research has benefited greatly from the use of various animal models. Since *Mycobacterium tuberculosis* can infect a wide range of animals, researchers can choose the best model for their studies, based on the characteristics of each model and the question being addressed. In this chapter, the mouse, guinea pig, rabbit, and nonhuman primate models are discussed. Each model has its strengths and weaknesses, and the choice of the most appropriate model for a study depends on a variety of factors, including cost, available housing, and the question being addressed.

An important issue in performing animal-based research of tuberculosis is the need for biosafety level 3 (BSL3) containment. The BSL3 requirements, space, housing needs, and transmissibility are different for each animal model and probably play a major part in the choice of animal model. In general, mice are the most economical model in terms of housing costs, containment, and space while nonhuman primates are the most expensive and most difficult to house in BSL3 facilities. The route of infection can also be an important consideration. It is generally thought that since *M. tuberculosis* is usually transmitted via the respiratory route, aerosol infection most closely approximates the human situation. Aerosolization chambers are becoming more common for small animals, enabling more studies to be performed using this route. Inbred strains of mice and, to a lesser extent, rabbits are available, which enhances the reproducibility of studies performed with these models and reduces the number of animals needed compared to studies in outbred populations (such as nonhuman primates). Finally, the availability of certain reagents for conducting studies may also dictate the choice of model. Extensive immunologic reagents are available for both the mouse and nonhuman primate models, while there is still much work to be done in developing such reagents for guinea pigs or rabbits.

MOUSE MODEL

The mouse model provides an economical and easily manipulated tool with which to determine the role of specific host or bacterial components in the pathogenesis of tuberculosis. Indeed, data from the mouse model of tuberculosis have provided a great deal of insight into the dynamic interaction between this chronic persistent pathogen and the vertebrate host. In addition, it is a useful model for the initial screening of drugs and potential vaccines.

Acute-Infection Models

The use of acute-infection models allows the investigator to determine which components of the

JoAnne L. Flynn • Department of Molecular Genetics and Biochemistry, University of Pittsburgh School of Medicine, Pittsburgh, PA 15261. Andrea M. Cooper • Trudeau Institute, Inc., Saranac Lake, NY 12983. William Bishai • Center for Tuberculosis Research, Department of Medicine, Division of Infectious Diseases, Johns Hopkins School of Medicine, Baltimore, MD 21231-1001.

vertebrate response are essential for initial control of bacterial growth. Intravenous delivery of bacteria has the advantage of a large and reproducible challenge resulting in measurable host responses. In this model, bacteria are deposited throughout the spleen, liver, and lungs and grow progressively for 10 to 15 days, whereupon the acquired immune response is able to limit bacterial growth (66). However, intravenous infection is not the natural route of infection, and the immune responses necessary to control this systemic infection can be different from those required to control an aerogenic, low-dose infection. Specific host components for which this has been shown are the β_2-microglobulin molecule (20, 26, 62, 97), the CC chemokine receptor 2 ($CCR2^{-/-}$) (71, 85), CD40 (44), and interleukin-6 (IL-6) (40, 80).

There are further limitations with this model. During intravenous challenge, bacteria are deposited directly in the spleen, resulting in very rapid induction of the acquired T-cell response (8, 66). This rapid induction means that the role of innate immunity and the induction of acquired immunity in the lungs are not addressed. Similarly, following intravenous infection, bacteria are deposited throughout the interstitium of the lungs rather than within the alveoli of the lower lungs. As a result, the recruitment and migration of immune lymphocytes and monocytes to the site of infection may be different from that seen following a natural aerosol infection.

The aerosol route of infection appears, intuitively, to be more appropriate for the study of tuberculosis since it most closely mimics natural infection. Indeed, when this route of infection is used, the result is that as is thought to happen naturally, bacteria are deposited directly in the alveolar space and establish foci of infection at specific sites (61, 72). The use of specialized equipment to deposit bacteria in the lower respiratory tract via the generation of small bacteria-containing aerosolized droplets has been developed over many years. A low dose inoculum (50 to 100 CFU per mouse) delivered to the lungs results in steady bacterial growth, reaching a plateau of between 10^5 and 10^6 bacilli by ~1 month postinfection (Fig. 1), as the immune response peaks in the lungs.

Chronic- or Latent-Infection Models

The development of a chronic infection is common to most mammals infected with *M. tuberculosis* (17). In humans, latent infection is defined as *M. tuberculosis* infection with no signs of active disease. Latent infection can reactivate and progress to active tuberculosis. Humans can also experience chronic tuberculosis, which can recur even in treated individuals. Murine models of chronic or latent infection

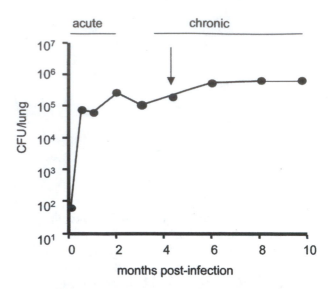

Figure 1. Course of *M. tuberculosis* infection in mice. C57BL/6 mice were infected with ~50 CFU of *M. tuberculosis* via an aerosolization chamber. At various times postinfection, the mice were euthanized and lung CFU were determined by plating homogenates on 7H10 plates. The acute phase lasts for up to 2 months postinfection, and the chronic phase begins after 3 months of infection. An arrow designates the time point where an interruption in the immune response could be experimentally performed to study reactivation of the infection.

have been developed to study the role of both the immune response and bacterial virulence factors in the development and maintenance of bacterial persistence.

Chronic tuberculosis in mice can be generated by low-dose infection (67, 76), while very low-level bacterial burdens can be achieved by treating infected mice with antimycobacterial drugs (55–57). Using the chronic-infection model, studies have highlighted the critical role of CD4 T cells, tumor necrosis factor alpha, (TNF-α), and nitric oxide in maintaining control of bacterial growth (reviewed in reference 23). Similarly, the ability of *M. tuberculosis* to respond to the immune response has been addressed using this model and appears to require specific signal transduction pathways (23) and expression of enzymes that allow the use of diverse carbon sources (58). These bacterial responses are not induced in the absence of gamma interferon (IFN-γ), a key product of the acquired protective immune response (58, 87).

Antimycobacterial drug treatment of infected mice has also been used as a model of latent tuberculosis. The Cornell model (in reference to the site of the development of this model [55–57]) has been used by numerous groups to study vaccines, reactivation, and drugs (reviewed in reference 23). The strengths of this model are that very small or undetectable numbers of bacteria can be produced and that reactivation of these bacteria in response to immunologic suppression can occur. This is desirable, since it can model the human situation. However, latent tuberculosis in humans does not require drug intervention, and the use of antibiotics may have substantial effects on development of the immune response, as well as on the bacterial population. This model is also subject to numerous variables, making reproducibility a problem (81).

Key Findings

The murine model has been instrumental in confirming the absolute requirement for T cells (53, 64), IFN-γ (13, 24), nitric oxide (9, 54), TNF-α (1, 4, 25), and IL-12 (12, 14) in mediating survival following *M. tuberculosis* infection. The necessity for at least some of these components in protecting humans from mycobacterial disease has been shown for CD4 T cells (increased susceptibility to disease when coinfected with human immunodeficiency virus [HIV] [74]), the IFN-γ/IL-12 pathway (severe mycobacterial infections in patients lacking components of these pathways [41, 69]), and TNF-α (increased risk of reactivation tuberculosis and extrapulmonary tuberculosis in patients treated with TNF-α-neutralizing compounds, [37]).

In addition to identifying the components of the response that are essential for the control of any level of infection with *M. tuberculosis,* the murine model has been used to characterize immune components that contribute to control of the infection but may not be required for survival. Understanding how these components of the response contribute to disease or protection may result in the identification of novel, currently suboptimal host responses that may be artificially augmented by vaccination. The CD8 T-cell response is a prime example of this type of response since, although these cells do not appear to be essential for control of bacterial growth, they are clearly activated and functional during *M. tuberculosis* infection (reviewed in reference 43). However, it is difficult to fully test the contribution of CD8 T cells to control of infection in the mouse, since mice lack a key antimycobacterial component of CD8 T cells, granulysin (91).

It also is becoming clear that the immune response to *M. tuberculosis,* at least in the most commonly used C57BL/6 mouse strain, is more robust than necessary (85). There is a substantial macrophage and lymphocyte recruitment to the lungs following infection, and quite high levels of IFN-γ are produced. However, reduction of this response does not necessarily lead to lack of control of the infection. In fact, there is a balance between bacterial numbers in the lungs and the immune response necessary to control this load. This is an important feature of the mouse model and should be considered carefully when one is analyzing knockout mice for phenotype. Even if bacterial numbers are the same in the lungs of knockout and control animals, there is still an opportunity to learn about the immune response to *M. tuberculosis*. If lung cell populations or functions in these knockout animals are impaired, but not enough to affect bacterial numbers, this can still be a significant finding. In the human situation, a suboptimal response may be the difference between a latent infection and active disease.

Granuloma Development

Tuberculosis results not only from bacterial infection but also from the immunopathological events that may compromise pulmonary function. In the C57BL/6 mouse, the granulomatous response following a low-dose aerosol challenge begins between days 20 and 30 postinfection and starts with accumulations of macrophages followed by a lymphocytic infiltrate; neutrophils can be seen but are not common (76). The murine granuloma contains organized CD4 T-cell aggregates, with more dispersed CD8 T cells located at the periphery. B cells are also present within the granuloma (30) and can be seen as tight clusters within the lungs. The structure of the granuloma is quite different from that of human granulomas, although the function of the granuloma (i.e., control of infection and prevention of dissemination) appears to be similar. Whereas the human granuloma is much more structured and organized, the murine granuloma in the lungs is composed of clusters and aggregates of cells. However, disrupting the granuloma structure, for example by TNF-α neutralization, abrogates control of the infection and contributes to substantial, severe pathology (reviewed in reference 96).

The role of the bacteria in initiating the mononuclear granuloma is currently being addressed using the murine model of infection. Recently it has been reported that bacterial mutants lacking either the gene for sigH (a sigma factor) (36) or a gene required for cyclopropanation of mycolic acid (29) fail to induce substantial pathological granulomas. These observations support the long held hypothesis that specific components of *M. tuberculosis* are highly inflammatory and contribute to the immunopathological consequences of infection.

Usefulness of the Model

The most useful aspect of the murine model of tuberculosis is its extreme versatility. Hypotheses specifically addressing the mechanisms by which both host and pathogen affect disease development can be addressed directly using this model. With the low-dose aerosol model of infection, the virulence and persistence of various *M. tuberculosis* mutants and their ability to cause lung pathology can be examined, and the interaction of *M. tuberculosis* factors with host factors can begin to be dissected. This is a powerful use of the murine model, in that a large number of mutants can be tested and compared for various phenotypes.

One important factor in using the aerosol model to assess the pathogenesis of *M. tuberculosis* is the use of bacterial cultures with high viability. Specifically, if late-log- or stationary-phase cultures are used, the 100 viable bacteria delivered to the lung during low-dose aerosol challenge will be accompanied by many dead bacteria. The presence of excess bacterial products from these dead bacteria will significantly alter the development of pulmonary lesions (63). To address this issue, bacterial cultures to be used for infection of animals should be grown to mid-log phase only (78). Similarly, if mutant bacteria are being compared with wild-type or parent strains for virulence or pathogenesis, the different cultures should be generated under identical conditions and compared prior to challenge for the relative numbers of live and dead bacteria.

The murine model allows the determination of the mechanisms by which T cells are activated, differentiated, and maintained during mycobacterial disease. By understanding how T-cell responses are generated during disease, we will be better able to modulate specific responses by vaccination or immunotherapy. Recent studies have identified the frequency and persistence of antigen-specific T cells during chronic mycobacterial infection (101), while others have determined the effect of mycobacterial infection on the phenotype, epitope specificity, and longevity of T-cell responses to model antigens (22). The identification of epitopes for protective mycobacterial antigens such as the mycolyl transferase Ag85 family and the ESAT-6 protein has also proved useful in determining the phenotype of T cells induced by vaccination (6, 21, 34). The use of model antigens to determine the effect of mycobacteria on T-cell activation has also recently highlighted the ability of *M. tuberculosis* and its components to drive a strong Th1 T-cell response (32) and to act as a potent adjuvant (75).

The resources required to test drugs in mice are much less extensive than those required for other animals, and thus this model provides an excellent tool for preliminary screening of drugs. Drug candidates identified by in vitro techniques can be tested rapidly against virulent *M. tuberculosis* bacteria that are proliferating in vivo, using any one of the infection mod-

els, although the low-dose aerosol model is used most frequently. A new model that utilizes mice lacking IFN-γ can more rapidly assess the activity of drugs against bacteria that are proliferating in vivo (45). The prevalence of latently infected humans has also spurred investigation into drugs active against bacteria physiologically adapted to persist in humans. While these studies are focused on identifying potential drug targets, the efficacy of new drugs against bacteria in a physiological state induced by an active immune response can be assessed in either of the chronic-infection models discussed above.

The power of the murine model in vaccine development lies in the ability to screen a large number of vaccines at limited cost and to be able to determine how the vaccine mediates any protective effects. The disadvantage is that the nature of the protection induced in a murine model may not be applicable to the human disease. The murine model allows the determination of how the route of vaccination, type of adjuvant, and specific antigen affect the ability of memory T cells to accumulate at the site of challenge. Understanding these aspects of vaccine-induced protection is crucial to the design of effective vaccines. For example, it was shown that the route of BCG vaccination, while able to alter the size and location of the initial response to vaccination, did not change the size and location of the response to challenge (70). In addition to understanding how vaccines can be effective against pulmonary disease, the murine model allows the efficacy of combined immunotherapy and chemotherapy regimens to be addressed. Specifically, vaccine protocols have been integrated with chemotherapeutic regimens to determine whether vaccination can limit the incidence of recrudescent disease following completion of drug therapy (46).

Limitations of the Model

Despite the many advantages of the murine model, its major weakness lies in the differences between disease progression in this mammal and disease progression in the human. A key difference is the large number of bacteria and evidence of dispersed pathological consequences in the lungs following even a low-dose infection in mice (76). In humans, *M. tuberculosis* infection resulting in antigen-specific cellular responses is often not accompanied by obvious pathological responses in the lungs, although a granuloma probably forms, and most humans do not progress to active disease. The mouse does not present with true latent infection, and the granuloma structure is quite different from that of human granulomas. In addition, certain aspects of the human system, such as the nonclassical antigen-presenting molecules CD1a,

CB1b, and CD1c and the toxic molecule of CD8 T cells, granulysin, are absent in mice. Conversely, while reactive nitrogen intermediates produced by inducible nitric oxide synthase are clearly essential in the control of murine tuberculosis, their role in human tuberculosis is still controversial. While these limitations should be considered when interpreting and extrapolating data to human disease, they do not negate the usefulness of this very tractable model.

GUINEA PIG MODEL

Guinea pigs have an important place in the history and future of tuberculosis research. Robert Koch used guinea pigs to establish Koch's postulates and to identify the tubercle bacillus as the etiologic agent of tuberculosis (38, 39). Guinea pigs are extremely susceptible to infection with M. tuberculosis and to progression to disease (65), and they were used for many of the seminal animal experiments in studies of tuberculosis. The guinea pig model of experimental tuberculosis remains an important tool for the identification of effective antituberculosis chemotherapy and vaccines, as well as for the characterization of mycobacterial virulence factors (15, 59, 60, 68, 88).

Some aspects of the lung pathology of infected guinea pigs are quite similar to those observed in humans (15, 59, 68). The granuloma in the lungs of guinea pigs infected with virulent M. tuberculosis consists largely of mononuclear cells and generally undergoes necrosis as the infection progresses. Necrosis, which causes tissue damage, is characteristic of the human granuloma and probably plays an important role in the immunopathology of tuberculosis. This necrosis may lead to liquefaction and cavitation; these latter pathological changes, critical to the respiratory transmission of M. tuberculosis, are not observed in the guinea pig. Necrosis of the granuloma is generally seen in mice only as a consequence of large bacterial numbers rather than as an immunopathologic phenomenon.

For vaccine development, reduction or prevention of tissue damage is an important goal; this aspect can be assessed in the guinea pig model. Another feature of the guinea pig granuloma is the existence of Langhans' multinucleated giant cells. These giant cells form as macrophages fuse and are often seen within human granulomas. Thus, the guinea pig granuloma exhibits many characteristics typical of its human counterpart.

A difference from humans is the inherent susceptibility of guinea pigs, indicating that the immune response which functions so well to contain the infection in the majority of infected humans is deficient in guinea pigs. An understanding of the exquisite susceptibility of M. tuberculosis-infected guinea pigs to progressive disease may provide clues about the more successful immune response of humans. This feature makes it an excellent model for vaccine testing.

The guinea pig experimental tuberculosis model has been well characterized (reviewed in reference 60). Guinea pigs can be efficiently infected by aerosolizing an extremely small number of bacilli (60, 77). The procedure used to deliver a low dose of bacilli directly into the lungs has been standardized. An aerosolization chamber designed by Smith and colleagues and built at the University of Wisconsin in the 1960s (100) was used to deliver low doses of bacteria to guinea pigs. At the sites of primary infection in the lungs, the bacilli grew exponentially for the first 21 days. Toward the end of this period of rapid growth, hematogenous spread from the primary foci of infection to other organs, as well as to the lungs, occurred. The bacterial burden reached 10^5 to 10^6 CFU in the tissues and then stabilized. All animals succumbed to the infection, characterized by progressive pulmonary tuberculosis.

The invariably fatal course of disease progression in guinea pigs provides a reliable readout for protection by a vaccine candidate or efficacy of drugs. Compared to the ~1-unit log decrease in peak lung bacillary load achievable by BCG vaccination in the mouse, the 2- to 3-log-unit drop in the bacillary load in BCG-vaccinated guinea pigs provides a substantially wider dynamic range for the assessment of vaccine efficacy (60, 68). In addition, pathologic changes and survival time post-challenge are used to monitor vaccine effectiveness.

One unique feature of the guinea pig model is that it allows differentiation between primary and secondary tuberculous lesions, the latter being the result of hematogenous spread (33, 89). Secondary lesions do not appear until after 18 days postinfection and can be differentiated from primary sites of infection by radiographs of the infected lungs. Since one goal for effective prevention or treatment of tuberculosis is reduction of secondary dissemination and since M. tuberculosis virulence correlates with its propensity to disseminate, the guinea pig model provides a unique system for the evaluation of vaccine and chemotherapeutic candidates as well as mechanisms involved in disease pathogenesis.

The limitations of the guinea pig model include the expense of maintaining guinea pig colonies in a biocontainment facility compared to the expense of housing mice. The limited availability of immunologic reagents for guinea pig experimentation makes it difficult to assess immunologic factors involved in protection in vaccine studies or in pathogenesis in this model, although efforts to develop these reagents are under way (35, 59, 60).

RABBIT MODEL

Selected because of its innate resistance to tuberculosis, mimicking that seen in humans, the rabbit has been used as a model of human tuberculosis since the early 20th century (47). The rabbit model was studied intensely for over 40 years by Lurie and colleagues until the 1960s (reviewed in reference 48). Yamamura conducted extensive studies of cavitary tuberculosis in rabbits from 1954 until the late 1980s (reviewed in reference 103). Since that time, the rabbit model has been used by Dannenberg and colleagues (reviewed in reference 17), and more recently other groups have used rabbits to address questions about tuberculosis (5, 11, 93). Among the attributes of the natural history of rabbit tuberculosis are caseation, cavitation, and containment in a potential latency-like state. The size and natural resistance of the rabbit to tuberculosis have permitted its use to evaluate bacterial virulence and dissemination, the genetics of resistance to tuberculosis, and the efficacy of vaccines.

Pathologic Features

Caseous necrosis in the form of small, spherical tubercles is a hallmark of human tuberculosis; indeed, it is the pathologic entity from which the disease derives its name. Pulmonary granulomas in infected rabbits bear a close pathologic resemblance to those seen in humans. Indeed, the rabbit model has provided the basis of our current understanding of the time course of caseation and of the cellular fluxes that contain the initial proliferation of *M. tuberculosis* in the lungs (16).

Following aerosol infection by *M. tuberculosis*, rabbits mount an immune response composed of an initial burst of neutrophils that ingest but do not destroy the bacilli. Subsequently, both resident macrophages and monocyte-derived macrophages appear at the site of infection and phagocytose large numbers of tubercle bacilli. The infected macrophages are surrounded by a spherical shell of additional uninfected macrophages. These cellular responses are bactericidal and reduce mycobacterial counts, which peak at 1 week, by about 30% by the second week. At 2 weeks, some of the initially infected macrophages have begun to adopt the morphology of epithelioid cells; these dying cells form the eosinophilic centers of the emerging caseous center. The periphery is composed of mature, activated macrophages plus neutrophils recruited in response to the centrally located

debris. By 4 weeks, the process has reduced the bacterial burden to 5 to 10% of the maximal level, and many more mature macrophages are seen at the periphery of the caseous lesion. Multinucleated giant cells (so-called Langhans' cells) are seen at the periphery, and for the first time lymphocytes appear at the periphery, along with plasma cells and fibroblasts. Small capillaries begin to infiltrate the caseous tubercle at this stage. By 6 weeks, multinucleated giant cells appear both at the periphery and in the center, and the rare remaining bacilli are found primarily at the margin between the caseous center and the periphery with activated macrophages. By 8 weeks, the centrally located macrophages have undergone necrosis and very few live bacilli may be found. The caseous center is bounded by a thick rim of lymphocytes. The tubercles range in size from 1 to 5 mm in the rabbit lung (47, 48). Color Plate 10 shows various features of granulomas in the rabbit.

The experimental pathology of rabbit caseous tubercles has clearly underscored the fact that the formation of primary tubercles is a highly effective host bactericidal mechanism. The maturation of tubercles described above is mirrored by a steep decline in the recovery of viable *M. tuberculosis* bacilli after 1 week. Moreover, the appearance of disintegrating epithelioid macrophages at the center of the tubercle at 4 to 6 weeks correlates with the onset of tuberculin sensitivity. Caseation may be the result of acquired cell-mediated immunity to *M. tuberculosis*, since it correlates in time with tuberculin skin test reactivity and is highly effective in killing the majority of bacteria and containing the remaining few survivors. Animal species which do not display classic caseous tubercles also do not reduce the bacterial load in the tissues to a paucibacillary contained state as is observed in humans (28).

A second hallmark of human tuberculosis is the development of the pulmonary cavitary lesion with accompanying pulmonary tissue destruction. The pulmonary cavitary lesion is a major cause of both human morbidity and disease transmission. There is verdant bacterial growth in the liquefied contents, and, in the process of expansion, erosion into bronchi and blood vessels leads to the spread of high titers of tubercle bacilli. Rabbits can also develop cavitary tuberculosis, as noted by several prominent investigators in the 1940s and 1950s (73, 90, 92, 99).

The process of cavitation in lesions in rabbit lungs is typically observed following infection or reinfection with *Mycobacterium bovis* (reviewed in reference 19). The process begins 8 to 12 weeks following infection and is characterized by a softening of the caseous lesions, with reinvasion of the lesions by mononuclear cells and neutrophils. For reasons which are poorly understood, the cellular response is unproductive and, in fact, leads to cell death, disintegration, and further softening of the lesions. As capillaries invade the lesions, they thrombose, and ultimately the softening process evolves into liquefaction and production of a pulmonary cavity. While, in general, *M. tuberculosis* aerosol infections are contained and *M. bovis* infections progress to cavitary disease, the time course and degree of disease show interanimal variability in outbred rabbits after aerosol infection.

Yamamura et al. used the rabbit model to develop a short-term reproducible model of cavitary tuberculosis following transthoracic injection of bacilli or bacterial extracts (103, 105). As evidence that the cavitation process was due to a hypersensitivity reaction, Yamamura et al. observed that transthoracic injection of heat-killed bacilli produced cavities in 40 to 85% of sensitized rabbits (depending on the dose) but failed to do so in nonsensitized rabbits. Immunosuppressive agents such as 6-mercaptopurine and azathioprine suppressed cavity formation in sensitized rabbits (104).

Converse et al. studied the process of cavitation by using the rabbit aerosol infection model with the *M. bovis* Ravenel strain (10, 11). They observed that low-dose aerosol infection with fewer than 1,000 bacilli typically produced one to five cavities in about 80% of rabbits 33 weeks after infection, although some rabbits had large numbers of cavitary lesions. High-dose infection with about 4,000 to 6,000 bacilli led to rapidly progressive and lethal cavitary disease, with between 5 and ca. 40 cavities observed between 5 and 18 weeks (10). Dissemination within the lungs, with primary lesions leading to secondary ones, was observed, and it was estimated that the Ravenel S strain (ATCC 35720) produced one tubercle for about every 20 to 100 organisms inhaled (11). Immunomodulators such as live attenuated vaccines have been tested in the aerosol cavitation rabbit model; however, since groups of only six rabbits were used, no statistically significant differences in the numbers of primary caseous lesions, the numbers of cavitary lesions, or tuberculin responsiveness could be detected (11).

Use of the Model

As discussed above, on infection with *M. tuberculosis*, rabbits develop caseous tubercles that generally contain the infection. Bacterial abundance and histopathologic evidence of disease peak in the first 8 weeks after *M. tuberculosis* aerosol infection, and this is followed by a decline in the inflammatory process and a dramatic reduction in the numbers of bacteria. The rabbits convert to a positive tuberculin

skin test. This ability to contain the infection and prevent progression to fulminant tuberculosis, in conjunction with immunologic evidence of acquired immunity, matches the observed course of tuberculosis in humans who meet the diagnostic criteria for latent *M. tuberculosis* infection. Rabbits may then serve as a model system for latency, although at present there is little published literature on this approach. Lurie et al. showed convincingly that immunosuppression with corticosteroids blocks the ability of rabbits to contain *M. tuberculosis*, leading to both larger numbers of tubercles and increased tubercle size after aerosol infection; it is therefore likely that steroids and other forms of immunosuppression could be employed as reactivating agents in such a rabbit latency model (50).

In view of the resistance of rabbits to lethal tuberculosis, the large size of rabbit lungs, and the reduction in bacterial numbers as tubercle formation progresses, traditional time-to-death methods and CFU enumeration in whole-organ homogenates are not particularly valuable parameters in comparing the virulence of different mycobacterial strains in rabbits. Instead, an approach toward quantifying local disease at the level of the caseous tubercle has been used in the rabbit model. In this approach, parameters can include numbers of caseous tubercles (the classic Lurie tubercle count method), tubercle size, tubercle diameter, and histological grade of tubercle inflammation (17). Moreover, with sophisticated aerobiology instrumentation, Dannenberg and colleagues have been able to quantify both the density of bacteria in the inhaled mist and the respiratory rate and volume of individual rabbits and hence to calculate the number of bacilli inhaled (although this number may differ from the number of bacilli implanted in the alveoli). For example, these methods have been used to determine that on a per-bacterium basis, *M. bovis* is 50- to 2,000-fold more virulent than *M. tuberculosis* in producing pulmonary tubercles in rabbits (19) and also that *M. tuberculosis* CDC 1551 may be less virulent for rabbits than H37Rv on the basis of tubercle size and bacterial count per tubercle (5). Despite the availability of these approaches, little has been done to compare the virulence of specific *M. tuberculosis* or *M. bovis* mutants in rabbits.

Kaplan and colleagues have developed the rabbit as a model of tuberculous meningitis and have exploited the model further to compare the ability of bacterial strains to disseminate beyond the meninges to other organs (93). For example, 8 and 21 days following intrathecal inoculation, *M. bovis* Ravenel was found to disseminate in larger numbers to the lungs, liver, and spleen compared with the *M. bovis* mutants BCG Montreal and BCG Pasteur. The group also assessed the immunopathogenesis of meningeal infection in rabbits and showed that *M. bovis* Ravenel elicited higher levels of TNF-α in the cerebrospinal fluid than did the BCG strains. Other studies have revealed that the TNF-α inhibitor thalidomide can reduce the disease burden and pathologic damage in rabbit experimental tuberculous meningitis, suggesting that the agent may be a valuable adjuvant to therapy (94, 95).

Genetics of Resistance to Tuberculosis

Lurie et al. used the tubercle count method to assess the resistance of inbred rabbit strains to a standard challenge with *M. tuberculosis* H37Rv (51, 52). Susceptible inbred rabbit strains C, FC, Ca, and CaC required ratios of 70 to 100 bacilli inhaled to produce a single tubercle, while resistant rabbit strains such as race III demonstrated ratios of 1,000 inhaled bacilli per tubercle. The group also conducted cross-breeding experiments between the inbred strains and showed that resistance to tuberculosis did not segregate as a single allele but, rather, was polygenic. Lurie's inbred rabbits were relatively infertile and are now extinct. Currently available New Zealand White rabbits are relatively resistant to tuberculosis but do not display the same uniformity in their responses to aerosol challenge observed in the inbred strains.

Importantly, resistant rabbit strains produced smaller tubercles and showed ~10-fold fewer CFU per caseous tubercle at necropsy (2). Histopathologic evaluations of the susceptible and resistant rabbits demonstrated greater recruitment of macrophages to the margins of the caseous tubercles in resistant animals. The degree of macrophage bactericidal activity appeared greater in these animals, with a corresponding reduction in the levels of detectable bacteria by both staining and culture. Of note, while susceptible rabbit strains succumbed to *M. bovis* infection, they did not develop cavities; only resistant rabbits developed cavitary disease. Thus, the more exuberant immunologic response to *M. tuberculosis* infection in the resistant rabbits also contributed to the tissue destruction and cavitary disease observed on high-dose *M. bovis* challenge. This pattern in the rabbit model parallels the observation that relatively immunodeficient humans such as those infected with HIV also rarely demonstrate cavitary tuberculosis but, rather, display a disseminated form of the disease with high bacterial loads and blunted tubercle formation (31).

Vaccines

Based on the principle that successful vaccination may not block primary infection but, rather, prevents the progression of disease, testing of vaccine efficacy in the rabbit has focused on acquiring a similar degree of disease control to that seen in Lurie's resistant rabbits. Since resistant rabbits show smaller and fewer tubercles 5 to 8 weeks after *M. tuberculosis* challenge than do susceptible rabbits, the usual outcome parameters for vaccine efficacy testing in the rabbit model have been the tubercle count, the mean tubercle diameter, and the number of cultivable bacteria per lesion about 5 weeks after challenge. Early experiments testing intradermal vaccination with the Phipps BCG strain 10 to 11 weeks prior to aerosol challenge with H37Rv showed that at 5 weeks after challenge, resistant race III rabbits had nearly 80% fewer tubercles than unvaccinated controls, while susceptible FC rabbits showed only a 15% reduction (49). Thus, the resistant host genotype gains the most by vaccination whereas the susceptible host (which is more in need of acquired resistance) benefits the least. More recent experiments with outbred New Zealand White rabbits show that even without the advantage of inbred rabbits, it is possible to use the tubercle count method with standard rabbit group sizes (six to eight rabbits) to show the superiority of BCG and *M. microti* over placebo (18). However, use of the tubercle count method with outbred rabbits to demonstrate a statistically significant advantage of a new vaccine over BCG will probably require rather large groups (15 to 20 rabbits).

NONHUMAN PRIMATE MODEL

Nonhuman primates have been used in tuberculosis research for many decades, although cost and containment requirements have reduced the use of this model substantially in the last 30 years. The monkey model can resemble human tuberculosis more closely than any other model, and there has been a resurgence of interest in this model. A few laboratories have recently been using macaques for studies of tuberculosis.

Active tuberculosis can be fatal in monkeys. An actively infected monkey can transmit infection to other animals in the facility, and this can lead to massive outbreaks of tuberculosis. Outbreaks cause substantial damage, in terms of lost research, containment, animal testing and monitoring, and euthanasia. All nonhuman primate colonies have strict control programs to limit the introduction of *M. tuberculosis*-infected monkeys, including repeated tuberculin testing during the 31- to 90-day quarantine period. However, tuberculin testing does not identify all infected monkeys, depending on the stage of infection. Aggressive control programs and better husbandry practices have greatly reduced the incidence of tuberculosis outbreaks in research colonies. However, the introduction of *M. tuberculosis* into a monkey facility for the purpose of performing research on tuberculosis must be handled very carefully, and redundant measures to prevent the spread of infection to monkeys and to workers are essential. BSL3 containment of *M. tuberculosis* in a nonhuman primate facility is expensive and challenging.

Macaques are commonly used in research. For studies with *M. tuberculosis*, both rhesus (*Macaca mulatta*) and cynomolgus (*M. fasicularis*) macaques have been used. Although aerosol infection is possible (3, 86), specialized equipment is necessary, and standardizing a dose delivered to the monkeys can be difficult. Delivery of organisms via the trachea or via a bronchoscope into the lungs is more commonly and easily performed. In one study, a dose-response curve was generated using cynomolgus monkeys, with doses ranging from 10^1 to 10^5 CFU of *M. tuberculosis* (98). All monkeys infected with higher doses (10^3 to 10^5) showed signs of disease and succumbed to tuberculosis between 3 and 29 weeks postinoculation. However, a subset of monkeys infected with 10 to 100 CFU apparently controlled the infection up to the time of euthanasia and showed only minimal lung disease on necropsy. This study suggested that low-dose infection could lead to a model that mimicked human infection and suggested the possibility that a latent infection could be achieved in this model.

Our own data using cynomolgus monkeys indicate that low-dose infection results in a spectrum of disease, including rapid and fulminant tuberculosis, active or chronic disease, and latent infection (7). Latent infection in monkeys is defined as infection (conversion of skin test to tuberculin positive) that does not cause clinical signs of illness for at least 6 to 9 months, with the infection contained in a few small granulomas in the lungs. Approximately 40% of the cynomolgus monkeys that we have infected with a low dose of *M. tuberculosis* (~25 bacilli of strain Erdman) present with latent infection.

There are numerous reports of tuberculosis cases in closed primate colonies, strongly suggesting that natural *M. tuberculosis* or *M. bovis* infections in monkeys can result in latent infection and can reactivate and cause active disease. Spontaneous reactivation of latent infection in our experimentally infected monkeys has occurred between 9 months and 2.5 years postinfection. Three cases of reactivation occurred shortly after latently infected monkeys were moved to a new BSL3 facility, suggesting that stress is one potential factor for reactivation of latent infection. Reactivation resulted in fulminant disease, in some cases with cavities apparent in the apical lung

lobes by radiography and at necropsy. This model presents the potential for experimental modulation of the immune response to induce reactivation of latent disease, as well as for the study of latent organisms, pathology, and immune responses. The nonhuman primate represents the only true animal model of experimental latent tuberculosis.

Available data regarding *M. tuberculosis* or *M. bovis* outbreaks in nonhuman primate colonies suggested that cynomolgus macaques were less susceptible to tuberculosis than were rhesus macaques. A recent study compared these two macaque species with respect to BCG-induced immunity to an *M. tuberculosis* challenge of 3,000 CFU, a relatively high dose (42). Unimmunized cynomolgus and rhesus macaques both developed progressive tuberculosis, although the cynomolgus macaques were somewhat more resistant. However, BCG immunization was much more protective in cynomolgus macaques than in rhesus macaques. These data suggest that both species will be useful in studying the immunology and pathogenesis of tuberculosis, as well as in testing vaccine candidates.

The pathology of tuberculosis in monkey lungs is strikingly similar to that in humans. The granulomas have a classical structure, with macrophages and multinulcleated giant cells surrounded by lymphocytes; granulocytes and fibroblasts are also observed. Caseation of granulomas and the presence of granulomas with necrotic centers but otherwise healthy tissue are commonly seen (Color Plate 11). Liquefaction and cavity formation are also observed in the lungs of monkeys with advanced disease (42) and in reactivation tuberculosis (7). Granulomas can also be fibrotic or solid, and these types of granulomas were observed more commonly in animals with less extensive disease, possibly representing resolving or successful granulomas. Calcification of granulomas was also observed in chronically or latently infected monkeys. As in humans, there is a spectrum of granuloma types within the lungs of monkeys with active tuberculosis. Disseminated disease is observed in some monkeys, with visible lesions in the spleen or liver and occasionally in other organs (7).

Monitoring the course of tuberculosis in monkeys can be challenging. Mammalian tuberculin, rather than purified protein derivative, is generally used for tuberculin skin testing, but the response to this is variable, even in monkeys with active disease. In our experience, all monkeys convert to a positive skin test within 6 weeks of infection, but the test often gives negative responses after that time. Therefore, this test seems to be most useful in the early stages of infection. The currently available diagnostics are not sufficient for reliable detection of latent or even active infection in monkeys. Chest radiographs can detect lung lesions and provide information about the severity of disease, but a latent infection is unlikely to be detected by this technique. However, a surrogate marker of disease or protection does not exist, just as is the case in human tuberculosis. The monkey may be a good model to search for a surrogate marker, since the full spectrum of human disease can be recapitulated on experimental infection of the monkey. The immunology of tuberculosis can be studied in the monkey model because the reagents exist already, due to cross-reactivity of human reagents as well as to the development of macaque-specific reagents by researchers in the simian immunodeficiency virus (SIV) field.

Nonhuman primates provide a useful model for testing vaccines that have given promising results in other models, although monkeys are too expensive for the initial screening of vaccine candidates. It seems reasonable that a vaccine demonstrating protection in monkeys would have a higher probability of providing protection in humans, although proof of this awaits clinical trials. The immune responses involved in protection could be investigated more easily with monkeys than with immunized humans, particularly because the peripheral blood, which is the sample most readily available from humans, may not be the best site to study immunity manifested in the lungs.

Nonhuman primates also provide a good model for studying drugs against tuberculosis. There is a long history of using monkeys for this purpose (27, 82–84). It has been demonstrated that 6 to 12 months of multidrug chemotherapy is effective in monkeys with active disease, although relapse rates over time have not been well studied (102). The monkey model may be useful in studies of new drugs that may reduce the duration of therapy as well as the rate of relapse. This model, with human-like pathology and granulomas and the potential for latent infection, represents an excellent opportunity to test the ability of drugs to penetrate the granulomatous environment or affect bacilli in latent disease.

One unique feature of the nonhuman primate model is the opportunity to study the interaction of SIV (a model for HIV) and M. tuberculosis. Coinfection with M. tuberculosis and HIV is a substantial problem worldwide, since tuberculosis is a major killer of AIDS patients. SIV infection of nonhuman primates is an excellent model of AIDS. Understanding the particular susceptibility of HIV-positive persons to tuberculosis, as well as the interaction between HIV and M. tuberculosis, with respect to modulating each infection, can be approached by using the macaque model. There have been limited studies in this area so far, but this is likely to be an important

use of the macaque model. Our studies and others showed that the extent of immunocompromise and the ability to control the virus have a major impact on the course of M. tuberculosis infection in monkeys. Monkeys with substantially deficient immune systems (due to SIV) prior to M. tuberculosis infection do not control the infection and rapidly succumb to fulminant tuberculosis. However, SIV-positive monkeys in which the viral infection is well controlled and CD4 T-cell levels are reasonable also seem capable of controlling M. tuberculosis infection, at least for a number of months (79; unpublished data). This model can also be used to study the effects of SIV or other immunocompromising regimens on latent M. tuberculosis infection (J. L. Flynn, unpublished data). Since tuberculosis is a leading cause of death in AIDS patients, this model will facilitate the study of the interaction of two important pathogens, HIV and M. tuberculosis.

The advantages of the nonhuman primate model include the similarity to human tuberculosis, in terms of spectrum of disease and pathology, and, unlike the guinea pig or rabbit model, the abundance of reagents for research. This translates into obtaining results that are more directly applicable to the human situation. The disadvantages are the high cost of nonhuman primate research, biosafety containment, and the outbred nature of the animals. The last of these is, however, similar to humans, and although this may cause more variability in experiments, it is a more realistic situation. Cost and biocontainment are serious obstacles to nonhuman primate research in tuberculosis. Monkeys with tuberculosis are contagious to other animals, including monkeys, and to humans, posing a serious risk in an animal facility. Biocontainment in a BSL3 facility is necessary, which achieves isolation of infected animals from other monkeys and personnel. Workers must don protective gear, including respirators, when in contact with the monkeys. The cost of nonhuman primate research is related to the actual cost of the monkeys, the need for veterinary care and veterinary technicians on a regular basis, and the space needed per animal. Thus, this model, which is quite attractive in many aspects, remains difficult to integrate into many research institutions.

CONCLUSIONS

In summary, animal models have been used to great advantage in tuberculosis research for more than a century. The increasing sophistication of the animal models will lead the way to new findings of great importance in tuberculosis. Each model has strengths and limitations. The choice of animal model is dependent primarily on the question to be asked by the researcher but also on practical considerations of cost, availability, space, and biosafety requirements.

Acknowledgments. J.L.F. acknowledges the assistance of Philana Ling Lin with the figures. W.B. acknowledges the assistance of Mark Yoder, Yukari Manabe, and Arthur M. Dannenberg, Jr. Research by J.L.F. is supported by NIH grants (AI37859, AI47485, AI50732, and HL075845) and the American Lung Association (grant CI-016-N). A.M.C. is supported by NIH grants (AI41922 and AI46530). W.B. is supported by NIH grants F32 AI 054087 (to Mark Yoder), and R01 HL71554 and awards from the Sequella Global Tuberculosis Foundation and the Ellison Medical Foundation.

REFERENCES

1. **Adams, L. B., C. M. Mason, J. K. Kolls, D. Scollard, J. L. Krahenbuhl, and S. Nelson.** 1995. Exacerbation of acute and chronic murine tuberculosis by adminstration of a tumor necrosis factor receptor-expressing adenovirus. *J. Infect. Dis.* **171:**400–405.

2. **Allison, M. J., P. Zappasodi, and M. B. Lurie.** 1962. Host-parasite relationships in natively resistant and susceptible rabbits on quantitative inhalation of tubercle bacilli. Their significance for the nature of genetic resistance. *Am. Rev. Respir. Dis.* **85:**553–569.

3. **Barclay, W. R., W. M. Busey, D. W. Dalgard, R. C. Good, R. W. Janick, J. E. Kasik, E. Ribi, C. E. Ulrich, and E. Wolinsky.** 1973. Protection of monkeys against airborne tuberculosis by aerosol vaccination with bacillus Calmette-Guérin. *Am. Rev. Respir. Dis.* **107:**351–358.

4. **Bean, A. G. D., D. R. Roach, H. Briscoe, M. P. France, H. Korner, J. D. Sedgwick, and W. J. Britton.** 1999. Structural deficiencies in granuloma formation in TNF gene-targeted mice underlie the heightened susceptibility to aerosol *Mycobacterium tuberculosis* infection, which is not compensated for by lymphotoxin. *J. Immunol.* **162:**3504–3511.

5. **Bishai, W. R., A. M. Dannenberg, Jr., N. Parrish, R. Ruiz, P. Chen, B. C. Zook, W. Johnson, J. W. Boles, and M. L. Pitt.** 1999. Virulence of *Mycobacterium tuberculosis* CDC 1551 and H37Rv in rabbits evaluated by Lurie's pulmonary tubercle count method. *Infect. Immun.* **67:**4931–4934.

6. **Brandt, L., M. Elhay, I. Rosenkrands, E. B. Lindblad, and P. Andersen.** 2000. ESAT-6 subunit vaccination against *Mycobacterium tuberculosis. Infect. Immun.* **68:**791–795.

7. **Capuano, S. V. I., D. A. Croix, S. Pawar, A. Zinovik, A. Myers, P. L. Lin, S. Bissel, C. Fuhrman, E. Klein, and J. L. Flynn.** 2003. Experimental *Mycobacterium tuberculosis* infection of cynomolgus macaques closely resembles the various manifestations of human *M. tuberculosis* infection. *Infect. Immun.* **71:**5831–5844.

8. **Cardona, P. J., A. Cooper, M. Luquin, A. Ariza, F. Filipo, I. M. Orme, and V. Ausina.** 1999. The intravenous model of murine tuberculosis is less pathogenic than the aerogenic model owing to a more rapid induction of systemic immunity. *Scand J. Immunol.* **49:**362–366.

9. **Chan, J., K. Tanaka, D. Carroll, J. L. Flynn, and B. R. Bloom.** 1995. Effect of nitric oxide synthase inhibitors on murine infection with *Mycobacterium tuberculosis. Infect. Immun.* **63:**736–740.

10. **Converse, P. J., A. M. Dannenberg, J. E. Estep, K. Sugisaki, Y. Abe, B. H. Schofield, and M. L. M. Pitt.** 1996. Cavitary tuberculosis produced in rabbits by aerosolized virulent tubercle bacilli. *Infect. Immun.* **64:**4776–4787.

11. **Converse, P. J., A. M. Dannenberg, T. Shigenaga, D. N. McMurray, S. W. Phalen, J. L. Stanford, G. A. W. Rook, T. Koru-Sengul, H. Abbey J. E. Estep, and M. L. M. Pitt.** 1998. Pulmonary bovine-type tuberculosis in rabbits: bacillary virulence, inhaled dose effects, tuberculin sensitivity, and *Mycobacterium vaccae* immunotherapy. *Clin. Diagn. Lab. Immunol.* **5:**871–881.

12. **Cooper, A. M., A. Kipnis, J. Turner, J. Magram, J. Ferrante, and I. M. Orme.** 2002. Mice lacking bioactive IL-12 can generate protective, antigen-specific cellular responses to mycobacterial infection only if the IL-12 p40 subunit is present. *J. Immunol.* **168:**1322–1327.

13. **Cooper, A. M., D. K. Dalton, T. A. Stewart, J. P. Griffen, D. G. Russell, and I. M. Orme.** 1993. Disseminated tuberculosis in IFN-γ gene-disrupted mice. *J. Exp. Med.* **178:**2243–2248.

14. **Cooper, A. M., J. Magram, J. Ferrante, and I. M. Orme.** 1997. Interleukin 12 (IL-12) is crucial to the development of protective immunity in mice intravenously infected with *Mycobacterium tuberculosis. J. Exp. Med.* **186:**39–45.

15. **Dai, G., S. Phalen, and D. N. McMurray.** 1998. Nutritional modulation of host responses to mycobacteria. *Front Biosci.* **3:**E110–E122.

16. **Dannenberg, A. M., Jr.** 1993. Immunopathogenesis of pulmonary tuberculosis. *Hosp. Pract. (Off. Ed.)* **28:**51–58.

17. **Dannenberg, A. M., Jr., and F. M. Collins.** 2001. Progressive pulmonary tuberculosis is not due to increasing numbers of viable bacilli in rabbits, mice and guinea pigs, but is due to a continuous host response to mycobacterial products. *Tuberculosis* **81:**229–242.

18. **Dannenberg, A. M., W. R. Bishai, N. Parrish, R. Ruiz, W. Johnson, B. C. Zook, J. W. Boles, and L. M. Pitt.** 2001. Efficacies of BCG and vole bacillus (*Mycobacterium microti*) vaccines in preventing clinically apparent pulmonary tuberculosis in rabbits: a preliminary report. *Vaccine* **19:**796–800.

19. **Dannenberg, A. M. J.** 2001. Pathogenesis of pulmonary *Mycobacterium bovis* infection: basic principles established by the rabbit model. *Tuberculosis* **81:**87–96.

20. **D'Souza, C. D., A. M. Cooper, A. A. Frank, S. Ehlers, J. Turner, A. Bendelac, and I. M. Orme.** 2000. A novel nonclassic beta2-microglobulin-restricted mechanism influencing early lymphocyte accumulation and subsequent resistance to tuberculosis in the lung. *Am. J. Respir. Cell Mol. Biol.* **23:**188–193.

21. **D'Souza, S., V. Rosseels, M. Romano, A. Tanghe, O. Denis, F. Jurion, N. Castiglione, A. Vanonckelen, K. Palfliet, and K. Huygen.** 2003. Mapping of murine Th1 helper T-cell epitopes of mycolyl transferases Ag85A, Ag85B, and Ag85C from *Mycobacterium tuberculosis. Infect. Immun.* **71:**483–493.

22. **Dudani, R., Y. Chapdelaine, H. van Faassen, D. K. Smith, H. Shen, L. Krishnan, and S. Sad.** 2002. Multiple mechanisms compensate to enhance tumor-protective CD8⁺ T-cell response in the long-term despite poor CD8⁺ T-cell priming initially: comparison between an acute versus a chronic intracellular bacterium expressing a model antigen. *J. Immunol.* **168:**5737–5745.

23. **Flynn, J. L., and J. Chan.** 2001. Tuberculosis: latency and reactivation. *Infect. Immun.* **69:**4195–4201.

24. **Flynn, J. L., J. Chan, K. J. Triebold, D. K. Dalton, T. A. Stewart, and B. R. Bloom.** 1993. An essential role for interferon-γ in resistance to *Mycobacterium tuberculosis* infection. *J. Exp. Med.* **178:**2249–2254.

25. **Flynn, J. L., M. M. Goldstein, J. Chan, K. J. Triebold, K. Pfeffer, C. J. Lowenstein, R. Schreiber, T. W. Mak, and B. R. Bloom.** 1995. Tumor necrosis factor-α is required in

the protective immune response against *M. tuberculosis* in mice. *Immunity* 2:561–572.

26. Flynn, J. L., M. M. Goldstein, K. J. Triebold, B. Koller, and B. R. Bloom. 1992. Major histocompatibility complex class I-restricted T cells are required for resistance to *Mycobacterium tuberculosis* infection. *Proc. Natl. Acad. Sci. USA* 89:12013–12017.

27. Francis, J. 1956. Natural and experimental tuberculosis in monkeys with observations on immunization and chemotherapy. *J. Comp. Pathol.* 66:123–135.

28. Francis, J. 1958. *Tuberculosis in Animals and Man: a Study in Comparative Pathology.* Cassell & Co., Ltd., London, United Kingdom.

29. Glickman, M. S., J. S. Cox, and W. R. Jacobs, Jr. 2000. A novel mycolic acid cyclopropane synthetase is required for cording, persistence, and virulence of *Mycobacterium tuberculosis*. *Mol. Cell* 5:717–727.

30. Gonzalez-Juarrero, M., O. C. Turner, J. Turner, P. Marietta, J. V. Brooks, and I. M. Orme. 2001. Temporal and spatial arrangement of lymphocytes within lung granulomas induced by aerosol infection with *Mycobacterium tuberculosis*. *Infect. Immun.* 69:1722–1728.

31. Havlir, D. V., and P. F. Barnes. 1999. Tuberculosis in patients with human immunodeficiency virus infection. *N. Engl. J. Med.* 340:367–373.

32. Hickman, S. P., J. Chan, and P. Salgame. 2002. *Mycobacterium tuberculosis* induces differential cytokine production from dendritic cells and macrophages with divergent effects on naive T-cell polarization. *J. Immunol.* 168:4636–4642.

33. Ho, R., J. S. Fok, G. E. Harding, and D. W. Smith. 1978. Host-parasite relationships in experimental airborne tuberculosis. VII. Fate of *Mycobacterium tuberculosis* in primary lung lesions and in primary lesion-free lung tissue infected as a result of bacillemia. *J. Infect. Dis.* 138:237–241.

34. Huygen, K., E. Lozes, B. Gilles, A. Drowart, K. Palfliet, F. Jurion, I. Roland, M. Art, M. Dufaux, J. Nyabenda, J. De Bruyn, J. P. van Vooren, and R. D. Lays. 1994. Mapping of TH1 helper T-cell epitopes on major secreted mycobacterial antigen 85A in mice infected with live *Mycobacterium bovis* BCG. *Infect. Immun.* 62:363–370.

35. Jeevan, A., T. Yoshimura, G. Foster, and D. N. McMurray. 2002. Effect of *Mycobacterium bovis* BCG vaccination on interleukin-1β and RANTES mRNA expression in guinea pig cells exposed to attenuated and virulent mycobacteria. *Infect. Immun.* 70:1245–1253.

36. Kaushal, D., B. G. Schroeder, S. Tyagi, T. Yoshimatsu, C. Scott, C. Ko, L. Carpenter, J. Mehrotra, Y. C. Manabe, R. D. Fleischmann, and W. R. Bishai. 2002. Reduced immunopathology and mortality despite tissue persistence in a *Mycobacterium tuberculosis* mutant lacking alternative sigma factor, SigH. *Proc. Natl. Acad. Sci. USA* 99:8330–8335.

37. Keane, J., S. Gershon, R. P. Wise, E. Mirabile-Levens, J. Kasznica, W. D. Schwieterman, J. N. Siegel, and M. M. Braun. 2001. Tuberculosis associated with infliximab, a tumor necrosis factor alpha-neutralizing agent. *N. Engl. J. Med.* 345:1098–1104.

38. Koch, R. 1882. Aetiologie der Tuberculose. *Berl. Klin. Wochenschr.* 19:221–230.

39. Koch, R. 1932. Die Aetiologie der Tuberculose. Translation by Berna Pinner and Max Pinner with an introduction by Allen K. Krause. *Am. Rev. Tuberc.* 25:285–323.

40. Ladel, C. H., C. Blum, A. Dreher, K. Reifenberg, M. Kopf, and S. H. E. Kaufmann. 1997. Lethal tuberculosis in interleukin-6-deficient mutant mice. *Infect. Immun.* 65:4843–4849.

41. Lammas, D. A., J. L. Casanova, and D. S. Kumararatne. 2000. Clinical consequences of defects in the IL-12-dependent interferon-gamma (IFN-gamma) pathway. *Clin. Exp. Immunol.* 121:417–425.

42. Langermans, J. A. M., P. Andersen, D. van Soolingen, R. A. W. Vervenne, P. A. Frost, T. van der Laan, L. A. H. van Pinsteren, J. van den Hombergh, S. Kroom, I. Peekel, S. Florquin, and A. W. Thomas. 2001. Divergent effect of bacillus Calmette-Guérin (BCG) vaccination on *Mycobacterium tuberculosis* infection in highly related macaque species: implications for primate models in tuberculosis vaccine research. *Proc. Natl. Acad. Sci. USA* 98:11497–11502.

43. Lazarevic, V., and J. Flynn. 2002. CD8⁺ T cells in tuberculosis. *Am. J. Respir. Crit. Care Med.* 166:1116–1121.

44. Lazarevic, V., A. J. Myers, C. A. Scanga, and J. L. Flynn. 2003. CD40, but not CD40L, is required for the optimal priming of T cells and control of aerosol *M. tuberculosis* infection. *Immunity* 19:823–835.

45. Lenaerts, A. J., V. Gruppo, J. V. Brooks, and I. M. Orme. 2003. Rapid in vivo screening of experimental drugs for tuberculosis using gamma interferon gene-disrupted mice. *Antimicrob. Agents Chemother.* 47:783–785.

46. Lowrie, D. B., R. E. Tascon, V. L. D. Bonato, V. M. F. Lima, L. H. Faccioli, E. Stavropoulos, M. J. Colston, R. G. Hewinson, K. Moelling, and C. L. Silva. 1999. Therapy of tuberculosis in mice by DNA vaccination. *Nature* 400:269–271.

47. Lurie, M. B. 1932. The correlation between the histological changes and the fate of living tubercule bacilli in the organs of tuberculous rabbits. *J. Exp. Med.* 55:31.

48. Lurie, M. B. 1964. *Resistance to Tuberculosis: Experimental Studies in Native and Acquired Defense Mechanisms.* Harvard University Press, Cambridge, Mass.

49. Lurie, M. B., P. Zappasodi, E. Cardona-Lynch, and A. M. J. Danneberg. 1952. The response of intracutaneous inoculation of BCG as an index of native resistance to tuberculosis. *J. Immunol.* 68:369–387.

50. Lurie, M. B., P. Zappasodi, A. M. J. Danneberg, and E. Cardona-Lynch. 1953. The effect of cortisone and ACTH on the pathogenesis of tuberculosis. *Ann. N.Y. Acad. Sci.* 56:779.

51. Lurie, M. B., P. Zappasodi, A. M. Dannenberg, Jr., and G. H. Weiss. 1952. On the mechanism of genetic resistance to tuberculosis and its mode of inheritance. *Am. J. Hum. Genet.* 4:302–314.

52. Lurie, M. B., P. Zappasodi, and C. Tickner. 1955. On the nature of genetic resistance to tuberculosis in the light of the host-parasite relationships in natively resistant and susceptible rabbits. *Am. Rev. Tuberc.* 72:297–329.

53. Mackaness, G. B. 1968. The immunology of antituberculous immunity. *Am. Rev. Respir. Dis.* 97:337–344.

54. MacMicking, J., R. J. North, R. LaCourse, J. S. Mudgett, S. K. Shah, and C. F. Nathan. 1997. Identification of nitric oxide synthase as a protective locus against tuberculosis. *Proc. Natl. Acad. Sci. USA* 94:5243–5248.

55. McCune, R. M., F. M. Feldman, and W. McDermott. 1966. Microbial persistence. II. Characteristics of the sterile state of tubercle bacilli. *J. Exp. Med.* 123:469–486.

56. McCune, R. M., F. M. Feldmann, H. P. Lambert, and W. McDermott. 1966. Microbial persistence I. The capacity of tubercle bacilli to survive sterilization in mouse tissues. *J. Exp. Med.* 123:445–468.

57. McCune, R. M., R. Tompsett, and W. McDermott. 1957. The fate of *Mycobacterium tuberculosis* in mouse tissues as determined by the microbial enumeration technique. II. The conversion of tuberculous infection to the latent state by the administration of pyrazinamide and a companion drug. *J. Exp. Med.* 104:763–802.

58. McKinney, J. D., K. Honer zu Bentrup, A. Miczak, B. Chen, W.-T. Chan, D. Swenson, J. C. Sacchettini, W. R. Jacobs, Jr., and D. G. Russell. 2000. Persistence of *Mycobacterium tuberculosis* in macrophages and mice requires the glyoxylate shunt enzyme isocitrate lyase. *Nature* 406:735–738.

59. McMurray, D. 2001. Disease model: pulmonary tuberculosis. *Trends Mol. Med.* 7:135–137.

60. McMurray, D. N. 1994. Guinea pig model of tuberculosis, p. 135–147. *In* B. R. Bloom (ed.), *Tuberculosis: Pathogenesis, Protection, and Control.* American Society for Microbiology, Washington, D.C.

61. Middlebrook, G. 1952. An apparatus for airborne infection of mice. *Proc. Soc. Exp. Biol. Med.* 80:105–110.

62. Mogues, T., M. E. Goodrich, L. Ryan, R. LaCourse, and R. J. North. 2001. The relative importance of T-cell subsets in immunity and immunopathology of airborne *Mycobacterium tuberculosis* infection in mice. *J. Exp. Med.* 193:271–280.

63. Moreira, A. L., L. Tsenova, M. H. Aman, L. G. Bekker, S. Freeman, B. Mangaliso, U. Schroder, J. Jagirdar, W. N. Rom, M. G. Tovey, V. H. Freedman, and G. Kaplan. 2002. Mycobacterial antigens exacerbate disease manifestations in *Mycobacterium tuberculosis*-infected mice. *Infect. Immun.* 70:2100–2107.

64. North, R. J. 1973. Importance of thymus-derived lymphocytes in cell-mediated immunity to infection. *Cell. Immunol.* 7:166–176.

65. Opie, E., and J. Aronson. 1927. Tubercle bacilli in latent tuberculous lesions and in lung tissue without tuberculous lesions. *Arch. Pathol.* 4:1–21.

66. Orme, I. 1987. The kinetics of emergence and loss of mediator T lymphocytes acquired in response to infection with *Mycobacterium tuberculosis. J. Immunol.* 138:293–298.

67. Orme, I. M. 1988. A mouse model of the recrudescence of latent tuberculosis in the elderly. *Am. Rev. Respir. Dis.* 137:716–718.

68. Orme, I. M., D. N. McMurray, and J. T. Belisle. 2001. Tuberculosis vaccine development: recent progress. *Trends Microbiol.* 9:115–118.

69. Ottenhof, T. H., D. Kumararatne, and J. L. Casanova. 1998. Novel human immunodeficiencies reveal the essential role of type-1 cytokines in immunity to intracellular bacteria. *Immunol. Today* 19:491–494.

70. Palendira, U., A. G. Bean, C. G. Feng, and W. J. Britton. 2002. Lymphocyte recruitment and protective efficacy against pulmonary mycobacterial infection are independent of the route of prior *Mycobacterium bovis* BCG immunization. *Infect. Immun.* 70:1410–1416.

71. Peters, W., H. M. Scott, H. F. Chambers, J. L. Flynn, I. F. Charo, and J. D. Ernst. 2001. Chemokine receptor 2 serves an early and essential role in resistance to *Mycobacterium tuberculosis. Proc. Natl. Acad. Sci. USA* 98:7958–7963.

72. Ratcliffe, H. L., and V. S. Palladino. 1953. Tuberculosis induced by droplet nuclei infection: initial homogeneous response of small mammals (rats, mice, guinea pigs, and hamsters) to human and to bovine bacilli, and the rate and pattern of tubercle development. *J. Exp. Med.* 97:61–68.

73. Ratcliffe, H. L., and W. F. Wells. 1948. Tuberculosis of rabbits induced by droplet nuclei infection. *J. Exp. Med.* 87:575–584.

74. Raviglione, M. C., D. E. Snider, and A. Kochi. 1995. Global epidemiology of tuberculosis: morbidity and mortality of a global epidemic. *JAMA* 273:220–226.

75. Rha, Y. H., C. Taube, A. Haczku, A. Joetham, K. Takeda, C. Duez, M. Siegel, M. K. Aydintug, W. K. Born, A. Dakhama, and E. W. Gelfand. 2002. Effect of microbial heat shock proteins on airway inflammation and hyperresponsiveness. *J. Immunol.* 169:5300–5307.

76. Rhoades, E. R., A. A. Frank, and I. M. Orme. 1997. Progression of chronic pulmonary tuberculosis in mice aerogenically infected with virulent *Mycobacterium tuberculosis. Tubercle Lung Dis.* 78:57–66.

77. Riley, R. L., C. C. Mills, F. O'Grady, L. U. Sultan, F. Willstadt, and D. N. Shivpuri. 1962. Infectiousness of air from a tuberculosis ward. *Am. Rev. Respir. Dis.* 85:511–525.

78. Roberts, A. R., A. M. Cooper, J. T. Belisle, J. Turner, M. Gonzalez-Juarrero, and I. M. Orme. 2002. Murine models of tuberculosis. *Methods Microbiol.* 32:433–462.

79. Safi, H., B. J. Gormus, P. J. Didier, J. L. Blanchard, D. L. Lakey, L. N. Martin, M. Murphey-Corb, R. Vankayalapati, and P. F. Barnes. 2003. Spectrum of manifestations of *Mycobacterium tuberculosis* infection in primates infected with SIV. *AIDS Res. Hum. Retroviruses* 19:585–595.

80. Saunders, B. M., A. A. Frank, I. M. Orme, and A. M. Cooper. 2000. Interleukin-6 induces early gama interferon production in the infected lung but is not required for generation of specific immunity to *Mycobacterium tuberculosis* infection. *Infect. Immun.* 68:3322–3326.

81. Scanga, C. A., V. P. Mohan, H. Joseph, K. Yu, J. Chan, and J. L. Flynn. 1999. Reactivation of latent tuberculosis: variations on the Cornell murine model. *Infect. Immun.* 67:4531–4538.

82. Schmidt, L. H. 1955. Induced pulmonary tuberculosis in the rhesus monkey: its usefulness in evaluating chemotherapeutic agents. *Trans. Conf. Chemother. Tuberc.* 14:226–231.

83. Schmidt, L. H. 1956. Some observations on the utility of simian tuberculosis in defining thetherapeutic potentialities of isoniazid. *Annu. Rev. Tuberc. Pulm. Dis.* 74:138–153.

84. Schmidt, L. H. 1966. Studies on the antituberculous activity of ethambutol in monkeys. *Ann. N.Y. Acad. Sci.* 135:747–758.

85. Scott, H. M., and J. L. Flynn. 2002. *Mycobacterium tuberculosis* in chemokine receptor 2-deficient mice: influence of dose on disease progression. *Infect. Immun.* 70:5946–5954.

86. Shen, Y., D. Zhou, L. Qiu, X. Lai, M. Simon, L. Shen, Z. Kou, Q. Wang, L. Jiang, J. Estep, R. Hunt, M. Clagett, P. K. Sehgal, Y. Li, X. Zeng, C. T. Morita, M. B. Brenner, N. L. Letvin, and Z. W. Chen. 2002. Adaptive immune response of Vγ2Vδ2+ T cells during mycobacterial infections. *Science* 295:2255–2258.

87. Shi, L., Y. J. Jung, S. Tyagi, M. L. Gennaro, and R. J. North. 2003. Expression of Th1-mediated immunity in mouse lungs induces a *Mycobacterium tuberculosis* transcription pattern characteristic of nonreplicating persistence. *Proc. Natl. Acad. Sci. USA* 100:241–246.

88. Smith, D. W., V. Balasubramanian, and E. Wiegeshaus. 1991. A guinea pig model of experimental airborne tuberculosis for evaluation of the response to chemotherapy: the effect on bacilli in the initial phase of treatment. *Tubercle* 72:223–231.

89. Smith, D. W., D. N. McMurray, E. H. Wiegeshaus, A. A. Grover, G. E. Harding. 1970. Host-parasite relationships in experimental airborne tuberculosis. IV. Early events in the course of infection in vaccinated and nonvaccinated guinea pigs. *Am. Rev. Respir. Dis.* 102:937–949.

90. Steenken, W., Jr., E. Wolinsky, P. S. Pratt, and W. J. Costigan. 1953. Effect of antibacterial agents on chronic pulmonary tuberculosis in rabbits: a roentgenographic, pathologic, and bacteriologic study. *Trans. Annu. Meet. Natl. Tuberc. Assoc.* 49:218–220.

91. Stenger, S., D. A. Hanson, R. Teitelbaum, P. Dewan, K. R. Niazi, C. J. Froelich, T. Ganz, S. Thoma-Uszynski, A. Melian, C. Bogdan, S. A. Porcelli, B. R. Bloom, A. M. Krensky, and R. L. Modlin. 1998. An antimicrobial activity

of cytolytic T cells mediated by granulysin. *Science* 282: 121–125.

92. Takeda, K., and K. Shinpo. 1942. On the meaning of the allergic tissue reaction as regards the development of pulmonary tuberculosis. *Kekkaku* 20:208–221, 275–290, 472–489.

93. Tsenova, L., A. Bergtold, V. H. Freedman, R. A. Young, and G. Kaplan. 1999. Tumor necrosis factor alpha is a determinant of pathogenesis and disease progression in mycobacterial infection in the central nervous system. *Proc. Natl. Acad. Sci. USA* 96:5657–5662.

94. Tsenova, L., K. Sokol, V. H. Freedman, and G. Kaplan. 1998. A combination of thalidomide plus antibiotics protects rabbits from mycobacterial meningitis-associated death. *J. Infect. Dis.* 177:1563–1572.

95. Tsenova, L., B. Mangaliso, G. Muller, Y. Chen, V. H. Freedman, D. Stirling, and G. Kaplan. 2002. Use of IMiD3, a thalidomide analog, as an adjunct to therapy for experimental tuberculous meningitis. *Antimicrob. Agents Chemother.* 46:1887–1895.

96. Tufariello, J. M., J. Chan, and J. L. Flynn. 2003. Latent tuberculosis: mechanisms of host and bacillus that contribute to persistent infection. *Lancet Infect. Dis.* 3:578–590.

97. Turner, J., C. D. D'Souza, J. E. Pearl, P. Marietta, M. Noel, A. A. Frank, R. Appelberg, I. M. Orme, and A. M. Cooper. 2001. CD8- and CD95/95L-dependent mechanisms of resistance in mice with chronic pulmonary tuberculosis. *Am. J. Respir. Cell Mol. Biol.* 24:203–209.

98. Walsh, G. P., E. V. Tan, E. C. de la Cruz, R. M. Abalos, L. G. Villhermonsa, L. J. Young, R. V. Cellona, J. B. Nazareno, and M. A. Horwitz. 1996. The Philippine cynomolgus monkey (*Macaca fascularis*) provides a new nonhuman primate model of tuberculosis that resembles human disease. *Nat. Med.* 2:430–436.

99. Wells, W., and M. B. Lurie. 1941. Experimental airborne disease: quantitative natural respiratory contagion of tuberculosis. *Am. J. Hyg.* 34:21.

100. Wiegeshaus, E., D. N. McMurray, A. A. Grover, G. E. Harding, and D. W. Smith. 1970. Host-parasite relationships in experimental airborne tuberculosis. III. Relevance of microbial enumeration to acquired resistance in guinea pigs. *Annu. Rev. Respir. Dis.* 102:422–429.

101. Winslow, G. M., A. D. Roberts, M. A. Blackman, and D. L. Woodland. 2003. Persistence and turnover of antigen-specific CD4 T cells during chronic tuberculosis infection in the mouse. *J. Immunol.* 170:2046–2052.

102. Wolf, R. H., S. V. Gibson, E. A. Watson, and G. B. Baskin. 1988. Multidrug chemotherapy of tuberculosis in rhesus monkeys. *Lab. Anim. Sci.* 38:25–33.

103. Yamamura, Y. 1958. The pathogenesis of tuberculous cavities. *Adv. Tuberc. Res.* 9:13–37.

104. Yamamura, Y., Y. Ogawa, and H. Yamagata. 1968. Prevention of tuberculous cavity formation by immunosuppressive drugs. *Am. Rev. Respir. Dis.* 98:720–723.

105. Yamamura, Y., S. Yasaka, M. Yamaguchi, K. Endo, H. Iwakura, S. Nakamura, and Y. Ogawa. 1954. Studies of the experimental tuberculosis cavity: the experimental formation of the tuberculous cavity in the rabbit lung. *Med. J. Osaka Univ.* 5:187–197.

Tuberculosis and the Tubercle Bacillus
Edited by Stewart T. Cole et al.
© 2005 ASM Press, Washington, D.C.

Chapter 37

Tuberculosis Vaccine Preclinical Screening and Development

IAN M. ORME AND ANGELO A. IZZO

Experimental-animal models of tuberculosis began to emerge shortly after the discovery of the bacterium itself. Koch performed studies with mice, rabbits were soon found to be susceptible, and an early clinical test consisted of inoculating guinea pigs with sputum to determine if this body fluid contained live bacilli.

With the exception of experimental *Mycobacterium bovis* infections in cattle, animals are not the primary host. Despite this, *M. tuberculosis* grows well in many mammalian species, and as a result models involving mice and guinea pigs, as well as, to a lesser extent, rabbits and primates, have provided a substantial amount of information regarding the immune response to this organism (39–41, 48, 55, 60, 67, 68).

As we have stressed before, models are not the real thing. In many cases, information provided by models clearly parallels that observed in humans, but there are some observations that do not, particularly in the realm of pathological responses. As a result the onus is on the animal modelist to carefully evaluate results that validate information that can be extrapolated to the human disease state. In that regard, there are at least three areas in which model validation can be determined fairly accurately. It is becoming increasingly clear that the great majority of information obtained from animal models regarding the basis of the acquired or adaptive response parallels that found in humans. The Th1 cytokine response in mice has been shown to be essential to protection, and genetic deficiencies in humans lead to similar susceptibility. CD4 cells can transfer immunity in mice, and mice lacking CD4 cells by gene disruption cannot control infection; similarly, humans lacking adequate numbers of these cells due to infection with human immunodeficiency virus are highly susceptible both to primary disease and to reactivation of latent tuberculosis (8, 12–16, 19, 20, 22, 24–27, 47, 77, 79). A more recent series of experiments have investigated the role of innate immunity, and it is clear that the array of Toll-like receptors expressed by human macrophages, including those that seem to be specifically triggered by mycobacterial ligands, are also expressed and triggered in a similar way by mouse macrophages (33, 70).

The second area involves the pathology of disease, and here model validation is weaker because the pathologic process in various models does not always parallel that seen in humans. All model animals studied to date develop granulomatous reactions in the lungs, but only the guinea pig develops the serious necrosis and mineralization that can be observed in humans (40). Rabbits develop liquefied cavities, but the disease process is very rapid, and the relative susceptibility of this animal to *M. tuberculosis* and *M. bovis* still remains unclear, with the most severe reactions being observed only with the latter bacterium (3, 9, 10, 17, 38, 72). Other models include the cow, in which there is a potent mineralization event that can totally calcify the entire lesion, and the primate, which can develop diffuse pulmonary tuberculosis detectable by radiography.

The third area, i.e., how animal models can be used to test new vaccines, is the topic of this chapter. If one is an optimist, one can argue that the animal models are fully validated because they predict that the only vaccine fully tested in humans, BCG, will have a positive effect and that this will be mediated via CD4 Th1 T-cell responses. If one is a pessimist, one can point to all the problems seen with BCG vaccination in humans, particularly the variation in efficacy, and lament the fact that there have been no vaccine trials since the advent of BCG upon which to further validate the usefulness of animal models. At the end of the day, however, no new vaccine candidate is likely to be tested in humans without at least some animal model data indicating a potentially positive outcome, with further information showing that the vaccine itself is probably safe. The most cost-

Ian M. Orme and Angelo A. Izzo • Department of Microbiology, Immunology and Pathology, Colorado State University, Fort Collins, CO 80523.

effective screening models available are the mouse and the guinea pig, and results using these models are described below.

BRIEF DESCRIPTION OF MOUSE AND GUINEA PIG MODELS

The primary models that are currently used in the preclinical screening program for vaccine candidates are (i) the low-dose aerosol mouse model and (ii) the low-dose aerosol guinea pig model (Fig. 1). The mouse model uses the well-characterized C57BL/6 strain and is a short-term (30-day interval between vaccination and challenge) standardized model in which mice are vaccinated, rested for about 30 days, and then challenged with a low-dose aerosol of virulent *M. tuberculosis*. The mice are then sacrificed about 4 weeks later, and the numbers of CFU in the lungs and spleen

are determined. Each vaccine candidate is assessed for its ability to reduce the bacterial load to a level statistically lower than that produced by the saline control. As a positive control, BCG is used; it gives about a 1-log-unit reduction in this model.

The 30-day assay is also used in the guinea pig model, but we are now also fairly routinely observing long-term survival of these animals. If guinea pigs are left unprotected after about 30 days, they develop "classical" granulomas similar to those seen in humans with active tuberculosis. These granulomas become increasingly necrotic and mineralized, after which the guinea pigs begin to lose weight and then die.

The course of infection in the lungs of guinea pigs following low-dose aerosol exposure to virulent *M. tuberculosis* has been documented (9, 10, 75). The number of *M. tuberculosis* bacilli increases progressively during the first 3 weeks and then plateaus into a chronic state, during which there is worsening

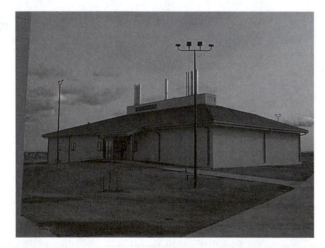
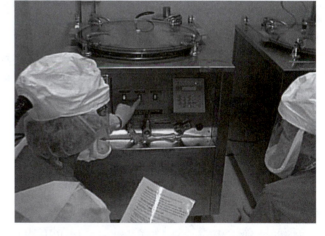
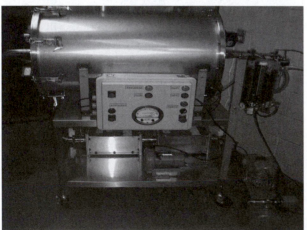
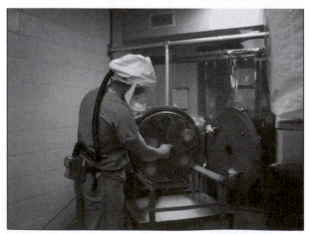

Figure 1. The BHRB building at Colorado State University (top left) is a biosafety level 3 facility in which much of our vaccine testing is performed. Mouse aerosol exposures are performed using a Middlebrook apparatus (top right), whereas guinea pigs are infected using an instrument manufactured by the University of Wisconsin at Madison (bottom).

pathology characterized by multiple sites of cellular infiltration, necrosis, and fibrosis. Under these conditions, the survival time for a guinea pig is approximately 25 weeks. The survival of guinea pigs vaccinated with BCG and then challenged with a low-dose aerosol of virulent *M. tuberculosis* is significantly greater than that of animals inoculated with saline (Fig. 2); this longer survival is associated with improved lung pathology and less tissue involvement.

STATUS OF THE NATIONAL INSTITUTES OF HEALTH SCREENING PROGRAM

The National Institutes of Health preclinical tuberculosis vaccine screening program was established to identify novel vaccines that will eventually be used throughout the world to combat tuberculosis. The program was established to allow investigators to submit their vaccine candidates for testing by using either or both of the animal models. Thus far, the program has tested vaccine candidates in both the mouse and guinea pig models, with a stronger emphasis on the former, mainly due to the greater amount of information and reagents available. However, with the increased knowledge of the guinea pig infection model and increasing availability of reagents, the number of vaccine candidates tested in the guinea pig model is already beginning to increase markedly.

At the time of writing, over 125 individual vaccine candidates have been tested at Colorado State University in over 300 separate experiments. To date, the program has been successful in identifying a number of vaccine candidates (1, 6, 7, 36, 45, 49–54, 56, 61, 76), some of which are in the process of progressing to clinical trials.

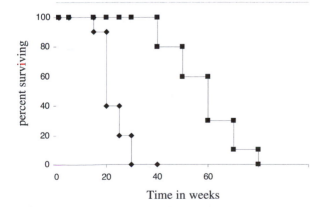

Figure 2. Survival of guinea pigs following low-dose (ca. 20 bacilli) aerosol exposure. Animals injected with saline live about 25 weeks (♦), whereas those vaccinated with BCG live about a year on average (■).

BASIS OF THE IMMUNE RESPONSE INDUCED BY VACCINATION

As described elsewhere in this book, a wealth of information regarding the host response to *M. tuberculosis* has been gained from using the mouse model. Indeed, it is from experiments with the mouse model that we have learned a great deal about the immune response in general, including the role of the major histocompatibility complex in presenting antigens, the nature of the T-cell receptor, the definition of T-cell subsets, the roles of cytokines and chemokines, and so forth. Because of this knowledge, along with all the specific reagents provided by mainstream immunology, we have been able to comprehensively dissect the immune response of the mouse to tuberculosis.

As a result, we now know that the immune response takes a finite time to recognize and detect the presence of bacilli deposited in the lungs by aerosol exposure (11). There is now good evidence that at some point early during this process, bacteria are engulfed by dendritic macrophages and transported to the adjacent lung lymph nodes or the lymphoid tissues lining the bronchial tree (4, 28, 29, 34). As a result of this process, both CD4 and CD8 primary T-cell subsets become sensitized by specific antigens presented both by conventional class II and class Ia major histocompatibility complex molecules and by class Ib (CD1-mediated) molecules (22, 32, 44, 62, 66).

The presence of the infection in the lung tissues sets up a local inflammation, creating chemokine gradients and blood vessel adhesion molecule expression, which facilitate the influx of granulocytes (which are short-lived and therefore not sustained) and monocytes from the bloodstream. These latter cells differentiate into epithelioid cells, establishing the basic structure of the subsequent granuloma, and are soon followed by the influx of large numbers of T cells. In the mouse, CD4 T cells penetrate the centers of the granuloma and tend to aggregate whereas CD8 cells tend to accumulate around blood vessels and assume a more peripheral distribution around the granulomas themselves (30) (Color Plate 12). To date, the reason for this is unknown.

As a result of this cellular influx and the subsequent production of gamma interferon (IFN-γ), the growth of the infection is curtailed and the animal enters into a chronic disease state wherein the bacterial load is static or rises very slowly over a considerable period. The stability of this chronic state differs between inbred mouse strains (31, 42, 43, 73), and our laboratory has advanced various explanations for this (Fig. 3); however, the suggestion by certain groups that this chronic disease state in the mouse

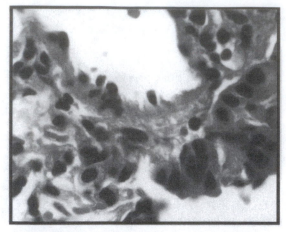

Bronchial epithelia degeneration

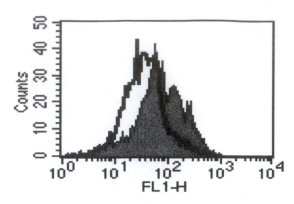

Poor expression of T cell adhesion markers

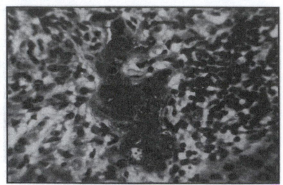

Massive IL-10 accumulation

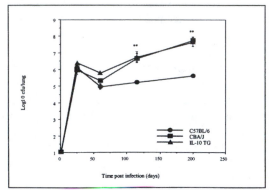

IL-10 Tg mice reactivation prone

Figure 3. Some explanations of why certain mouse strains, such as CBA/J, are prone to reactivation or regrowth of pulmonary infection about 150 days after aerosol exposure. These include bronchial epithelial degeneration (top left), failure to up-regulate the expression of adhesion molecules such as ICAM-1 on responding T cells (top right; open trace, CBA/J; filled trace, C57BL/6), and accumulation of large amounts of interleukin-10 (IL-10) in macrophages in lung lesions. C57BL/6 mice rendered transgenic (Tg) overexpressors of IL-10 behave like reactivation-prone strains in terms of the course of the infection (bottom).

models a state of latent tuberculosis is almost certainly erroneous.

It has been shown by our colleagues in mainstream immunology that exposure of naïve T cells to their specific antigen triggers their differentiation into an effector state, characterized by clonal expansion, cytokine secretion, and modulation of an array of cell surface markers (many of which control their circulatory abilities). Once the source of antigen is removed, some cells enter a state of memory immunity and are ready to rapidly respond to recall antigen.

It remains unclear whether or how this process occurs in mice infected with tuberculosis. Much of what is known in mainstream immunology has been determined from experiments with transgenic mice (such as those that can respond only to ovalbumin), and so factors such as the sheer inflammatory nature of the response to mycobacteria and the fact that the organism, and therefore the source of antigen, is not cleared will clearly compound the issue. In fact, Bevan has suggested in a recent commentary (2) that the chronic nature of diseases such as tuberculosis totally precludes the establishment of a stable memory T-cell population. Recent results from our laboratory support his conclusions (Fig. 4), by showing that CD4 and CD8 cells harvested from the lungs of mice at various stages of the chronic disease process at all times predominantly express a $CD44^{hi}$ $CD62L^{lo}$ activated effector phenotype (37).

The purpose of vaccination is to establish a long-lived state of heightened resistance to challenge infection, which in practical terms means many recirculating memory T cells capable of rapidly entering sites of inflammation in the lungs. In our vaccine models in the mouse, the primary characteristics of this are a reduction in the bacterial load relative to unvaccinated

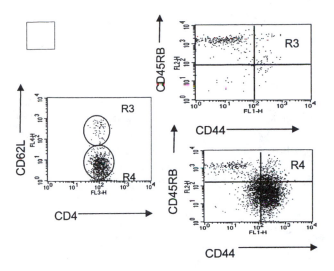

Figure 4. CD4 cells in the lungs express an activated/effector phenotype even well into the chronic stage of the disease process.

controls and the appearance in the lungs of T cells that stain positive for intracellular IFN-γ.

The question now becomes whether these are valid goals, or at least measurements, or whether there is more to it. Recent studies by Wu et al. (78) have suggested that counting IFN-γ-positive cells does not give a direct prediction of the subsequent memory response, since memory cells in fact arise from the IFN-γ-negative population. This is unsettling, because it implies that looking at cells shortly after vaccination for IFN-γ as a surrogate marker may be invalid. Moreover, if a vaccine strongly induces a state of memory, then current information suggests that it must switch to an effector phenotype when entering the lungs. This can certainly happen, but exactly how this is controlled is not currently understood.

If IFN-γ is not a surrogate marker, then maybe it can still be a guide. Our working hypothesis is that different vaccine formulations may result in different ratios of effector and memory cells after inoculation. Certain materials (CpGs, for example) can enhance the IFN-γ response to mycobacterial subunit vaccines, but this does not appear to result in better protection and often can diminish it. Other vaccines (such antigen 85A [Ag85A] DNA) have no effect on the initial postaerosol bacterial load but clearly have long-term beneficial effects on lung immunopathology (1). Thus, a possible interpretation of these observations is that certain vaccines may induce strong early protection (many IFN-γ-positive cells, reductions in bacterial load) but with most cells tending to be relatively short-lived whereas others are better at inducing a stable memory response (Fig. 5) In the latter case, therefore, there would initially be too few IFN-γ-positive cells to have any major effect on the bacterial load but there would be better production by the vaccine of more antigen-specific (initially) IFN-γ-negative T cells that would be active later and would have a longer-lived phenotype.

It is not even clear if such cells would be truly memory cells, at least in terms of the expected phenotypes. Of course, those defined in models of viral immunity (CD8 memory) or in transgenic mouse systems (Th2) may not even apply to a real-life, Th1-inducing chronic bacterial infection. For instance we have noticed that mice that have been infected with *M. tuberculosis* and then given chemotherapy, our standard method of generating "memory-immune" mice, retain a significant population of CD4 T cells in the lungs, with an effector phenotype. Thus, the rules established in mainstream immunology for less

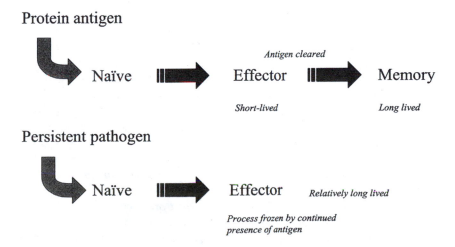

Figure 5. The possible fates of antigen-specific T cells may be different for chronic infectious diseases such as tuberculosis in comparison to T cells induced into individual protein antigens.

threatening antigens, such as ovalbumin, may not apply to serious and persistent complex pathogens.

IMMUNOPATHOLOGY OF THE IMMUNE RESPONSE

Although it is obvious that it is the pathological processes in the lungs that can kill humans infected with tuberculosis, until recently there was not much information from animal models. A sequential study with the mouse low-dose aerosol model provided the important information that although the bacterial load in the lungs of C57BL/6 mice does not appreciably change for a considerable time, there is a progressive and dynamic change in the pathology of the lungs (46, 64).

It takes about 80 to 100 days for the granulomatous response in the mouse lungs to develop. This structure is rich in lymphocytes in mouse strains such as C57BL/6, which is reactivation resistant, whereas in reactivation-prone mice such as the CBA/J strain, lymphocytes are more sparse (73). However, even in C57BL/6 mice, from about day 100 onwards, the lesions stain less densely, indicating that T cells are being gradually lost; the reason for this has yet to be explained. Rather than result in collapse of the granuloma, however, there is a substantial fibrotic response that seems to maintain its integrity. As time goes by, however, there is increasing necrosis and tissue degeneration, until the animal dies.

We have recently defined four stages in the guinea pig model (75) (Fig. 6). In the first, small lesions, which contain macrophages, a few lymphocytes, and clusters of eosinophils, develop (usually close to airways). Then, by about day 15 to 20, these lesions are much larger, the eosinophil clusters have disappeared, and there is an obvious necrotic core that is brightly eosinophilic when stained. The third stage represents the "classical" granuloma. There is a large necrotic core, then a mantle of mostly activated (foamy) macrophages, a second layer very rich in lymphocytes (a random mixture of CD4 and CD8 cells), and an outer layer of fibrous material. The lymphocytes show no evidence of aggregation (as seen in the mouse), and very few are in a state of apoptosis (in our opinion, an in vitro phenomenon). Acid-fast bacteria can be detected in an extracellular state on the rim of the necrotic core, and in the adjoining macrophages. The third stage can be seen about a month after infection by aerosol, and it then slowly degenerates over the next 70 to 100 days or so into a final stage. Here, much of the lesion has mineralized, and the size of this structure has apparently compressed the foamy macrophage layer around it. The lympho-

cyte layer has become disorganized by this point and is not readily identifiable.

It would be useful to monitor these pathologic events over time, not only to better understand them but also to use such data to try to explain the modes of action of certain types of vaccines. At the pathological level at least, we cannot even say as yet exactly how BCG works. We have recently attempted to try to address this by using magnetic resonance imaging (MRI). In the example shown here (Color Plate 13) guinea pigs were exposed to approximately 20 to 30 bacilli by aerosol and euthanized 35 days later. The lungs were inflated and fixated and then cut into whole-organ 2-mm-wide slices. These were analyzed by MRI, and stacking software was used to generate three-dimensional images. In the example shown, there are about 28 visible lesions, fairly evenly distributed throughout the lung and of similar size. There is also a single patch of what appears to be a site of infection in the pleura.

It is interesting to compare these results with the established dogma, which holds that primary lesions are established in the lungs and the organisms begin to grow. Because the immune response has not yet mobilized, some bacilli escape (hematogenous dissemination) and seed other areas of the lung where the ventilation/perfusion ratio is more favorable (i.e., where more oxygen is available) (68). As the immune response to the infection peaks, the exuberant T-cell response ("excessive delayed-type hypersensitivity") results in central tissue destruction, causing the resultant necrosis (18). The granulomas in the lungs stabilize, but eventually some type of immunosuppressive event triggers reactivation and dissemination of the infection, killing the animal about 20 to 25 weeks after aerosol exposure.

Our observations may suggest a completely different story. The necrotic core is a very early event, far earlier than any evidence of acquired immunity or delayed-type hypersensitivity. We think that the core comes about from degeneration or degranulation of the eosinophil clusters seen very early in the lesions. As these clusters break down, they leave obvious patches of eosinophilic material consisting of hydrolytic enzymes that digest the surrounding cells, allowing these areas to coalesce into the central necrotic core. This probably sets up a vicious cycle in which local capillaries are destroyed and the area becomes hypoxic, causing the intial core to grow larger. At least initially, this has no effect on the host protective response, which carries on around it.

Our preliminary studies using MRI indicate that BCG vaccination of guinea pigs significantly reduces the size but not the initial numbers of granulomas, consistent with the classical studies of Smith, Mc-

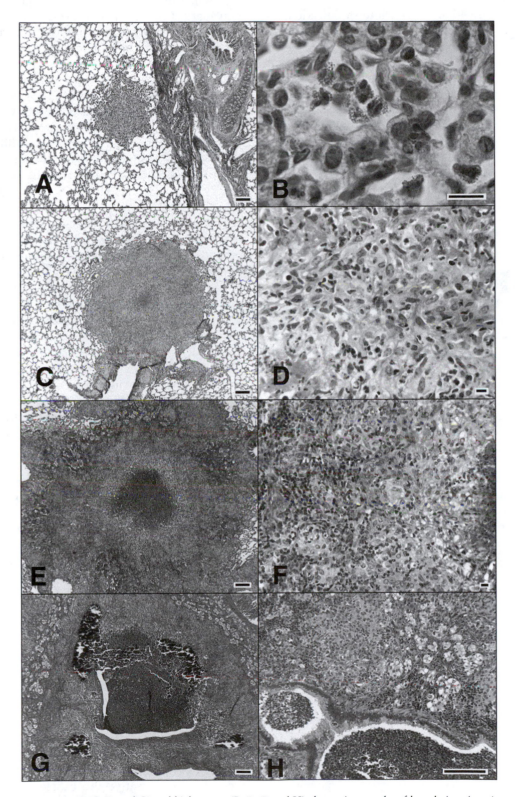

Figure 6. Low-power (A, C, E, and G) and high-power (B, D, F, and H) photomicrographs of lung lesions in guinea pigs 10 (A and B), 20 (C and D), 30 (E and F), and 90 (G and H) days after aerosol exposure to *M. tuberculosis*. As described in the text, a "classical" granuloma develops over the first 30 days and then degenerates into a highly mineralized mass that erodes out through adjacent vessels. Reprinted from reference 72a.

Murray, and others. In unprotected animals, lesion numbers increase 40 to 60 days into the infection, indicating secondary lesion establishment. This is after peak immunity has been expressed, which represents a major enigma. As for an immunosuppressive event triggering the end stages of the disease process, we would suggest instead that the mineralizing granuloma core becomes so large that it compresses the tissue layers outside it, where the acid-fast bacilli can be detected, to the extent that they are forcibly pushed or eroded into surrounding airways or large blood vessels. If so, this would suddenly cause substantial bacterial dissemination, causing a "shock-like" tumor necrosis factor alpha-mediated response by the immune system, resulting in rapid weight loss and death.

IMPROVING THE WAYS IN WHICH WE MEASURE VACCINES

People do not contract tuberculosis by appointment 30 days after receiving a vaccination. And yet, despite this, most of our assays are geared toward the short-term. The primary reason for this is economics; conducting long-term studies with the animal models, even with mice, is a very expensive procedure. Moreover, in such assays, animals occupy housing space for very long periods. It should also be remembered that in long-term survival assays with the guinea pig model, in which we have observed some of the most promising data to date, the aerosol challenge was still administered soon after the cessation of vaccination. Obviously, therefore, to be really sure that a vaccine has some degree of longevity, one has two choices. The first is to conduct studies of the most promising vaccines in which the interval between vaccination and subsequent challenge is sequentially increased (in guinea pigs, this interval can be up to 18 to 24 months) to determine if the vaccine still protects the animals. The second is to find some sort of surrogate marker that predicts with confidence that a given vaccine has certain properties that ensure that its protective efficacy is long-lived. To date, this latter option does not exist.

A second area in which the developmental process needs improvement is that of vaccine safety. The problems can range from a lump at the injection site (a problem we have seen with certain adjuvants) to exacerbation of the host response to infection in a nonbeneficial manner to outright pathological events in the lungs, leading to death (71). Despite the enthusiasm of certain laboratories, we are probably not quite at the stage yet where we can go from a decent result with a SCID mouse straight into experiments with people.

While much of our emphasis (and models, for that matter) has been concentrated on prophylactic vaccines, it would be enormously beneficial to develop vaccines that could be used therapeutically in people who already have tuberculosis or are suspected of having a latent form of the disease (21, 23). However, to date, the results of experiments attempting to use therapeutic or postexposure vaccines have generally been disappointing (63, 74). There are probably several reasons why this is so difficult; they include the possibilities (i) that the host response is already operating at maximum capacity and the immunity generated to the vaccine cannot add anything, (ii) that the vaccine is stimulating immunity to antigens that are not actually being presented at that time (the wrong antigens are being targeted, or antigen processing in the granulomas is being inhibited), or (iii) that the T cells induced by the vaccine simply cannot penetrate the already well-formed granuloma either for simple physical reasons or due to inappropriate expression of adhesion molecules or the correct integrins. In fact, one must conclude that this is a woefully underresearched area of the field.

As for vaccines against latent tuberculosis, our experience to date suggests that the murine model completely fails to deliver. It is very hard to establish a latent state and even harder to actually prove that one has been achieved. The so-called Cornell model has been suggested, but there has never been any thorough analysis of what actually happens in this model (other than ways to trigger bacterial regrowth [65]), and our own data suggest that experiments to date have no statistical power. Finally, one considerable worry is that "anti-latent" vaccines might have the reverse effect and may trigger latent disease rather than sterilize lesions. This type of "Koch reaction" may be akin to our experience with the Hsp60 and Ag85A DNA vaccines, which induced severe necrosis in mice when given as therapeutic vaccines (71).

A further issue is less a matter of safety and more one of efficacy, and it pertains to the general observation that the BCG vaccine does not work very well in people already presensitized by exposure to environmental mycobacteria (EM) such as the ubiquitous *M. avium*. This has been debated periodically through the years, and experiments with animal models have unfortunately given ambiguous or contradictory information (35, 57–59, 69). A key element seems to involve the viability of the EM; if alive, then it can in fact contribute positively to protective immunity to *M. tuberculosis*; however, as recently shown, it can also act to inhibit the proliferation of a subsequent vaccination with BCG (5). It seems fair to say at this point that the jury is still out and that the generation of positive or negative effects with EM depends entirely on the protocol used. What is obvious however, is that this event is still poorly understood. With the current enthusiasm for attenuated live vaccines based on BCG or *M. tuberculosis* itself, this is a serious issue that needs to be resolved. Fortunately, such EM effects may be less important in interfering with other classes of vaccines including DNAs and subunit non-living vaccines.

Acknowledgments. This work was supported by NIH grants AI-75320, AI-40488, AI-054697, and AI-45707. We are very grateful to our many colleagues in the Mycobacteria Research Laboratories at CSU for their contributions to the vaccine program and to the many investigators who continue to provide us with highly innovative vaccine candidates. We are also grateful to Susan Kraft and Randy Basaraba for providing the MRI image.

REFERENCES

1. Baldwin, S. L., C. D'Souza, A. D. Roberts, B. P. Kelly, A. A. Frank, M. A. Lui, J. B. Ulmer, K. Huygen, D. M. McMurray, and I. M. Orme. 1998. Evaluation of new vaccines in the mouse and guinea pig model of tuberculosis. *Infect. Immun.* 66:2951–2959.

2. Bevan, M. J. 2002. Immunology: remembrance of things past. *Nature* 420:748–749.

3. Bishai, W. R., A. M. Dannenberg, Jr., N. Parrish, R. Ruiz, P. Chen, B. C. Zook, W. Johnson, J. W. Boles, and M. L. Pitt. 1999. Virulence of *Mycobacterium tuberculosis* CDC1551 and H37Rv in rabbits evaluated by Lurie's pulmonary *Tubercle* count method. *Infect. Immun.* 67:4931–4934.

4. Bodnar, K. A., N. V. Serbina, and J. L. Flynn. 2001. Fate of *Mycobacterium tuberculosis* within murine dendritic cells. *Infect. Immun.* 69:800–809.

5. Brandt, L., J. Feino Cunha, A. Weinreich Olsen, B. Chilima, P. Hirsch, R. Appelberg, and P. Andersen. 2002. Failure of the *Mycobacterium bovis* BCG vaccine: some species of environmental mycobacteria block multiplication of BCG and induction of protective immunity to tuberculosis. *Infect. Immun.* 70:672–678.

6. Brandt, L., and I. Orme. 2002. Prospects for new vaccines against tuberculosis. *BioTechniques* 33:1098, 1100, 1102.

7. Brooks, J. V., A. A. Frank, M. A. Keen, J. T. Bellisle, and I. M. Orme. 2001. Boosting vaccine for tuberculosis. *Infect. Immun.* 69:2714–2717.

8. Caruso, A. M., N. Serbina, E. Klein, K. Triebold, B. R. Bloom, and J. L. Flynn. 1999. Mice deficient in CD4 T cells have only transiently diminished levels of IFN-gamma, yet succumb to tuberculosis. *J. Immunol.* 162:5407–5416.

9. Converse, P. J., A. M. Dannenberg, Jr., J. E. Estep, K. Sugisaki, Y. Abe, B. H. Schofield, and M. L. Pitt. 1996. Cavitary tuberculosis produced in rabbits by aerosolized virulent *Tubercle* bacilli. *Infect. Immun.* 64:4776–4787.

10. Converse, P. J., A. M. Dannenberg, Jr., T. Shigenaga, D. N. Mc-Murray, S. W. Phalen, J. L. Stanford, G. A. Rook, T. Koru-Sengul, H. Abbey, J. E. Estep, and M. L. Pitt. 1998. Pulmonary bovine-type tuberculosis in rabbits: bacillary virulence, inhaled dose effects, tuberculin sensitivity, and *Mycobacterium vaccae* immunotherapy. *Clin. Diagn. Lab. Immunol.* 5:871–881.

11. Cooper, A. M., J. E. Callahan, M. Keen, J. T. Belisle, and I. M. Orme. 1997. Expression of memory immunity in the lung following re-exposure to *Mycobacterium tuberculosis*. *Tubercle Lung Dis.* 78:67–73.

12. Cooper, A. M., D. K. Dalton, T. A. Stewart, J. P. Griffin, D. G. Russell, and I. M. Orme. 1993. Disseminated tuberculosis in interferon gamma gene-disrupted mice. *J. Exp. Med.* 178:2243–2247.

13. Cooper, A. M., A. Kipnis, J. Turner, J. Magram, J. Ferrante, and I. M. Orme. 2002. Mice lacking bioactive IL-12 can generate protective, antigen-specific cellular responses to mycobacterial infection only if the IL-12 p40 subunit is present. *J. Immunol.* 168:1322–1327.

14. Cooper, A. M., J. Magram, J. Ferrante, and I. M. Orme. 1997. Interleukin 12 (IL-12) is crucial to the development of protective immunity in mice intravenously infected with *Mycobacterium tuberculosis*. *J. Exp. Med.* 186:39–45.

15. Cooper, A. M., A. D. Roberts, E. R. Rhoades, J. E. Callahan, D. M. Getzy, and I. M. Orme. 1995. The role of interleukin-12 in acquired immunity to *Mycobacterium tuberculosis* infection. *Immunology* 84:423–432.

16. Corbett, E. L. 2003. HIV and tuberculosis: surveillance revisited. *Int. J. Tuberc. Lung Dis.* 7:709.

17. Dannenberg, A. M., W. R. Bishai, N. Parrish, R. Ruiz, W. Johnson, B. C. Zook, J. W. Boles, and L. M. Pitt. 2000. Efficacies of BCG and vole bacillus (*Mycobacterium microti*) vaccines in preventing clinically apparent pulmonary tuberculosis in rabbits: a preliminary report. *Vaccine* 19:796–800.

18. Dannenberg, A. M., Jr. 1994. Roles of cytotoxic delayed-type hypersensitivity and macrophage-activating cell-mediated immunity in the pathogenesis of tuberculosis. *Immunobiology* 191:461–473.

19. Davies, P. D. 2003. The world-wide increase in tuberculosis: how demographic changes, HIV infection and increasing numbers in poverty are increasing tuberculosis. *Ann. Med.* 35:235–243.

20. Flynn, J. L., and B. R. Bloom. 1996. Role of T1 and T2 cytokines in the response to *Mycobacterium tuberculosis*. *Ann. N.Y. Acad. Sci.* 795:137–146.

21. Flynn, J. L., and J. Chan. 2003. Immune evasion by *Mycobacterium tuberculosis*: living with the enemy. *Curr. Opin. Immunol.* 15:450–455.

22. Flynn, J. L., and J. Chan. 2001. *Immunology* of tuberculosis. *Annu. Rev. Immunol.* 19:93–129.

23. Flynn, J. L., and J. Chan. 2001. Tuberculosis: latency and reactivation. *Infect. Immun.* 69:4195–4201.

24. Flynn, J. L., J. Chan, K. J. Triebold, D. K. Dalton, T. A. Stewart, and B. R. Bloom. 1993. An essential role for interferon gamma in resistance to *Mycobacterium tuberculosis* infection. *J. Exp. Med.* 178:2249–2254.

25. Flynn, J. L., M. M. Goldstein, K. J. Triebold, J. Sypek, S. Wolf, and B. R. Bloom. 1995. IL-12 increases resistance of BALB/c mice to *Mycobacterium tuberculosis* infection. *J. Immunol.* 155:2515–2524.

26. Frucht, D. M., and S. M. Holland. 1996. Defective monocyte costimulation for IFN-gamma production in familial disseminated *Mycobacterium avium* complex infection: abnormal IL-12 regulation. *J. Immunol.* 157:411–416.

27. Frucht, D. M., D. I. Sandberg, M. R. Brown, S. M. Gerstberger, and S. M. Holland. 1999. IL-12-independent costimulation pathways for interferon-gamma production in familial disseminated *Mycobacterium avium* complex infection. *Clin. Immunol.* 91:234–241.

28. Gonzalez-Juarrero, M., and I. M. Orme. 2001. Characterization of murine lung dendritic cells infected with *Mycobacterium tuberculosis*. *Infect. Immun.* 69:1127–1133.

29. Gonzalez-Juarrero, M., T. S. Shim, A. Kipnis, A. P. Junqueira-Kipnis, and I. M. Orme. 2003. Dynamics of macrophage cell populations during murine pulmonary tuberculosis. *J. Immunol.* 171:3128–3135.

30. Gonzalez-Juarrero, M., O. C. Turner, J. Turner, P. Marietta, J. V. Brooks, and I. M. Orme. 2001. Temporal and spatial arrangement of lymphocytes within lung granulomas induced by aerosol infection with *Mycobacterium tuberculosis*. *Infect. Immun.* **69:**1722–1728.

31. Gruppo, V., O. C. Turner, I. M. Orme, and J. Turner. 2002. Reduced up-regulation of memory and adhesion/integrin molecules in susceptible mice and poor expression of immunity to pulmonary tuberculosis. *Microbiology* **148:**2959–2966.

32. Gumperz, J. E., and M. B. Brenner. 2001. CD1–specific T cells in microbial immunity. *Curr. Opin. Immunol.* **13:**471–478.

33. Heldwein, K. A., and M. J. Fenton. 2002. The role of Toll-like receptors in immunity against mycobacterial infection. *Microbes Infect.* **4:**937–944.

34. Henderson, R. A., S. C. Watkins, and J. L. Flynn. 1997. Activation of human dendritic cells following infection with *Mycobacterium tuberculosis*. *J. Immunol.* **159:**635–643.

35. Hernandez-Pando, R., L. Pavon, K. Arriaga, H. Orozco, V. Madrid-Marina, and G. Rook. 1997. Pathogenesis of tuberculosis in mice exposed to low and high doses of an environmental mycobacterial saprophyte before infection. *Infect. Immun.* **65:**3317–3327.

36. Huygen, K., J. Content, O. Denis, D. L. Montgomery, A. M. Yawman, R. R. Deck, C. M. DeWitt, I. M. Orme, S. Baldwin, C. D'Souza, A. Drowart, E. Lozes, P. Vandenbussche, J. P. Van Vooren, M. A. Liu, and J. B. Ulmer. 1996. Immunogenicity and protective efficacy of a tuberculosis DNA vaccine. *Nat. Med.* **2:**893–898.

37. Junqueira-Kipnis, A., P. J., Turner, M. Gonzalez-Juarrero, O. C. Turner and I. M. Orme. 2004. Stable T-cell population expressing an effector cell surface phenotype in the lungs of mice chronically infected with *Mycobacterium tuberculosis*. *Infect. Immun.* **72:**570–575.

38. Manabe, Y. C., A. M. Dannenberg, Jr., S. K. Tyagi, C. L. Hatem, M. Yoder, S. C. Woolwine, B. C. Zook, M. L. Pitt, and W. R. Bishai. 2003. Different strains of *Mycobacterium tuberculosis* cause various spectrums of disease in the rabbit model of tuberculosis. *Infect. Immun.* **71:**6004–6011.

39. McMurray, D. N. 2000. A nonhuman primate model for preclinical testing of new tuberculosis vaccines. *Clin. Infect. Dis.* **30**(Suppl 3):S210–S212.

40. McMurray, D. N., F. M. Collins, A. M. Dannenberg, Jr., and D. W. Smith. 1996. Pathogenesis of experimental tuberculosis in animal models. *Curr. Top. Microbiol. Immunol.* **215:**157–179.

41. McMurray, D. N., G. Dai, and S. Phalen. 1999. Mechanisms of vaccine-induced resistance in a guinea pig model of pulmonary tuberculosis. *Tubercle Lung Dis.* **79:**261–266.

42. Medina, E., and R. J. North. 1996. Evidence inconsistent with a role for the Bcg gene (Nramp1) in resistance of mice to infection with virulent *Mycobacterium tuberculosis*. *J. Exp. Med.* **183:**1045–1051.

43. Medina, E., and R. J. North. 1998. Resistance ranking of some common inbred mouse strains to *Mycobacterium tuberculosis* and relationship to major histocompatibility complex haplotype and Nramp1 genotype. *Immunology* **93:**270–274.

44. Moody, D. B., M. Sugita, P. J. Peters, M. B. Brenner, and S. A. Porcelli. 1996. The CD1-restricted T-cell response to mycobacteria. *Res. Immunol.* **147:**550–559.

45. Orme, I. M. 1999. Beyond BCG: the potential for a more effective TB vaccine. *Mol. Med. Today* **5:**487–492.

46. Orme, I. M. 1998. The immunopathogenesis of tuberculosis: a new working hypothesis. *Trends Microbiol.* **6:**94–97.

47. Orme, I. M. 1987. The kinetics of emergence and loss of mediator T lymphocytes acquired in response to infection with *Mycobacterium tuberculosis*. *J. Immunol.* **138:**293–298.

48. Orme, I. M. 2003. The mouse as a useful model of tuberculosis. *Tuberculosis* **83:**112–115.

49. Orme, I. M. 1999. New vaccines against tuberculosis. The status of current research. *Infect. Dis. Clin. North Am.* **13:**169–185, vii–viii.

50. Orme, I. M. 1997. Progress in the development of new vaccines against tuberculosis. *Int. J. Tuberc. Lung Dis.* **1:**95–100.

51. Orme, I. M. 1995. Prospects for new vaccines against tuberculosis. *Trends Microbiol.* **3:**401–404.

52. Orme, I. M. 2001. The search for new vaccines against tuberculosis. *J. Leukoc. Biol.* **70:**1–10.

53. Orme, I. M. 2000. Tuberculosis: recent progress in basic immunity and vaccine development. *Kekkaku* **75:**97–101.

54. Orme, I. M. 1999. Vaccination against tuberculosis: recent progress. *Adv. Vet. Med.* **41:**135–143.

55. Orme, I. M., P. Andersen, and W. H. Boom. 1993. T cell response to *Mycobacterium tuberculosis*. *J. Infect. Dis.* **167:**1481–1497.

56. Orme, I. M., and J. T. Belisle. 1999. TB vaccine development: after the flood. *Trends Microbiol.* **7:**394–395.

57. Orme, I. M., and F. M. Collins. 1986. Crossprotection against nontuberculous mycobacterial infections by *Mycobacterium tuberculosis* memory immune T lymphocytes. *J. Exp. Med.* **163:**203–208.

58. Orme, I. M., and F. M. Collins. 1984. Efficacy of *Mycobacterium bovis* BCG vaccination in mice undergoing prior pulmonary infection with atypical mycobacteria. *Infect. Immun.* **44:**28–32.

59. Orme, I. M., and F. M. Collins. 1983. Infection with *Mycobacterium kansasii* and efficacy of vaccination against tuberculosis. *Immunology* **50:**581–586.

60. Orme, I. M., and A. M. Cooper. 1999. Cytokine/chemokine cascades in immunity to tuberculosis. *Immunol. Today* **20:**307–312.

61. Orme, I. M., D. N. McMurray, and J. T. Belisle. 2001. Tuberculosis vaccine development: recent progress. *Trends Microbiol.* **9:**115–118.

62. Porcelli, S. A., and R. L. Modlin. 1999. The CD1 system: antigen-presenting molecules for T cell recognition of lipids and glycolipids. *Annu. Rev. Immunol.* **17:**297–329.

63. Repique, C. J., A. Li, F. M. Collins, and S. L. Morris. 2002. DNA immunization in a mouse model of latent tuberculosis: effect of DNA vaccination on reactivation of disease and on reinfection with a secondary challenge. *Infect. Immun.* **70:**3318–3323.

64. Rhoades, E. R., A. A. Frank, and I. M. Orme. 1997. Progression of chronic pulmonary tuberculosis in mice aerogenically infected with virulent *Mycobacterium tuberculosis*. *Tubercle Lung Dis.* **78:**57–66.

65. Scanga, C. A., V. P. Mohan, H. Joseph, K. Yu, J. Chan, and J. L. Flynn. 1999. Reactivation of latent tuberculosis: variations on the Cornell murine model. *Infect. Immun.* **67:**4531–4538.

66. Sieling, P. A., D. Chatterjee, S. A. Porcelli, T. I. Prigozy, R. J. Mazzaccaro, T. Soriano, B. R. Bloom, M. B. Brenner, M. Kronenberg, P. J. Brennan, and R. L. Modlin. 1995. CD1-restricted T cell recognition of microbial lipoglycan antigens. *Science* **269:**227–230.

67. Smith, D. W., V. Balasubramanian, and E. Wiegeshaus. 1991. A guinea pig model of experimental airborne tuberculosis for evaluation of the response to chemotherapy: the effect on bacilli in the initial phase of treatment. *Tubercle* **72:**223–231.

68. Smith, D. W., and G. E. Harding. 1977. Animal model of human disease. Pulmonary tuberculosis. Animal model: experimental airborne tuberculosis in the guinea pig. *Am. J. Pathol.* **89:**273–276.

69. Stanford, J. L., M. J. Shield, and G. A. Rook. 1981. How environmental mycobacteria may predetermine the protective efficacy of BCG. *Tubercle* **62:**55–62.

70. Stenger, S., and R. L. Modlin. 2002. Control of *Mycobacterium tuberculosis* through mammalian Toll-like receptors. *Curr. Opin. Immunol.* **14:**452–457.

71. Taylor, J. L., O. C. Turner, R. J. Basaraba, J. T. Belisle, K. Huygen, and I. M. Orme. 2003. Pulmonary necrosis resulting from DNA vaccination against tuberculosis. *Infect. Immun.* **71:**2192–2198.

72. Tsenova, L., A. Bergtold, V. H. Freedman, R. A. Young, and G. Kaplan. 1999. Tumor necrosis factor alpha is a determinant of pathogenesis and disease progression in mycobacterial infection in the central nervous system. *Proc. Natl. Acad. Sci. USA* **96:**5657–5662.

72a. Turner, O. C., R. J. Basaraba, A. A. Frank, I. M. Orme. 2003. Granuloma formation in mouse and guinea pig models of experimental tuberculosis, p. 65–84. *In* D. L. Boros (ed.), *Granulomatous Infections and Inflammations.* ASM Press, Washington, D.C.

73. Turner, J., M. Gonzalez-Juarrero, B. M. Saunders, J. V. Brooks, P. Marietta, D. L. Ellis, A. A. Frank, A. M. Cooper, and I. M. Orme. 2001. Immunological basis for reactivation of tuberculosis in mice. *Infect. Immun.* **69:**3264–3270.

74. Turner, J., E. R. Rhoades, M. Keen, J. T. Belisle, A. A. Frank, and I. M. Orme. 2000. Effective preexposure tuberculosis vaccines fail to protect when they are given in an immunotherapeutic mode. *Infect. Immun.* **68:**1706–1709.

75. Turner, O. C., R. J. Basaraba, and I. M. Orme. 2003. Immunopathogenesis of pulmonary granulomas in the guinea pig after infection with *Mycobacterium tuberculosis. Infect. Immun.* **71:**864–871.

76. Ulmer, J. B., D. L. Montgomery, A. Tang, L. Zhu, R. R. Deck, C. DeWitt, O. Denis, I. Orme, J. Content, and K. Huygen. 1998. DNA vaccines against tuberculosis. *Novartis Found. Symp.* **217:**239–253.

77. Wolday, D., B. Hailu, M. Girma, E. Hailu, E. Sanders, and A. L. Fontanet. 2003. Low CD4+ T-cell count and high HIV viral load precede the development of tuberculosis disease in a cohort of HIV-positive ethiopians. *Int. J. Tuberc. Lung Dis.* **7:**110–116.

78. Wu, C. Y., J. R. Kirman, M. J. Rotte, D. F. Davey, S. P. Perfetto, E. G. Rhee, B. L. Freidag, B. J. Hill, D. C. Douek, and R. A. Seder. 2002. Distinct lineages of T(H)1 cells have differential capacities for memory cell generation in vivo. *Nat. Immunol.* **3:**852–858.

79. Yun, H. J., C. C. Whalen, A. Okwera, R. D. Mugerwa, and J. J. Ellner. 2003. HIV disease progression and effects of tuberculosis preventive therapy in HIV-infected adults. *Ann. Epidemiol.* **13:**577–578.

INDEX